Obstetric Nursing

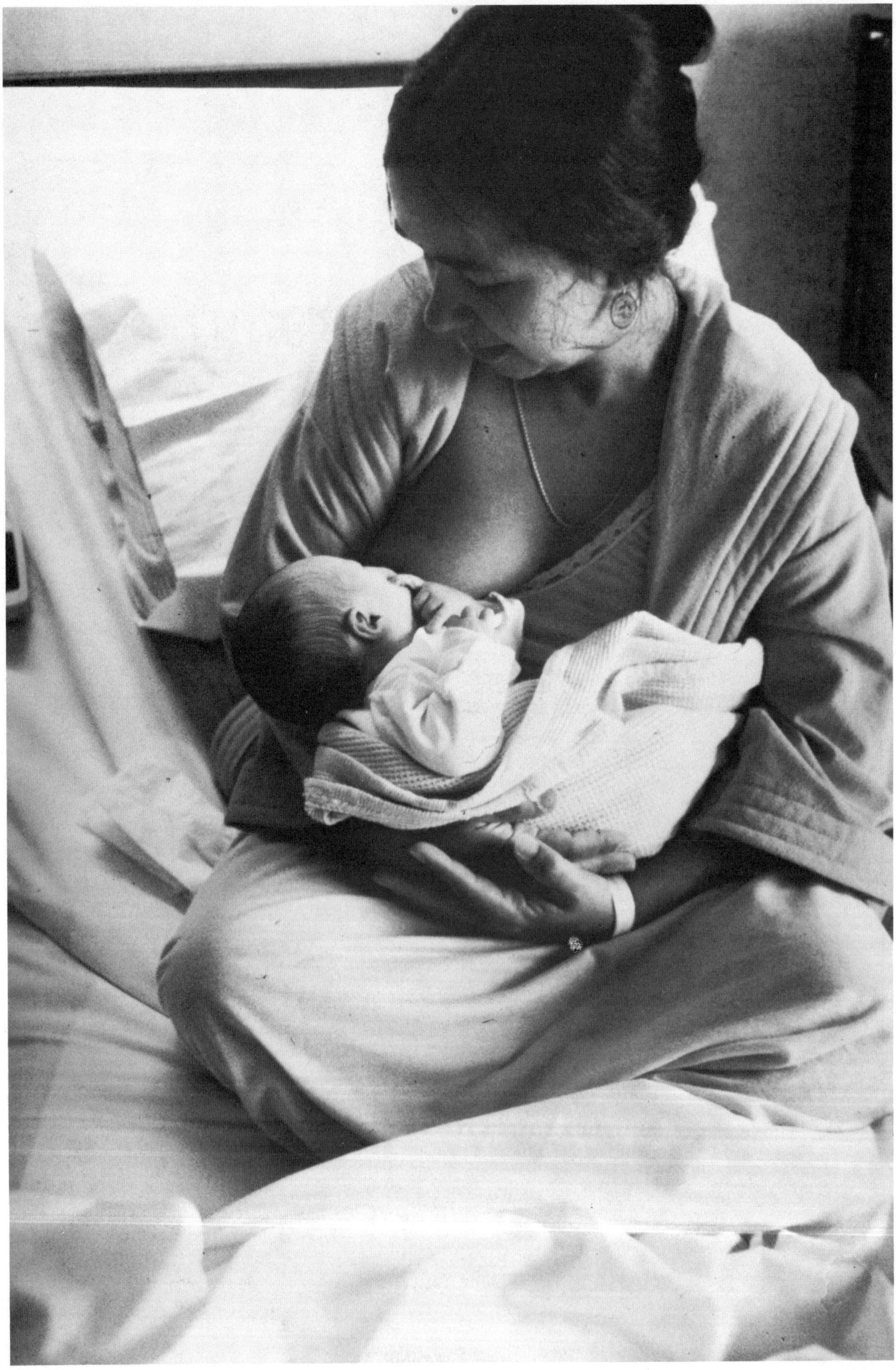

Obstetric Nursing

Eighth Edition

Erna E. Ziegel, R.N., M.A.
Emeritus Associate Professor,
University of Wisconsin-Madison
School of Nursing
Madison, Wisconsin

Mecca S. Cranley, R.N., Ph.D.
Associate Professor, Perinatal Nursing,
University of Wisconsin-Madison
School of Nursing
Madison, Wisconsin

Macmillan Publishing Company
NEW YORK

Collier Macmillan Canada, Inc.
TORONTO

Collier Macmillan Publishers
LONDON

Printed in the United States of America

Macmillan Publishing Company
866 Third Avenue, New York, New York 10022

Collier Macmillan Canada, Inc.
Collier Macmillan Publishers • London

Library of Congress Cataloging in Publication Data
Ziegel, Erna.
Obstetric nursing.

Includes bibliographies and index.
1. Obstetrical nursing. I. Cranley, Mecca S.
II. Title. [DNLM: 1. Obstetrical nursing.
2. Pregnancy—Nursing texts. WY 157 X66o]
RG951.V3 1984 610.73′678 83-25576
ISBN 0-02-431570-2

Printing: 1 2 3 4 5 6 7 8 Year: 4 5 6 7 8 9 0 1 2

Preface

In preparing the eighth edition of *Obstetric Nursing,* we have been particularly aware of the American Nurses Association's definition of nursing as "the diagnosis and treatment of human responses to actual or potential health problems." Although it is not a new concept, this definition has refocused nursing on those aspects of health care that are uniquely its own. We have attempted to reflect this refocus in chapter headings as well as in content.

This edition, as did the seventh edition, reflects an emphasis on the role of nurses as integral members of professional teams that deliver health care of increasing excellence. The nurse, with greater responsibility for health care, is in a key position to influence the kind of maternity care that will enable individuals and families to achieve their goals for health and for family unity. The nurse will serve the best interests of childbearing families when she continually pursues excellence through knowledge of the scientific basis for childbirth care—biologic, medical, and behavioral. He or she can then provide families with the sensitive care and homelike atmosphere they desire before, during, and after birth.

In their practices, nurses have the opportunity to be colleagues of both client and physician. Patient advocacy can involve defending patient's rights. It can also involve patient education, providing women with information about all of their options and helping them make the best choices for themselves.

Believing the above, we have made an effort to include in this edition a balance of physiologic, technical, and psychosocial information—both the *science* and the *art* of perinatal nursing are essential to good care. The nurse must apply this knowledge in a logical, systematic fashion to the individual women and families who seek nursing care. This systematic approach traditionally is named the nursing process.

Every effort has been made to avoid any bias toward one gender or another. Fetuses, infants, nurses and physicians are recognized as being both female and male. Occasionally, it is less awkward to use a conventional grammatical form rather than the more cumbersome his/her or he/she. The indulgence of the reader is requested in this matter.

It is our hope that the nurses who read this book will be stimulated to synthesize the information into nursing care plans that meet the best interests of their patients, to make pertinent and insightful adaptations of care, and to seek new knowledge to enhance their professional practice. We expect some of our readers will be new to perinatal nursing. We hope they will be excited by the possibilities for a fulfilling, professional practice in the care of mothers, infants, and families. Some readers no doubt will be advanced students or experienced practitioners. For them, we have tried to include a depth of information that will enrich their practice and stimulate them to greater learning. Perinatal nursing is a dynamic, rapidly changing field. Excellent nurses will continually read and study to maintain their skills at the cutting edge of innovative practice.

Erna E. Ziegel
Mecca S. Cranley

Acknowledgments

No task as large and complex as producing a textbook can be accomplished by two persons alone. We want to take this opportunity to thank the many individuals who assisted us both morally and materially in this undertaking. We are particularly indebted to our colleagues in nursing and to our students who made valuable suggestions regarding content. Dorothy M. Patteson critiqued the chapters on the newborn based on her wealth of expertise as a teacher and practitioner of neonatal nursing. Sue A. Frazier, Associate Professor of Nursing, University of Wisconsin–Madison, revised three of the labor chapters and ably assisted with the review of galleys and pages.

Illustrations are a particularly challenging aspect of assembling a book. We thank the several families who shared their family albums and made themselves available for photographs. Barbara Decker, R.N., C.N.M., Director, Nurse Midwifery Program, Columbia University, provided invaluable aid in arranging for a number of photographs from the Presbyterian Hospital of the City of New York.

The nimble fingers of our typists, Barbara Schutz and Gloria Barsness, enabled us to meet almost all the many deadlines.

Special recognition is due the very able staff at Macmillan, in particular our editor, Carol Wolfe, and the production supervisor, Toni A. Scaramuzzo. Carol managed to use just the right blend of encouragement and harassment to keep us on schedule, while Toni's attention to detail and calm good humor made the tedium of production much more bearable.

Dr. Cranley wishes to give credit to her family: to husband, Edward, and daughter, Martha, who provided some of the artwork for the line drawings and to all the other members of the Clan Cranley, who like to see their names in print as partial compensation for all the time Mom was away from home "doing the book." Thanks Patrick, Elizabeth, Paul, Anne, Philip, and Peter!

Erna E. Ziegel
Mecca S. Cranley

Contents in Detail

Part One Scientific Foundations of Perinatal Care

PART ONE

Scientific Foundations of Perinatal Care

CHAPTER

1

Introduction to Perinatal Nursing

DEFINITION

Three terms are often used interchangeably to describe the specialized area of nursing practice focused on meeting the health and illness needs of childbearing families. These are *obstetric nursing, maternity nursing,* and *perinatal nursing*. Although similar in meaning, each evokes a somewhat different connotation.

The term *obstetric nursing* originated from the medical practice model to designate the nursing care of pregnant women from conception until six weeks post partum. Although the medical counterpart does not include the care of newborns, obstetric nursing has traditionally included the infant during the first few days after birth. Before the majority of births took place in hospitals, the obstetric nurse frequently cared for the mother and infant in the home, often living-in for several weeks.

Adoption of the term *maternity nursing* during the early post-World War II era was an attempt to move away from the medical model and to use a term that directs the focus toward the recipient of care rather than the provider. It has come to imply a broader meaning of the care of the woman and her offspring that includes an emphasis on the interpersonal relationships between mother and infant and between mother and family.

Perinatal nursing is the newest term and is currently used by the American Nurses' Association to designate a specialized area of maternal and child health nursing. This area of nursing practice focuses on diagnosing and treating the responses (both physiologic and psychosocial) of whole families to the childbearing continuum: from planning the pregnancy through the first three months following the birth of the infant.

PHILOSOPHY

The beliefs or philosophy of perinatal nursing practice must be affirmed by the individual nurse. They emerge from the nurse's values and beliefs about life, people, families, and health and are colored by his or her own life experiences. The following statements of beliefs are those of the authors, and as such they influence not only their nursing practice but also the contents of this text.

- The individual woman has the ultimate responsibility for her own health care. The role of the nurse is to identify areas where health promotion, illness prevention, or treatment are indicated and to advise, counsel, and educate. For example, the nurse may diagnose a knowledge deficit with respect to pregnancy and childbirth and suggest antepartal classes or initiation of one-to-one teaching. The woman herself, however, must make the choice to attend or not attend classes or to participate or not in the teaching-learning process. In another example, the nurse carefully explains the need for supplemental iron during pregnancy and the most efficacious way to take the iron. Each woman has the right to refuse to take the iron in spite of understanding what the nurse has told her.

- In circumstances when harm may occur to others because of an individual's choice, society may intervene on behalf of itself or others. Examples of this are the mandatory immunization laws and those that require reporting of child abuse. Many ethical and legal issues arise in this area when there are two or more conflicting "rights" as well as because of the difficulty in defining the harm, particularly when it is potential harm.
- Childbearing occurs in a family context. Each member affects the other and is affected by the experience of pregnancy, birth, and the addition of a new family member. Perinatal nurses must be aware of the family dynamics and, as much as possible, work to facilitate healthy adaptation of the entire family system.
- Childbearing is a developmental process. The nurse must be knowledgeable about human development and facilitate an environment that assists both individuals and families to grow cognitively and psychosocially as well as physically.
- The developmental, and occasionally situational, crises inherent in childbearing enhance the family's openness to learning. Health teaching done during this time often has benefits lasting well beyond the childbearing year.

FACTORS INFLUENCING PERINATAL NURSING PRACTICE

The practice of perinatal nursing, like that of any profession, is substantially influenced by a number of factors both within the profession itself and in the larger society. The following list is intended to be illustrative rather than exhaustive.

Societal Factors

Licensure

The various states, as a part of their regulatory function, strive to protect the public from unsafe practitioners of nursing by setting minimum standards and requiring licensure to practice as a professional nurse. Through the state nurse practice acts, a definition is established to describe what constitutes professional nursing practice.

Economics

In the free-enterprise, fee-for-service health care system in the United States, the fiscal resources of a given woman or family influence their general health and nutrition as well as the quality and quantity of health care available to them. In addition, the overall economic climate in the society as a whole has an impact. During the early 1980s, in a time of recession and high unemployment, a growing number of families are without health insurance. Many of these families are likewise ineligible for the traditional forms of public assistance. As a result, fewer women receive early and continuous antepartal care, and many authorities predict an increase in perinatal morbidity and mortality unless remedial measures are taken.

Culture

Perinatal care must be not only available and affordable but also acceptable to the people for whom it is intended. Failure to take into account the individual's cultural views and values will quickly make the care unacceptable. Culture is intended here in its broadest meaning, that is, the totality of socially transmitted attitudes and behaviors that characterize a group of people.

Third-Party Payment

Nursing practice is also influenced by the extent to which private and public insurance companies are willing to reimburse nurses directly for services rendered. As long as nurses must remain employees of agencies or physicians in order to be paid, practice will have certain constraints, particularly with respect to contracting between nurse and patient.

Professional Factors

ANA Social Policy Statement

In 1980, the American Nurses' Association enunciated a comprehensive position defining nursing and its scope of practice, its relationship to other health disciplines, and to society. This definition of nursing as the diagnosis and treatment of human responses to actual or potential health problems has given nurses and others a new perspective on the profession. It has served to clarify those aspects of health care that are distinctly nursing as opposed to medicine, social work, and so on.

According to the Policy Statement there are four defining characteristics of nursing practice. The first is the *phenomena,* the human responses. These are of two types:

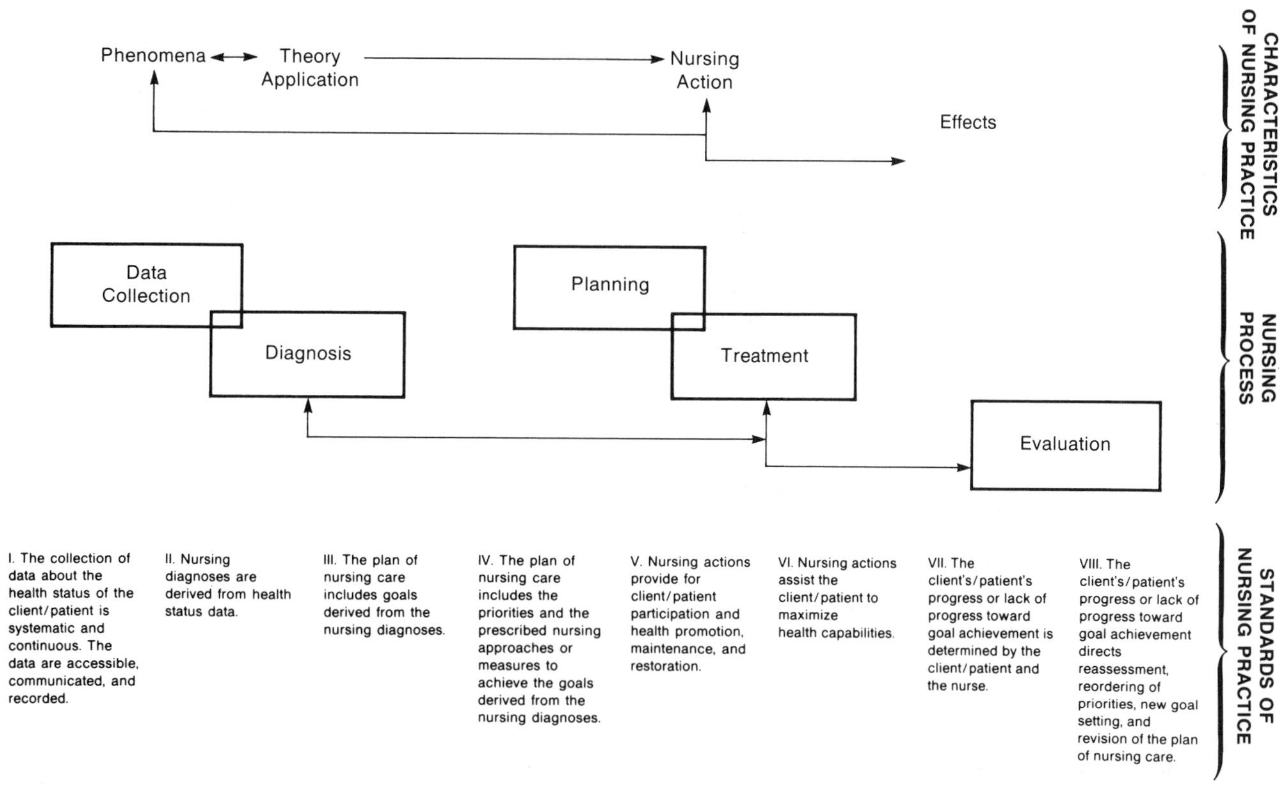

Figure 1–1. Defining characteristics of nursing practice: relationship to the nursing process and the standards of nursing practice. (Reprinted with permission from Nursing: A Social Statement. Kansas City, Mo.: American Nurses' Association, 1980.)

> 1. The reactions of individuals and groups to actual health problems (health-restoring responses), such as the impact of illness-effects upon the self and family, and related self-care needs; and
> 2. Concerns of individuals and groups about potential health problems (health-supporting responses), such as monitoring and teaching in populations or communities at risk . . . .[1]

Having identified or diagnosed the phenomenon, nurses use *theory,* the second defining characteristic, to understand the phenomenon within the domain of nursing practice. This theory is partly unique to nursing and partly derived from a wide variety of other disciplines. Theory also directs *nursing actions,* the third defining characteristic. Actions are directed toward improving or correcting conditions, preventing illness, and promoting health. They include technical skills as well as interpersonal skill and intellectual competencies. The fourth and final defining characteristic is *effect.* Nursing actions are, of course, intended to produce beneficial effects. The evaluation of effects is crucial and is carried out by assessing individual patient outcomes as well as those of groups of patients. In addition, systematic research which rigorously tests the relationships between specific phenomena and nursing actions is needed to increase the understanding of nursing practice.

The relationship between the characteristics of nursing, the nursing process, and nursing practice standards is shown in Figure 1–1.

Generalist Versus Specialist Practice

Perinatal nursing practice may differ depending on the educational and experiential background of the nurse. According to *A Statement on the Scope of Maternal and Child Health Nursing Practice,*

> The practice of the maternal and child health nursing generalist is characterized by the application of generic nursing skills to a specified clientele. Nurse generalists have had generic nursing preparation with additional inservice or continuing education in specialized areas . . . . These specialized areas of practice include, for example, labor and delivery; neonatal, postpartum, and prenatal nursing. . . .
>
> The practice of the maternal and child health nursing specialist is characterized by expertise in . . . perinatal nursing. . . . The nursing specialist explores and tests scientific theories on which the practice of . . . nursing is based, and

[1]*Nursing: A Social Policy Statement,* American Nurses' Association, Kansas City, Mo., 1980, pp. 9–10.

Table 1-1. Examples of Health Care Settings Where Perinatal Nurses Practice.

Setting	*Area of Practice*	*Level of Practice*
Family planning clinics	Contraceptive care and counseling	Primary care
Physician's offices or clinics	Antepartum Postpartum	Primary care Primary care
Public health departments	Home visits and/or public health clinics for Antepartum Postpartum Newborn care Family planning	Primary care
Birth centers	Antepartum Labor and delivery	Primary care
Hospitals	Labor and delivery Postpartum Newborn care	Primary and secondary care
Perinatal centers	High-risk antepartum (inpatient and ambulatory) Intrapartum intensive care Newborn intensive care High-risk postpartum Inservice and outreach education	Tertiary care
State health departments	Consultant to providers of perinatal health and to executive and legislative branches of government about perinatal health needs	
Colleges and universities	Teacher of perinatal nursing Researcher	

uses investigative skills to systematically study and solve complex problems in their specialty area. The . . . [perinatal] nursing specialist has educational preparation at the master's level.[2]

The Health Care Setting

Perinatal nurses practice in both ambulatory and institutional settings. Nurses providing primary health care work chiefly in ambulatory settings. They are concerned with health promotion and illness prevention. Nursing activities include health assessment, case-finding, anticipatory guidance, teaching, counseling, and treatment of common deviations from health. Low-risk antepartal clinics are common examples of this type of care, as is the care of normal birth and postpartum families with healthy newborns.

Nurses providing care for women experiencing complications of pregnancy or for premature, sick, or developmentally disabled infants practice chiefly in institutional settings. In general, these patients require nursing skills that incorporate more technology than does primary care. In addition, as the pathology becomes more complex, a greater degree of collaboration among different health care disciplines is important.

[2]American Nurses' Association, Kansas City, Mo., 1980, p. 11.

Table 1-1 contains a partial list of settings where perinatal nurses may practice.

Ethical Issues in Perinatal Practice

The ANA Code

There are many situations in perinatal nursing practice where decisions cannot be made on the basis of scientific information alone. These situations require reference to ethical or moral considerations. Ethics is a branch of philosophy which deals with the principles that guide moral behavior. Ethics is the *why* behind the *oughts* and *shoulds* of the moral code. The *ANA Code for Nurses* is one available guide to ethical decision making.

When a person becomes a professional nurse, he or she accepts the responsibility to adhere to the profession's code of conduct. Over the years this code has changed as nursing has changed. The emphasis has shifted from personal ethics to professional ethics. In addition, the issue of to whom nurses are responsible has been redefined. Earlier versions held that the nurse was responsible to and obeyed the physician; present versions hold the nurse accountable directly to the patient/client. The Code reflects the basic philosophy of nursing practice—respect for human dignity and protection of the patient. It also describes the appropriate conduct with respect to collaboration and consultation with other professions, as well as the nurse's responsibility to the profession of nursing itself (See Table 1-2).

The Scope of Perinatal Ethical Issues

Although the ANA Code provides a guideline for acceptable professional nursing practice behaviors, it is not helpful in answering all of the myriad ethical questions that arise in day-to-day practice. Perhaps no other area of nursing practice encompasses so many major bioethical dilemmas. Included among these are overriding issues of informed consent and the right to life as well as issues of contraception, sterilization, genetic research and manipulation, *in vitro* fertilization, artificial insemination, abortion, treatment of tiny premature infants and infants with congenital malformations, life-support technology and when to use it, and the risk-benefit of unproven technology or research protocols. Questions also arise concerning the allocation of scarce resources. For instance, would society be better served if the millions of dollars spent on newborn intensive care were redirected to strong antepartal care programs? If two infants need one respirator, which one receives care? And who decides? If a woman can choose to abort a fetus because he has Down's syndrome, can she also choose to abort a normal male fetus because she prefers to have a daughter? And, if the nurse's views on abortion differ from the client's, what are the nurse's obligations to give counseling and care?

Table 1-2. The American Nurses' Association Code of Ethics for Nurses

1. The nurse provides services with respect for human dignity and the uniqueness of the client unrestricted by considerations of social or economic status, personal attributes, or the nature of the health problems.
2. The nurse safeguards the client's right to privacy by judiciously protecting information of a confidential nature.
3. The nurse acts to safeguard the client and the public when health care and safety are affected by the incompetent, unethical, or illegal practice of any person.
4. The nurse assumes responsibility and accountability for individual nursing judgments and actions.
5. The nurse maintains competence in nursing.
6. The nurse exercises informed judgment and uses individual competence and qualifications as criteria in seeking consultation, accepting responsibilities, and delegating nursing activities to others.
7. The nurse participates in activities that contribute to the ongoing development of the profession's body of knowledge.
8. The nurse participates in the profession's efforts to implement and improve standards of nursing.
9. The nurse participates in the profession's efforts to establish and maintain conditions of employment conducive to high quality nursing care.
10. The nurse participates in the profession's effort to protect the public from misinformation and misrepresentation and to maintain the integrity of nursing.
11. The nurse collaborates with members of the health professions and other citizens in promoting community and national efforts to meet the health needs of the public.

The answers to these troubling questions will not be found in this chapter any more than in the ANA Code. Indeed, it is beyond the scope of this chapter even to present a comprehensive discussion of the questions. For most issues there is no simple, generally accepted answer. This is why they present dilemmas. The subject of ethics is raised here to alert the reader to the magnitude of this issue as an essential component of professional nursing practice and to encourage nurses to study ethics as a means of enriching their practice as care-givers and decision-makers.

A Systematic Approach to Ethical Decision Making

Even straightforward ethical principles have a way of becoming extremely complex in application. The nurse may be clear about what she believes, but when she is in the middle of a situation complicated by conflicting values and points of view on the part of patients and colleagues, perhaps where the well-being of one individual may be seen as competing with that of another and where time is a critical factor, the result often may be confusion, frustration, and indecision. Certainly, this outcome will occur more frequently if the nurse has not given the issue any previous thought and is very unclear about her own beliefs. While it is not possible to avoid all uncertainty and confusion about ethical issues, some steps can be made to ameliorate the problem.

Values Clarification

Central to acting as an ethical person is the awareness of and comfort with one's own beliefs and values. This is an important reason for studying ethics. An individual's training in his or her family, church, and community forms the basis for values and biases. The ability to make moral judgments is dependent upon cognitive development, as well as upon concepts and facts about particular situations. Increasingly, professional schools of all disciplines, including nursing, are including courses of ethics in their curricula.

One reason for being aware of one's values is to determine the limits of ability to provide care for patients who have opposing values. A nurse with a strong sense of the importance of "paying your own way" may be intolerant of so-called "welfare mothers" and thus unable to give supportive care. Referral to a nurse colleague might be a reasonable solution.

A sense of relative certainty about one's values also will limit the sense of confusion experienced when confronted with differing views. Individuals secure in their own beliefs are usually freer to be tolerant of others' views because their own are not threatened.

Information Gathering

Good ethical decisions must take into account all relevant facts. These facts include the scientific information about such things as diagnosis and prognosis, as well as the values and feelings of all the patients and professionals involved. The scientific facts are learned in professional education, both basic preparation and continuing study. The information about feelings and values must be gathered for each situation.

Framework for Study

A rational approach to any problem-solving suggests the desirability for a systematic, logically progressing process. Researchers employ the scientific method of solving problems; nurses rely on the nursing process. Even a casual observer will note the extraordinary degree of similarity between the two. Utilizing basically the same principles of systematic inquiry a number of authors have developed frameworks for ethical decision making. One of these, described by Thompson and Thompson, is quoted in Table 1–3.

Rehearsal

Because on-the-spot decisions, however difficult, sometimes may be required in practice, it is advantageous for nurses to examine critical situations involving ethical dilemmas in the security of a classroom or conference. Here "practice" in decision-making about real or fictional case studies allows time for reflection and discussion. Having had some experience in this kind of activity, real-life situations may be less perplexing. In the practice setting, it is beneficial for a group representing various professions—nursing, medicine, law, ethics—to engage periodically in such an exercise.

SUMMARY

Perinatal nursing is a special area of maternal-child nursing directed toward meeting the needs of families during the childbearing year from conception through the fourth trimester. Perinatal nurses, either generalists or specialists, practice in a variety of health care settings. Their practice is influenced by a variety of societal as well as intraprofessional factors.

The complexity of modern health care technology has created many new areas of ethical uncertainty. The perinatal nurse needs knowledge of ethics as well as science to make responsible decisions about his or her own actions and to facilitate clients' decisions.

Table 1–3. Guidelines for Identifying and Analyzing Ethical Dilemmas in Nursing Practice*

1. Review the situation as presented and
   a. Determine what health problems exist;
   b. Identify what decision(s) need to be made;
   c. Separate the ethical components of the decisions from those decisions that can be made solely on a scientific knowledge base;
   d. Identify all the individuals/groups who will be affected by the decision(s).
2. Decide what further information is needed before a decision on a course of action can be made, and gather this information.
3. Identify the ethical issues involved in the situation as presented. Discuss the historical, philosophical, and religious bases for each of these issues.
4. Identify your own values/beliefs (moral stand) regarding each of these ethical issues and your professional responsibilities dictated by the Code for Nurses.
5. Identify the values/beliefs operant in the other people involved in the situation. Use knowledge of historical, philosophical, and religious bases of ethical issues to enhance understanding of other people's moral stands on the issues.
6. Identify the value conflicts, if any, in the situation.
7. Discuss who is best able to make the needed decision(s) and identify the nurse's role in the decision-making process. (Who owns the problem?)
8. Identify the range of decisions/actions that are possible and the anticipated implications of same for all people involved in the situation. Identify how closely the suggested actions conform to the Code for Nurses.
9. If appropriate, decide on a course of action as the nurse in the situation and follow through.
10. In retrospect, evaluate/review the results of the actions or decisions and keep in mind for future situations of this type.

*J. B. Thompson, and H. O. Thompson, *Ethics in Nursing,* Macmillan, New York, 1981.

REFERENCES AND SUGGESTED READINGS

A Statement on the Scope of High-Risk Perinatal Nursing Practice, American Nurses' Association, Kansas City, Mo., 1980.

A Statement on the Scope of Maternal and Child Health Nursing Practice, American Nurses' Association, Kansas City, Mo., 1980.

Code for Nurses with Interpretive Statements, American Nurses' Association, Kansas City, Mo., 1976.

Fost, N., Counseling families who have a child with a severe congenital anomaly, *Pediatrics,* 67(3): 321–24, 1981.

Fromer, M. J., *Ethical Issues in Health Care.* Mosby, St. Louis, 1981.

McCormick, R. A., The quality of life, the sanctity of life, *Hastings Cent. Rep.* 8(1): 30–36, 1978.

Nursing: A Social Policy Statement, American Nurses' Association, Kansas City, Mo., 1980.

Smith, S. J., and Davis, A. J., Ethical dilemmas: Conflicts among rights, duties and obligations, *Am. J. Nurs.,* 80: 1463–66, 1980.

Steinfels, M. O., New childbirth technology: A clash of values, *Hastings Cent. Rep.* 8(1): 9–12, 1978.

Thompson, J. B., and Thompson, H. O., *Ethics in Nursing,* Macmillan, New York, 1981.

CHAPTER

2

Anatomy and Physiology of the Female Reproductive Organs

THE FEMALE REPRODUCTIVE ORGANS, their anatomic structure, and their physiological function will be described in this chapter. The anatomy and physiology of the male reproductive system will be considered in the chapter that follows.

ANATOMY OF THE FEMALE REPRODUCTIVE ORGANS

The female reproductive organs are divided into two groups, the internal organs and the external genitalia. These organs, as well as other related structures, the bladder, urethra, rectum, pelvic diaphragm, and perineum, because of their close proximity, and the breasts, because of their functional relationship, will be discussed. The bony pelvis, in and below which the reproductive organs are situated, is described in Chapter 16, where the pelvis is considered as the birth canal or passage through which the fetus moves during the birth process.

External Organs

The external genitalia of the female, collectively, are commonly called the *vulva;* occasionally the term *pudendum* is used for this group of organs. The vulva includes all the externally visible organs, situated between the thighs, extending from the area over the symphysis pubis to the base of the perineal body, which lies in front of the anus. The following structures are included in the vulva; mons pubis, labia majora, labia minora, clitoris, vestibule, urinary meatus, vaginal opening, and glandular structures.

Mons Pubis (Mons Veneris)

The mons pubis, which constitutes the upper aspect of the vulva, is the firm cushion of adipose and connective tissue that lies over the symphysis pubis and the adjoining pubic bones (Fig. 2–1). The overlying skin contains many sebaceous glands and after puberty is abundantly covered with short, crinkly hair.

Labia Majora (Singular: Labium Majus)

The labia majora are the two longitudinal, heavy ridges of adipose and connective tissue, covered with skin, that form the lateral boundaries of the vulva (Fig. 2–1). They are continuous with and extend downward on

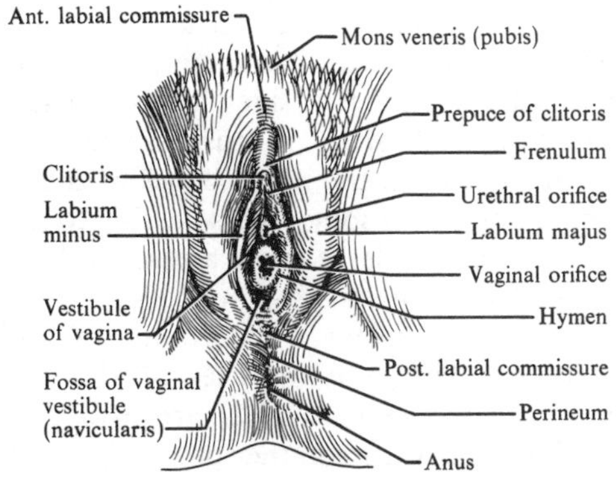

Figure 2–1. Female external genitalia. (Reprinted with permission from Ben Pansky, *Review of Gross Anatomy,* 4th ed. New York: Macmillan, 1979.)

each side from the mons veneris, gradually becoming narrower, and disappearing into the base of the perineal body posteriorly. The labia majora usually lie in close apposition, covering the structures between them, but they may gape in women who have had children.

Each labium has an inner and an outer surface. After puberty the outer aspect is covered with hair, which becomes more sparse toward the perineum. The inner surface of the labium is moist and has the appearance of a mucous membrane; it has numerous sebaceous glands, but is not covered with hair. The labia contain an abundance of blood vessels. Varicose veins sometimes develop and may become markedly enlarged during pregnancy.

Labia Minora (Singular: Labium Minus)

The labia minora are two thin cutaneous folds lying between, and parallel to, the labia majora; they may be completely covered by the labia majora or may project from between them (Fig. 2–1). Resembling the inner surface of the labia majora, they are reddish in color, have the appearance of a mucous membrane, are moist, contain numerous sebaceous glands, and do not have a hair covering. The labia minora contain a number of blood vessels. An abundance of nerves makes them very sensitive.

Anteriorly each labium minus divides into two parts for a short distance and then joins at an angle with the other labium to form a double ridge of tissue around the clitoris, one ridge above and one below the clitoris. The labia minora thus form a hoodlike covering for the clitoris, termed the *prepuce* (Fig. 2–1), and a band of tissue below it, termed the *frenulum* of the clitoris. Like the labia majora, the labia minora taper as they extend posteriorly, where they join below the vaginal opening into a thin, flat, transverse fold of tissue called the *fourchet*.

Clitoris

The clitoris is a small, cylindrical body located at the upper aspect of the vulva in the area where the labia minora join anteriorly (Fig. 2–1). The clitoris is the homologue of the penis of the male and, similar to it, is composed of erectile tissue, contains many blood vessels and nerves, and is extremely sensitive. The clitoris is 2 to 3 cm in length, but is almost entirely covered by the labia. Only the anterior end, the glans, is visible under the prepuce and above its frenulum. These tissues sometimes draw together over the end of the clitoris, cover it, and give this area the appearance of the opening to an orifice. This resemblance to an opening may cause confusion with the urethral orifice unless both are carefully identified and an attempt to insert a catheter here for bladder catheterization causes considerable discomfort.

Vaginal Vestibule

The vestibule is the triangular area that becomes visible when the labia minora are spread apart; the clitoris is at the apex of this triangle and the fourchet at its base. The orifices of the urinary meatus, Skene's (paraurethral) ducts, vagina, and Bartholin's (vulvovaginal) glands are located in the vestibule. A depressed space in the tissue between the vaginal opening and the fourchet, termed the *fossa navicularis,* may be seen at the posterior end of the vestibule, but it is usually obliterated after childbirth.

Urinary Meatus

The external urinary meatus, although not a part of the female genital organs, is described with the vulva because of its anatomic location. It is situated in the midline of the vestibule below the clitoris and above the vaginal orifice (Fig. 2–1). The urinary meatus varies considerably in appearance, ranging from an easily identifiable opening to a puckered elevation of tissue that appears to have no orifice. Separation of the labia minora, followed by slight upward traction on the labia, will usually reveal a triangular opening in the puckered membrane that surrounds the meatus.

The *paraurethral (Skene's) ducts,* which have a very small caliber, open just on each side of the urethral meatus. These ducts may become infected by the gonococcus.

Vaginal Opening and Hymen

The vaginal orifice is in the lower portion of the vestibule (Fig. 2–1). It is partly covered by the *hymen,* a membranous tissue which varies considerably in thickness and size in different women. The opening in the hymen is somewhat circular in outline; it may be so large that the vaginal orifice is almost completely open, or it may be very small and nearly close the orifice. The hymen may be quite elastic and stretch considerably with distention, or it may tear easily. After childbirth the remnants of the hymen are seen as small tags of mucous membrane around the vaginal orifice; these are termed *caruncülae myrtiformes*.

Bartholin's Glands

Bartholin's glands, the largest of several vulvovaginal glands, are compound, racemose, mucus-secreting glands. They are situated at the base of the labia majora, and their ducts open into the vestibule just outside the lateral margins of the vaginal orifice (Fig. 2–1). Their muscus secretion keeps the inner surfaces of the labia moist and provides lubrication to the vaginal orifice and canal, especially during coitus. Secretion is considerably increased during sexual excitement. These glands are normally small and are not palpable, but a gland may become so large as to distend a considerable part of the labium if it becomes infected or cystic.

The Pelvic Diaphragm and the Perineal Region

Pelvic Diaphragm

The pelvic diaphragm, made up of muscles and their fascial covering, stretches across the lowermost part of the pelvic cavity like a hammock. It almost completely closes the abdominal and pelvic cavities and serves as a slinglike support for the abdominal and pelvic organs. The urethra, vagina, and anal canal pass through this diaphragm to their external openings. In addition to the major supportive function of the pelvic diaphragm, its muscle fibers are important in assisting with constriction of the vagina, the rectum, and the anus.

The pelvic diaphragm is composed of two pairs of muscles, the levator ani and the coccygeus muscles (Fig. 2–2). The *levator ani,* the largest and most important component of the pelvic diaphragm, is in actuality a paired muscle, but the two sides join so closely that it functions as a single sheet of muscle. This broad, thin muscle stretches from the pubic bones to the spines of the ischial bones, with some fibers passing to the coccyx and the sacrum. The levator ani are often described as consisting of three parts—the pubococcygeus, iliococcygeus, and puborectalis muscles, all of which are closely joined. The other muscles of the pelvic diaphragm, the *coccygeus* muscles, are also paired and closely joined. They arise at the spines of the ischia and insert into the coccyx and lower part of the sacrum. The coccygeus muscles assist the levator ani in giving support to the abdominal and pelvic viscera.

Perineum

The perineum is the area between the thighs that extends from the pubic area to the coccyx and lies below and superficial to the pelvic diaphragm. The perineum is made up of several pairs of muscles and their fascia, among which are the bulbocavernosus (sphincter vaginae), the transverse perineal muscles, and those forming the anal sphincters (Fig. 2–3). The pelvic diaphragm and the muscles and fascia of the perineum are closely associated in structure and in function; the structures in the perineum reinforce the diaphragm by providing support and assisting in constricting the orifices that pass through it.

Perineal Body

The perineal body is a wedge-shaped mass of fibromuscular tissue that extends upward from the perineum and occupies the area between the vagina and the rectum. The lower and outer surface of this body, representing the base of the wedge, lies between the vaginal and anal openings and is covered with skin. This

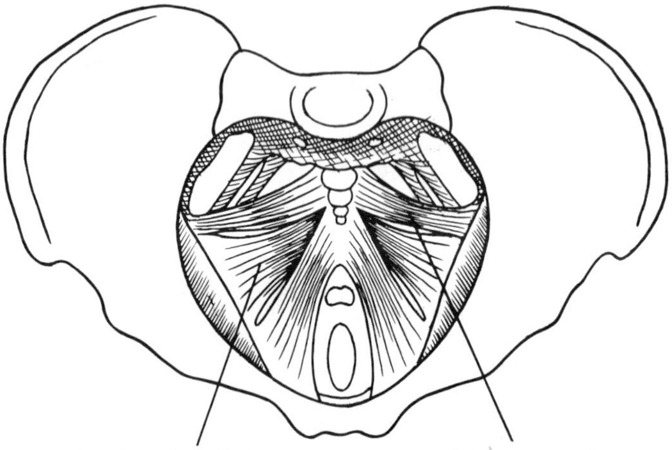

Figure 2–2. Levator ani and coccygeus muscles as seen from above.

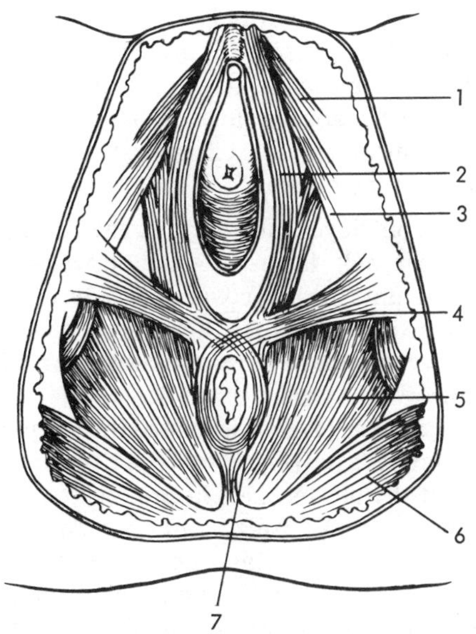

Figure 2–3. Dissection showing the muscles of the vulvar area and the pelvic floor. 1, 3. Ischiocavernosus. 2. Sphincter vaginae. 4. Transversus perinei. 5. Levator ani. 6. Gluteus maximus. 7. External and sphincter.

external surface, or base, is often called the perineum of the female and is the area referred to when the woman is said to have sustained a perineal laceration or incision.

The perineal body is about 4 cm in width and depth and is continuous, deep into the pelvis, with the rectovaginal septum. The levator ani and a number of muscles of the perineum, including the sphincter ani, meet and fuse in the center of this body.

The perineal body is stretched and flattened when the vagina is distended as the fetus passes through the birth canal during delivery. Although this mass of tissue, largely made up of muscle, stretches to a considerable degree during the birth of an infant, it nonetheless is often lacerated, or it is incised to prevent tearing and to facilitate delivery. An incision or a laceration of more than minor extent must be repaired to reestablish the support that this structure gives to the pelvic organs. (See Chapter 21 for further discussion of perineal lacerations and episiotomy and for perineal repair.)

Internal Reproductive Organs

The internal female reproductive organs are contained in the true pelvic cavity and comprise the *uterus* and *vagina* in the center, an *ovary* and a *fallopian tube* on each side, together with their various ligaments, blood vessels, lymph supply, and nerves and a certain amount of fat and connective tissue (Fig. 2–4).

Uterus

The uterus (womb) is the organ in which the fetus develops and from which menstruation occurs. It is a muscular structure that contains a cavity lined with mucous membrane. The uterus is situated in the pelvic cavity between the bladder and the rectum; it joins with a fallopian tube on each side near its upper part, and its lower end (the cervix) projects into the vagina (Figs. 2–4 and 2–5).

The uterus has the shape and approximate size of a somewhat flattened, inverted pear. Its size varies in different women, but measurements approximate 7.5 cm (3 in.) in length, 5 cm (2 in.) in width at the upper part, and 2.5 cm (1 in.) in anteroposterior diameter. It weighs approximately 60 gm (2 oz). The uterus enlarges tremendously during pregnancy, attaining a length of 30 to 35

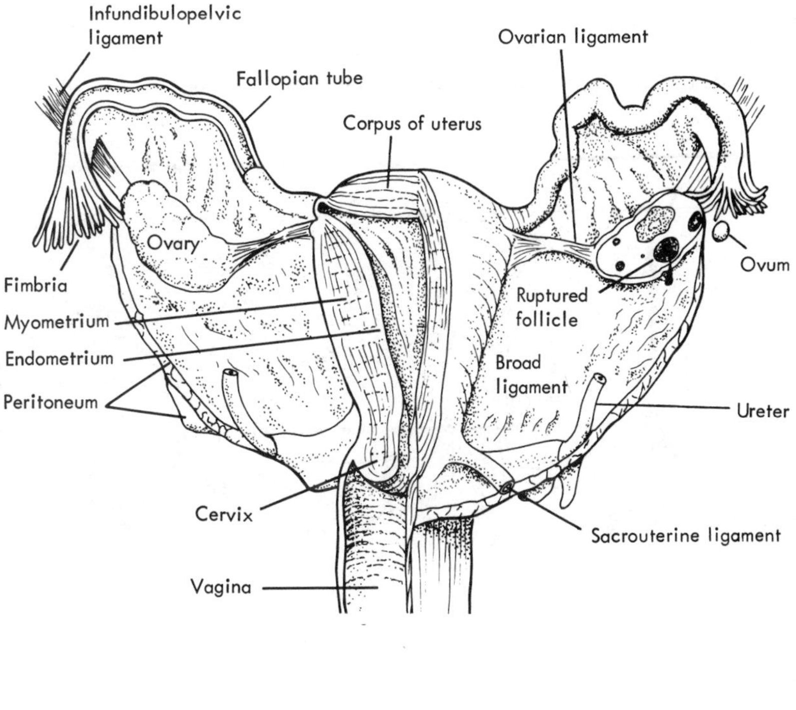

Figure 2–4. Uterus and associated organs. (Reprinted with permission from Sigmund Grollman, *The Human Body: Its Structure and Physiology,* 4th ed. New York: Macmillan, 1978. Copyright Sigmund Grollman, 1978.)

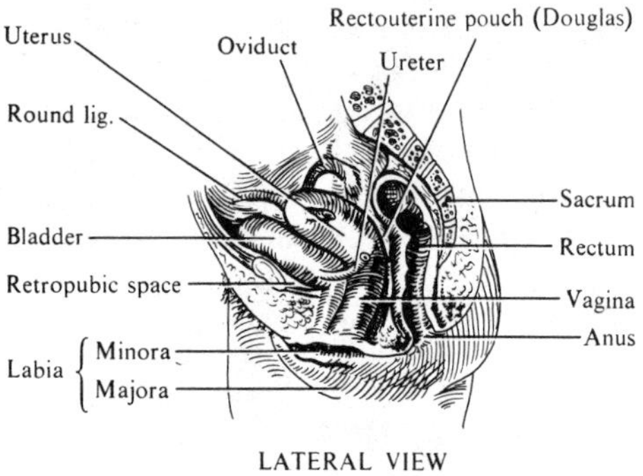

Figure 2-5. Lateral view of female pelvic organs. (Reprinted with permission from Ben Pansky. *Review of Gross Anatomy,* 4th ed. New York: Macmillan, 1979, p. 381.)

cm (12 to 14 in.), a width of 20 to 25 cm (8 to 10 in.), and a weight of approximately 1000 gm (2 lb). After pregnancy the uterus returns almost, but not entirely, to its former size and shape.

The uterus is comprised of two parts: an upper triangular part termed the *corpus,* or *body,* and a lower cylindrical, and smaller, part designated the *cervix,* or *neck* (Fig. 2–4).

CORPUS The corpus narrows from above downward. Its upper, rounded portion, above the points of entrance of the fallopian tubes, is termed the *fundus uteri,* and the lower, narrowed portion where the corpus meets the cervix is called the *isthmus* (Fig. 2–6). The isthmus is significant during pregnancy when it forms the lower uterine segment; the remainder of the corpus makes up the upper uterine segment.

The cavity of the corpus of a nonpregnant uterus is small, since the major part of the corpus consists of thick muscular tissue and its anterior and posterior walls lie close together. The uterine cavity is somewhat triangular in shape with an opening at each of the three angles. The openings at the *cornua,* or two upper angles, join with the fallopian tubes, and the lower opening leads into the cavity of the cervix, which in turn opens into the vagina (Fig. 2–6).

The corpus of the uterus is a firm, hard mass, consisting of irregularly disposed, involuntary (nonstriated) muscle fibers, connective tissue, elastic fibers, nerves, and blood vessels and an inner lining of mucous membrane. It consists of three layers: the serous, the muscular, and the mucous.

1. The serous layer, also termed the *perimetrium,* is the external layer. It is derived from the peritoneum, which covers the uterus front and back, except along the lower part of the anterior wall, where it is reflexed up over the bladder (Fig. 2–6).
2. The muscular layer, designated the *myometrium,* is the middle layer (Fig. 2–4). It makes up the largest part of the uterus. This layer consists of muscular tissue through which are interspersed blood vessels, lymphatics, and nerves. The arrangement of the muscle fibers in the uterus is unique. They run longitudinally, circularly, spirally, and crisscross in every direction, forming a veritable network. Strong intermittent contractions of this muscular layer during labor dilate the cervical canal to permit the fetus to pass through it and also serve as a major force in advancing the infant through the birth canal during delivery. Contraction of these unusually arranged muscle fibers around open blood vessels is the chief factor in prevention of hemorrhage after delivery of the placenta.
3. The mucous, internal layer, which lines the uterine cavity, is called the *endometrium* (Fig. 2–4). It is a pinkish, velvety, highly vascular mucous membrane which contains numerous uterine glands and is covered with ciliated columnar epithelium. This layer undergoes constant cyclic changes during the reproductive period and varies in thickness from 1 to 5 mm, depending on the phase of the cycle. These changes are described under "The Menstrual (Endometrial) Cycle" on subsequent pages. This internal layer is continuous with the lining of the fallopian tubes and with the lining of the cervix.

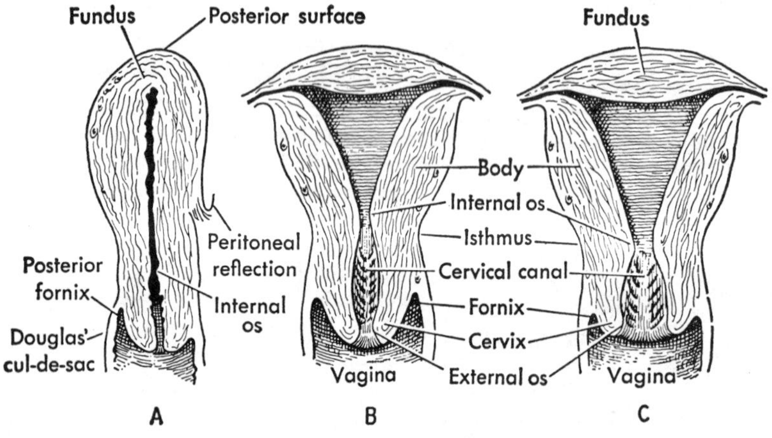

Figure 2-6. Diagrams of sections of virgin and multiparous uteri. *A.* Anteroposterior section. *B.* Lateral section of a virgin uterus. *C.* Lateral section of a multiparous uterus. Since Douglas' cul-de-sac lies beyond the upper portion of the posterior wall of the vagina, it is through the posterior fornix that pathology in the cul-de-sac often can be determined by palpation, by cul-de-sac puncture, or by insertion of a culdoscope for visualization.

CERVIX The cervix, which constitutes the smaller part of the uterus, measures from 2.5 to 3 cm long, about one third the length of the corpus. It is approximately an inch in diameter. About one half of the cervix protrudes into the vagina (Figs. 2-4 and 2-6). The attachment of the vagina at about the midpoint divides the cervix into two parts, a supravaginal and an infravaginal portion.

The cavity of the cervix, known as the *cervical canal,* is spindle-shaped, being expanded between its two somewhat constricted openings, the internal orifice or *internal os* above, by which it opens into the cavity of the uterine body, and the external orifice or *external os* below, opening into the vagina (Fig. 2-6). The external os, only a few millimeters in diameter, is a small round opening in the woman who has not borne children, but after childbirth is converted into a small transverse opening, bounded in front by the *anterior lip* and posteriorly by the *posterior lip* of the cervix. It is through the cervical canal that the fetus passes during birth. Under the influence of strong uterine muscle contractions the cervix dilates sufficiently to permit a full-term infant to pass through it and thereafter returns to its original size and shape, with the exception of the change in the external os noted above.

The cervix consists largely of connective tissue, but contains some muscle fibers and elastic tissue. It has many blood vessels. The cervical canal is lined with a single layer of ciliated columnar epithelium, which contains numerous glands extending into the stroma of the cervix. These glands secrete a mucus with complex properties that vary considerably during the different phases of each ovarian cycle, as described below. Near the external os the cervical lining changes to squamous epithelium, similar to the lining of the vagina.

BLOOD SUPPLY The uterus has an excellent blood, lymph, and nerve supply. The abundant blood supply reaches the uterus principally through the uterine arteries from the internal iliac (hypogastric) arteries, but also to some extent through the ovarian arteries from the aorta. The arteries follow a tortuous course, and many of the branches anastomose. Arteries from both sides of the uterus are united by a branch vessel in the area where the cervix and corpus of the uterus meet, thus forming an encircling artery at this site. A deep cervical tear during delivery of an infant may break this vessel and result in profuse bleeding. Veins in the uterus are also large and tortuous. The uterine and ovarian veins empty into the internal iliac (hypogastric) veins and then into the common iliac veins.

POSITION The uterus normally occupies an oblique or almost horizontal position in the body, with the corpus pointed forward. It is also slightly anteflexed, being somewhat bent forward on itself. In this position the fundus lies above the bladder, and the cervix points downward and backward toward the sacrum (Fig. 2-5). However, the position of the uterus is not firmly fixed, and it is easily subject to variations. A distended bladder may push the uterine body backward; a full rectum, forward. Changes of body posture may alter the position of the uterus, and during pregnancy it rises upward.

LIGAMENTS The major support to the uterus comes from the muscles and fascia of the pelvic diaphragm, to which it is attached at the junction of the cervix and corpus. Several pairs of ligaments, described below, give additional support and help to maintain the uterus in its forward inclination.

The *broad ligaments,* one on each side, are in reality one continuous structure that is formed by a fold of the peritoneum, which drops down over the uterus, investing the corpus, part of the cervix, and part of the posterior wall of the vagina (Fig. 2-4). It unites on each side of the uterus to form a broad, flat membrane extending laterally to the pelvic wall, dividing the pelvic cavity into an anterior and posterior compartment, containing, respectively, the bladder and rectum. Between the folds of the broad ligament are situated the ovaries and ovarian ligaments, the fallopian tubes, the round ligaments, the cardinal ligaments, blood vessels, lymphatics, nerves, and a certain amount of muscle and connective tissue.

The *cardinal ligaments,* one on each side, are a part of the broad ligaments, making up their lower borders. They are bands of dense connective tissue attached to the supravaginal part of the cervix and extending to the lateral wall of the pelvis. These ligaments, along with the pelvic diaphragm and the perineum, keep the uterus from prolapsing by providing support from below.

The *round ligaments,* one on each side, are fibromuscular cords composed of muscle prolonged from the uterus and a small amount of connective tissue. They contain blood and lymph vessels and nerves. They extend upward and forward from their uterine origin just below and in front of the tubal entrance, pass through the inguinal canal, and merge into the mons veneris.

The *uterosacral ligaments,* again one on each side, extend backward from the cervix, pass on each side of the rectum, and insert at the posterior wall of the pelvis (Fig. 2-4). They connect the cervix with the fascia covering the sacrum and aid in keeping the uterus in its normal position by exerting traction on the cervix.

The *anterior ligament* is a portion of the peritoneum that forms a fold between the bladder and the uterus. The *posterior ligament* is formed in the same manner by a deep fold of peritoneum between the uterus and the rectum.

Vagina

The vagina is a musculomembranous canal which extends from the lower part of the vulva to the cervix and thus connects the external and internal reproductive organs (Fig. 2–5). It serves as the organ of copulation and as the passageway for menstrual blood and for the fetus during birth.

The axis of the vagina is pointed toward the first sacral vertebra, thus in the erect position of the body it is directed upward and backward from the vulva to the cervix, to which it joins at an angle (Fig. 2–5). Attachment to the cervix is near its midpoint. The cervix thus protrudes into the vagina for 1.0 to 1.5 cm (about 1/2 in.) at almost a right angle, with the external os pointing backward. The posterior wall of the vagina is about 8 to 9 cm (3.2 to 3.6 in.) long. The anterior wall is shorter, because of the angle of its attachment, measuring 6 to 7 cm (2.4 to 2.8 in.) in length (Fig. 2–5).

The vagina consists of a muscular layer, a loose connective tissue layer, and a mucous layer. It is abundantly supplied with blood vessels and lymphatics. The mucous layer is a thick, heavy, mucous membrane which normally lies in small transverse folds or corrugations called *rugae.* These folds are obliterated and the lining is stretched into a smooth surface as the canal distends during delivery; the folds may disappear after childbirth. The epithelial cells of the mucosa undergo changes in response to hormonal stimulation, showing different characteristics during the various phases of ovarian function. The mucosal cells contain a considerable amount of glycogen.

There are no glands in the vagina. The small amount of whitish secretion present in the vagina is derived from the epithelial cells, the mucus-secreting glands in the cervix, and from the bacteria that normally inhabit the vagina and their by-products. Nonpathogenic organisms are normally present in the vagina; among these the Döderlein bacilli are prevalent and important to maintenance of normal secretion and acidity. During the childbearing years of life the vaginal secretion is normally acid, with a pH ranging from 4.0 to 5.0. This acidic reaction is believed to be due to lactic acid resulting from breakdown of glycogen by the Döderlein bacilli. The pH varies with ovarian activity; the acidity is somewhat reduced by alkaline cervical secretions before the onset of menstruation and by menstrual flow during menstruation.

The vagina is somewhat flattened, since the anterior and posterior walls lie in apposition toward the middle; on cross section it resembles the letter H. The bore of the vaginal canal ordinarily permits introduction of a vaginal speculum for visualization of the cervix or introduction of one or two fingers for palpation of the pelvic organs. The vagina is capable of a great deal of distention, as is evident from the tremendous stretching it undergoes during the birth of a child. Tissue changes occurring during the pregnancy permit such distention. The levator ani muscle, through which the vagina passes, serves to constrict the vaginal opening to some extent, and the sphincter vaginae provides slight sphincter action, but the vagina is not tightly closed by a sphincter as are the urethral and anal openings.

The upper end of the vagina, which forms a circular cuff around the cervix, ends in a blind vault. This vault, or space between the cervix and vaginal wall, is termed the *fornix* (Fig. 2–6). It is in actuality a potential space, since the tissues lie in apposition; however, they are easily spread apart. For convenience of description, the fornix is divided into four sections or fornices: the anterior, the posterior, and the two lateral fornices. The posterior fornix is considerably deeper than the anterior, because the vagina is about 2 cm (3/4 in.) longer posteriorly than anteriorly and it is attached higher up on the posterior wall of the cervix than on its anterior wall (Fig. 1–6). The fornices are important in pelvic examination, since the internal pelvic organs usually can be quite readily palpated through their relatively thin walls.

Other pelvic organs lie in close proximity to the vagina. The bladder and the urethra are situated immediately above it anteriorly. Posteriorly, the middle portion of the vaginal wall lies close to the rectum; at its lower end the perineal body and the rectovaginal septum separate the vagina and the rectum; and at its upper end a blind pouch in the peritoneal cavity, known as *Douglas' cul-de-sac,* lies between the vagina and the rectum (Figs. 2–5 and 2–6). In this cul-de-sac area the peritoneum is separated from the vagina by only a thin muscular wall.

Fallopian (Uterine) Tubes

The fallopian tubes, also known as oviducts, are two slender muscular tubes that extend laterally from the cornua of the uterine cavity, one from each side, to the ovaries (Fig. 2–4). They provide the passageway through which ova reach the uterus. After passing through the uterine muscle wall, the tubes extend between the folds of the upper margin of the broad ligaments, taking a somewhat tortuous course in an upward and outward direction. Their length varies from 7 to 14 cm (2.8 to 5.6 in.). Thickness also varies; at the juncture with the uterus the lumen of the tubes is so small as to admit the introduction of only a fine bristle, but there is a slight gradual increase in width distally.

The uterine tubes consist of a serous layer, made up of peritoneal covering, a muscular layer, and an inner mucous membrane, which lies in longitudinal folds (Fig. 2–4). The inner surface is lined by a single layer of epithelium composed in part of ciliated cells and in part of nonciliated, secretory cells. Rhythmic contractions of the musculature of the tube and probably also movement of the cilia effect transport of ova and sperm in the tubes. Activity of tubal mucosa and muscle undergoes cyclic changes in response to the hormonal changes of the ovarian cycle.

Each fallopian tube is described in several parts: the portion that passes through the muscular wall of the uterus is termed the *interstitial;* the *isthmus* is immediately adjacent to the uterus; the *ampulla* is the expanded lateral portion; and the wide distal opening is called the *fimbriated end* or *infundibulum*. The distal, or fimbriated, end of the tube is a funnel-shaped opening surrounded by fringelike projections called *fimbriae* (Fig. 2-4). One of the fimbria, the *fimbria ovarica,* which has the form of a shallow gutter, or groove, extends to, or almost to, the ovary. The fimbriated ends of the fallopian tubes open into the peritoneal cavity. There is thus a small, but continuous opening from the vulva to the peritoneal cavity through the irregularly constructed muscular canal which passes through the vagina, the uterus, and the fallopian tubes. This canal is lined throughout its entire length with continuous mucous membrane.

Ovaries

The ovaries, the sex glands (gonads) of the female, are two small, flattened, oval-shaped organs, located one on each side of the uterus. They are attached to the back of the broad ligaments below the fimbriated end of the fallopian tubes (Fig. 2-4). The longest of the fimbria from each tube, the fimbria ovarica, reaches to, or nearly to, the ovary. Each ovary is attached to the lateral wall of the uterus by the *ovarian ligament* and to the pelvic wall by the portion of the broad ligament that continues beyond the fallopian tube; this portion is termed the *infundibulopelvic* or *suspensory ligament* (Fig. 2-4). The position of the ovaries is not fixed and will vary with positional changes of the uterus.

An ovary is usually described as having the size and shape of an almond; each is about 4 to 5 cm long, 2 cm wide, and 1 cm thick, and has a weight of 2 to 5 gm. It presents a glistening, more or less irregular, roughened surface externally, and is a dull white color. Size and external appearance of the ovaries vary according to the maturity of the woman, since the ovaries undergo constant change until after the menopause.

The ovary consists of two parts: a central portion or *medulla,* and an outer layer or *cortex*. The medulla is composed of connective tissue, blood and lymph vessels, and nerves. Embedded in the cortex, between connective tissue, are numerous minute follicles, each of which contains an oocyte, the germ cell of the female. These have been produced during the first five to six months of fetal life, at which time further development of germ cells ceases, and the individual's full quota of oocytes is established. It is estimated that there are 200,000 or more primary oocytes present in each ovary at birth; many of these undergo degenerative changes early in life, leaving an estimated number of 50,000 or more in each ovary at the beginning of adolescence. During reproductive years, the follicles containing the oocytes are present in varying stages of development between a primary state, when the follicle is designated a *primary follicle,* and the mature stage, when it is termed *a graafian follicle*. Growth and development of the follicles are described below under "The Ovarian Cycle."

The ovaries perform two vital functions: (1) they produce, mature, and extrude ova, and (2) they elaborate internal secretions or hormones. Because of this latter function, they are included in the group of glands classified as the endocrine, or ductless, glands of the body. Ovarian function will be described in detail subsequently.

Related Pelvic Organs

The bladder and the rectum are contained in the pelvic cavity and lie in close proximity to the reproductive organs. Thus pressure from one organ may exert an effect on another. A full bladder or full rectum may interfere with a satisfactory examination of the reproductive organs. Pressure exerted during pregnancy by the enlarged uterus is felt in both the rectum and bladder at certain stages of pregnancy and may at these times cause a feeling of urgency to evacuate their contents frequently.

Bladder and Urethra

The urinary bladder is a musculomembranous sac that serves as a reservoir for urine. It is situated behind the symphysis pubis and in front of the uterus and the vagina (Fig. 2-5). Urine is conducted into the bladder by the *ureters,* two slender tubes, one on each side, that pass downward from the kidney pelves. The ureters pass across the brim of the bony pelvis, to the posterior part of the bladder, which they enter somewhat obliquely, at about the level of the cervix (Fig. 2-4). Pressure of an enlarged pregnant uterus on the ureters may be a contributing factor to pyelitis, sometimes a complication of pregnancy.

The bladder empties through the *urethra,* a short tube about 3.8 cm (1 1/2 in.) long that terminates in the *urinary meatus*. The meatus is a small opening situated in the middle of the vestibule between the clitoris and the vaginal orifice (Fig. 2-1).

Rectum

The rectum, the lowest segment of the intestinal tract, is situated behind and to the left of the uterus and vagina (Fig. 2-5). It extends downward from the sigmoid flexure of the colon to its termination in the anal opening. The *anus* is a deeply pigmented, puckered opening situated 4 to 5 cm (1 1/2 to 2 in.) below the vaginal orifice. It is provided with bands of circular muscles, the *internal* and *external sphincter ani.* Normal contraction and relaxation of these muscles make possible retention and expulsion of rectal contents. The skin covering the surface of the body extends upward into the anus, where it becomes highly vascular, and merges into the mucous membrane lining of the rectum. Veins of the lower rectum and anal canal sometimes become engorged and inflamed during pregnancy, as a result of pressure exerted by the greatly enlarged uterus. The distended veins, called *hemorrhoids,* not infrequently protrude from the anus and may become very painful.

The Breasts

The breasts are large, specially modified skin glands of the compound racemose or grape-cluster type, embedded in fat and connective tissue, and abundantly supplied with nerves and blood vessels (Fig. 2–7). They are situated quite remote from the pelvic organs, but because of the intimate functional relation with these organs, the breasts of the female may be regarded as accessory glands of the reproductive system. Their function is to secrete, in the parturient woman, suitable nourishment for the human infant during the first months of life.

The breasts are symmetrically placed, one on each side of the chest, and occupy the place between the second and sixth ribs, extending from the margin of the sternum almost to the midaxillary line. A bed of connective tissue separates them from the underlying muscles and ribs. The breasts are usually hemispheric or conical in shape, but vary in size and shape at different ages and with different individuals, particularly in women who have borne and nursed children, when they tend to become pendulous.

A nipple protrudes from the apex of each breast for a distance of 0.6 to 1.3 cm (1/4 to 1/2 in.). The nipples are composed largely of sensitive, erectile tissue and become more rigid and prominent during pregnancy and at menstrual periods. The nipple surfaces are pierced by the orifices of the milk ducts, which are 15 to 20 in number (Fig. 28–1, Chapter 28).

The breasts are covered with delicate, smooth skin, except for the *areolae,* the circular, pigmented areas 2.5 to 10 cm (1 to 4 in.) in diameter that surround the nipples. The areolae are darker in brunettes than in blonds, and in all women become darker during pregnancy, gradually becoming paler again after delivery. The surface of the nipples and of the areolae is roughened by small, shotlike lumps or papillae known as the *tubercles of Montgomery* (Fig. 28–1). This roughness becomes more marked during pregnancy, since the papillae then become larger. The tubercles are sebaceous glands that secrete a lipoid material which lubricates the nipples and thus helps to protect them during the infant's sucking.

The small breasts of the child begin to develop markedly at puberty due to hormonal stimulation. During pregnancy, hormones influence additional growth, as well as stimulate the secretion of milk after delivery of a baby.

The mammary glands first appear in the human embryo at 6 weeks as thickened bands of raised ectoderm. As the fetus grows the mammary glands continue to develop until at full-term birth they have become rudimentary mammary buds and nipples. Each breast consists of 15 to 20 epithelial tubules surrounded by connective tissue. Sometimes the glandular tissue of the newborn is developed sufficiently to secrete a small amount of fluid for a few days after birth. This is the result of stimulation from a high level of estrogens in the mother's blood, which crosses the placenta to the fetus. During infancy and childhood there is little development of the breasts other than normal growth along with the rest of the body.

In early puberty the breasts undergo extensive changes and rapid growth, characterized by a complex branching and lengthening of the mammary ducts. The nipples enlarge and the areolae become pigmented. Each breast is made up of 15 to 20 lobes of ductal systems, and each lobe has an excretory duct that opens into the nipple. A large amount of connective tissue and adipose tissue sur-

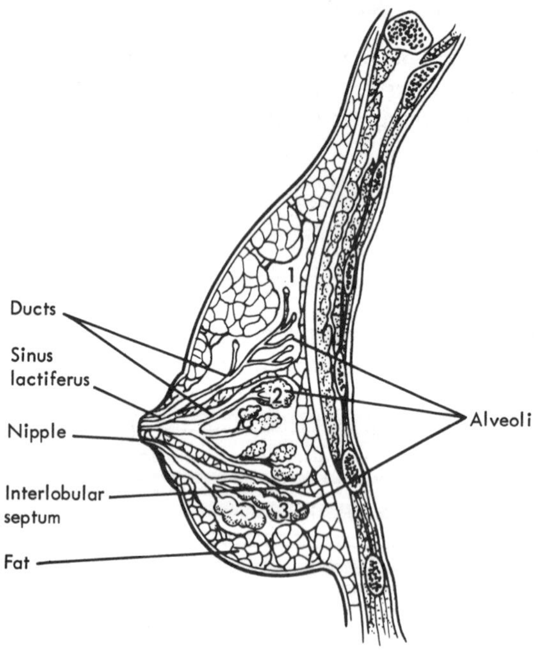

Figure 2–7. Cross section of mammary gland, showing the development of the alveolar system under different conditions. *1.* Nonpregnant woman. *2.* Middle pregnancy. *3.* During lactation. [Reprinted with permission from Sigmund Grollman, *The Human Body: Its Structure and Function,* 4th ed. New York: Macmillan, 1978, Copyright Sigmund Grollman, 1978.]

rounds each ductal system. True alveolar (secretory) cells are not formed in this first period of rapid growth and development.

Mammary growth is controlled by hormones. The combined influence of the ovarian hormones, estrogen and progesterone, and the anterior pituitary hormones, somatotropin (growth hormone) and prolactin, bring about normal growth of the breasts, providing that normal metabolism of the mammary cells is maintained by insulin. It is believed that estrogens are responsible for development of the mammary ducts, and progesterone stimulates lobuloalveolar development.

At the end of puberty the breasts reach a size that is characteristic for the individual woman. There is little change until pregnancy, when major changes take place, especially in development of secretory tissue (described in Chapter 8). Still other changes occur during lactation, when the glandular tissue secretes milk (Chapter 28).

Under hormonal influence the breasts continue internal changes during the first years after puberty until they reach maximum development. These changes alternate between proliferation and involution according to the alternating blood levels of hormones during the menstrual cycles. In the two-week period after ovulation, while progesterone predominates, the epithelial glandular tissue proliferates. Under the influence of adrenocorticoids, insulin, somatotropin, prolactin, estrogen, and progesterone, the ducts lengthen and branch, some lobuloalveolar development takes place, and increased vascularization and blood flow occur. The breasts may feel somewhat tender and heavy during this time.

With the onset of menstruation, and for the two weeks following, the ovarian hormonal influence is different. Estrogen levels are relatively higher than progesterone. During this period there is a regression in some of the cellular changes that took place in the previous two-week period. Involution of glandular tissue does not regress to the state of the previous proliferation, however, and there is always some advancement until the breasts have reached their maximum postpuberty development. An understanding of the cycling of the ovarian hormones, described below, will be helpful in understanding their influence on breast development.

PHYSIOLOGY OF THE REPRODUCTIVE SYSTEM

During childhood the reproductive system undergoes gradual growth, along with other parts of the body, but it does not become physiologically mature until sometime during adolescence. About the age of 9 to 11 years the reproductive organs begin to undergo rapid development and in another three to five years they are physiologically capable of carrying out their reproductive function. This development is completed earlier today than in past generations and is accompanied by rapid physical growth of the entire body.

The period of adolescence and puberty will be described before function of the mature system is considered.

Discussion of adolescence and puberty and the physical and endocrinologic changes in the reproductive system applies, in general, to both sexes, and these changes will be presented as similar to the time of full maturation of the system.

Adolescence

Adolescence is the period of physiologic and psychologic growth and development during which an individual gradually progresses from the physical and emotional characteristics of a child to full maturation of the body and the traits and capabilities of an adult. It is the transitional period of development between childhood and adulthood. The adolescent period covers a span of several years. It is characterized by continuing growth processes that lead to somatic and sexual maturation and psychologic maturity. It is considered to begin with puberty, which of itself begins at variable times in different individuals, and to extend over a span of several years until sexual development reaches the adult stage. Thus age at which adolescence begins and the rate of progression to adulthood vary, depending on constitutional traits, genetic influences, and other factors.

Major issues during adolescence concern (1) biologic effects, in which hormonal changes lead to both physical and emotional changes in the individual; (2) body-image changes as the body rather quickly matures to adult proportions; and (3) conflicts, confusion, and ambivalence over the kind of behavior this new individual wishes to adopt.

Adolescence is thus a period of emotional growth of considerable magnitude as well as a time of many physiologic changes. An adolescent changes from a dependent child to a more independent individual, with an expanding social awareness requiring many social adjustments. An adolescent's ties with other persons change; these ties become strong with other adolescents of both sexes and are of a less dependent nature with parents. A striving for independence is strong in the adolescent, but this is interspersed with intervals of dependence. Periods of modesty, self-consciousness, uncertainty, and awkwardness are common during the adjustments the adolescent necessarily must make to rapid increase in body size and in sexual development. Confused feelings and attitudes regarding sex role arise. Understanding, support, and guidance by adults throughout the variety of changes that take place in adolescents can contribute much to their emotional growth.

Puberty

Puberty may be defined as a series of physiologic events that take place over a period of several years and that result in sexual maturity of the individual and his/her capacity to reproduce. Puberty is sometimes considered synonymous with early adolescence. Puberty cannot be dated as beginning at a specific time. It is instead a series of events—a phase of development—that takes place over a period of three to five years, beginning usually between 9 and 14 years of age. Genetic and environmental factors appear to have an influence on its onset.

The changes of puberty are dependent upon a number of interrelated factors, but especially rely upon changes in the function of the endocrine glands. It is at this time that the anterior pituitary gland begins secretion of appreciable amounts of gonadotropic hormones, which thereafter gradually rise to adult levels. These hormones, in turn, gradually stimulate the gonads to produce hormones and to mature germ cells. The typical sex hormones secreted by the gonads, estrogen in the female and testosterone in the male, stimulate growth and development of adult sexual characteristics. Among pubertal developments are accelerated growth of the body, rapid growth of the genital organs, development of pubic and axillary hair, menstruation and ovulation in the female, and spermatogenesis in the male.

The changes in hormonal milieu lead to changes in psychologic perspectives as well as to distinct physiologic events.

Although the onset of puberty is variable, it follows quite a similar course in both males and females. There is some age difference as to when changes appear, but the sequence of events tends to be the same in all individuals.

Physical Changes of Puberty

The usual sequence of sexual development in girls and the average age at which these changes are first seen are listed in Table 2-1. If sexual change in a girl begins before the age of 8, her development is considered precocious, and if it does not begin by age 12 to 13, it is considered delayed. Average age and sequence of development in boys are listed in Table 3-1, page 36.

An initial change at the beginning of puberty in girls is growth of the bony pelvis and widening of the hips due to both actual growth and increased deposition of fat. Certain changes in the breasts also appear early, but at first only in the areolar area which becomes puffy and pigmented. The breast tissue first appears as a nodule under the areola, then later extends outward and continues enlargement. The ovaries also begin to enlarge.

Breast development usually precedes appearance of pubic hair. With continued breast development and growth of pubic hair, appearance of axillary hair, growth of the external genitalia, development of the vagina toward adult characteristics, and a thick white vaginal discharge also occur.

Table 2-1. Average Age and Sequence of Sexual Development—Girls*

Age (years)	
9–10	Growth of bony pelvis Hyperemia and pigmentation of areola
10–11	Breast-budding Pubic hair
11–12	Growth of internal and external genitalia Changes in vaginal smear Further growth of breasts Axillary hair
12–13	Pigmentation of nipples Menarche
13–14	Ovulation
14–15	Acne Deepening of voice
16–17	Arrest of skeletal growth

* Reprinted with permission from S. Douglas Frasier, *Pediatric Endocrinology*, Grune & Stratton, New York, 1980, p. 148.

There is an acceleration of growth during adolescence. In girls this usually begins soon after the appearance of pubic hair, and it reaches its greatest increase in the year preceding the menarche. In general, then, girls grow most rapidly between 12 and 13 years of age.

The first menstrual period, termed the *menarche*, usually appears after axillary hair is noted. The average age for the first menstruation in girls in the United States is 12 3/4 years. Age of menarche varies widely, however, and it may range from 9 to 17 years. Menstrual periods are often not well established at the beginning, and they may occur at irregular intervals during the first one to two years. These periods are likely to be anovulatory at first and occur as a result of changes in estrogen levels rather than following a complete hormonal cycle and progesterone withdrawal.

Ovulation usually does not begin for one to two years after the menarche. Following ovulation, the menstrual periods become ovulatory, as described later in this chapter.

After the menarche, development of the breasts and the reproductive tract and of the pubic and axillary hair continues to full development.

Endocrinologic Changes of Puberty

Pubertal maturation and sexual development in both sexes, and thereafter continuing function of the mature reproductive tracts, all depend upon a control system that involves the extrahypothalamic central nervous system, the hypothalamus, the anterior pituitary, and end organs (the gonads). This system, which regulates hormonal synthesis and secretion and through these hormones gonadal development and function, is largely self-regulating. There is an interrelationship between the various component parts of the system that controls what hormones are secreted, when they are put out, and how much is produced. Certain stimuli lead to the secretion of a specific hormone and yet other stimuli will at certain points exert an inhibitory effect (also called a negative feedback). All levels of control are involved in regulation of the hormonal influence on gonadal function. Figure 2–8 provides a schematic representation of the interrelationship of the organs of the system.

PREPUBERTY All levels of the gonadal control system are functional in the child. The gonads, which will mature at puberty, are functionally quiet until that time, but they are capable of mature function in the prepuberty period. The child has low concentrations of gonadotropins and of gonadal hormones in the blood, and a negative feedback apparently exists between the gonads, the anterior pituitary, and the hypothalamus.

Maturation of the control system, which regulates gonadal function, takes place during puberty. The function of the different parts of the control system change in a sequence that eventually brings about adult characteristics and function of the reproductive system. The mechanisms by which many of these changes take place are not known.

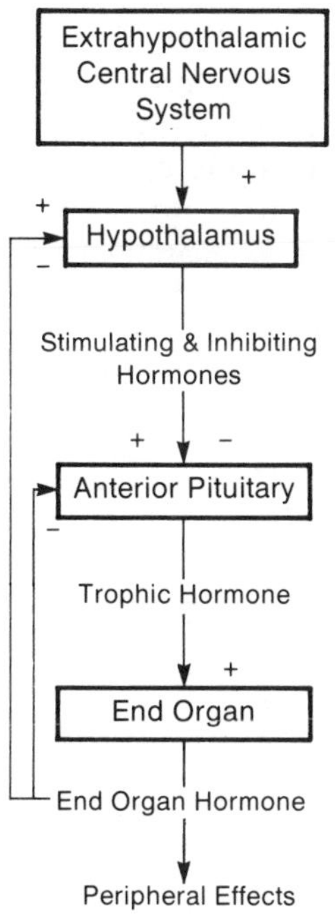

Figure 2–8. Schematic representation of the regulatory mechanisms for the synthesis and secretion of hormones with a hypothalamic, pituitary, end-organ control system. (Reproduced with permission from S. Douglas Frasier, *Pediatric Endocrinology,* New York: Grune and Stratton, 1980, p. 14.)

In brief, the maturational changes are as follows. At the onset of puberty the hypothalamic response changes. The hypothalamus becomes more responsive to neural input from the central nervous system, and the extreme sensitivity of the hypothalamus to the negative feedback influence of the gonadal hormones decreases. The hypothalamus no longer responds to the low level of circulating gonadal hormones with the same sensitivity that it did in the prepuberty period. The result of the changes is an increased secretion of gonadotropin-releasing hormone (GnRH), which, in turn, stimulates the anterior pituitary to increase synthesis of gonadotropins, known as follicle-stimulating hormone (FSH) and luteinizing hormone (LH).

The increasing gonadotropins now stimulate further development of the gonads. The gonads begin to secrete increasing amounts of steroids, which stimulate development of the secondary sex characteristics. There is an interrelationship between these various component parts that controls how much of the several hormones is produced and at what times.

As maturation is taking place, the daily secretion of the gonadotropins and the gonadal hormones increases with advancing puberty. When all changes have taken place and adult responses are achieved at all levels, the maturational process can be considered complete. Function of the mature hormonal system in the female will be described below. That of the mature male reproductive process will be presented in Chapter 3.

The Adrenal Cortex

The adrenal cortex is very important in the pubertal maturation process. It is the major source of androgen in the female. Adrenal androgen secretion stimulates the growth of pubic and axillary hair, as well as the characteristic spurt in body growth, with a distinct increase in height and a still more marked increase in weight. Adrenal androgens increase prior to increasing activity of the hypothalamic–anterior pituitary-gonadal system, and this activity continues to increase during puberty.

Function of the Mature Female Reproductive Cycle

After the ability to reproduce has been attained, the reproductive organs of the female go through a series of cyclic changes each month throughout the childbearing years, with the exception of alterations during pregnancy and lactation. The many changes in each cycle include development of a graafian follicle, ovulation, formation of a corpus luteum, production of ovarian hormones, changes in the epithelial lining and secretions of the reproductive tract, and menstruation. Normal function of the reproductive organs is dependent on a complex interrelationship between the hypothalamic gonadotropin-releasing hormone, the gonad-stimulating hormones from the anterior pituitary gland, and the ovarian hormones, as previously described.

THE OVARIAN CYCLE

The ovarian cycle consists of the series of changes in an ovary that are repeated at monthly intervals. These changes are under the influence of anterior pituitary gonadotropic hormones. Main phases of the cycle include the development of a graafian follicle, ovulation, and formation of a corpus luteum. The results of ovarian changes are the maturation and extrusion of an ovum, making one available for fertilization at monthly intervals, and the production of ovarian hormones.

Primary Follicle

The formation of each woman's full quota of ova is complete before birth. These *immature* or *primary oocytes,* as they are called, are single cells scattered throughout the connective tissue of the ovarian cortex. An oocyte is sometimes referred to as an ovum, although it is technically not an ovum until it has reached full maturation. Each oocyte is surrounded by a single layer of flattened cells. This structure of an oocyte and its surrounding single layer of epithelial cells is termed a *primary follicle* (Fig. 2-9). It is estimated that at birth each ovary contains 200,000, or even a larger number, of immature follicles closely packed together and separated by thin bands of connective tissue. Many of these disappear in early life by an atretic process, so that perhaps 50,000 or a somewhat larger number of oocytes are present in each ovary when puberty is reached.

Some of the immature follicles are always in a process of development toward a more mature state. Up to the age of puberty they develop mainly in the deeper portion of the cortex and do not reach the surface of the ovary and rupture, as does the mature follicle during reproductive years. After a certain stage of development has been reached, these partly matured follicles go through retrogressive changes. At birth the ovary is largely cortex, but the cortex gradually becomes thinner as the follicles go through development and then disappear.

Graafian Follicle

From the time ovulation begins during puberty until the menopause, some of the primary follicles, under the influence of follicle-stimulating hormone from the anterior pituitary gland, develop to full maturation. When a follicle matures, remarkable changes take place (1) in the oocyte, (2) in the cells of the follicle, and (3) in the connective tissue adjacent to the follicle.

As soon as a primary follicle begins maturation, two layers of cells derived from the adjacent ovarian stroma develop around it. The outer layer of cells is known as the *theca externa* and the inner layer the *theca interna.* The theca interna seems to be important in the formation of the hormone estrogen, which is derived from the follicle. The theca interna cells develop a granular appearance due to fat and a yellow pigment. They are known as *theca lutein cells,* and have a role in the formation of the corpus luteum and in degeneration of follicles that do not develop to full maturity.

The single layer of cells of the primordial follicle, the layer surrounding the oocyte, proliferates during maturation of the follicle, with the result that the oocyte is surrounded by several layers of epithelial cells instead of only one layer. Fluid develops between the follicular cells, and, as this fluid accumulates in the center of the follicle, it forms a vesicle (Fig. 2-9). This fluid, known as *follicular fluid* or *liquor folliculi,* contains the ovarian follicular hormone *estrogen*. The epithelial lining of the

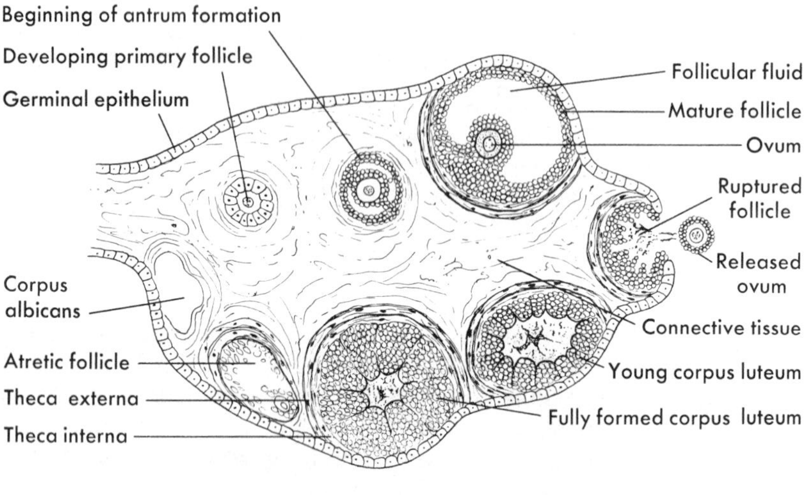

Figure 2-9. Diagrammatic view of the ovary showing ovum in various stages of maturation. (Reprinted with permission from Marjorie A. Miller, Anna B. Drakontides, and Lutie C. Leavell, *Kimber-Gray-Stockpole's Anatomy and Physiology,* 17th ed., New York: Macmillan, 1977.)

follicle, which encloses the oocyte and the follicular fluid, having now developed to several layers of thickness, is termed the *membrana granulosa* (Fig. 2–9). This lining is much thicker at one point than in any other area; at this thickened point it forms a mass of cells in which the oocyte is included. This mass is called the *discus proligerus* or *cumulus oophorus* (Fig. 2–9).

The structure described above constitutes a *graafian follicle,* named for Dr. Reijnier de Graaf, who first described it (Fig. 2–9). In the course of its maturation, the graafian follicle expands toward the surface of the ovary, where it resembles a clear blister. When fully developed and about to rupture, this blisterlike protrusion on the surface of the ovary measures 10 to 15 mm (roughly 1/2 in.) in diameter.

While the changes described above are taking place in the follicle, the oocyte grows and increases considerably in size; its diameter may reach a length of 0.2 mm. During this growth period yolk granules, known as *deutoplasm,* are being deposited in the cytoplasm to be available for nutriment during the early days of embryonic development, should fertilization occur. Just before rupture of the graafian follicle, the oocyte undergoes the first of the two maturational cell divisions that must take place in all germ cells before they are ready for fertilization. Maturation of germ cells is described on pages 43–45.

Maturation of a follicle, and finally rupture and extrusion of the ovum, occur regularly each month during the years from puberty to the menopause, except during pregnancy, and probably also during lactation, when this process is suspended. Several follicles begin to develop, but usually only one reaches maturity each month (Fig. 2–10). The others, after reaching partial

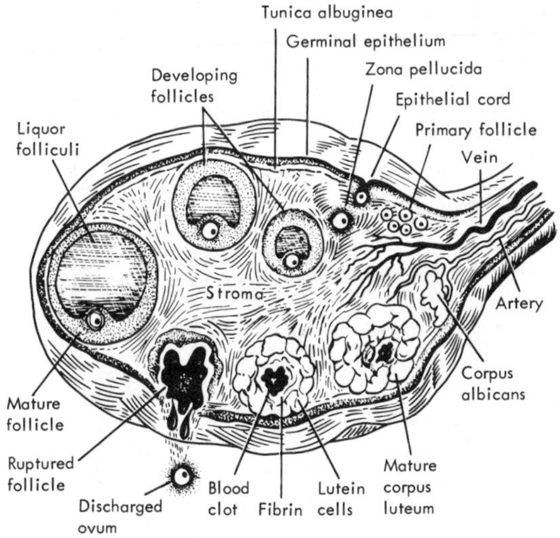

Figure 2–10. Cross section of ovary, showing the stroma and associated structures. [Reprinted with permission from Sigmund Grollman, *The Human Body: Its Structure and Physiology,* 4th ed. New York: Macmillan, 1978. Copyright Sigmund Grollman, 1978.]

development, undergo an atretic process. Occasionally, however, more than one follicle matures and ruptures at the same time, and if each extruded ovum is fertilized, this results in double-ovum twins or treble-ovum triplets.

Ovulation

When a graafian follicle, with its enclosed maturing oocyte, reaches the surface of the ovary, its wall becomes thinner and it finally ruptures. The follicle contents, the follicular fluid and the oocyte which has become separated from the discus proligerus, are extruded. This process of extrusion of a maturing oocyte from the ovary through rupture of a graafian follicle is called ovulation (Fig. 2–10). The ovum, with some adherent epithelial cells, is discharged near the fimbriated end of the fallopian tube, which it usually enters (Fig. 5–6, page 64).

Ovulation is the dividing period between two phases of an ovarian and a menstrual cycle. The preovulatory period, during which a graafian follicle and its hormone estrogen develop, is commonly termed the *follicular phase.* The postovulatory period, during which the corpus luteum and its hormones develop, is designated as the *luteal phase.*

The time of ovulation is approximately 14 days before the end of a cycle, which means about 14 days before the first day of the next menstrual period. In a 28-day cycle ovulation therefore will occur at approximately the middle of the cycle or usually between the twelfth and sixteenth days. In cycles that are shorter or longer than the average of 28 days, ovulation will occur before or after the middle of the cycle since the postovulatory period remains fairly constant at approximately 14 days.

Several signs and symptoms may give evidence that ovulation will or has probably taken place. Some are recognizable only after ovulation has occurred and thus do not predict when the follicle will rupture.

The cervical mucus alters considerably under estrogen stimulation as the graafian follicle proceeds in its development. This mucus reaches its maximum changes at ovulation and after ovulation returns to the characteristics prior to the stimulation by estrogen. The characteristics of cervical mucus and examinations for evidence of ovulation are described on page 27 and in Chapter 7.

Midcycle abdominal pain, known as *mittelschmerz,* may be felt by some women near the time of ovulation. This discomfort may vary in intensity or in its regularity of appearance, and many women rarely or never experience it.

Midcycle vaginal bleeding, amounting to no more than spotting, is also noted by some women at the time of ovulation.

A shift in basal body temperature occurs at approximately the time of ovulation or shortly thereafter. The body temperature is relatively higher during the postovulatory than the preovulatory phase of the cycle. A rise of a fraction of a degree takes place rather abruptly at this shift. Often there is a sharp drop just before the rise. Once risen, the higher temperature level is maintained until at or near the next menstrual period, when it again drops. The basal body temperature shift is a useful clinical method of determining the approximate time of ovulation. The woman is instructed to take her temperature daily, immediately after waking in the morning and before arising. She records these daily readings on a graph in order to visualize the pattern they are taking (Fig. 2–11).

Corpus Luteum

After ovulation the cavity of the ruptured graafian follicle is replaced by a compact mass of tissue termed the *corpus luteum* (yellow body), so named because of its yellow color (Fig. 2–10). The corpus luteum functions as an endocrine organ. It produces a typical or main hormone *progesterone* and also secretes the follicular hormone *estrogen.*

Rapid changes take place in development of the corpus luteum; these are under the influence of the luteinizing hormone of the anterior pituitary gland. After extrusion of the oocyte and the follicular fluid with ovulation, the walls of the follicle collapse; its cavity becomes smaller; and the space that remains is filled with a small blood clot, which is soon absorbed. Granulosa cells that remained adherent to the follicle wall and cells from the theca interna begin invasion of the clot-filled follicle (Fig. 2–10). The granulosa cells increase in size and number and assume a yellowish tint due to a yellowish pigment; these cells are then termed *granulosa lutein cells.* Connective tissue and blood vessels arising from the theca interna grow into the structure between the lutein cells.

The corpus luteum continues activity and growth for about eight days and reaches a diameter of 10 to 20 mm at the end of that time. Its course thereafter is determined by whether or not the ovum has been fertilized. If fertilization has not taken place, which is the common event, retrogressive changes begin after about the eighth day. This structure is then termed the *corpus luteum of menstruation.* Degenerative changes are rapid; secretory activity decreases; menstruation begins in about six days; and regression of the corpus luteum is soon complete. The degenerated cells are absorbed, and the corpus luteum is replaced by connective tissue. Late in its regressive phase, when the corpus luteum takes on a dull white appearance, it is termed a *corpus albicans* (Fig. 2–10).

If the ovum has been fertilized, existence and activity of the corpus luteum, which is now termed the *corpus luteum of pregnancy,* continue for approximately three months. It becomes larger than the corpus luteum of menstruation and may occupy as much as one third of the ovary. The corpus luteum apparently functions at its

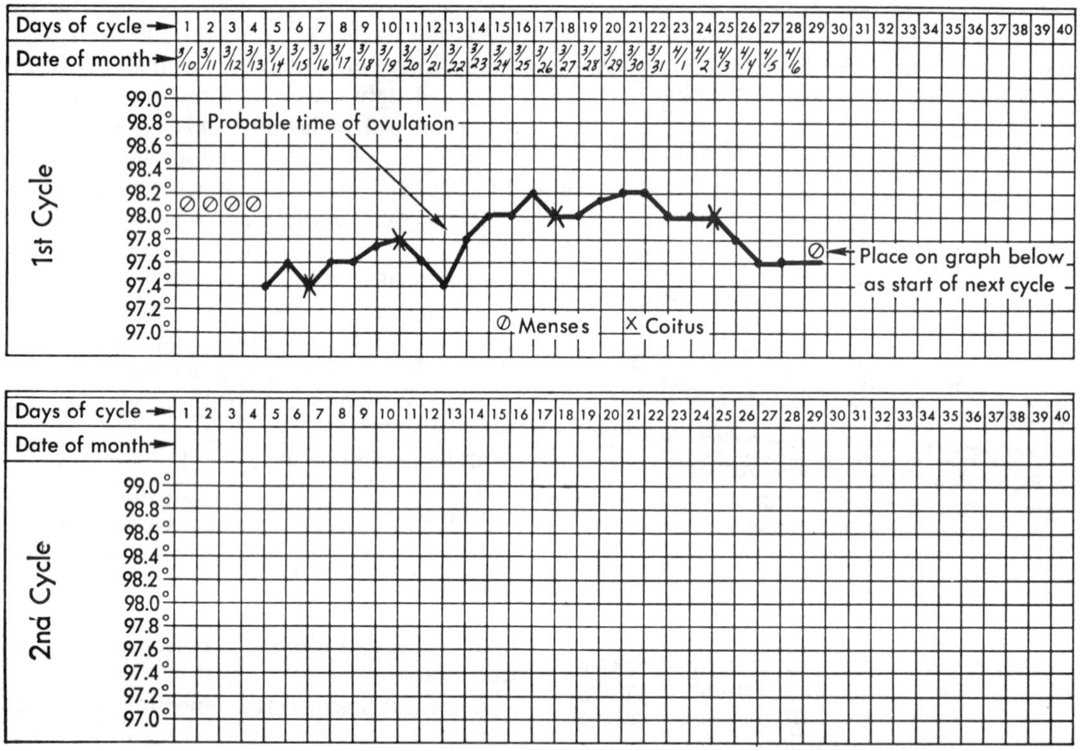

Figure 2–11. Basal body temperature record which may be used to determine the approximate time of ovulation.

highest level during the first two months of pregnancy, continues good function for another few weeks, and then, at about the third month of pregnancy, begins to undergo retrogressive changes and decrease in secretory activity. The placenta begins production of the corpus luteum hormones at a very early stage of development, secretes substantial amounts of hormones by the third month of pregnancy, and assumes the corpus luteum function as that structure regresses.

Follicular Atresia

The majority of primordial follicles that begin development do not reach maturity; they degenerate without rupture and disappear by a process termed *atresia*. When partly grown, the follicles undergo retrogressive changes, during which the oocyte undergoes cytolysis; the follicular fluid absorbs; and the follicle cells change until the structure takes on the characteristics of a degenerated corpus luteum. This atretic process begins during fetal life and continues until after the menopause. It is particularly active before puberty and during pregnancy.

The reason for the lavish provision of at least 200,000 or more oocytes for each woman, who uses only a few hundred in the course of her life, is not known. Whatever the purpose of this enormous supply, it makes possible the removal of a considerable amount of ovarian tissue, in case of disease, without loss of reproductive ability, provided the remaining tissue is normal.

The Hypothalamic–Anterior Pituitary–Ovarian Cycle Interrelationship

The central nervous system, hypothalamus, anterior pituitary gland, and ovaries are all closely interrelated in the reproductive process. Interaction among hormones released into the bloodstream from these organs follows a monthly cyclic pattern in which the proportion of each hormone present in the blood varies at different periods in each cycle. Levels of one hormone influence production of the others. The level of these hormones at different periods of the cycle in turn produces the cyclic changes that occur in all of the female reproductive organs each month, such as ovulation, changes in cervical secretion, changes in the endometrial lining, and menstruation.

CNS and Hypothalamus Control

Certain stimuli activate specialized neurons in the brain to release neurotransmitter molecules that reach neurosecretory cells in the hypothalamus, which is located at the base of the brain. These stimuli may be sensory from the external environment and/or humoral from the internal environment, such as a change in hormone levels.

When the hypothalamus receives the neurotransmitter message, it responds by releasing the appropriate releasing factor. The hypothalamus synthesizes and releases several different neurohormones that stimulate pituitary secretion; among these are a thyrotropin-releasing factor and a corticotropin-releasing factor. In responding to a message concerning the reproductive cycle, the hypothalamus discharges a gonadotropin-releasing factor (GnRF), which is a small polypeptide hormone composed of 10 amino acids. These hormones from the hypothalamus reach the anterior pituitary gland in high concentration through a short local circulatory system of small blood vessels, the portal vessels of the hypothalamopituitary stalk.

Pituitary Gonadotropic Hormones

The GnRF causes the anterior lobe of the pituitary gland to discharge two gonadotropic hormones. These are large glycoproteins called follicle-stimulating hormone (FSH) and luteinizing hormone (LH), which enter the bloodstream and are carried to the gonads where they exert their influence (Fig. 2–12).

In the female the two gonadotropic hormones act together in stimulating the ovaries, but each also has a specific effect. Although both hormones are present in fairly large amounts in the early part of a cycle, FSH is the hormone that causes growth and maturation of an ovarian follicle, changing it into a graafian follicle. As the follicle grows, its hormone-secreting cells increase the level of the estrogens, principally estradiol (Fig. 2–13).

The gonadotropin LH reaches a midcycle peak level about the time the graafian follicle and its enclosed oocyte are mature. The declining FSH level resurges at this time (Fig. 2–13). The surge of hormones, mainly LH, is responsible for triggering ovulation within 24 hours of this peak production.

After ovulation the empty follicle is changed to a corpus luteum. LH stimulates these new luteal cells to produce the ovarian hormone progesterone in increasing amounts. At this time ovarian hormonal production is reversed from a predominance of estrogens to a predominance of progesterone (Fig. 2–13).

Ovarian Hormones

The ovaries produce two steroid hormones, estrogen and progesterone, which exert a major influence on preparation of the endometrium for implantation of a fertilized ovum. In addition, these hormones have an effect on many other systems, including bone, muscle, blood, and metabolic processes. These two hormones are also pro-

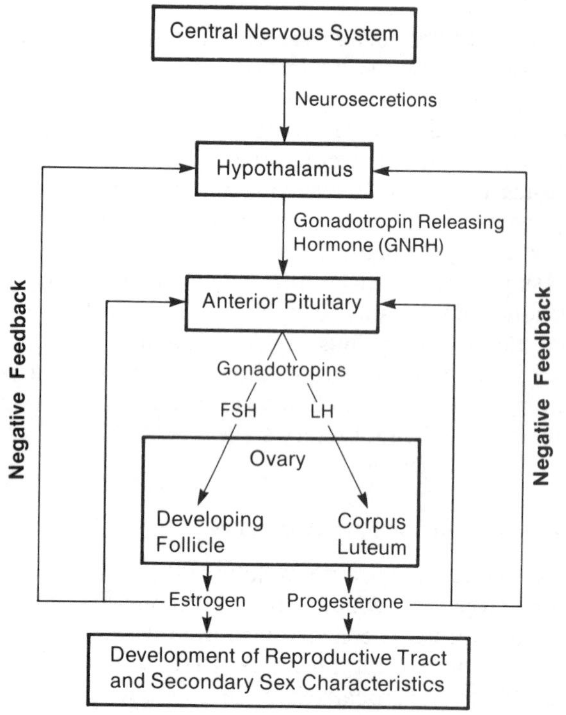

Figure 2–12. A diagram to show the interrelationship of the structures involved in the mature female reproductive process. The influence of the CNS, stimulated by external or internal stimuli, upon the hypothalamus, is shown. Further influence upon the anterior pituitary, the ovary, and the reproductive organs can be noted. Also shown is the feedback of the ovarian steroids to the anterior pituitary gland and to the hypothalamus.

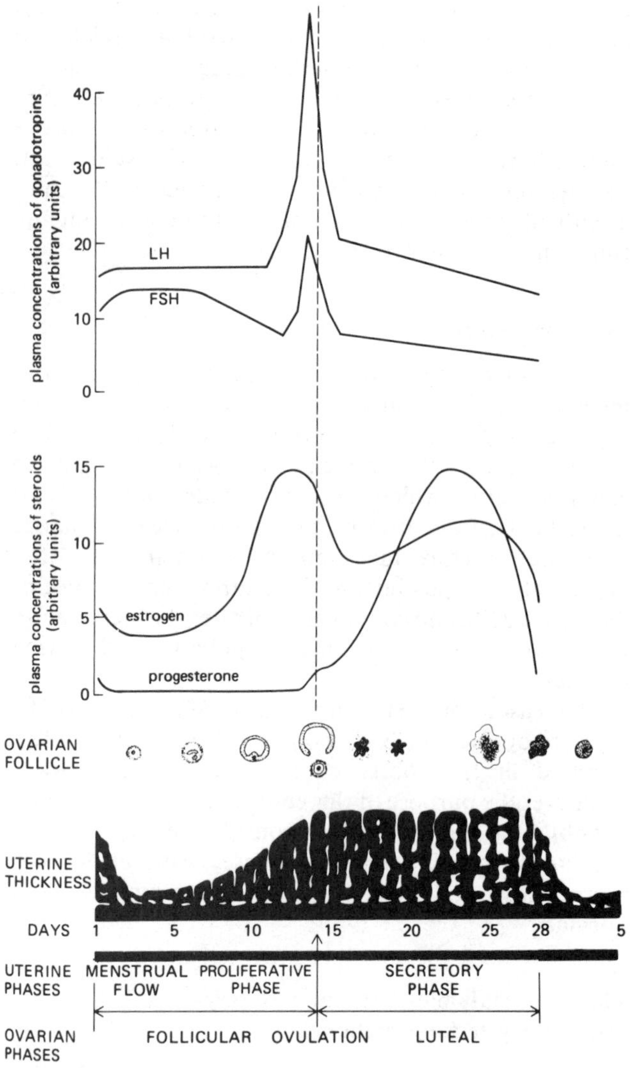

Figure 2–13. Summary of plasma hormone concentrations, ovarian events, and uterine changes during the menstrual cycle. (Reproduced with permission from Arthur J. Vander; James H. Sherman; and Dorothy S. Luciano. *Human Physiology. The Mechanisms of Body Function,* 3rd ed. New York: McGraw-Hill, 1980.)

duced in abundance by the placenta; their production and actions in pregnancy are described in Chapter 8.

Estrogen

Estrogen, which may be considered the characteristic female sex hormone, is important to growth and development of the reproductive organs and the mammary glands and to their maintenance in a normally mature state. It is also obligatory for the maturation of secondary female sex characteristics. Estrogen stimulates many of the cyclic changes in the reproductive organs; changes in cervical secretions and growth of the endometrium during the follicular phase of each menstrual cycle are described below. In addition to influence on the reproductive organs, estrogen is involved in a number of systemic processes, such as fluid and electrolyte balance and body temperature, described in Chapter 8.

Estrogen is responsible for (1) changing the cervical mucus to favor migration of sperm, (2) stimulating mobility of the fallopian tubes to propel matured ova through the tube, and (3) bringing about proliferation of the endometrium as one phase in its preparation for implantation of a fertilized ovum.

Estrogen plays a major role in growth of the uterus during pregnancy, and it influences a number of metabolic processes during that time. Along with progesterone, it is important to ensure proper function of the uterus and development of the breasts in pregnancy. Production and function of estrogen in pregnancy are further described in Chapter 8.

Estrogen is produced in increasing amounts in the first half of a cycle with a surge of hormone production at midcycle. Thereafter the level diminishes. The surge of estrogens at midcycle signals the hypothalamus, which in turn induces the surge of LH that will trigger ovulation and initiate development of a corpus luteum (Fig. 2–13).

Progesterone

The corpus luteum secretes its typical hormone progesterone in large amounts (Fig. 2–13) and also some estrogen.

Progesterone is a progestational hormone, which induces changes in the endometrium to prepare the uterus for implantation of a fertilized ovum and maintenance of a pregnancy. This hormone, along with estrogen, is responsible for many of the cyclic changes in the reproductive tract, and is necessary for complete development of the mammary glands. Progesterone also has some effect on metabolic processes, such as its influence on basal body temperature, described on page 115, and has considerable influence on a number of body processes during pregnancy. Its production and function in pregnancy are described in Chapter 8.

After proliferation of endometrium under the influence of estrogen, progesterone causes the secretory changes necessary for pregnancy. The endometrium becomes spongy and highly vascular with an increased glandular secretion by the twentieth day of a cycle, ready for implantation and nourishment of a fertilized ovum (Fig. 2–13).

When a fertilized ovum imbeds in the endometrium, progesterone maintains the pregnancy through support of the endometrium in its secretory state. It also reduces the contractions that normally recur in the uterine muscle, thereby allowing the fertilized ovum to implant and develop, protected against expulsion.

If the ovum is not fertilized, the luteal cells decrease their production of progesterone. In 4 to 5 days the endometrium, no longer receiving adequate support from the diminishing amount of progesterone, sloughs off, and menstruation occurs (Fig. 2–13). Buildup of endometrium and its regression leading to menstruation is described below.

CYCLIC CHANGES IN THE CERVIX AND THE VAGINA

The cyclic changes in the ovaries have been described above. Simultaneous with, and in response to, changes in the ovarian cycle, all the other reproductive organs undergo cyclic variations. As with the ovarian cycle, changes in other organs may be divided into those that appear in the follicular cycle and those that develop during the luteal phase. Ovulation is the dividing event.

Of all the changes, alterations in the endometrium during the menstrual cycle are most apparent; those of the cervix can be observed readily; others are more obscure. These cyclic changes take place in response to the level of ovarian hormones in the body. The changes that are easily detected clinically can be studied for assessment of hormone secretion, for evidence of normal ovarian function, and for indication of ovulation. Of the many changes that take place in the reproductive system, only a few will be described below.

Cervical Mucus

The cervical mucus is a complex secretion at all times, but, in addition, varies considerably in its characteristics during the course of each ovarian cycle. Estrogen stimulation during the preovulatory or follicular phase of a cycle causes increased activity of the cervical glands and changes in their secretion. These changes are progressive, reach their maximum at the time of ovulation, and then regress, returning to the characteristics of the beginning of the cycle.

During much of the ovarian cycle cervical mucus is relatively scant in amount, opaque in appearance, and viscous in consistency. In midcycle, corresponding to the ovulatory period, cervical mucus is considerably increased in amount, is clear in appearance, and of low viscosity. A thin, clear mucus secretion from the vagina may be noted at this time. The pH of cervical mucus, which may be slightly below 7.0 before and after ovulation, rises to near 7.5 at the time of ovulation. Changes in the cervical mucus during the ovulatory period make it most receptive to sperm at this time, enhancing sperm penetration of the mucus and migration through it.

Cervical mucus can be examined and evaluated for its qualities to determine the approximate time of ovulation and to assess ovarian function. Two properties which easily can be investigated clinically are termed spinnbarkheit and ferning or arborization. These properties develop under estrogen stimulation, are maximal at ovulation, and decrease after progesterone appears.

Spinnbarkheit relates to the elasticity of cervical mucus, a property that permits it to be drawn into a long, thin strand. Spinnbarkheit can be measured by placing a drop of mucus on a glass slide and then drawing it out into a thread with another slide, a cover glass, or a small wooden spatula. Elasticity of cervical mucus increases progressively during the follicular phase and reaches a maximum at the time of ovulation. Threads of mucus from 15 to 20 cm in length can be drawn from cervical mucus examined at ovulation as compared to threads from 1 to 2 cm long when estrogen stimulation of the cervical glands is minimal.

Fern pattern or *arborization* refers to the pattern into which cervical mucus dries when it is under estrogen stimulation. Examination for this characteristic aids in assessment of ovulation time. To observe cervical mucus for ferning, a drop of mucus is spread on a glass slide, allowed to dry, and examined microscopically for pattern. The pattern of dried cervical mucus results from crystallization of the sodium chloride in the mucus and is determined by the environment (the other components of the mucus) from which the sodium chloride crystallizes. When the concentration of sodium chloride in the mucus is relatively high, ferning takes place. Ferning is dependent upon estrogen stimulation, which increases the content of sodium chloride in the mucus, provided the mucus is not simultaneously under progesterone influence. Progesterone lowers the sodium chloride content of the mucus, and when progesterone is present, ferning does not occur. The presence of a ferning pattern of cervical mucus is thus determined by the hormones present.

The fernlike pattern of cervical mucus progressively increases during the preovulatory phase, becoming more full and complete, and it is most pronounced about the time of ovulation. The fernlike pattern is replaced by a cellular pattern when progesterone appears, beginning one or two days after ovulation. This cellular pattern persists during the postovulatory period.

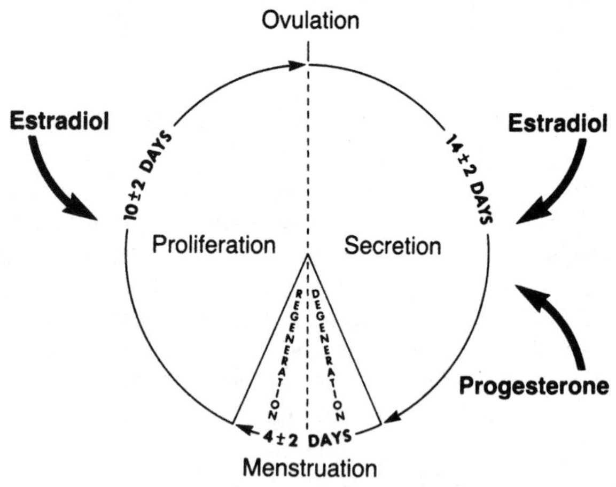

Figure 2–14. Influence of hormones on phases of the human endometrial cycle. (Reprinted with permission from Alex Ferenczy and Leon Speroff. How to date the endometrial cycle. *Contemp. OB/Gyn.*, Medical Economics Company, 18:115–136 *passim*, (Nov.) 1981.)

Vaginal Mucosa

The mucosal cells and the secretions of the vagina undergo regular cyclic changes during each ovarian cycle, with the type of epithelial cells and the content of the secretions dependent upon the level of estrogen and progesterone. The vaginal epithelium thickens under the influence of estrogen, and the glucose excretion is maximal at the time that the estrogen level is highest, about the time of ovulation. Vaginal smears may be used to estimate estrogen activity.

The Menstrual (Endometrial) Cycle

As the ovary undergoes cyclic changes, so the endometrial lining of the uterus also undergoes a series of changes, repeated at monthly intervals. These endometrial changes are under the influence of ovarian hormones and thus progress concurrently with changes in the ovarian cycle. As the amount and kind of ovarian hormones change during the cycle, the endometrial characteristics typical of each ovarian hormonal action appear. Since the ovarian cycle is under the influence of anterior pituitary gonadotropic hormones, there is a close correlation between the pituitary gonadotropic hormones, the ovarian cycle and its hormones, and the endometrial (menstrual) cycle.

The endometrial cycle can be described in three main phases (Fig. 2–14):

1. The follicular or preovulatory phase, during which the endometrium grows under the influence of estrogen
2. The luteal or postovulatory phase, during which there is a progressive increase in secretory activity of the endometrium, as it is influenced by progesterone as well as estrogen
3. The menstrual phase, during which regression and partial desquamation of the endometrium occur as a result of regression of the corpus luteum and withdrawal of its hormones

The Follicular Phase

The follicular phase immediately follows a menstrual period. It coincides with the preovulatory period of the ovarian cycle, at which time the graafian follicle develops and produces increasing amounts of estrogen (Fig. 2–13). Under the influence of estrogen the endometrium, which was partly desquamated during the preceding menstrual period, regenerates and grows. This follicular phase, during which proliferation of endometrium takes place, may be termed the *proliferative phase* of the cycle.

At the beginning of the follicular phase the endometrium is from 1 to 2 mm thick, and its glands are short, straight, and narrow. During this phase cells proliferate; the uterine glands increase in size; and the mucosa reaches a thickness of about 3 mm by the end of the period of proliferation.

The Luteal Phase

The luteal phase begins after ovulation and coincides with the period of corpus luteum development and progesterone secretion (Fig. 2–13). In response to progesterone the glands of the endometrium begin to secrete; this phase therefore can be termed the *secretory phase* of the cycle.

The luteal phase is characterized by increasing endometrial secretory activity, as well as continuing increase in thickness. The glands become longer, wider, and tortuous, and they secrete large quantities of glycogen. Vascularity increases and the arterioles become coiled and tortuous. The stroma increases and becomes edematous.

At the end of the luteal phase the endometrium is soft, velvety, and edematous and measures 4 to 6 mm in thickness. This vascular, spongy, glycogen-rich endometrium is ready for implantation and nourishment of a fertilized ovum. Because of this preparation for pregnancy, the luteal phase also can be termed the *progestational phase*. If pregnancy occurs, endometrial development continues under the influence of progesterone to an even thicker tissue which is termed the *decidua* of pregnancy. When pregnancy does not occur, the endometrium regresses, along with the corpus luteum.

The Menstrual Phase

The menstrual phase is a period of regression during which the previously well-developed endometrium becomes ischemic, degenerates, and desquamates with moderate bleeding. This phase coincides with regression of the corpus luteum and withdrawal of its hormones, progesterone and estrogen (Fig. 2–13).

The menstrual phase begins several days before the actual onset of menstrual bleeding and can be divided into a premenstrual and menstrual period. During the few days preceding menstruation, concurrent with corpus luteum regression, circulation in the endometrium decreases, and shrinkage due to loss of tissue fluids and secretions takes place. There is a period of vasoconstriction, then relaxation of, and bleeding from, the vessels, and thereafter desquamation of the upper layers of tissue begins. Bleeding and tissue loss continue during the next several days, which are termed the menstrual period. Regeneration begins in the lower layer of the endometrium even before the menstrual phase is completed.

Menstruation normally recurs throughout the childbearing period, from the time it begins during puberty to the menopause, except during pregnancy and lactation. Although menstruation is usually preceded by ovulation and corpus luteum formation, periodic bleeding without prior ovulation sometimes occurs. Such anovulatory periods are physiologically different from true menstrual periods, but do not necessarily vary much clinically.

The interval from the onset of one menstrual period to the onset of the next period is termed the *menstrual cycle*. A cycle usually is considered to be 28 days in length, but there are many variations from this, not only in different women, but also in the same individual. Such variations in interval usually range between 21 and 32 days. Regularity of menstrual periods may be disturbed temporarily, or the periods may be completely absent for a few months, as a result of a marked change in a woman's daily regime of living due to either physical or emotional factors. After adjustment to the disturbing cause, gradual resumption of normal menstrual periods follows.

The duration of a menstrual period is usually from four to six days, but lengths from two to eight days are considered within normal range.

The amount of menstrual flow varies from 60 to 180 ml (2 to 6 oz), but actual blood loss is less, usually from 30 to 60 ml (1 to 2 oz). In addition to blood, the menstrual discharge consists of fragments of endometrium, secretions from uterine glands, and mucus. The menstrual flow is scant at the beginning, gradually increases, is usually greatest on the second day, and then gradually diminishes. Menstrual discharge is ordinarily dark red in color. It normally does not clot. The rather offensive odor from menstrual discharge is caused by decomposition of blood and increased secretions from the sebaceous glands of the vulva.

Clinical Aspects and Premenstrual Syndrome

A menstrual period may be preceded and/or attended by a certain amount of emotional and physical disturbance. A few days before bleeding begins, certain premonitory signs are frequently noticed. Common signs are abdominal distention, headache, backache, breast fullness, and premenstrual tension, characterized by depression or anxiety.

Although many women may observe little or no physical change during menstruation, others are somewhat uncomfortable at this time. They may be tired and may have less endurance and resistance than usual. Headaches, with a sense of fullness, dizziness, and heaviness, are sometimes accompaniments. Backache is a frequent source of distress. Abdominal discomfort may vary from an uncomfortable sense of dragging heaviness to pain. There may be pain in the hips and thighs. Occasionally there is a loss of appetite or nausea. Slight bladder irritability and a tendency to constipation may be noted. If breast changes occur, they are much the same as, though slighter than, those occurring during pregnancy. The breasts may become firmer and somewhat increased in size; a burning, tingling sensation and soreness may accompany these changes. The nipples may be turgid and prominent, and the pigmented areas may temporarily become darker. The skin over other parts of the body sometimes changes in appearance, possibly accompanied by circles under the eyes and pimples. Some women are pale and others are flushed during their menstrual period.

In addition to the physical discomfort that may be coincident with menstruation, there is sometimes evidence of emotional and nervous instability. This may be characterized by irritability, lack of poise and control, and a state of depression or of tension. Drowsiness and mental sluggishness are not uncommon.

The disturbances accompanying menstruation, described above, vary widely in different women, and in the same woman at different times and under different conditions. Several symptoms may persist with more or less severity throughout the menstrual life of one woman, while perhaps only one or two occasionally will disturb another. Discomfort usually begins from one to several days before the menstrual flow appears, is at its height during the following day, and then subsides steadily and progresses to a feeling of well-being. Many women feel better at the end of their menstrual period and during the days immediately following than at any other time during the cycle.

It is believed that an attitude that regards menstruation as a normal physiologic process often reduces its discomforts. When discomfort appears to be greater than that which normally may be expected to accompany menstruation, a medical examination is indicated.

Under normal circumstances it is seldom necessary for a woman to depart markedly from her usual mode of living during a menstrual period. Exercise in moderation and all other normal activities can be performed as usual.

Personal hygiene during menstruation is not necessarily different from daily hygiene at any other time. Frequent bathing and frequent changes of perineal pads are important. Many women use a vaginal tampon to absorb the menstrual flow. The tampon is comfortable when worn properly, has certain advantages over the perineal pad, and in most instances there is no objection to its use. The tampon eliminates the bulk and irritation of the external pad. It overcomes the problem of the unpleasant odor that accompanies the menstrual flow, since menstrual discharge is almost entirely odorless unless exposed to air. Women must be cautioned to change vaginal tampons frequently to minimize risk of toxic shock syndrome.

Heat to the abdomen and lumbar region, warm baths, rest and quiet, and good posture usually will give relief from menstrual discomfort. Cold baths are not advisable during painful menstruations since they may increase distress. If the woman understands that premenstrual tension and general irritability may appear, she more readily may accept this discomfort and plan according to her ability to cope with it.

Menstrual Irregularities

The most common menstrual irregularities are as follows. *Dysmenorrhea* is painful menstruation. *Menorrhagia* is an abnormally copious menstrual flow. *Metrorrhagia* is bleeding between the menstrual periods. *Amenorrhea* is absence of menstruation. Common causes are pregnancy, lactation, and endocrine disturbances.

Menstrual irregularities require medical attention. Endocrine disturbances often can be corrected. Pathologic conditions require early diagnosis and treatment, this being especially important for diagnosis and treatment of malignancy.

Summary of the Cyclic Interrelationships of Events in the Female Reproductive Process

The hypothalamus, the gonadotropic hormones of the anterior pituitary, the ovarian hormones, maturation of an ovum, ovulation, and preparation of the endometrium for a fertilized ovum are all very finely integrated.

At the beginning of a cycle, follicles in the ovary develop in response to an increase in FSH and LH from the pituitary gland. As these follicles grow toward maturation, they produce increasing amounts of estrogens, which cause the endometrium to proliferate. The ovum develops simultaneously (Fig. 2–13).

When follicular development nears its maximum and estrogen production is high, FSH secretion decreases somewhat, but LH secretion gradually increases. At the maximal estrogen level there are a moderate surge of FSH and an enormous surge of LH, which stimulate ovulation (Fig. 2–13). Usually only one of the follicles reaches complete maturity and ruptures. This rupture, termed ovulation, marks the dividing period between the preovulatory or follicular phase and the postovulatory or luteal phase.

The luteinizing hormone influences development of the corpus luteum and, concomitantly, the production of progesterone as well as estrogen. These hormones stimulate the endometrial glands to secrete abundantly; this is called the secretory phase.

After ovulation, just past midcycle, estrogen and progesterone feed back to the hypothalamus and the anterior pituitary to suppress secretion of FSH and LH (Fig. 2–12), thereby preventing further follicle development and ovulation.

After 8 to 10 days, the corpus luteum degenerates, unless pregnancy has occurred; its hormones are gradually withdrawn; the endometrium regresses; and menstruation takes place. When the corpus luteum hormones decrease in the late luteal phase, a stimulus to the hypothalamus and the anterior pituitary brings about a rise in FSH and LH. These hormones then stimulate development of another cycle even before menstruation from the last cycle has taken place. Apparently, if an ovum has not been fertilized, a signal to the brain initiates the series of events that will lead to another series of hormonal production (Fig. 2-12). Feedback between the ovarian hormones and the hypothalamus, with its gonadotropic-releasing factor, appears to regulate synthesis and release of FSH and LH. The anterior pituitary and its hormones appear to regulate the sequence of events surrounding ovulation.

The above-described cycle changes continue from puberty to menopause, with the exception of interruptions during pregnancy and lactation. Both the ovary and the endometrium are in a constant state of change, and each day is different from the preceding one. This is also true, to a less apparent degree, of the other reproductive organs. Although the changes described above have been presented in phases, they are not so distinctly divided, but rather are on a continuum, and one phase may begin before another ends.

If the mature ovum that was expelled from the graafian follicle at midcycle is fertilized, a new series of events must take place to prevent menstruation and expulsion of the embryo. An uninterrupted supply of progesterone is necessary to maintain endometrial attachment.

A blastocyst soon develops from the fertilized ovum. Even before implantation into the endometrium, the outer cells of this blastocyst, the trophoblastic cells, produce a hormone called human chorionic gonadotropin (HCG). This hormone, which is very similar to LH in function and structure, signals the corpus luteum to continue producing progesterone. With continuing production of progesterone, the events of menstruation and the beginning of a new cycle are suspended.

The corpus luteum is limited in its ability to survive and produce, but by about the fifth week the placenta begins to take over production of progesterone. Soon thereafter the corpus luteum does not appear to be essential to maintenance of pregnancy. Placental production of HCG is described in Chapter 8 and its production of the hormone progesterone in Chapter 8.

The Climacteric or Menopause

The *climacteric,* frequently termed the *menopause* and sometimes called "the change of life," is the period of life at which ovarian function gradually decreases and eventually stops. Menopause, which means the permanent cessation of menstruation, is one of the easily distinguishable signs of the climacteric. Menopause is only one of the physiologic changes of the climacteric, but it is the term that is commonly used for all or any part of this transitional period.

The climacteric occurs ordinarily between the ages of 45 and 50, but there is a considerable variation of time. In some women menstruation normally ceases before the age of 45, while in others it continues after age 50. The climacteric is not abrupt; it involves a change covering a period of several years.

Just as adolescence is a normal developmental process during which ovarian activity begins and becomes well established, so the climacteric is a normal retrogressive change in which there is a gradual physiologic decline in ovarian activity. A period of anovulatory function, with follicular development and estrogen secretion, but without ovulation, may precede cessation of activity. During the climacteric, ovulation stops and the childbearing period ends; menstruation ceases; the reproductive organs undergo atrophic changes; and the body makes adjustments to hormonal alterations. The climacteric is a physiologic process, and the entire organism is gradually prepared for cessation of ovarian function, both physically and psychologically. Since the transition of the climacteric is made slowly, it should not be greatly disturbing, but women often experience a certain amount of nervous instability, and some discomfort from "hot flashes," until a physiologic adjustment has been made.

As menopause approaches, menstruation often occurs irregularly; the flow sometimes temporarily increases slightly, but usually begins to diminish in amount. Menstrual periods may stop abruptly, but the process is more likely to be gradual, with periods of fairly regular menstrual cycles alternating with periods of amenorrhea. Eventually menstruation does not reappear.

Vasomotor changes—hot flushes of the face and neck, sweats, and flashes of heat that may involve the entire body—are the most characteristic symptoms of the climacteric. Severity of these symptoms varies, being almost absent in some women, moderate in others, and severe in a few. Other effects of menopause are vulvovaginal changes. Atrophy of the epithelium, which may become traumatized easily, vaginal dryness, and pruritus may cause discomfort.

During the reproductive years there is a close interrelation between pituitary gonadotropic and ovarian hormone production. The decrease in ovarian function during the climacteric disturbs this relationship and may, for a variable period of time, result in an imbalance in the relationship. The vasomotor phenomena that often accompany the climacteric may be produced by an excess of gonadotropic hormones, or the symptoms may be caused primarily by the decrease in estrogens. The reason is not quite clear. There is an upset in the feedback mechanism. The close interrelationship of these hormones with the CNS also may have an influence on some of the symptoms attributed to the menopause.

Many women have little or no discomfort during the climacteric, but if or when symptoms become severe enough to merit the risks, estrogen replacement therapy may be used to treat the estrogen deficiency. Estrogen may be administered only during the period of transition, until adjustment to the changes in endocrine function have been made, or it may be continued longer. It is used in the lowest therapeutic dose possible. An increased incidence of osteoporosis in postmenopausal women is one reason for prophylactic estrogen therapy. Reports linking the use of estrogen to endometrial carcinoma make prophylactic use risky, especially in anything more than minimal dose.

Unfortunately, many unrelated symptoms are often ascribed to the menopause, with the result that symptoms of serious organic disease may be attributed to it erroneously. Excessive menstrual flow, for example, may be accepted as normal prior to menopause and accordingly neglected. A change in menstruation, with increased or prolonged bleeding, cannot be accepted as a normal forerunner of menopause, and any bleeding, however slight, occurring after the menopause demands medical attention.

REFERENCES AND SUGGESTED READINGS

Caldwell, Laura Ryan, Questions and answers about the menopause, *Am. J. Nurs.*, 82:1100–1101, (July) 1982.

Calkins, Evan, Aging of cells and people, *Clin. Obstet. Gynecol.*, 24:165–79, (Mar.) 1981.

Frasier, S. Douglas, *Pediatric Endocrinology*, Grune & Stratton, New York, 1980, Chap. 5.

Miller, Marjorie A.; Drakontides, Anna B.; and Leavell, Lutie C., *Kimber-Gray-Stockpole's Anatomy and Physiology*, 17th ed., Macmillan, New York, 1977, Chap. 25.

Montagu, Ashley, The adolescents' unreadiness for pregnancy and motherhood, *Pediatr. Ann.*, 10:507–11, (Dec.) 1981.

Nelms, Bobbie Crew, What is a normal adolescent? *MCN*, 6:403–406, (Nov./Dec.) 1981.

Pearson, Linda, Climacteric, *Am. J. Nurs.*, 82:1098–1102, (July) 1982.

Tichy, Anna M., and Malasanos, Lois J., The physiological role of hormones in puberty, *MCN*, 1:384–88, (Nov./Dec.) 1976.

Vander, Arthur J.; Sherman, James H.; and Luciano, Dorothy S., *Human Physiology. The Mechanisms of Body Function*, 3rd ed., McGraw-Hill, New York, 1980, Chap. 16.

CHAPTER

3

Anatomy and Physiology of the Male Reproductive System

ANATOMY OF THE MALE REPRODUCTIVE ORGANS

The male reproductive system consists of the testes (sex glands) in which the male germ cells and the sex hormones are formed; a series of ducts, continuous with one another, through which spermatozoa are transported from the testes to the exterior; accessory glands that produce secretions important to sperm nutrition, survival, and transport; and the penis which serves as the organ of copulation.

Testes

The testes, the sex organs, or gonads, of the male are two slightly flattened, ovoid, glandular bodies suspended by bilateral spermatic cords (Fig. 3–1). The spermatic cords originate just above the inguinal canal, pass through the canal, and down into the scrotum. The testes, epididymides, and parts of the spermatic cords are enclosed, supported, and protected in the *scrotum,* a pouchlike, double-chambered structure made up of skin, fascia, and muscle (Fig. 3–1).

Similar to the ovaries of the female, the glandular reproductive organs of the male have a twofold function. They produce germ cells, called *spermatozoa,* and they serve as an endocrine gland, producing a typically male hormone, called *testosterone.*

The testes are formed in the peritoneal cavity during fetal development and then normally migrate through the inguinal canal and into the scrotum during the eighth or ninth month of fetal life, or occasionally soon after birth. Descent into the scrotum by the age of puberty is essential for normal spermatogenesis, which is adversely affected by the relatively higher temperature within the body. Each testis is a mass of narrow, coiled tubules, called *seminiferous tubules* (Fig. 3–2). Partial septi, extending from a fibrous capsule covering the testis, divide its substance into a large number of wedge-shaped lobules. Each lobule contains three or four seminiferous tubules. These tubules are from 1 to 3 ft long; the combined length of the many tubules in one testis equals almost 1 mile.

As the seminiferous tubules leave the lobules near their apexes, they join together with adjacent tubules to form ducts. These ducts come together to form a network of ducts, the *rete testis,* from which they lead out and converge into a single coiled tube, the epididymis.

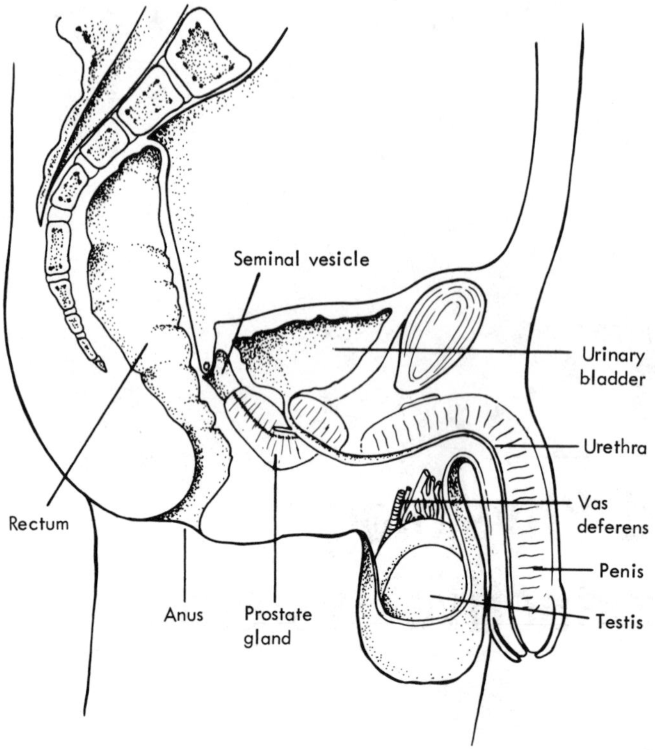

Figure 3–1. Male reproductive system. Sagittal section. (Reprinted with permission from William B. Youmans, *Human Physiology,* rev. ed. New York: Macmillan, 1954.)

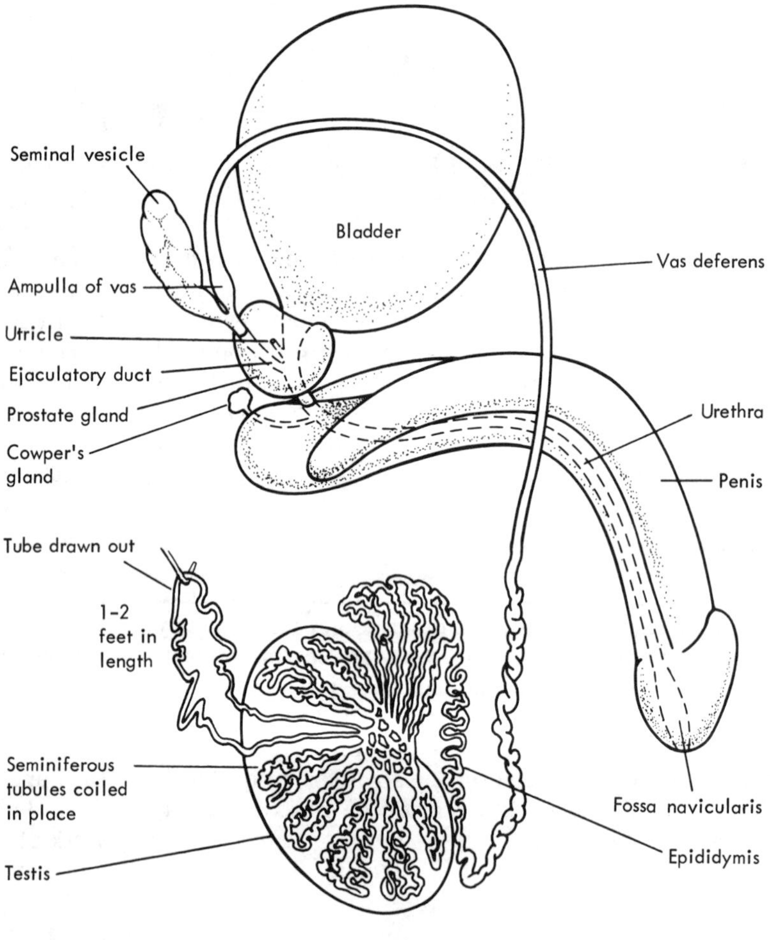

Figure 3–2. Diagrammatic representation of the testis, showing its duct system and the relation of the ducts to the accessory sex glands and penis. (Reprinted with permission from Sigmund Grollman, *The Human Body: Its Structure and Physiology,* 4th ed. New York: Macmillan, 1978. Copyright Sigmund Grollman, 1978.)

Epididymides

The epididymides (sing., epididymis) are bilateral narrow bodies, situated along the upper posterior part of each testis. Each contains a narrow, tortuous tubule approximately 20 ft in length (Fig. 3-2). This tubule serves as the area to which the spermatozoa that have been released into the seminiferous tubules are conveyed, and where they may remain for about three weeks. Here they are retained until physiologic maturation is complete and until they become motile. As the tubule of the epididymis leaves this body, it becomes known as the vas deferens.

Vasa Deferentia (Ductus Deferentia, Seminal Ducts)

The vasa deferentia (sing., vas deferens) are bilateral ducts, approximately 18 in. long, which continue from each epididymis, and, after a devious course, terminate in the bilateral ejaculatory ducts, which open into the urethra (Figs. 3-1 and 3-2). A vas deferens ascends from each testis through a spermatic cord, passes through the inguinal canal, enters the pelvic cavity, and after coursing upward and medially, passes downward to the base of the bladder where it widens into an ampulla. This terminal end joins with a duct from the seminal vesicle, and they become the ejaculatory duct. In addition to functioning as a part of the long excretory duct from the testis, the vas deferens serves as a storage site for sperm.

Seminal Vesicles

The seminal vesicles are two membranous pouches, situated between the lower part of the bladder and the rectum (Figs. 3-1 and 3-2). Through a short duct each vesicle joins the terminal end of a vas deferens and with it becomes an ejaculatory duct.

Ejaculatory Ducts

The ejaculatory ducts are paired, narrow, short tubes formed by the joining of the terminal ends of the vasa deferentia and the ducts from the seminal vesicles. These two ducts descend between the lobes of the prostate gland and open into the urethra into which they discharge sperm and secretions from the seminal vesicles and the epididymides (Fig. 3-2).

Prostate Gland

The prostate gland is located just below the bladder and surrounds the upper portion of the urethra (Figs. 3-1 and 3-2). It generally is described as being the size and shape of a chestnut. It secrets a thin, complex fluid that is discharged into the urethra through many small tubules that open into it.

Bulbourethral Glands (Cowper's Glands)

The bulbourethral glands are two small peasized bodies located below the prostate gland, within the pelvic floor. They secrete an alkaline, viscous fluid that is emptied into the urethra through a small duct from each gland.

Penis

The penis is the male organ of copulation. Semen is ejaculated through it into the vagina of the female during intercourse, and active spermatozoa in the semen can enter the cervix and travel to the fallopian tubes where fertilization of an ovum may take place.

The penis is a cylindrical organ composed of three elongated masses of cavernous erectile tissue; two of these columns lie paired and anteriorly, and one lies medially and ventrally to the other two. The urethra passes through the medial column of tissue and opens at the tip of the penis. This organ is enclosed in fascia and is covered with skin (Figs. 3-1 and 3-2). Relatively large spaces in the cavernous tissue usually become distended with blood during sexual stimulation, causing this organ, which is otherwise flaccid, to become firm and erect.

A slight enlargement at the end of the penis, called the *glans penis,* contains the urethral opening and many very sensitive nerve endings. The skin of the penis extends over its end, covers the glans, and becomes folded upon itself. This is called the *prepuce* or *foreskin* (Fig. 3-1) and is the portion that is surgically removed when a circumcision is performed.

The male urethra, which extends from the neck of the bladder to the orifice in the glans of the penis, serves two purposes. It conveys urine from the bladder and, at separate times, transmits semen containing spermatozoa to outside the body.

PHYSIOLOGY OF THE MALE REPRODUCTIVE SYSTEM

Adolescence and Puberty

The changes that take place in the period between childhood and maturity of the body are much the same for boys and girls, the same except for the actual physical development. Pubertal maturation and development toward sexual maturity, as it applies to both sexes, and the endocrinologic changes that take place during this time have been described on pages 19-21. Development specific to the male is presented below.

Physical Changes in Puberty in Boys

The usual sequence of sexual development during puberty and the age at which these various changes appear are listed in Table 3-1.

Table 3–1. Average Age and Sequence of Sexual Development—Boys*

Age (years)	
10–11	First growth of testes
11–12	Pigmentation and thinning of scrotum Growth of penis
12–13	Prostate activity Pubic hair
13–14	Rapid growth of testes and penis Subareolar breast tissue
14–15	Axillary hair "Down" on upper lip Voice change
15–16	Mature spermatozoa
16–17	Facial and body hair Acne
18–21	Arrest of skeletal growth

*Reprinted with permission from S. Douglas Frasier, *Pediatric Endocrinology*, Grune & Stratton, New York, 1980, p. 149.

The earliest physical changes of puberty in boys are testicular growth and thinning and pigmentation of the scrotal skin. Growth of the penis begins soon after testicular enlargement, and growth of the genital organs then continues. These early changes in boys may not be noticed readily, but measurements of lengths and circumferences of organs are helpful in recognizing them. Pubic hair begins to appear after genital growth has started. Next prostatic growth and secretory activity begin. There also may be some enlargement of the areolar breast area.

In boys, axillary hair does not appear until approximately the middle of puberty. Then fine hair appears on the upper lip. Deepening of the voice also occurs at this time. The acceleration of growth seen in adolescents begins after puberty is progressing well, usually when pubic hair has begun to develop. The maximum growth period usually coincides with the appearance of axillary hair, generally between 14 and 16 years of age. Boys often continue to grow beyond the age of 18 years.

Mature spermatozoa and therefore fertility develop soon after midpuberty in most boys, usually at the age of 15 to 16 years.

There is a wide variability in the age at which puberty begins and the rate at which it progresses, but the changes that take place will be the same in the end under normal conditions. When a boy has attained full physical maturity, he has developed adult facial and body hair, and his voice has completed the change to adult.

The Adrenal Cortex

The adrenal cortex, an important source of androgens, is important in pubertal maturation. Blood levels of adrenal androgens rise prior to increased activity of the hypothalamic–anterior pituitary-gonadal system, and they continue to increase during puberty. The influence of increasing adrenal androgens is not as evident in men as it is in women, because of the testosterone that is being produced in the male.

Function of the Mature Male Reproductive Organs

The Testes

The two major functions of the testes are hormone secretion and spermatogenesis. In the male, as has been described above for the female, the CNS, the hypothalamus, and the anterior pituitary gland are closely integrated with function of the reproductive organs. The CNS sends out a neurotransmitter to the hypothalamus to discharge a releasing factor. This gonadotropin-releasing factor (GnRF) causes the anterior pituitary to discharge the two gonadotropic hormones which then stimulate the testes to produce testosterone and mature sperm (see Fig. 3–4).

Hormone production is carried out by specialized cells, known as Leydig cells. A framework of connective tissue between the seminiferous tubules in the testes contains these specialized cells, called *interstitial cells* or *Leydig cells.* These cells produce the male sex hormone, *testosterone,* under the influence of the pituitary gonadotropic hormones. Testosterone is necessary for normal development and activity of the male genital organs, development and maintenance of masculine secondary sex characteristics, and normal spermatogenesis.

Spermatogenesis also takes place in the lining of the seminiferous tubules.

The lining of the seminiferous tubules contains two types of cells important for sperm production. (The terms *sperm* and *spermatozoa* will be used interchangeably; sperm may be considered as a shortened term for spermatozoa.) Many of the lining cells are germinal epithelium or *spermatogenic cells,* which produce immature germ cells, spermatogonia, continuously after sexual maturity. Thus, the male produces billions of spermatozoa in a lifetime. This process differs from formation of oogonia in the ovaries, in that the latter activity ceases during fetal life, and the full quota of immature germ cells is established before birth. A significant depletion of germ cells, characteristic of the ovaries, never occurs in the testes.

Other cells in the lining of the seminiferous tubules, called *Sertoli cells,* are supportive in function. These cells are tall and extend from the basement membrane of the tubules to the lumen. They provide a place for the germ cells that have reached the spermatid stage to attach and receive nutritive material during their further development into spermatozoa (Fig. 3–3). Spermatozoa that have matured become detached from the Sertoli

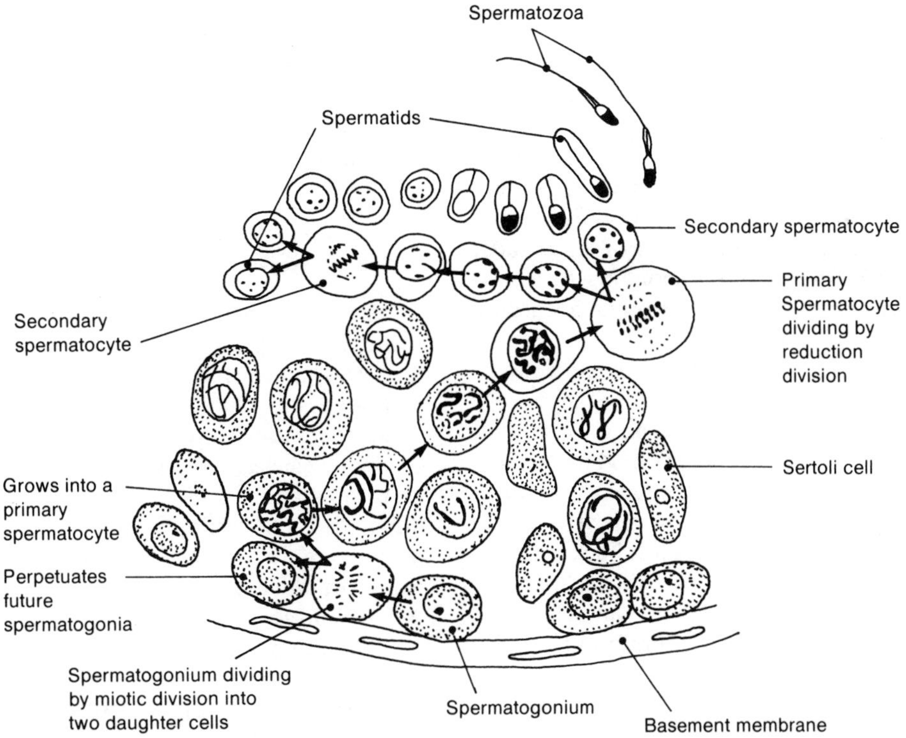

Figure 3–3. Enlarged section of a portion of a seminiferous tubule, showing spermatogonia at different stages of development. Top of illustration indicates lumen into which are discharged mature sperm cells. (Reprinted with permission from Sigmund Grollman, *The Human Body: Its Structure and Physiology,* 4th ed. New York: Macmillan, 1978. Copyright Sigmund Grollman, 1978.)

cells, are released into the lumen of the seminiferous tubules, and are conveyed through this duct system to the epididymis. These sperm are not motile at this stage of development and are believed to be transported by mechanical pressure from more sperm released into the tubules and possibly by movement of cilia in the tubular lining.

Maturation of germ cells in the male is not cyclic, as in the female, but rather is a continuous process. Many germ cells, in various stages of development, are always present in the lining of the seminiferous tubules and are released into the lumen when they have reached the spermatozoan stage of development (Fig. 3–3). A great number are constantly matured and released, in contrast to maturation and release of one germ cell from the ovaries during each monthly cycle.

The testes begin their function of producing mature germ cells and sex hormones at approximately midpuberty, between 14 and 16 years. The testes continue to function into advanced years, or throughout life in many individuals. Whereas cessation of ovarian function occurs during the fourth or fifth decade of life, testicular function ordinarily does not show a sharp decline or cessation at a definite age. A very gradual decline in function with advancing age may result in decreased or incomplete spermatogenesis and also a lowering of hormone production, but often without evidence of distinct change.

The Hypothalamic-Anterior Pituitary-Gonadal Interrelationship

The testes, similar to the ovaries, are under the influence of the pituitary gland for normal function, both for spermatogenesis and for hormone production. The pituitary gonadotropic (gonad-stimulating) hormones, which are the same in both sexes, are named according to their influence on the ovaries, but they also influence testicular function.

The follicle-stimulating hormone (FSH), the hormone that stimulates growth of ovarian follicles, stimulates spermatogenesis from the germinal cells in the lining of the seminiferous tubules. The hormone known as the luteinizing hormone (LH), named for its influence in the female on the corpus luteum, stimulates the interstitial cells (Leydig cells) in the testes to produce testosterone. The luteinizing hormone, because of its influence on the interstitial cells, has sometimes been called the interstitial cell-stimulating hormone (ICSH), especially when referred to in the male. In the female, both of the pituitary gonadotropic hormones are involved in ovarian hormone secretion; only one, LH, is believed to influence testicular hormone secretion. However, both gonadotropic hormones are necessary for sperm development. Although FSH is primarily the spermatogenic hormone, LH is necessary for spermatogenesis, since adequate development of sperm cannot take place without a normal level of testosterone.

In the male as in the female, there is a reciprocal relationship between the gonadotropic hormones of the anterior pituitary gland and the hormones of the gonads, with the activity of either gland responding to an increase or a decrease in the activity of the other, according to a feedback mechanism (Fig. 3-4).

In the interrelationship of the hormones the amount of testosterone synthesis by the Leydig cells is dependent upon the amount of LH in the blood, and the secretion of LH is controlled by the action of the gonadal hormones on the hypothalamus and the anterior pituitary. High blood levels of a hormone may switch off production of the other, and low levels switch it back on.

Although it is not certain, it appears that a hormone termed *inhibin* influences the feedback on release of FSH. Inhibin is released from the seminiferous tubules

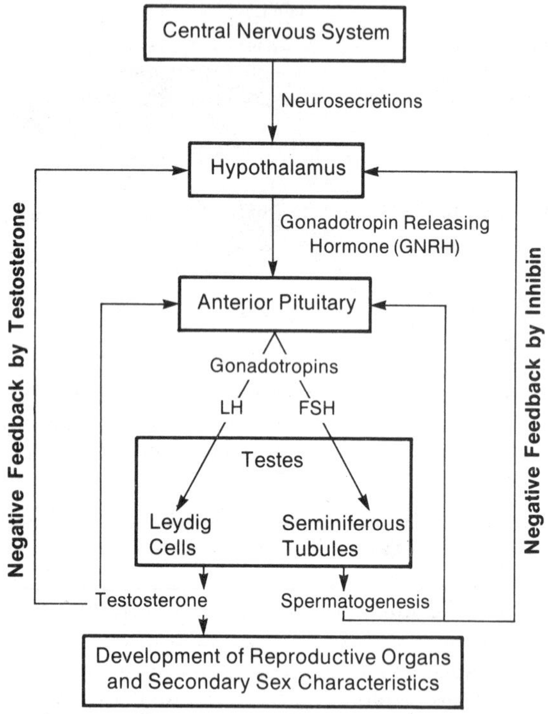

Figure 3-4. A diagram to show the interrelationship of the structures involved in the mature male reproductive process. The CNS, stimulated by external or internal stimuli, influences the hypothalamus to produce a gonadotropin releasing hormone. The anterior pituitary responds with gonadotropins, which then influence the testes to produce testosterone and to develop mature sperm. A feedback mechanism from testosterone to the hypothalamus and the anterior pituitary and from inhibin to those organs is also shown.

and under its influence the secretion of FSH is apparently reduced.

Figure 3-5 shows the influence of the various component parts of the hypothalamus-anterior pituitary-Leydig cell axis and of the hypothalamus-anterior pituitary-seminiferous tubule axis.

Semen and Secretions from the Male Accessory Glands

Semen is a viscous, slightly yellowish or grayish fluid consisting of spermatozoa, produced and released from the testes, and suspended in secretions derived from the male accessory glands. The seminal fluid, or plasma, is a complex mixture of secretions produced primarily by the seminal vesicles, the prostate gland, and the bulbourethral glands, and to a smaller extent by the epididymides. The combined secretion of the several glands provides a fluid that serves as a medium for sperm transport and as a substance favorable to sperm fertility.

The *seminal vesicles secrete a slightly yellowish, complex fluid* that contains, among a number of substances, a rich supply of fructose. This fluid is discharged during ejaculation and becomes available to the sperm at that time, when both are simultaneously being discharged from the vasa deferentia. This secretion increases the bulk of the seminal plasma (the fluid in which the sperm are suspended), thus adding to the fluid medium in which sperm are transported. The high fructose content in the secretion is an important source of nutritive material, which enables the sperm to develop good motility and fertilizing ability.

The *secretion from the prostate gland* is also added to the semen during ejaculation, being discharged at the same time that sperm are discharged from the vasa deferentia. This secretion is a further addition to the bulk of the semen, and also adds substances important to sperm for good motility and fertility. Finally, the *bulbourethral glands contribute an alkaline viscous fluid* to the semen that is believed to aid in neutralization of the acidic vaginal secretions.

Among the many components of seminal fluid are water, fructose, sodium, potassium, chloride, bicarbonate, acid-soluble phosphate, proteins, citric acid, acid phosphatase, and proteolytic enzymes. The pH of semen varies from 7.35 to 7.50. Its phosphate and bicarbonate components provide a buffer action that protects sperm from the acidity of vaginal secretions. The function of the glands that secrete the seminal fluid, and the concentration of some of its substances, are dependent upon and closely related to androgenic activity.

Semen is ejaculated from the male genital tract in an average volume of 3 ml. Each milliliter of semen normally contains from 50 to 150 million spermatozoa, with a range from below 40 to over 160 million. A count of 20

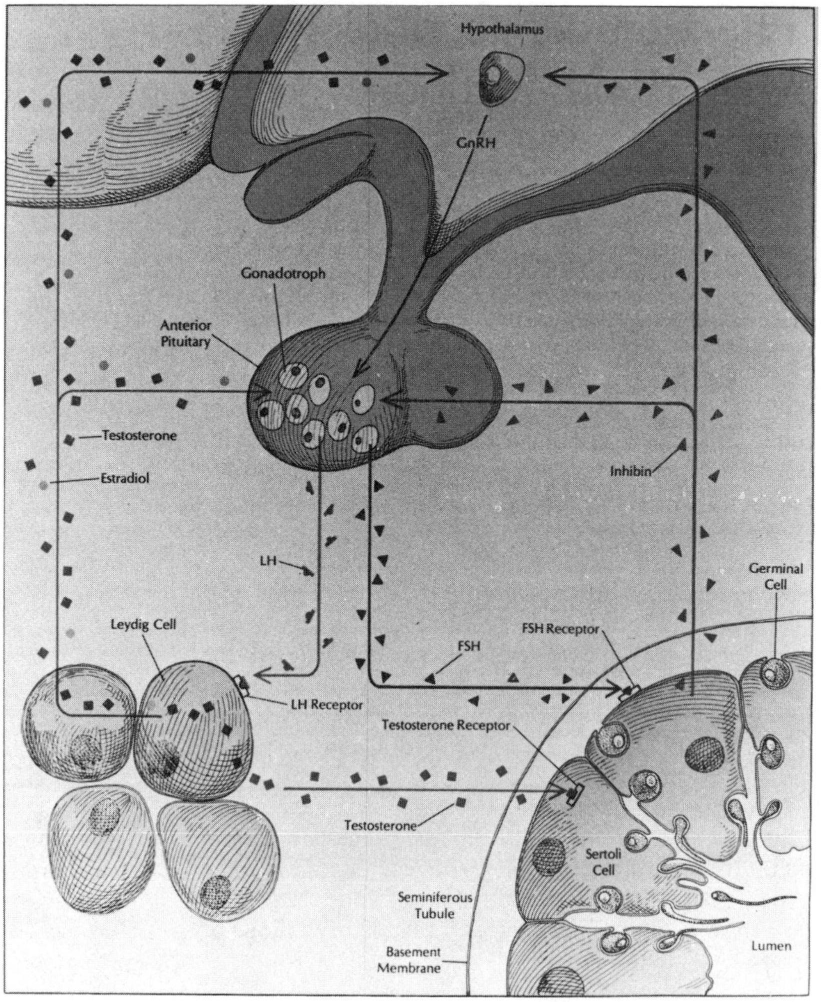

Figure 3-5. The hypothalamus and pituitary serve both to control and to integrate the two major testicular functions, steroid secretion (left) and spermatogenesis (right). Hypothalamic gonadotropin-releasing hormone (GnRH) mediates pituitary release of LH and FSH. When LH binds to specific membrane receptors on testicular Leydig cells, a series of reactions is entrained, eventuating in secretion of testosterone and estradiol. The sex steroids, in turn, act on brain and anterior pituitary, where they exert control of gonadotropin release via negative feedback mechanisms. Testosterone secreted by the Leydig cells binds to cytoplasmic receptors in the Sertoli cells of the seminiferous tubule, a critical event in spermatogenic differentiation. Binding of FSH to its membrane receptors on the Sertoli cells also is important for induction of spermatogenesis. Inhibin, released from Sertoli cells, reduces FSH secretion. (Reprinted with permission from C. Wayne Bardin, The neuroendocrinology of male reproduction. *Hosp. Pract.,* 14:65–75 (Dec.) 1979. Drawing by Bungi Tagawa.)

million or less sperm per milliliter is considered to be unfavorable for fertility. Semen analysis for fertility assessment includes, in addition to sperm count per milliliter, examination of sperm morphology, degree of motility, percentage of motile sperm, and volume of ejaculate.

Route of Sperm Through the Male Reproductive System

Spermatozoa develop from the spermatogenic cells in the lining of the seminiferous tubules of the testes. When mature, they separate from the Sertoli cells to which they have been attached, fill the tubules, and are pushed into the epididymides where they accumulate until they reach physiologic maturity and become motile. They may remain there for several weeks. From the epididymides they enter the vasa deferentia, which also serve as a storage site.

Sperm transport through the epididymides and the vasa deferentia is accomplished by their own motility, cilia on the tubular lining, and muscular contraction of the tubules, with the relative significance of each not certain. Passage of sperm from the lower ends of the vasa deferentia through the ejaculatory ducts, into the urethra, and to the exterior of the body occurs during ejaculation. During this reflex act, at the climax of coitus, involuntary muscle contractions, chiefly those of the perineum, forcibly eject the sperm and the secretions of the accessory glands (the semen) through the urethra. As the sperm are discharged from the vasa deferentia into the urethra, the secretions of the bulbourethral glands, the prostate, and the seminal vesicles are added in rapid succession and provide the sperm with the vehicle and the nutritive and protective substances that these glands supply. The route of the sperm and the points at which glandular secretions are added to the semen can be traced in Figure 3-2.

Spermatozoa can live in the ducts of the male reproductive tract for several weeks, but once they are discharged to the exterior, their life is short. They may survive in the female reproductive tract for two to three days, but their ability to fertilize is lost even sooner. When sperm are not ejaculated, they disintegrate and are reabsorbed from the reproductive tract.

SUMMARY

The complex interrelationship of the organs involved in reproduction is similar in many respects in both male and female. In both sexes, the series of events that lead to maturation of germ cells and production of hormones begins with the onset of puberty. The initiating factor is not exactly clear. Changes that start the process appear to be in the hypothalamus. Evidence suggests that an increase in gonadotropin-releasing factor is responsible for the onset of puberty and its subsequent events. An increase in GnRF then stimulates the anterior pituitary to produce gonadotropic hormones.

The series of interrelationships of the hormones begins with specialized nerve cells in the brain. In response to stimuli they send a neurotransmitter to the hypothalamus, which causes the pituitary to discharge two gonadotropic hormones, FSH and LH. These two hormones, similar in both sexes, are carried to the gonads by the bloodstream.

The gonadotropic hormones stimulate the ovaries to produce two hormones, estrogen and progesterone, and maturation and release of an ovum each month. In the male, they stimulate production of one hormone, testosterone, and maturation and release of millions of sperm.

The sex hormones influence a number of target cells. Under hormone influence in the female, release of a mature ovum is coordinated with changes in the cervix, which permit passage of sperm, changes in the fallopian tubes to assist ovum transport, and development of the endometrium for implantation. In the male the sex hormone influences maturation and transport of spermatozoa and the components of the secretions that make up the semen as a medium for transport.

The process described above is cyclic in the female and noncyclic in the male. Also, this process ends between ages 45 and 50 years in the female, but continues throughout life in the male.

REFERENCES AND SUGGESTED READINGS

Bardin, C. Wayne, The neuroendocrinology of male reproduction, *Hosp. Prac.,* 14:65–75, (Dec.) 1979.

Frasier, S. Douglas, *Pediatric Endocrinology,* Grune & Stratton, New York, 1980, Chap. 5.

Grollman, Sigmund, *The Human Body. Its Structure and Physiology,* 2nd ed., Macmillan, New York, 1978, Chap. 15.

Miller, Marjorie A.; Drakontides, Anna B.; and Leavell, Lutie C., *Kimber-Gray-Stockpole's Anatomy and Physiology,* 17th ed., Macmillan, New York, 1977, Chap. 25.

Nelms, Bobbie Crew, What is a normal adolescent? *MCN,* 6:403–406, (Nov./Dec.) 1981.

Vander, Arthur J.; Sherman, James H.; and Luciano, Dorothy S., *Human Physiology. The Mechanisms of Body Function,* 3rd ed., McGraw-Hill, New York, 1980, Chapter 16.

CHAPTER

4

Genetics and Genetic Counseling

BASIC KNOWLEDGE OF genetic mechanisms and of cell reproduction is important in order to understand the normal growth and development of the embryo/fetus as well as genetic disorders which may have a profound impact on the perinatal patient. Genetic factors may reduce fertility, significantly influence the course of pregnancy, or cause spontaneous abortion, premature birth, or neonatal disease.

The importance of genetic disorders cannot be overlooked. On the average, every couple has a 3 to 5 percent risk of having a child with a major malformation, while women over 35 and men over 55 have considerably higher risks. It is estimated that half of spontaneous abortions result from genetic abnormalities and that one third of all hospitalized pediatric patients have a genetic disease. Approximately 80 percent of mental retardation in the United States is the result of a genetic condition.

This chapter will describe chromosomes, genes, and the manner in which this genetic material is replicated, divided, and transmitted to new generations. Several of the more common genetic disorders will be discussed, along with the application of this knowledge to the role of the nurse in the genetic counseling of families.

CHROMOSOMES

All of the genetic material of an individual is contained in the nucleus of each cell packaged into *chromosomes*. The chromosomes, so named because of their ability to take up certain dyes, are composed of deoxyribonucleic acid (DNA) and complex nucleoproteins. Chromosomes occur in pairs, with each cell of a normal human being containing 23 pairs or 46 chromosomes. Twenty-two of these pairs are the same in both men and women and are referred to as *autosomes*. The twenty-third pair, the sex chromosomes, is made up of two X chromosomes in the female and one X and one Y chromosome in the male. One member of each pair is derived from the mother and the other from the father. With the exception of sex chromosomes in the male, each member of the pair is similar to the other member in size and shape and is said to be *homologous* with the other member.

Each individual chromosome has a characteristic size and shape. Each is a rodlike structure, either straight or bent, and has, somewhere along its length, an area of constricture. This constricture is called the *centromere* (Fig. 4-1), and the portions above or below this point are called *arms*. The centromere is situated in a different position in different chromosomes, but it is in a constant position in any one chromosome. In some chromosomes the centromere is placed near the center, and in others it is located near one of the ends.

Chromosomes have been identified, grouped, and numbered on the basis of decreasing size, position of the centromere, and length of arms above and below the centromere. Specially prepared and enlarged pairs of chromosomes of a single cell may be photographed or drawn, placed in order of decreasing size, and numbered

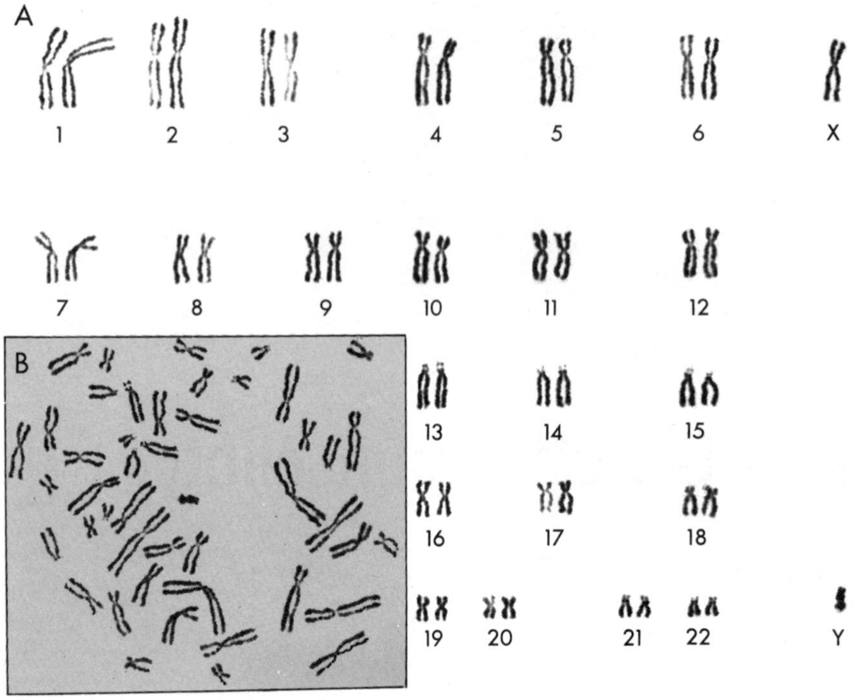

Figure 4–1. Normal human male chromosomes as they appear during metaphase. Cell division has been arrested by treatment with colchicine; hypotonic salt solution then is added to swell and disperse the chromosomes and make them more visible. B. Inset: chromosomes as they appear under the microscope following this treatment. A. Karyotype: chromosomes are paired and arranged according to a standard classification based on the size, position of the centromere, and other characteristics. The normal human has 22 somatic pairs (autosomes) plus two sex chromosomes (an X and Y in males, two X's in females).

from 1 to 23. Such a picture is called a *karyogram* or *karyotype* of the cell from which the preparation was made. Karyotypes are used in the diagnosis of chromosomal abnormalities.

A more precise identification of individual chromosomes is possible with the use of banding techniques. It has been found that certain stains or dyes bind differentially, giving the stained chromosome a striped appearance. Although the exact mechansism for the banding is conjectural, the pattern of the bands is consistent for any one chromosome. These patterns, unique for each chromosome, make it possible to distinguish all 23 pairs of human chromosomes and are significant in identifying abnormal chromosome complements, especially structural variations. Even the addition or deletion of small amounts of chromosomal material can be detected with banding techniques, making much greater diagnostic precision possible.

GENES

Tens of thousands of genes are located on each chromosome. Each gene has its own unique chemical structure and, according to that structure, directs an aspect of development or function. A gene is matched by a corresponding gene on the other chromosome of the pair. Thus, genes, like chromosomes, appear in pairs. Those that occur at the same position or *locus* on homologous chromosomes are concerned with the same trait and are said to be *alleles*.

The alleles may be *alike*, producing the same effect on a particular body characteristic, or they may be *different*, with each controlling a contrasting variation of the same characteristic.

When a pair of genes or alleles is alike in an individual, he is said to be *homozygous* for that trait. When the alleles differ, the individual is *heterozygous* for the trait influenced by those genes. When the individual is heterozygous, one of the two genes of the pair may be *dominant* to the other and exert its influence strongly enough to mask the other. The gene of a pair that is unexpressed is *recessive*. A recessive gene can be carried for many generations and ultimately may find expression when a mating occurs that matches it with another gene recessive for the same trait.

In the female the genes carried on the X chromosome occur in pairs as do those carried on all autosomes. However, the Y chromosome does not contain corresponding genes. This difference has important implications for the transmission of genetic disorders coded for by the genes on the X chromosome. These will be described under X-linked inheritance.

Genotype

Genotype is a description of the genetic makeup (kinds of genes) of an individual with respect to a given characteristic. Genes are assigned letters for symbols (see Fig. 4–4). A capital letter is traditionally used to designate a gene that is dominant and a lowercase letter for one that is recessive. If the letters *D* (dominant) and *d* (recessive) are used for genes governing a particular characteristic, then individuals with a *DD* pair would be of homozygous genotype for the dominant genes, those with *dd* would be homozygous for the recessive genes, and those with *Dd* would be heterozygous.

Phenotype

An observable physical or chemical characteristic, one that develops under the control of an individual's genotype, is termed his *phenotype* for that characteristic. Observation of a characteristic often does not reveal the genotype, but may provide a clue. When the observable characteristic is known to be produced by a dominant gene, at least one of the genes of the pair is dominant. From the example given above it could be a *DD* or *Dd* genotype. If the phenotypic characteristic is known to be governed by a recessive gene, then both of the individual's genes are recessive, from the example above, a *dd* genotype.

CELL DIVISION

Mitosis

Somatic or body cells replicate themselves by mitosis, a process whereby the cell materials, including genes and chromosomes, duplicate themselves and then separate into two new cells known as daughter cells. Because each daughter cell is identical or equal to the parent cell, this form of cell division is sometimes referred to as *equational division*. Although mitosis is a continuous process, it is divided into stages for descriptive purposes. These stages are illustrated in Figure 4–2.

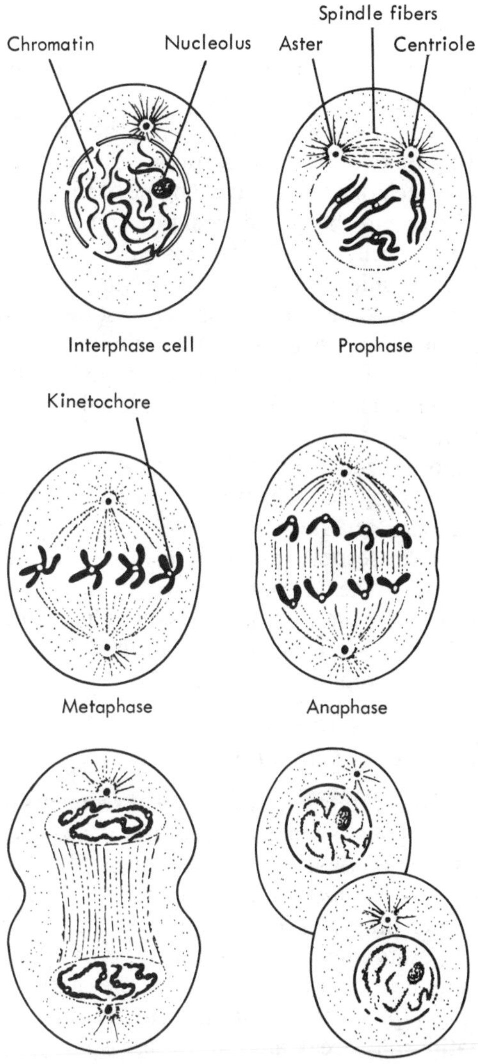

Figure 4–2. Schematic summary of mitosis in animal cells, showing chromosomes, spindle, and asters. [Reprinted with permission from Karl F. Guthe, *The Physiology of Cells*. New York: Macmillan, 1968. Copyright Karl F. Guthe, 1968.]

Meiosis

Meiosis is the special process by which germ cells (ovum and sperm) divide and mature. In contrast to mitosis, it is a *reduction division* which reduces the number of chromosomes in the cells from a diploid set (23 pair or 46 chromosomes) to a haploid set (only 23 chromosomes). This reduction process is necessary to keep the number of chromosomes in the cells of each new human being constant, since the nuclei of two germ cells unite during fertilization.

Meiosis takes place in two successive stages termed the first and second meiotic division, with the second division rapidly following the completion of the first.

First Meiotic Division

In the first meiotic division the chromosomes duplicate to form two chromatids joined at a centromere. Each duplicated chromosome then *pairs* with its homologue. These pairs of homologous chromosomes arrange themselves side by side with one member of the pair on either side of the equatorial plane of the cell. As the cell divides, one member of each pair of chromosomes goes to each daughter cell. Chance alone determines which member of the chromosome pair goes into each daughter cell as well as which daughter cell will be fertilized (if any). Thus, several offspring of the same parents will most likely inherit different characteristics.

The two daughter cells produced by the first meiotic division each contain the 23 chromosomes in their doubled state with the identical chromatids still joined by the centromere. They are thus ready to immediately undergo the second meiotic division.

Second Meiotic Division

The second division is shorter and less complicated than the first and resembles mitosis in many ways. Similar to mitosis, a spindle forms; the chromosomes consisting of two identical chromatids joined at a centromere attach on the equatorial plane of the spindle; the centromeres and chromatids separate and go to opposite poles of the cell, and the cytoplasm divides. One difference from mitosis is that the chromosomes enter the second meiotic division in a duplicated state as two identical chromatids, this duplication having taken place early in the first meiotic process. A second difference is the number of chromosomes involved in the division, 23 rather than 46.

To summarize, the first meiotic division divides the paired homologous chromosomes between two cells, each receiving one member of each pair or 23 chromosomes. The second division divides the identical chromatids of the 23 chromosomes in each of the two cells resulting from the first division. The result of the maturation divisions is the formation of four haploid cells from one diploid cell (Fig. 4–3).

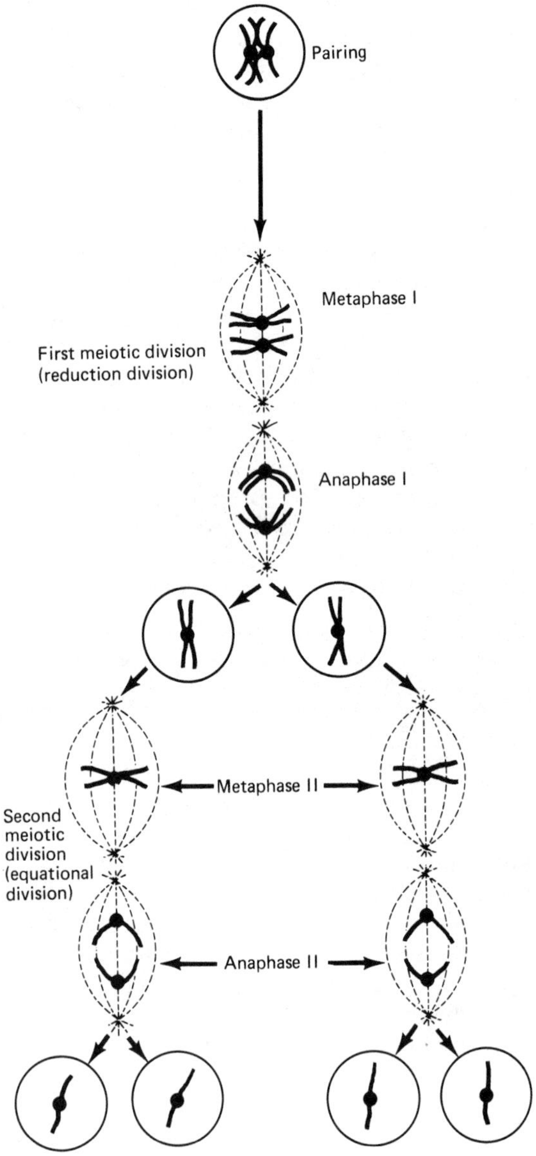

Figure 4–3. Schematic diagram of meiosis showing one chromosome. The original cell gives rise to four haploid cells or gametes. Not all of the steps recognized by cytologists are shown.

Crossing-Over of Chromosome Parts

Crossing-over refers to an exchange of segments between two homologous chromosomes as they are paired during the first meiotic division. In the process of pairing, the chromatids of homologous chromosomes tend to twist around each other. As the chromosomes move apart, the point or points where chromatids have crossed over each other may not separate as readily as the centromeres or as easily as the parts that are not closely entwined. The chromatids may break apart at the crossover points and the broken off segments may interchange and combine with the homologous chromatid involved in the crossover (Fig. 4-4).

An interchange of chromosome parts at crossover does not change the number of, or the position of, genes in the chromosomes. Genes each have their own particular position on a chromosome; homologous genes occur at corresponding positions on homologous chromosomes. When the chromosomes pair, they do so very precisely, with homologous chromosomes coming together so that all corresponding parts of the chromosomes lie exactly side by side. Crossing-over, therefore, will involve exchange of exactly the same parts of homologous chromosomes and exchange of the genes involved in those particular segments of the chromosomes.

Crossing-over changes the distribution of maternal and paternal chromatin material within the germ cell before it divides. The reshuffling or interchange of genes between any two homologous chromosomes produces two chromosomes that are different from the original two in the pair but which are still homologous. Together the two chromosomes of a pair have the same amount and kind of genetic material that they had before crossover, but as they separate, they will carry to each gamete a different genetic material than they would have carried if crossover had not taken place.

Crossing-over is an important feature of meiosis. It provides an additional opportunity for redistribution of maternal and paternal genes in the mature germ cells and thus another possibility for variation in the characteristics a germ cell may carry.

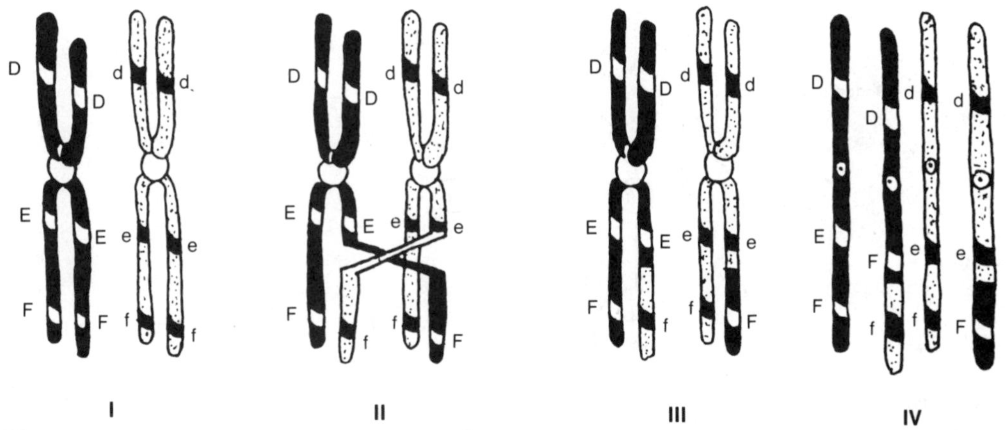

Figure 4–4. Diagram illustrating a single crossover of pieces of chromosomes with their genes, represented by the bars and letters respectively. In IV the two chromosomes have separated into four different combinations of genes in the haploid products.

Gametogenesis

The germ cells of both males and females mature by means of meiosis. However, there are several differences between oogenesis (maturation of an ovum) and spermatogenesis (maturation of sperm).

Spermatogenesis is a process that occurs continuously in the seminiferous tubules from puberty until senescence. A primary spermatocyte undergoes first meiotic division to form two secondary spermatocytes, each containing 23 chromosomes. Each of the two secondary spermatocytes then divides to form two spermatids, thus resulting in four haploid spermatids from a single primary spermatocyte. The spermatids subsequently differentiate into the highly motile spermatozoa. Hundreds of primary spermatocytes may be undergoing meiosis simultaneously in order to produce the large number of mature sperm present in the adult male reproductive tract at any one time (Fig. 4–5).

Oogenesis does not take place entirely during sexual maturity, but rather begins many years before, during fetal life. Prior to birth of the infant, the primary oocytes enter the first meiotic division. However, the process is then arrested to be completed during sexual maturity when ordinarily one oocyte will progress through complete maturation during each ovarian cycle.

When meiosis is resumed, the primary oocyte divides into two secondary oocytes, each with 23 chromosomes but a very unequal amount of cytoplasm. The smaller of the two which contains very little cytoplasm is known as the *first polar body*. It is a functionless cell which may undergo a second division or may simply degenerate.

The large secondary oocyte begins the second meiotic division probably just after ovulation but may not complete this stage until the entrance of the sperm at fertilization. As in the first division, the distribution of cytoplasm is very uneven with one daughter cell, the ovum, receiving most of the cytoplasm. The remaining smaller cell is termed the *second polar body*. Thus, oogenesis results in one functional cell and three polar bodies (if the first polar body divides), in contrast to spermatogenesis which results in four functional cells (Fig. 4–6).

At the time of fertilization the diploid number of chromosomes is restored as the 23 chromosomes of the sperm are joined with the 23 chromosomes of the ovum to form a new organism, the zygote.

MECHANISMS OF INHERITANCE

Those characteristics and genetic disorders which are controlled by a single gene follow the classic Mendelian patterns of inheritance. Over 2,000 disorders caused by a single gene have been identified. These are catalogued in a comprehensive reference by Victor A. McKusick, *Mendelian Inheritance in Man*. A discussion of the four basic patterns of Mendelian inheritance is included here.

Autosomal Dominant Inheritance

Genes that code for autosomal dominant inheritance are located on 1 of the 22 autosomes. The term *dominant* implies that only one member of the gene pair need carry the trait since it will mask the expression of the second gene. Thus, an individual need receive only one dominant gene from either parent in order to inherit the characteristic or disorder. Dominant traits are transmitted from generation to generation by both sexes and are equally likely to affect males and females. The offspring of affected individuals have a 50 percent chance of being affected themselves. Stated another way, on the average, one half of the offspring of affected individuals will inherit the trait or disorder. Those offspring who do not inherit the trait have no risk of having affected children

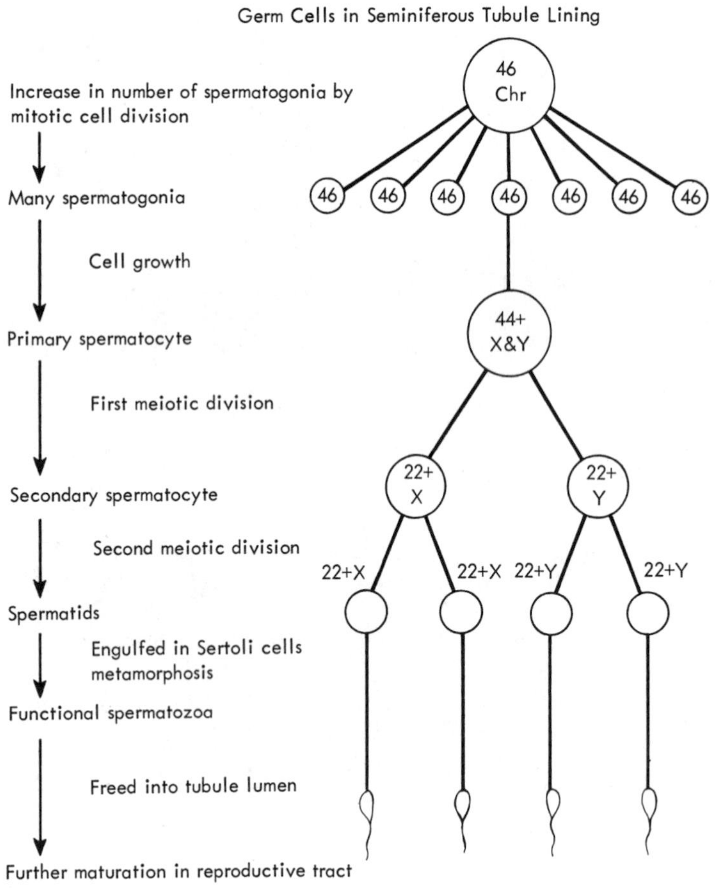

Figure 4–5. Diagram illustrating maturation of spermatozoa.

since they do not possess the gene. A family pedigree that illustrates the inheritance pattern of autosomal dominance is shown in Figure 4–7. Possible offspring of a couple in which one has an autosomal disorder is diagrammed in Figure 4–8.

Ordinarily a person who possesses a gene for an autosomal dominant disorder will manifest symptoms of that disorder and those without signs or symptoms can be assumed not to possess the gene. However, in some situations a person may carry the gene without any apparent manifestations. In this case the gene is said to have *incomplete penetrance.* When clinical manifestations are present, they may vary in severity. This is known as *variable expressivity*.

Some examples of autosomal dominant disorders are Huntington's chorea, achondroplasia, which is the most common form of dwarfism, osteogenesis imperfecta, and adult polycystic kidney disease.

Autosomal Recessive Inheritance

Genes for this inheritance pattern also are located on the autosomes. Unlike the dominant pattern, autosomal recessive inheritance requires that both members of a gene pair must code for the same trait or disorder. In order to inherit the trait an individual must receive two genes for that trait, one from the mother and one from the father. Parents of individuals affected by an autosomal recessive trait who are themselves normal are known to be *carriers* of the trait. They each possess one "normal" gene and one affected gene which is masked by the dominant, normal gene. A family pedigree that illustrates an autosomal recessive inheritance pattern is shown in Figure 4–9A.

On the average, when two carriers of an autosomal recessive disorder mate, one fourth of their children will be affected, one fourth will be normal, and one half will be heterozygous carriers. An important point to remember is that each pregnancy is a new event which is subject to the same probabilities without regard to the outcome of previous pregnancies. Thus, having one affected child does *not* mean that the next three will be unaffected. Possible outcomes from the matings of two carriers of an autosomal recessive trait are illustrated in Figure 4–9B.

It is common for unaffected siblings of someone with an autosomal recessive disorder to seek counseling about their own risks of having an affected child. Even though they are likely to be carriers (probability equals two thirds), their risk of having an affected child is less than 1

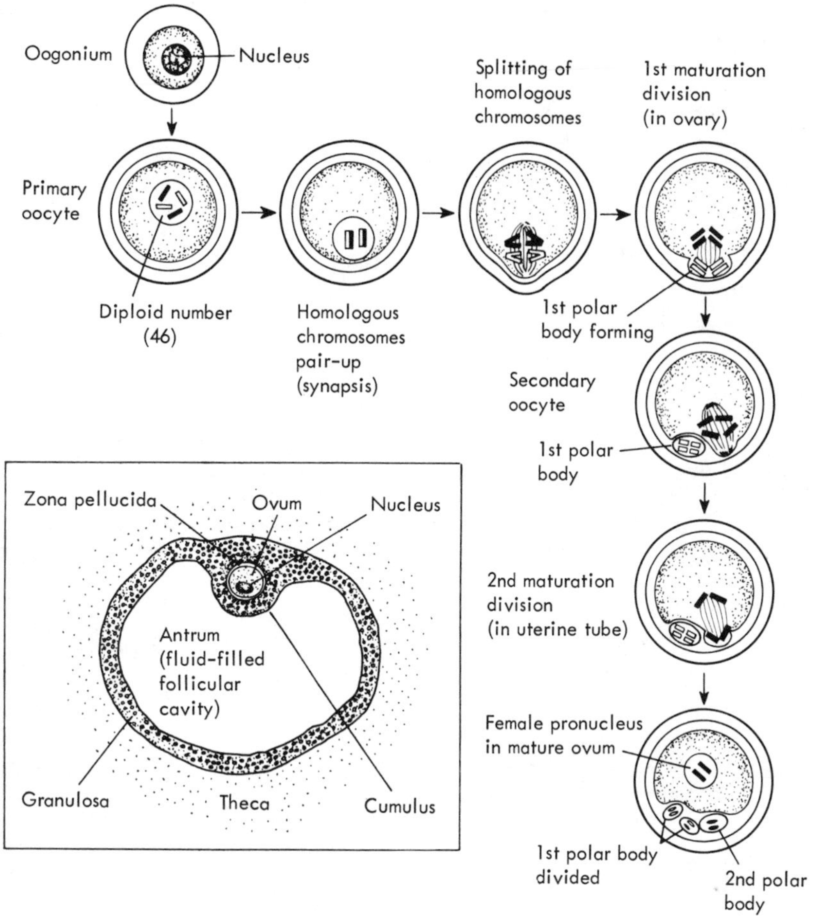

Figure 4-6. Diagram illustrating oogenesis, showing the reduction in chromosomes to form a mature female ovum. For simplification only two pairs of homologues are included. Insert illustrates the mature ovum located within the graafian follicle. [Reprinted with permission from Sigmund Grollman, *The Human Body: Its Structure and Physiology,* 4th ed. New York: Macmillan, 1978. Copyright Sigmund Grollman, 1978.]

percent. This is because any one autosomal recessive gene is fairly rare in the general population, making it quite unusual for two carriers to mate and have children. In fact, each person is probably the carrier for four or five deleterious autosomal recessive disorders. However, each gene is so individually rare that the likelihood of a mating of two carriers of the same gene is quite remote.

There are some circumstances that increase the likelihood of a mating of two persons with the same recessive genes. Since persons in the same family are more likely to carry the same genes, matings between related individuals (*consanguineous matings*) have a higher risk for producing offspring with autosomal recessive disorders. Some autosomal recessive disorders are almost exclusively limited to certain ethnic or racial groups. Thus, two people of black African origin are more likely to be carriers of sickle cell anemia, and two

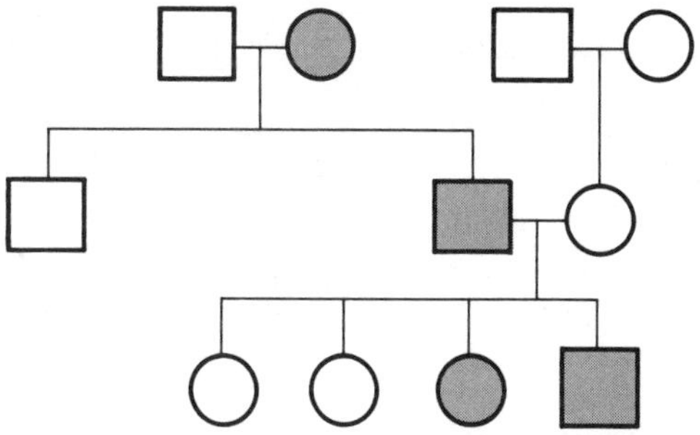

Figure 4-7. Family pedigree showing an *autosomal dominant* inheritance pattern. Only one dominant gene need be inherited from either parent. Males and females are equally likely to be affected. Non-affected individuals cannot pass on the trait since they do not possess the gene.

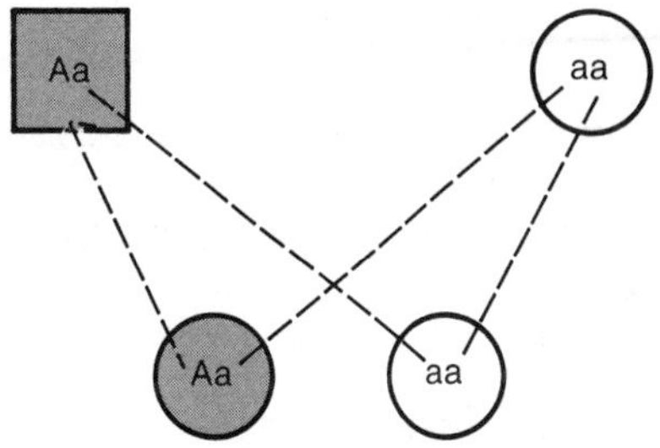

Figure 4-8. Diagram showing possible offspring of a couple where the father possesses an *autosomal dominant* trait. If the dominant gene (represented by A) is inherited, the child will also have the trait; if the recessive gene (a) is inherited the child will not have the trait. It is apparent that the recurrence risk for an autosomal dominant trait is 50%; e.g., an average 1/2 of the offspring will inherit it.

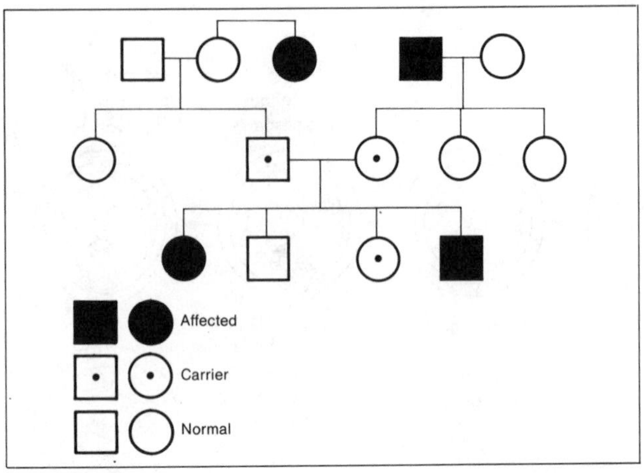

Figure 4–9A. Family pedigree showing an *autosomal recessive* inheritance pattern. Neither parent possesses the trait but both must be carriers. Although the occurrence risk for a recessive trait is 25%, one-half of this couple's children are affected.

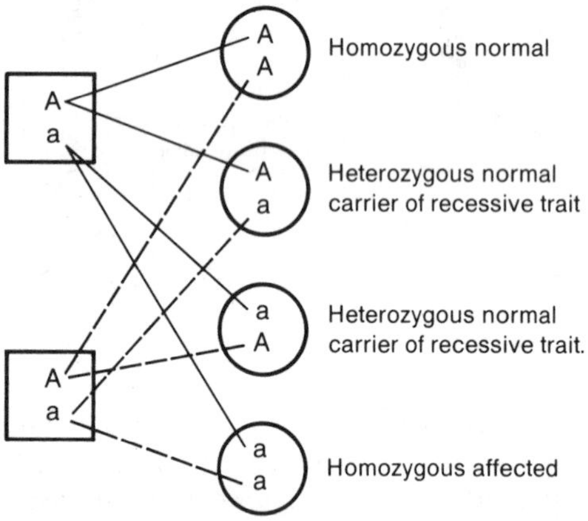

Figure 4–9B. Diagram showing the possible offspring of a couple where both parents are carriers of an autosomal recessive trait. The offspring is not affected unless a recessive gene is inherited from each parent. Recurrence risk is 25%; 50% of offspring will be carriers.

descendants of the eastern European Ashkenazi Jewish population are at higher risk for being carriers of Tay-Sachs disease.

Although there are tests to detect some carrier states, usually the birth of an affected child is the first time a couple is aware that they are carriers of an autosomal recessive disorder.

X-Linked Recessive Inheritance

This inheritance pattern is controlled by genes that are located on the X chromosome. Like recessive genes on autosomes, these X-linked genes do not express themselves as long as they are balanced by a "normal" and dominant gene on the other X chromosome. Therefore, females will not be affected unless both X chromosomes carry the same recessive gene. Males, on the other hand, have only one X chromosome. Since the Y chromosome does not have genes to match those on the X chromosome, all genes on the X chromosome in the male are expressed whether they are dominant or recessive.

Almost all individuals affected by X-linked recessive disorders are males who receive the gene from their mothers who are carriers and almost always normal themselves. A female carrier has an overall risk of 25 percent (1-in-4 chance) of having an affected child with any given pregnancy. However, if the child is a male, there is a 50 percent risk (1-in-2 chance), and if the child is female, there is virtually no risk of her being affected, although she has a 50 percent chance of being a carrier like her mother. A family pedigree illustrating X-linked recessive inheritance is shown in Figure 4–10. Possible outcomes of matings in such a family include affected males and carrier females.

Examples of X-linked recessive disorders include hemophilia, Duchenne's muscular dystrophy, and deutan color blindness. Very occasionally, an X-linked recessive disorder is observed in a female. This could happen if an affected male mated with a carrier female. It also could occur in a female with Turner's syndrome where there are 45 rather than 46 chromosomes and only one sex chromosome, a single X. In this case all genes on the single X chromosome are expressed in the same way that they are in the male. In addition, some female carriers may exhibit some of the manifestations of the disorder, but this is quite unusual.

X-Linked Dominant Inheritance

These very rare disorders occur equally in males and females since only one dominant gene need be present in order to produce the condition. This mode of inher-

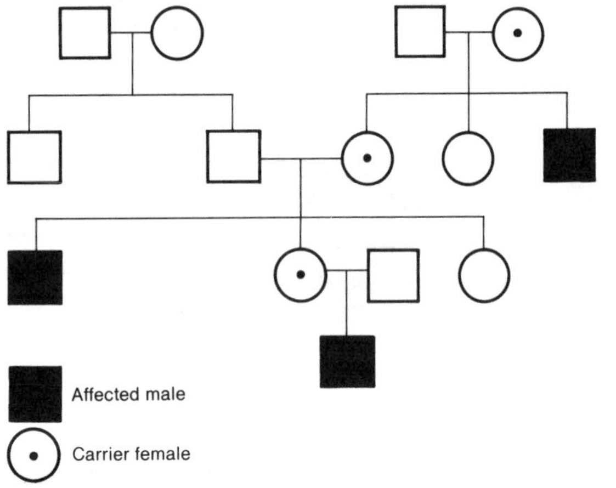

Figure 4–10. A family pedigree illustrating an *X-linked recessive* inheritance pattern. Only males are affected since they have no genes on the Y chromosome to balance the affected gene on the X which, of course, is always inherited from the mother.

itance can be distinguished from autosomal dominant because the family pedigree will demonstrate an absence of male-to-male transmission. Since a father contributes only a Y chromosome to his sons, he obviously cannot transmit any X-linked disorders. However, all of his daughters will receive the trait since they all receive one of their X chromosomes from him. An affected female has a 50 percent risk (1-in-2 chance) of transmitting the disorder, and the risk is the same whether the child is male or female.

Two examples of these rare X-linked dominant disorders are ornithine transcarbamylase deficiency (a urea cycle defect) and a vitamin D–resistant form of rickets.

MUTATIONS

Sometimes an individual will clearly manifest the signs and symptoms of a single gene defect without any identifiable family pedigree. In such a situation the individual may represent a new gene mutation. A mutation is a heritable change in the structure of the genetic material in a gene. This variation changes the genetic code and results in an alteration in the kind of protein that is synthesized or in the amount that is produced. Mutations may involve (1) a loss of part of a DNA molecule (deletion); (2) an addition of a new base (insertion); or (3) a variation in the sequential intramolecular arrangement of the bases (substitution).

It is important to note that a mutation is a *heritable* change. Unless it is passed on to an offspring it cannot be accepted as a mutation since its genetic implication cannot be established.

As a chemical substance, DNA is subject to chemical reactions with other substances which change its structure and, often, the genetic code. This is most likely to occur during replication of the DNA molecule as the long strands of nucleotides separate to form two new molecules. At this time mutagens (substances which cause mutations) may bring about alterations in the base-pair sequences by substituting, adding, or deleting bases to the DNA molecule. Other mutagens, such as ionizing radiation, cause changes by altering the covalent structure of the DNA, thereby leading to chromosomal breakage.

Mutations may appear to arise spontaneously or they may be attributable to certain factors in the environment, such as radiation or pharmacologic agents. In either event the exact duplication of the DNA is altered and the genes carry a set of instructions that differ from those of the original cell. A mutation may cause only a very slight variation in a body characteristic, or it may produce a major alteration. A significant number of mutations are thought to be lethal and therefore are never detected in offspring, since they result in early embryonic death. Most mutations that involve a change from function to nonfunction are recessive and therefore will not be detected unless there is a chance mating with another individual carrying an identical mutant gene. Needless to say, this may not occur for many generations, if ever. Some mutations have barely detectable effects; a few may be useful; others are undesirable and harmful.

On rare occasions, somatic cell mutations can be detected. When mutation occurs in such a cell it gives rise to a clone of cells that differ from the nonmutant surrounding cells. Usually this difference can be detected only if there is a visible change such as in pigmentation. Because somatic cell mutations are not transmissible to offspring, it is difficult to determine their genetic implications, if any.

MULTIFACTORIAL INHERITANCE

Many familial diseases, including some of the more common congenital malformations, are not the effect of a single gene. Rather, they result from several genes working together and sometimes from a combination of several genes plus environmental factors. The number of genes involved in any given disorder and the exact nature of the influencing environmental factors are unknown.

Recurrence risks for multifactorial disorders are determined by the statistical study of thousands of affected families in particular populations. For example, if all families with one parent having a cleft lip were surveyed, it would be found that approximately 4 percent of their children also had a cleft lip. Thus, a particular couple with one parent having a cleft lip could be counseled that the risk of their child having a cleft lip is 4 percent. Recurrence risks for malformations resulting from multifactorial inheritance are generally in the 3 to 7 percent range.

Congenital malformations with this inheritance pattern include neural tube defects (anencephaly, myelomeningocele, and so forth), cleft lip and palate, clubfoot, some types of congenital heart disease and pyloric stenosis. Also included are diseases such as cancer, maturity onset diabetes mellitus, hypertension, ischemic heart disease, and schizophrenia.

CHROMOSOMAL ABNORMALITIES

Alterations in the normal number or structure of chromosomes occur with a frequency of about 1 in 150 newborns. The addition of a complete set(s) of chromosomes is known as *polyploidy*. *Triploidy* refers to the presence of 69 or a triple set of chromosomes; *tetraploidy* is 92 or a quadruple set of chromosomes. *Aneuploidy* is a term used to describe the addition or subtraction of a single chromosome or several chromosomes rather than a complete set. The most common example of aneuploidy is *trisomy* in which there are three of a particular chromosome rather than the usual two. Another relatively common example is *monosomy*—only one of a particular chromosome pair. Sometimes it happens that an individual will have two or more kinds of cells, each with a different number of chromosomes. This is known as *mosaicism* and results from an error in cell division after fertilization.

Beside additions or absences of whole chromosomes or sets of chromosomes, there can be alterations in the structure of a chromosome. Segments of chromosomes may break off and be lost, or they may reattach in an inverted position or even to another chromosome. Most structural changes, perhaps all, are reciprocal; a broken end attaches to another broken end. Such a change or moving around of chromosomal material is known as a *translocation*. If no material is lost, merely rearranged, it is said to be a *balanced translocation*. There is probably no such thing as a completely balanced translocation since all involve breakage of chromosomes. However, the amount of material lost apparently may be so small as to be insignificant.

Autosomal Abnormalities

Trisomies

The possible variations in number and structure of chromosomes are infinite. However, many of these alterations are incompatible with life and result in early embryonic death. The autosomal abnormalities most commonly observed in liveborn infants are the trisomies 21, 18, and 13. The incidence and clinical characteristics of these disorders are shown in Table 4–1.

The occurrence of a trisomy results from an abnormal segregation of chromosomes during meiosis. Instead of the chromosome pair dividing evenly so that each member goes to a separate daughter cell, both members of a pair go to one daughter cell with none going to the other. This failure to segregate properly is known as *nondisjunction*. If it occurs during the first meiotic division, it is termed *primary nondisjunction;* whereas if it occurs during the second meiotic division, it is called *secondary nondisjunction*. If the gamete containing the two chromosomes of the same pair is fertilized by a gamete with the normal chromosomal complement, the resulting zygote will have three chromosomes of one kind, hence, the name trisomy. Figure 4–11 illustrates how this occurs.

The factors responsible for nondisjunction are poorly understood. One of the most commonly associated factors is advanced maternal age, usually defined as maternal age greater than 35. More recently, advanced paternal age also has been implicated, although most studies report the critical paternal age to be greater than 55, suggesting that this is probably not a significantly large factor.

One occurrence of nondisjunction in an individual increases the risk of the same thing happening again. The reasons for this remain unclear.

Translocations

A small percentage (about 5 percent in trisomy 21 or Down's syndrome) of trisomy patients do not demonstrate the typical 47 chromosome karyotype. Although

Table 4–1. Incidence and Characteristics of the Three Human Trisomies that Occur in Liveborn Infants

Trisomy	*Incidence*	*Characteristics*
13 Patau's syndrome	Varies with studies—1 in 4,000 to 1 in 10,000 livebirths*	Marked mental retardation Delayed physical development Hypertelorism, eye defects, cleft lip and palate, polydactyly, micrognathia, malformed ears, dermatoglyphic abnormalities Lifespan: one half die by 1 month of age, survival rare beyond 3 years
18 Edward's syndrome	1 in 1,000 livebirths*	Marked mental retardation Hypertonicity, malformed ears, micrognathia, congenital heart defects, rocker-bottom feet, marked increase in digital arches
21 Down's syndrome	1 in 600–700 livebirths* Maternal age 30: 1/800 35: 1/300 40: 1/100 45: 1/55	Variable mental retardation—moderate to severe Short stature Short, broad fingers and toes Round face with epicanthal folds and long tongue Unusual finger and palm points, including simian crease (a single transverse palmar crease)

*Incidence increases with parental age.

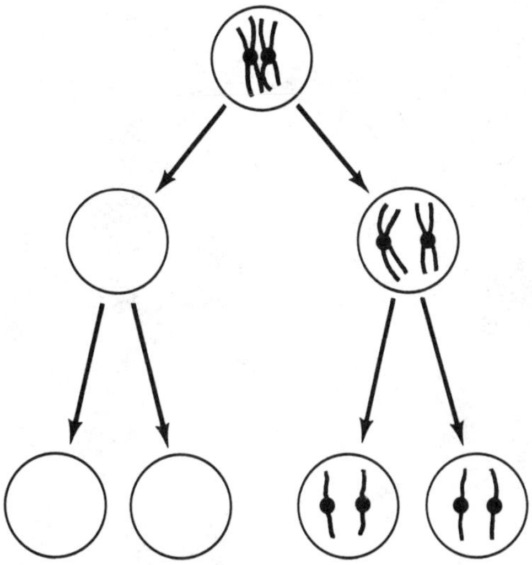

First division nondisjunction

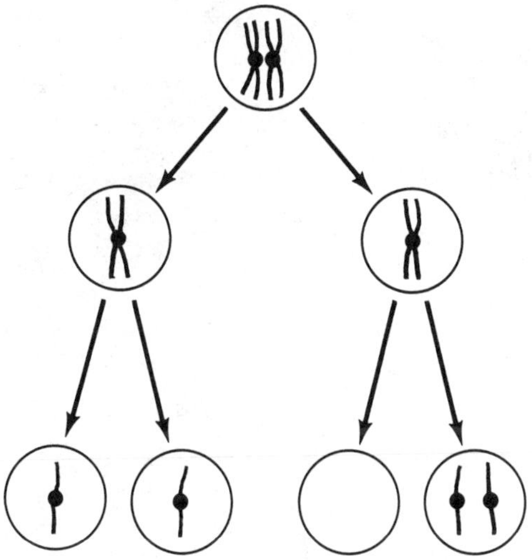

Second division nondisjunction

Figure 4–11. First and second division nondisjunction are diagrammed. Such accidents of meiosis result in offspring having too many or too few chromosomes. The most commonly recognized example is Down's syndrome where nondisjunction of chromosome 21 results in the individual having three no. 21 chromosomes and 47 rather than 46 total chromosomes.

they appear to have only 46 chromosomes, there is additional chromosomal material attached to one of the chromosomes so that the total amount of genetic material is the equivalent of 47 chromosomes. The only difference is the way in which it is arranged or packaged. This phenomenon is known as the translocation type of trisomy. The most common of these are the D/G and G/G translocations in which an extra G or 21 chromosome is attached to either a D or a G chromosome causing Down's syndrome (trisomy 21). (See Figure 4–12A, B, C.)

Whether a trisomy results from nondisjunction or translocation is of no clinical significance since the effect on the individual is the same. However, it is of great importance for genetic counseling since a translocation carrier parent has a substantial risk of having subsequent children with the same trisomy. The actual risk varies with the type of translocation, the age and sex of the parent. The recurrence risk for female carriers of D/G translocation is 10 to 15 percent for any given pregnancy, while a male carrier of the same translocation has a 2 to 3 percent risk of recurrence.

Deletion Syndromes

With the advent of sophisticated banding techniques, the number of identified syndromes associated with the deletion or absence of genetic material has increased. One of the more commonly encountered disorders is the *cri du chat,* or cat's cry, syndrome, so named because of the characteristic high-pitched catlike cry that occurs in infancy. This syndrome is the result of the deletion of the short arm of chromosome 5. The clinical picture of these children is one of profound mental retardation, failure to thrive, hypotonia, microcephaly, and a variety of other anomalies. Parents of these children are candidates for genetic counseling since about 15 percent of cases reveal one of the parents to be a balanced translocation carrier with a high recurrence risk.

Sex Chromosomal Abnormalities

Abnormalities of the sex chromosomes occur with a frequency of about 1 in 400 liveborn infants. They are more common in phenotypic males than in phenotypic females. In general, they are not characterized by the major anomalies that are seen with autosomal abnormalities. Most abnormalities center around body stature and sexual development.

Understanding of the diagnosis of sex chromosome abnormalities is assisted by knowledge of the *Lyon hypothesis.* This hypothesis states that in any one mammalian cell only one X chromosome is active. In males the single X chromosome is always active, whereas in females one of the two X chromosomes is inactivated at an early stage of embryonic development. In any given cell the choice of which X remains active is purely a matter of chance. Once inactivated the chromosome continues to replicate at mitosis but remains inactive in all subsequent cell cycles. The inactivated X chromosome forms a small, dark chromatin body called the *sex chromatin,* or *chromatin-positive body,* or *Barr body.* The number of Barr bodies in a cell nucleus is always one less than the number of X chromosomes. Thus, normal

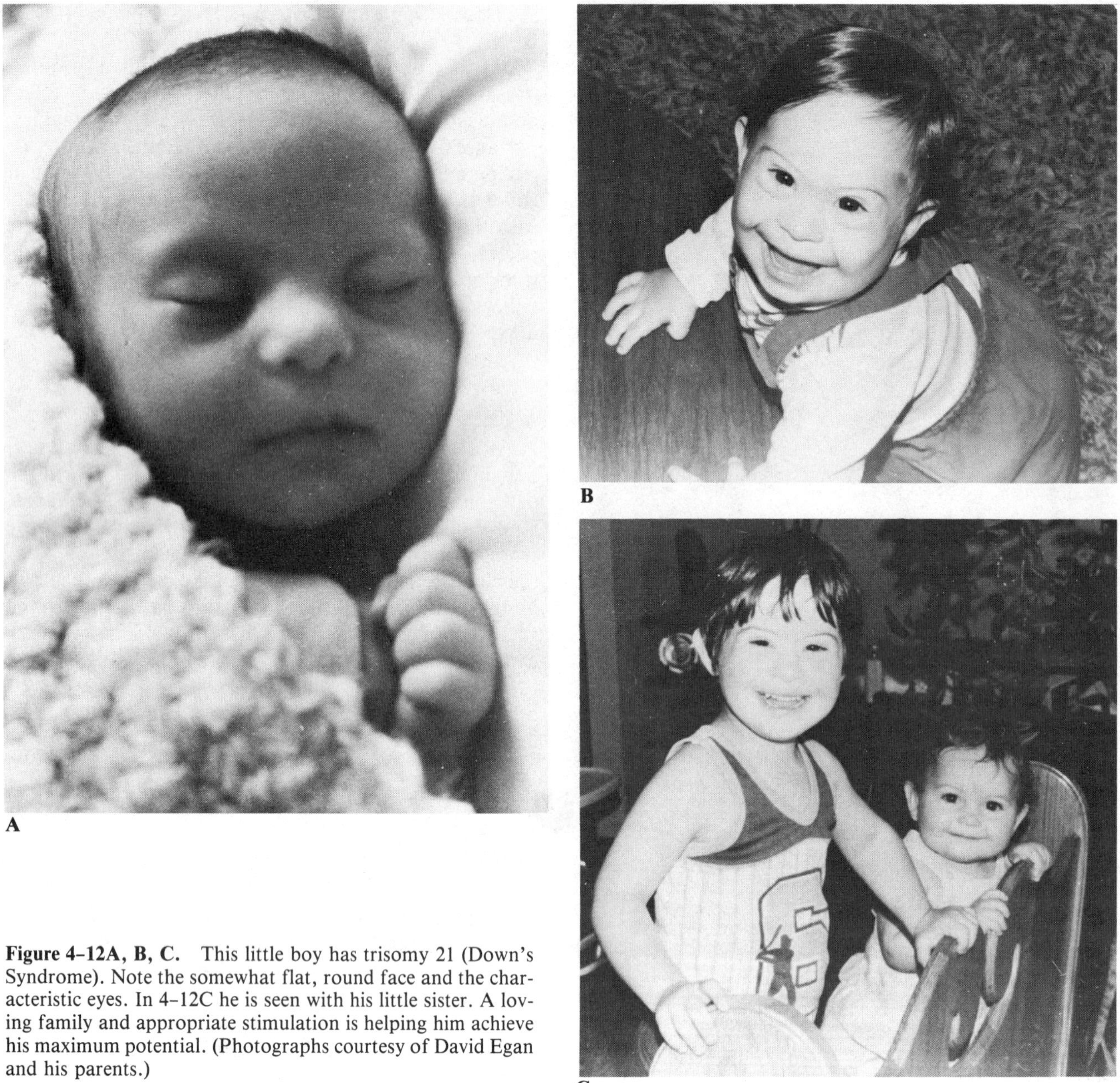

A

B

C

Figure 4–12A, B, C. This little boy has trisomy 21 (Down's Syndrome). Note the somewhat flat, round face and the characteristic eyes. In 4–12C he is seen with his little sister. A loving family and appropriate stimulation is helping him achieve his maximum potential. (Photographs courtesy of David Egan and his parents.)

males have no Barr bodies, while normal females have one.

Epithelial cells taken from the lining of the cheek readily may be examined for the number of Barr bodies whenever there is reason to suspect a sex chromosome anomaly.

Table 4–2 describes the more commonly recognized sex chromosome abnormalities.

Inborn Errors of Metabolism

Disorders characterized by a defect in metabolism are known collectively as *inborn errors of metabolism*. They result from the absence of or change in a protein, usually an enzyme. Although individual disorders may be very rare, taken together they are not rare.

Ideally, an accurate diagnosis of an inborn error of metabolism should be made early in the neonatal period. Successful therapy is available for an increasing number of these disorders if treatment is begun early. One example of this is the dietary treatment of phenylketonuria (PKU) and galactosemia. Diagnosis is equally important for those disorders for which there is no effective treatment so that genetic counseling can be recommended. Almost all inborn errors of metabolism are either recessive or X-linked recessive and therefore carry a substantial recurrence risk.

Prenatal diagnosis is now available for many of the in-

Table 4–2. Commonly Recognized Sex Chromosome Abnormalities

Syndrome	*Incidence*	*Chromosomal Pattern*	*Clinical Characteristics*
Turner's	1 in 2,000 female births	45 XO (no second X or Y)	Phenotypically female Short stature Webbed neck Infantile genitalia Lack of secondary sex characteristics Mental development within normal range Sterile
Triplo-X (metafemales or superfemales)	1 in 1,000 female births	47 XXX	Phenotypically female Normal physical development May be mentally retarded or of normal intelligence Fertile—offspring normal
XYY	1 in 1,000 male births	47 XYY	Phenotypically male Unusually tall Normal physical and mental development Fertile—offspring usually normal
Klinefelter's	1 in 500 male births	47 XXY	Phenotypically male, somewhat eunuchoid Longer than average limbs, underdeveloped genitalia, sparse body hair Often of low intelligence Sterile

born errors of metabolism for which the underlying biochemical defect has been identified. When this is the case, parents may be offered the option of amniocentesis and selective abortion. An outline of some of the inborn errors of metabolism is found in Table 4–3.

GENETIC COUNSELING

Genetic counseling, the ultimate practical application of the science of human genetics, is a social and sometimes a medical service to families. The purpose of genetic counseling is to provide families with information about the risk of occurrence or recurrence of a particular genetic disorder in their family, as well as information about available alternatives so they can make the reproductive decisions that are best for them. An overall societal goal of genetic counseling is to reduce the incidence and the impact of genetic disease.

Indications for Counseling

When family histories or other screening procedures indicate the presence of genetic disorders or when a couple's anxieties about inherited disorders is very high, genetic counseling should be recommended. In general, three categories of genetic disorders suggest a need for action in terms of health teaching, counseling, or direct intervention. In the first category are those genetic disorders that have special implications for the course of the pregnancy itself. The second category consists of disorders that can be predicted to affect the fetus and may suggest the desirability of prenatal diagnosis. The third, and largest, category contains those diseases of a hereditary nature that are likely to affect the parents and/or their offspring in later life, for example, cardiovascular disease.

The first category of genetic diseases includes such common genetic factors as Rh and ABO blood incompatibilities. Polygenic or multifactorial conditions such as diabetes mellitus, hypertension, and heart disease also belong to this category. Other genetic disorders present in the mother may present so great a risk that the advisability of pregnancy is seriously questioned. Such disorders include Marfan's syndrome, sickle cell anemia, and acute intermittent porphyria. Others require only slight modifications in care. Achondroplasia, for example, will almost always necessitate a cesarean birth because of the abnormal pelvis structure. Otherwise pregnancy progresses normally.

A number of genetic disorders are beginning to be found in pregnancy simply because newer advances in the treatment of these diseases are permitting individuals to reach reproductive age in better states of health. One such example is phenylketonuria. Because of early screening and dietary treatment, many PKU children are now adults having their own children. Women with PKU who wish to bear children should reinstitute a low phenylalanine diet prior to conception and continue it through gestation. If this is not done, the fetus will suffer mental retardation from intrauterine exposure to the

TIMETABLE OF HUMAN PRENATAL DEVELOPMENT
1 to 6 weeks

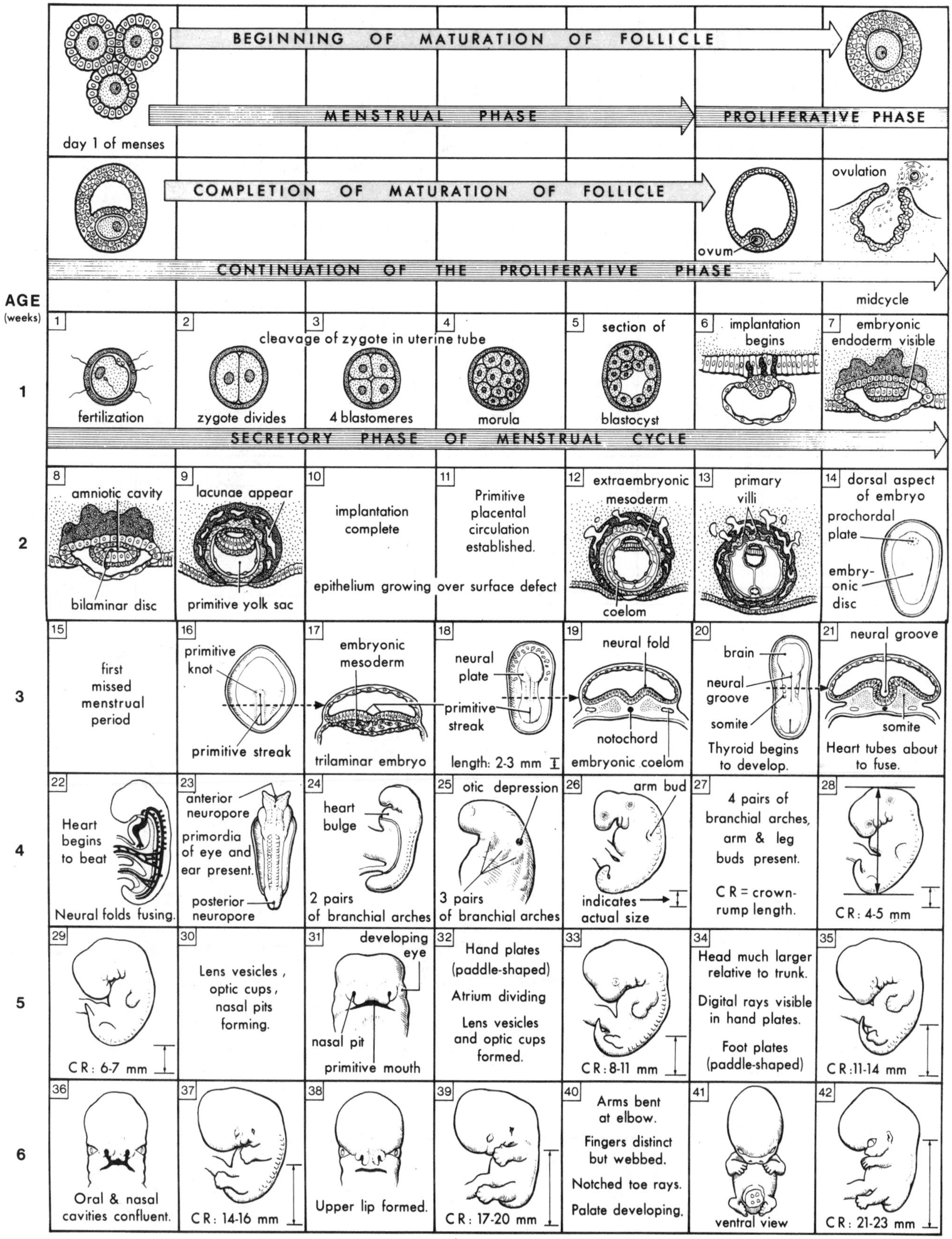

BEGINNING OF MATURATION OF FOLLICLE
day 1 of menses
MENSTRUAL PHASE
PROLIFERATIVE PHASE
COMPLETION OF MATURATION OF FOLLICLE
ovum
ovulation
CONTINUATION OF THE PROLIFERATIVE PHASE
midcycle
AGE
(weeks)
1
1
fertilization
2
cleavage of zygote in uterine tube
zygote divides
3
4 blastomeres
4
morula
5
section of
blastocyst
6
implantation begins
7
embryonic endoderm visible
SECRETORY PHASE OF MENSTRUAL CYCLE
2
8
amniotic cavity
bilaminar disc
9
lacunae appear
primitive yolk sac
10
implantation complete
epithelium growing over surface defect
11
Primitive placental circulation established.
12
extraembryonic mesoderm
coelom
13
primary villi
14
dorsal aspect of embryo
prochordal plate
embryonic disc
3
15
first missed menstrual period
16
primitive knot
primitive streak
17
embryonic mesoderm
trilaminar embryo
18
neural plate
primitive streak
length: 2-3 mm
19
neural fold
notochord
embryonic coelom
20
brain
neural groove
somite
Thyroid begins to develop.
21
neural groove
somite
Heart tubes about to fuse.
4
22
Heart begins to beat
Neural folds fusing.
23
anterior neuropore
primordia of eye and ear present.
posterior neuropore
24
heart bulge
2 pairs of branchial arches
25
otic depression
3 pairs of branchial arches
26
arm bud
indicates actual size
27
4 pairs of branchial arches, arm & leg buds present.
C R = crown-rump length.
28
CR: 4-5 mm
5
29
CR: 6-7 mm
30
Lens vesicles, optic cups, nasal pits forming.
31
developing eye
nasal pit
primitive mouth
32
Hand plates (paddle-shaped)
Atrium dividing
Lens vesicles and optic cups formed.
33
CR: 8-11 mm
34
Head much larger relative to trunk.
Digital rays visible in hand plates.
Foot plates (paddle-shaped)
35
CR: 11-14 mm
6
36
Oral & nasal cavities confluent.
37
CR: 14-16 mm
38
Upper lip formed.
39
CR: 17-20 mm
40
Arms bent at elbow.
Fingers distinct but webbed.
Notched toe rays.
Palate developing.
41
ventral view
42
CR: 21-23 mm

TIMETABLE OF HUMAN PRENATAL DEVELOPMENT
7 to 38 weeks

AGE (weeks)							
7	43 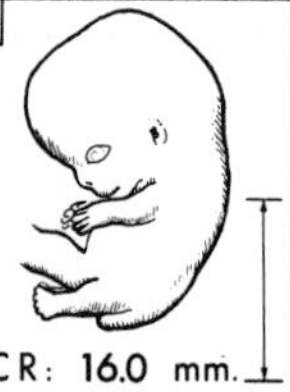 CR: 16.0 mm.	44 Stage 18 begins 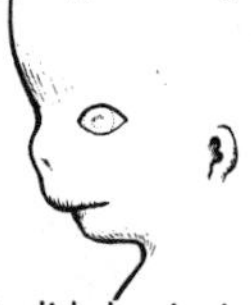 Eyelids beginning	45 Tip of nose distinct. Toe rays appear. Ossification may begin. CR: 17.0 mm	46 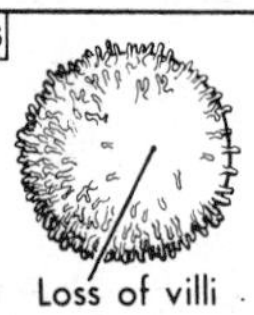 Loss of villi. Smooth chorion forms.	47 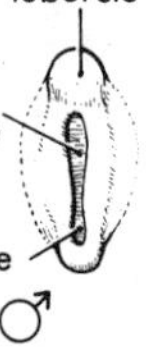 genital tubercle; urogenital membrane; anal membrane; ♀ or ♂	48 Stage 19 begins. Trunk elongating ana straightening	49 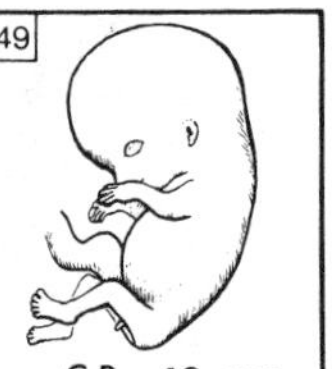 CR: 18 mm
8	50 Upper limbs longer & bent at elbows. Fingers distinct	51 Anal membrane perforated. Urogenital membrane degenerating. Testes and ovaries distinguishable.	52 Stage 21 begins 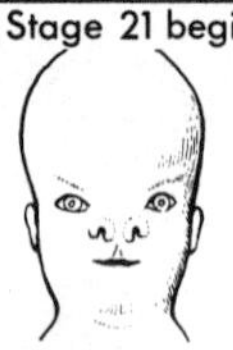	53 Stage 21. External genitalia still in sexless state but have begun to differentiate.	54 Stage 22 begins 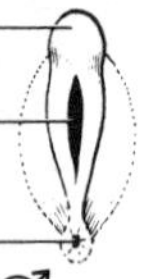 genital tubercle; urethral groove; anus; ♀ or ♂	55 Beginnings of all essential external & and internal structures are present.	56 Stage 23 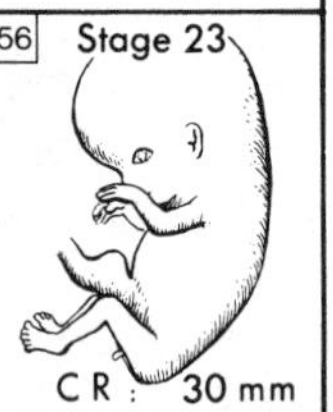 CR: 30 mm
9	57 beginning of fetal period	58 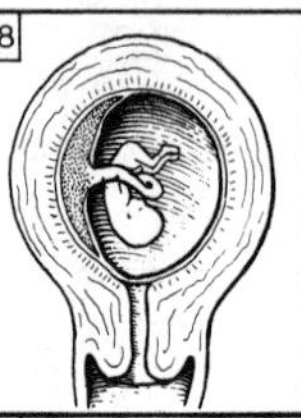	59 Genitalia show some ♀ characteristics but still easily confused with ♂.	60 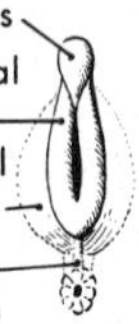 phallus; urogenital fold; labioscrotal fold; perineum; ♀	61 Genitalia show fusion of urethral folds. Urethral groove extends into phallus.	62 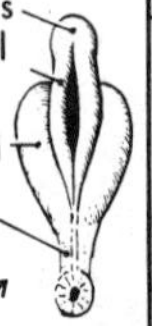 phallus; urogenital fold; labioscrotal fold; perineum; ♂	63 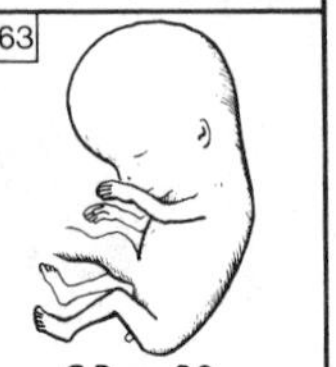 CR: 50 mm
10	64 Face has human profile. Note growth of chin compared to day 44.	65 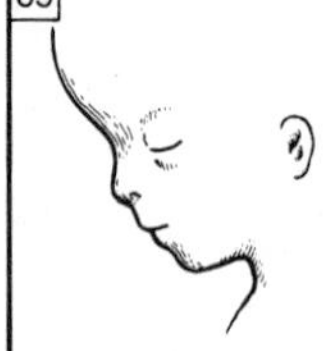	66 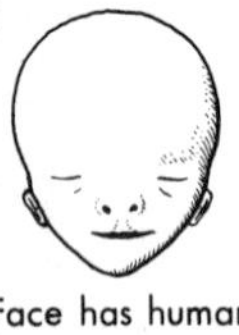 Face has human appearance.	67 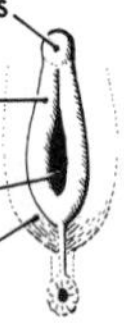 clitoris; labium minus; urogenital groove; labium majus; ♀	68 Genitalia have ♀ or ♂ characteristics but still not fully formed.	69 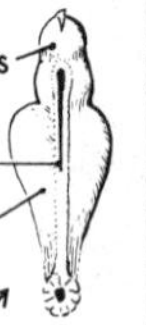 glans penis; urethral groove; scrotum; ♂	70 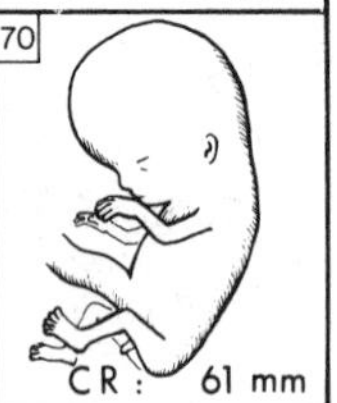 CR: 61 mm

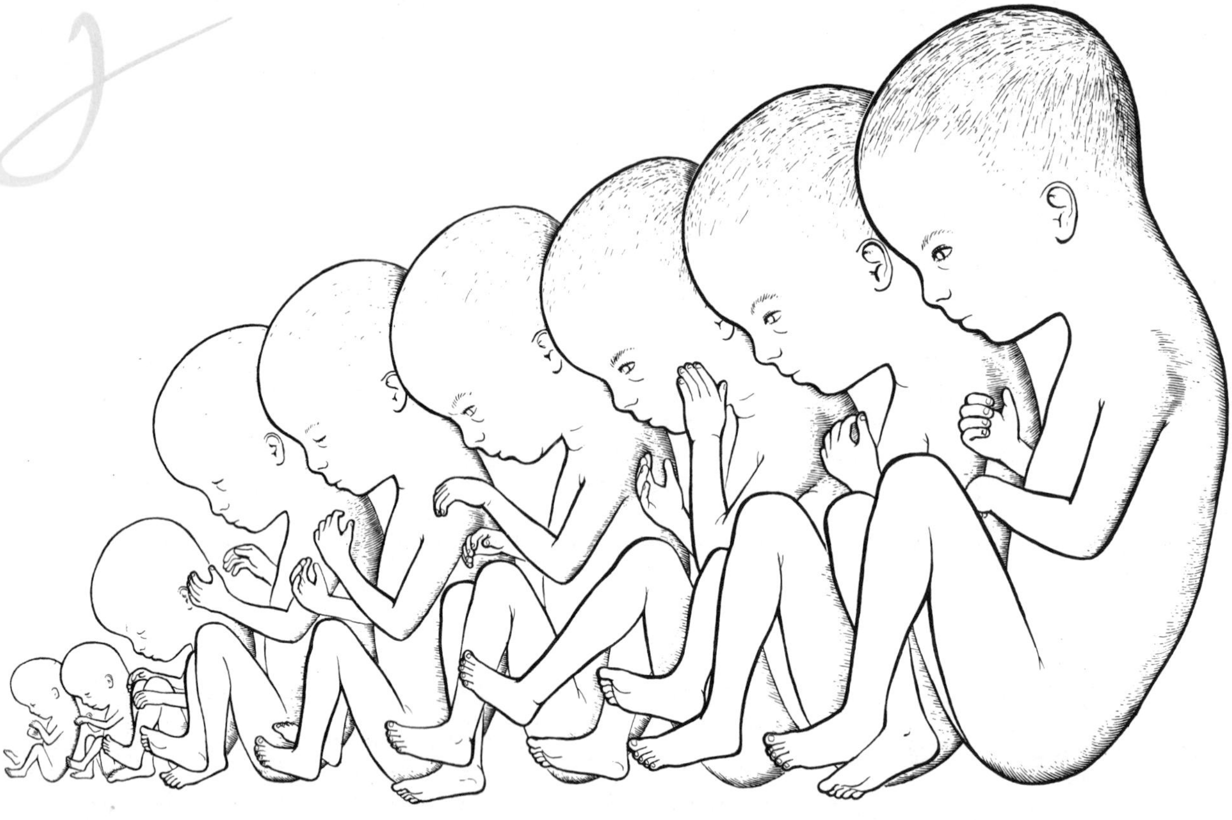

11 12 16 20 24 28 32 36 38 FULL TERM

midline cord called the notochordal process. This cord grows between the ectoderm and endoderm until it reaches the prochordal plate, which is located at the cranial end of the germ disc and is the site of future development of the mouth.

A cellular rod, called the *notochord,* develops from the notochordal process (Fig. 5–7). This notochord forms a midline axis in the human embryo and is the basis of the axial skeleton. The skull and the vertebral column develop around the notochord.

As the notochord develops, the embryonic cells over it thicken to form the neural plate. This plate soon develops a neural groove with neural folds on each side, and by the end of the third week the neural folds close and fuse. This changes the neural plate into the neural tube (Figs. 5–7 and 5–8). The neural tube will develop into the central nervous system—the brain and the spinal cord.

Development of Somites

The mesoderm on each side of the notochord and the neural tube, called the *paraxial mesoderm,* thickens to form two longitudinal columns. By the end of the third week, these columns of mesoderm begin to divide and become segmented to eventually form 42 to 44 pairs of cuboidal bodies of mesoderm, known as *somites.* The word somite is from the Greek *soma,* meaning a body. The somites form distinct surface elevations. They appear first in the occipital area and then gradually continue to develop caudally (Fig. 5–8).

Between 20 and 30 days of development, called the *somite period,* the stage of development of an embryo often is described by the number of somites present. About 38 pair form during this time; the last few pair form soon after the somite period.

Development proceeding from the somites includes most of the axial skeleton and associated musculature—the vertebrae, ribs, and muscles of the axial skeleton and the dermis of the skin. Spinal nerves enter the portions of the somites that will form the muscles.

Development of the Intraembryonic Coelom

The *intraembryonic coelom* first appears at the end of the third week as a number of small, isolated, coelomic spaces within the mesoderm. These spaces soon coalesce to form a horseshoe-shaped cavity, which is called the intraembryonic coelom. During the second month of development this coelom will be divided into the cavities of the human body—the pericardial cavity containing the heart, the pleural cavity containing the lungs, and the peritoneal cavity containing the viscera below the diaphragm.

The Early Cardiovascular System

Blood vessels begin to form early in the third week in the yolk sac, allantois, connecting stalk, and chorion, and shortly thereafter in the embryo. Primitive plasma and blood cells then develop from the endothelial cells of the vessels. Primitive paired heart tubes form from mesenchymal cells before the end of the third week, and they soon begin to fuse into the primitive heart tube.

By the end of the third week, the heart tubes have joined with blood vessels in the embryo, the connecting stalk, the yolk sac, and the chorion. A primitive cardiovascular system, with circulation of blood, has started by the end of the third week (Fig. 5–7). The circulatory system of the embryo must begin to function very early to transport the nourishment and oxygen that are taken up from the maternal blood through the chorionic villi.

Summary of Development During the Third Week

At the end of the third week of development, the embryo measures approximately 2.0 mm in length, and the entire product of conception has a diameter of approximately 15 mm. This is a tremendous increase in size of the ovum from the time of fertilization, but much more impressive is the complexity of its development. By the end of the third week, the fertilized ovum has progressed into a complex, multicellular mass ready to proceed rapidly with development of body form that will make it recognizable as a human with differentiation and growth of all internal organs and systems. The circulatory system already has a good start at this time in its continuing development.

THE EMBRYONIC PERIOD

The fourth to eighth weeks of development, known as the embryonic period, constitute a very important period in human development. It is the time during which all major internal and external structures develop to a significant degree, and it is a critical time, during which exposure to developmental disturbances may cause congenital malformations, ranging anywhere from very mild to severe and life-threatening.

Figure 5–7B. The embryonic period ends at the end of the eighth week; by this time, the beginnings of all essential structures are present. The fetal period, extending from the ninth week until birth, is characterized by growth and elaboration of structures. Sex is clearly distinguishable by 12 weeks. The above 9- to 38-week fetuses are about half actual size. (Reproduced with permission from Keith L. Moore, *The Developing Human, Clinically Oriented Embryology,* 3rd ed. Philadelphia: Saunders, 1982.)

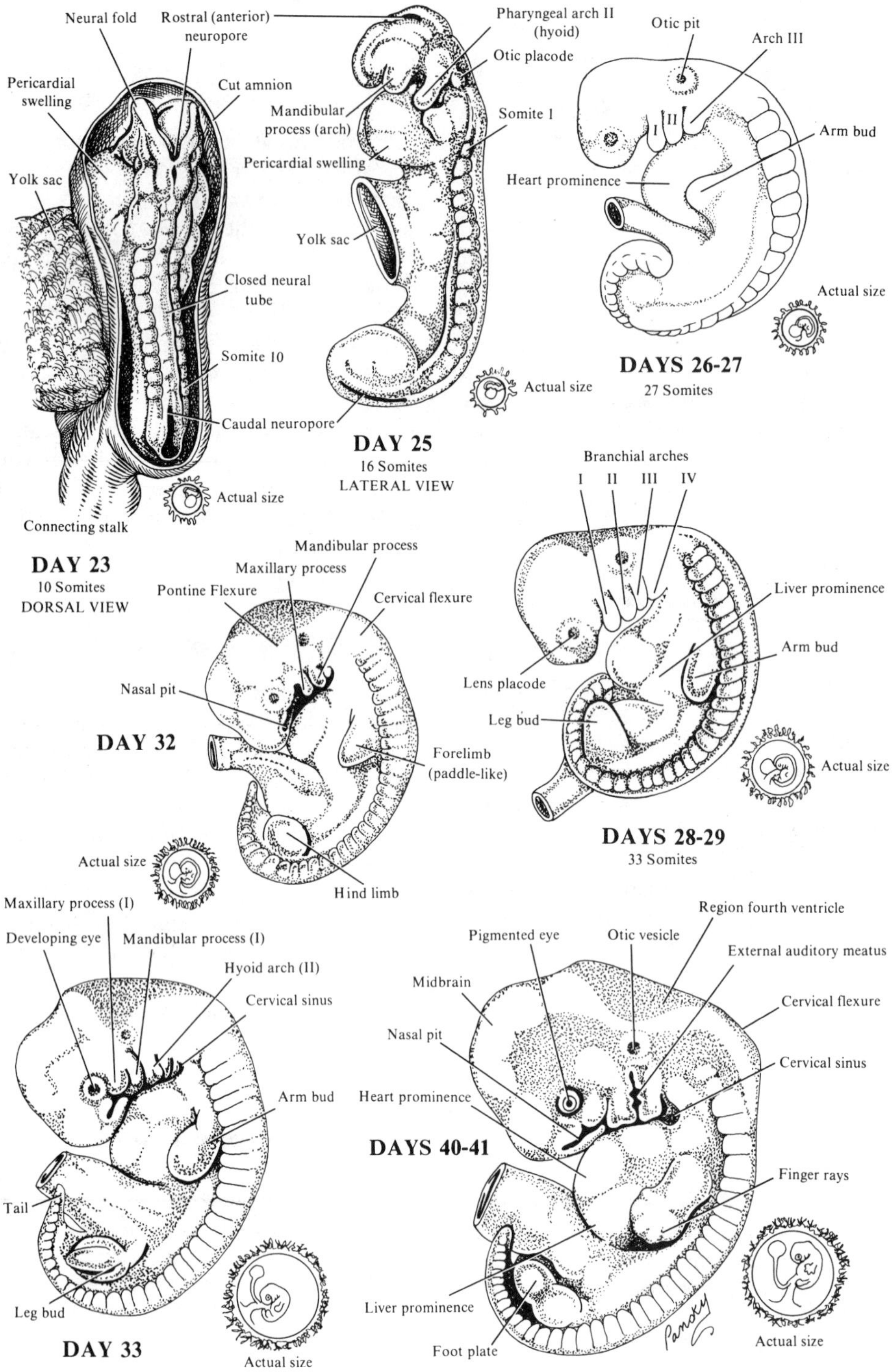

Figure 5–8. Diagrams of growth and development of embryos from days 23 to 41 (approximately weeks three through six). Note the drawings of the actual size of the embryo within the chorionic vesicle. (Reprinted with permission from Ben Pansky, *Review of Medical Embryology*. New York: Macmillan, 1982.)

The Derivatives of the Three Germ Layers

The three primary germ layers, described in the preceding pages, which give rise to all tissues and organs of the body, differentiate into specific structures during the embryonic period. The main derivatives of each germ layer are as follows:

Ectoderm

The ectodermal germ layer, the outer layer of cells, gives rise to structures that help the body to maintain contact with the outside. The ectoderm gives rise to the formation of the central nervous system (the brain and spinal cord), the peripheral nervous system, the sensory epithelium of the eyes, ears, and nose, and the skin including the hair, nails, and sebaceous and sweat glands. In addition, the pituitary gland, the mammary glands, and the enamel of the teeth are formed from the ectoderm (Table 5–1).

Mesoderm

The mesodermal germ layer, the middle layer of cells, provides all the supporting structures of the body, the cardiovascular system, the urogenital system, the serous membranes, and the spleen. The somites, important bodies of mesoderm, which develop in the very early embryo, give rise to cartilage and bone, muscle, connective tissue, and subcutaneous tissue of the skin. The mesoderm also gives rise to all of the vascular system—the heart, arteries and veins, lymph vessels, and blood and lymph cells. The urogenital system develops from mesoderm; this includes the kidneys, the gonads (ovaries and testes), and the ducts of this system with the exception of the bladder. In addition, the serous membrane lining of the body cavities (pericardial, pleural, and peritoneal) and the spleen and the suprarenal glands are derivatives of the mesoderm (Table 5–1).

Endoderm

The endodermal germ layer, the inner layer of cells, provides most of the epithelial lining of the body tracts. It gives rise to the epithelial lining of the gastrointestinal tract, the respiratory tract, the urinary bladder and urethra, and the tympanic cavities and eustachian tubes. In addition, the endoderm forms the parenchyma of the tonsils, thyroid, parathyroids, thymus, liver, and pancreas (Table 5–1).

The Fourth Week of Development

The fourth week is one of beginning development of body organs and systems, a period of rapid growth, and a time of remarkable change in body form. This week can be considered the beginning of organogenesis of most body organs and systems. Also, within the short span of this one week the body grows very rapidly, and body form changes significantly.

Organogenesis

The very beginnings of some of the major organs are present in primordial form by the end of the third week, but they are very difficult to identify at that time. During the fourth week, however, organogenesis begins quickly and proceeds rapidly. The major organs and systems begin to appear in more definitive form at this time, and distinct changes take place each day. Among organs and systems beginning during week four are the neural tube, otic placodes, optic vesicles, lens placodes, lung buds, esophagus, stomach, liver, pancreas, and nephric ducts. Highlights of development in the fourth week and continuing progress in the weeks thereafter are shown in Figure 5–7 *A* and *B* and Table 5–2.

The Somites and the Pharyngeal Arches

The somites, which began to appear late in the third week, continue to develop during the fourth week. They

[Text continues on page 78.]

Table 5–1. Organs and Tissues of the Body Arising from Each of the Primary Germ Layers

Ectoderm Derivatives	*Mesoderm Derivatives*	*Endoderm Derivatives*
Central nervous system	Bone and cartilage	Epithelial lining of respiratory tract
Peripheral nervous system	Connective tissue	Epithelial lining of gastrointestinal tract
Sensory epithelium of ear, nose and eye	Muscles—smooth and striated	Epithelial lining of urinary bladder and urethra
Skin (epidermis) and its appendices—hair, nails, sebaceous glands, sweat glands	Cardiovascular and lymphatic systems	Epithelial lining of tympanic cavities and eustachian tubes
	Blood and lymph cells	
Mammary glands	Kidneys and gonads and their ducts	Thyroid, parathyroids
Pituitary gland	Subcutaneous tissues of the skin	Liver
Enamel of the teeth	Serous membrane lining of the pericardial, pleural, and peritoneal cavities	Pancreas
		Thymus
	Spleen, suprarenal gland, adrenal cortex	Tonsils

Table 5–2. Stages in the Development of the Embryo and Fetus

System	*3rd Week*	*4th Week*	*5th Week*
External appearance	Trilaminar germ disc with developing neural folds	Change from disc to tubular shape. Head and tail folds developing. Head at right angles to body. Pericardial and hepatic elevation on ventral surface. Umbilical cord begins to take form. Limb buds appear. Embryonic body cavity developing	Head much larger than trunk. Limb buds grow. Extremities become recognizable. Digital rays visible in hand plates. Hands and feet paddle-shaped. Face developing toward human form
Approximate length	2–3 mm CR	4–5 mm CR	11–14 mm CR
Approximate weight			
Cardiovascular system	Heart tubes form. Intraembryonic blood vessels appear. Blood vessels form in yolk sac. Primitive plasma and blood cells derived from yolk sac. Primitive circulatory system begins to function	Primitive heart is beating. Aortic arches formed. Hematopoiesis in yolk sac and chorion	Heart becomes 4-chambered. Hematopoiesis reaches maximum in yolk sac, decreases in chorion, and begins in liver. Formation of aorta and pulmonary arteries
Respiratory system		Laryngotracheal goove appears. Primary lung buds begin developing	Laryngotracheal tube separates from esophagus. Primary, secondary, and tertiary bronchi are formed
Body cavities		An embryonic body cavity is developing which extends from thoracic to pelvic region	Membranes form that separate the pleural, pericardial, and peritoneal cavities
Gastrointestinal system	Head fold encloses foregut. Tail fold encloses hindgut. Cloacal membrane is formed. Liver bud appears	Primitive mouth and tongue formed. Esophagus and stomach appear. Primitive gut develops. Midgut is connected to yolk sac. Liver develops rapidly and distends ventral body wall. Pancreatic bud appears. Gallbladder and bile ducts appear	Tongue and mouth continue development. Stomach modified in shape and position. Intestinal tract elongates and herniates into umbilical cord. Liver begins hematopoiesis. Pancreas becomes definitive. Parathyroid and thymus begin
Musculoskeletal system	Notochord is formed. First pair of somites forms	30–35 pairs of somites present. Arm and leg buds present. Vertebral column begins to form	Somite formation completed. Somites begin differentiation into three layers which will give rise to dermis of skin, muscles, vertebral column, and ribs
Nervous system	Primitive streak appears. Neural plate and groove form	Neural folds expand, close over, and fuse above the deepening neural groove, forming a neural canal. Three primary brain vesicles and spinal cord develop. Primary beginning of cranial nerves	Cerebrum and cerebellum appear. Most brain centers and fiber tracts begin to differentiate. Cranial nerves developing. Spinal nerves formed
Urinary system		A rudimentary, transitory, nonfunctional pronephros ("forekidney") develops. This is quickly followed by a mesonephros (midkidney) which may function for a short while. Urorectal septum beginning to form; it will later divide the cloaca into two parts	Permanent kidneys appear. More transitory nephrons develop, some with glomeruli. Urorectal septum advances and divides the cloaca into a urogenital sinus and a rectal sinus. Genital tubercle (same in male and female) develops

Table 5–2. Stages in the Development of the Embryro and Fetus (Cont.)

System	*3rd Week*	*4th Week*	*5th Week*
Specific organs	Thyroid begins to develop	Pharynx develops. Primordia of eye, ear, and nose are present. Inner ears beginning. Embryonic body cavity developing	Parathyroid glands and thymus appear. Thyroid and pharynx continue development. Adrenal cortex developing. Optic cups and primitive retina develop. Primitive nasal cavities appear. Primordia of spleen appears—weeks 5 and 6
Skin Teeth	A single layer of ectodermal cells covers embryo		Periderm develops
Reproductive system	Genetic sex is determined at fertilization. Primordial germ cells appear in the wall of the yolk sac	Primitive germ cells migrate to floor and walls of hindgut	Gonadal ridges form. Ovaries or testes are not distinguishable

System	*6th Week*	*7th and 8th Weeks*	*9th to 12th Weeks*
External appearance	Dorsal portion of body straightens. Head still large. Fingers and elbows established. Fingers webbed. Toe rays notched. Face develops rapidly. Upper lip forms. Eyes rotate forward. Nose develops a tip. Ear pinnas become well defined	Becomes recognizable as a human being. Head is almost as large as rest of the body. Eyelids appear and extend over the cornea. Large heart and liver bulge the ventral body. External nares become plugged. Ear pinnas form elevation. Form of jaws is clear. Sex not recognizable. Legs short, thighs small	Head still large but now only one half of body length. Face has a more human appearance, still broad with eyes widely separated and ears low set. Neck becomes well defined. Eyelids close and fuse. Upper limbs longer and bent at elbows. Fingers distinct. Legs short. External genitalia sex not distinguishable. Skin pink and very thin
Approximate length	14–16 mm CR	28–30 mm CR	8–9 cm CR
Approximate weight		2–3 gm	45 gm
Cardiovascular system	Basic form of heart established. Arterial and venous systems continue development. Vena cava takes form. Hematopoiesis mainly in liver. CV system now similar to adult type with exception of ductus venosus, patent foramen ovale, and ductus arteriosus	Liver is major site of hematopoiesis. Lymph vessels begin to form a continuous system. Primordia of lymph nodes appear	Heartbeat can be detected by electronic means. Hematopoiesis increases in liver. Lymphocytes appear in lymph nodes. Pulmonary lymphatics appear
Respiratory system	Several lung bud divisions present	Nasal passageways form. General structure of system becomes established. Basic structure of larynx complete. Bronchi continue to divide. Lining epithelium does not yet have cilia or glands. Nostrils closed by epithelial plugs	Nasal mucosa develops glands and cilia. Larynx develops cilia. Lungs have acquired definitive shape. Bronchi and bronchioles continuing to form
Body cavities	Membranes continue to form which separate the pleural, pericardial, and peritoneal cavities	Paired canals, communications between the pericardial and peritoneal cavities, now close.	The diaphragm is developing and "moving" into its final position.
Gastrointestinal system	Lips defined. Muscle of tongue differentiated. Salivary glands appear. Division of nasal and oral cavities	Salivary glands differentiate. Segments of gut grossly identifiable. Rectum takes form. No	Taste buds appear on tongue. Palate fuses. Herniated midgut loop returns to abdominal cavity

(Continued)

Table 5-2. Stages in the Development of the Embryro and Fetus (Cont.)

System	*6th Week*	*7th and 8th Weeks*	*9th to 12th Weeks*
	continues. Rotation of intestinal tract continues. Intestinal villi appear. Liver grows rapidly and becomes the major site of hematopoiesis	glands in mucosa of gut. Midgut loop still herniated. Gallbladder and bile duct patent; no bile formed. Pancreatic enzymes and insulin not yet produced. Anal canal closed to exterior by an anal membrane	from the umbilical cord in week 10. Glands begin to develop in esophagus, stomach, duodenum, and jejunum. Anal membrane perforates in week 9, and anus becomes patent
Musculoskeletal system	Skull fairly well developed. Differentiation of almost all muscles is complete or nearly so. Cartilage centers appear in many of the bones. Fingers and elbows are established. Digital rays of feet develop	Continuing differentiation and growth of body muscles. Perineal muscles and special eye muscles appear. Development of ossification centers in bones. Marrow begins to form in the humerus	Differentiation of facial muscles takes place. Ossification centers continue to develop in bones. Bone marrow begins to form in bones other than humerus. Bone marrow becomes an important site of hematopoiesis. Some movement is possible by the end of this period
Nervous system	Simple reflex pathways established. Tactile stimulation can evoke a generalized muscular response. Cranial nerves continue development. General pattern of the autonomic system is established	Cerebral hemispheres develop. Spinal cord extends the length of the spine. General pattern of sympathetic nervous system well established and beginning to function	Cerebral cortex still relatively primitive, but development will now proceed rapidly. New nerve cells forming
Urinary system	Subdivisions of renal pelves becoming established. Division of cloaca complete	Prior temporary kidney tubules (the midkidney) degenerate. New generations of nephrons appear. Urogenital membrane is perforated. Metanephros begins function. Bladder and urethra separate from rectum	Early temporary nephritic tubules continue to degenerate. Development of permanent tubule is underway. Permanent kidneys are present with pelves, calyce collecting tubules, and ureters well defined. Urine is being formed by the kidneys
Specific organs	Pharynx, thyroid, and thymus quite well developed. Eyes, ears, and nose develop more distinct structures such as retina, semicircular canals	Primordia of tonsils appear. Eyelids grow over surface of eye. Lymphocytes seen in thymus. Optic and olfactory nerve fibers grow toward brain. Inner ear nearly reaches adult form	Thyroid begins to function. Hypothalamus producing several kinds of releasing hormones. Testosterone produced by 10 weeks
Skin Teeth	Epidermis begins to differentiate. Tooth development begins as dental laminae. Deciduous teeth begin as toothbuds	The surface ectodermal cells form a protective layer called periderm. Bud stage of deciduous teeth appears	Eyelids become sealed. Skin is pink and very thin. Collagenous and elastic tissue fibers develop in dermis. Nails begin development—fingernails earlier than toenails. Toothbuds for permanent teeth appear. Mammary glands and nipples appear
Reproductive system	Germ cells continue migration and reach the gonadal ridges where they will later become the sperm or ova in the sex glands. Bilateral müllerian ducts appear. Primordia of the external genitalia appear	Müllerian ducts fuse. External genital tubercle continues growth. External genitalia still undifferentiated. Gonads become recognizable as testes in the male; ovaries not identifiable until week 10	Müllerian ducts complete fusion in female and degenerate in male. Ovaries become identifiable—week 10. Primordia of uterus, tubes, and vagina appear in female. Primordia of prostate, bulbourethral glands, and penile urethra are formed in male. External genitalia may show sex characteristics by week 12

Table 5-2. (Cont.)

System	*13th to 16th Weeks*	*17th to 20th Weeks*	*21st to 24th Weeks*
External appearance	Head about one third of total body length. Head erect, eyes more frontal, eyelids fused, ears stand out from head, and ear pinna well developed. A characteristic chin develops. Body growth is rapid in this period. Extremities become proportional to each other and to trunk. Fingernails develop. Mammary glands and nipples appear. Sex definitely becomes identifiable. Scalp hair appears	Proportions of head, trunk, and extremities very near normal. Chin, eyes, ears, nose placed normally. Eyebrows and hair on head visible. Skin covered with lanugo hair and vernix caseosa	Skin deep pink to reddish color and wrinkled, covered with lanugo hair and with vernix caseosa. Blood in capillaries is visible beneath the skin. Body thin. Eyes still closed. Fetus is capable of crying
Approximate length	14 cm CR	18–19 cm CR	34 cm CH
Approximate weight	200 gm	450 gm	800 gm
Cardiovascular system	Blood formation begins in spleen	Fetal heart becomes audible with stethoscope at 18–20 weeks. Hematopoiesis: production by yolk sac insignificant, by liver and spleen at their maximum, bone marrow beginning	Hematopoiesis begins in sternum
Respiratory system	External nares become patent by week 16. Glands and cilia appear progressively in bronchi. Weak respiratory movements take place. Amniotic fluid begins to accumulate in respiratory tree by the end of this period	The sinuses begin to form. Bronchioles dividing into more and smaller canals. Pulmonary alveolar ducts developing. Lung tissue becomes very vascular	Vascularity of lung increasing. Respiratory movements fairly well developed. Bronchioles continuing to divide into more and smaller canals. Pulmonary alveolar ducts continue to develop. Surfactant production in lungs begins
Gastrointestinal system	Tongue becomes functional. Glands of mouth, esophagus, stomach, and duodenum continue development. Intestinal muscles established and peristalsis appears. General structure of colon established. Weak sucking movements take in amniotic fluid. Meconium beginning to collect in intestines. Bile secretion begins. Islets of Langerhans differentiate. Digestive enzymes appearing	Fetus actively sucks and swallows amniotic fluid. Stomach muscles begin to form. Active peristaltic movements take place in tract. Pancreas secretes insulin	Glands of stomach begin function. Pancreas produces proteolytic enzymes. Sucking reflex quite well developed. Fetus swallows large amounts of amniotic fluid
Musculoskeletal system	Skeletal muscles become active and functional and lead to active fetal movements. Tongue becomes functional. Intestinal muscles established by week 14. Weak sucking and respiratory movements take in amniotic fluid. Primary ossification centers are present in all long bones at beginning of this period. Skeleton will show on x-ray film at week 14	Muscular activity increases progressively. Mother begins to feel fetal movements. More and more ossification centers appear. Calcification of teeth begins. Toenails developing	Movements stronger. Capable of crying
Nervous system	New nerve cells continue to form. Cerebellum, hypophysis, and spinal cord continue development. Sucking and swallowing and grasp reflex appearing. 10–18 weeks is major period of new nerve cell formation	CNS myelination begins. Myelination of spinal cord begins. Grasp reflex is good but not strong	Rapid brain growth begins now and continues to 18 months postnatal. Layers of cerebral cortex established. Rapid multiplication of fibrous network of supporting substance for nerves and cells of

(*Continued*)

Table 5–2. Stages in the Development of the Embryro and Fetus (Cont.)

System	*13th to 16th Weeks*	*17th to 20th Weeks*	*21st to 24th Weeks*
			brain. Myelination takes place. Synapses between branching nerve cells grow rapidly
Urinary system	Permanent nephritic tubules continue to differentiate	Permanent metanephros tubules continue to develop. Each collecting tubule undergoes repeated branching, forming more collecting tubules. Continuing secretion of urine voided into amniotic fluid	Renal pelves establish subdivisions
Specific organs	Retina continues development. Ear pinnas take adult form. Parathyroids show differentiation. Pituitary gland differentiates and is able to synthesize hormone. Suprarenal medulla begins function	Spleen begins production of erythrocytes. Pancreas begins to function	—
Skin Teeth	Epidermis well developed. Eyelashes and glands in eyelids appear. Hair papillae and sebaceous gland buds for scalp and body appear. Skin ridge patterns begin. Hair papillae for scalp and body appear	Lanugo hair covers entire body, vernix caseosa forms, hair on head and eyebrows visible. Sweat glands begin to develop. Melanocytes developing	Sebaceous gland secretions become chief constituent of vernix caseosa. Periderm begins to slough off
Reproductive system	Ovaries and testes descend in the body. Internal reproductive organs definitely show form and sex but major development is still necessary. External genitalia definitely show sex	Leydig cells appear in testes. Primary follicles appear in ovaries. External genitalia reach definitive form. Vaginal lumen develops	Active mitosis of oogonia

System	*25th to 28th Weeks*	*29th to 32nd Weeks*	*33rd to 36th Weeks*
External appearance	Skin pink and wrinkled but deposit of fat beneath the skin is now proceeding. Skin is well covered with vernix. Hair on head quite abundant. Eyes have reopened. Eyelashes present. Fetus is capable of surviving if born prematurely	Body still thin. Skin still appears old and wrinkled. Lanugo hair begins to disappear, especially from face. Subcutaneous fat deposition accelerated beginning at week 30. Fingernails reach fingertips. Toenails by week 30. Nipple buds visible	Body usually filled out fairly well by fat deposits. Lanugo hair disappearing—vernix caseosa present, especially in skin folds. Toenails reach tips of toes. Flat breast areola visible. Ears fairly firm—return slowly from folding. Skin pink and smooth
Approximate length	37 cm CH	42.5 cm CH	47 cm CH
Approximate weight	1100 gm	1600 gm	2600 gm
Cardiovascular system	—	Erythropoiesis ends in spleen. Bone marrow becomes major site	Erythropoiesis decreasing to low level in liver
Respiratory system	Beginning of terminal sac period. The capillary networks grows closer to the air sacs. Primitive alveoli or saccules form from the alveolar ducts. Pulmonary lining cells change into flat, thin cells, and blood and lymph capillaries are closer to lining. Lungs developed sufficiently to permit exchange of gas	—	Beginning surge of stable surfactant in lungs at week 34. The lining of the air sacs is becoming very thin and is showing further indentation. Abundant fetal pulmonary fluid present in potential air spaces

Table 5-2. (Cont.)

System	*25th to 28th Weeks*	*29th to 32nd Weeks*	*33rd to 36th Weeks*
Gastrointestinal system	Intestines contain an increased amount of meconium	The fetus can suck food if born prematurely, but may tire easily	Insulin production is well developed. Liver becomes proportionately smaller with decrease in hematopoiesis. Sucking and swallowing becoming coordinated
Musculoskeletal system	——	Fingernails reach fingertips	Toenails reach tips of toes. Cartilage developing in ear, but ear still returns slowly from folding
Nervous system	Capable of crying. CNS sufficiently matured to direct rhythmic breathing and to control body temperature. Sucking reflex weak but quite well developed	Reacts to auditory stimuli. Suck and swallow may be coordinated by week 32. Continuing development of reflexes. Moro reflex present	Rooting reflex good. Sucking reflex strong. Grasp reflex strong—may lift baby off bed. Sucking and swallowing reach better integration
Urinary system	——	Nephrons are continuing development	Glomerular filtration and tubular activity continue to improve
Specific organs	——	Fetus apparently hears sounds *in utero*	Responsive to different tastes
Skin Teeth	Eyes begin opening in this period and are open by week 28. Eyebrows and eyelashes present	Lanugo hair begins to disappear. Nipple buds visible. Skin appears thin and old and wrinkled	Lanugo hair almost gone, mainly present on shoulders and upper back. Moderate amount of silky hair on head. Plantar creases fine and indistinct at week 34 and show indentation on anterior one third of soles at week 36. Flat breast areola of 1–2 mm
Reproductive system	Beginning descent of testes through the inguinal canal	Active mitosis of oogonia continuing—none after birth	Labia majora widely separated. Scrotum small—few rugae. Testes make further descent in inguinal canal or into scrotal sac

System	*37th to 40th Weeks*
External appearance	Skin smooth, white or bluish pink in color. Body becomes plumper. Moderate to large amount of hair. Chest becomes prominent. Mammary gland begins to protrude in both sexes. Fingernails grow to beyond fingertips. External genitalia show further development
Approximate length	48–49 cm CH
Approximate weight	2950–3200 gm
Cardiovascular system	Almost all of blood formation takes place in the bone marrow
Respiratory system	Lung development and surfactant production sufficient to permit good function at birth. Bronchioles and alveoli still developing. Development of characteristic alveoli begins and continues until 8 years of age

(*Continued*)

Table 5–2. Stages in the Development of the Embryo and Fetus (Cont.)

System	*37th to 40th Weeks*
Gastrointestinal system	Development of hepatic enzymes is still somewhat immature
Musculoskeletal system	Bones of skull are firm and close together at suture lines. Fingernails extend beyond fingertips. Cartilage in ears thickening so that they become firm and erect. Growth and maturation of bone and deposit of calcium continue until adulthood. Skeletal muscles will continue maturation postnatally
Nervous system	Myelination and branching of nerve cells and synapses started earlier. Will continue into postnatal life. Cortical activity has begun. Many reflexes are well developed
Urinary system	Function of the kidneys is fairly adequate, but they will continue to develop postnatally both in structure and in function
Specific organs	Mammary glands may be enlarged and may secrete. Skin shows varying degrees of keratinization
Skin Teeth	Mammary glands protrude and have a raised areola of 4 mm or greater. Plantar creases become deeper and extend over most of foot by week 40. Fingers and toes have well-developed nails
Reproductive system	Labia majora develop so that they completely cover labia minora by weeks 38 to 40. Scrotum becomes fuller with many more rugae. Testes have descended into scrotum or are palpable in inguinal canal

form distinct surface elevations that can be counted and used to estimate the age of an embryo up until the end of the fourth week (Fig. 5–8).

Appearance of the pharyngeal (branchial) arches is a significant feature of the fourth week. By midweek, the first and second (the mandibular and the hyoid) branchial arches become visible. The third pair of branchial arches appears two days later, and the fourth pair is present by the end of the fourth week. These arches appear as distinct ridges on the future face and neck region of the embryo (Fig. 5–8).

Change in Body Form

The flattened, disc-shaped embryo of the third week changes into a C-shaped, tubular structure during the fourth week. This occurs because of rapid growth, which produces a tripling in size, and a process called *folding*. With rapid growth, especially of the neural tube, infolding in both the longitudinal and the transverse planes takes place. A folding ventrally in the longitudinal plane of both the cranial and the caudal regions of the embryo produces a head fold and a tail fold. This occurs as the brain grows cranially and overhangs ventrally, and the tail region projects over the cloacal membrane with dorsal and caudal growth of the neural tube.

Transverse folding of the embryo, which occurs simultaneously with longitudinal folding, produces right and left lateral body folds. With rolling of the edges of the embryonic disc ventrally, the transverse folding gives the embryo a rounded body form. Thus, at the beginning of the fourth week, the embryo was a flat disc. With infolding during the fourth week, the body becomes curved, and by the end of the week, the continuous longitudinal folding has produced an embryo with a C-shaped curve (Fig. 5–8).

Other notable changes during the fourth week are as follows: (1) in the folding process, a part of the yolk sac becomes incorporated into the embryo, and it gives rise to the primitive gut; (2) with the curving of the embryo, the heart produces a large ventral prominence; and (3) toward the end of the fourth week, the arm buds become recognizable as swellings along the embryo's trunk. Leg buds will appear two or three days later, early in the fifth week (Figs. 5–7 and 5–8).

By the end of the fourth week, the chorionic sac which surrounds the fetus is 20 mm or slightly larger in diameter, and it is large enough to begin bulging the uterine mucosa out into the uterine cavity. The sac has two walls, an outer wall, or chorion, covered with villi, and a smooth inner wall, the amnion, and it contains amniotic fluid which surrounds the embryo. The placenta has begun development, and the umbilical cord is taking form from the body stalk (Fig. 6–3). The embryo measures 4 to 5 mm (0.2 in.) from crown to rump.

The Fifth Week of Development

The fifth week of development mainly involves continuation of the organogenesis that took place on a broad scale in the fourth week. Those organs that started development in the fourth week continue rapid growth and differentiation. Also, several structures that have not yet made their appearance will do so in week five. Among these are the cerebrum, cerebellum, pulmonary bronchi, spleen, pancreas, cardiac septa, ureteric buds, gonadal ridges, and genital tubercle.

An important feature of week five is extensive head growth, brought about mainly by rapid brain growth. Growth of the head exceeds considerably growth of other regions of the embryo, and the head will be larger than the trunk by the end of the period.

In external appearance the embryo does not show the marked changes of earlier weeks, but there are some distinct differences visible. Obvious differences from the fourth week are the large relative head size, development of the primitive mouth cavity and other structures that will contribute to development of the face, and marked changes in the limbs. The extremities show considerable development in the fifth week, especially the arms. The elbow and wrist regions become identifiable, and digital ridges show where the fingers will develop. The legs will soon begin to show similar regional differentiation, but progress is later (Figs. 5–7 and 5–8).

Among other developments during the fifth week are changes in the cardiovascular system, which are marked by septation of the heart, and in the gastrointestinal system, where rotation of the stomach around its longitudinal axis takes place and the midgut begins to elongate and to herniate into the umbilical cord. This is a normal and necessary occurrence because there is not enough room for the growing gut in the abdomen. The liver and kidneys are taking considerable room at this time.

The length of the embryo by the end of the fifth week is from 11 to 14 mm, and the chorionic sac has a diameter of approximately 50 mm.

The Sixth Week of Development

The sixth week of development is marked mainly by growth and differentiation of the established organs and systems. Almost all body structures have begun their development previous to this time.

In external appearance the embryo's head is much larger relative to the trunk than previously, and the head is more bent over the heart prominence because of bending of the brain (the cervical flexure) in the cervical region. The face shows continued rather rapid growth and development. The eyes are rotating forward and seem more prominent; the external auditory meatus and pinna develop; the nose becomes elevated above the face and develops a tip; and the mandibular and maxillary processes grow and mold the face (Figs. 5–7 and 5–9).

The trunk has begun to straighten, and the somites are no longer visible toward the end of the week. The extremities are changing considerably, showing lengthening and flexing. Finger and toe development is visibly progressing.

The intestines have now entered the proximal end of the umbilical cord and have produced a herniation of the midgut, causing a large swelling in the umbilical cord. The intestines will return to the abdominal cavity during the tenth week. Communication between the primitive gut and the yolk sac has now been reduced to a small tube, namely, a small yolk stalk.

During the sixth week the cloaca is divided by a membrane into the urogenital area anteriorly and the rectum and upper anal canal posteriorly. Primary germ cells, which are migrating from the yolk sac, reach the genital ridges during the sixth week.

The Seventh and Eighth Weeks of Development

The embryo is showing many human characteristics by this time. The head is still large in comparison to the rest of the body, but it is more rounded and erect and the neck region is more distinctly noticeable. Facial features are more distinct. The upper limbs have lengthened and have bent at the elbows. The fingers and toes are well developed. The body is covered with a thin skin (Figs. 5–7 and 5–9).

The central nervous system is developing well and neuromuscular development is sufficient to permit occasional fetal movements. The abdomen protrudes less, but the intestine is still in the umbilical cord. The gonads

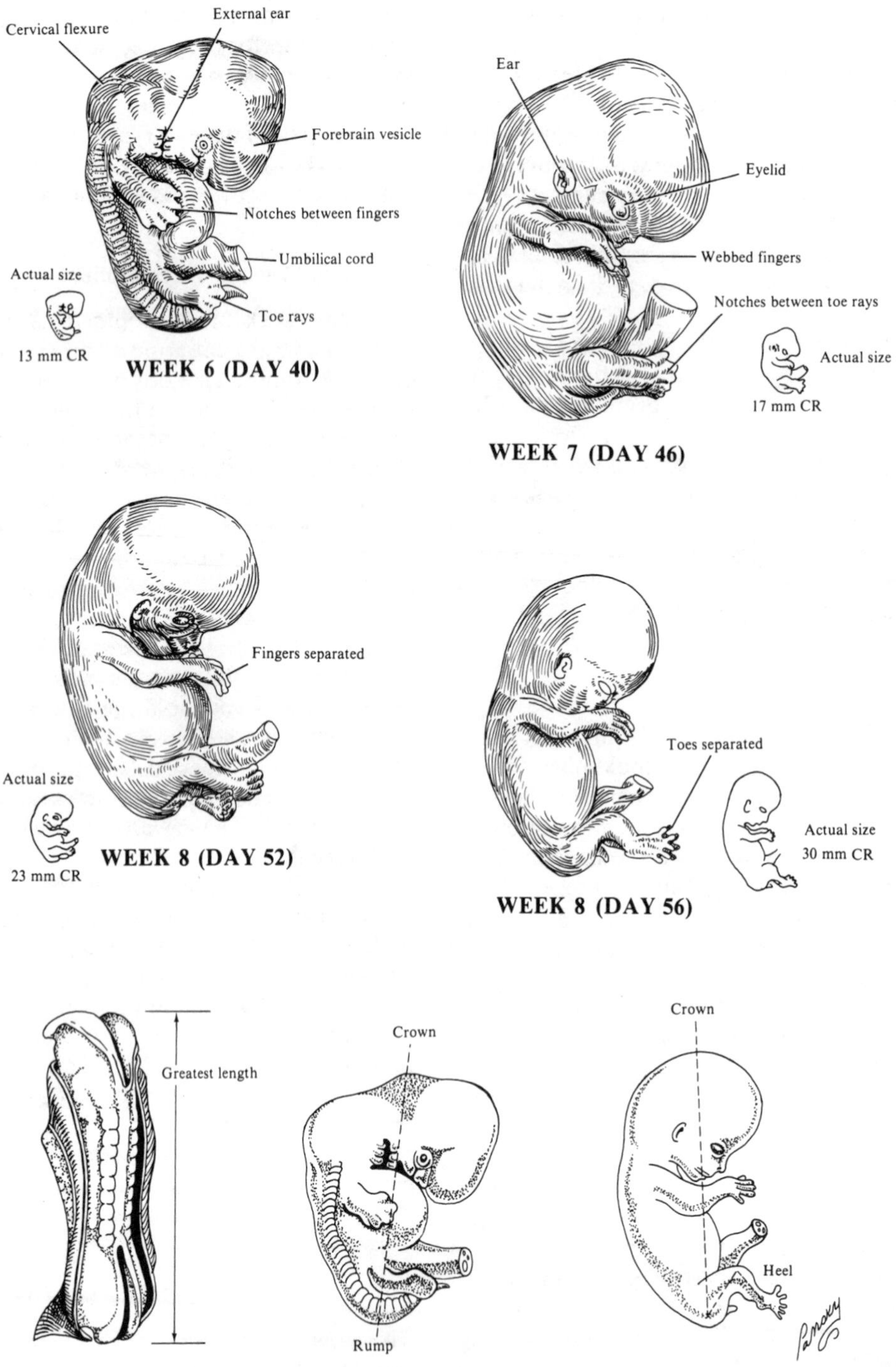

EMBRYONIC MEASUREMENTS

Figure 5-9. Diagrams of growth and development of embryos during weeks six, seven, and eight. Note the actual size of the embryos during this stage of development. (Reprinted with permission from Ben Pansky, *Review of Medical Embryology*. New York: Macmillan, 1982.)

begin to acquire sexual characteristics in this time period. If the embryo is under the influence of a Y chromosome, the indifferent gonads will begin development into testes during the seventh week. They become identifiable at this time. If there is no Y chromosome influence, the gonads will develop into ovaries, but they do not become identifiable until the tenth week. The external genitalia may have begun to differentiate at this time, but it is not yet possible to determine sex from their appearance.

All essential internal and external organs are present by the end of the eighth week of development, and the embryonic period generally is considered to end at this time. The embryo now weighs approximately 5 gm, and its crown-rump length is about 30 mm.

THE FETAL PERIOD

The fetal period usually is considered to begin with the ninth week; it ends with birth of the infant. By the ninth week, all essential structures have been established, and the embryo has developed into a recognizable human being. Development during the fetal period is primarily concerned with growth and maturation of the tissues that appeared in the embryonic period. Development does not proceed as rapidly as it did in the embryo. Some systems develop to the stage where they are already functioning quite efficiently before birth (example, cardiovascular system); others are ready to begin function soon or immediately after birth; still others must continue maturation after birth. The extent of maturation of the systems at the time of birth determines the ability of the fetus to survive if born prematurely. Much depends upon the extent of maturation of the respiratory system.

Nine to Twelve Weeks of Development (Third Lunar Month)

Growth in body length is accelerated during this period; total fetal length doubles from the ninth through the twelfth weeks. Growth of the head slows down considerably. The head constitutes about one-half of the total length of the fetus at the beginning of this period and only a little over one third by the end of the twelfth week. The head becomes more round, and the neck is well defined. The face becomes less broad; the eyes come closer together and the ears are less low set. The eyes have lids, which fuse during the ninth week and do not reopen until the sixth lunar month. Teeth are forming under the gums (Fig. 5–10).

The arms have almost reached their final relative length. The legs are still short and the thighs small at the ninth week, but they develop considerably in this period. Fingernails begin to appear in the tenth week. Centers of ossification are present in most of the bones, and bone marrow is beginning to form.

The lungs take definitive shape, although their development continues throughout intrauterine life and on into childhood. The kidneys begin urine secretion, but kidney development is still immature and will continue into childhood. The digestive system develops more completely. Nasal septum and palate fusion is completed. The intestinal coils that have been looped in the umbilical cord return to the abdominal cavity during the tenth week. The anal canal becomes patent when the membrane that has been covering the anus becomes perforated in the ninth week. Nucleated red blood cells predominate in the blood, and the liver becomes very active in blood formation.

The external genitalia begin to show more distinct sex differentiation by the end of the ninth week and show mature form by the end of the twelfth week. The ovaries become identifiable during the tenth week.

By the end of the twelfth week, the fetus weighs about

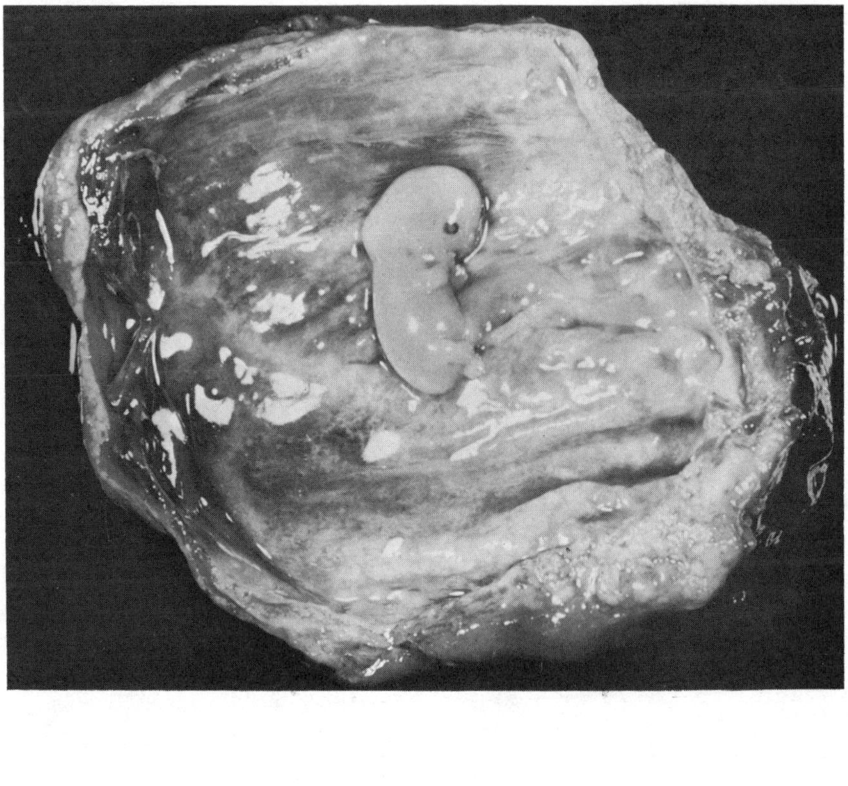

Figure 5–10. Embryo in amniotic sac. This photograph is of a spontaneous complete abortion at 10 weeks gestation. (Courtesy of Dr. Madeline J. Thornton.)

45 gm (1 1/2 oz) and measures from 8 to 9 cm (3 to 3.5 in.) from crown to rump.

Thirteen to Sixteen Weeks of Development (Fourth Lunar Month)

Growth is very rapid in the fourth lunar month as well as in the previous month. The size of the fetal head in relation to his body decreases with growth. By the sixteenth week, the head and body have become a more proportionate size. The legs have now become a normal length, and the extremities have become proportional to each other and to the trunk (Fig. 5–11). Scalp hair appears. Mammary glands and nipples begin to grow. Sex is definitely identifiable. Bones are ossifying well, and the skeleton will show on an x-ray film by the fourteenth week. The digestive system develops more completely. The fetus can swallow by the end of this period, and he begins to take in the amniotic fluid, which he will swallow in large amounts for the remainder of his intrauterine life. A tarry fecal material, called meconium, is beginning to collect in the intestines. Bile secretion is beginning.

The respiratory system is developing well. The external nares become patent. The fetus now begins to make weak respiratory-like movements.

Neuromuscular development increases rapidly during the fourth month. The fetus moves easily and becomes active, although his mother does not feel these movements because he is still very small and his movements are weak. The fetus responds to stimulation, and some of his reflexes, such as the grasp reflex, are developing.

By the end of this time period, the fetus is about 14 cm (6 in.) long and weighs about 200 gm (7 oz).

Seventeen to Twenty Weeks of Development (Fifth Lunar Month)

Growth slows somewhat at this time, but the fetus is becoming very active. Fetal movements are becoming stronger. It is usually sometime during the fifth lunar month, though occasionally earlier, that movements are first felt by the mother. This early detection of fetal movement by the mother is commonly referred to as *quickening,* or perception of life (Table 5–2).

It is during the fifth lunar month, usually between 18 and 20 weeks, that the fetal heartbeat can first be heard through a stethoscope placed against the mother's abdomen. Use of ultrasound equipment permits detection of heart movement much earlier, ordinarily by 10 weeks' gestation.

The fetus now actively sucks and swallows amniotic fluid. The kidneys continue to secrete urine, which is voided into the amniotic fluid. The bone marrow is now becoming the primary site of hematopoiesis, and the spleen is beginning production of erythrocytes.

Rapid brain growth begins in the fifth lunar month and continues into the postnatal period. Myelination of the spinal cord begins.

The fetal skin is less transparent. A downy hair, termed *lanugo,* covers the entire body. *Vernix caseosa,* a greasy, cheesy substance consisting of secretion of the sebaceous glands of the skin, makes its appearance. It covers the skin from now until birth. Eyebrows and hair on the head become visible.

By the twentieth week, the fetus is about 25 cm (10 in.) long from crown to heel and weighs about 450 gm (16 oz).

Twenty-one to Twenty-four Weeks of Development (Sixth Lunar Month)

By the end of the twenty-fourth week, the skin is markedly wrinkled, but there is a beginning deposit of fat beneath it, which produces a substantial weight gain. The body is better proportioned, but it is thin, and the head is still large compared with the rest of the body. Growth in the fetus proceeds more rapidly at the head end than the caudal end. Thus, the fetal head constitutes a large part of the body throughout embryonic and fetal development. The skin is varying shades of pink to red because blood is visible in the capillaries. The skin is covered with lanugo hair and vernix caseosa (Table 5–2).

The fetus now swallows large amounts of amniotic fluid. Movements have become stronger, and the infant is capable of crying by 24 weeks and possibly earlier. Respiratory movements have become fairly well developed. Surfactant production in the lungs is beginning toward the end of the sixth lunar month.

By the end of 24 weeks, the fetus is about 34 cm (13 in.) long and weighs about 800 gm (1 lb, 12 oz). If born at this time, it will attempt to survive, but often dies shortly after birth.

Twenty-five to Twenty-eight Weeks of Development (Seventh Lunar Month)

By the end of the twenty-eighth week, the fetus still appears thin and scrawny; the skin is reddish, is somewhat wrinkled, and is well covered with vernix caseosa and with lanugo hair; eyebrows and eyelashes are present; hair on head is usually quite abundant. The eyes, which has been closed since the third lunar month, now begin to unseal and are open by 28 weeks (Table 5–2).

The central nervous system is sufficiently matured to maintain rhythmic breathing and to control body temperature, if the body is not severely stressed. The infant is now capable of crying quite well. The sucking reflex, though weak, is quite well developed.

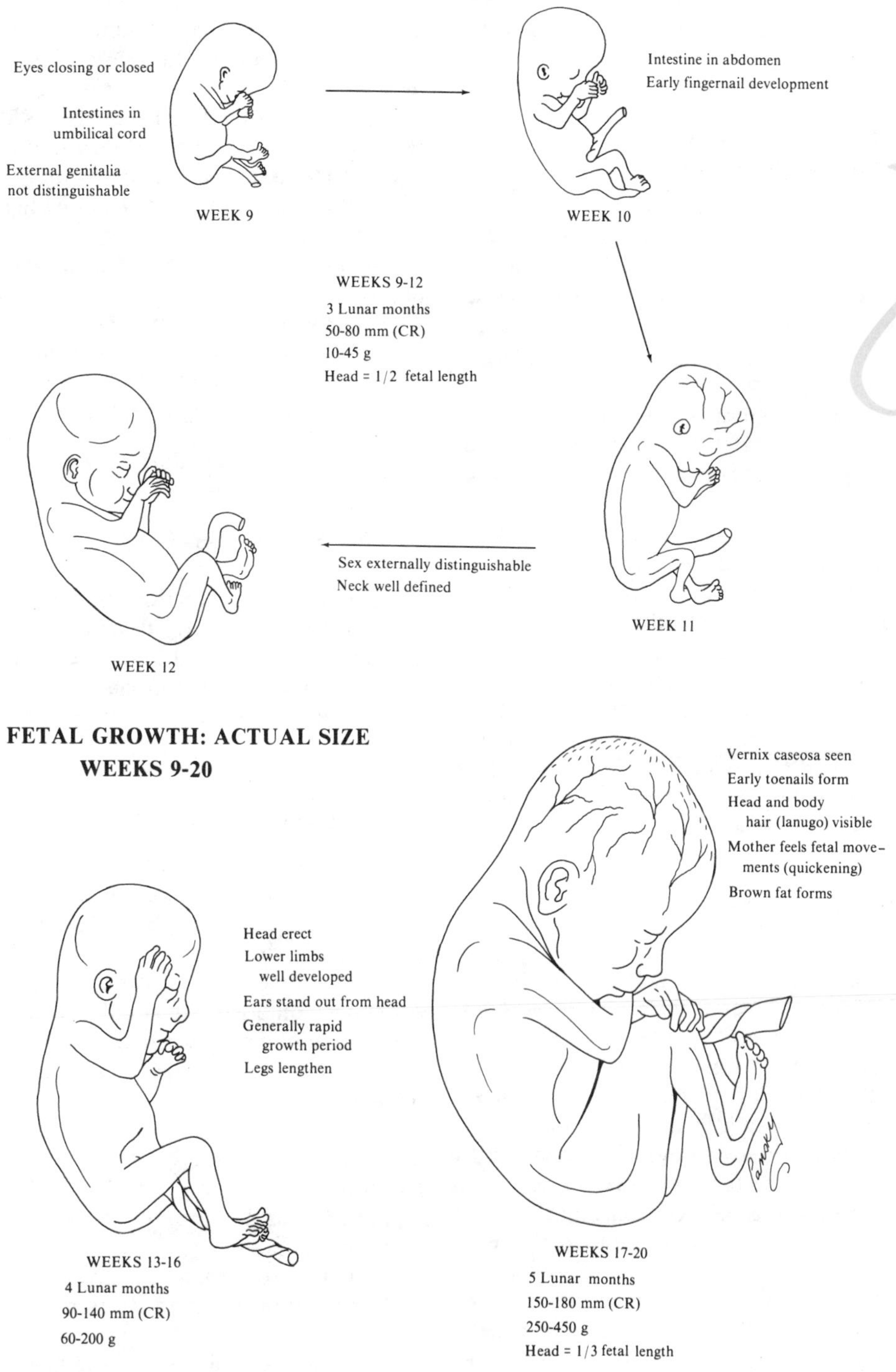

Figure 5-11. Diagram of growth and development of a fetus from the ninth through the twentieth week. (Reprinted with permission from Ben Pansky, *Review of Medical Embryology*. New York: Macmillan, 1982.)

The respiratory system is sufficiently developed to permit exchange of gases. Surfactant production may be sufficient to permit adequate lung expansion. However, if the fetus is born at this time, he may have severe respiratory distress and may not be able to maintain continuing respirations.

If the fetus is born at the end of seven lunar months, he may move well and cry quite vigorously, and his organs may be sufficiently developed to make his chances for survival not entirely unfavorable. An infant of this developmental stage, however, is very immature and extrauterine survival may not be possible.

niotic fluid is completely replaced about once every three hours.

The continual circulation of amniotic fluid may involve several possible sites for its removal. The amnion may actively remove the fluid, the fetal skin may absorb it, and absorption from the gastrointestinal tract may play a major role. The relative importance of any of these sites is not known.

Amniotic fluid consists of over 98 percent water and between 1 and 2 percent organic and inorganic solids. The composition of the fluid changes as pregnancy advances. In the first half of pregnancy the fluid is essentially the same composition as maternal plasma, but with a lower protein concentration. Later in the pregnancy the fluid becomes progressively hypotonic, presumably from the addition of very hypotonic fetal urine.

The amniotic fluid contains electrolytes, glucose, lipids, proteins, enzymes, hormones, and an increasing concentration of urea, uric acid, and creatinine as the end of pregnancy approaches. It also contains fetal urine and secretions from the respiratory tract. Variable amounts of particulate matter also accumulate in the amniotic fluid. There are desquamated fetal cells, sebaceous material, epithelial cells, lanugo and scalp hair, and vernix caseosa. The fluid is fairly clear except for the flecks of solid material cast off from the fetal skin.

The volume of amniotic fluid increases as pregnancy advances. The volume increases at a rate of about 25 ml per week from 11 to 15 weeks and at a rate of 50 ml per week from 15 to 28 weeks. There is an average volume of 50 ml at 12 weeks, 400 ml at midpregnancy, and a variable volume with a mean of 850 ml in the last trimester of pregnancy. Volume reaches a peak of about 1000 ml at 38 weeks and then begins to decrease somewhat. In the woman who progresses to a postterm pregnancy, the fluid may be well below the mean of 850 ml by 42 or 43 weeks' gestation.

An excessive amount of amniotic fluid, called polyhydramnios, or an unusually small amount of fluid, termed oligohydramnios, is sometimes present. These conditions may be associated with congenital anomalies in which the fetus cannot swallow fluid, or cannot produce urine, or in which the membranes produce excessive amounts of fluid, or various other conditions. Sometimes there is no apparent defect with polyhydramnios or oligohydramnios.

Amniotic fluid serves a variety of purposes, all of which appear to be directed mainly toward providing an optimal environment for the fetus during intrauterine development. The fetus begins to swallow amniotic fluid by the fourth month of development, and it has been calculated that by the time he reaches full term, he swallows as much as 500 ml per day. This may indicate that the fluid is important to fetal metabolism. The fluid helps to dispose of secretions from the kidneys and the respiratory tract. The fluid permits the fetus to move with ease in the uterus. It protects him against possible injury, by equalizing the pressure of any sudden force, and it keeps him at a uniform temperature. By acting as a water wedge, forced down by uterine contractions at the time of labor, the fluid may be important in dilating the cervix.

Since the amniotic fluid contains cells and secretions that originate with the fetus, analysis of the fluid gives valuable information concerning fetal health and maturity. When necessary for diagnosis, a sample of fluid can be withdrawn through a needle introduced into the amniotic cavity through the abdominal and uterine walls. Removal of fluid and the examinations that may be performed on it are described in Chapter 13.

THE PLACENTA

The placenta (afterbirth), vital to fetal life, is formed as a special organ to serve the fetus. It serves as lungs, intestinal tract, and kidneys for the fetus throughout intrauterine life, functioning as an organ for exchange of nutrients and waste products between mother and fetus. It also functions as an endocrine organ, producing hormones that will serve the fetus and that are necessary to maintenance of the pregnancy. The health, and sometimes survival, of the fetus is dependent on how efficiently the placenta functions throughout pregnancy.

The placenta's unique functional characteristics include such diverse activities as transport of oxygen and metabolites from mother to fetus, elimination of waste products from the fetus to the maternal circulation, and production of protein and steroid hormones for the needs of the fetus and the pregnancy.

Placental Growth

The amount of yolk accompanying the human ovum is very small, and the fetus is soon dependent on the mother for nutrition. The embryo receives nutritive material from the mother as soon as it reaches the uterine cavity. Even before implantation, the trophoblasts serve as a membrane through which nutritive material in the uterine cavity reaches the embryonic cells. This early supply comes from the secretion of the uterine glands, which are rich in glycogen. After implantation of the embryo, the products of the cells that were broken down by the erosive trophoblasts during entry of the blastocyst into the endometrium—blood, glandular secretion, and tissue fluids—surround the vesicle. These nutritive substances reach the embryonic cells by diffusion.

After the above two stages of nourishment, the placenta and its circulation begin to develop. Villi begin to form over the chorion during the second week of embryonic development, and they involve more and more of the endometrium (Figs. 6–2 and 6–3). These villi arise

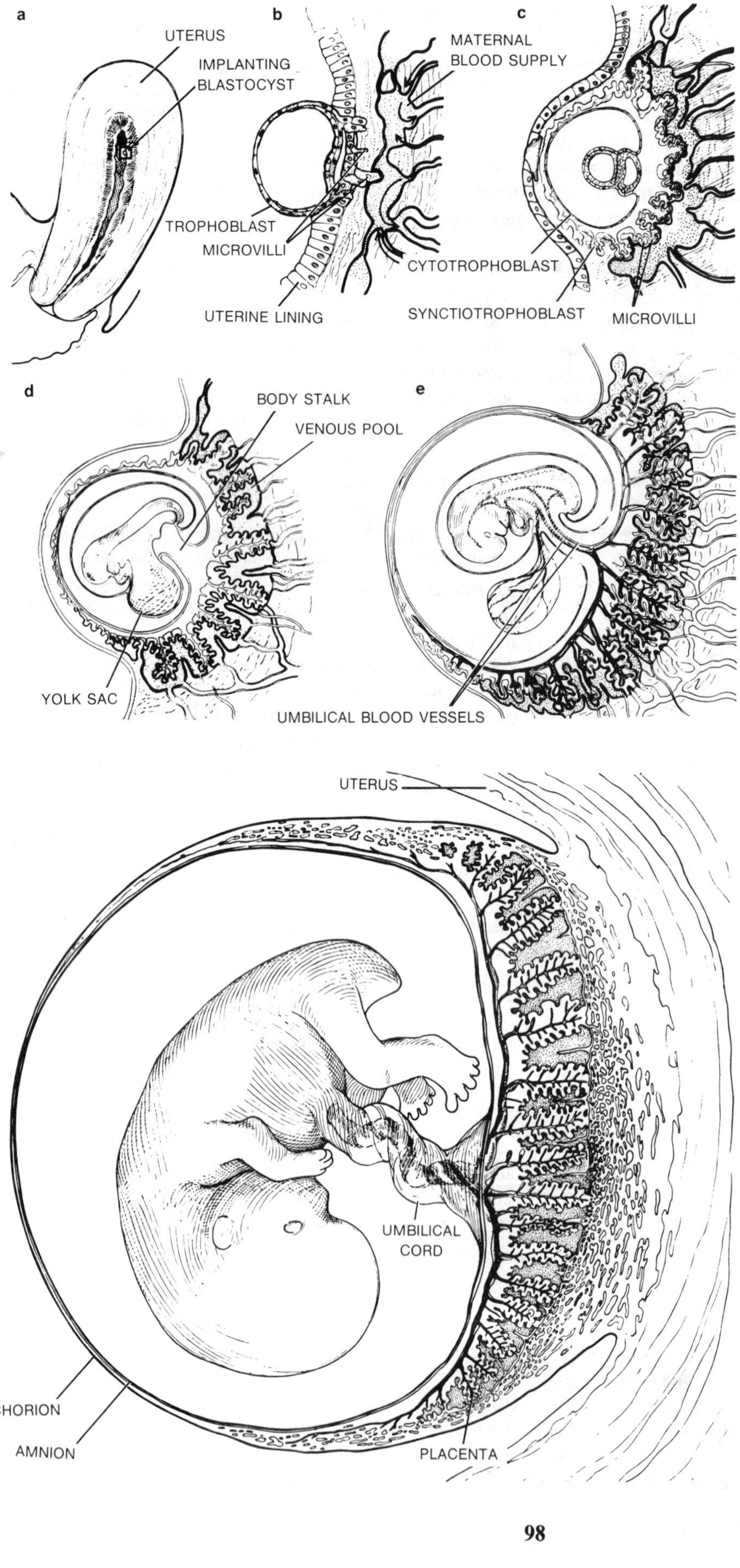

Figure 6–3. (a) Development of the human placenta is portrayed in the sequence of drawings on these two pages. The sequence starts with the implantation of the blastocyst in the wall of the uterus. (b) When the part of the blastocyst containing the inner cell mass first makes contact with the endometrium, or uterine lining, the trophoblast (the cell layer that will develop into the placenta) begins to form the small, fingerlike projections called microvilli, which extend into the endometrial lining. (c) As the invasion proceeds the trophoblast differentiates into two layers, the outer syncytiotrophoblast, which leads the advance into the endometrium, and the cytotrophoblast, which forms a complex system of projections that eventually push through the syncytiotrophoblast into the pools of maternal blood that collect in the path of the invading cells; before long the blastocyst becomes completely buried in the endometrial tissue. (d) During the invasion phase the trophoblast and the developing fetus continue to be connected by the body stalk, a structure that at a later stage of development will become the umbilical cord. (e) At about the fifth week of pregnancy the branched projections of the cytotrophoblast are penetrated by fetal blood vessels originating in the arteries in the umbilical cord. The cytotrophoblast spreads laterally during this period, finally joining other embryonic membranes to form the outermost shell known as the chorion; the final differentiation of the trophoblast to form the placenta gives rise to inner decidual membranes that actually enclose the amniotic fluid in which the fetus will grow. (Reproduced with permission from Peter Beaconfield; George Birdwood; and Rebecca Beaconfield, *The Placenta. Sci. Am.*, 243:94–102, (Aug.) 1980. Copyright August, 1980 by Scientific American, Inc. All rights reserved.)

from the trophoblasts. As the trophoblasts proliferate, they differentiate into two layers: an inner cellular layer of trophoblasts called the *cytotrophoblast* or *Langhans' layer* and an outer layer called the *syncytiotrophoblast,* which is a layer of protoplasm without cell margins (Fig. 6–3*c*). Isolated spaces, called lacunae, appear in the syncytiotrophoblast during the second week (Fig. 6–2). These lacunae soon become filled with (1) blood from opened-up maternal capillaries, and (2) secretions from eroded maternal glands. This fluid in the lacunae provides nourishment to the embryo.

Development of villi continues rapidly and an extensive network of lacunar spaces, filled with maternal blood from small vessels opened by trophoblastic cells, is soon formed (Fig. 6–3). An overall intervillous space is thus derived from the lacunae that began development in the second week. These spaces enlarge through further erosion by the trophoblasts. Together they form a large blood-filled sinus, known as the *intervillous space,* located between the chorionic plate and the decidua basalis. This space, which does not have clearly defined boundaries, connects the maternal arterial input with the venous outflow (Fig. 6–4). The space becomes more and more occupied with chorionic villi as pregnancy progresses until the space becomes more virtual than real.

Growth continues and maternal blood begins to flow through the intervillous space, entering from the arterial capillaries of the endometrium that have been opened by trophoblastic cells and returning through opened venous capillaries (Fig. 6–4). A maternal circulation, a rather primitive uteroplacental circulation, thus is established around the chorionic vesicle in a period of slightly over three weeks, and there is continual replacement of blood in the intervillous space.

Blood vessels appear in the villi very soon after they are formed. Blood vessels simultaneously begin to form in the yolk sac and the connecting stalk, and very soon blood vessels, heart tubes, and primitive plasma and blood cells develop in the embryo. Isolated vessels then fuse and form a network to establish a circulation between the embryo and the chorionic vesicle and the embryo and the yolk sac. By the end of the third week after fertilization, blood is flowing through vessels connecting the villi and the embryo. Thus, within less than one month, both a fetal and a maternal circulation have been established. Exchange of nutritive material and waste takes place between the maternal blood circulating in the intervillous space and the fetal blood circulating in the villi that dip into this space.

At the end of the first month of development the chorionic villi lying over the decidua basalis have developed into an early placenta. The placenta, developing at the site of implantation, is partly fetal and, to a smaller extent, maternal in origin. It arises jointly from the chorion frondosum and the underlying decidua basalis. The free villi of the chorion frondosum grow and branch, increasing the absorptive surface; the anchoring villi that serve to attach the chorionic vesicle to the decidua grow and multiply, and the decidua basalis increases in thickness.

As the placenta grows, enlarges, and takes on its characteristic shape, the roof is called the chorionic plate. This is the side of the placenta that faces the amniotic cavity. The major branches of the umbilical artery and the umbilical veins course through the chorionic plate. The floor of the placenta, which is the side next to the uterine wall, is called the basal plate. It is periodically indented by septa. The septa may not reach the area of the chorionic plate, so separation is not complete.

During the fourth and fifth months of development, the septum formation takes place in the placenta, dividing it into a number of compartments called

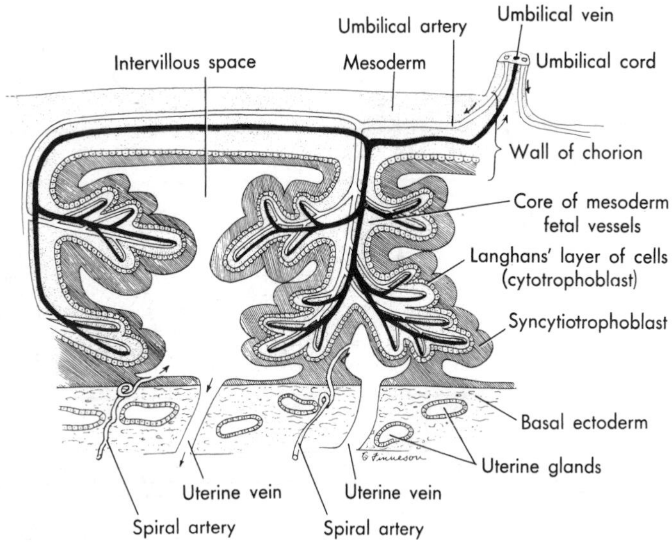

Figure 6–4. Schematic drawing of the structure of the villi in an early stage of development. The capillaries of the fetal circulation are separated from maternal blood in the intervillous spaces by surrounding layers of mesoderm, cytotrophoblast, and syncytiotrophoblast. After the fifth month only a single layer, the syncytiotrophoblast, lies between the fetal capillary wall and the maternal blood. Note the umbilical cord containing one umbilical vein and two arteries. Two uterine arteries and two veins are shown. (Reprinted with permission from Marjorie A. Miller, Anna B. Drakontides, and Lutie C. Leavell, *Kimber-Gray-Stockpole's Anatomy and Physiology,* 17th ed. New York: Macmillan, 1977.)

cotyledons. The septa separate the placenta into 15 to 30 units, or large cotyledons, which are further subdivided into smaller units. The septa develop when the decidua projects into the intervillous spaces. The projections of decidua do not reach as far as the chorionic plate, and separation of the cotyledons is therefore incomplete. Since the cotyledons are only partly divided from one another, contact between the intervillous spaces in the different cotyledons is not interrupted, and maternal blood can flow from one unit into the other.

As pregnancy advances, the placenta continues to enlarge. It covers nearly one third of the internal surface of the uterus at any stage of its development (Fig. 6–3*f*). Although the placenta is growing throughout pregnancy, its growth is not as rapid as that of the fetus. Before the fourth month of gestation, the placenta is heavier than the fetus; at the fourth month the weights of the placenta and the fetus are approximately equal; and at full term, the weight of the placenta is about one sixth to one seventh that of the fetus.

To meet the demands of the increasingly greater size of the fetus as compared to that of the placenta, the villi increase in size and complexity by branching in a treelike fashion beginning in the third week of development. With the villi internally supplied with a circulatory system that carries fetal blood and externally surrounded by maternal blood, the ever increasing branches of villi enlarge the surface area through which exchange can take place. Most of the bulk of the placenta is made up of the chorionic villi and the blood in the intervillous space. In addition to the expanding surface area of the villi, exchange is also increased as pregnancy advances by progressive thinning and permeability of the membranes making up the villi.

Placental Circulation

As implied above, the placenta contains both a fetal and a maternal circulation. Fetal blood flows to the placenta through two umbilical arteries, which branch and divide until they terminate in the innumerable chorionic villi dipping into the intervillous space. This blood returns to the fetus through a single umbilical vein (Fig. 6–4).

On the maternal side of the circulation, blood spurts into the intervillous space of the placenta from the spiral arteries and drains back into uterine veins (Fig. 6–4). Maternal arterial blood from the spiral arteries enters the intervillous space in "spurts" that are produced by the maternal arterial blood pressure. The entering blood is propelled into the intervillous space, which has a low pressure, in funnel-shaped streams, which are driven high up toward the chorionic plate (Fig. 6–5). As the head of pressure is reduced the blood disperses laterally. When this happens, blood flows around the chorionic villi, enhancing metabolic exchange through the capillaries of the villi. Continuing influx of arterial blood exerts pressure on that which is already in the intervillous space, pushing it out. The blood drains out through peripherally located endometrial veins, and from there into the uterine and pelvic veins (Fig. 6–5).

Each cotyledon (lobe) of the placenta is supplied by a spiral artery, which carries the maternal blood through the myometrium and the basal plate and then enters the intervillous space in a centrally located, relatively empty space in the cotyledon. This permits the jets of maternal blood to enter the middle of the cotyledon where there is a space that is relatively empty of villi. Among factors that influence flow of blood in the intervillous space are intermittent uterine contractions of the Braxton-Hicks

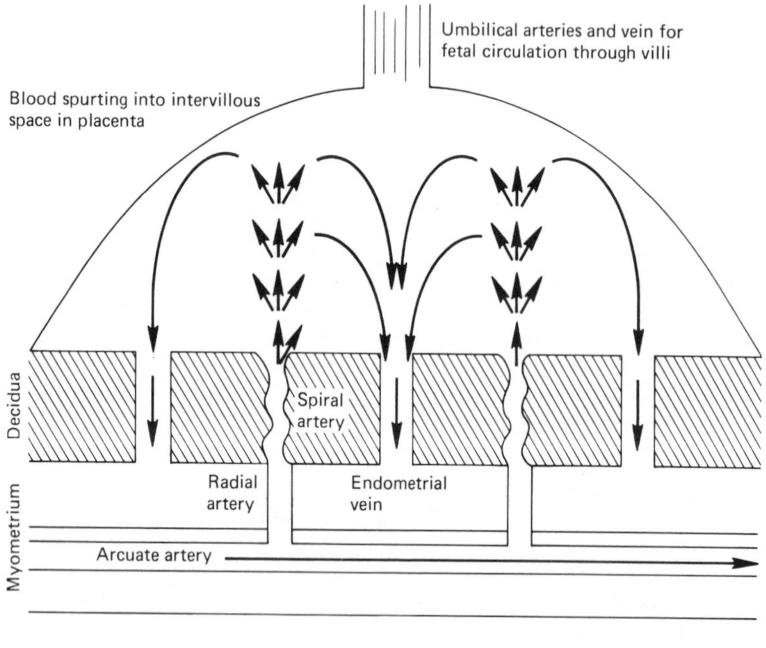

Figure 6–5. Diagrammatic representation of the maternal circulation in the placenta. Blood spurts into the intervillous space of the placenta from the spiral arteries and drains back into endometrial veins. Reference should be made to Figure 6–4 to visualize how the fetal circulation relates to the maternal circulation in the placenta.

quality (Chap. 9). These contractions temporarily compress veins, preventing drainage of blood. Then, when the uterine muscle relaxes, drainage of blood from the intervillous space takes place rapidly. Other factors are shown in Figure 6–6.

It is estimated that the intervillous space can hold about 150 ml of blood at any one time and that from 500 to 700 ml of maternal blood circulates through the placenta every minute, permitting a replacement of the blood in the intervillous space every two to three minutes. The fetal circulation through the placenta is estimated to be from 300 to 400 ml per minute.

The total absorbing surface of the villi of a full-term placenta is very large, with estimates of this surface as high as 10 square yards. Owing to a copious maternal circulation through the placenta, an extensive absorbing area, and a large volume of fetal blood flowing through the villi, the exchange of substances between the two bloodstreams is usually very efficient.

It is apparent that the maternal and fetal bloodstreams are in close relation, being separated by only the thin tissues that form the walls of the villi and the walls of the blood vessels within the villi. This arrangement makes it possible for the villi to discharge their function of receiving nourishment for the embryo from the maternal blood and releasing to the mother waste products from the fetal blood.

Transfer of Substances Across the Placenta

Transfer of substances from mother to fetus and from fetus to mother takes place through the chorionic villi. These villi, dipping into the intervillous space which is continuously filled with blood, can take from and give substances to the maternal blood according to the needs of the fetus (Fig. 6–4). From the time the first fetal blood vessels appear in the early floating villi, until the infant is born, when many complex villi make up the placenta, there is a constant exchange of nutriment and waste material between the maternal and fetal blood. The maternal blood in the intervillous space gives to the fetal blood in the villi the oxygen and other substances necessary to nourish and build the growing body. It receives the broken-down products of fetal metabolism. The waste is carried by the maternal bloodstream to the mother's lungs and kidneys for excretion. Adequate exchange across the placenta between maternal and fetal circulation is essential to normal growth and development of the fetus. The placenta is a very active organ. Its growth is ongoing, at least until near the end of pregnancy, and its function changes when necessary as pregnancy advances in order that it may adequately serve the fetus.

Three microscopic tissue layers separate the fetal and maternal circulation, and it is across this placental "membrane" that exchange takes place. The tissue layers of this membrane consist of (1) a first layer, the trophoblast which covers the villi and consists of a layer of cytotrophoblast and a layer of syncytiotrophoblast; (2) a second layer of connective tissue; and (3) a third layer composed of the endothelium of the fetal capillaries (Fig. 6–4). As maturation of the villi continues, the placental membrane becomes progressively thinner until finally only a very thin layer of tissue separates the maternal and fetal blood.

Transfer of substances across the biologic membrane in the placenta may take place by six different mechanisms: simple diffusion, facilitated diffusion, active transport, pinocytosis, bulk flow, and breaks in the placental villi. Different from other organs of the body,

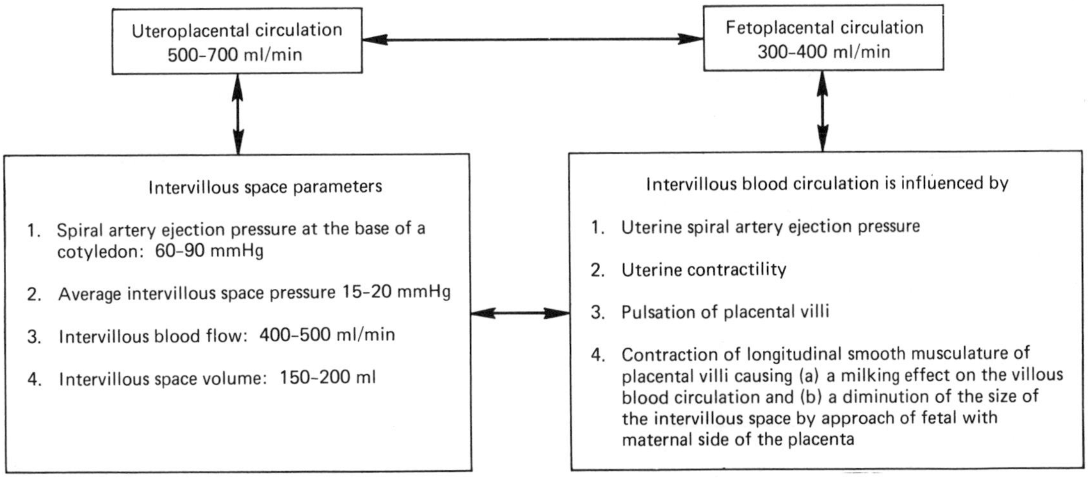

Figure 6–6. Parameters and interrelationships of uteroplacental circulation near term. The figures listed in this chart represent average values as derived from various reports in the literature; they serve only to give an idea of the uteroplacental and fetoplacental circulatory interrelationships near term. (Reproduced with permission from Nicholas S. Assali (ed.); Volume I in *Maternal Disorders. Pathophysiology of Gestation*. New York: Academic Press, 1972, p. 159.)

Table 7-1. Summary of Common Tests of Infertility

Factor	*Test*	*Expected Findings*	*Interventions if Abnormal*
Male	Semen analysis	Semen volume 1–4 ml Semen pH 7.2–7.8 Sperm concentration ≥ 20 million/ml Sperm motility > 50% Sperm morphology > 60% normal	Correct underlying cause if known (e.g., infection, obstruction) Clomiphene Artificial insemination
Female Cervical	Postcoital test (examination of cervical mucus 2 to 8 hours after intercourse)	Number of sperm present; 2–20/hpf Characteristics of mucus; 2 cm *spinnbarkheit* Sperm-mucus interaction	Clomiphene to increase sperm Estrogen if mucus deficient Partner or donor insemination
Tubal	Hysterosalpingogram	Tubal patency Contour of endometrial cavity	Surgical correction
	Laparoscopy	Tubal patency Visualization of pelvis including tubal walls, and tubal and fimbrial motility	Surgical correction
Ovulation	Basal body temperature (BBT)	Ovulation marked by increase in BBT of approximately 1° F (0.5° C)	Clomiphene
	Endometrial biopsy	Evidence of luteal (progesterone) simulation of the endometrium	Progesterone
	Serum progesterone	3 mg/ml suggests ovulation	Clomiphene
Uterine	Endometrial biopsy Hysterosalpingogram Pelvic examination	Evidence of luteal (progesterone) stimulation of the endometrium Rule out abnormalities of structure, myomas, and so on	Surgical correction

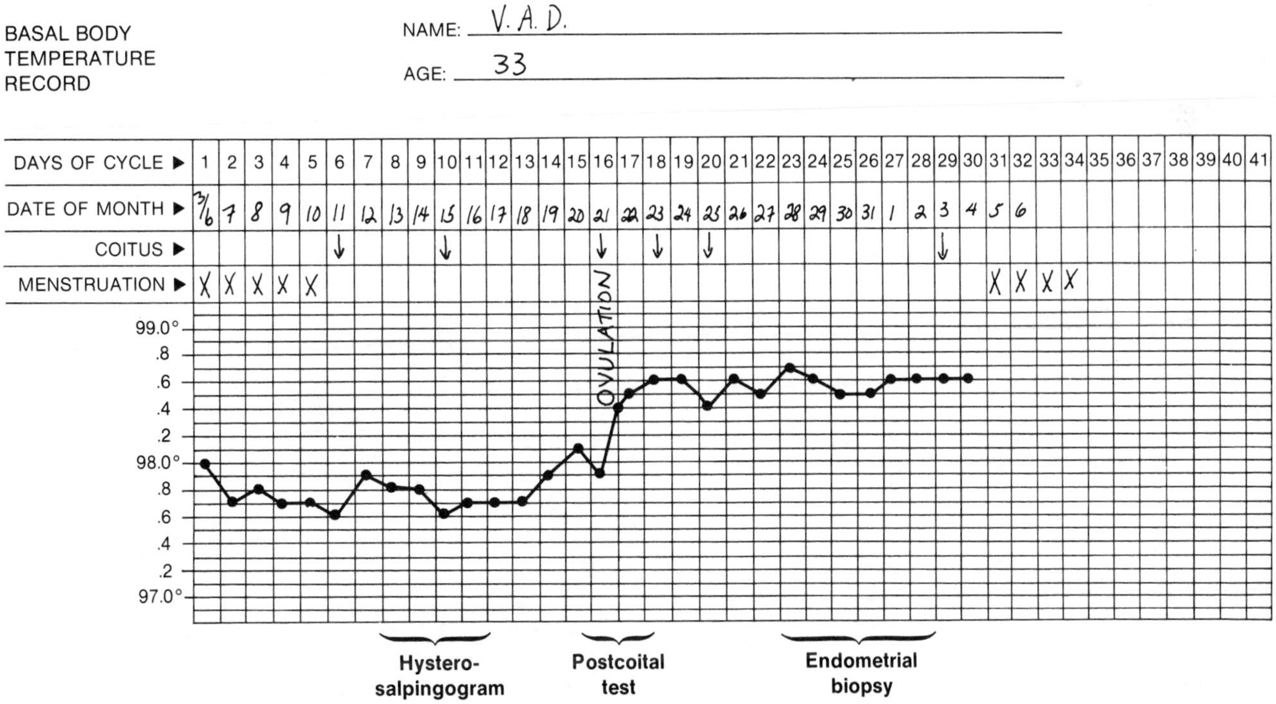

Figure 7-1. Timing of the more common infertility tests in relationship to the phases of the menstrual cycle. Shown here on a basal body temperature (BBT) graph.

refers more specifically to the temporary prevention of pregnancy and gives rise to the terminology of contraceptive methods which are used in order to accomplish this temporary prevention. The term *birth control* has been attributed to Margaret Sanger, a nurse, who in the 1910s began a historic fight for the right of families to limit their size, the right of women to health, and the right of children to the love they may expect through being wanted, planned-for children.

Before any individual or couple uses any method of contraception, two decisions must be made: first, a decision to use some form of family planning to prevent or postpone conception, and second, the choice of the method that is most acceptable and workable for the particular individuals concerned. Unless both of these decisions are made freely and with clear understanding of all the implications, the effectiveness of any method will be compromised. Health professionals, therefore, have the obligation to present information about all of the various methods in a manner that can be understood by each client. Attempts to influence the client's decision based on the nurse's or physician's own values are never appropriate.

Among the factors which are likely to influence the decision to use contraception are the following:

Sociocultural: Current trends in family size; effect of the size of the family in which the individuals grew up; stress of a society upon the importance of children; stress any particular society or culture places upon the importance of having a male child to perpetuate the family name; belief of a direct correlation between number of children and proof of virility.

Occupational-economic: The possibility of lengthy separation until the husband's military obligations have been met; economic resources being channeled into the couple's completion of schooling; priority placed on establishing a career; economic ability to provide prospective children with food, clothing, shelter, medical and dental care, and future education.

Religious: All major religious bodies endorse the basic concept of family planning.

Physical: General health of both partners but especially the woman; existence of genetic disorders in the family.

Marital-psychologic: Stability of the couple's relationship; beliefs about the effect of children on marital happiness.

Having arrived at the decision to utilize family planning, still other factors influence the selection of a particular method. In general, these factors reduce to the acceptability of the method to the individuals involved. Variables that contribute to the acceptability of a method include its cost, its effectiveness, and the ease of using it. Previous experience with a method as well as the extent to which it is used by friends or other members of the family also will have an impact. Women who are hesitant to touch their genitalia will not be likely to choose a method that requires such manipulation for its use. Those who object to "unnatural" drugs or devices will eliminate still other methods from their consideration. The frequency of sexual intercourse also may be a deciding factor. Someone who anticipates infrequent coitus may elect a more episodic means of conception control than those who have an ongoing sexual relationship. In some cases, religious affiliation may limit the acceptable ways of avoiding pregnancy. Publicity in the popular press concerning possible side effects and questions of safety may influence many decisions. Furthermore, there are medical contraindications for a number of methods that may preclude their consideration by certain couples. As an example, women with hypertension or a history of thromboembolic disease should not use oral contraceptives.

Because of the multiplicity of the variables involved in decision making, it should be clear that "selling" someone a particular method is likely to result in reduced effectiveness in the long run. Even though the professional may feel the client's objections to a method to be irrational, the decision must be made independently by the person who is going to use the method.

Effectiveness of a Contraceptive Method

Failure in a contraceptive method is usually caused by defects in the method itself, human error of the individuals using the method, or a combination of the two. Possible method defects will be noted in the discussion of the specific contraceptive methods. The dominating factor in human error is the strength of a couple's motivation to prevent a pregnancy. Motivation directly affects the degree of regularity with which the contraceptive is used. Without consistent use, any method will fail; irregular use of a method constitutes a major reason for contraceptive failure due to human error. Influences of human error, such as the couple's degree of acceptance of the procedure involved may be counterbalanced by their motivation. The other major reason for failure of a contraceptive method owing to human error is the improper handling of the technique involved. This may result from an inadequate knowledge of reproductive anatomy and physiology, inaccurate understanding of the method itself and how it works, or an inability to master the skills required by the technique.

Although frequently stated in terms of percentages, it is customary to calculate the clinical effectiveness (use effectiveness) of a contraceptive method according to the pregnancy rate per 100 years of exposure. This is done by means of a formula developed in the early 1930s by Raymond Pearl. After having one child, couples not using a contraceptive method average an approximate pregnancy rate of 80 per 100 years of exposure. The effectiveness of a contraceptive method is considered to be high if the pregnancy rate is below 10 per 100 years of exposure, moderate if between 10 and 20, and low if more than 20.

Contraceptive Methods

Since time immemorial people have tried to prevent conception. A wide variety of instruments have been used, ranging from potions, magic, tampons, and penal sheaths of various materials such as handkerchiefs and Saran wrap, to coins, collar buttons, stones, bottle caps, jewelry, carbonated beverages in a bottle released under pressure, or anything else a person thinks will prohibit the spermatozoa from reaching the ovum if it is inserted into the vagina or uterus. This can lead to tragic results such as mutilation or sterility due to infection. It is important to be aware that such dangerous nonmedical and futile attempts are still being made so that efforts may be directed toward finding and guiding such individuals to medical help.

Natural Family Planning

Natural family planning methods, sometimes referred to as *fertility awareness,* are based on the principle that women are fertile only on certain days during the menstrual cycle. These days, which surround the time of ovulation, are known as the *fertile period,* or the *unsafe period,* depending on whether the perspective is one of trying to conceive or trying to avoid conception. Intercourse during this period is quite likely to result in conception, whereas abstinence will prevent conception from occurring.

The obvious problem is determining the day of ovulation and so being able to define accurately the unsafe period. The various natural methods differ in the techniques used to identify this period. At this time, all methods leave something to guess work, although this is currently an active area of research.

THE CALENDAR RHYTHM METHOD The calendar rhythm method is the simplest of the fertility awareness techniques. The unsafe period is calculated mathematically using the length of previous menstrual cycles as a basis. Before initiating the calendar rhythm method, a woman should have an accurate record of 6 to 12 consecutive cycles. Based on the fact that ovulation is known to occur 12 to 16 days prior to the onset of menstruation, the fertile phase is calculated to extend from the eighteenth day before the end of the shortest cycle through the eleventh day before the end of the longest cycle. Thus, a woman whose previous 12 cycles had varied from 28 to 35 days would have a fertile period extending from day 10 through day 24 of each cycle (see Fig. 7–2). Abstinence from intercourse during this entire period would be necessary in order to prevent conception. Unfortunately, no woman has assurance that her cycle will remain the same, since it often will be sensitive to change in her routine, strong emotions, physical illness, and other factors.

THE BASAL BODY TEMPERATURE The basal body temperature method utilizes a temperature graph to indicate the time of ovulation and therefore the safe

SUNDAY	MONDAY	TUESDAY	WEDNESDAY	THURSDAY	FRIDAY	SATURDAY
				1	2 Menstruation begins	3
4	5	6	7	8	9	10
11	12 X	13 X	14 X	15 X	x 16 Estimated date of ovulation	17 X
18 X	19 X	20	21	22	23	24
25	26	27	28	29	30 Menstruation begins	31

Figure 7–2. The rhythm method for a 28-day menstrual cycle. The days marked X are considered "unsafe" days; days on which pregnancy may occur. The estimated day of ovulation is 14 days prior to the next menstrual period. In a 28-day cycle this would be day 14 of the menstrual cycle. Two days should be allowed on either side of day 14 for variations of the time of ovulation from month to month —days 12, 13, 15, and 16 are thus considered unsafe. If ovulation occurred on day 16, day 17 would be unsafe because of ovum survival. If ovulation occurred on day 12, days 10 and 11 would be unsafe because of sperm survival until day 12. In a 28-day menstrual cycle fertilization of an ovum is thus a possibility from day 10 through day 17.

period. The cycles of estrogen and progesterone are responsible for sequential changes in basal body temperature. During the follicular phase (first half of the menstrual cycle), the temperature is approximately one degree lower than during the luteal phase following ovulation. If a woman takes her temperature each morning before rising from bed and graphs it on a chart, the time of ovulation can be noted by observing the rise in basal temperature (Fig. 7-3). It must be recognized that temperature variations also may be the result of an illness, sleeplessness, alcohol ingestion, emotional upset, or other factors. Although basal body temperature does not permit prediction of ovulation, the rise in the reading does identify the safe, luteal period after ovulation. Abstinence should be continued until the temperature has remained elevated for three days. This method is often used in conjunction with the calendar rhythm method for a more precise estimation of the time of ovulation.

THE OVULATION METHOD The ovulation method is also known as the *Billings' method* after John and Lyn Billings, two Australian physicians who introduced the method into the United States. Dr. John Billings describes this method thoroughly in his book written for the lay person, *Natural Family Planning: The Ovulation Method.* This method depends upon cyclic changes in the consistency of cervical mucus. In response to rising estrogen levels, the mucus undergoes distinct changes at the time of ovulation. It increases in amount, making the vagina feel more moist and lubricated, and it becomes slippery and stretches without breaking (*spinnbarkheit*). The consistency is not unlike that of egg white. Following ovulation, progesterone causes the mucus to become thicker and to decrease in amount.

Billings recommends that this method be taught from woman to woman, and many communities have organized lay groups for this purpose. After using the method herself for a time, a woman is likely to be able to give practical suggestions and support to other women.

When starting to use this method, abstinence is necessary for the entire first cycle while the woman learns to distinguish the types of mucus. She observes the degree of wetness of the labia and vagina and tests the stretchability (*spinnbarkheit*) of the mucus by pulling it between two fingers. With practice, she will be able to predict ovulation from the characteristics of the mucus. After the first learning cycle, abstinence is necessary during the fertile phase of each cycle and every other day during the proliferative or follicular phase to enable the woman to detect the fertile mucus.

This method has an advantage over the two previously mentioned methods in that it allows prediction of ovulation and can be used by women with irregular cycles as well as by lactating and premenopausal women.

THE SYMPTOTHERMAL METHOD The symptothermal method utilizes a combination of all of the above techniques plus other symptoms of ovulation. This method emphasizes the joint responsibility of couples for observ-

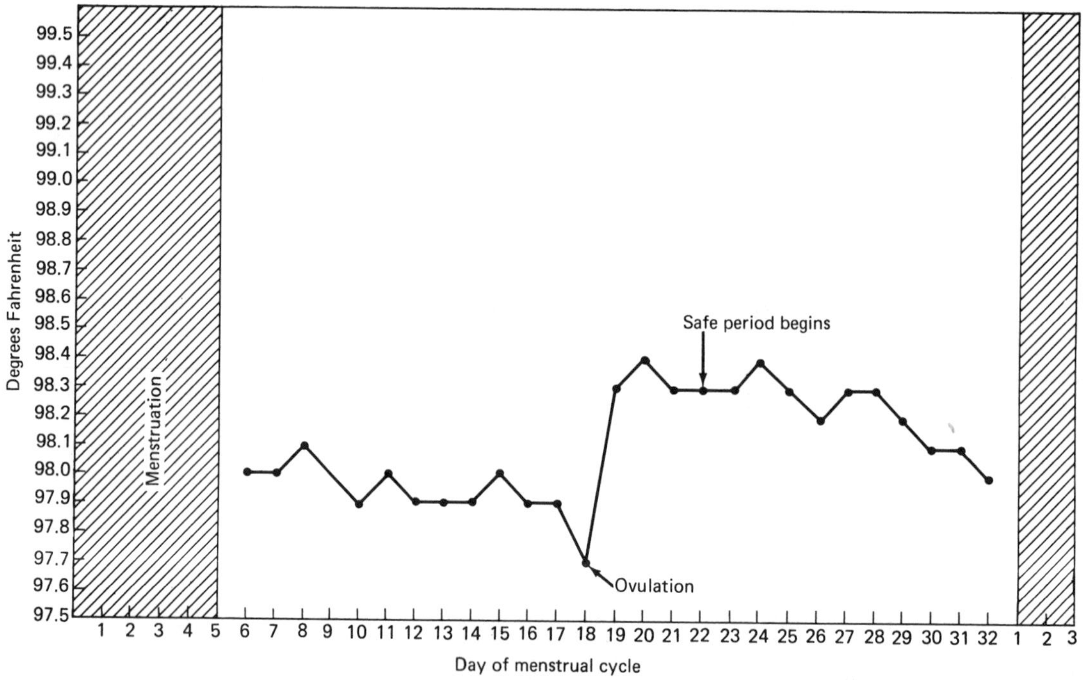

Figure 7-3. A graph of basal body temperature for a woman with a 32-day menstrual cycle. The ovum is considered to be degenerated after 72 hours of sustained temperature increase; thus the safe period begins on day 22 of this cycle.

ing and recording the pertinent symptoms and for interpreting the results. Practicing this method requires both partners to develop extraordinary sensitivity to the physiology of the woman's body. Taught from couple to couple, the instruction includes emphasis on communication and expression of affection by means other than intercourse.

In addition to the day of the cycle, temperature, and mucus, couples using this method observe changes in the dilation and consistency of the cervix and such secondary symptoms as *mittelschmerz,* abdominal bloating, vulvar swelling, increased libido, and spotting. A complete discussion of this method is contained in *The Art of Natural Family Planning* by John and Sheila Kippley.[2]

All the methods of natural family planning have the advantage of avoiding chemicals and foreign bodies and so may be the only acceptable alternative to total abstinence for some people. To the extent that they heighten the awareness of the woman's body and increase communication between partners, they also may enrich the relationships of those who practice natural family planning. Without a strong commitment to both the relationship and the prevention of conception, sexual fulfillment may be sought elsewhere and/or conception control will not be effective.

Mechanical Methods

The mechanical contraceptive methods are those that provide a mechanical barrier between the spermatozoa and ovum or between fertilization and implantation. The mechanical methods most often utilized in the United States are the condom, the diaphragm, and the intrauterine contraceptive devices. Another mechanical method, the cervical cap, is more frequently used in other countries. As the cervical cap is, in some respects, similar in concept to the diaphragm, it will be described briefly at the end of the segment pertaining to the diaphragm.

CONDOM The condom is a thin, elastic, and strong sheath of rubber or collagenous material which is unrolled down over the erect male penis. When the male ejaculates, the semen is caught in the condom, thereby preventing its being deposited in the vagina.

Three techniques in using the condom will enhance its efficacy:

1. The condom must be in place before the male penis approaches the female genitalia because of the possibility of spermatozoa being in male urethral coital secretions.
2. When using a plain-ended condom, an overlap allowance of one-fourth to one-half inch should be made for collection of the semen, thereby decreasing the possibility of the condom breaking at the time of ejaculation.
3. As the penis becomes flaccid following ejaculation, it is important that the male withdraw from the vagina immediately following ejaculation while securely holding the edge of the condom so that there is no leakage of semen out the open end of the condom and to prevent the condom from slipping off into the vagina while withdrawing.

If correctly used, the only other reason for possible failure would be due to defects in the condom itself. Defects include weakness of material, causing the condom to break from the force of ejaculation, or minute (pinpoint) holes in the condom that would render it ineffective. Condoms made in the United States are under the supervision and quality control of the Food and Drug Administration of the federal government and are unlikely to have imperfections. It is possible to test a condom by overdistending it with water or air and checking for leakage. However, having done this, there is the possibility that such stretching may have weakened the condom for actual use. Although it is possible to reuse a condom if given proper care, a precaution against breakage during sexual intercourse would be to use a condom only once and throw it away.

There is some discrepancy in the literature as to the effectiveness rate of the condom, with pregnancy rates from 5 to 15 per 100 years of exposure being stated. This discrepancy may be due to variations in the population samples and whether or not the sample included irregular as well as regular users of the condom method of contraception. It might be safe to say that the effectiveness rate of the condom is in the low 90s percentile but probably increases in effectiveness to the mid-90s percentile when correctly used, used in conjunction with a spermicidal preparation such as the contraceptive jellies, creams, or foams, and used consistently with each sexual intercourse.

Condoms, sometimes known as "rubbers," "safes," "sheaths," or "prophylactics," are readily available without prescription and may be purchased dry or lubricated. The cost varies with the make but generally is not exorbitant.

Side effects are limited to possible perineal and vaginal irritation if the condom is not lubricated and there are insufficient female coital secretions or if there is a reaction to the lubricant on the condom. In either situation, contraceptive foam, cream, or jelly, which should be used anyway, is a good substitute. Although the condom is a most widely used method of contraception (either totally, sporadically, or in conjunction with another method such as the spermicidal preparations), many couples do have negative feelings toward it. Some

[2] Kippley, John, and Kippley Sheila, *The Art of Natural Family Planning*. Harper & Row, New York, 1974.

feel the condom dulls sensation, others object to a possible interruption of sexual foreplay to put the condom on, and still others feel that it creates a barrier between them at a time when they desire the feeling of "oneness" which can be attained during sexual intercourse. An additional problem is that the condom has often been associated with prostitutes and disease prevention. Thus, a husband may feel negative and/or a wife feel insulted unless they are reeducated for a change in mental associations and attitudes.

DIAPHRAGM The dome-shaped diaphragm is made of somewhat thicker rubber than the condom and has a flexible metal spring encased in the rubber rim. This allows the diaphragm to be compressed for ease in insertion and yet retain its shape and provide a snug fit against the vaginal tissues when in place and no longer compressed. The concept is that when the diaphragm is properly positioned with the dome side down, the cervix is covered by the diaphragm, thereby preventing spermatozoa from gaining access to the cervical os.

The dome of the diaphragm is approximately an inch and a half deep in its apex. As each woman is individual in vaginal size and contour, the diameter of a diaphragm may vary from 5 1/2 to 10 cm. In addition, there are three types of diaphragms which differ only in the construction of the metal spring. The type of diaphragm to be used depends upon normal or unusual vaginal size or contour and normal or mild displacements of the uterus or adjacent structures. Owing to difficulty or impossibility in fitting, a diaphragm is medically contraindicated for women with severe anteflexion, retroversion, retroflexion, or prolapse of the uterus, or with severe rectocele or cystocele. It is, therefore, essential for the woman to seek medical help for a pelvic examination, evaluation of pelvic structures, determination of the proper size and type of diaphragm, and instructions in using a diaphragm.

The proper position of the diaphragm, which is inserted into the vagina either digitally or with the mechanical inserter, is as follows: posteriorly, the rim of the diaphragm fits behind the cervix into the posterior vaginal fornix; anteriorly, the rim of the diaphragm rests snugly against the soft tissues posterior to the symphysis pubis; and the entire circumference of the diaphragm rests against the vaginal walls. This, then, effectively covers the cervix. It is important that after the woman has inserted the diaphragm she check to make sure it is properly positioned. Proper positioning of a diaphragm is not possible if the diaphragm no longer fits owing to change in size, shape, or position of the pelvic structures. Therefore, a woman should be rechecked for fit and possible change in size or type of diaphragm a few weeks after initial sexual experience, after each childbearing experience, and in the event of any weight gain or loss in excess of 20 lb.

The application of a spermicidal jelly or cream to the diaphragm greatly enhances its effectiveness as a contraceptive method and provides a double protective method. The spermicidal preparation, which is made specifically for use with a diaphragm, is applied to the rim and either the inside or the outside of the diaphragm in such a way as to completely cover the area before insertion. As it takes about six hours for the spermicidal preparation and/or vaginal secretions to immobilize and kill all the spermatozoa, the diaphragm must be left in place for at least six hours following coitus. The woman may then, but not before, douche. One half of the douche is taken before removing the diaphragm and the other half may be taken after its removal if she so desires. If sexual intercourse is repeated within six to eight hours, the diaphragm is left in place and an applicator full of spermicidal preparation inserted.

It is also important that the woman receive instructions on how to remove the diaphragm. Removal is accomplished by the woman inserting her finger into her vagina, bearing down, grasping the upper edge of the diaphragm posterior to the symphysis pubis, and pulling it down and out. She should compress the sides of the diaphragm as it comes out. This is also done for insertion in order to reduce the diameter and make the insertion and removal procedures more comfortable. Pelvic models are most useful in teaching a woman how to insert and remove a diaphragm. This is followed by practice on herself under supervision after the size and type of her diaphragm are determined.

It is possible for a diaphragm to become dislodged during sexual intercourse. Such a possibility is a potential cause of failure and the inherent limitation of the diaphragm method of contraception. Other major reasons for failure of the diaphragm as a contraceptive method are improper positioning of the diaphragm and inconsistent use. The diaphragm should be periodically checked for wear, pinholes, and brittleness of the rubber. However, if properly cared for through washing, drying, and dusting with cornstarch following removal, a diaphragm should be usable for at least a year, depending on use.

The pregnancy rate for the diaphragm used in conjunction with a spermicidal preparation is approximately 3 per 100 years of exposure for consistent users. The pregnancy rate is much higher without the addition of the spermicidal preparation and in the event of poorly motivated, inconsistent use.

The cost of the diaphragm may be in addition to the medical help received and varies according to size up to approximately $14.00. The diaphragm usually comes in a kit containing the diaphragm, instruction pamphlet, mechanical inserter (optional in use of the method), and a tube of spermicidal jelly or cream. Periodic replenishing of the spermicidal preparation adds somewhat to the cost.

The diaphragm was for some time the "standard" contraceptive method. Of methods previously in common use, it had the lowest pregnancy rate for intelligent, highly motivated women. Some women find the techniques of the method too difficult to learn, since a good understanding of female reproductive anatomy is beneficial. Lack of acceptance of the diaphragm method of contraception is found in women who have a strong aversion to the self-intravaginal manipulation the method demands for insertion, checking position, and removal. Other women object to what they consider the nuisance of inserting the diaphragm, especially on a nightly basis as is frequently recommended for consistent conception protection. Although the diaphragm is usually not felt during sexual intercourse, some couples have the feeling of a barrier between them.

The *cervical cap,* while relatively unknown in the United States, is widely accepted and used in European countries. This discrepancy has been credited to its historical development and differences in cultural background relevant to mastering the technique of the method. The cervical cap is made of either rubber or a clear plastic, Lucite. The latter is known as the firm cervical cap and has the advantage over the rubber of being able to be worn for a number of days before removal.

The rounded, cone-shaped cervical cap fits over the cervix into the vaginal fornices. It stays in place due to a snug, but not tight, adherence to the vaginal fornices and a partial vacuum which is created between the dome of the cap and the cervix. The cervical cap is indicated in women who want a diaphragm-type of method, but, due to anatomic or functional reasons, cannot use a diaphragm. It is contraindicated for women with either an extremely long or short cervix, cervical erosions, nabothian cysts, deep cervical lacerations, or acute or subacute inflammatory conditions of the adnexae.

The pregnancy rate of the cervical cap is 7 to 8 per 100 years of exposure and is generally comparable to the effectiveness of the diaphragm combined with contraceptive jelly or cream method of contraception.

CONTRACEPTIVE SPONGE A product new to the United States in the autumn of 1983, the contraceptive sponge acts in three ways: it releases a spermicide; it serves as a barrier to sperm by blocking the cervical os; and it absorbs seminal fluid.

The round sponge is smaller and thicker than a diaphragm with an indentation on one side to fit over the cervix and a woven tape to facilitate removal hanging from the other side. One gram of nonoxynol-9 is incorporated into the sponge as a spermacide. After moistening with about two tablespoons of water it is inserted in a manner similar to the diaphragm. It is protective immediately upon insertion and for 24 hours following regardless of the frequency of intercourse.

This method of contraception appears to be somewhat less effective than the diaphragm; however, the convenience of being able to purchase it over-the-counter will probably make it popular with many women. Currently the cost is approximately $1.00 per sponge.

INTRAUTERINE CONTRACEPTIVE DEVICES Intrauterine contraceptive devices, variously abbreviated as IUCD or IUD, are made of a variety of materials, but usually of an inert plastic or stainless steel. Some have the addition of a layer of copper on the surface, usually in the form of a winding of fine copper wire. The qualities of the material used must be such that the device is noninflammatory in the normal uteus, flexible for insertion and removal, and able to retain its "memory" to resume its shape when in position.

IUDs are produced in a variety of shapes. Those most commonly used in the United States at this time are Lippes Loop, Saf-T-Coil, and the Cu-7. The IUDs also vary as to whether or not the device has a cervical appendage. A cervical appendage to the device in the uterus may take the form of "ties," a string, or an extension of the device itself in order to facilitate removal and enable a woman to check periodically to ascertain if the IUD is still in place. (See Fig. 7–4.)

The mechanism of action of the IUD is not known, although several theories have been advanced. One theory holds that the presence of a foreign body increases both uterine and fallopian tube contractions, thus speeding the progress of the ovum through the tube. Even if fertilization should occur, the ovum reaches the uterus prematurely, the endometrium is unready, and implantation cannot occur. A second possibility is that the endometrium forms cytotoxins in response to the foreign body, and these substances either attack the blastocyst directly or somehow interfere with implantation. Still another theory holds that the IUD stimulates the production of a substance that diminishes the motility and fertility of the sperm. Perhaps some combination of these mechanisms or some as yet undefined mechanism is actually responsible. In any case, it seems certain that the larger the surface area of the device, the lower the failure rate. Some researchers believe this to be the reason for the success of those devices that utilize a winding of copper wire, although there is some evidence that copper ions exert a contraceptive effect of their own.

Insertion of an IUD is medically contraindicated in the presence of pregnancy or suspected pregnancy, acute or subacute pelvic inflammatory disease, acute cervicitis, myomas that distort the uterine cavity, suspected uterine carcinoma, unexplained abnormal uterine bleeding or heavy menstrual flow, and in a woman with a history of postpartal endometritis or an infected abortion within the preceding six weeks.

The insertion of an IUD is a medical procedure requiring sterile technique. The procedure is preceded by a

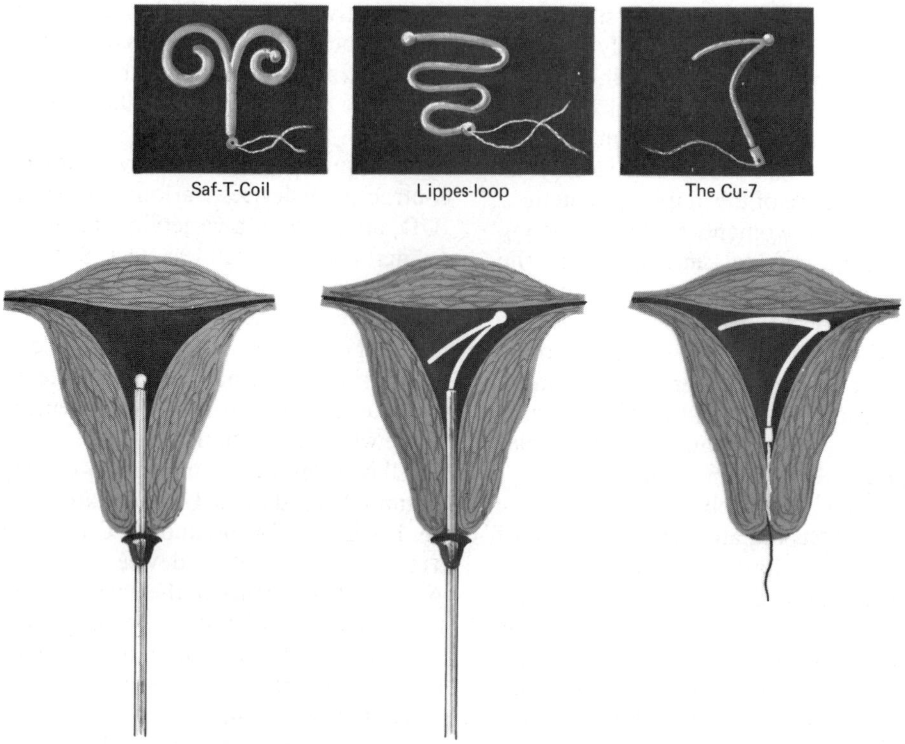

Figure 7–4. The three IUDs most commonly used in the United States are pictured above. Below is a schematic drawing of the insertion of a Copper 7. The IUD is pulled into the introducer forcing it into a straight line. After preparation of the patient, the uterus is sounded to minimize the risk of perforation. The introducer is then inserted just inside the internal cervical os. The IUD is extruded from the introducer tube into the uterine cavity where it resumes its original shape. The introducer is then withdrawn.

thorough pelvic examination, in part to determine the position of the uterus. A uterine probe is used to determine the direction and depth of the uterine cavity. The actual procedure for inserting an IUD will vary according to the device being inserted. Generally, a tenaculum or long Allis clamp will be used to grasp the cervix for the purpose of applying traction to straighten the cervicouterine canal. The woman may feel a short, sharp pain at this time. She also may feel a cramp when the uterine probe passes through the internal cervical os, another cramp when the inserter with the device passes through the internal cervical os, and, depending on the device used, another cramp when the IUD is positioned in the uterus.

Following insertion, women usually experience a varying amount of spotting or bleeding and cramps. Spotting may continue for a few days, and some women have a light intermenstrual bleeding during the first menstrual cycle postinsertion. Two or three longer and heavier menstrual periods are not uncommon postinsertion. The menstrual periods gradually may return to what a woman had before insertion or remain slightly more heavy. Cramps usually vary from being light and of brief duration in multiparas to being severe and lasting several days in nulligravidas who may require analgesics. Other side effects include the possibility of syncope, which most often occurs only in nulligravidas immediately postinsertion, and an unresolved question regarding the incidence of pelvic inflammatory disease with the IUDs. A general feeling among authorities at this time is that the incidence of pelvic inflammatory disease is essentially the same as that in the general population without an IUD, but necessary data are lacking for any definite conclusions. Perforation of the uterus is rare. There is no evidence for believing that the IUDs are carcinogenic, cause ectopic pregnancies, or increase the incidence of prematurity or malformations in the limited number of infants born of women with an IUD *in situ*. It is sometimes necessary for an IUD to be removed and a different size of the same device or a different device used. If this does not effectively alleviate the situation, a different contraceptive method is recommended. The usual reasons for removal are severe, unremitting cramps and heavy bleeding.

Research and statistics compiled in relation to the IUDs generally emphasize pregnancy rates, expulsion rates, removal rates for various reasons, and continuation rates. The pregnancy rate of the IUDs have varied from 1 to 5 per 100 years of exposure depending on the size and shape of the device. Unrecognized expulsion of an IUD, more common in the young nulligravida, contributes to failure of an IUD as a contraceptive method.

IUDs are, however, second only to the oral contraceptives ("pills") in effectiveness and have the advantage of not needing daily or monthly thought and supplies.

The cost of IUDs from the manufacturer varies according to the type of device. They usually come to the physician in a set including inserters. Added to this is the cost of a medical visit and a Papanicolaou smear.

Psychologically, again, some women who are adverse to inserting their finger into their vagina may object to checking themselves after each menstrual period if they have a device with a cervical appendage. The couple would need to resolve any moral or religious conflict for themselves. A very favorable psychologic reaction has been that the intrauterine contraceptive device method of conception protection is quite apart from the sexual act itself.

Spermicidal Preparations

The spermicidal preparations are those that contain a spermicidal ingredient that inactivates spermatozoa, combined with an inert base as the vehicle. The nonreactive base constitutes the bulk of such a preparation and also serves as a mechanical block to the cervical os. Most of the spermicidal preparations have an acid pH of 4.5, thereby ensuring a vaginal environment that is hostile to the mildly alkaline spermatozoa-containing semen. This is particularly important in the area of the external cervical os as the cervical secretions are slightly alkaline at the time of ovulation and therefore receptive to the spermatozoa.

These preparations are made, and are so designated, to be used alone, i.e., not in conjunction with a diaphragm. As a group they must exhibit certain common features: high ability to immobilize and kill spermatozoa, widespread vaginal distribution of the contraceptive method with the initial thrust of the penis, and the formation of a surface film that withstands coital activity. The spermicidal preparation is inserted near the cervix. Subsequent distribution over the cervix and throughout the vagina is accomplished through coital movements. Possible contraceptive failure due to inadequate distribution of the spermicidal preparation is inherent in the method.

Patient directions for all the spermicidal preparations, except the sponge and foam method, include the following imperative principles for effective use: reapplication of the method if sexual intercourse does not occur within one hour from the time of insertion, reapplication of the method before each sexual intercourse, reapplication of the method if the woman gets up, or walks around, or goes to the bathroom after insertion but before sexual intercourse, and no douching until at least six hours after sexual intercourse. Douching before six hours have elapsed may dilute or remove the spermicidal preparation before complete inactivation of the spermatozoa has occurred, thereby rendering the method ineffective.

The spermicidal preparations generally have higher failure rates than any of the mechanical methods, perhaps due to a less well-motivated group of patients as to routine use. On the other hand, women who lack motivation in attaining consistent use of the mechanical methods may be more regular in their use of a spermicidal preparation, thus affording greater conception protection for these women than would other methods. Spermicidal preparations are readily available in drug stores without prescription and are easy to use.

The cost of the spermicidal preparations varies according to type and brand, but generally it is not prohibitive.

The major complaint of couples using spermicidal preparations has been one of "messiness." This relates to both the type of product (with the exception of the vaginal foam tablet and the suppository) and postcoital leakage of all the spermicidal preparations to a greater or lesser degree. A reduction in postcoital leakage, owing to a smaller amount by weight, constitutes one of the advantages of the aerosol foam as a spermicidal preparation. At the other end of the spectrum, the sponge and foam method has considerable relative "messiness." The suppository is the least esthetic of all the spermicidal preparations since when adequately dissolved it drains freely over the perineum during coitus as well as postcoitally. If this is annoying to the woman, her sexual pleasure may be diminished. Postcoital drainage can be controlled by placing tissues or a clean towel between the legs against the perineum. This will absorb moisture and make the woman more comfortable. Some couples also have a negative feeling toward a certain amount of "clock watching."

In addition to the foregoing, each spermicidal preparation has features specific to it alone, as mentioned in the following enumeration of the methods.

JELLIES AND CREAMS The jellies and creams are tubed products which come in a kit containing an applicator and instructions. It is important that the instructions be followed so an adequate amount of the preparation is inserted to prevent dilution of the agent by the vaginal secretions. In order to deposit the spermicidal preparation near the cervix, it is recommended that the woman, who is lying down, insert the applicator in a down and backward direction the full length of the vagina and then withdraw it about 1/2 inch before pushing the plunger.

AEROSOL FOAM The aerosol foam is a variation of the cream spermicidal preparation in which the agent has been compressed into a container under pressure with a gas such as Freon. Foam is released when the applicator is pressed against the container, and the remainder of the procedure is the same as that for the jellies and creams.

VAGINAL FOAM TABLETS The vaginal foam tablet is a round, flat, white, 1-gm tablet that contains a spermicide, a bacteriostatic agent, and ingredients that produce a carbon dioxide foam when the tablet is moistened. While lying down, the woman moistens the tablet with a little water or saliva. She waits a moment to see or hear if it fizzes, then immediately inserts it into her vagina, pushing it as far as she can with her finger. If the tablet does not fizz when moistened, it should be discarded and another tablet used. An interval of five minutes must be allowed between insertion and sexual intercourse in order for the foaming action to occur which distributes foam throughout the vagina. Additional foaming action and dissolution of the tablet come at the time of ejaculation.

A complaint related to the vaginal foam tablet has been an irritative vaginal reaction and a "burning" sensation felt by both husband and wife during the foaming process. Women with an aversion to inserting their finger into their vagina may object to this method.

Although the vaginal foam tablet generally has been considered one of the least effective of the spermicidal methods, it is well accepted by poorly motivated, low socioeconomic, minimally educated groups because of the simplicity of technique involved. As such, it may be more effective for these women than other methods, owing to greater willingness to use it, thereby yielding increased regularity of conception protection.

SUPPOSITORIES It is extremely important that products advertised for "feminine hygiene" are not mistaken for the spermicidal suppositories used as a contraceptive method. The cone-shaped contraceptive suppositories contain a spermicidal ingredient incorporated into a cocoa-butter or glycerogelatin base. They have a melting point of slightly below body temperature which makes them a poor choice of method in areas with a combination of hot weather and lack of refrigeration. As the average melting time of the suppository at body heat is around 10 minutes, a suppository should be inserted into the vagina at least 15 minutes before coitus. This waiting period may be objectionable to some couples. The suppository is considered to be one of the least effective of the spermicidal preparations.

SPONGE AND FOAM The sponge and foam method of contraception involves a small water moistened sponge to which a spermicidal powder or liquid is applied. The sponge then is squeezed gently to form a foam and inserted into the vagina with as little loss of content as possible throughout the procedure.

There is an almost total reserve foaming power which allows for sexual intercourse to take place any time within six hours after insertion at which time foam is generated by the coital movements. If more than six hours elapse from the time of insertion to the time of sexual intercourse, the sponge is removed, and additional spermicidal powder or liquid is applied and reinserted. The sponge must not be removed until at least six hours after sexual intercourse. If later or repeated coitus is desired before this six hours have elapsed, a second, smaller sponge is inserted in front of the first sponge.

The sponge and foam method is one of the least effective of the spermicidal contraceptive methods. However, the method is simple and some women seem to gain confidence that an effective method is being used when they see the foam-filled sponge.

Oral Contraceptives

Basically, two types of oral contraceptive therapy are in widespread use: the combination and the sequential. Both types provide a regular cyclic menstruation and are thought to inhibit ovulation.

The combination type of oral contraceptive was the first type to be developed and derives its name from the fact that each pill consists of a combination of synthetic preparation of an estrogen and a progestogen. The main variations among the different formulations of the combined oral contraceptives are the dosages, relative proportion of the estrogenic and progestogenic components, and which estrogenic substance (ethinyl estradiol or mestranol) is used with which of the available progestogens. These variations result in a spectrum of pills with somewhat different minor side effects, which, in addition to the choice of the sequential type, allows for a certain amount of changing of the pill to best accommodate the individual woman's adjustment to the hormonal therapy.

The sequential type of oral contraceptive also derives its name from its formulation and administration. Sequential therapy consists of two different pills to be taken during the menstrual cycle. The first type of pill consists of an estrogenic substance only for three fourths of the pill-taking sequence. The pills taken for the remainder of the pill-taking sequence (usually five days) are a combination of the estrogen with a progestogen. The thinking underlying the development of the sequential oral contraceptive was twofold: (1) that the sequential administration of estrogen and a progestin more closely approximates the physiologic production of hormones by the ovaries, and (2) the later knowledge that estrogen alone could produce the antifertility action. The progestin is added to control the bleeding caused by the administration of estrogen alone and to produce a predictable withdrawal bleeding.

The mechanism of action of the oral contraceptives is not completely understood. It has long been known that suppression of the production of the pituitary gonadotropins (specifically, for contraception, the follicle-stimulating hormone and luteinizing hormone) can be effected by any of the sex hormones: progesterone, estrogen, and androgen. The administration of synthetic steroid preparations effectively inhibits the development of a graafian follicle and the subsequent event of ovulation, without which there is no ovum to be fertilized. However, the antifertility effect of steroids is not dependent on inhibition of ovulation. Other possible methods of action are under investigation and include hypotheses on the effect of hormonal contraception on ovarian responsiveness to gonadotropic stimulation, biogenesis and/or catabolism of ovarian hormones, factors within the fallopian tubes, spermatozoa capacitation, and endometrial changes.

The "menstruation" of a woman on oral contraceptives is actually a pseudomenstruation produced by the administration and then withdrawal of the hormonal substances and more appropriately termed "withdrawal bleeding." The characteristics of the withdrawal bleeding differ between the combination and sequential types of therapy owing to the different action each type has upon the endometrium. The combined estrogen-progestin oral contraceptives produce stromal edema, predeciduation, and some degree of glandular involution yielding in a few cycles a thin, hypoplastic-appearing endometrium. This accounts for the characteristic shorter duration and scantier flow noticed by women taking the combination contraceptive pills. In contrast, the sequential type of therapy yields an anovulatory pattern during the estrogen phase and an incomplete progestational endometrium transformation during the combined estrogen-progestin phase. Therefore, neither the predeciduation or thinning out of the endometrium occurs and a woman taking the sequential contraceptive pills will not notice as much change in her "menstruation."

As already mentioned, the minor side effects a woman may experience while taking the oral contraceptives depend on a combination of her individual biochemical and physiologic response to the formulation of her pills and the properties of the progestin being utilized. For example, the progestin norethindrone in one of the combination type of pills is androgenic in character. In contrast, the progestin norethynodrel in another one of the combination type of pills has estrogenic characteristics. Thus, for example, a woman inclined toward hirsutism might have an exacerbation of these tendencies on the former type of pills and would probably be more satisfied with the use of the latter type. The minor side effects experienced by women on oral contraceptives have often been compared to those of early pregnancy, e.g., nausea, fatigue, breast tenderness. Much of the literature on the minor side effects is based on the extensive research conducted with the first oral contraceptive: a 10-mg pill. Subsequent reduction of dosage has effected a responsive reduction in the incidence and severity of the minor side effects. Intermenstrual ("breakthrough") bleeding is not uncommon and usually can be controlled with dosage or pill prescription changes.

The continuing major issue in the utilization of the oral contraceptive methods is the question of their safety. Of particular concern is the possibility of existing relationships between the hormonal contraceptive formulations and thromboembolic phenomena; endocrine and metabolic effects, especially diabetes and liver function; cervical carcinoma; and heart disease. Oral contraceptives are generally contraindicated for women with a history of thromboembolic disease or hepatic disorders and premenopausal women who have a diagnosis of breast cancer. Diabetics, women with hypertension, and those over age 40 also should use some other form of contraception. The continuing research on the safety of the oral contraceptives is not minimized by the awareness that final evaluation of them as the most effective of all the contraceptive methods must be weighed carefully. The dangers of childbirth for an individual woman as well as the health and social benefits for families and society that can be accrued through widespread oral contraceptive programs must be considered.

The oral contraceptives are virtually 100 percent effective if taken as directed. A woman on the combination therapy is much less likely to become pregnant if she forgets one or even two pills than is the woman who forgets one pill on the sequential therapy. This probably accounts for the slightly higher pregnancy rates for the sequential in contrast to the combined oral contraceptives.

A woman is more apt to remember to take her pills if she puts them next to or on something which is part of her daily routine, e.g., toothbrush, alarm clock, coffee pot, dining table, and so forth. The drug companies also have devised innumerable aids for remembering to take the pills in the packaging of their products. These include calendar packs, dial packs, and punch packs which give the day or date of each pill that is to be taken. The original pills were to be taken for 20 days starting on day 5 of the menstrual cycle. The woman usually would start her withdrawal bleeding two or three days after the twentieth pill and start her pills again on day 5 after her period started. These are still the most common directions for the oral contraceptive pills. However, it has been recommended in working with women for whom such a system of counting might be confusing that the woman take her 20 pills, stop for her "menstruation," and start taking her next package of 20 pills on the same day a week later as the day she stopped taking pills. Some drug companies have incorporated this idea into their packaging of pills with 21 days of pills and seven days without: three weeks on and one week off. The woman then would be starting and stopping her pills on the same day throughout the months. This enables the woman to choose the days of the week on which menstruation will occur. For example, by starting the 21 pills on a Saturday she will never have her period on a weekend.

A more recent development is the packaging of 28 days of pills in which the last 7 pills are hormonal placebos. The idea behind the packages of 28 pills is that this enables the woman to get into the habit of taking a pill every day, thereby reducing the chance of her either forgetting her pill or being confused as to whether any particular day is a day during which she should take a pill.

The oral contraceptive pills vary slightly in amount of expense per month, depending on brand and dosage, but for many women cost is not prohibitive.

Psychologically, there has been a diverse reaction to the oral contraceptives. One is fear, owing to the large volume of publicity they have received, much of it based on the thus far unresolved questions of safety and subsequent rumor. The other reaction has been very favorable, based on the ease of using this contraceptive method, its being unrelated to the act of sexual intercourse, and its high effectiveness rate.

Folklore

The following are so-called contraceptive methods of long-standing reputation which because of a basic fallacy in concept and low efficacy might well be labeled as folklore.

DOUCHES Douching following sexual intercourse as a contraceptive method is one of the most prevalent erroneous ideas. The concept is that if a woman douches immediately following ejaculation, she will flush the semen out of the vagina before the spermatozoa can enter the uterus. However, the majority of spermatozoa are contained in the first few drops of the ejaculate and are into the cervical canal within 90 seconds following the usual depositing of the semen at the cervical os. Since it is highly unlikely that a woman could douche within this period of time, the entire concept is rendered invalid.

A pregnancy rate in excess of 30 per 100 years of exposure has been stated in various reports for couples using this method, which is better than no contraceptive method at all. However, such low efficacy scarcely can recommend the douche as a very reliable method of contraceptive.

COITUS INTERRUPTUS Coitus interruptus, more commonly known as withdrawal or "being safe," is based on the fact that the male can feel when he is about to ejaculate. The method relies on the male withdrawing his penis from the vagina at this moment and ejaculating outside of it, thereby preventing the spermatozoa from being in a location where they could conceivably reach a mature ovum. Such an action demands split-second timing and idealistic self-control by the male, who may not always be psychologically able to withdraw at the climax of sexual intercourse. In addition, if the male is a fraction of a second too late in withdrawing and the first drop or two of semen is deposited in the vagina or if he ejaculates on the external female genitalia, the method may be rendered invalid.

Coitus interruptus is a method that many couples have used at least occasionally and is recommended in the absence of a more reliable contraceptive method. Although some couples have been satisfied with coitus interruptus as a contraceptive method and have used it successfully, it has been noted for many family planning failures. There also has been some objection to coitus interruptus as limiting full sexual gratification.

BREAST-FEEDING Following delivery there is a period of six to eight weeks of amenorrhea which may be prolonged to as much as a year by breast-feeding. Because they are not menstruating, many women may believe that they cannot become pregnant. However, ovulation very frequently occurs prior to the reestablishment of menses. Therefore, although conception is less likely to occur while a woman is breast-feeding fully, this is not a totally reliable means of contraception.

FEMALE RESERVE Some people believe that a woman may not become pregnant unless she has an orgasm at the time of intercourse. This piece of folklore therefore advises the woman to hold back her orgasm and she will not conceive. This belief is totally untrue.

Sterilization

Surgical sterilization of both men and women is available as a means of permanent contraception. For couples where the wife is in the age range of 30 to 44, sterilization is the most common method of contraception (Presser and Bumpass, 1972).[3] The operations are approximately equally divided between men and women.

Male sterilization is effected by vasectomy—the severing of the vas deferens. This destroys the pathway of the sperm from the testicles to the urethra. The procedure may be done on an outpatient basis under local anesthetic. A small incision is made over each spermatic cord, and the vas is ligated and severed. A scrotal support is recommended for approximately one week. Since ten or more ejaculations are required to eliminate all sperm from the proximal tract, the couple should be advised to

[3] Presser, H. B. and Bumpass, L. L., The acceptability of contraceptive sterilization among U. S. couples: 1970, *Family Planning Perspectives*, 4(4): 18, 1972.

use some form of contraceptive until a negative sperm count is obtained.

This procedure has no physiologic effect on sexual potency; however, many men are reluctant to undergo sterilization because they feel it may somehow diminish their "manhood." Couples contemplating sterilization need information and, perhaps, counseling to assist in their decision-making.

The most common method of female sterilization is tubal ligation in which the fallopian tubes are ligated or severed (or both) so that the ovum is unavailable for fertilization. This procedure requires one to two days of hospitalization and, usually, a general anesthesia. Women often elect to have this procedure done during the first two days after giving birth since they are already in the hospital and need not worry about child care and other issues involved in a second hospitalization. There is a question as to whether or not this is an optimal time psychologically. The loss of the childbearing period of life nearly always evokes some degree of regret and grieving, regardless of how thoughtfully the decision was made. This, coupled with the physical discomforts of surgery, intrude upon the energy needed to continue attachment to a new infant and reintegration of a family.

Couples should clearly understand the permanent nature of both sterilization procedures. Although microsurgery techniques are successful in reuniting fallopian tubes, the pregnancy rate after such surgery is quite low—about 15 percent.

Future Methods

It is a well-recognized, noncontroversial fact that the ideal contraceptive method, combining the features of 100 percent effectiveness, 100 percent safety, no side effects, ease of use with no interference with sexual intercourse, and acceptability to all religions, has not yet been developed. Intensive research continues both in exploration of possible new methods, and in perfecting already existing methods, based on studies of the cause of side effects, possible relationships with disease (safety), and mechanisms of action.

Of vital importance is the development of a so-far elusive method of being able to accurately predict the time of ovulation at least four days prior to the event. Such a development would revolutionize the rhythm method and ease the current religious controversy.

The ongoing research with the intrauterine contraceptive devices yields modifications in existing devices relative to size and material used. New shapes are periodically introduced which, with modifications, are all geared toward ease of insertion and a decrease in expulsion rates, pregnancy rates, and bleeding. Still to be resolved is the question of the role of the transcervical appendage in the development of infection.

Research is being done in the area of ovulation-inhibiting methods or, more broadly, with steroid compounds that act as antifertility agents but not necessarily by means of inhibiting ovulation. One such hormonal contraceptive formulation is the "one-a-month pill," consisting of the combination of a long-acting estrogen and progestogen. Another is the long-acting injectable formulation. This is composed of a long-acting progestogen either alone or in conjunction with a long-acting estrogen. Investigations are being made of injections given every month, every three months, and every six months. Time-release pellets for intradermal implantation are also under investigation. The main difficulties with these formulations are their irreversibility, amenorrhea, and irregular uterine bleeding. A supplement of a short cycle of an oral estrogen each month decreases the incidence of irregular uterine bleeding and produces a satisfying withdrawal bleeding. The latter is of particular importance for many women who, despite their considering menstruation "the curse" or "sickness," feel it is evidence of their femininity and assurance of their not being pregnant.

Another area of research involves the search for a male contraceptive. Most efforts are directed at finding a suitable combination of progesterone, which inhibits spermatogenesis, and testosterone, which will offset the undesirable side effects such as decreased libido. Unlike female contraception, which interrupts a relatively predictable cycle, male contraceptives must suppress a continuous process of spermatogenesis. So far, no male contraceptive has been approved for general use in any country.

REFERENCES AND SUGGESTED READINGS

Bernstein, Judith, and Mattox, John H., An overview of infertility, *JOGN Nurs.,* 11(5):309–14, 1982.

Chapler, F. K., Uterine and tubal surgery for infertility and habitual abortion, in R. M. Pitkin and J. R. Scott (eds.), *Yearbook of Obstetrics and Gynecology,* Yearbook Medical Publishers, Chicago, 1977.

Dickerson, Janet, Oral contraceptives: Another look, *Am. J. Nurs.* 83: 1392–98, (Oct.) 1983.

Hastings-Tolsma, M. T. The cervical cap: A barrier contraceptive, *MCN,* 7:382–86, 1982.

Huxall, Linda Kay, Update on IUD's, *MCN,* 5(3):186–90, 1980.

McCusker, M. Peter, The subfertile couple, *JOGN Nurs.,* 11(3):157–62, 1982.

Moghissi, K., The cervix in infertility, *Clin. Obstet. Gynecol.,* 22:27–42, 1979.

Peach, Ellen Hammerlund, Counseling sexually active very young adolescent girls, *MCN,* 5(3):191–95, 1980.

Pepperell, R. J.; Hudson, Bryan; and Wood, Carl (eds.), *The Infertile Couple,* Churchill Livingstone, New York, 1980.

PART TWO

Pregnancy

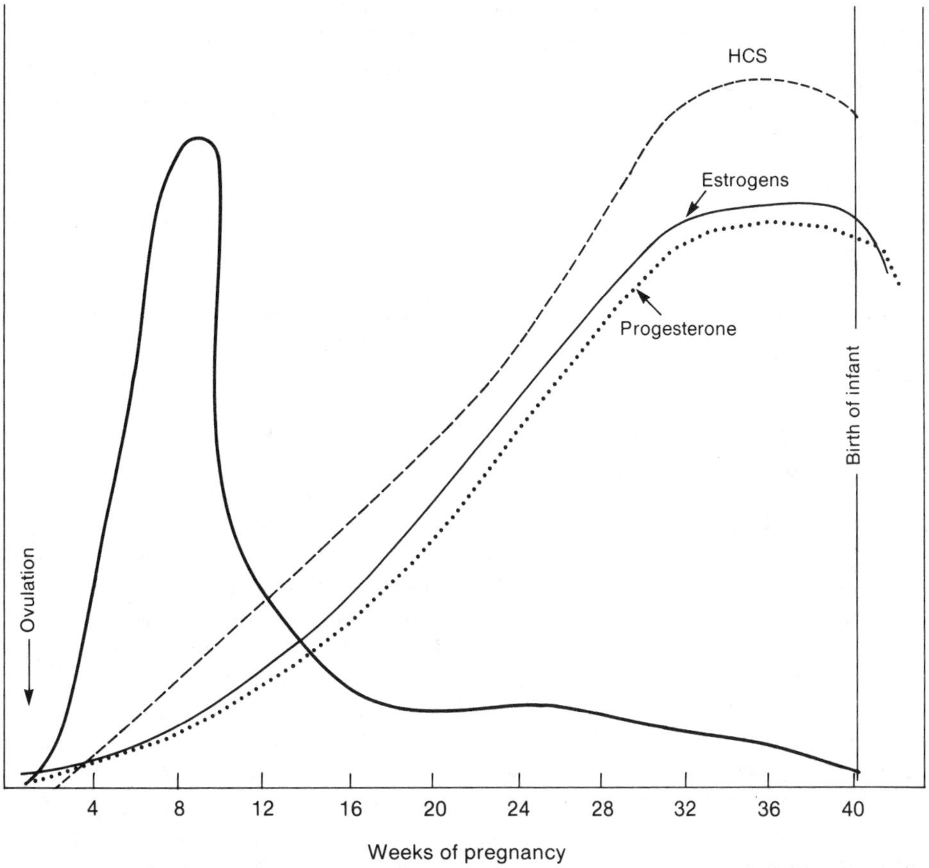

Figure 8-8. Relative concentrations of the major placental hormones present during the course of pregnancy.

should closely reflect the rate of production. Serial determinations of blood levels of HCS are sometimes used as one means of monitoring placental function and fetal well-being. HCS disappears very rapidly after separation of the placenta.

HCS appears to be an important metabolic hormone of pregnancy, affecting carbohydrate and fat metabolism so as to assure a good supply of nutrients for the fetus. It has two opposing effects on carbohydrate metabolism, promoting secretion of insulin and also antagonizing the insulin, diminishing its peripheral effectiveness. This tends to raise the blood sugar and contribute to a diabetogenic state in pregnancy. HCS induces mobilization of free fatty acids. This action appears to favor growth of the fetus by providing the mother with a source of energy that decreases her utilization of carbohydrates and increases glucose availability to the fetus. HCS also has some effect on protein metabolism, reducing the mother's use of breakdown products and enhancing amino acid availability to the fetus.

HCS influences breast growth and development in pregnancy, thus assisting in preparation for milk secretion, but actual lactogenic properties have not been demonstrated in humans. The hormone has disappeared from the circulation by the time lactation begins. HCS also may stimulate the acromegaloid changes, or coarsening in features, that some women develop in pregnancy.

HUMAN CHORIONIC THYROTROPIN A recently described protein placental hormone is human chorionic thyrotropin (HCT). The exact structure and the determination of maternal serum levels of the hormone remain to be defined, but it appears to have thyrotropic properties, with some similarity to pituitary thyroid-stimulating hormone.

The physiologic role of HCT is not well defined. It may play a role in the thyroid function changes observed in pregnancy, such as enlargement of the thyroid gland and increase in maternal thyroid activity.

OTHER PROTEIN PLACENTAL HORMONES Human chorionic corticotropin (HACTH), an ACTH-like substance, recently has been demonstrated in the placenta. Its physiologic role, if any, is presently not known.

The placenta may be able to produce many pituitary-like and hypothalamic-like protein hormones. Recent studies have suggested that the placenta can synthesize hypothalamic-like gonadotropin-releasing hormone

(GnRH), human chorionic follicle-stimulating hormone (HCFSH), human uterotropic placental hormone (HUTPH), and probably others. The placenta also may be the origin of some of the serum enzymes that are elevated in pregnancy, and it may secrete certain plasma proteins during pregnancy.

The same protein hormones, HCG, HCS, and HCT, that are secreted in normal pregnancy appear to be elaborated by all varieties of trophoblastic tissue. They are not restricted to trophoblasts and have been found in certain malignancies.

Steroid Hormones

The placenta synthesizes large quantities of steroid hormones—progesterone, estradiol, estrone, and estriol—during pregnancy and secretes these hormones into the fetal and the maternal circulations. The normal course of pregnancy appears to depend on the secretion of placental steroids (Fig. 8-9). The role these steroids play in the development and well-being of the fetus is not yet clear.

After fertilization of an ovum, the life of the corpus luteum is prolonged for several weeks. This corpus luteum of pregnancy and the hormones it produces are necessary for maintenance of the pregnancy until the placenta is able to produce sufficient steroid hormones.

In the normal ovulatory menstrual cycle, the corpus luteum secretes progesterone and estradiol for about 12 days. Then the corpus luteum degenerates rapidly, hormone production stops, and menstruation begins. When the ovum of such a cycle becomes fertilized, a different

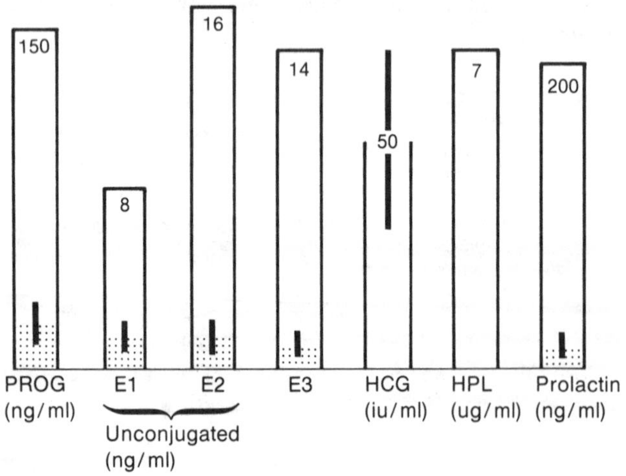

Figure 8-9. Serum hormone levels in advanced pregnancy. Nonpregnant values (stippled) fluctuate with the menstrual cycle. PROG = progesterone; E1 = estrone; E2 = estradiol; and E3 = estriol. Note that there is a massive and sustained increase in each of the hormones listed. (Reproduced with permission from Leslie Iffy and Harold A. Kaminetzky (eds.), *Principles and Practice of Obstetrics and Perinatology,* vol. I, New York: Wiley, 1981, p. 693).

series of events takes place. The blastocyst, resulting from the fertilized ovum, produces chorionic gonadotropin, which maintains the corpus luteum, changing it into the corpus luteum of pregnancy, and stimulating it to continue producing progesterone and estradiol for at least another four weeks. By the end of this four-week period, the pregnancy has reached the eighth menstrual week of gestation, and the placenta is able to produce a sufficient amount of hormones.

PROGESTERONE Progesterone is the important hormone in the maintenance of pregnancy. The placenta produces a very large amount of progesterone during normal pregnancy. The level of progesterone in the plasma and in urinary excretion as pregnanediol, the main metabolite of progesterone, increases steadily during gestation (Figs. 8-7 and 8-8). Only a very small amount of the total production of progesterone comes from the ovary after the first few weeks of pregnancy. In the first several weeks of gestation, progesterone from the corpus luteum is vital to maintenance of the pregnancy. It has been shown that corpus luteum hormone production is essential for the first seven weeks of pregnancy (five weeks after fertilization). Thereafter, placental production of progesterone is adequate and increasing. The placenta becomes the main source, and the corpus luteum is no longer essential to the outcome of the pregnancy. The corpus luteum may produce hormones throughout pregnancy, but its role is not important five weeks after fertilization of the ovum.

In production of progesterone by human placental tissue during pregnancy, serum cholesterol is brought to the placenta by the maternal circulation and converted to progesterone. A precursor from the fetus does not seem essential as is true with production of estrogens. Since only maternal cholesterol is necessary for production of progesterone, its synthesis does not seem to be associated with fetal well-being as described below for estriol synthesis.

Placental production of progesterone increases steadily during pregnancy, reaching a level of 250 to 350 mg per day toward the end of pregnancy. Ten percent of the hormone is secreted into the fetal circulation and 90 percent into the maternal circulation. Although the maternal excretion of the metabolite pregnanediol is quite high during pregnancy, the maternal plasma level of progesterone rises steadily from 40 to 160 ng/ml during the pregnancy. Even though the fetus receives considerably less progesterone from the placenta than the mother does, the fetal plasma level of the hormone is much higher than the mother's.

Progesterone, generally regarded as the hormone that preserves pregnancy, is responsible for some of the characteristic changes of pregnancy.

Under the influence of progesterone, in the second half of the menstrual cycle, the endometrium is changed from proliferative to secretory, the stroma becomes edematous, and the glycogen content of the endometrial cells increases. With these changes, the endometrium is ready for implantation and nourishment of the blastocyst.

A major function of progesterone during pregnancy is believed to be its quieting effect on uterine myometrial contractions. By reducing muscle tone in the uterus and decreasing the inherent contractility of the muscle, the blastocyst is allowed to implant and develop, and it is protected against expulsion by uterine myometrial activity. Administration of progesterone to women with uterine contractions in early pregnancy with a threatened abortion or at any other stage of pregnancy is not advised, however, unless a deficiency in progesterone production can be demonstrated. Although the progesterone theoretically decreases uterine contractions, there is no good evidence that it has been useful in treating threatened abortion, and there is concern that it may harmfully decrease uterine blood flow. Administration of progesterone also may affect fetal development adversely.

Progesterone is believed to have a relaxing effect on smooth muscles in several other parts of the body in pregnancy. Poor muscle tone might explain slow emptying of the stomach, regurgitation and heartburn, and constipation, all common occurrences in pregnancy. Similarly, the relaxation and dilation of the ureters in pregnancy may be an effect of progesterone.

Progesterone is believed to have an influence on the central nervous system that results in a listless, sleepy feeling which makes concentration on work difficult. This is a common complaint of women in early pregnancy. Also, the woman is very easily fatigued in the first trimester.

There is evidence that progesterone induces hyperventilation in pregnancy, which reduces alveolar and arterial P_{CO_2}. This effect may be brought about by a progesterone influence on the respiratory center.

The large amount of progesterone in pregnancy appears to have a number of metabolic effects. The reason for many of these influences is obscure. There is a suggestion that the considerably large amount of fat the mother stores in pregnancy may be governed by progesterone. This hormone also may influence the rate of protein catabolism and the lowering of amino acids in the plasma. Progesterone influences fluid and electrolyte homeostasis in pregnancy. It enhances sodium and chloride excretion in pregnancy, which then results in a compensatory rise in aldosterone to overcome the effects of progesterone and prevent a dangerous sodium loss. Another general metabolic effect is the rise in basal body temperature after ovulation in each normal menstrual cycle. If conception occurs, the elevated temperature of 0.4 to 0.6° C is maintained until midpregnancy when it returns to normal.

Progesterone, along with estrogen and other hormones, is responsible for growth of the breasts; progesterone is thought to be necessary for alveolar development.

Progesterone action often appears to be combined with the estrogens or it may be modified by the estrogens, which have an opposing influence and probably balance its action. An example of combined action is the influence of both hormones on breast development. The quieting effect of progesterone on the myometrium as opposed to the enhancement of uterine muscular activity by estrogen is an example of opposing hormonal influence with a balancing of action. The large amount of progesterone produced in pregnancy also influences other hormone production, sometimes being matched by large amounts of other hormones, as, for example, by secretion of aldosterone in large amounts.

ESTROGENS In the mature, nonpregnant woman estrogens are produced cyclically by the ovary. In pregnancy the principal source of an ever increasing level of estrogens in the body is the placenta. The ovary does not appear to be an important source of estrogens after the first few weeks of pregnancy. In nonpregnant women the ratio of urinary estriol to estrone plus estradiol is about equal. In pregnancy there is a very large increase in the ratio of estriol to the other estrogens. This disproportionate rise in estriol excretion in pregnancy is from a second independent pathway for estriol biosynthesis—the placenta.

Production of estrogens in the placenta is different than in the ovary in that its biosynthesis depends primarily on an increasing supply of a steroid precursor that is produced mainly by the fetal adrenals. Enzyme systems necessary for the production of estrogens are present in the fetal liver and the fetal adrenal glands and in the placenta.

Estrone and estradiol are synthesized in placental tissue by conversion of precursors derived from the maternal and fetal adrenals and carried to the placenta by the maternal and fetal bloodstreams. These hormones then are secreted into both the maternal and fetal circulations, with the bulk going into the maternal bloodstream (Fig. 8-9).

Estriol is synthesized by the placenta, largely from fetal-derived precursors; approximately 90 percent of the precursors are fetal. The estrogen precursor from the fetal adrenal goes to the fetal liver where it is hydroxylated. From there it passes to the placenta where it is changed by an enzyme and converted to estriol (Fig. 8-10). The placenta also receives a precursor from the maternal adrenal, which accounts for about 10 percent of the estriol excreted in late pregnancy. All the other precursors needed arise in the fetal adrenals.

The estriol that is formed in the placenta is secreted into both the maternal and the fetal circulations.

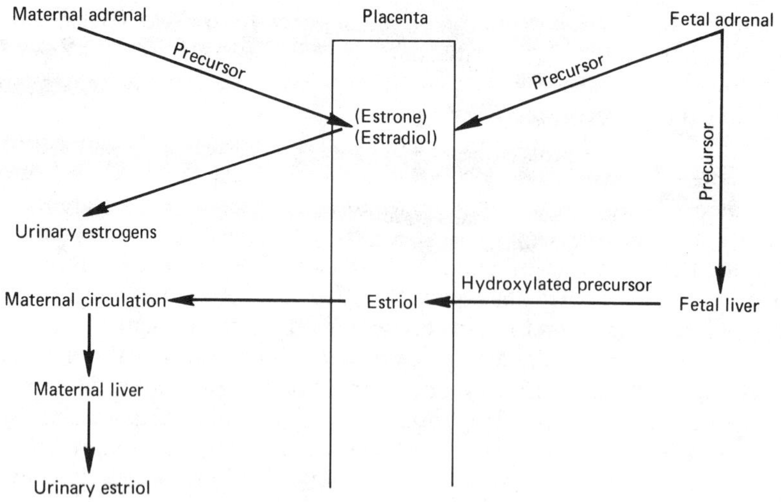

Figure 8–10. Simplified scheme of biosynthesis of placental estrogens in pregnancy.

Estrogens formed in the placenta and secreted into the maternal circulation are excreted in the maternal urine, but they first must be conjugated in the maternal liver (Fig. 8–10).

It is apparent that there is considerable interdependence between the fetus and the placenta in the production of estrogens. The production and excretion of the hormone are dependent on the integrity of the fetal adrenal, the fetal pituitary gland which appears responsible for development of the fetal adrenal, the fetal liver, and the placenta, and excretion in the mother's urine involves prior conjugation in the maternal liver.

Placental production of estrogens, largely estriol, is high. This is reflected in maternal urinary estriol excretion, which rises progressively in pregnancy. The tremendous rise in estrogen production in pregnancy reflects increasing production of precursors by the fetal adrenals. The fetal adrenal glands grow rapidly and by four months of fetal life have reached a size that is larger than the fetal kidneys. The glands are very active in steroid metabolism, providing the hormonal precursors to the placenta for estrogen and progesterone production. The fetal adrenals rapidly decrease in size as full-term growth is approached and continue a rapid involution after birth.

Urinary excretion of estriol rises slowly until about the twelfth week of gestation and then increases more rapidly in a steady upward curve (Fig. 13–3, Chap. 13). Since estriol originates predominantly in the fetal-placenta unit and adequate function of both fetus and placenta is necessary for its production, measurement of maternal urinary estriol level may be used as one clinical index of the well-being of the fetus and the placenta. A single measurement of urinary estriol excretion does not accurately reflect the status of the fetal-placental unit because variations in estriol production occur normally from day to day, but readings daily or several times weekly are valuable. Serial measurements are necessary with the expectation that there will be fluctuations in values, but the trend will be constantly upward. Falling values of 50 percent or more would indicate fetal-placental impairment. Use of estriol studies as one measure of assessment of fetal status in high-risk pregnancies is described in Chapter 13.

Many phenomena of pregnancy have been attributed to estrogens, but clear evidence of their action on many processes, at least in the human, is lacking. Many of the functions attributed to estrogens seem to be combined with progesterone action. It seems that the two hormones may exert an influence on a number of processes, such as development of the uterus and the breasts, at different stages in the development of these organs, and that both hormones are necessary for their adequate function. Also estrogens often appear to oppose the influence of progesterone and thus balance the end result.

It generally is believed that a major role of estrogens is control of growth and function of the uterus. After implantation of the blastocyst, estrogens bring about the hyperplasia and hypertrophy of the uterine muscle that permit the growth of the uterus necessary to accommodate the growing fetus. Estrogens also have the effect of enhancing the activity of the myometrium, the opposite effect of progesterone. Estrogens bring about vasodilation of the myometrium, important to good uterine blood flow. Paradoxically, progesterone appears to constrict arterioles. A proper ratio, of some unknown quantity, of estrogen to progesterone appears to be important to uterine muscle tone and to uterine blood flow.

Estrogens may have a softening effect on the substance between the fibers of collagen tissues of the cervix which permits easy stretching of the cervix in late pregnancy. Changes in connective tissue also may bring about the increased mobility of the nipples of the breasts that occurs in pregnancy and also permit striae (stretch marks) in the skin to develop over several parts of the body.

Estrogen, along with progesterone, is important to development of the breasts, with estrogen believed to be responsible for development of the alveolar ducts.

Estrogen has an influence on the respiratory center. It seems that, while progesterone lowers the threshold of the respiratory center to carbon dioxide, estrogen increases the sensitivity of the center.

A number of generalized metabolic effects are attributed to the influence of estrogens, at least in part. Estrogens appear to be responsible for some of the changes in the blood picture in pregnancy. The fall in total plasma proteins, mostly in serum albumin; the increase in a variety of serum-binding proteins, which bind with increased hormones of other glands such as the thyroid; the rise in fibrinogen concentration; and the characteristic leukocytosis of pregnancy are attributed to estrogen influence.

Changes in a number of other endocrine glands in pregnancy occur as a result of estrogens.

In closing this discussion on placental hormones, it can be said that much has been learned in recent years about the biochemistry of many of the hormones and also of some of their biologic actions, some of this from animal studies. Conclusions from animal evidence cannot, however, be transferred easily to the human. Thus many important questions remain concerning placental hormones. The physiologic function of the large amount of hormones is as yet not clearly understood in such important aspects of pregnancy as control of uterine muscle contractions and uterine blood flow, action in onset and control of labor, influence on general metabolic function, and maintenance of electrolyte balance.

Although the fetus is intimately involved in production of the placental hormones, very little is known about their role in fetal development.

The Thyroid Gland

The thyroid gland shows increased vascularity, hyperplasia, and a tendency to moderate enlargement in pregnancy, and the serum concentration of thyroid hormones, thyroxine (T_4) and triiodothyronine (T_3), is increased during gestation. Changes in thyroid function in pregnancy suggest hyperthyroidism, but in actuality thyroid hormone activity remains normal, and the normal pregnant woman remains euthyroid.

In pregnancy the general picture of thyroid activity is modified by the hormones of pregnancy. Estrogens increase the thyroid-binding globulin in the blood by a considerable amount and progesterone is associated with a low level of arterial Po_2, which in turn is associated with a low level of free hormone. As thyroid hormone is released from the thyroid gland into the plasma, most of it is bound to a thyroid-binding globulin and becomes inactive. It then acts as a storage source for ready availability. The free or unbound circulating hormone, the metabolically active hormone, is not increased above nonpregnant normal values. Thus, in pregnancy the total amount of hormone is increased, but the free amount is normal, remaining relatively constant, and the peripheral thyroid activity remains normal.

The usual clinical criteria of hyperthyroidism can be misleading in pregnancy, and interpretation of thyroid function tests is difficult. There is a rise in BMR of 15 to 20 percent in pregnancy, but most of this increase in oxygen consumption is caused by metabolic activity of the fetus and the increased maternal tissues. A rapid pulse and warm skin are normal pregnancy changes. The bound thyroid hormone, measured as protein-bound iodine (PBI), or in other tests that measure bound hormone, shows increased levels in pregnancy, similar to levels in hyperthyroidism, but these values do not reflect the free hormone level in the same way as they do in the nonpregnant state. The only useful test of thyroid function in pregnancy is one that ascertains the amount of free hormone by determining the free thyroxine concentration (FT_4) in the serum or by calculation of the free thyroxine index (FTI) of the serum.

Available evidence suggests that thyroxine (T_4) crosses the placenta but does so with some difficulty. Crossing-over may change with duration of pregnancy and with aging of the placenta, but exact changes are not clear.

Radioactive iodine is not used in pregnancy for studying thyroid function through measurement of uptake in the thyroid gland, or for treatment of hyperthyroidism, because of its radiation effects, particularly to the fetus. Iodine quickly crosses the placenta. The fetal thyroid gland has a very special affinity for iodine. It readily takes up the iodine and concentrates it in the gland in large amounts beginning as early as the twelfth week of gestation.

When antithyroid drugs must be used for treatment of hyperthyroidism, the mother is closely monitored by frequent thyroid function studies to keep the drug used at an optimal level, one that keeps her at an upper range of normal values. Antithyroid drugs cross the placenta, and they have the potential of adversely affecting fetal thyroid function, inducing fetal hypothyroidism and causing goiter in the fetus. When drugs have been used to treat the mother, the infant is monitored closely for both early and delayed signs of drug influence.

The Parathyroid Glands

Parathyroid hyperplasia occurs during pregnancy, suggesting increased hormone production. The reason for such increased function is not clear. Parathyroid hormone has an important function in calcium metabolism, and it has been hypothesized that the hyperparathyroidism occurs as a physiologic response to the demands of the growing fetus on maternal calcium stores.

The Adrenal Glands

The blood levels of cortisol (free and bound) and of aldosterone are increased considerably in pregnancy, and there are major changes in their metabolism. Plasma levels of cortisol rise progressively. An increase in the plasma level of cortisol-binding globulin results in a considerable increase in the circulating level of bound cortisol, but there is also a rise in free cortisol (the metabolically active hormone), approaching two or three times normal. There appears to be evidence that the increase in cortisol in pregnancy may be the result of a slowed rate of metabolism and prolonged half-life of the hormone as well as, or instead of, increased production.

The clinical effects of increased plasma cortisol are uncertain but appear to show some evidence of mild adrenocorticol hyperfunction. Maternal carbohydrate metabolism may be affected by the increased level of cortisol, which induces mobilization of protein and fat when food carbohydrate is not available. It increases the synthesis of glucose by the liver from the amino acids that become available and thus contributes to the tendency to hyperglycemia in pregnancy.

In addition to the effect on glucose metabolism, the adrenocorticol hyperactivity is thought to be one of the predisposing factors in the development of striae in the skin, the stretch marks of pregnancy. It is also thought that increased cortisol may suppress inflammatory reactions in pregnancy.

Another hormone of the adrenal glands, aldosterone, is increased greatly in pregnancy. It is secreted in response to the threat of sodium loss, which is promoted by progesterone and increased glomerular filtration. Aldosterone secretion increases as necessary to maintain sodium balance, as described on page 156.

Prostaglandins (PGs)

Prostaglandin is a generic term for a number of closely related fatty acid derivatives of prostanoic acid. The different members of the groups of prostaglandins are designated by letters, numbers, and Greek letters as, for example, PGE_2 and PGF_2. PGs are widely distributed in the body, and they have a great variety of actions. Some of these actions are of special interest to reproductive physiology, and some of their biologic activity is related to many nonreproductive physiologic mechanisms.

Prostaglandins originally were isolated from seminal fluid, which has a high concentration of these substances, but they are now known to be widely distributed in all tissues of the body including lungs, kidneys, brain, and reproductive organs. They occur in amniotic fluid, decidua, and in umbilical and placental vessels. The uterine endometrium and myometrium produce PGs, and the placenta probably does also.

PGs have a potent stimulating effect on the contractility of the myometrium at any stage of pregnancy.

A greater than usual amount of PGs is found in the amniotic fluid in women prior to onset of labor and in the blood after labor begins. This suggests a relationship of these agents to spontaneous abortion and spontaneous labor. Applying this action of these substances clinically, PGs are widely used to terminate midtrimester pregnancy and to a lesser extent to induce labor.

Uterine contractions sometimes have episodes of incoordination and hypertonic action with the use of prostaglandins.

Administration of PGs is associated with a number of side effects of which increased intestinal motility and frequent episodes of vomiting and diarrhea are very distressing. Currently, use of PGs for termination of pregnancy in the second trimester seems to be a reasonable alternative to other methods. There is an ongoing search for a compound that will have fewer disadvantages than those named above when it is used clinically.

Relaxin

Relaxin is a hormone produced only by the corpus luteum of pregnancy. It is not produced by the fetus, and it does not cross the placenta. The exact function of relaxin in the human is quite obscure, but it is thought to play a role in the softening of cartilage in the pelvic joints, in promoting relaxation of pelvic ligaments, and in relaxation of smooth muscles.

Pituitary Prolactin (PRL)

Prolactin has only recently been identified as a separate pituitary hormone—separate from human growth hormone, which has some prolactinlike activity.

Prolactin has many known functions in birds and mammals, but at present the only certain action in humans is its role in preparation of breasts for lactation and initiation of lactation and possibly maintenance of breast milk secretion. Its action also apparently influences the considerable breast growth and development of the alveolar system that take place in pregnancy, possibly in conjunction with chorionic somatomammotropin.

An increased level of prolactin is first observed in pregnancy between the fifth and eighth weeks' gestation. There is then a steady rise of prolactin to a maximum by the end of pregnancy, reaching a mean level of 200 ng/100 ml or more. The normal serum prolactin level is below 20 ng/ml.

If the level of prolactin alone was the stimulating factor for lactation it could be expected that the rise in prolactin in pregnancy would result in lactation. There is reason to believe that the high level of steroid hormones in pregnancy, especially progesterone, blocks prolactin action until these hormones decrease postdelivery. By the time breast engorgement occurs in the postpartum period, the level of prolactin has already decreased to one half the concentration it was at the time of delivery.

In women who do not nurse their infants, serum levels of prolactin are back to about prepregnancy levels in three weeks. In women who do nurse, prolactin levels also decrease and reach about 20 ng/ml in four weeks, but each sucking stimulus produces large, transient increases within 15 to 30 minutes, which again fall back to the baseline in about the same length of time. After three to four months' nursing the infant no longer produces the transient increases. The level of prolactin apparently does not need to be elevated for lactation to continue after it is well established.

Prolactin is present in the amniotic fluid and the fetus, as well as in the mother. Amniotic fluid contains a high concentration of prolactin in the first trimester; the level then progressively decreases. High levels of the hormone are found in the fetus and newborn. There is some evidence that the prolactin present in fetal plasma is of fetal pituitary rather than maternal origin. The possible role of prolactin in the fetus and newborn is not known.

CHANGES IN THE CARDIOVASCULAR SYSTEM

Some of the most significant and extensive adaptations in maternal physiology during pregnancy occur in the cardiovascular system. Circulatory system adjustments are important to both mother and fetus. They protect the mother's normal functions by adapting her body to the demands of pregnancy, performing a major function in meeting her metabolic needs. They provide for adequate fetal growth and development by assuring efficient delivery of nutrients and removal of wastes. The cause of the altered circulation in pregnancy is obscure and may be multifactorial. At present, it seems reasonable to suppose that the dramatic changes in hormonal production in early pregnancy play an important part in bringing about circulatory adaptations.

Blood Volume—Plasma and Erythrocytes

The maternal blood volume increases considerably in pregnancy. It begins to expand by the tenth to twelfth week of gestation, reaches a maximum volume over nonpregnant levels by 32 to 34 weeks of pregnancy, and then plateaus and remains constant until delivery. Blood volume returns to the nonpregnant level within two to three weeks after delivery (Fig. 8–11).

The increase in total blood volume during pregnancy averages 30 to 40 percent, but the range is wide and varies from only a moderate amount to nearly a double volume in different individuals. The increase in amount of blood in the body is between 1 and 1 1/2 liters. This hypervolemia of pregnancy serves to fill the greatly enlarged vascular system of the uterus and the expanded venous capacity of the legs. It meets the demands of the pregnant uterus and helps to protect the mother and the fetus against the poor venous return from the lower extremities that is common in pregnancy.

The increase in blood volume during pregnancy results from an increase in both plasma and erythrocyte volumes, but the increase in plasma volume is greater than that of the red cell mass (Fig. 8–11). Although there is considerable increase in erythrocyte production during pregnancy (an average increase of 250 to 450 ml of red blood cells, depending upon the amount of iron available), the disproportionate increase in plasma volume leads to a decrease in hemoglobin and

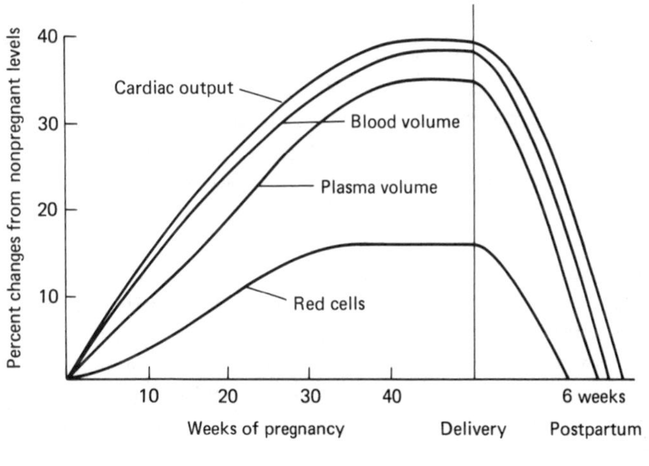

Figure 8–11. Changes in blood volume, plasma volume, red cell volume, and cardiac output during pregnancy and in the puerperium. The curves were constructed from various reports in the literature. They serve to illustrate the trend of changes rather than absolute values. (Reproduced with permission from Nicholas S. Assali (ed.), *Maternal Disorders.* Volume I in *Pathophysiology of Gestation.* New York: Academic Press, 1972, p. 280.)

erythrocyte concentrations, thus a fall in hematocrit value during pregnancy.

The above changes in the blood picture in pregnancy have often been called "physiologic anemia of pregnancy." This is an erroneous statement, since the physiologic blood changes do not result in a true anemia. Anemia, however, may be present during pregnancy from another cause, usually iron deficiency. There does seem to be some increased liability to iron-deficiency anemia during pregnancy, and it must be considered when hematocrit value, hemoglobin level, and erythrocyte count fall below the minimum levels of normal.

An anemia, rather than a change due to increased blood volume, is suggested when the hematocrit value is less than 34 percent, or the hemoglobin level drops below 11 gm/100 ml of blood, or the red blood cell count is less than 3,750,000/ml blood. Medicinal iron is administered prophylactically to meet the demand for iron that is created by the increased erythropoiesis or it is started at the appearance of anemia. Iron administration will increase the likelihood of the pregnant woman having a normal level of hemoglobin and erythrocytes at the end of pregnancy. Iron requirements in pregnancy are discussed on page 200.

Leukocytes

The white blood cell count generally rises during pregnancy. The count varies considerably during normal pregnancies, ranging from 5,000 to 15,000 per mm^3. Most of the increase in WBCs is in polymorphonuclear neutrophils; there is very little change in the lymphocyte count.

Other Hematologic Changes

Other hematologic changes in pregnancy are listed in Appendix 3, Table 1.

Cardiac Output

Cardiac output, the volume of blood distributed by the heart to the body per minute, increases tremendously during pregnancy. This rise in cardiac output is important in meeting not only the demands of the enlarging uterus and growing placenta, but also those of other organs with increased functions, as, for example, the kidneys.

It generally has been thought that increases in cardiac output during pregnancy progressed at approximately the same rate as increases in blood volume, and that return to nonpregnant levels within the first six weeks after delivery also followed the blood volume pattern.

Information has been accumulating that strongly suggests that the increase in cardiac output in pregnancy is much faster than previously thought. Cardiac output appears to show a dramatic increase very early in pregnancy (Fig. 8–11). It appears to increase 20 to 25 percent above nonpregnancy levels within the first trimester of pregnancy and thereafter to continue to rise slowly to approximately 35 percent above nonpregnant levels. This rise is maintained to the end of pregnancy.

The increase in cardiac output during pregnancy is brought about by an increase both in the heart rate and in stroke volume, that volume of blood that is expelled from the left ventricle with each beat.

Increased cardiac output during pregnancy imposes an increased work load on the mother's heart. Since this work load is proportional to the cardiac output and the mean arterial blood pressure, which is altered very little during pregnancy, the basal work of the heart will have increased 30 to 35 percent by the beginning of the second trimester of pregnancy.

Added to the increase in basal work load is the additional work of physical activity, since the pregnant woman's activity demands more work of the heart than does the identical activity performed by the nonpregnant woman, especially as pregnancy advances and maternal weight increases. The normal heart of a healthy mother is not affected by this additional work load, but if the pregnant woman has heart disease, the added work may cause cardiac complications, especially between the twenty-eighth and thirty-fifth weeks of gestation, when blood volume reaches its peak and cardiac load reaches a high level.

During labor and delivery and the immediate puerperium, there are sudden changes in hemodynamics. Cardiac output is difficult to study during labor but is known to increase. Up to 300 ml of blood is expelled from the uterus with each uterine contraction, temporarily increasing systemic blood volume and raising cardiac output. There is a definite but lesser increase in cardiac output during labor in the intervals between contractions.

Immediately after delivery there is also a rise, at least transient, in cardiac output, as the contracted uterus expels blood from the uterine vessels into the systemic circulation. In addition, pressure of the heavy uterus on the abdominal and pelvic veins is relieved as the uterus is emptied, blood flow from the lower extremities is improved, and venous return to the heart is increased. At the same time that the amount of circulating blood is increased by the above changes, it is modified to a variable degree by blood loss at the time of delivery. A loss of 200 to 300 ml, the amount associated with a normal delivery, reduces the volume of blood that would otherwise be available to the circulation. Larger blood loss can markedly reduce total blood volume. Cardiac output quickly decreases in the postpartum period, returning to the nonpregnant level within a few weeks.

Heart Rate

Heart rate is difficult to study during pregnancy because of the influence of many stimuli, but there is fairly general agreement that there is a distinct increase in pulse rate early in pregnancy, in the first trimester. Thereafter, the pulse rate may rise gradually even more to an overall increase in rate of at least 15 beats per minute over nonpregnant levels by late pregnancy. This means a rise from a nonpregnant mean of 70 beats per minute to a rate of approximately 85 beats per minute by late pregnancy. Many minor stimuli may temporarily increase the heart rate.

Position and Size of the Heart

Alterations in the heart during pregnancy involve a change in position of the heart, altered cardiac sounds, a slight increase in cardiac filling volume, and possibly slight hypertrophy or dilation of the heart, or both, resulting from the increased volume. As the diaphragm is progressively elevated during pregnancy, the heart is gradually pushed upward and to the left and rotated forward (see Fig. 8–15). With this shift, changes in cardiac outline can be expected, and the apical impulse moves upward and laterally. The amount of change depends upon the size and position of the uterus and the extent to which it pushes on the diaphragm.

Auscultatory changes are common during pregnancy. Systolic murmurs over the base of the heart are common, some cardiac sounds are accentuated, and split sounds may develop. Changes in heart sounds and development of murmurs become evident in the first half of pregnancy, and most disappear one week after delivery. The physiologic changes in heart sounds and in size and position of the heart during pregnancy are sometimes difficult to interpret, since they may be altered sufficiently to be considered pathologic when they are present at any other time.

Blood Pressure

There is fairly general agreement that arterial blood pressure readings during pregnancy are somewhat below nonpregnant levels (Fig. 8–12). Evidence from studies on arterial blood pressures suggests that the blood pressure falls early in pregnancy (first trimester), generally reaches its lowest readings in the second trimester, and then rises slightly and progressively for the remainder of pregnancy toward the nonpregnant level.

Changes in blood pressure during pregnancy are more marked in the diastolic than in the systolic readings. Whereas the fall in the systolic reading in early pregnancy may be only a few millimeters of mercury, the diastolic reading may be from 10 to 15 mm lower. Subsequent rise of blood pressure in later pregnancy toward nonpregnancy levels is also more obvious and distinct in the diastolic readings.

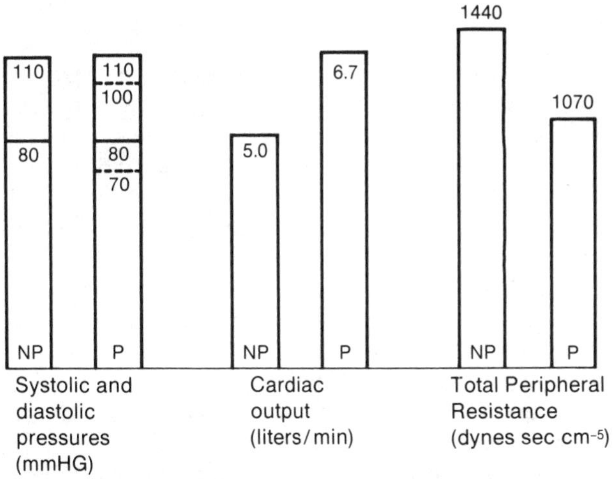

Figure 8–12. Arterial pressures, cardiac output, and total peripheral resistance in nonpregnant (NP) and late pregnant (P) women. Note that arterial pressures drop by about 10 mm/Hg by mid-term (as shown by the dotted lines) but return to nonpregnant levels near term. Cardiac output is already elevated by the end of the first trimester. (Reproduced with permission from Leslie Iffy and Harold A. Kaminetzky (eds.), *Principles and Practice of Obstetrics and Perinatology*, vol. I. New York: Wiley, 1981, p. 678.)

Posture is likely to have some influence on blood pressure readings. Compression of the aorta and/or the inferior vena cava by the pregnant uterus may influence venous return and cardiac output and, consequently, the blood pressure reading.

The lowering of blood pressure during pregnancy results from a lowered vascular tone (a lower generalized systemic vascular resistance) and from the presence of the placental circulation, which is considered a low-resistance system. It is possible that, during the second trimester, the lowered vascular tone and a relative hypovolemia, caused by a rapidly increasing uteroplacental vascular space, combine to reduce the blood pressure to its lowest level.

Knowing that there is a normal lowering of blood pressure during pregnancy has important clinical implications for observation and diagnosis. A woman with chronic hypertension may be normotensive during part of her pregnancy because of the physiologic fall, and her blood pressure may be at a low level when she presents for antepartum care. Then when her pressure rises significantly, diagnosis is difficult if there is no prepregnancy record. Also a blood pressure of 140/90, which often has been considered the upper limit of normal, is likely to be too high for some women. Judgment of the significance of a rise in blood pressure in pregnancy should be related to the individual's previous readings rather than to an absolute figure.

Systemic Vascular Resistance

Systemic vascular resistance, the resistance offered by the vascular bed to the flow of blood, is decreased during pregnancy. Studies have shown that there is a considerable decrease in the midpregnancy period. This fall in systemic vascular resistance is responsible for the decrease in arterial blood pressure during pregnancy, and it probably also facilitates the increase in cardiac output (Fig. 8–12). Although a number of factors may act to reduce peripheral vascular resistance in pregnancy, the two changes that exert the major effects are peripheral blood vessel dilation and the addition of the placental vascular system to the maternal circulation.

The placental vascular bed acts as a low-resistance network and takes on a relatively large portion of the maternal cardiac output. Uterine veins increase enormously in size and number during pregnancy. Uterine vascular resistance is greatly decreased during pregnancy, being at least ten times less than in the nonpregnant state. This marked decrease in uterine vascular resistance facilitates the tremendous increase in uterine blood flow during pregnancy, and it is also responsible for a considerable fall in systemic vascular resistance.

Pregnancy-associated changes in blood vessels lead to a generalized, progressive, peripheral blood vessel dilation during gestation. There is relaxation of most or all smooth muscles during pregnancy, and this includes the muscular coat of all blood vessels. The vascular tone, maintained by the smooth muscle fibers, is thus decreased; the vessels have looser walls, an increased ability to dilate, and increased capacity. This capacity for vasodilation is probably a major factor in a greatly increased peripheral blood flow in pregnancy.

Since the total peripheral vascular resistance is dependent upon all factors that affect peripheral blood flow, the vasodilation in pregnancy, which leads to an increased caliber of the terminal arteries, arterioles, and capillaries, is an important factor in the decrease in total peripheral vascular resistance.

Within a week after delivery the uterine blood flow, the uterine vascular resistance, the cardiac output, and the systemic vascular resistance all return to their nonpregnant levels.

Regional Increases in Blood Flow

Uterus

The uterus with its tremendous growth, its greatly enlarged blood vessels, and its development of the placental circulation to serve the fetus is a major target of an increased blood flow in pregnancy. Uterine blood flow increases tremendously, progressively becoming greater until it reaches a peak of 20 to 40 times nonpregnant values by the end of pregnancy. Measurements of uterine blood flow are very difficult, but estimates from observations that have been made indicate that there is a steady increase during gestation. It is estimated that the uterine blood flow is around 200 ml/min by 28 weeks' gestation, and at term pregnancy the average from a wide range of figures is 500 ml/min (Fig. 8–13). This increased blood flow in the uterus is of prime importance in providing adequate oxygen and nourishment for the fetus and for the uterine tissues.

The increment in blood flow to the uterus during pregnancy is derived from the increment in cardiac output. It is facilitated by the low-resistance network of the uteroplacental circulation, which results in at least a tenfold decrease in uterine vascular resistance during pregnancy.

Skin

There is considerable evidence that blood flow in the skin is greatly increased in pregnancy, especially in the hands and feet. Clinically, pregnant women feel warm, frequently complain of heat, and feel quite comfortable in cold weather and cold rooms. Their skin feels warm to touch and their hands are often clammy.

Increased blood flow in the skin has been estimated to be around 500 ml/min (Fig. 8–13). Blood flow in the hands is probably six to seven times greater than in the nonpregnant state; flow in the feet is smaller but definitely increased. Increased blood flow to the skin begins early in pregnancy. Its purpose is elimination of heat from the body, dissipating heat generated by the fetus and by increased metabolism. The increased flow is brought about by peripheral vasodilation and also some increase in the number of capillaries. As a result of the increased blood flow, there is a considerable increase in skin temperature during pregnancy. Finger temperature

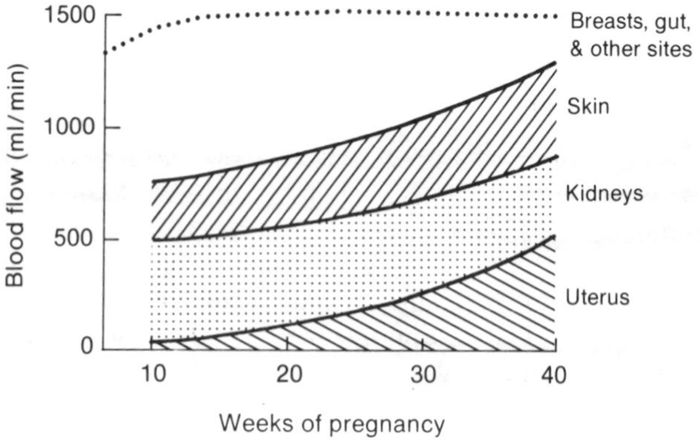

Figure 8–13. Distribution of increased cardiac output during pregnancy. (Reproduced with permission from Frank Hytten and Geoffrey Chamberlain, eds., *Clinical Physiology in Obstetrics*. Oxford: Blackwell Scientific Publications, 1980, p. 28.)

reaches nearly physiologic maximum levels in late pregnancy.

As a result of the dilation and increased number of capillaries, pregnant women may develop vascular spiders and palmar erythema. Hemangiomas that are present may increase in size and new ones may form, especially on the face and hands. Increased growth of fingernails of pregnant women has been reported, probably the result of increased blood flow. Hair growth has not been reported as increased in rate, but its character of growth has been found to be changed. It appears that in pregnancy the percentage of actively growing hair is greater and that fewer hairs are ready to fall out. There are then more overaged hairs by the end of pregnancy, and these fall out in large numbers in the puerperium.

The nasal mucous membranes also appear to have an increased blood flow in pregnancy, causing congestion of the mucosa. The vasodilation brings about a tendency to nosebleeds, and it may cause blockage of narrow nasal passages.

Kidneys

The kidneys are an important target of increased blood flow during pregnancy. This increase begins early in pregnancy, and the flow is up to 400 ml/min above nonpregnancy levels by the beginning of the second trimester (Fig. 8-13). The purpose of the increased blood flow to the kidneys is to enhance elimination, beginning early in pregnancy.

Breasts

The changes in the breasts in early pregnancy that include sudden enlargement, engorgement, sensation of tingling and heat, and dilated veins suggest that blood supply is considerably increased. Growth of the breasts during pregnancy surely would indicate that there would be a need for an increase in blood flow.

The Alimentary Canal

Measurements of blood flow to the alimentary canal during pregnancy have not been carried out, but the apparent increased efficiency of digestion and absorption of foods may mean an increased blood supply.

Summary Comments on Increased Blood Flow

The increased cardiac output in pregnancy is distributed to a number of regions in the body. The mechanisms that control regional blood flow changes are not clear and are probably complex. A major change appears to be vasodilation, with a lowering in peripheral vascular tone. Increased blood flow to the uterus is necessary for local growth needs and for needs of the fetus. Increased flow to the breasts is probably, at least in part, caused by growth of tissue. Two other major regional increases, that of the kidneys and of the skin, serve to enhance elimination from the body. There may be other important areas of increased flow that are unknown at this time. The regional blood flow increases described above all begin early in pregnancy and reach their maximum early, with the exception of the uterus, which continues a gradual, progressive increase up to the end of pregnancy (Fig. 8-13).

Venous Pooling and Venous Pressure

Venous pooling, the capacity of the venous system of the lower part of the body, is expanded by several times above normal during pregnancy, especially when the woman is in an upright position. Pregnancy-associated changes in blood vessels lead to a progressive increase in venous distensibility as well as to the progressive peripheral blood vessel dilation described above. The change takes place early in pregnancy. The looser walls of the veins permit a progressive increase in the capacity of the veins of the lower extremities to store blood. The velocity of venous blood flow may then be reduced considerably.

Under ordinary circumstances, in nonpregnant persons, the walls of veins, which are thin and flaccid, will yield to small pressure changes and easily increase their storage capacity. During pregnancy, this capacity for distensibility is greatly increased. Small increments of internal pressure will augment the capacity of the veins enormously. This means that the tendency to venous pooling on standing, which is present in all individuals, is aggravated in pregnancy. Venous capacity and venous pressure in the legs increase progressively throughout gestation, often becoming marked toward the end of pregnancy, as the enlarging uterus exerts more and more pressure on major abdominal and pelvic veins.

Both changes in the blood vessels themselves and mechanical factors appear to influence the distensibility of the veins. Although the hypervolemia of pregnancy tends to keep circulation normal by filling the enlarged vascular area in the legs, venous pooling does contribute to circulatory problems, such as postural hypotension, by reducing the amount of blood returned to the heart.

Venous pressure in the legs show a marked increase during pregnancy. Pressures in the femoral and other leg veins are high. In the nonpregnant individual, venous pressure tends to be nearly equal in all parts of the body when the individual is in the horizontal position. During pregnancy, however, venous pressure in the legs is several times higher than in the upper extremities, even when the woman lies horizontally. This increase in femoral venous pressure is the result of venous obstruction brought about by mechanical pressure of the heavy

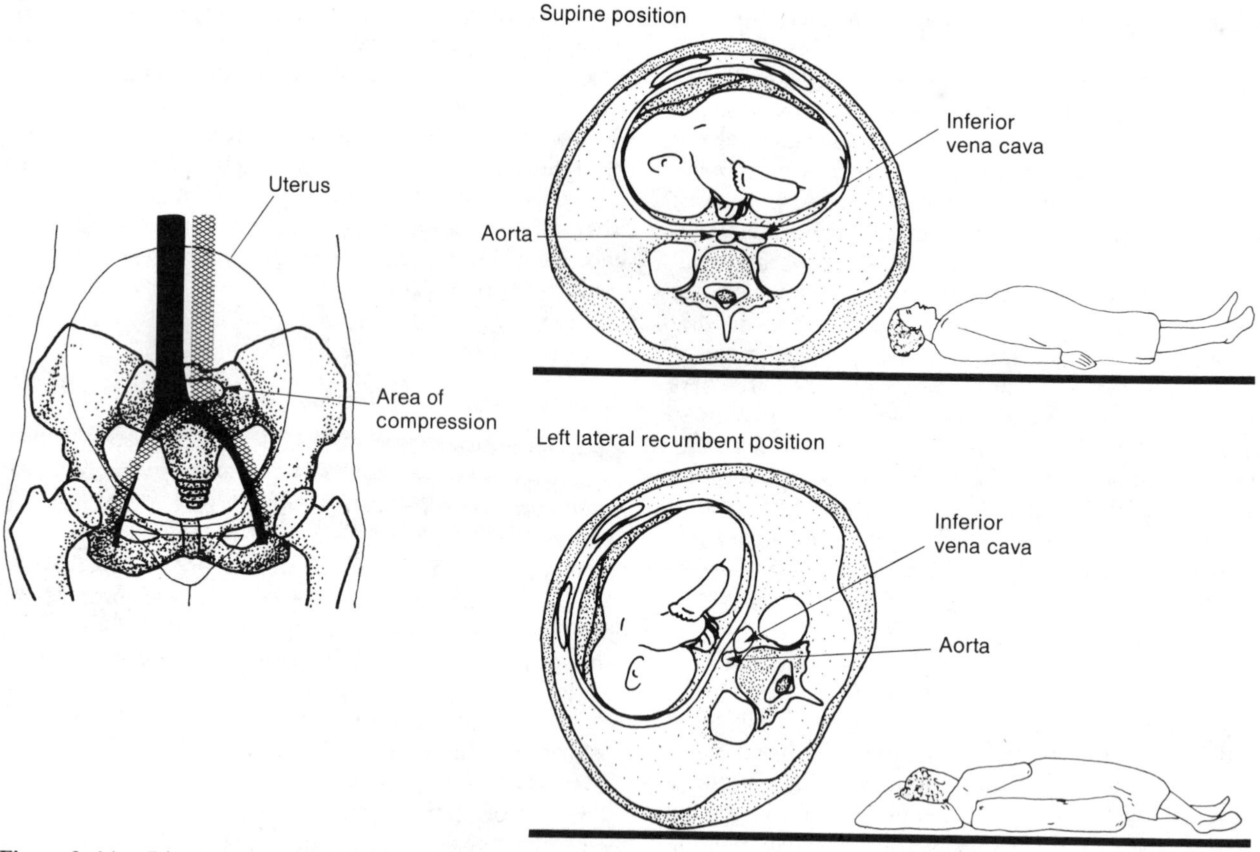

Figure 8–14. Diagram depicting the way in which the pregnant uterus can compress the inferior vena cava and/or the aorta when the woman lies in a supine position. A lateral recumbent position, preferably on the left side, tilts the heavy uterus off of the major vessels and favors optimum cardiac output. Compression of the vessels may result in hypotension in the woman as well as symptoms of nausea, clammy skin, and dizziness. This is referred as the "vena caval syndrome." Fetal distress may also occur as a result of uteroplacental insufficiency.

uterus on the iliac veins and the inferior vena cava and by pressure of the fetal head on the iliac veins (Fig. 8–14).

High venous pressure in the legs and stagnation of blood contribute to the edema of the feet and legs common to pregnancy, and to increased incidence of varicosities. After delivery, the high pressure in the femoral veins drops abruptly.

Venous problems with *thrombosis* and *varicosities* may result, at least in part, from the venous dilation, increased capacity of the veins, sluggish blood flow, and increased venous pressure. Venous thrombosis, which sometimes develops after birth of the infant and occasionally during pregnancy, is described in Chapter 25.

Easy distention of the walls of the veins, along with the pressure and stagnation of blood that accompany venous pooling in the legs, contributes to an increased incidence of problems with varicose veins and hemorrhoids in pregnancy. These problems arise from both preexisting varicose veins and from veins that develop incompetent valves during pregnancy. Vulvar varicosities, a problem unique to pregnancy, may also develop.

The veins return to normal during the first month after delivery, although some residual effects from venous problems may remain.

Edema of the Legs

When any individual stands or sits for long periods of time, the normally higher venous pressure in the legs, as opposed to the upper part of the body, increases capillary pressure in the legs. This results in a shift of fluid from the blood to the extravascular space and subsequently to edema of the feet and legs.

In the pregnant individual, the much higher than normal venous pressure in the legs, brought about by pressure of the heavy uterus on major abdominal and pelvic veins, increases capillary pressure. Also, a fall in plasma colloid oncotic pressure permits fluid to escape from the capillaries. Shift of fluid from the blood to the extravascular space in the legs is therefore much greater than normal in pregnancy. Dependent edema of the legs is very common and may be considered normal in pregnancy. Edema may be confined to the feet and ankles, or it may extend up the legs to the thighs, and it may include the vulva.

To minimize lower extremity edema, the pregnant woman who must stand or sit a considerable amount of time should walk around frequently to improve circulation, through the massaging action of the muscles close to the veins. The edema also lessens when the effect of gravity is reduced. Sitting down with the feet resting on a chair or elevation of the feet for a short time several times daily may provide considerable relief of discomfort from swelling. Edema fluid from the lower extremities is redistributed when the woman lies down and frequently is mobilized and excreted to some extent while she is recumbent, especially in the lateral position.

Postural Hypotension and Fainting

As described above, when a recumbent person stands up, there is a normal tendency for blood to pool in the dependent distensible veins in the legs. This tends to decrease return of venous blood to the heart, diminish cardiac output, and lower the systemic arterial pressure. Under normal circumstances, compensatory factors will quickly counteract the effects of gravity and restore the circulation to normal.

With a greater than normal tendency to venous pooling in a pregnant woman upon assuming the upright position, compensatory mechanisms may not be able to restore adequate circulation quickly, especially when a large uterus has already exerted pressure on major veins and caused considerable pooling of blood while the woman was recumbent. With decreased blood return to the heart and decreased cardiac output as a result of the pooling, marked hypotension and fainting may occur when the pregnant woman stands up. Severe oliguria may also occur.

Supine Hypotension Syndrome

A supine hypotensive syndrome, accompanied by dizziness, faintness, pallor, tachycardia, sweating, and nausea, will occur in some pregnant women when they lie on their backs. In the supine position, the inferior vena cava and the major pelvic veins are compressed to varying degrees by pressure of the heavy pregnant uterus (Fig. 8–14). This results in the same pathophysiologic circulatory abnormalities as those that occur in assuming the upright position. There is pooling of blood in the lower extremities, a decrease in venous return to the heart, fall in cardiac output, and hypotension. It is possible for a very large amount of the circulating blood to be collected in the legs. The blood pressure may drop precipitously and hypotension, accompanied by shock-like signs and symptoms, may become severe. Evidence of fetal distress will most likely also be elicited almost immediately. Prompt checking of fetal heart action is important when maternal signs of hypotension appear.

Whenever signs of supine hypotension occur, it is very important for maternal and fetal well-being, as well as for maternal comfort, to have the mother turn to her side immediately. Such a change of position will remove pressure from the inferior vena cava and quickly restore the pooled blood to the circulation. A mother is likely to recognize that turning to her side will relieve her faintness. If she becomes distressed while on her back during an examination or a treatment, she must be permitted to change her position immediately.

Since compression of major veins by the enlarged uterus will vary, all pregnant women do not develop signs of hypotension when they lie on their backs. Severe venous pooling may not occur when pressure on major abdominal veins is not great. The degree of pressure may depend upon the amount of pressure exerted by the abdominal wall or by a greatly enlarged uterus, or it may be determined by variations in position. A tight abdominal wall places more pressure on the uterus and the veins than a relaxed one. A uterus considerably distended with a large fetus or a large amount of amniotic fluid is likely to exert more pressure than one of moderate enlargement. There is less likelihood of pressure on the vena cava when the woman lies on a soft flexible mattress than when she lies on a hard table.

Effects of Autonomic Block

Increased activity of the autonomic nervous system in pregnancy provides good control over the vasomotor tone of the circulatory system. This good tone possibly tends to counteract to some degree the increased vein distensibility and venous pooling. Blockage of the autonomic nervous system with spinal anesthesia or with drugs also blocks the increased venomotor tone present in pregnancy and leaves pregnant women especially susceptible to hypotension and circulatory shock.

Blockage of the autonomic nervous system leaves the veins with very little or no tone and greatly increases their capacity. Pooling of blood in the legs can become severe. Under such circumstances, even a small amount of compression of abdominal and pelvic veins by the uterus can lead to a great amount of venous pooling and severe hypotension. In administration of spinal anesthesia to a pregnant woman, it is essential to take measures that will prevent or minimize hypotensive problems. One such step is to position the woman on her side to prevent or reduce pooling of blood in the legs.

Advantages of the Lateral Position in Pregnancy

Regardless of whether or not a pregnant woman has signs of hypotension when she lies supine, it can be assumed that an enlarged uterus will compress the major abdominal and pelvic vessels (inferior vena cava, abdominal aorta, and iliac vessels) to some degree when she lies on her back. Such interference with circulation may reduce cardiac output significantly and be deleterious to both mother and fetus.

In the supine position an enlarged uterus may compress the aorta as well as the inferior vena cava. As a result, pressure in the uterine arteries and other vessels distal to the compression is reduced. When the mother lies supine, measurement of blood pressure in the brachial artery does not provide a good estimate of pressure in the uterine and other arteries that lie distal to compression of the aorta. It is likely that the uterine arterial blood pressure is significantly lower than that in the brachial artery. Thus, even when the blood pressure is normal in the brachial arteries, it is likely to be low in the uterine arteries with the pregnant woman in the supine position. This decreased pressure results in decreased tissue perfusion, including poor placental perfusion. If, for some reason, the mother also has systemic hypotension, the arterial pressure distal to compression of the aorta may be markedly lowered. Perfusion of tissue may then be greatly reduced and be very harmful to both mother and fetus.

When a pregnant woman turns to her side (preferably left side) from a supine position, obstruction of the major abdominal veins is relieved, the pooled blood in the lower extremities quickly returns to the systemic circulation, and cardiac output and general circulation are improved. Blood flow to the placenta and the uterine tissues is significantly improved and maternal kidney function is greatly enhanced. It has been observed that there may be a 30 to 50 percent increase in cardiac output and in uterine and renal blood flow when a woman changes from the supine to the lateral position.

To assure that neither the inferior vena cava nor the abdominal aorta will be compressed, that maternal circulation will be good, and that blood flow to the placenta will be adequate for fetal well-being, it is highly desirable for a pregnant woman to lie on her side rather than on her back at all times that she is recumbent. If, in addition, she has complications that may result in hypotension, such as bleeding or conduction anesthesia, the lateral position is especially important.

CHANGES IN THE RESPIRATORY SYSTEM

Respiratory adjustments are made in pregnancy to provide for both maternal and fetal needs. The fetus must obtain oxygen and eliminate carbon dioxide through the mother, and the maternal oxygen requirements rise in response to the increase in tissues in the uterus and the breasts and to the greater metabolic activity of the maternal body in pregnancy.

Anatomic Changes

Capillary engorgement of the respiratory tract is common in pregnancy. The nose, nasopharynx, larynx, trachea, and bronchi become swollen. Nose breathing is difficult, nosebleed occurs easily, and voice changes frequently become apparent. Congestion of the larynx in pregnancy may adversely affect the voice of singers. Mild upper respiratory infections easily produce inflammatory manifestations in pregnancy.

Even before there is much upward pressure of the enlarging uterus, the level of the diaphragm rises by as much as 4 cm in pregnancy, and there is an equal decrease in the length of the lungs. At the same time, the effect of this shortening is satisfactorily offset by a broadening of the chest as the anteroposterior and transverse diameters increase by 2 cm. The lower ribs flare out progressively in pregnancy, and the substernal angle widens about 50 percent, from approximately 68 degrees in the first trimester to 103 degrees by the end of pregnancy. There is a 5- to 7-cm increase in thoracic cage circumference during pregnancy (Fig. 8–15).

Expansion of the thoracic cage is made possible, at least in part, by relaxation of the ligamentous attachment of the ribs, a change similar to that which takes place in other joints in the body. The ribs do not always return to their prepregnancy position after delivery. Changes in the chest begin early in pregnancy, before there is any significant enlargement in uterine size, and they are therefore not entirely produced by mechanical pressure.

Diaphragmatic movement is not decreased by encroachment of the full-term uterus. Breathing has been found to be more diaphragmatic and less costal at any stage of pregnancy than it is in nonpregnant women.

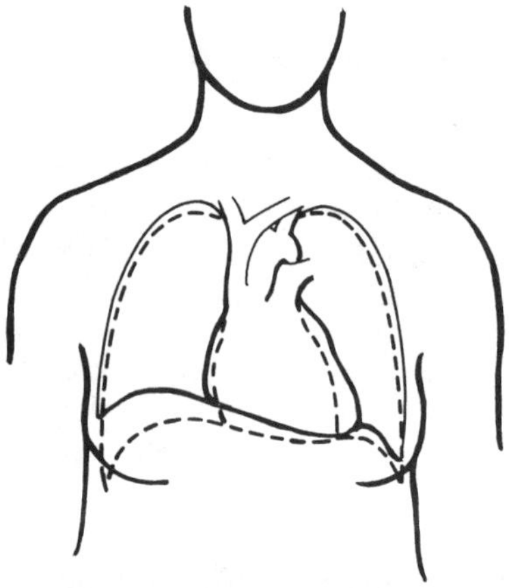

Figure 8–15. Changes in the position of the heart, lungs, and thoracic cage in pregnancy. Broken line: Nonpregnant. Solid line: Change that occurs in pregnancy.

Lung Function

Vital capacity, the maximum volume of gas that can be expired after a maximum inspiration, and *maximum breathing capacity,* the maximum voluntary ventilation, are not significantly altered in normal pregnancy. There is, however, a rearrangement in pregnancy of the various components of lung function. Beginning at the first trimester there is a progressive increase in *tidal volume,* the volume of gas inspired or expired with each breath (the amount of gas that is exchanged with each breath), and there is a slight rise in respiratory rate, from 14 to 16 per minute. The pregnant woman increases her ventilation mainly by breathing more deeply and only slightly by increased respiratory rate. The increase in tidal volume and slight rise in respiratory rate mean that the volume of gas expired per minute, the *minute ventilation,* increases to a peak level of close to 50 percent above normal by the end of pregnancy (Fig. 8–16). Clinically, this rise means hyperventilation.

Another progressive change during the second half of pregnancy is a considerably smaller *functional residual capacity,* the volume of gas that remains in the lungs at the end of a normal expiration. This means that the lungs of a pregnant woman are more collapsed and contain less residual gas at the end of a normal expiration than the lungs of a nonpregnant woman (Fig. 8–17). Since the functional residual capacity is the volume of gas with which the tidal air must mix, the changes in pregnancy mean that an increased tidal volume of air is taken into a smaller volume of gas in the lungs. This means much more efficient gas mixing. The *alveolar ventilation* thus increases 65 to 70 percent (Fig. 8–17).

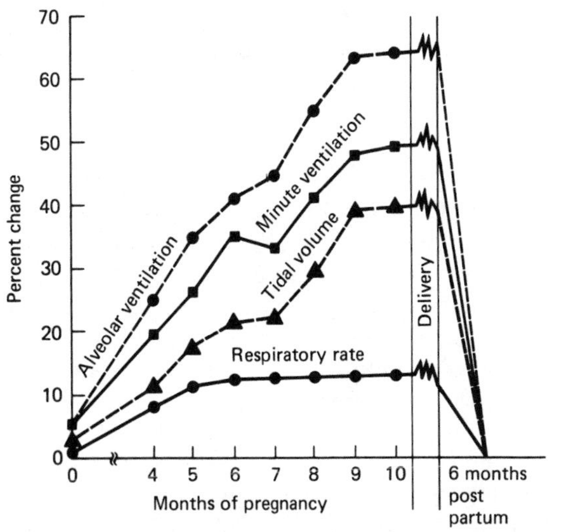

Figure 8–16. Changes in respiratory parameters during pregnancy. The curves for rate, tidal volume, and minute ventilation were developed from data of Cugell et al. Since the respiratory rate increases to a much lesser degree than tidal volume, percent increase in alveolar ventilation is greater than the percent increase in minute ventilation. (Reproduced with permission from John J. Bonica, *Fundamental Considerations.* Volume I in *Principles and Practices of Obstetric Analgesia and Anesthesia.* Philadelphia: Davis, 1967, p. 32.)

More rapid changes of gas in the lungs mean that very rapid, deep breathing, as might occur during the stress of a labor contraction, could lower arterial P_{CO_2} and raise

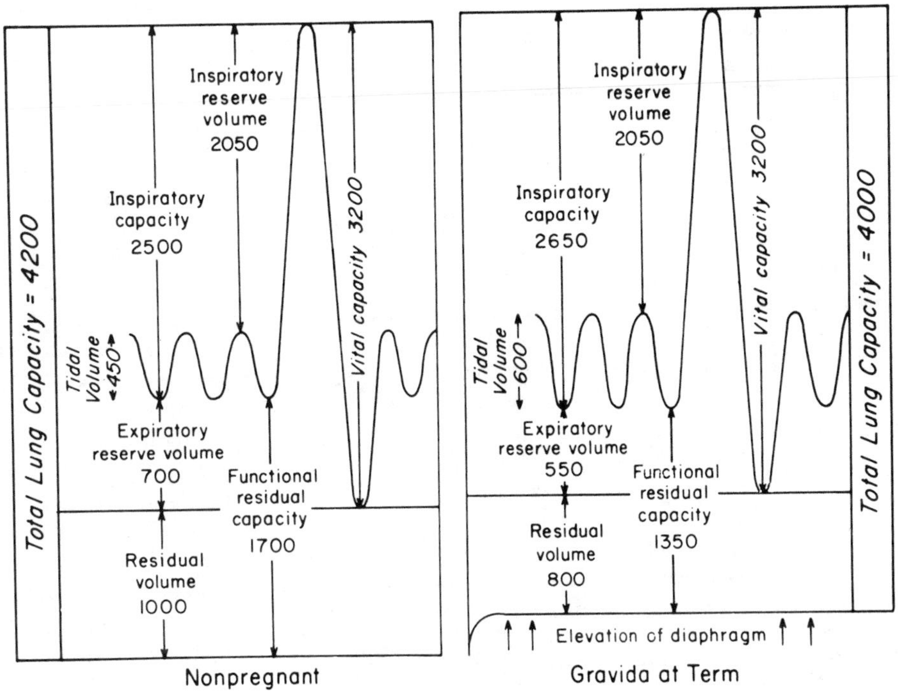

Figure 8–17. Pulmonary volumes and capacities in the nonpregnant state and in the gravida at term. (Reproduced with permission from John J. Bonica, *Fundamental Considerations.* Volume I in *Principles and Practices of Obstetric Analgesia and Anesthesia.* Philadelphia: Davis, 1967, p. 32.)

pH values to harmful levels. It also means that induction of and recovery from inhalation anesthesia are more rapid than in the nonpregnant woman.

Oxygen Consumption

Oxygen consumption in pregnancy, usually studied as basal metabolic rate, is difficult to determine, and studies have often been unsatisfactory. However, it has been estimated that a rise of 15 percent, or approximately 30 cc of oxygen per minute above nonpregnant oxygen consumption, seems to be reasonable and in accord with the increase in oxygen-carrying capacity of the blood.

A large part of the increment in oxygen consumption, at least as pregnancy advances, is related to the products of conception, the fetus and placenta. The increased metabolic activities of some parts of the mother's body, increased cardiac, respiratory, and renal work, and increased tissues of the uterus and the breasts account for the rest of the rise in oxygen consumption (Fig. 8–18).

Hyperventilation (Overbreathing)

A state of hyperventilation exists during pregnancy, beginning as early as the first trimester. Nonpregnant persons ordinarily do not hyperventilate until their Pco_2 reaches approximately 60 mm Hg. Pregnant women hyperventilate at a normal Pco_2 level (38 to 40 mm Hg).

Overbreathing is not related to changed mechanics of breathing and is not necessary for adequate ventilation. Although oxygen consumption increases during pregnancy (approximately 15 percent), minute ventilation increases much more, up to 50 percent above normal by the end of pregnancy. In addition, ventilation is more effective. With alveolar ventilation increasing up to 65 to 70 percent, it is approximately four times greater than the increase in oxygen consumption. Thus, there is considerable hyperventilation in pregnancy. The increased ventilation is evidence of overbreathing, or a response of the body to a stimulus other than need.

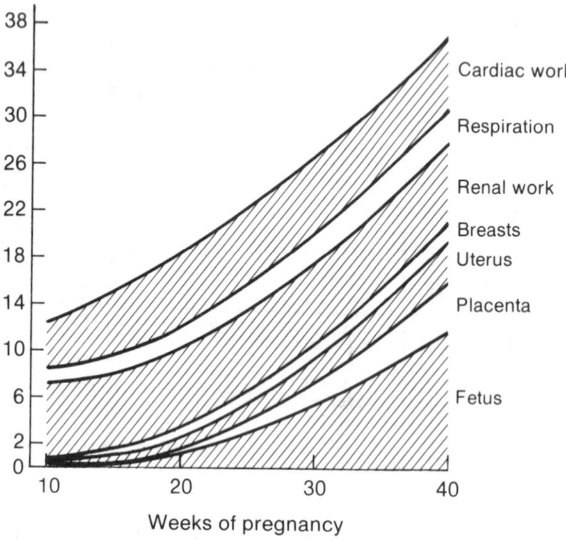

Figure 8–18. Partition of the increased oxygen consumption of pregnancy amongst the organs concerned. (Reproduced with permission from Frank Hytten and Geoffrey Chamberlain, eds., *Clinical Physiology in Obstetrics.* Oxford: Blackwell Scientific Publications, 1980, p. 91.)

Hyperventilation appears to be stimulated by a lowered threshold of the respiratory center to carbon dioxide, a response which is very likely brought about by the action of progesterone on the respiratory center. The respiratory center is also more sensitive, a reaction that may be influenced by estrogen. To some extent the hyperventilation and the changes that accompany it (such as a lowering of alveolar Pco_2) are a continuation of changes found in the luteal (progestational) phase of each menstrual cycle.

Carbon Dioxide Output

Overbreathing causes carbon dioxide to be washed out of the lungs, and because of this the alveolar concentration of carbon dioxide is significantly lower in the pregnant than in the nonpregnant woman. Accompanying this is a lowering of the arterial carbon dioxide tension from approximately 38 to 30 to 32 mm Hg.

As the arterial Pco_2 level changes, there is a transient respiratory alkalosis. Then renal excretion of bicarbonate appears to compensate for the lowered arterial carbon dioxide tension. Thus, the decrease in arterial Pco_2 is accompanied by a parallel decrease in plasma bicarbonate, causing the pH to readjust to a normal nonpregnant level.

Dyspnea

Approximately 60 to 70 percent of normal pregnant women develop dyspnea, a conscious need to breathe. Dyspnea should be differentiated from hyperventilation, which is effortless breathing. Shortness of breath is a common complaint of pregnant women. Exaggerated breathlessness may be evident on exertion, such as exercise, but the sensation of dyspnea is also often present at rest and not when moving about. It may be episodic and it is likely to begin to occur in the first trimester.

The cause of dyspnea is obscure. It appears to be unrelated to the mechanics of breathing, but may be caused by changes in respiratory center sensitivity. It is believed that the lowered alveolar Pco_2 may contribute to dyspnea. Dyspneic women may have a tendency to hyperventilate more excessively than those who are nondyspneic, and they may either be more sensitive to progesterone or have a higher level of this hormone.

Although dyspnea is usually physiologic, it may at

times be important to look for a pathologic reason. Common causes of dyspnea in pregnancy, other than excessive hyperventilation, include severe anemia, pulmonary edema, severe acidosis, and excessive pressure on the diaphragm as with hydramnios.

CHANGES IN THE URINARY SYSTEM

The kidneys, vital as excretory organs, have the very important function of maintaining the internal environment of the body in a relatively constant homeostatic state and in an optimal condition for the efficient functioning of body cells. They maintain electrolyte balance, control acid-base balance, regulate the extracellular fluid volume, excrete waste products, and conserve essential nutrients. To accomplish these very important functions approximately 1000 to 1200 ml of blood (about 500 to 600 ml of plasma) normally flow through both kidneys per minute. This is 20 to 25 percent of the total cardiac output. About 125 ml of plasma is filtered through the 2,000,000 glomeruli in one minute (170 to 180 liters per 24 hours). The glomerular filtrate, which is essentially protein-free plasma removed from the blood, is greatly modified, and, through a very complex process of tubular reabsorption and tubular secretion, most of the filtrate is selectively reabsorbed and other substances are secreted (excreted from the blood).

Tubular function includes all of the processes that change glomerular filtrate into urine. This includes the reabsorption of almost all of the filtered water, electrolytes, amino acids, inorganic salts, and other solutes. Unneeded substances are not absorbed, and others that are unwanted or are waste products are actively excreted by the renal tubule cells. Thus, the constancy of the internal environment of the body is maintained, and the volume of the filtrate is reduced from the 180,000 ml, which pass through the glomeruli in 24 hours, to about 1500 ml of fluid, which is excreted as urine during the 24-hour period.

Renal function is greatly altered in normal pregnancy. During pregnancy the mother's kidneys must handle the increased metabolic and circulatory demands of the maternal body and also excretion of fetal waste products. In addition, there is a tremendous increase in stimuli that may affect renal function. Mechanisms that maintain homeostasis are changed, and renal function and water and electrolyte distribution are altered considerably. Values from clinical tests of renal function and any seemingly pathologic changes in function therefore must be considered in light of the physiologic changes that are normally peculiar to pregnancy.

Anatomic Changes

The kidneys apparently increase slightly in size during pregnancy, probably due to hypertrophy and hyperemia. Also, the kidney pelves and the ureters, down as far as the pelvic brim, become dilated, starting as early as the tenth week of gestation. The ureters have been found to be of normal caliber below the pelvic brim. Dilation of the ureters is accompanied by hypertrophy and hyperplasia of the ureteral smooth muscle. Later in pregnancy, dilation of the renal pelvis and the ureter becomes more pronounced on the right side than on the left. Kinking of the ureters, often acute, has been found to occur on both sides.

The volume of urine contained in the renal pelves and ureters is greatly increased in pregnancy because of their dilation. This means that there is considerable lag between the time urine is formed and the time it enters the bladder. This easily distorts clearance tests, particularly if the urine flow rate is low at the time of the test. If the urine flow is slow, the urine that is retained in the dilated kidneys and ureters and in the bladder may contain substances that were filtered through the glomeruli many hours previously.

For accurate testing, as much of the urine as possible that is produced in a unit of time should be obtained for analysis. Unless this is done, errors may be significant even when 24-hour urine specimens are collected. Inaccuracies caused by retained urine can be reduced in two ways: by producing a fairly adequate urinary flow with an increase in fluid intake (a water load) an hour before the beginning and the end of a test, and by requesting the woman to lie in the lateral recumbent position as much as possible during the collection period.

Stagnation of urine due to dilation of the urinary tract also may be a factor in frequent urinary tract infections. There is an increased incidence in both asymptomatic bacteriuria and acute pyelonephritis in pregnancy. In addition to stagnation, the excretion of a large number of nutrients in the urine in pregnancy, especially glucose, provides a very favorable environment for bacterial growth.

The cause of dilation of the renal collecting system is not clear. For many years it was believed that there was atony of tissues, largely a hormonal effect, possibly typical of smooth muscle relaxation in general, attributed to a progesterone effect. This concept has not been entirely discarded, although there is some evidence to the contrary. Some believe that the dilation is a purely mechanical effect and may be so even when it occurs early. There has been evidence that the ureters may be compressed by dilated blood vessels which lie in close proximity. Later the enlarging uterus compresses the ureters as they pass over the pelvic brim, placing more pressure on the right side than the left, possibly owing to uterodextrorotation. Also, the left side is believed to be somewhat protected by the sigmoid colon.

The bladder becomes elevated in pregnancy as the uterus enlarges, and the trigone area becomes somewhat hypertrophic. The trigone area may become stretched so much that the ureterovesical valves become incompetent. When this happens, there is a predisposition to ascending urinary tract infection. The bladder wall and mucosa may become hyperemic, with the size and tortuosity of the blood vessels increasing. This accompanies the changes in other tissues in the pelvis.

Renal Plasma Flow (RPF) and Glomerular Filtration Rate (GFR)

Renal plasma flow (RPF) and glomerular filtration rate (GFR) are markedly increased in pregnancy. A rapid rise is evident very early in pregnancy, by the end of the first trimester, and is sustained to term (Figs. 8-19 and 8-20). According to data currently available, it seems that the rise in blood flow through the kidneys is from a nonpregnant level of a mean of 1000 ml/min to a level that is between 25 to 50 percent higher. The renal plasma flow, which is the volume of plasma flowing through the kidneys every minute, seems to rise by about 225 ml/min, from a level of 500 to 600 ml/min to between 700 and 900 ml/min. The glomerular filtration rate, which is the amount of plasma filtered by the glomeruli of both kidneys per minute, rises from a nonpregnant level of 100 to 125 ml/min to as high as 140 to 170 ml/min, a rise of about 50 percent.

As the renal plasma flow increases approximately 35 percent, the GFR rises to as much as 50 percent. The greater rise in glomerular filtration over that of plasma flow means that the filtration fraction, the proportion of the renal plasma flow that is filtered by the glomeruli, is greater than the nonpregnant level. The serum protein concentration in plasma is lower in pregnancy by about 1 gm per 100 ml. Such a change decreases the plasma oncotic pressure by about 20 percent, and it is likely that this decreased colloid oncotic pressure permits increased filtration of plasma in the kidneys.

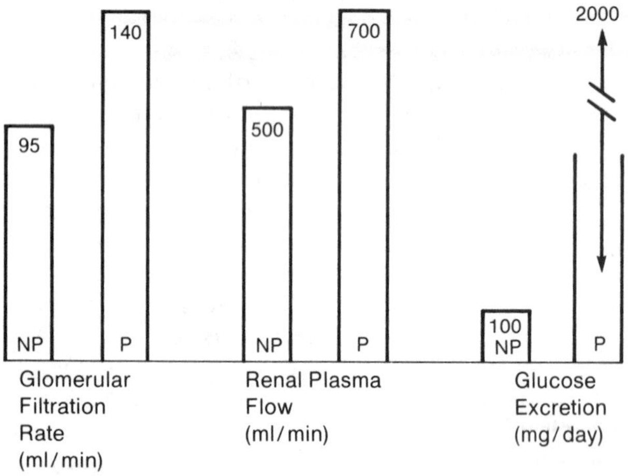

Figure 8-19. Glomerular filtration rate, RPF, and urinary excretion of glucose in nonpregnant (NP) and late pregnant (P) women. The filtered load is increased substantially during pregnancy. Nonpregnant women generally excrete no more than 100 mg glucose per day, but even normal pregnant women may excrete much larger amounts sporadically, ranging from 100 to above 2,000 mg/day. (Reproduced with permission from Leslie Iffy and Harold A. Kaminetzky (eds.), *Principles and Practices of Obstetrics and Perinatology*, Vol. I. New York: Wiley, 1981, p. 687.)

The cause of the increases in renal blood flow and glomerular filtration in pregnancy is not known. It has been suggested that, with the rise in cardiac output early in pregnancy and the decrease in total peripheral vascular resistance, the resistance to blood flow through the kidneys may be specifically lowered and the flow easily increased. Progesterone and possibly estrogen may have an effect. Human growth hormone is known to increase renal plasma flow and glomerular filtration. This hormone remains at normal levels during pregnancy, but human chorionic somatomammotropin (HCS), a hormone present early in pregnancy and having similarities to growth hormone, has been considered a possible cause of increasing renal blood flow and glomerular filtration. Another consideration is that the increase in extracellular fluid volume in pregnancy may bring about an increase in renal hemodynamics.

Effect of Posture on Renal Function

Renal function of women in late pregnancy is considerably altered by position. The supine and the upright positions both bring about a reduction in renal blood flow and glomerular filtration and in excretion of water and sodium and chloride (Fig. 8-20). The rate of excretion may be less than half in either the supine or standing position. As described on page 147, women in late pregnancy are very likely to pool a large amount of blood in their legs. When they lie supine, the heavy uterus compresses the inferior vena cava and the aorta, and when they sit or stand quietly, the uterus compresses the common iliac veins. In either case, venous return from the legs is impaired, the effective blood volume is decreased, cardiac output falls, and blood pressure falls.

A compensatory change in response to decreasing circulating blood volume and decreasing cardiac output is renal vasoconstriction. This response provides a better blood flow to areas more vital than the kidneys, but it also means a considerable reduction in renal blood flow and in glomerular filtration. Whenever renal function must be improved during gestation, it is essential that the pregnant woman lie in bed on her side, preferably her left side, as much as possible.

Diurnal Pattern of Renal Function

The normal nonpregnant individual has a lower excretion of water and electrolytes during the night than in the daytime. This pattern of urinary output is an established

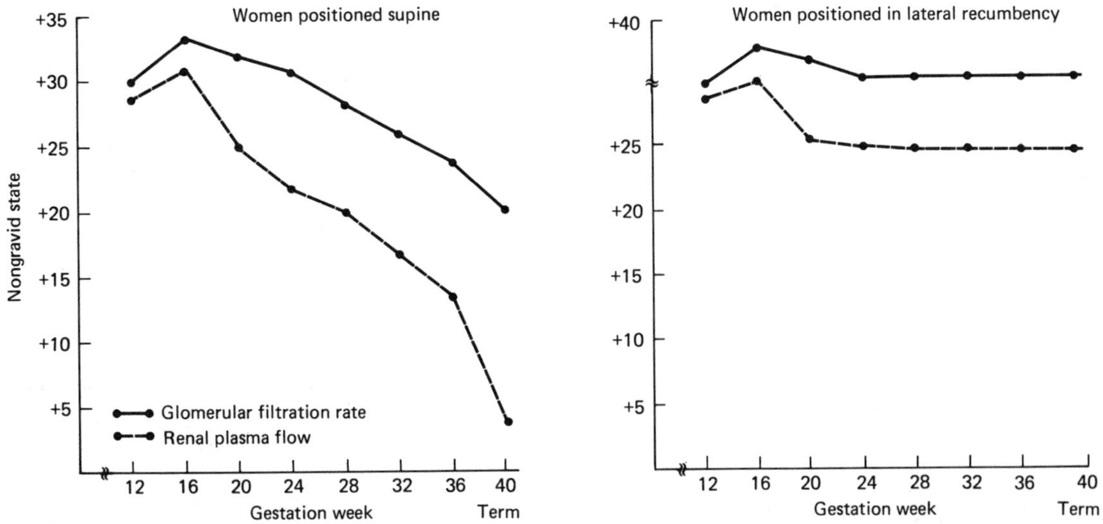

Figure 8-20. Renal hemodynamics in pregnancy. Increases in parameters of renal hemodynamics occur early in pregnancy and are sustained to term if subjects are tested in lateral recumbency. (Reproduced with permission from Marshall D. Lindheimer and Adrian I. Katz, "Managing the Patient with Renal Disease," *Contemp. Ob/Gyn* 3(1): 49–55 (Jan.) 1974, p. 51.)

periodic alteration that is not merely a reflection of difference in fluid intake. In ambulatory pregnant women this usual pattern of urinary output is reversed. During the day pregnant women tend to collect fluid as dependent edema. At night, when they lie down, they mobilize this extracellular fluid and excrete it. Excretion of sodium and water thus is increased at night. This change in pattern of urinary output also leads to the common problem of nocturia in pregnant women.

Clearance of Waste Products

Creatinine, urea, and uric acid are excreted more effectively in pregnancy than in the nonpregnant state, owing to enhanced renal clearance. Since there is essentially no change in the production of these products in pregnancy, the result of this increased clearance is a lower level of nitrogenous breakdown products in the blood than in nonpregnant women. In addition, the normal increase in plasma volume in pregnancy may lower the serum urea nitrogen and serum creatinine values somewhat. Concentrations of plasma urea nitrogen, creatinine, and uric acid are reduced to about two thirds of nonpregnant levels. Thus, values that are considered normal in nonpregnant women may signify decreased renal function in pregnancy. Concentrations of serum urea nitrogen over 13.0 mg percent or of serum creatinine over 0.8 mg percent are at the upper levels, or above, the normal values for pregnancy and require further evaluation of renal function.

Renal Sodium Excretion

The content of sodium in the body is kept within narrow limits by the regulatory functions of the kidneys. Under normal circumstances, threats to sodium balance are countered by quick physiologic adjustments, which keep the extracellular fluid (plasma and interstitial fluid) constant in volume and osmolarity. This is necessary since any distortion in the composition of these extracellular fluids would soon have disastrous results.

Since sodium is freely filtered at the glomeruli and actively absorbed by the tubules, the amount of sodium excreted in the urine is the difference between the amount filtered and the amount reabsorbed. It could be assumed then that sodium excretion may be increased by an increase in GFR or by a decrease in reabsorption, or by a combination of both. Ordinarily, however, tubular reabsorption is quickly adjusted to the rate of glomerular filtration to maintain sodium in careful balance. More than 99 percent of the sodium filtered by the glomeruli is reabsorbed.

A number of factors control GFR and tubular reabsorption, but regulation of reabsorption seems to be of major importance. Reabsorption must be, and is, quickly adjusted to changes in the filtered load of sodium so that it keeps pace with that which is filtered out. Increases in sodium intake, or losses of sodium from the body, are accompanied by changes in tubular reabsorption. Thus, sodium and water balances, the balance between their intake and output, depend critically on tubular reabsorption.

In normal persons regulatory mechanisms are very precise and sodium balance varies very little despite marked changes in dietary intake or in losses due to sweating, vomiting, or diarrhea. Sodium balance may, however, become upset in disease or under certain circumstances in which sodium-retaining factors or sodium-losing factors are disrupted so that they operate out of proportion to normal.

Regulation of sodium excretion and sodium retention, a very complicated process under normal circumstances, appears to be even more so in pregnancy. Sodium-retaining factors and sodium-losing factors are changed sufficiently in pregnancy to bring about a tendency to sodium depletion. This can become a major problem if an inadequate amount of dietary sodium is ingested in pregnancy or if diuretics are used.

There is actually a very gradual cumulative retention of sodium during pregnancy, a total of 500 to 900 mEq, but this amount is only enough to meet the special needs of pregnancy and does not change the maternal electrolyte balance. This retained sodium is necessary to meet the requirements of the developing fetus and to provide for the mother's increased interstitial and intravascular fluid volumes. Considering the usual increase in extracellular fluids in pregnancy, it is apparent that additional sodium must be retained to permit expansion of fluid volume and to maintain an isotonic state.

Factors Tending to Promote Renal Excretion of Sodium

Of the several factors that tend to promote renal excretion of sodium in pregnancy, the increased GFR and an increase in progesterone levels have the greatest influence. These tend to produce considerable sodium loss.

INCREASE IN GLOMERULAR FILTRATION The tremendous rise in GFR in pregnancy, up to levels of 50 percent above nonpregnant values, results in a similar increase of filtered load of sodium. If this were not accompanied by an equal increase in tubular reabsorption of sodium, severe sodium depletion would quickly occur. The ability of the kidney to adjust to a large increase in reabsorption of sodium so that it can match the enhanced filtration of sodium is a major adaptation of pregnancy.

PROGESTERONE Progesterone may significantly promote sodium excretion. It antagonizes the effect of aldosterone, which enhances sodium reabsorption, and thus interferes with reabsorption. Since progesterone is greatly increased in pregnancy, anywhere from 10- to 100-fold, it can exert considerable influence.

PHYSICAL FACTORS A decrease in both plasma albumin and vascular resistance in pregnancy may tend to enhance excretion of sodium. The low serum colloid oncotic pressure in pregnancy may tend to reduce reabsorption.

Factors Tending to Enhance Sodium Reabsorption

A compensatory mechanism, the renin-angiotensin-aldosterone system, that works toward overcoming sodium loss by enhancing its reabsorption, functions very well in pregnancy. Thus, the influence of the increased GFR and the increased progesterone level in producing considerable sodium loss is offset by increased activity of the renin-angiotensin-aldosterone system. With such activity, there is a marked increase in aldosterone secretion in normal pregnancies, an increase of severalfold. The aldosterone enhances sodium reabsorption and thus prevents excessive sodium wasting while the increased GFR is filtering it out in large amounts.

THE RENIN-ANGIOTENSIN-ALDOSTERONE SYSTEM Renin is a proteolytic enzyme secreted into the blood by the kidneys, specifically by the cells of a specialized area of each nephron known as the juxtaglomerular apparatus, which is located in the walls of the renal afferent arterioles. It acts on a circulating renin substrate causing the formation of angiotensin. Angiotensin, the major regulator of aldosterone secretion, stimulates secretion of aldosterone by the adrenal cortex. Aldosterone enhances the tubular reabsorption of sodium, returning it to the circulation.

The marked increase in plasma renin activity and in aldosterone secretion in normal pregnancy apparently is not excessive but is an adaptation that is ready to prevent sodium depletion. It appears to be a compensatory response to the threat of sodium loss and to the need to retain additional sodium to meet the needs of the fetus and of the additional maternal extracellular fluids. Thus, aldosterone secretion is regulated by normal mechanisms in pregnancy and increases only as necessary for maintenance of sodium balance.

As in normal nonpregnant persons, aldosterone secretion is easily influenced by changes in dietary sodium intake; its secretion increases with sodium deprivation and decreases with high salt intake. The difference is in the much greater levels of the hormone in pregnancy at all levels of dietary sodium intake. The renin-angiotensin-aldosterone system thus apparently adjusts to sodium restriction or to increased needs of pregnancy, but could possibly be severely stressed if necessary adjustments were prolonged or severe.

OTHER HORMONES Estrogen, which is considerably increased in pregnancy, tends to induce sodium retention. Other hormones tending to decrease sodium excretion are placental HCS, increased prolactin levels in pregnancy, and increased plasma cortisol concentration.

Effect of Posture on Sodium Excretion

The supine and upright positions tend to decrease renal excretion of sodium and water. The fall in GFR in these positions is accompanied by an equal fall in sodium excretion (Fig. 8–20). In addition to this influence of posture, it appears that the supine and upright positions also cause an active reabsorption of sodium, independent of glomerular filtration. It has been suggested that the reduction in effective circulating plasma volume in these positions stimulates reabsorption of sodium.

Summary Comments on Renal Sodium Excretion

In summary, pregnancy results in a tendency to sodium depletion rather than excessive sodium retention. Restriction of dietary sodium or administration of diuretics in pregnancy may stress the renin-angiotensin-aldosterone mechanism and exaggerate the normal sodium-depletion tendency. If this became severe, it could cause excessive volume depletion and could even result in poor placental perfusion.

Excretion of Water

The capacity of the kidneys to deal with a water load changes as pregnancy progresses. The ability to excrete water is excellent in early pregnancy. This is also a time of thirst for many pregnant women. There is then a decline, and in later pregnancy excretion of a water load is considerably below the nonpregnant average. There is evidence to suggest that the ability to excrete a water load decreases in late pregnancy because the water then pools in the lower extremities and does not trigger a diuretic response. It is only mobilized when the woman lies down. It has also been suggested that there may be a new lower level of osmolarity in late pregnancy, or that increased oxytocin secretion in late pregnancy may cause some antidiuresis.

As with sodium excretion, the excretion of water is decreased in the upright and the supine positions. Also the nonpregnant diurnal variation is reversed, and excretion of both sodium and water is greater at night during pregnancy.

Glucosuria

Under normal conditions almost all glucose filtered through the glomeruli is reabsorbed by the tubules and only minute amounts can be detected in the urine. Normally there is so little glucose in the urine that for clinical purposes it may be considered absent. Normal pregnancy, however, is frequently associated with glucosuria. Reabsorption of glucose in pregnancy is apparently not as efficient as reabsorption of sodium, and the glucose that is not absorbed is excreted in the urine. The amount of sugar lost can vary considerably from day to day, and individual urine specimens may be positive or negative to glucose at irregularly intermittent times (Fig. 8-19).

Glucosuria in pregnancy seems to be due, in part, at least, to an increase in the filtration of glucose brought about by the increased GFR in pregnancy and an inability of the renal tubules to increase reabsorption as much as the glomerular filtration increases. More glucose is filtered out with the plasma filtrate and presented to the renal tubules than they can reabsorb.

There is also some evidence that maximum tubular glucose reabsorption may be lower in pregnant than in nonpregnant women. This would mean that pregnant women have a somewhat lower blood sugar value than nonpregnant women at which reabsorption no longer takes place or at least is decreased. Sugar may then be excreted into the urine rather than be reabsorbed back into the bloodstream at blood values of considerably less than 160 to 180 mg/100 ml of blood (the values up to which reabsorption normally takes place). Such a loss of sugar appears to be a waste by the kidneys, but the same is true of amino acids and water-soluble vitamins and a number of other nutrients. The reason for such increased excretion by the kidneys and the apparent waste is not known.

The urine of pregnant women is tested for glucose at each antepartum visit. A dip stick, to which a reagent specific for reaction with glucose is affixed, is used for the testing. It is dipped into freshly voided urine, and the reagent is checked for a color change that will take place if glucose is present. The results are read by comparing the color change in the reagent with a color chart, which is read as negative, or light, medium, or dark, signifying varying degrees of positive reaction. The results are qualitative, indicating negative or the presence of glucose in relative amounts from small to large. Approximately 0.1 gm of glucose per 100 ml of urine is detectable.

Although glucosuria is common in normal pregnancy, it should not be ignored. The possibility of diabetes mellitus must be considered. All pregnant women, however, whether or not they have glucosuria should be screened for diabetes by blood testing according to the regimen described in Chapter 9.

Proteinuria

Proteins (albumin, globulin) are abnormal constituents of the urine. Proteinuria is an important sign of renal disease, and it is commonly present in preeclampsia. Measurement of urinary protein excretion is therefore one of the most valuable tests of renal function. Although trace amounts of protein normally may be found in concentrated urine, it is difficult to detect in such small amounts. Protein excretion is abnormal in nonpregnant women when the total daily excretion exceeds 150 mg. Normal pregnant women may excrete slightly more because of their increased glomerular blood supply and their tendency to lordosis, but an amount over 250 mg per day is considered excessive.

Since proteinuria is an important sign of abnormal

renal function and a characteristic sign in preeclampsia, measurement of urinary protein excretion is an essential test in pregnancy for both discovery of renal disease and detection of preeclampsia. The urine of pregnant women therefore is examined for protein at each antepartum visit.

A rapid, convenient, and sensitive method of detecting protein in urine is based on a color-producing reaction between albumin and a reagent dye at the end of a dip stick. The albumin reagent stick is a very satisfactory semiquantitative measure of small amounts of protein in the urine.

The reagent end of the dip stick is dipped into *freshly voided* urine, or the mother is asked to pass the reagent end of the stick through a stream of urine. A clean, midstream-voided specimen should be used to reduce the chance of contamination of the urine with vaginal discharge. The dip stick is read by comparison with a color chart. The protein reagent's color change may read negative, or trace (5 to 20 mg of albumin per 100 ml of urine), or present in 30, 100, 300, or 1000 or more mg of protein (albumin) per 100 ml of urine. When the dip stick reaction to protein is more than a trace, a 24-hour urine specimen may be necessary to assess accurately the total daily excretion.

Clinical Tests of Renal Function

Clinical tests of renal function and for evidence of renal disease include complete urinalysis, testing of urine for glucose and protein, and evaluation of glomerular filtration rate by creatinine clearance or urea clearance tests if this seems indicated.

Microscopic Examination

Microscopic examination of the urine is valuable in detecting renal disease. A morning, first-voided specimen is preferable, since it will be more concentrated than urine voided at other times of the day. Casts, red blood cells, white blood cells, and epithelial cells are abnormal constituents of the urine, are interpreted as evidence of renal lesions, and require further investigation. Testing for the presence of glucose and protein has been described above.

Glomerular Filtration Test

A commonly used clinical test for evaluation of glomerular filtration consists of measurement of blood creatinine and creatinine clearance in the urine. Measurement of plasma creatinine is made at the same time that urine is collected for the test because clearance is calculated from the amount excreted within a unit of time and its concentration in the plasma. Measurement of blood urea and urea clearance in the urine may be used in assessment of renal function, but these measurements are influenced by a number of factors that may influence results adversely and make interpretation difficult.

Creatinine is cleared primarily by glomerular filtration, whereas urea clearance measures a composite of glomerular and tubular function. Creatinine clearance is a practical measure of GFR and therefore of renal function. It can be followed serially if necessary during pregnancy. With normal renal function, the results of urea clearance tests in pregnancy should be expected to average 30 to 50 percent above normal, nonpregnant values. Normal creatinine clearance in the nonpregnant person is approximately 100 ml/min; normal pregnancy values will be 140 to 150 ml/min.

Other Clinical Function Tests

The phenolsulfonphthalein (PSP) test for renal plasma flow is invalid during pregnancy. Owing to the dilated ureters and the increased dead space of the urinary tract during pregnancy, there is often a lag in the appearance of the dye in the bladder. An apparent below-normal excretion of PSP is not meaningful because excretion of the dye may be normal but seem to be impaired, owing to the lag in appearance.

Urine concentration-dilution tests are occasionally used to measure kidney function. These tests are likely to give misleading results in pregnancy because of the diurnal pattern of urinary flow. Even when fluids have been properly withheld to test the ability of the kidneys to concentrate urine, mobilization of edema fluid at night causes the urine to be more dilute in the morning than in the nonpregnant state. If such tests are done during pregnancy, the woman should be in bed and lie in the lateral recumbent position in order to assure normal kidney function.

Summary of Renal Function

Alterations in the renal system in pregnancy include both anatomic and functional changes. Dilation of the kidney pelves and ureters brings about changes that result in stagnation of urine. Stasis of urine may interfere with accurate urine testing, and it is a factor in the tendency to urinary tract infections in pregnancy.

Renal plasma flow and glomerular filtration rate increase markedly in pregnancy and bring about a great increase in filtration of a number of substances such as metabolic waste products, nutrients, and electrolytes.

Unless reabsorption of many of these substances is also increased, there will be a greater than normal output, and a deficit will quickly occur.

Enhanced renal clearance in pregnancy means more effective excretion of waste products, creatinine, urea, and uric acid. As a result, blood level values of these products in pregnancy are normally two thirds of nonpregnant values and urine clearance tests of waste products in pregnancy should average 30 to 50 percent above normal nonpregnant values.

Enhanced renal clearance also means rapid clearance of sodium and water and of glucose and other nutrients. Tubular reabsorption must increase and keep pace with filtration of these substances to prevent their rapid depletion in the body.

Sodium is a substance that is freely filtered at the glomeruli, being promoted by increased GFR and an increase in progesterone, which antagonizes the effect of aldosterone. A quick adjustment in the reabsorption of sodium, equal to the amount filtered, is critical to maternal homeostasis. To overcome the increased excretion of sodium, a compensatory mechanism, the renin-angiotensin-aldosterone system, produces aldosterone in large amounts. The aldosterone enhances tubular reabsorption of sodium as necessary to prevent sodium depletion.

There is a tendency toward sodium depletion in pregnancy and yet also a need to accumulate a total of 500 to 900 mEq of sodium during pregnancy for fetal needs and for expansion of maternal fluid volume. Although aldosterone production adjusts to need, restriction of dietary sodium or use of diuretic drugs may unduly stress the system, interfere with sodium reabsorption, and exaggerate sodium depletion.

Water excretion is excellent in early pregnancy, but later declines. In late pregnancy water pools in the lower extremities and excretion is below nonpregnant averages.

The supine and upright positions (sitting and standing) reduce GFR and excretion of both water and sodium. In these positions, pooling of blood in the legs and decreasing circulating blood volume bring about renal vasoconstriction and a reduced renal blood flow. Pregnant women with edema thus may be advised to lie on their side, preferably left, to improve excretion of fluid and sodium.

Glucosuria is common in pregnancy and may be present intermittently. It is caused in part by increased GFR and an inability of the renal tubules to reabsorb all that is filtered. Maximum tubular reabsorption also may be lowered in pregnancy so that spillage of glucose begins at a lower blood sugar value than in nonpregnant persons. Glucosuria, although common, requires evaluation.

Proteinuria is abnormal in pregnancy, signifying the presence of preeclampsia, renal disease, or urinary tract infection. Measurement of urinary protein excretion is a very valuable test of renal function, and the urine should be examined for protein at each antepartum visit.

CHANGES IN BODY WEIGHT

Components of, and Extent of, Normal Weight Gain

An increase in body weight is one of the metabolic changes of pregnancy. The total weight gain of a well-nourished pregnant woman at 40 weeks' gestation is usually between 10 and 12.5 kg (22 and 27.5 lb); the average is 11 kg (24 lb). Whether or not such a gain is optimal is not certain, nor is it known if specific gains are likely to be optimal for all persons. Some healthy individuals with a normal pregnancy will gain considerably more than the above average.

The weight gain of pregnancy includes weight of the fetus of approximately 3400 gm (7 1/2 lb), placenta of about 650 gm (1 1/2 lb), and amniotic fluid of 800 to 1000 gm (1 3/4 to 2 1/4 lb). The increase in uterine muscle accounts for approximately 900 gm (2 lb), and an increase in the glandular tissue of the breasts adds from 400 to 500 gm (1 lb). The increase in maternal blood volume during pregnancy adds a weight of approximately 1300 to 1500 gm (3 to 3 1/4 lb), and an increase in extracellular fluid toward the end of pregnancy adds another 1500 gm (3 1/4 lb) or more to the total weight gain in pregnancy (Fig. 8–21).

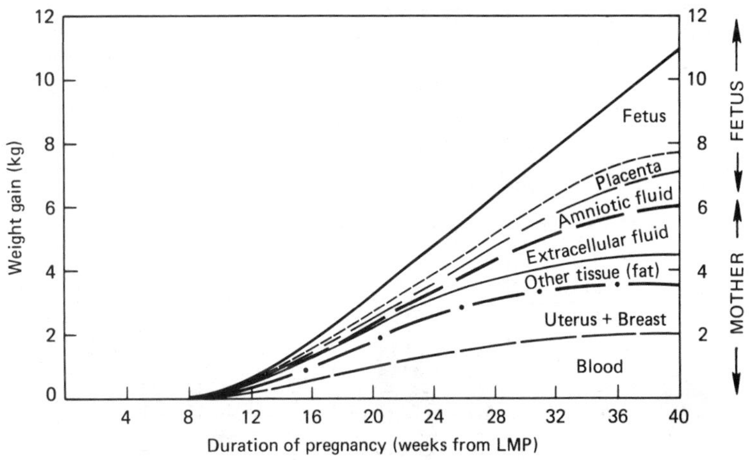

Figure 8–21. Patterns and components of average maternal weight gain during pregnancy. (Reproduced with permission from Roy M. Pitkin, "Nutritional Support in Obstetrics and Gynecology." *Clin. Obstet. Gynecol.* 19(3): 489–513 (Sept.) 1976, p. 491.)

Growth of the products of conception, growth of the maternal organs of reproduction, and increases in maternal blood volume and extracellular fluid account for approximately 9000 gm (20 lb). It is apparent from the components of weight gain listed above that a gain of 9 kg (20 lb) is the minimum that should be expected at term pregnancy. A gain of less than 9 kg (20 lb) means that the mother must be catabolizing her own tissues to some degree.

The weight gain not accounted for by the increases named above appears to consist mainly of maternal stores of fatty tissue.

In enumerating the components of weight gain above, an increase of extracellular fluid was listed as accounting for an average of 1500 gm (3 1/4 lb) of the total weight. If the woman develops clinical edema, even when it is slight, she may have as much as 5 liters (11 lb) or even more of extra fluid in her tissues. Such retention of tissue fluid may add considerably to her weight in the last weeks of pregnancy. This weight, however, is quickly lost after delivery.

Weight gain during pregnancy follows a slightly sigmoid upward trend (Fig. 8-22). There is little gain during the first trimester, rapid increase during the second trimester, and a slightly slower increase during the third trimester. With an average weight gain of 11 kg (24 lb), the gain may be about 1 to 1 1/2 kg (2 1/4 to 3 1/4 lb) during the first trimester, 5 to 6 kg (11 to 13 lb) during the second trimester, and 4 to 5 kg (9 to 11 lb) during the third trimester. At 20 weeks a gain of about 3 3/4 kg (8 lb) can be expected, and at 30 weeks approximately 8 kg (18 lb) normally will have been gained. During the second half of pregnancy a gain of 350 to 450 gm (3/4 to 1 lb) per week will keep the weight gain within a favorable range. A weight gain of only 1000 gm (2 1/4 lb) per month is not adequate, and one of 3000 gm (6 1/2 lb) per month may be excessive for many women.

About 5 kg (11 lb) of the weight gain of pregnancy are lost at the time of delivery of the fetus, placenta, and amniotic fluid. Another 2 to 2 1/2 kg (4 1/2 to 5 1/2 lb) are lost in the immediate puerperium, largely due to release and elimination of the extracellular fluid in the tissues. A still further reduction occurs during the succeeding weeks when the mother's body returns to approximately its prepregnant state. Most women, especially if they breast-feed their infants, continue to lose weight for at least three months after delivery, and all but a small number eventually lose all of the weight they gained dur-

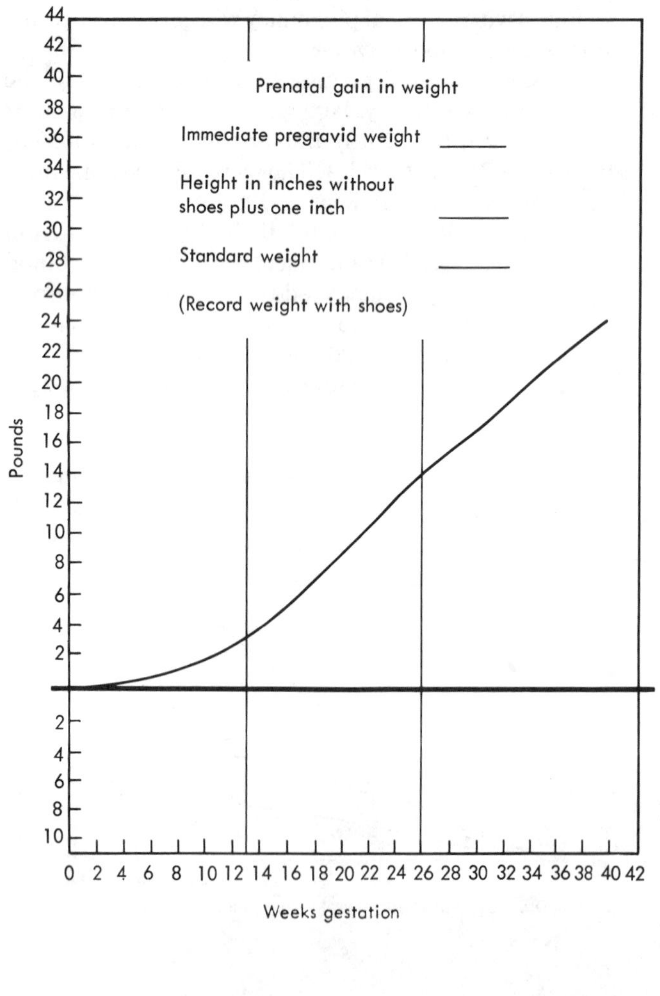

Figure 8–22. Pattern of normal prenatal gain in weight. Use of a grid with pounds listed along the vertical sides and weeks gestation along the lower horizontal line will be very helpful in assessing the pregnant woman's weight gain pattern. Each weight measurement is recorded and observed for its trend in relation to the weights recorded at previous measurements.

ing pregnancy. If there has been an excessive amount of fat storage and it is not lost between pregnancies, it may contribute to later obesity.

Body Fat Storage

Fat storage appears to be one of the normal physiologic processes of pregnancy. In women with an average weight gain, the stores of fat may account for 2300 to 3300 gm (5 to 7 1/4 lb). Fat deposition begins early in pregnancy and slows late in pregnancy (Fig. 8–21). Most of the fat deposit apparently has been stored by 30 weeks' gestation, and little more is laid down thereafter. Weight gain after 30 weeks' gestation is from growth of the products of conception and from fluid retention. It appears that when the nutritional needs of the fetus increase in the latter weeks of pregnancy, the storage of body fat is considerably slowed.

The reason for storage of body fat in pregnancy is not known exactly. There seems to be some evidence that progesterone may provide the mechanism for storage. It is believed that the body fat serves as a potential energy supply which could be used in late pregnancy. Such use probably would become necessary only in a society where women work hard until the end of pregnancy. Theoretically such storage of body fat might protect mother and fetus during times of starvation or excessive physical exertion. For women in a relatively affluent society, such storage may not be necessary, but diet restriction to control fat storage is likely to be unwise in pregnancy. However, if fat storage becomes excessive and is not lost in the puerperium, it may become a significant component of excess weight later in life.

If the mother nurses her infant, the fat deposit of pregnancy may be used for some of the energy requirements of lactation.

Generalized Edema

One of the metabolic alterations of pregnancy is an increased tendency of the body to retain water in all of its tissues. Total body water increases continuously throughout pregnancy. This includes water accumulated in the products of conception, the added maternal tissues and the blood, and water in the maternal extracellular tissue spaces. The extravascular, extracellular fluid may or may not be clinically apparent as edema. When edema does develop, it is usually not evident until after 30 weeks' gestation, and it is likely to be most obvious in the last few weeks of pregnancy.

A certain amount of edema seems to be a normal physiologic accompaniment of pregnancy. It is often confined to the lower extremities (see page 148) but also may be perceptible elsewhere, as in the face and hands, probably noticed mainly by tightness of the rings. An *abnormal* amount of generalized fluid retention is often associated with preeclampsia as described in Chapter 14.

It has been estimated that women with no evidence of clinical edema, or with leg edema only, have an increase of 2 1/2 to 3 liters of body water that cannot be accounted for in the fetal tissues and the added maternal tissues and blood. When generalized, although only slight, edema develops, there appears to be an excess of body water that averages about 5 liters at term. This excess or surplus body water is assumed to be mainly fluid in the extracellular spaces. Retention of surplus water and edema will be reflected in the weight gain of the pregnant woman. Retention of even several liters of extracellular fluid may mean 2000 to 4000 gm (4 to 8 lb) of additional weight.

Although edema of the legs is common in late pregnancy, there is some evidence to suggest that the fluid in the legs represents only a small part of the total extracellular fluid increase in pregnancy. There is some reason to believe that much of the extracellular fluid is held in the skin. It is considered probable that estrogens bring about an increased mobility and distensibility of connective tissue in the body, and that the skin, which has large amounts of connective tissue, can hold much of the excess fluid. This may or may not appear as clinical edema.

In late pregnancy, especially when edema of the lower extremities is common, there may be fairly large diurnal variations in body fluid. Edema of the legs often decreases considerably after a period of rest in bed. Some of this change may be the result of redistribution of fluid, but often there is also a diuresis, especially when the woman assumes the lateral recumbent position.

Reversal of water retention, with release of accumulated extracellular fluid, occurs during the first few days after delivery. Diuresis is apparent during the first day or two post partum, and weight loss is greater during the first week of the puerperium than in the succeeding weeks.

CHANGES IN THE GASTROINTESTINAL TRACT

Changes in the digestive tract during pregnancy are signified by nausea and possibly vomiting in early pregnancy; heartburn and eructations; flatulence; and constipation, which may be most troublesome during the latter part of pregnancy. The appetite may be very capricious during the early weeks of pregnancy or it may be increased. Cravings for, or aversions to, certain foods without apparent reason are common. *Pica,* a craving for unusual substances that are not considered food, such as chalk, laundry starch, or clay, also is present sometimes.

Nausea and *vomiting* are very common disturbances in early pregnancy, occurring to some degree in about 50 percent of expectant mothers. The symptoms vary from the slightest feeling of nausea when the woman first raises her head in the morning to persistent and frequent vomiting, which then assumes a serious condition. Nausea and/or vomiting may appear at any time of the day but is most common in the early morning upon arising. Nausea and vomiting will usually disappear at the end of the first trimester.

There may be changes in the mouth tissues in pregnancy. The gums often become swollen. Some women develop a pregnancy *gingivitis,* characterized by edematous spongy gums, which bleed easily and may show some detachment. The edema is believed to be a part of the general change in the connective tissue ground substance that is caused by the estrogens in the body. Pregnancy usually does not affect the teeth adversely, but an occasional woman has an increase in dental caries in pregnancy.

Pyrosis (heartburn), a painful retrosternal burning sensation, often described as a feeling of burning first in the stomach and then rising into the throat, and eructations are fairly common. Heartburn is caused by frequent regurgitations of acidic gastric contents into the esophagus. This influx of secretions may be the result of changed position and general relaxation of the stomach in pregnancy and, along with it, relaxation of the cardiac sphincter, especially when intraabdominal pressure is raised. To decrease discomfort from heartburn it is advisable to avoid foods that tend to cause distress or to limit their intake. These include fatty foods, chocolate, citrus fruits, and coffee. It is also wise to eat small meals and to avoid lying flat immediately after eating.

Gastric secretion is reduced in pregnancy, a relative hypochlorhydria is present, and gastric tone and mobility are slowed. Thus, food is retained in the stomach longer. The enlarging uterus causes the stomach to be displaced upward and to rotate to the right. The large bowel and the cecum are also displaced upward, and the rest of the intestinal tract is pushed to the sides and behind the uterus (Figs. 8–5 and 8–6). The appendix is usually displaced upward and laterally.

A *general relaxation of tone* of the entire gastrointestinal tract is characteristic of smooth muscle relaxation in pregnancy and appears concomitant with relaxation of smooth muscle of other parts of the body such as the uterus, the ureters, and the blood vessels. Large amounts of progesterone apparently contribute to this muscle relaxation. It is felt that the relaxation of the gastrointestinal tract may contribute to the common occurrences of nausea and constipation in pregnancy.

Constipation appears to be present in at least one half of all pregnant women. It may become a considerable problem, especially for the woman who previously had a tendency to constipation. Bowel relaxation is considered a major cause of constipation in pregnancy, but impaired tone of the stretched abdominal muscles also may be a contributing factor. Decreased mobility of the gastrointestinal tract also may permit gas to accumulate in the bowel to an uncomfortable extent.

Digestion and absorption of foods seem to be very efficient in pregnancy and apparently are not adversely influenced by the poor tone of the intestinal tract.

CHANGES IN CARBOHYDRATE METABOLISM

Pregnancy is associated with considerable change in carbohydrate metabolism. The following discussion of these changes begins with a brief account of some of the basic mechanisms in carbohydrate metabolism in the nonpregnant individual. This is followed by a description of how these mechanisms are altered by several factors in pregnancy.

Carbohydrate Metabolism in the Nonpregnant Individual

The intermittent ingestion of food and the steady requirement of the body for energy make some mechanism for metabolic homeostasis essential. Such homeostasis is achieved by a series of complex processes that function to keep the blood glucose level within a range of 70 to 110 mg per 100 ml of blood. The blood glucose is maintained at a relatively constant and appropriate level by metabolism and storage of the foods that are absorbed; by hormones, mainly insulin; and by liberation of glucose into the circulation by the liver to counterbalance the amount of glucose that is taken out of the blood by the tissues.

The level of blood glucose at any given time is the balance between sources of glucose to the blood and the demands made on it by the tissues. A change in one direction or the other toward hypoglycemia or hyperglycemia is normally counteracted by mechanisms that bring the blood sugar back to a normoglycemic range. As glucose is taken out of the circulation by the tissues, more glucose, although not necessarily a similar amount, is added through liberation by the liver. Many individuals, however, will experience hypoglycemia after a short fast that can be corrected by eating. The liver is the principal regulator of the blood sugar level. The blood sugar level has an important regulatory influence on protein and fat metabolism as well as carbohydrate metabolism.

Glucose is supplied to the blood from three general sources: (1) absorption of food carbohydrate from the small intestine, (2) breakdown of glycogen that is stored in the liver to glucose, and (3) formation of glucose by the liver from certain amino acids and a very small amount of glycerol. Glucose, obtained from breakdown of glycogen which has been stored in the liver, is liberated at times when food carbohydrate is not available. The glycogen reserve in the liver is a short-term source of blood glucose because it can be depleted within 24 hours if food is not taken. Manufacture of glucose by the liver from amino acid and glycerol precursors maintains the blood sugar when glycogen stores become exhausted and over a more sustained period of time.

Glucose is removed from the blood by (1) the cells that utilize it for energy, (2) the liver for storage as glycogen, and (3) conversion to fat for storage.

Immediately after a meal the blood sugar rises to 120 to 130 mg per 100 ml of blood. After several hours the blood glucose level is back to 70 to 100 mg percent and is maintained at that level between meals, even though glucose is constantly used by the tissues. When a glucose load from food comes to the liver and into the circulation, it is soon removed from the blood by utilization for cell energy and by conversion into stores of glycogen and fat. This assures that the blood sugar level does not stay elevated for very long and that stores are built up for later use.

In normal individuals the plasma insulin level rises and falls in response to increases and decreases in blood sugar. Increased blood glucose levels stimulate the beta cells of the islets of Langerhans in the pancreas to secrete insulin. In this way, insulin regulates use and storage of food supplies. As the blood glucose level rises with a meal, the plasma insulin level also rises. Absorption of a glucose load from the gastrointestinal tract is accompanied by a relatively large spurt of insulin, which is secreted in response to the hyperglycemia and to some undetermined intestinal factor.

Insulin stimulates the various processes that will lower the blood glucose level. It stimulates the tissues to utilize glucose as a major source of energy. An important and fundamental effect of insulin is to facilitate the entry of glucose into tissue cells and thus make possible the utilization of glucose by muscle and adipose tissue. Insulin also stimulates conversion of glucose to glycogen and to fat, each to be stored for later use. With these processes functioning adequately, production of glucose from protein and fat is not necessary at this time, and protein is conserved, being made available for repair and growth of tissue. Insulin thus serves to promote storage of carbohydrate, protein, and fat during the hours of an abundant supply.

When the supply of glucose from food is diminished, there is a decrease in insulin secretion as well. Thus, the plasma insulin level falls between meals. Low levels of insulin cause decreased use of glucose by muscle and adipose tissue cells; most tissues then begin to increase their utilization of fatty acids for their metabolic needs. Lipolysis of adipose tissue stores is very sensitive to drops in insulin; this then provides for an accelerated release of fatty acids for use for tissue energy. A decrease in insulin also shifts protein synthesis to a certain degree of protein breakdown. The amino acids thus released may then be used by the liver as precursors for synthesis of glucose.

The glucose synthesized by the liver is used mainly to meet the energy requirements of the brain. Other tissues are utilizing fatty acids for energy. They use only a minimal amount of carbohydrates during hypoinsulinemia. Central nervous system tissue depends on a continuous supply of glucose from the blood. These cells do not store glycogen, but glucose is indispensable to them for their fuel and to their function. Utilization of glucose by brain cells is not dependent upon insulin as it is for many other cells of the body, therefore the plasma insulin level is not important to them.

In certain circumstances, when there are insufficient carbohydrate supplies, metabolism of fatty acids may become excessive while meeting the body's energy needs and ketone bodies may accumulate in the tissues. As fatty acids are oxidized, formation of ketone bodies takes place. Ordinarily the rate of fat catabolism and ketone body formation is such that the ketone bodies are promptly and completely oxidized by the peripheral tissues. When fatty acid breakdown becomes excessive, formation of ketone bodies in the liver exceeds the rate by which the peripheral tissues can oxidize and dispose of them. Ketone bodies—beta-hydroxybutyric acid and acetoacetic acid—then accumulate in the blood and tissues and are also excreted in the urine. An accumulation of ketones in the blood above normal concentration is termed ketosis.

One condition in which ketone bodies increase to excess is fasting, a time during which the rate of catabolism of fatty acids is high in order to meet the body's energy needs. Such starvation ketosis can be corrected by an intake of carbohydrate. The carbohydrate will replenish the liver glycogen and restore normal carbohydrate metabolism, it will inhibit output of fatty acids, and the glucose will stimulate utilization of ketone bodies by the peripheral tissus.

Starvation ketosis differs from ketosis in a person with diabetes, who has an adequate supply of carbohydrates that cannot be properly utilized because of an inadequate supply of insulin. Excess fatty acid catabolism and ketone formation then take place. Diabetic ketosis is corrected by administration of insulin, whereas starvation ketosis requires only carbohydrates. A diabetic, however, could also develop starvation ketosis if carbohydrate intake was not adequate. The results of both ketotic processes are the same on the developing fetus and should be avoided.

Carbohydrate Metabolism in Pregnancy

The fetus is totally dependent on the mother for his nutrition, and he receives a continuous supply of glucose from her for his energy needs. Also, in pregnancy large amounts of hormones that interfere with the action of insulin make their appearance. These two major factors, plus several others of lesser importance, alter carbohydrate metabolism and make adjustments a necessity.

Tendency to Hypoglycemia

FETAL GLUCOSE NEEDS The fuel requirements of the fetus are met entirely by glucose obtained from the mother. The fetus uses glucose (1) for his maintenance energy needs, (2) to provide the energy necessary to synthesize proteins for his growth, (3) as a precursor in the synthesis of fat, and (4) for formation of his own glycogen stores. It has been estimated that the fetus utilizes glucose for his oxidation and synthesis needs at the rate of 6 mg per kilogram of body weight per minute, which is two to three times greater than that used by an adult per kilogram per minute.

Blood glucose level in the fetus is 20 to 30 mg per 100 ml of blood lower than maternal blood glucose. This would permit transfer of glucose by simple diffusion, but it is believed that glucose is transferred across the placenta from mother to fetus at a faster rate and that facilitated diffusion takes place at a fairly rapid rate. Insulin does not cross the placenta, but the fetus has his own insulin by 12 weeks of age. He can utilize maternal glucose independent of maternal insulin, and he can respond with his own insulin production, at least to some degree, to the amount of available glucose and amino acids.

Amino acids are actively transported across the placenta from the maternal to the fetal circulation. This results in a lowered level of blood amino acids in the mother. Since the mother uses amino acids, especially alanine, as precursors for glucose formation by the liver when she is in a fasting state, the fetus is drawing glucose precursors as well as glucose from the mother.

There is a distinct lowering of fasting blood glucose values in the mother beginning fairly early in pregnancy. As early as 15 weeks' gestation the mother's blood sugar values after an overnight fast are 15 to 20 mg lower per 100 ml of blood than after a similar fast in a nonpregnant individual. Blood sugar level drops even a greater amount if the mother is without food for a longer period of time, and hypoglycemia then becomes significant.

GLUCOSURIA Loss of glucose in the urine is a possible factor in lowering blood sugar. An increased glomerular filtration rate in pregnancy means that an increased amount of glucose is filtered out. If the renal tubules cannot increase reabsorption of glucose at the same rate that it is filtered, some glucose will be lost in the urine. It is thought that maximum glucose tubular reabsorption may be lower in pregnancy than at other times. This would mean that glucose could be lost at a lower blood glucose level in pregnancy than in the nonpregnant state. Glucosuria is present intermittently in many pregnant women.

Tendency to Ketosis

Since insulin production is lowered as blood sugar is lowered, the mother whose blood sugar is falling will also have a fall in plasma insulin levels. Pregnancy exaggerates and accelerates the response to fasting. Both blood glucose and plasma insulin levels fall more rapidly than in the nonpregnant woman. This precipitates an acceleration of the processes that lead to ketosis during fasting.

The lowered insulin levels bring about utilization of fatty acids for energy and release of amino acids as described above. Metabolism of an excessive amount of fatty acids, especially in the absence of carbohydrates, results in release of a large number of ketone bodies. Blood levels of beta-hydroxybutyric acid and acetoacetic acid are two to four times higher in pregnancy after an overnight fast than in the nonpregnant individual.

Ketone bodies are transferred across the placenta, and they may help to meet fuel requirements in the fetus if the glucose supply is limited, but this may not be without danger. There is some evidence that use of ketones by the fetus, or possibly some of the metabolic changes that accompany ketosis, have an adverse effect on fetal brain development.

Tendency to Hyperglycemia

Maternal peripheral tissues become progressively resistant to the hypoglycemic effects of insulin in the course of pregnancy. This progressive insulin antagonism is the result of increased secretion of hormones, primarily by the placenta, that interfere with the action of insulin. Secretion of hormones increases as pregnancy advances and as the placenta grows, making their effect most noticeable in the latter half of pregnancy. Four hormones appear to exert a major influence on carbohydrate metabolism in pregnancy.

HUMAN CHORIONIC SOMATOMAMMOTROPIN HCS is known to exert a significant anti-insulin effect. It augments insulin secretion but diminishes its peripheral effectiveness. By diminishing the effect of insulin, HCS reduces utilization of glucose by the mother. It also causes a marked increase in mobilization of fatty acids from fat depots, and it appears to have some anabolic effect on protein metabolism.

HCS has been described as a hormone that enhances utilization of fatty acids by the mother and reduces her utilization of glucose and protein breakdown. In this way it enhances glucose and amino acid availability to the fetus, providing for a constant flow of these nutrients from mother to fetus. This promotion of lipid metabolism by HCS, together with hypoinsulinemia, also leads to increased production of ketone bodies.

HCS is secreted in increasing amounts in pregnancy, and its concentration in maternal plasma is especially high in the last trimester. Some studies have shown a rise in HCS during nutritional deprivation.

ESTROGEN AND PROGESTERONE The placental sex hormones, estrogen and progesterone, are secreted in increasing amounts in pregnancy. The exact influence of these hormones is not clear, but it appears that both augment insulin secretion and at the same time act as insulin antagonists.

CORTISOL Maternal carbohydrate metabolism may be influenced by increasing plasma levels of cortisol in pregnancy. This rise in cortisol has generally been attributed to a rise in the metabolically inactive bound hormone, but it is not known if the bound hormone is completely inactive. Also, recent studies have indicated that the concentration of free cortisol promotes insulin secretion, but at the same time antagonizes peripheral insulin action. Cortisol induces mobilization of protein during fasting, thus increasing glucose production in the liver and contributing to hyperglycemia. Cortisol also contributes to mobilization of fat during fasting.

Maternal Increasing Insulin Requirement

A constant increase in hormones antagonistic to insulin as pregnancy progresses means that more and more insulin is needed to regulate the storage and utilization of the body's energy supplies and keep the blood sugar below a hyperglycemic level. There is a significant need for increased insulin by the middle of pregnancy, and the need is even greater in the last trimester when placental hormones reach peak concentrations.

As more insulin is needed in pregnancy to overcome the hormonal anti-insulin effects, the beta cells produce more and more insulin to attempt to maintain homeostasis of carbohydrate metabolism. The anti-insulin effects of the hormones are matched by insulin production.

Anti-insulin effects do not appear to be present in the first trimester of pregnancy. When exogenous insulin is used by diabetics, its hypoglycemic effects appear to be slightly increased in the first trimester. Thereafter, however, the effect of insulin diminishes considerably and progressively.

Requirement for an increasing amount of insulin secretion in pregnancy places a stress on the beta cells, but they are usually able to meet the demand. For the woman who has a tendency toward a disordered carbohydrate metabolism, the stress of providing more and more insulin may become too great during the latter half of pregnancy. She may develop hyperglycemia and have an abnormally high two-hour postprandial blood sugar. She is then identified as having gestational diabetes, described in Chapter 15. The purpose of blood sugar screening in late second trimester of pregnancy as noted on page 185 is to identify the clients in whom the challenge to insulin production becomes too great.

For the pregnant diabetic, the increasing production of anti-insulin hormones and increasing need for insulin require very frequent monitoring and insulin dosage adjustment throughout pregnancy to maintain homeostasis.

Although the increase in insulin production in pregnancy brings the postprandial plasma insulin level up, the fasting insulin level still tends to be quite low. This occurs because of the tendency toward fasting hypoglycemia, which is present at all times during pregnancy.

Summary of Carbohydrate Metabolism

Fuel metabolism in pregnancy is associated with marked alterations. There is an overall tendency to fasting hypoglycemia in pregnancy, which is characterized by low blood sugar, a lowered level of circulating amino acids, an increase in free fatty acids, a low level of plasma insulin, and an increase in ketone bodies. This metabolic condition has been described as one of "accelerated starvation," since it rapidly shows the characteristic responses to starvation.

Pregnancy is also said to have a diabetogenic influence on the mother. Her peripheral tissue response to insulin is decreased and two-hour postprandial blood glucose levels tend to be in the upper limits of normal.

The two seemingly opposite conditions of tendency to hypoglycemia and tendency to hyperglycemia are the result of the fetus continuously taking food supplies from the maternal circulation, producing a hypoglycemic state, and the placenta producing hormones that interfere with the action of insulin, especially in the last half of pregnancy. The beta cells produce an increasing amount of insulin to counterbalance the hormonal influence.

In the normal pregnant woman an equilibrium usually exists between the various factors that alter carbohydrate metabolism, and she remains nearly normoglycemic. If the client has a tendency to disordered carbohydrate metabolism, she may show an abnormal glucose tolerance as pregnancy progresses.

With the tendency to hypoglycemia in pregnancy, it is important to minimize the likelihood of starvation ketosis and its possible adverse effects on the fetus. Caloric restrictions or weight reduction programs should not be imposed on the mother at any time during pregnancy. It is advisable for her to eat food at fairly regular times; to avoid long periods of fasting, such as an overnight fast plus omitting breakfast; and to maintain a minimal intake of 150 gm of carbohydrate per day even when it may seem necessary for her to slow her rate of weight gain.

After delivery, placental anti-insulin hormones are rapidly metabolized and excreted from the body. Insulin requirements are quickly decreased. In the normal woman a physiologic adjustment in carbohydrate metabolism is apparently made without difficulty. For the diabetic, insulin sensitivity is considerably increased immediately after delivery. Her requirements for insulin probably fall well below prepregnancy levels in the first days of the puerperium. From there, adjustments in insulin dosage are made according to blood and urine glucose determinations.

CHANGES IN THE MUSCULOSKELETAL SYSTEM

Changes in the skeleton of pregnant women are characterized by softening of the pelvic cartilages and increased mobility of the joints of the sacroiliacs, the sacrococcygeal, and the symphysis pubis. There is a marked relaxation of ligaments, probably the effect of both estrogens and relaxin.

The increased size and weight of the uterus during pregnancy shift the center of gravity forward, increasing the normal amount of lordosis as an effort is made to balance the body. If the abdominal muscles are relaxed and in poor tone before pregnancy, the abdomen may protrude markedly as the uterus enlarges. This is followed by a great increase in the forward tilt of the pelvis, an increased strain at the sacroiliac joints, and marked lordosis.

Occasionally the marked lordosis may lead to anterior flexion of the neck and slumping of the shoulders and possibly aching and weakness of the upper extremities.

Change in posture during pregnancy, progressive lordosis, and increased mobility and instability of the pelvic joints tend to cause tripping and falling, result in a waddling gait, and commonly lead to backache. See Chapter 11 for discussion of backache in pregnancy.

CHANGES IN THE SKIN

Skin changes in pregnancy consist of increased blood flow, appearance of vascular spiders, increased coloration of pigmented areas, appearance of striae, and possibly increased activity of the sebaceous and sweat glands and the hair follicles. The increase in blood flow, the possible appearance or increase in size of vascular spiders and hemangiomas, and increase in hair follicle activity have been described on page 146.

During the latter part of pregnancy, irregular, wavy, slightly depressed streaks or striations frequently develop in the skin of the abdomen and sometimes also in the skin of the breasts, hips, and upper part of the thighs. These striations are termed *striae gravidarum.* Fresh striae are pale pink or bluish in color. After delivery, they take on the silvery, glistening appearance of scar tissue. In a woman who has borne children, there may be both new and old striae, those resulting from former pregnancies are silvery and shining and are termed *striae albicantes,* while the fresh striae are pink or blue (Fig. 8–23).

Two factors are involved in the formation of striae, and it appears that both factors need to be present. The skin is primed for separation of its collagen fibers by hormones of pregnancy, and the primed skin then gets tension (stretch) placed on it by the enlarging uterus.

Estrogens, corticosteroids, and relaxin, hormones that are formed in increasing amounts in pregnancy, produce changes in the connective tissue of the skin. Under this hormonal influence, the cohesive force between the collagen fibers of the skin relaxes, allowing the fibers to separate easily. When the primed skin is subjected to stretching, some of the collagen fibers pull apart, resulting in a thinning of the skin (striae), which appear pinkish or bluish, depending on the vascular bed.

Striae develop in areas of maximum stretch: the abdomen, breasts, and thighs. Subcutaneous fat increases in pregnancy and stretches the skin above it. Considerable weight gain in pregnancy, obesity from the beginning of pregnancy, unusual stretching of the abdominal skin, and fluid retention and generalized edema are all likely to increase stretching of the skin. Some women are much more susceptible than others to separation of the connective tissue of the skin; thus, some women have many striae and others with a similar amount of stretching have few or none.

Abdominal striae in nonpregnant women occasionally may be associated with abdominal distention, a marked increase in fat, or an abdominal tumor. Those on the hips and thighs may be due to normal postpubertal changes.

As a result of increased coloration, the nipples and areolar areas of the breasts grow darker. The umbilical area becomes more pigmented. The *linea alba,* a whitish line that divides the abdomen longitudinally from sternum to symphysis pubis, becomes darker and is then known as the *linea nigra.* This line grows progressively paler after delivery (Fig. 8–23).

Brownish, irregularly shaped blotches sometimes appear on the face and in a masklike distribution around the eyes and over the nose and cheekbones. These are

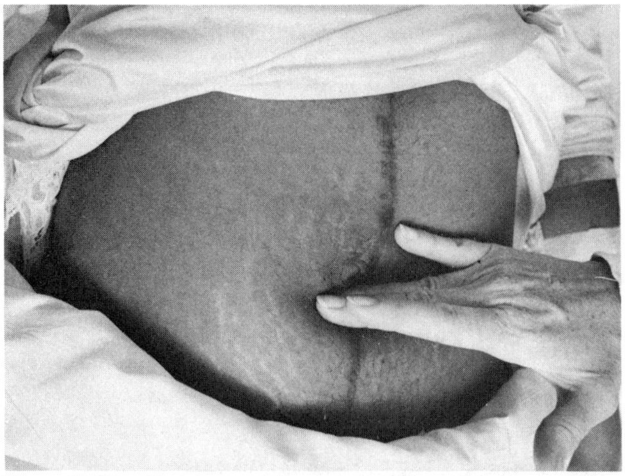

Figure 8–23. Pregnant abdomen showing striae gravidarum (lower right quadrant) and linea nigra. The nurse is palpating the uterus prior to measuring fundal height (See Chapter 9). [Courtesy of The Presbyterian Hospital in the City of New York. Photo by Elizabeth Marshall.]

termed *chloasma,* or mask of pregnancy. Dark circles under the eyes are common.

Changes in skin pigment are probably brought about by a pituitary hormone, the *melanocyte-stimulating hormone (MSH).* The blood level of this hormone is greatly increased in pregnancy beginning with the second month of gestation. Estrogen and progesterone have also been reported to stimulate deposition of melanin.

The pigmented areas on the breasts and abdomen usually do not return completely to their original color. The mask of pregnancy usually disappears or at least becomes considerably lighter.

SUMMARY

Pregnancy brings about dramatic alterations in maternal physiology that involve every system of the body. A number of these changes have been described in this chapter; many others have not been discussed.

Many physiologic adaptations of pregnancy begin very early, earlier than often appears necessary, and a number of them appear to be greater than essential to meet any immediate need. An example of a change that goes beyond the demands of pregnancy is the nearly 50 percent increase in respiratory minute volume, which is more than adequate to meet the 15 percent increase in oxygen consumption. Another example is the storage of fat early in pregnancy as a potential energy source in case of later need. Often the alterations of pregnancy appear to be exaggerated, perhaps to serve as safeguards.

The mechanisms that cause the dramatic changes in maternal physiology sometimes can be explained, at least partially. At other times the cause of the adaptations is not at all clearly understood. There is reason to believe that many of the alterations in pregnancy are triggered by hormones from the fetoplacental unit and are controlled by the fetus. Many of the adaptations of pregnancy represent changes important to adequate fetal development. In general, it probably can be said that the responses in the mother appear to work toward both facilitating growth and development of the fetus and safeguarding her own welfare.

A summary of the important changes in the maternal body during pregnancy and some of the implications that these changes have for maternal care are listed in Table 8–1.

Table 8–1. Clinically Significant Physiologic Changes of Pregnancy

Physiologic Changes	*Clinical Implications for Patient Care*
CHANGES IN THE REPRODUCTIVE ORGANS	
Uterus	
Marked increase in size	Uterus takes up more and more space in abdomen, pushes intestines and other organs upward and laterally
	Abdominal support may give some relief for lordosis and backache
	Height of fundus is measured at each antepartum visit to assess normal growth
	Early enlargement a probable sign of pregnancy
Muscle contractions become more pronounced as pregnancy advances	Braxton-Hicks contractions may become quite noticeable to mother toward latter part of pregnancy
Blood supply increases from 20 to 40 times	
Ligaments hypertrophy and elongate	Mother may have round ligament pain. Suggest rest and position changes for comfort

(*Continued*)

Table 8–1. Clinically Significant Physiologic Changes of Pregnancy (Cont.)

Physiologic Changes	*Clinical Implications for Patient Care*
CHANGES IN THE REPRODUCTIVE ORGANS	
Cervix	
Increased vascularity and edema. Glands proliferate. Becomes softer, shorter, and more elastic and has increased secretions. Canal becomes plugged with mucus	Softening and bluish color—presumptive sign of pregnancy. Mucous plug is expelled early in labor
Vagina	
Increased vascularity. Connective tissue becomes looser. Vaginal discharge more profuse	Presumptive sign of pregnancy. Vaginal douches ordinarily contraindicated in pregnancy. May be necessary to assess if discharge is normal or caused by pathogens
Vulva and Perineum	
Edema and increased vascularity. Vulvar varices may develop	Elevate hips as indicated for relief of varices
CHANGES IN THE BREASTS	
Increase considerably in size, firmness, and vascularity beginning early and continuing progressively. Feel tender, tingly, and heavy. Nipples and areolae become larger and darker. Colostrum fills alveoli and ducts in third trimester	Explain reason for tenderness and heaviness to the woman. Need for a well-fitted supportive bra. A presumptive sign of pregnancy. May need to wear a pad for leaking from breasts
CHANGES IN THE ABDOMEN	
Gradual distention and change in contour as the enlarging uterus pushes into the abdominal cavity. The abdominal muscles support much of the weight of the fetus. Striae gravidarum are likely to develop	Mother feels pressure on the diaphragm and on the abdominal organs. Explain distention and pressure. Mother may be more comfortable while wearing a maternity girdle
CHANGES IN THE ENDOCRINE GLANDS	
Placental Hormones	
Human chorionic gonadotropin (HCG)	Produced only during pregnancy. Necessary to maintenance of corpus luteum in early pregnancy, thus, necessary to maintain pregnancy. HCG is the pregnancy hormone basic to any of the hormone pregnancy tests. Thought to stimulate testosterone production by the fetal testes; necessary for fetal sex differentiation.
Human chorionic somatomammotropin (HCS) / Human placental lactogen (HPL)	Produced only during pregnancy
A metabolic hormone of pregnancy affecting carbohydrate, fat, and protein metabolism	Makes glucose available for fetal energy needs. Influences need for frequent checks of maternal insulin requirements in diabetics. Makes it important to check for gestational diabetes in third trimester of pregnancy. Has an influence on breast growth and development. May stimulate acromegaloid changes in pregnancy
Several other placental hormones	Role is not well known
Steroid Hormones	
Progesterone Placental production increases steadily during gestation	Important to maintenance of pregnancy. Responsible for many characteristic changes in pregnancy. Among these are quieting effect on uterine muscle contractions, relaxing effect on smooth muscle in other parts of body, development of breasts for lactation, deposition of body fat, fluid and electrolyte homeostasis
Estrogens Placental production of the hormone, largely of estriol, increases steadily during gestation	Many phenomena of pregnancy attributed to estrogens, often in combined action with progesterone. Among these are hyperplasia and hypertrophy of the uterus and of the breasts, increased circulation to these organs, and bodily metabolic effects

Table 8-1. (Cont.)

Physiologic Changes	*Clinical Implications for Patient Care*
CHANGES IN THE ENDOCRINE GLANDS	
	Measurement of maternal urinary estriol excretion is used as a clinical index of fetal and placental well-being. Must be done serially
The Thyroid Gland	
Total amount of hormone increased, but the free or unbound (metabolically active) is not increased. Much of the hormone is bound (inactive) but ready if needed	Clinical criteria and thyroid function tests may show results similar to hyperthyroidism but do not have the same meaning in pregnancy as in the nonpregnant. To evaluate, it is necessary to determine the free thyroxine concentration in the serum
Radioactive iodine cannot be used for diagnosis or treatment in pregnancy	Iodine crosses the placenta quickly, and the fetal thyroid has a special affinity for it
Antithyroid drugs cross the placenta	Fetus may be adversely affected. Drug must be monitored closely to keep at optimal level. Newborn must be closely monitored for early and late signs of hypothyroid function and/or goiter
Adrenal Glands	
Cortisol (free and bound) is considerably increased	May influence carbohydrate metabolism and contribute to maternal hyperglycemia. May predispose to development of striae
Aldosterone is greatly increased	Maintains sodium balance in body
Prostaglandins	
Widely distributed in the body. Produced by uterine endometrium and myometrium and probably by placenta	Appears that there is a relationship between these agents and spontaneous abortion and spontaneous labor. Widely used to terminate midtrimester pregnancy. May be used to induce labor
Pituitary Prolactin	
A pituitary hormone that begins to increase at the fifth week and continues to term	Acts as a stimulant to lactation, but this does not occur until after delivery of the fetus
CHANGES IN THE CARDIOVASCULAR SYSTEM	
Increase in blood volume of 1 to 1 1/2 liters during pregnancy	
Large plasma volume increase	Increased tendency to develop iron-deficiency anemia
Erythrocyte increase of 250 to 450 ml of RBC	Medicinal iron is usually administered to prevent anemia. Antepartum or postpartum blood loss may drastically change the necessary blood volume
Increase in leukocytes	
Increase in cardiac output beginning very early in pregnancy, and continuing up to 35% increase. Increase brought about by 1. Increase in heart rate 2. Increase in stroke volume	Imposes an increased work load on maternal heart. Normal heart of healthy woman usually not affected by increased work load. Woman with heart disease may develop complications
Hemodynamic changes during labor, delivery, and immediate post partum may produce sudden changes in cardiac output	Careful monitoring of cardiovascular system during periods of stress is necessary
Heart is pushed upward and to left Alterations in heart sounds and development of murmurs	Upon examination of heart, must distinguish between signs of normal changes in pregnancy and signs of heart disease
Blood pressure is lowered	A woman with hypertension may be normotensive during part of the pregnancy. A change in blood pressure during pregnancy must be compared and related to previous readings for adequate interpretation
Systemic vascular resistance decreased. Blood vessels have a greatly increased capacity for dilation	
Increased blood flow To uterus In skin	Body feels warm; skin temperature in increased. Pregnant woman usually feels comfortable in cool rooms and too warm in warm environment

(Continued)

Table 8-1. Clinically Significant Physiologic Changes of Pregnancy (Cont.)

Physiologic Changes	*Clinical Implications for Patient Care*
CHANGES IN THE CARDIOVASCULAR SYSTEM	
	May develop vascular spiders Hair and nails grow actively—results in loss of large number of overaged hair in puerperium
To nasal mucous membrane	Tendency to nosebleeds. Tendency to congestion of nasal passages
To kidneys	Enhances elimination
To breasts	Normally can expect to see dilated veins and to feel engorgement, tingling, and heat
To alimentary canal	
Venous pooling expanded several times above normal	Elastic stockings help to reduce pooling
Veins distend easily and peripheral blood vessels dilate	Constricting bands should not be worn
Capacity of veins in legs to store blood increases progressively. Venous pressure in legs is markedly increased	These changes contribute to circulatory problems: postural hypotension, edema of feet and legs, thrombosis, varicosities, hemorrhoids
Tendency to venous pooling on standing greatly increased	Blood flow from legs is sluggish
Edema of the legs very common; brought about by high venous pressure, resulting in increased capillary pressure and by reduced plasma oncotic pressure	Reduce effect of gravity—elevate legs on chair when possible Avoid long periods of standing or sitting—if necessary, walk about frequently to improve circulation
Postural hypotension and fainting, especially if pressure from a large uterus caused considerable pooling of blood while recumbent	Observe closely for signs of hypotension when a pregnant woman stands up from a recumbent position
Supine hypotensive syndrome with hypotension and shocklike symptoms may occur when pregnant woman lies on her back. The enlarged uterus places pressure on the inferior vena cava and the major pelvic veins and traps blood in the legs	Prevent pooling of blood in lower extremities. Woman should lie on her side, or turn to her side upon recognition of any symptoms. When supine position is necessary, the heavy uterus must be held toward the left side, removing pressure from the vessels. The fetus must be monitored for any ill effects from maternal hypotension
Use of spinal anesthesia—pregnant women are especially susceptible to hypotension	Careful monitoring. Positioning to minimize pooling of blood in legs
The lateral position is always advantageous in pregnancy for good perfusion of all maternal tissues and for good blood flow to the placenta. It removes pressure from the inferior vena cava, the aorta, and/or the iliac vessels	The lateral position, preferably on the left, will improve cardiac output, general circulation, and blood flow through the placenta
CHANGES IN THE RESPIRATORY SYSTEM	
Capillary engorgement and mucosal swelling of all of the respiratory tract are common	Nose breathing may be difficult. Nose bleeding occurs easily. Voice change may be noticeable. Respiratory infections may produce exaggerated inflammatory symptoms
Diaphragm rises and chest broadens during pregnancy. Breathing pattern is not affected by this change	Breathing becomes more diaphragmatic and less costal at each or any stage of pregnancy—either early or late. The increase in circumference of thoracic cage may require a larger size bra.
Breathing is somewhat deeper than nonpregnant state and respiratory rate slightly higher	
Exchange of gas in the lungs is more rapid than in nonpregnant state	Very rapid deep breathing, as in labor, could significantly lower arterial PCO_2 and raise pH. May be necessary to monitor the breathing and encourage the woman to breath more slowly. Induction with and recovery from inhalation anesthesia can be expected to occur more rapidly than in nonpregnant individual
Hyperventilation is common in pregnancy, beginning as early as first trimester. Appears to be caused by hormonal changes that produce increased sensitivity of the respiratory center and a lower threshold of this center to carbon dioxide	A feeling of breathlessness develops. Hyperventilation is not necessary for adequate ventilation. By lowering alveolar CO_2, hyperventilation reduces arterial PCO_2 and brings about a transient respiratory alkalosis. This results in renal adjustments of plasma bicarbonate to bring about a normal pH. Observe mother for hyperventilation in times of labor or other stress and encourage slower breathing

Table 8-1. (Cont.)

Physiologic Changes	*Clinical Implications for Patient Care*
CHANGES IN THE RESPIRATORY SYSTEM	
Dyspnea—many pregnant women develop dyspnea, a conscious effort to breath	Shortness of breath is a common complaint of pregnant women. This may occur at rest as well as with exertion. Suggest to mother to lie on back with arms extended above head and resting on the bed. Dyspnea is usually physiologic, but it may be necessary to search for a pathologic cause
CHANGES IN THE URINARY SYSTEM	
Kidney pelves and ureters become dilated, leading to stagnation of urine in collecting system	Reduce stagnation of urine when doing urine analyses 1. Increase urinary flow with increased fluid intake 2. Encourage lateral recumbent position Reduce stagnation of urine to decrease chance of urinary tract infection
Ureters may be compressed by dilated blood vessels and pressure of enlarging uterus on pelvic brim, especially on the right side	Use left lateral position to reduce urine stagnation
Trigone of bladder becomes hypertrophic and stretched, and valves become incompetent	Predisposition to ascending urinary tract infection. Routine urine cultures for screening in pregnancy are advisable
Renal plasma flow (RPF) increases approximately 35%	Lateral recumbent position enhances plasma flow
Glomerular filtration rate (GFR) increases approximately 50% beginning early in pregnancy	A creatinine clearance test can be used, if indicated, to test glomerular filtration rate
Excretion of water and sodium is higher in early than in late pregnancy, and at night than in daytime	Excretion is mobilized by recumbent position, preferably left lateral. Leads to nocturia in pregnancy
Clearance of waste products very efficient in pregnancy. Serum urea nitrogen and creatinine values are normally approximately 2/3 lower than in nonpregnant individual	Serum nitrogen and creatinine must be evaluated according to normal values for pregnancy
Regulation of sodium excretion and sodium retention is changed in pregnancy, with tendency to sodium depletion. A gradual cumulative retention of sodium is present in pregnancy to meet the special needs of the fetus and those of the maternal increased extracellular fluids. Retention of sodium totals 500 to 900 mEq in pregnancy	Restriction of dietary sodium or administration of diuretics in pregnancy may exaggerate sodium-depletion tendency and may cause excessive decrease in body fluid volume
Glucosuria common; may be intermittent	Urine is tested for glucose at each antepartum visit. Blood testing for diabetes is done on all pregnant women
Proteinuria abnormal; a sign of preeclampsia or of renal disease	Urine is examined for protein at each antepartum visit. Measurement of 24-hour urinary protein excretion may be indicated; a valuable test of renal function
CHANGES IN BODY WEIGHT	
Total weight gain by 40 weeks' gestation which is considered normal and average is 10 to 12.5 kg (22 to 27.5 lb). Weight gain follows a slightly sigmoid upward trend. Weight gain of only 1000 gm (2 1/4 lb) per month not considered adequate. Weight gain of 3000 gm (6 1/2 lb) per month may be excessive	Caloric restriction during pregnancy may have ill effects
BODY FAT STORAGE	
Fat deposition is normal in pregnancy; begins early and slows later	Dietary restriction to control fat storage is unwise
Stored fat serves as a potential energy supply for late pregnancy and lactation	Fat is usually lost during the puerperium. If fat storage is excessive and is not lost, it may contribute to obesity later
GENERALIZED EDEMA	
Edema appears to be a normal accompaniment of pregnancy after 30 weeks' gestation. May be present in lower extremities only, or also	An abnormal amount of generalized fluid retention is often associated with preeclampsia. Edema fluid may be excreted after a

(*Continued*)

Table 8-1. Clinically Significant Physiologic Changes of Pregnancy (Cont.)

Physiologic Changes	*Clinical Implications for Patient Care*
GENERALIZED EDEMA	
in face and hands. There may be considerable fluid in the skin, which is not clearly evident. Retention of fluid and edema may mean 4 to 8 lb of additional weight	period of bed rest, especially in lateral recumbent position. Diuresis and weight loss are great during first two days post partum
CHANGES IN THE GASTROINTESTINAL TRACT	
Nausea and vomiting, especially in first trimester	Adequate rest and relaxation. Eat crackers or toast and no liquids on awakening. Eat 6 small meals rather than 3 large ones. Avoid food that seems to distress. Concentrate on carbohydrate foods. Eat liquids and solids separately. Drug therapy should be used only when usual activities or nutrition is affected and only under medical supervision
Gingivitis—edematous spongy gums which bleed easily common	Gentle brushing with a soft-bristle brush. See dentist as symptoms require
Heartburn caused by frequent regurgitations of acidic gastric contents into esophagus	Eat frequent small meals rather than 3 customary larger ones. Possibly use an antacid preparation
Relaxation of muscle tone of all of GI tract	Food remains in stomach longer than usual. Increased risk of regurgitation
Displacement of abdominal organs by enlarging uterus	Stomach, large bowel, and appendix are displaced upward
Gastric secretion is reduced	Nausea, constipation, and accumulation of gas in bowel may result from decreased mobility
Constipation is common due to 1. Relaxation of bowel tone 2. Impaired tone of abdominal muscles Hemorrhoids may develop or worsen	Diet with ample bulk and fiber and fluids. Regular time for defecation. Fecal softeners and mild laxatives if necessary. Mineral oil contraindicated; cathartics and enemas should be avoided
CHANGES IN CARBOHYDRATE METABOLISM	
Carbohydrate metabolism is considerably altered due to 1. Fetal need for a continuous supply of glucose 2. Appearance of placental hormones that interfere with action of insulin	
Tendency to hypoglycemia, especially in state of fasting All fetal fuel requirements come from maternal glucose supply Fetus also draws glucose precursors (amino acids) from mother Glucosuria may result in maternal loss of blood glucose Fasting blood glucose values in mother are 15 to 20 mg lower than in nonpregnant state	Caloric restrictions and weight reduction program should not be imposed. Food should be eaten regularly to avoid long periods of fasting. Breakfasts should not be omitted, and evening snacks are advisable. Mother requires a minimum of 150 gm carbohydrate per day
Tendency to ketosis; may have an adverse effect on fetus. Blood glucose and plasma insulin levels fall quickly; fatty acids may be utilized and ketone bodies may accumulate	Avoid periods of fasting by taking food regularly. Assure adequate carbohydrates for energy requirements
Tendency to hyperglycemia; placental hormones exert an increasingly significant anti-insulin effect	More and more insulin is required as pregnancy progresses. Beta cells are stressed, but are usually able to meet the demand. Blood sugar screening is done in late second trimester to identify the woman who cannot produce sufficient insulin (who has gestational diabetes). Known diabetics must be monitored very frequently for their changing insulin needs in order to adjust dosage
CHANGES IN THE MUSCULOSKELETAL SYSTEM	
Softening of pelvic cartilages Increased mobility of the pelvic joints Relaxation of ligaments Abdominal muscles likely to be relaxed and in poor tone Increased lordosis	Tendency to tripping and falling. Tendency to backache. Waddling gait Preventive measures include concentration on improvement of posture, certain exercises, abdominal support, supportive shoes

Table 8-1. (Cont.)

Physiologic Changes	*Clinical Implications for Patient Care*
CHANGES IN THE SKIN	
Increased blood flow, vascular spiders, increased coloration of pigmented areas, increased activity of sebaceous and sweat glands, appearance of striae	Itching of skin may develop and be uncomfortable—tepid bathing, soda bicarbonate bath, no soap or a change of soap, application of oils or lotions may be helpful. Some women feel that rubbing the abdomen with oil or ointment is not only soothing, but possibly preventive of development of striae
Chloasma, mask of pregnancy, may appear	Pigmented areas become lighter or return to original color after pregnancy

REFERENCES AND SUGGESTED READINGS

Assali, Nicholas S. (ed.), *Pathophysiology of Gestation,* Vol. I, *Maternal Disorders.* Academic Press, New York, 1972.

Bonica, John J., Maternal respiratory changes during pregnancy and parturition, *Clin. Anesth.,* 10:1–19, 1973.

Bruce, Neville W., Gestational adaptation: major systems, in *Principles and Practice of Obstetrics and Perinatology,* Vol. I, Leslie Iffy and Harold A. Kaminetzky (eds.), Wiley, New York, 1981, Chap. 37.

Danforth, David N. (ed.), *Obstetrics and Gynecology,* 4th ed. Harper & Row, New York, 1982, Chap. 17 and 18.

Hytten, Frank, and Chamberlain, Geoffrey, *Clinical Physiology in Obstetrics,* Blackwell Scientific Publications, Oxford, 1980.

Kelley, Maureen, Maternal position and blood pressure during pregnancy and delivery, *Am. J. Nurs.,* 82:809–12, (May) 1982.

Lindheimer, Marshall D., Current concepts of sodium metabolism and use of diuretics in pregnancy, *Contemp. Ob/Gyn.,* 15:207–16, (May) 1980.

Martin, Chester, Physiologic changes during pregnancy: The mother, in E. J. Quilligan and Norman Kretchmer (eds.), *Fetal and Maternal Medicine,* Wiley, New York, 1980, Chap. 6.

Osathanondh, Rapin, and Tulchinsky, Dan, Placental polypeptide hormones, in Dan Tulchinsky and Kenneth J. Ryan (eds.), *Maternal-Fetal Endocrinology,* Saunders, Philadelphia, 1980, Chap. 2.

Page, Ernest, W.; Villee, Claude A.; and Villee, Dorothy B., *Human Reproduction,* 3rd ed., Saunders, Philadelphia, 1981, Chap. 11 and 13.

Pritchard, Jack A., and MacDonald, Paul C., *Williams Obstetrics,* 16th ed. Appleton-Century-Croft, New York, 1980, Chap. 9.

Ryan, Kenneth J., Placental synthesis of steroid hormones, in Dan Tulchinsky and Kenneth J. Ryan (eds.), *Maternal-Fetal Endocrinology,* Saunders, Philadelphia, 1980, Chap. 2.

Tulchinsky, Daniel, The role of maternal and fetal hormones in pregnancy, *Contemp. Ob/Gyn.,* 17:113–16 and 121–22, (June) 1981.

Weiss, Gerson, Relaxin—Can it be used to help control parturition? *Contemp. Ob/Gyn.,* 17:73–76, (Jan.) 1981.

CHAPTER

9

Maternal-Fetal Care—Data Collection and Assessment in Healthy Pregnancy

THE ANTEPARTUM PERIOD extends from conception until the onset of labor. The terms *prenatal* and *antepartum* are often used interchangeably. Strictly speaking, the meaning is not identical, but for practical purposes precise definition is not necessary. Antepartum means before labor. Prenatal means before birth and therefore includes the period of labor until the time of the infant's birth.

Antepartum care has traditionally been defined as the care given an expectant mother during her pregnancy. With increasing knowledge and sophistication in the science of fetology, the developing fetus has become as much the focus of care as the woman herself. In addition, the birth of an infant has an impact not only on the mother but also on the father, other siblings, and grandparents, requiring adjustments in all of their roles and relationships. For this reason, the nurse most properly should consider childbearing in the setting of the family to which the woman belongs and into which the infant will be introduced.

Although pregnancy is a biologically normal event, it is an unusual one in the life of a woman and as such requires some special adaptations for the promotion of her health and that of her fetus. Health professionals should view this time as an optimal opportunity for health promotion, preventive care, and client education. Often the woman has not had a complete physical examination or health history since childhood. In addition, instruction and counseling in many health-related areas are needed, such as pregnancy, nutrition, sexuality, and family relationships.

ANTEPARTAL HEALTH NEEDS

Pregnant women have several needs that the nurse must be prepared to meet during the course of gestation. These include:

1. Health history and physical assessment
2. Ongoing assessment of the mother's physiologic status and that of her fetus
3. Adequate nutrition to maintain the mother's health and assure optimal development of the fetus

4. Emotional/psychological support
5. Education and information concerning what is happening to the woman's body as well as immediate preparation for labor and delivery and care of an infant

The following seven chapters will explore in some detail the various aspects of antepartum care. Underlying the discussion is belief in the family-centered nature of pregnancy and childbearing, the importance of careful screening and continual vigilance in the areas of preventive health, and the necessity for well-informed clients who can be knowledgeable participants in the decision-making relative to care. Emphasis will be on the role of the nurse as a provider of health care in colleagueship with professionals from other disciplines.

DIAGNOSING PREGNANCY

Confirmation of the fact of pregnancy is the first task of antepartum care for the health professional as well as for the woman and her family. Some women "just know" that they have conceived; rare others have reportedly remained ignorant of the pregnancy until delivery. For most women, however, diagnosis of pregnancy is made because of the manifestations of certain signs and symptoms.

So many signs of pregnancy are known to women that the majority recognize pregnancy quite early, particularly if they have borne children before. However, they usually will seek confirmation of their opinion from other women or health professionals, probably as one way of working out the ambivalence so characteristic of early pregnancy.

Occasionally women approaching menopause, or others who intensely desire to be pregnant, may experience an imaginary or spurious pregnancy. This condition, known as *pseudocyesis,* is characterized by many of the signs and symptoms of true pregnancy but usually can be readily ascertained by bimanual examination, revealing an unenlarged uterus. Psychiatric assistance may be necessary to support the woman in accepting this diagnosis.

Signs of Pregnancy

Traditionally the signs of pregnancy are classified under three self-explanatory headings: *presumptive* signs and symptoms, *probable* signs, and *positive* signs. The absolutely positive signs cannot be detected until the sixteenth to twentieth week of gestation; the probable signs usually are available earlier, and the presumptive signs may be present at varying times.

Presumptive Signs and Symptoms

The presumptive symptoms, which consist largely of subjective symptoms observed by the woman herself and may be experienced at varying periods, are as follows.

CESSATION OF MENSTRUATION A menstrual period may be missed for any one of several causes, but in a healthy woman of the childbearing age, whose menses previously have been regular, missing two successive periods after intercourse is a strong indication of pregnancy. This is usually the first symptom noticed.

CHANGES IN THE BREASTS Early in pregnancy the breasts increase in size and firmness, and many women have a throbbing, tingling, or pricking sensation and a feeling of tension and fullness. The breasts may be so tender that even slight pressure is painful. The nipples are larger and more prominent, and along with the surrounding areolae, become darker. The veins under the skin are more apparent and the glands of Montgomery larger. If, in addition to these symptoms, it is possible to express a pale yellowish fluid from the nipples of a woman who has not had children, pregnancy may be strongly suspected. Practically all of these signs in the breasts can be due to causes other than pregnancy. A woman who has borne children may have milk present in her breasts for months after the birth of a baby even if she is not breastfeeding.

NAUSEA AND VOMITING "Morning sickness," as the name suggests, is nausea, sometimes accompanied by vomiting, which many pregnant women have immediately upon arising in the morning. It varies in severity from a mild attack when the woman first lifts her head to repeated and severe recurrences during the day, and even into the night. The morning nausea, lasting but a few hours, usually occurs daily for about six weeks, when it gradually disappears. When the vomiting is very severe and not relieved by simple remedies, it is termed "pernicious vomiting." Morning sickness may begin immediately after conception, but as a rule it starts about the sixth week of gestation and continues until the third or fourth month. It occurs in about half of all pregnancies and is particularly common among women pregnant for the first time. Many women go throughout the entire period of gestation without nausea and vomiting, while others are entirely comfortable in the morning and nauseated only during the latter part of the day.

FREQUENT MICTURITION There is usually a desire to void urine frequently during the first three or four months of pregnancy, after which the tendency disappears, but recurs during the later months. Frequency of urination largely is caused by reduction in the capacity of the bladder, due to crowding by pressure exerted on it by the enlarging uterus while both organs remain within the unyielding bony pelvis. Pressure on the outside of the bladder gives much the same sensation as is experienced when the bladder is distended with urine. After the uterus and bladder rise from the pelvic cavity into the abdomen, the uterus no longer crowds the bladder. During the last month or six weeks of pregnancy the fetal head presses on the bladder, and again there is a desire to void frequently.

OTHER SIGNS AND SYMPTOMS *Increased discoloration* of the pigmented areas of the skin and the appearance of abdominal striae are other presumptive signs.

Chadwick's sign, the dark bluish or purplish appearance of the vulval and vaginal lining, which is the result of the great increase in vascularity, is another early sign of pregnancy.

Quickening is the widely used term which designates the mother's first perception of fetal movements. This occurs about the sixteenth to eighteenth week of pregnancy. The sensation is comparable to a very slight quivering or tapping, or to the flutter of a bird's wings imprisoned in the hand. Beginning very gently, these movements increase in intensity as pregnancy progresses. They may become very troublesome toward the latter part of pregnancy, amounting then to sharp kicks and blows.

Women who have had children usually can be relied upon to distinguish between quickening and the somewhat similar sensation caused by the movement of gas in the intestines, but a woman pregnant for the first time may be deceived. Women often use the term "feeling life" when they feel the fetus move, and physicians and nurses frequently use this term when questioning the expectant mother about the perception of fetal movements.

Fatigue may be one of the most prominent complaints of the woman during the first trimester.

There are other possible symptoms of pregnancy, but their value is uncertain. Even the ones described above are not entirely dependable, but if two or more of them occur coincidentally, they probably indicate pregnancy.

Probable Signs

The probable signs of pregnancy are chiefly discoverable by the physician or nurse after careful examination. They also are numerous and uncertain, but some are quite dependable. All of the probable signs of pregnancy, like the presumptive symptoms, may be simulated in nonpregnant conditions; hence, the appearance of any one of them alone may not be deeply significant. Two or more occurring coincidentally consitute strong evidence of pregnancy.

ENLARGEMENT OF THE ABDOMEN Enlargement of the abdomen begins to be apparent about the third month of gestation. At this stage, the growing uterus may be felt through the abdominal wall as a tumor that steadily increases in size as pregnancy advances. Rapid enlargement of the abdomen in a woman of childbearing age, therefore, may be taken as fair, but not positive, evidence of pregnancy. Too much reliance cannot be placed on this sign, as the abdomen may be enlarged by a tumor, fluid, or a rapid weight gain.

CHANGES IN THE UTERUS Changes in the size, shape, and consistency of the uterus which take place during the first three months of pregnancy are very important indications of pregnancy. These are discoverable upon vaginal examination. The uterus is found to be considerably enlarged, somewhat globular in shape, and of a soft, doughy consistency.

About the sixth week, the so-called *Hegar's sign* is perceptible through bimanual examination. This is discovered when the fingers of one hand are pressed deeply into the abdomen, just above the symphysis pubis, and two fingers of the other hand are passed through the vagina until they rest in the posterior fornix, behind the cervix. The isthmus of the uterus, which may be felt between the fingertips of the two hands, is extremely soft and compressible. Occasionally the change in consistency is so marked that there appears to be no connection between the cervix, which is felt below the fingertips, and the body of the uterus, which lies above them. This sign, named for the man who first described it, is one of the most valuable signs of early pregnancy.

Softening of the cervix occurs, as a rule, about the beginning of the second month of pregnancy. In some cases, such as certain inflammatory conditions and in carcinoma, this sign may not appear. This softening of the cervix is often called *Goodell's sign.*

Painless uterine contractions, called *Braxton-Hicks* contractions, from their first observer, begin during the early weeks of pregnancy and recur at intervals of 5 to 10 to 20 minutes throughout the entire period of gestation. These contractions may be observed during the early months by bimanual examination and subsequently by placing the hand on the abdomen. One feels the uterus growing alternately hard and soft as it contracts and relaxes. At first the woman is not conscious of these contractions, but as pregnancy progresses she may become aware of a periodic tightening of her abdomen. As term approaches, Braxton-Hicks contractions are sometimes mistaken by the woman for beginning labor.

BALLOTTEMENT During the fourth and fifth months of gestation, the fetus can move freely in the amniotic fluid. If it is made to passively move in this fluid, it rebounds against the fingers. Ballottement is accomplished by giving a sharp or sudden push to the fetus and feeling it rebound in a few seconds to its original position. Such passive movements are among the most certain of the probable signs.

ABILITY TO PALPATE THE OUTLINE OF THE FETUS When the outline of the fetus can be distinguished by feeling and pressing the abdomen, it is a fairly reliable sign of pregnancy. Since a tumor occasionally may simulate the fetal head or other parts of the body, this sign alone is not considered reliable for positive diagnosis.

PREGNANCY TESTS Although pregnancy tests are quite reliable, they are not considered a positive sign of pregnancy, since both false-positive and false-negative results are possible, as well as laboratory errors.

The theory that something in the urine of pregnant women would cause plants to grow or seeds to germinate has been held since ancient time, but it was not until the twentieth century that any real scientific research was carried out. Several investigators discovered that the urine of pregnant women contained large amounts of a hormone that would stimulate the ovaries of animals to ovulate. This hormone, now known as *chorionic gonadotropin,* is one of the placental hormones elaborated by the chorionic villi. It is present in the blood and urine of pregnant women in fairly large concentration by the fifteenth day of pregnancy. The concentration increases, reaching a peak between 8 and 10 weeks of gestation. Then it slowly falls, reaching a low level between 14 and 18 weeks, after which it remains at a low level until separation of the placenta, when it disappears.

As a result of the early research, the first scientific test for pregnancy, known as the Aschheim-Zondek test, was demonstrated in 1928. In that test immature female mice were injected with urine from the woman in whom pregnancy was suspected. Further developments in pregnancy testing utilized rabbits, and in a later discovery the common North American male frog proved to be a very reliable test animal.

More recently *immunologic pregnancy tests,* dependent upon antigen-antiserum reaction, have replaced the biologic tests. These tests are based on the reaction of human urinary chorionic gonadotropin (HCG) to antiserum. The tests are easy to use clinically and are highly reliable, and the test material is readily available commercially.

For the immunologic pregnancy test, particles of latex coated with human chorionic gonadotropic hormone are used as the antigen. A drop of the urine to be tested is thoroughly mixed on a glass slide with a drop of antiserum against HCG. Next, two drops of a suspension of latex particles coated with HCG are added to the urine and antiserum mixture. After a few minutes of agitation, to ensure complete exposure of the latex particles, the slide is examined for agglutination. If the urine does not contain HCG, the antiserum is available to react with the HCG-coated latex particles and agglutination takes place. Visible agglutination is a negative test. If HCG is present in the urine, the hormone will neutralize the antiserum and prevent agglutination of the latex particles. Absence of agglutination means a positive pregnancy test (Fig. 9–1). Depending upon the commercial preparation used, the test results may be available in two minutes.

A hemagglutination inhibition test may also be used as a pregnancy test. For this test urine and antiserum are mixed, and a suspension of sheep erythrocytes coated with HCG is added. Results are not available for two hours.

Urine for a pregnancy test should be collected in a laboratory urine specimen bottle. Any container considered suitable for collection of a specimen at home is *not* satisfactory. Residue of former contents, which may remain in such a container even after careful washing, and traces of detergent may interfere with agglutination results and give erroneous values.

Soon after fertilization of an ovum the trophoblastic cells begin to secrete chorionic gonadotropin. Since con-

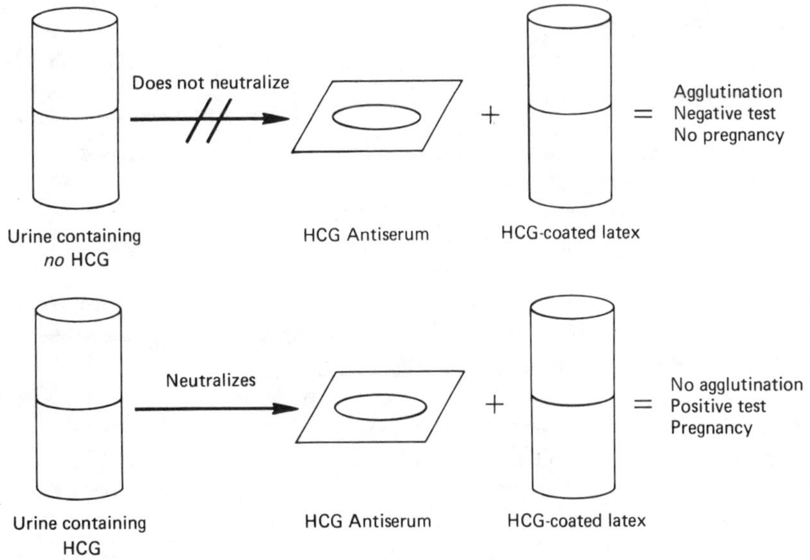

Figure 9–1. Diagram illustrating the mechanism of immunologic pregnancy tests.

ception would have taken place approximately two weeks after the last menstrual period, there may be sufficient chorionic gonadotropin in the urine to detect pregnancy by the time the woman realizes that she has missed her first menstrual period. The assurance of accuracy of a pregnancy test is high after six weeks have elapsed since the first day of the last menstrual period. The test is thus a fairly reliable means of diagnosis of early pregnancy.

False-negative pregnancy tests are more common than false-positive tests. False-negative results may be obtained when the test is done so early that there is insufficient hormone or when the urine is greatly diluted. A positive pregnancy test only indicates that chorionic gonadotropic hormone is present. This may or may not be produced by a normal pregnancy.

A pregnancy test may be a valuable aid in diagnosis of complications in which it is essential to know whether or not conception has occurred. Tumors and cysts can simulate or mask pregnancy, and this test may help in making a final diagnosis. The test is one of several findings that may confirm or rule out the suspicion of an ectopic pregnancy when a tubal mass is discovered, although a negative test does not exclude the possibility of an ectopic pregnancy. When an abortion has threatened, the test may be valuable in determining whether or not the placenta has separated and thus may be important when a decision must be made on further treatment.

The pregnancy test is very strongly positive in such abnormal conditions as hydatidiform mole and choriocarcinoma. On this basis it may be an aid in making the diagnosis and also in determining whether or not all abnormal tissue has been expelled or removed.

A radioreceptorassay of HCG is available for the diagnosis of pregnancy as early as two weeks after conception. Although it is not ordinarily necessary to have such an immediate diagnosis, it does have benefits for determining the presence of an ectopic pregnancy, in situations following infertility treatment or artificial insemination, or when the pregnancy would be high risk (to initiate early care of the diabetic, for example).

Pregnancy testing kits are available for over-the-counter purchase in pharmacies and supermarkets. Many women enjoy having this additional means of confirming their pregnancies without the "public" acknowledgment inherent in a clinic or office visit. Nurses should emphasize to their women clients that the home pregnancy test is not a substitute for an early antepartal health supervision visit.

Formerly a *hormone-induced withdrawal bleeding test* was sometimes used to differentiate early pregnancy from amenorrhea of a functional nature in a woman who previously had regular menses. This test is based on the physiologic effect on the development of the endometrium when the ovarian hormones, estrogen and progesterone, are administered. If the woman is not pregnant, the discontinuance of the medication after a few days results in endometrial desquamation and withdrawal bleeding or menstruation. If the woman is pregnant, the corpus luteum of pregnancy or, later, the placenta are producing sufficient hormones to maintain the decidua and no bleeding will occur. Both animal and clinical studies now suggest that there is a teratologic risk to the developing embryo when these hormones are administered during pregnancy, especially during the first trimester. Therefore, their use as an aid in the diagnosis of pregnancy is not warranted.

Positive Signs

The three positive signs of pregnancy are not apparent until the sixteenth to twentieth week of pregnancy. All emanate from the fetus.

HEARING AND COUNTING THE FETAL HEARTBEAT The fetal heartbeat is unmistakable evidence of pregnancy. The sound of the fetal heartbeat is usually likened to the ticking of a watch under a pillow. It should be counted and recorded. The rate varies from 120 to 160 beats per minute in different fetuses, but tends to remain at nearly the same rate in an individual fetus. To ensure that the fetal heart and not the maternal pulse is being counted, the mother's radial pulse may be palpated while counting.

With a stethoscope the fetal heartbeat is usually heard between 18 and 20 weeks' gestation. Ultrasonic equipment permits detection of heart movement by 10 weeks of gestation. Ultrasonic equipment is generally not necessary in normal pregnancy but may be used when auscultation of the fetal heart is questionable at a time when it could be expected to be audible. Figure 9–2 shows a midwife helping a woman listen to her baby's heart beat.

PERCEPTION OF ACTIVE MOVEMENT OF THE FETUS Active movement of the fetus is accepted as a second incontrovertible sign of pregnancy if the fetal movements are perceived by an objective observer other than the mother. Active fetal movements may be felt at intervals after the fifth month of pregnancy by placing a hand over the abdomen. They are very faint at first, but become strong later and are easily felt and sometimes seen.

ABILITY TO VISUALIZE THE FETAL SKELETAL OUTLINE BY X-RAY OR BY ULTRASOUND Because x-ray exposure of the fetus is not without risk, particularly early in pregnancy, it is advisable to avoid x-ray studies unless absolutely essential for diagnosis. This may be neccessary, however, in order to differentiate between a normal pregnancy and a tumor, or for diagnosis in a very obese woman. Since the fetal skeleton can be seen only

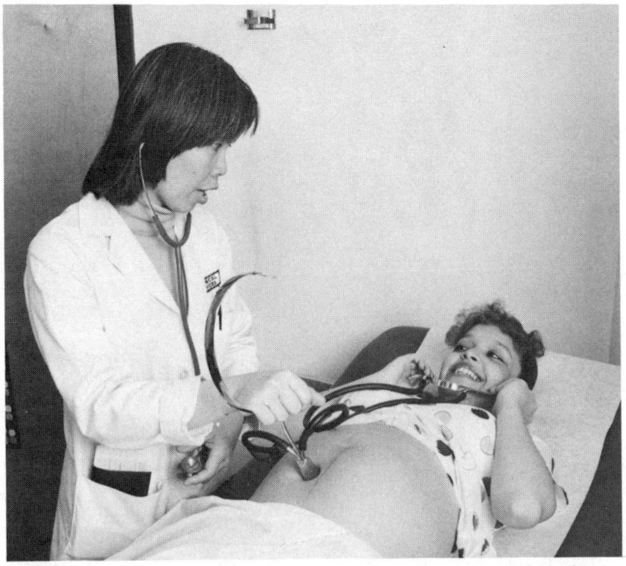

Figure 9–2. Mother listening to the heartbeat of her fetus. This is an important activity in helping her to form an attachment to her developing child during the pregnancy. [Courtesy of The Presbyterian Hospital in the City of New York. Photo by Elizabeth Marshall.]

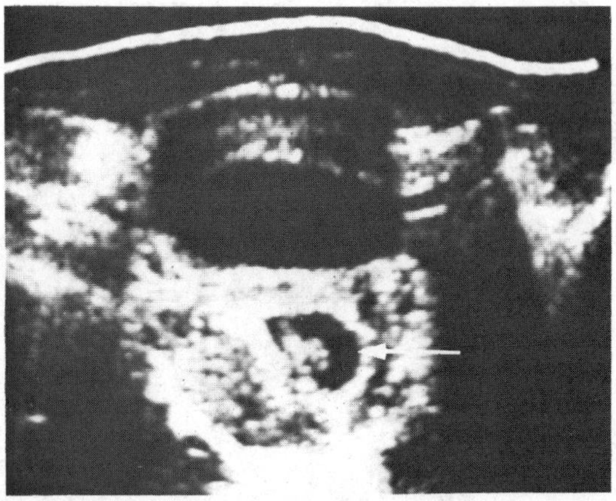

Figure 9–3. An ultrasound image during the first trimester of pregnancy. The arrow is pointing to the gestational sac and the embryo is seen as the white area in the dark sac. The large black area above the developing embryo is an ovarian cyst.

after some calcification has taken place, it is not visible before the fourteenth week, and usually 18 weeks is the earliest it can be seen with reasonable certainty.

With the use of *ultrasound,* pregnancy can be diagnosed as early as the sixth week of gestation when the gestational sac appears as a white ring in the fundus of the uterus (Fig. 9–3). Since there are no known ill effects of ultrasonography on the products of conception, this method not only permits earlier diagnosis but also appears to be safer.

ESTIMATING THE PROBABLE DATE OF DELIVERY

The exact duration of pregnancy cannot be ascertained, since the time when the ovum was fertilized is not known. It is impossible, therefore, to know the exact length of pregnancy, but labor usually begins about 10 lunar months, 40 weeks, or from 273 to 280 days after the onset of the last menstrual period.

The approximate date of delivery may be estimated by counting forward 280 days or backward 85 days from the first day of the last menstrual period. What is perhaps simpler, and gives approximately the same date, is to add seven days to the onset of the last period and count back three months. For example, if the last period began on June 3, the addition of seven days gives June 10, while counting back three months indicates March 10 as the approximate date on which the delivery may be expected. Designating the months by numbers the foregoing example would be as follows: 6/3 plus 7 days = 6/10 minus 3 months = 3/10. This method of computation, known as *Naegele's rule,* is probably as satisfactory as any, being accurate within 10 days before or after the estimated date in about two thirds of all deliveries.

Another method sometimes employed to determine the duration of pregnancy is to estimate the gestational age to which pregnancy has advanced by measuring the height of the uterine fundus. This may be done by palpating the abdomen and noting the height of the fundus in relation to other abdominal landmarks or by measuring the distance from the superior edge of the symphysis pubis to the top of the fundus, using either calipers or an ordinary tape measure (Fig. 9–4).

The growth of the uterus should be fairly uniform throughout pregnancy. When palpating the abdomen, it is observed that the fundus is palpable as a firm, rounded organ just above the symphysis pubis at approximately 12 to 14 weeks' gestation. By 16 weeks it is halfway between the symphysis and the umbilicus, and by 20 weeks it is at the level of the umbilicus. At 28 weeks' gestation the fundus is halfway between the umbilicus and the xiphoid process, and it is at the level of the xiphoid by about the 36th week. At the 40th week, or term, the fundus in primigravidas frequently sinks downward to about the position it occupied at the 32nd to 34th week (Fig. 9–5). This descent is more common among primigravidas, since the head enters the pelvis earlier than in the multigravida. In primigravidas this descent usually occurs in the last weeks of pregnancy, but in women who have had children the head may not enter the pelvis until the onset of labor.

Various formulas or rules have been devised to estimate the gestational age from measurements of fundal height. The most convenient rule of thumb to bear in mind, however, is that the distance in centimeters from the symphysis pubis to the top of the fundus, when measured with an ordinary tape measure, is approx-

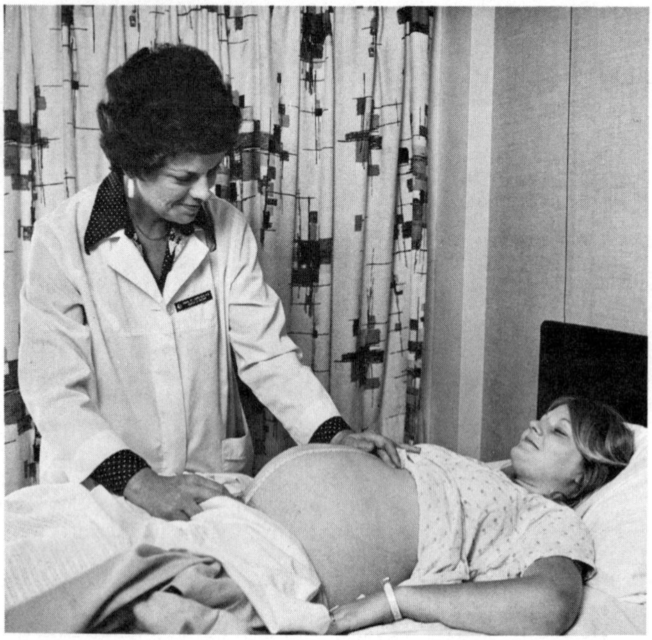

Figure 9–4. The nurse is measuring the height of the uterine fundus to determine the duration of pregnancy.

imately the same as the weeks of gestation. In other words, if the height of the fundus is 28 cm by tape measure, the weeks' gestation will also be approximately 28 (Fig. 9–6).

Still another method of estimating the duration of pregnancy is to count forward 22 to 24 weeks from the day on which the expectant mother first feels fetal movement. This experience, termed "quickening," usually occurs about the eighteenth to twentieth week, but is so irregular that it is unreliable as a basis for computation.

Dates when pregnancy tests are positive in relation to the last menstrual period and the time when fetal heart tones are first heard with an ordinary fetoscope also may be valuable information in estimating the gestational age and therefore the probable date of delivery.

All of these estimations may be further complicated by variations in the size of the fetuses and amounts of amniotic fluid at the same periods of gestation in different pregnancies, an unknown date of onset of the last menses, or conception occurring during a period of amenorrhea, as in the nursing mother. For this reason, no one piece of information is relied upon as a sufficient estimator; rather a combination of all available data is analyzed in order to arrive at the most reasonable assessment of gestational age. Occasionally it is necessary to utilize ultrasonic measurements of the fetal biparietal diameter and/or laboratory studies of fetal lung maturity to substantiate the expected date of confinement. This is particularly true in the case of high-risk pregnancies.

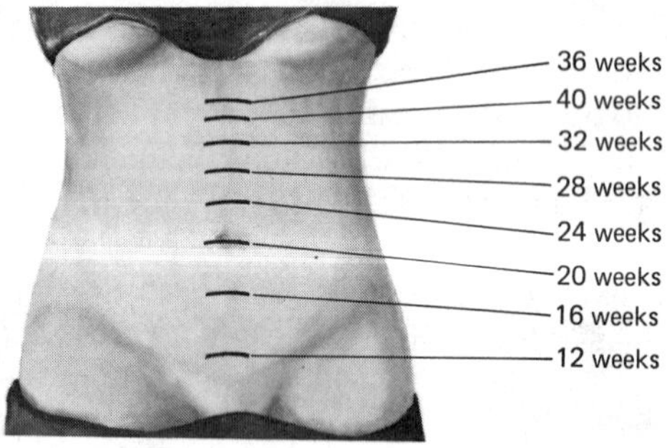

Figure 9–5. Height of the uterine fundus at each of the 10 lunar months of pregnancy.

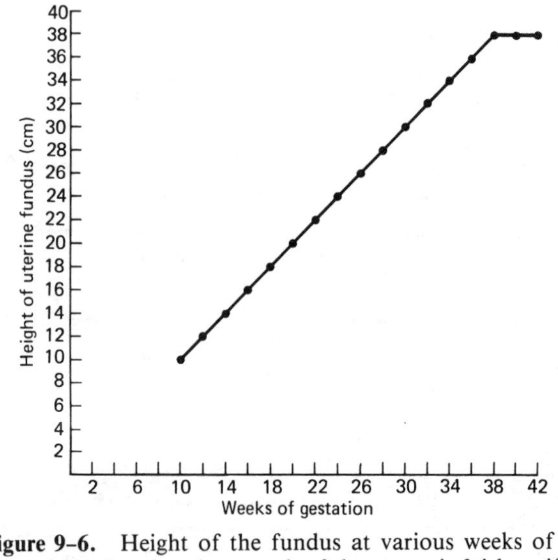

Figure 9–6. Height of the fundus at various weeks of gestation, showing that the growth of the uterus is fairly uniform throughout pregnancy.

INITIATING ANTEPARTUM CARE

As soon as a woman suspects herself to be pregnant she should make an appointment with a clinic or physician's office to initiate antepartum care for herself and her fetus. Although pregnancy is a normal physiologic process, the many changes taking place in the woman's body result in a narrower borderline between health and illness than is present when she is not pregnant. Prevention—or at least early detection—of abnormal signs, followed by prompt and efficient treatment, will avert many complications associated with childbearing, not only throughout the antepartum period but also during labor and delivery and afterward. Thus, antepartum care is essentially preventive care for mother and fetus.

The first antepartum visit should be primarily one of assessment for both the woman and the health professionals. This is the woman's opportunity to evaluate for herself the health care system she has entered. She should become aware of the basic philosophy of the health care providers, the number and qualifications of the personnel, general policies and procedures, and costs of care. The nurse has a responsibility to facilitate this introduction to the system. This often can be accomplished in informal conversation and by supporting the client in asking questions of others. The woman may wish to know if she will be examined by the same physician at each visit, if nurses will do some or all of the antepartum care including physical assessments, if the physician "approves" of natural childbirth, how frequently she will have to visit, and which hospital or maternity center she will use for delivery. The most satisfying childbearing experiences generally are provided in settings where the health professionals encourage the development of knowledge that enables clients to participate actively in making decisions about their own care.

Collection of Data

In addition to becoming acquainted with the office or clinic, the main purpose of the first antepartum visit is to determine the physiologic and psychosocial responses of the woman to pregnancy by means of a thorough health assessment. Three methods of data collection are utilized: the health history, the physical examination, and laboratory screening procedures.

The Health History

The health history is perhaps the most important of the three data collection methods. A carefully elicited history will provide not only objective facts but also valuable information concerning the client's beliefs and feelings and ways in which she prefers to be helped.

The interview for a health history should take place in a comfortable, homelike environment removed from the disquieting sight of examination tables and gleaming instruments. The presence of her husband or other supportive person may help the woman to feel more at ease and will make the family feel included and important (Fig. 9-7).

For a thorough review of history-taking procedures the reader is referred to one of the basic texts on this subject. Outlined below are selected portions of the history that are of particular importance to the perinatal practitioner.

1. Menstrual history
   A. Age at time of onset of menses (menarche)
   B. Regularity, interval, and duration of flow
   C. Dysmenorrhea or other complications
   D. Date of first day of last menstrual period

These data provide valuable gynecologic information. In addition, the nurse who is sensitive to affect and terminology can often pick up significant clues about the client's feelings about her own femininity and self-worth. This will be an important foundation for how she feels about herself as a pregnant woman and, ultimately, as a mother. For example, women who regard menstruation as a "curse" or who are repulsed by this bodily function may need special help to cope with the physical changes and increased body awareness that are characteristic of pregnancy.

The first day of the last menstrual period (LMP) is important in order to make use of Naegele's rule in estimating the expected date of confinement (EDC). Of equal importance in interpreting the estimated date of confinement is the information concerning the interval between menses. Naegele's rule is based on the presumption of a 28-day cycle with ovulation and fertilization occurring on approximately day 14 of the cycle. If an individual woman's cycle is not 28 days, this method of estimation will be less accurate. Although this is seldom

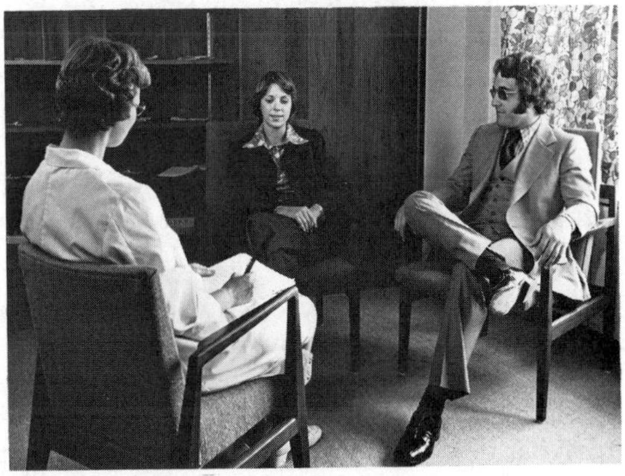

Figure 9–7. Nurse taking a health history from a couple at the woman's first antepartum visit.

DIET HISTORY (Page 2)

What beverages do you drink frequently (3 times a week or more)? Coffee ________ Tea ________ Milk ________
Soft drinks such as Coke ________ Fruit juice ________ Wine________ Beer ________
Other alcoholic drinks ________

List any foods you do *not* like:

Meat____

Vegetables ____

Fruits ____

Milk and dairy foods ____

Others ____

Are you presently taking any vitamins or iron or other minerals? ____

Are you allergic to any foods? No________ Yes________ List ____

____

Have you had cravings for any particular foods since you have been pregnant? ____________ If so, which foods?__________

____

Do you have cravings for starch, clay, or other substances?____

Are you bothered by nausea?________ indigestion? ________ "gas"? ________ constipation? ____________

loss of appetite? ________ excessive thirst? ________ excessive appetite? ________

Number of people in your household: Adults over 18 ____________
Children 12–18____________
Children under 12 ____________

Who does most of the cooking at your house? ____

Who does the grocery shopping? ____

How often is grocery shopping done? ____

Are you receiving either of the following: Food stamps?__________ WIC vouchers? __________

What questions do you have about your diet during pregnancy or about the diets of any of your family members? ____________

____

____

____

ticular attention can be directed toward helping them meet the dietary needs of pregnancy. Several groups of women at increased risk are discussed here.

1. Those who are underweight prior to conception (that is, their prepregnant weight was 10 percent or more below ideal weight for height and age). These individuals are more likely to have insufficient nutrient stores and to maintain these deficits throughout childbearing. They have an increased incidence of small-for-gestational-age infants.
2. Obese women (that is, their prepregnant weight was more than 20 percent above ideal weight for their height and age). It is not uncommon for the obese to be poorly nourished because of the kinds of foods they eat. These women will need special help in selecting quality foods rather than a quantity of calories and in resisting the temptation to try to lose weight during pregnancy.
3. Those who fail to gain weight during pregnancy or who gain 1 kg or less per month during the second or third trimester. The less the weight gain, the greater the risks of prematurity and small-for-gestational-age infants. These women should be helped to increase food intake and bring their weight gain up to normal.
4. Those who have excessive weight gains of 3 kg or more per month. Several obstetric complications, notably preeclampsia, traditionally have been attributed to excessive weight gain during preg-

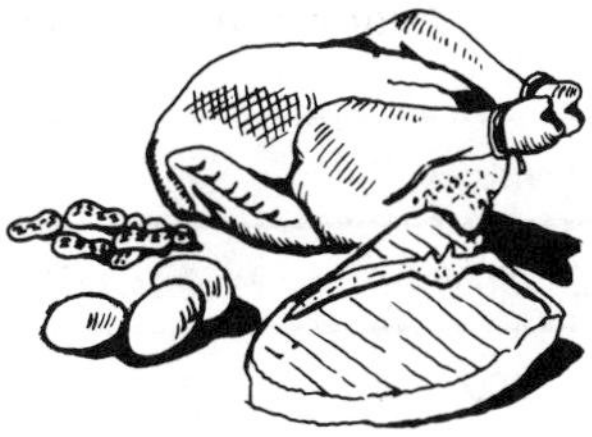

Meat Group: beef, veal, pork, lamb, poultry, fish, or eggs

3 or more servings per day
1 serving equals: 2–3 oz. lean meat
1/2 cup canned tuna
2 frankfurters
2 eggs
1 cup cooked diced peas, beans, or lentils
4 tablespoons peanut butter

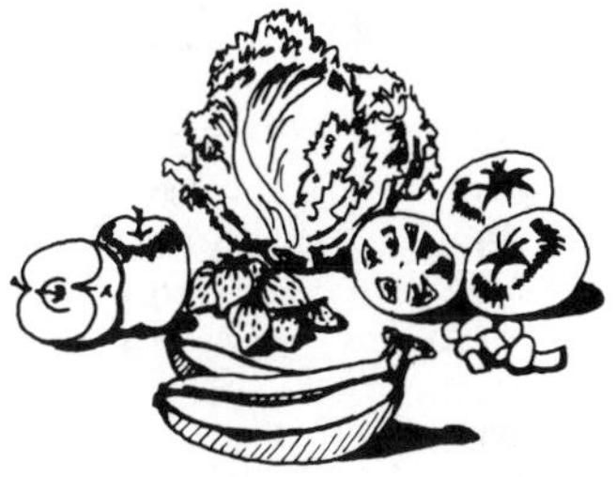

Fruit and Vegetable Group

4 or more servings including one good source vitamin C and one good source vitamin A
1 serving equals: 1/2 cup vegetable
1 apple, banana, orange, potato
1/2 grapefruit

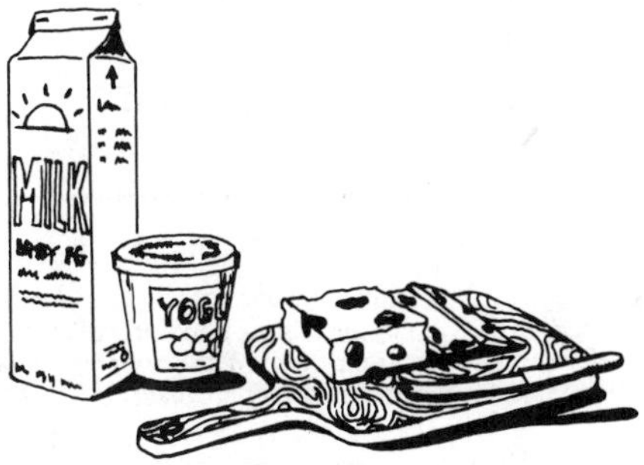

Milk Group

Adults — 4 or more cups
Under 17 — 6 or more cups
1 cup of milk equals: 1 cup buttermilk, yogurt, baked custard
2 inch cube of cheese
1-1/2 cups cottage cheese
1/3 cup dried milk powder

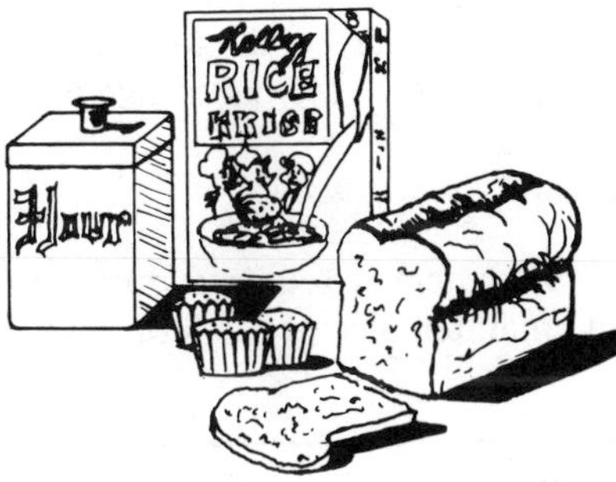

Cereal–Bread Group

4 or more servings (Include one serving of iron-enriched food daily)
1 serving equals: 1 slice bread
1 roll, muffin, pancake, waffle
1 ounce ready-to-eat cereal
1/2–3/4 cup cooked cereal, rice, macaroni, grits, cornmeal, spaghetti
If made with enriched flour count
1 taco shell, 1 wedge pizza crust, 1 doughnut, 1 serving of cake

Other Foods

Add variety and calories by using foods such as butter, margarine, salad dressing, jellies, candies, syrups, carbonated beverages, gravies, and sauces

Figure 10–2. Basic Four Food Groups as a guide to meal planning in pregnancy and lactation.

and Nutrition Board, National Academy of Sciences-National Research Council, recommends the intake of an additional 300 calories per day over and above the prepregnant diet throughout pregnancy. This exceeds the energy needs of early pregnancy and is less than that recommended for late pregnancy. However, a review of the literature suggests that this pattern is consistent with that of healthy women with good pregnancy outcomes who freely select their own food. It is believed that maternal fat stores deposited early in pregnancy are then utilized during the last half of pregnancy as well as during lactation.[1] Thus, the consistent increase of 300 kcal throughout gestation appears to be appropriate to meet the needs of the growing fetus. It should be noted that these increases are necessary for the energy expenditures of pregnancy alone. Additional dietary modifications

[1] J. C. King and S. Charlet, Current concepts in nutrition—pregnant women and premature infants, *Journal of Nutrition Education*, 10:158, 1978.

Table 10–1. Recommended Dietary Allowances (Food and Nutrition Board, National Academy of Sciences—National Research Council, 1980)

	Nonpregnant Females					
	*11–14 yr**	*15–18 yr†*	*19–22 yr†*	*23–50 yr†*	*Pregnancy*	*Lactation*
Energy (kcal)‡	2200	2100	2100	2000	+300	+500
Protein (gm)	46	46	44	44	+30	+20
Vitamin A (μg)	800	800	800	800	+200	+400
Vitamin D (μg)	10	10	7.5	5	+5	+5
Vitamin E (mg)	8	8	8	8	+2	+3
Ascorbic acid (mg)	50	60	60	60	+20	+40
Folacin (μg)	400	400	400	400	+400	+100
Niacin (mg)	15	14	14	13	+2	+5
Riboflavin (mg)	1.3	1.3	1.3	1.2	+0.3	+0.5
Thiamin (mg)	1.1	1.1	1.1	1.0	+0.4	+0.5
Vitamin B_6 (mg)	1.8	2.0	2.0	2.0	+0.6	+0.5
Vitamin B_{12} (μg)	3	3	3	3	+1	+1
Calcium (mg)	1200	1200	800	800	+400	+400
Phosphorus (mg)	1200	1200	800	800	+400	+400
Iodine (μg)	150	150	150	150	+25	+50
Iron (mg)	18	18	18	18	¶	¶
Magnesium (mg)	300	300	300	300	+150	+150
Zinc (mg)	15	15	15	15	+5	+10

*Weight, 46 kg (101 lb); height, 157 cm (62 in.).
†Weight, 55 kg (120 lb); height, 163 cm (64 in.).
‡The energy allowances are for women doing light work. There is a variation in energy needs of ± 400 kcal at any one age.
¶The increased requirements of pregnancy cannot be met by the iron content of habitual American diets nor by the existing iron stores of many women. Therefore, supplemental iron is recommended. Iron needs during lactation do not differ substantially from those of the nonpregnant woman. However, supplemental iron continued for two to three months post partum is advisable to replenish stores depleted by pregnancy.

may be needed to accommodate growth requirements of an adolescent pregnant woman, or in the presence of physical exercise, climatic differences, and so on.

Obviously, caloric intake will have to be individualized according to the needs of each pregnant woman. Probably the easiest method of evaluating the adequacy of caloric intake is to observe weight gain systematically during pregnancy. If this follows a pattern of accumulation of 1 to 2 kg (2 to 4½ lb) in the first trimester and then a fairly linear progression of 0.35 to 0.4 kg (0.77 to 0.88 lb) per week until term, the caloric intake is appropriate. For a more complete discussion of weight gain during pregnancy, see pages 159–61.

Proteins

Additional protein is required during pregnancy for growth and maintenance of the fetus and for formation

Table 10–2. Sample Meal Plans for Pregnancy

Meal	*Food Groups*	*Sample Meal*	*Vegetarian Meal (Ovolacto)*
Breakfast	Fruit—1 serving Grain product—1 serving Protein food—1 serving Milk—1 serving	Orange juice 2 Scrambled eggs Whole-wheat toast Milk	½ Grapefruit 2 Poached eggs on toast Milk Hot tea
Lunch	Protein food—1 serving Grain product—2 servings Fruits and vegetables—2 servings Milk—1 serving	Roast-beef sandwich Carrot and celery sticks Apple Milk	Peanut butter sandwich Vegetable soup Apricots Milk
Dinner	Protein food—1 serving Grain product—1 serving Fruits and vegetables—2 or more servings Milk—1 serving	Baked chicken breast Rice Tossed green salad Cranberry sauce Broccoli Ice cream	Macaroni and cheese Lima beans Tossed green salad Fresh-fruit cup Milk
Snack	Protein food or Milk or Fruits	Orange	Cheddar cheese Apple

of new maternal tissues. It has been estimated that about 950 gm of new protein is formed during pregnancy. Nearly one half of this amount is accumulated in the fetus; the remainder is needed for development of the placenta, growth of the uterus and the breasts, and increase in the maternal blood. From this estimate it is determined that about 950 gm of additional protein is needed during pregnancy to meet its demands.

The amount of protein deposited daily during pregnancy is relatively small during the first trimester and then gradually increases as the pregnancy advances. The average daily amount of protein added to the fetal and maternal tissues is computed to be 0.8, 4.4, and 7.2 gm for the first, second, and third trimesters, respectively, with some individual variation.

To meet the protein needs of pregnancy the Food and Nutrition Board of the National Research Council recommends an additional 30 gm of protein per day during pregnancy. This additional allowance takes into account individual variability of mothers and variability in the quality of protein ingested. If the expectant mother is an adolescent whose growth is not complete, the total recommended protein allowance for pregnancy may be too low for her. She will need protein to meet her own growth needs as well as the demands of pregnancy. This may raise her requirements for protein above the recommended allowance of 76 gm daily during pregnancy.

If the woman's intake is normally high, she may need to make little or no adjustment in her diet to meet the protein needs of pregnancy. For example, a diet that includes 1 qt of milk, ¼ lb of lean meat, 2 slices of bread, and 1-oz slice of chedder cheese furnishes approximately 76 gm of protein and thus meets most or all of the daily requirements of pregnancy. Animal proteins (meat, fish, eggs, milk) are said to have high biologic value, since they contain all of the eight essential amino acids and therefore furnish the best building materials available.

Most vegetables and cereal proteins are low in some of the essential amino acids, and some are also low in digestibility. These proteins are said to have low biologic value when eaten alone. However, if they are supplemented with animal protein, they make valuable additions to the diet, since they add variety and are usually less costly than animal protein. It can be seen that a vegetarian diet presents a real challenge to a woman to meet protein requirements. It is important that she have counseling about the specific amino acid content of various foods so that these can be combined to form a total diet of protein of high biologic value.

Carbohydrates and Fats

Carbohydrates and fats serve as important sources of food energy for the body. When it is necessary to increase or decrease caloric intake during pregnancy, this can best be done by altering carbohydrate and fat intake. When a decrease in caloric intake is desirable, the daily intake of fat, the most concentrated form of food energy, must be carefully considered. However, a moderate amount of fat is important in the pregnant woman's diet to provide her with essential fatty acids, and its intake should not be severely curtailed. Fat in the form of dairy products, meat, poultry, and fish will supply some important nutrients as well as energy. Carbohydrate in the form of milk, fruits, vegetables, and whole-grain cereals and breads will provide protective substances and bulk as well as energy.

Calcium and Phosphorus

Calcium and phosphorus are essential in the diet as tissue-building material. The requirement for these minerals is increased during pregnancy to meet the needs of the fetus. There is evidence that about 30 gm of calcium is required for pregnancy; all except about 2 gm is utilized by the fetus, mainly during the latter half of gestation at the time of calcification of the fetal skeleton. A good calcium intake will provide for the needs of the fetus and, in addition, permit the mother to store some calcium in preparation for lactation. Despite evidence of increased intestinal uptake and conservation of calcium during pregnancy, additional dietary calcium is important to meet the increased requirements.

The recommended increase of calcium during pregnancy is 400 mg per day, which raises the total daily recommended intake to 1200 mg. Increase in the phosphorus requirement is probably even greater than increase in calcium need, but when calcium requirements are met, the phosphorus will be adequately supplied. Foods that are high in calcium are also high in phosphorus.

Milk is the best food source of calcium and phosphorus; 1 qt of milk supplies 1200 mg of calcium. Since it is virtually impossible to ingest sufficient calcium without adequate milk, and since milk is an inexpensive source of many other dietary essentials (protein, carbohydrates, fats, vitamins, and fluid), many authorities consider milk to be an indispensable part of the diet for pregnancy. Milk may be used in any form, but, as it is difficult to use a whole quart in cooking, some should be taken as a beverage, as whole milk, low-fat milk, skimmed milk, buttermilk, or cocoa. Using skimmed milk instead of milk with fat is a means of reducing caloric intake should this be necessary because of a tendency toward excessive weight gain. Unless fortified with vitamin A, skimmed milk cannot be considered a source of vitamin A, but this vitamin can be supplied by other foods as necessary.

Rarely, individuals may be allergic to milk. In such instances nondietary calcium supplementation is required as well as dietary adjustments to insure adequate protein and calorie intake without drinking milk. Intolerance to the lactose in milk, which is not the same as an allergy, is due to a deficiency of the enzyme lactase and may be either congenital or acquired. Such deficiency is particularly common in blacks, American Indians, and orientals. Lactose intolerance may be treated by restricting dietary lactose (usually accomplished by avoiding milk and milk products) or by using commercial lactase to pretreat the milk.

If nondietary calcium supplementation is required, it is recommended that this be supplied by sources other than bonemeal (crushed animal bone available in powder, capsule, tablet, or wafer form) or dolomite (a form of limestone marketed as a calcium supplement). These two products contain lead and may contribute significantly to excessive lead blood levels. Pregnant and lactating women, as well as infants and children, are particularly susceptible to this problem.

Ingestion of large amounts of milk has been implicated in the tendency toward leg cramps experienced by some pregnant women. The rationale is that the high phosphorus content of milk results in high phosphorus concentration in blood and a relative hypocalcemia. According to this theory, treatment of leg cramps consists of curtailing milk consumption, supplementing the diet with nonphosphate calcium salts, and taking an aluminum antacid, which tends to remove some of the dietary phosphorus from the alimentary tract. This relationship remains controversial, however, since not all studies confirm these findings. For the woman bothered by leg cramps, this approach may be tried for relief.

The calcium needs of the pregnant teenager may not be met as easily as stated above. During the rapid growth period of puberty, a high level of calcium retention (approximately 400 mg/day) appears to be necessary for adequate mineralization of the skelton.[2] With the added burden of the developing fetal skeleton, the adolescent's calcium needs range between 1200 and 1600 mg/day with individual requirements being determined by her own rate of growth at the time of pregnancy. Foods other than dairy products contribute only from 200 to 300 mg of calcium daily. To assure that the pregnant teenager has an adequate calcium intake from food, she needs an extra glass of milk, or some other dairy products, in addition to the 1 qt of milk recommended for the adult woman during pregnancy. Emotional distress is likely to disturb calcium metabolism. In this event, it may be difficult for the teenager to meet the calcium requirements of her own body and those of her pregnancy.

Iron

The demands for iron are considerably increased during pregnancy. In the entire course of a pregnancy an additional 600 to 800 mg of elemental iron is required to meet fetal and increased maternal needs. About 300 mg, or more, of iron is transferred to the fetus and the placenta. The fetus needs iron to form hemoglobin and to build up a store of iron for the first three months after birth when an infant's iron intake from food is low. Up to 500 mg of iron is incorporated into maternal hemoglobin as the red blood cell volume expands. This large requirement of iron is to some extent offset by cessation of menstruation which reduces the woman's ordinary loss. There is an estimated saving of about 120 to 140 mg of iron due to the amenorrhea of pregnancy. Thus, the iron requirements increase from the average of 1.5 mg per day for the nonpregnant female of childbearing age to about 3.5 mg per day during pregnancy, with a range of need up to 6.0 mg per day. The additional requirements are greatest during the latter part of pregnancy and may be as high as 6.0 to 7.0 mg per day during the last four to five months of pregnancy.

Absorption of food iron varies both according to the type of food eaten and the individual eating it. On the average, healthy persons absorb approximately 10 percent of the iron ingested in food. For this reason the RDA of food iron must be ten times greater than the daily requirement to ensure sufficient absorption. The recommended allowance of food iron during pregnancy is 18 mg per day, the same as for the nonpregnant woman of childbearing age. This should be sufficient to permit the accumulation of iron stores which then would be available to meet *some* of the needs of pregnancy, assuming the woman's iron stores were adequate at the time of conception.

It is difficult to obtain an adequate amount of iron from food. Uusal diets contain about 6 mg of iron per 1000 calories and dietary surveys indicate that the ordinary American diet contains 10 to 15 mg of food iron daily.[3] Careful selection of food and use of foods enriched with iron can enhance this amount. Liver is an excellent source of iron; other organ meats, eggs, green leafy vegetables, and certain fruits, such as prunes, peaches, apricots, grapes, and raisins are good sources if eaten often. Iron-enriched cereals, breads, and flour can also significantly improve the iron intake. Even with all this, the iron intake will most likely be inadequate for pregnancy.

In addition to food, a potential source of iron for pregnancy is that stored in the reticuloendothelial cells of the bone marrow. However, most women of childbearing age have inadequate iron stores, so this backup system is not likely to be sufficient to meet the needs of pregnancy.

For the reasons suggested above, supplemental iron usually is required to meet the needs of gestation, especially during the latter half. Medicinal iron in the form of

[2] Bonnie S. Worthington, Joyce Vermeersch, and Sue Rodwell Williams, *Nutrition in Pregnancy and Lactation*, 2nd ed., Mosby, St. Louis, 1981, p. 147.

[3] Roy M. Pitkin, Nutritional support in obstetrics and gynecology, *Clin. Obstet. Gynecol.*, 19:489–513, (Sept.) 1976.

ferrous fumarate, ferrous sulfate, or ferrous gluconate may be prescribed as a prophylaxis against iron deficiency. Supplemental iron is not recommended, however, during the first trimester because of aggravation of gastrointestinal symptoms common during this period of gestation. In 1970 the Committee on Maternal Nutrition, National Academy of Sciences, National Research Council, recommended that all women receive 30 to 60 mg of ferrous iron as a daily oral supplement during the second and third trimesters, in order to build and protect their iron stores. It has been found that with the ingestion of supplemental iron the hemoglobin concentration at the end of pregnancy averages 12.0 gm or more per 100 ml of blood.

In women who do not receive iron supplements, the iron stores decrease as pregnancy advances because of the effective parasitism of the fetus. Without adequate stores or adequate intake, sufficient iron will not be available to increase the hemoglobin mass, and the maternal hemoglobin and hematocrit values will fall. Depletion of maternal iron stores may result in an iron deficiency of a nonanemic nature or in an iron-deficiency anemia. The infant of a mother with severe iron-deficiency anemia will have adequate neonatal hemoglobin, but he may have a low store of iron, thus placing him at risk for anemia later in infancy. Unless the mother loses an excessive amount of blood at or following delivery, some of the iron that was added to her own blood cells may later be available for her own supply.

INSTRUCTIONS FOR THE USE OF IRON SUPPLEMENTS In order for the pregnant woman to obtain the maximum benefit from her iron supplements, she should be advised of several facts. First, iron is most effective when taken on an empty stomach one hour before or two hours after a meal. Taking the iron with a glass of ascorbic acid–containing fruit juice such as orange or tomato juice is helpful since ascorbic acid favors iron absorption. If the iron causes stomach upset, it may be taken with a small amount of food; however, certain foods should not be taken at the same time as iron because they block absorption by forming less soluble or insoluble iron complexes. These foods include cheese, eggs, ice cream, milk, tea, and whole-grain breads and cereals.

The woman should be advised to expect that her stools normally will become black owing to the presence of unabsorbed iron. She also may experience a variety of gastrointestinal side effects such as constipation, diarrhea, heartburn, nausea, and vomiting. These are usually mild and can be remedied readily with dietary manipulation and/or a change to a different iron salt.

Finally, the woman should be reminded to keep iron and all medicines out of the reach of children. Iron poisoning is particularly dangerous in young children and is often caused by flavored vitamin and iron products and by pregnancy formulas. The ingestion by a small child of only three or four adult-dose tablets may be enough to produce serious poisoning. Suspected overdoses should be treated immediately with syrup of ipecac and the victim transported to the emergency room without delay.

Folacin

Folacin, a water-soluble vitamin normally stored in the body, is required in increased amount during pregnancy. Unless intake of folacin is ample, a moderate folacin deficiency may appear during the last trimester of pregnancy, caused by increasing demands of the growing fetus and depletion of maternal stores.

Folacin deficiency results in megaloblastic anemia. Such anemia may be induced by pregnancy when dietary intake is inadequate. A significant number of cases of megaloblastic anemia of pregnancy occur. Overt evidence is apparently less common in the United States than in other parts of the world.

An allowance of 800 μg (micrograms) of folacin per day, from dietary sources, is recommended during pregnancy. This is 400 μg above the normal needs of the nonpregnant woman. Pure forms of folacin are effective in much smaller doses. With dietary sources, the absorption of the total amount of ingested food folacin averages only 10 percent, with wide variations, in which absorption may be much higher.

Folacin occurs in a wide variety of animal and vegetable foods, particularly in glandular meats and green leafy vegetables. However, a considerable amount, and sometimes practically all, of the folacin in food may be lost in cooking. Dietary intake is likely to be inadequate in women who do not eat raw, green, leafy vegetables, or foods high in animal protein. Vitamin B_{12} appears to be important to folate metabolism. Vitamin B_{12} is quite stable during cooking and is provided adequately by a diet that includes animal protein.

Prophylactic administration of an oral folic acid preparation to all pregnant women may be desirable, but the optimal dose is controversial. However, if a multivitamin supplement is prescribed during pregnancy, it is considered advisable to use a preparation that includes folacin. When oral folic acid is administered prophylactically to pregnant women, a dose varying from 200 to 400 mg may be used daily throughout pregnancy. Vitamin supplementation should not be a substitute for helping the woman improve her general nutrition.

Iodine

In certain geographic regions, where soil and water are low in iodine content, the diet is likely to be deficient in this mineral. Pregnancy may require an increased amount of iodine. Lactation increases the need for iodine, since it is excreted in the milk. Iodized salt usually supplies this need adequately. Seafoods are another rich source of iodine.

Vitamin A

Need for vitamin A is increased to 1000 μg (micrograms) daily during pregnancy. This vitamin is essential to the nutritional well-being of the rapidly growing fetus, and furnishes the mother with good resistance to infection. It is fat-soluble and readily stored in the body. Whole milk, green leafy vegetables, yellow vegetables, fruits, and liver are the best sources of vitamin A. Vegetable sources should be used freely, especially if the woman drinks only skimmed milk, as it contains little vitamin A. Eating raw carrots for snacks is a convenient way to meet the daily requirement.

Mineral oil in the gastrointestinal tract interferes with the absorption of fat-soluble vitamins and also of calcium and phosphorus; therefore, it should not be used with foods (e.g., as an ingredient in salad dressing) and should never be taken as a laxative near a mealtime.

Vitamin D

Since vitamin D is necessary for proper utilization and retention of calcium and phosphorus, it is important during pregnancy. Vitamin D is present in significant amounts in only a few foods—fish, liver, whole milk, cream, butter, and eggs—and even then varies with the seasons. Some foods, especially milk, are enriched with vitamin D. Their use aids in meeting requirements. Vitamin D also is acquired by exposure to sunlight and for some persons this may be a good source.

Vitamin C

This water-soluble vitamin is poorly stored in the body and should be included in the diet daily for good nutrition. The recommended daily dietary allowance for pregnancy and lactation is increased above that of the woman's usual needs (see Table 10-1). Ascorbic acid is present in liberal quantity in fresh fruits (especially citrus), tomatoes, and raw green leafy vegetables. There is seldom a deficiency of ascorbic acid in the summer when fresh fruits and vegetables are readily available and used freely. With a daily intake of orange juice or tomato juice, it is possible to maintain an adequate intake of vitamin C during the winter months. Increased dietary ascorbic acid also promotes the absorption of iron.

Niacin

The recommended allowance for niacin is 6.6 mg per 1000 calories, but not less than 13 mg for caloric intakes of less than 2000 calories. The recommended allowance for pregnancy is increased by 2.0 mg, based on the increased energy need and caloric intake. Since the recommended caloric intake of the teenage expectant mother is higher than that for the adult, the niacin allowance is increased accordingly, being raised to 15 mg per day during pregnancy. Most diets in the United States supply an adequate amount of niacin.

Riboflavin

The increase in metabolic rate during pregnancy, owing to growth of the fetus and accessory structures, raises riboflavin requirements. An additional intake of 0.3 mg per day is considered to meet this requirement. The recommended allowance during pregnancy is thus raised to 1.6 mg per day. The requirement for riboflavin is met when 1 qt of milk, which contains 1.6 mg riboflavin, is consumed daily. Other foods, especially meat, will help to ensure an adequate intake of riboflavin.

Thiamin

Thiamin needs appear to be increased during pregnancy. The requirement has been established to be 1.5 mg per day. This is a 0.4 mg increase over the woman's ordinary allowance and is in accord with the slight increase in caloric requirements during pregnancy.

Whole-grain cereals and breads and enriched cereals and breads are the most important sources of food thiamin; lean pork is an especially good source. Milk is a fair source when it is consumed in quantity, such as 1 qt per day.

Vitamin B_6

Vitamin B_6 is actively transported by the placenta to the fetus, but it is not definitely known how much of the vitamin the mother needs to meet the fetal requirements. On the assumption that an additional 0.6 mg in the mother's diet would meet fetal requirements, a total of 2.6 mg of vitamin B_6 per day is considered a safe allowance for a pregnant woman.

Sodium

Additional sodium is needed during pregnancy to maintain the osmolarity of the expanding maternal interstitial and intravascular fluid volumes as well as to meet the requirements of the developing fetus. This additional sodium would appear to be supplied by the physiologic adjustments in tubular reabsorption (see pages 155-57). For this reason it is probably most appropriate neither to increase nor restrict sodium intake during pregnancy but simply to advise the woman to salt her food to taste.

Water

Under normal conditions thirst is a good guide to intake of water. It is not unusual for the woman to consume large quantities of fluid during the first trimester. Her extraordinary thirst is probably related to the rapidly changing physiology of her body, particularly the expanding blood volume.

Caffeine

Although caffeine is more appropriately classified as a drug, it is discussed here because of its presence in so many commonly consumed beverages. Large doses of caffeine have been associated with fetal wastage and malformations in laboratory animals. Epidemiologic studies of humans have found high caffeine intake, 600 mg per day or greater, to be related to a higher-than-expected incidence of fetal loss and small-for-gestational-age infants. Although no specific mechanism of action has been identified, it is believed that one factor may be the ability of caffeine to increase circulating levels of catecholamines. These hormones, through their vasoactive properties, decrease uteroplacental blood flow. High intake of caffeine is often associated with smoking, which may further compromise the developing fetus.

Pregnant women should be urged to keep their caffeine intake at least below 600 mg per day. The caffeine content of common beverages is shown in Table 10–3.

Table 10–3. Caffeine Content of Common Beverages*

Coffee	
Brewed†	125 mg/5-oz serving
Instant	66 mg/5-oz serving
Decaffeinated coffee	2–8 mg/5-oz serving
Tea	
Bagged†	
Black	38 mg/5-oz serving
Green†	27 mg/5-oz serving
Leaf tea†	
Black	35 mg/5-oz serving
Green	30 mg/5-oz serving
Instant tea (for iced tea)	40 mg/12-oz glass
Cocoa	12 mg/5-oz serving
Soft drinks	
Coca-Cola	65 mg/12-oz can
Dr. Pepper	60 mg/12-oz can
Mountain Dew	55 mg/12-oz can
Diet Dr. Pepper	55 mg/12-oz can
TAB	50 mg/12-oz can
Pepsi-Cola	43 mg/12-oz can
Diet-Rite Cola	32 mg/12-oz can

*This chart is compiled from M. L. Bunker and M. McWilliams, Caffeine content of common beverages, *J. Am. Dietet. Ass.*, 74:28–32, 1979, and D. M. Graham, Caffeine—Its identity, dietary sources, intake and biological effects, *Nutr. Rev.*, 36:97–102, 1978.

†This figure represents an average. The amount of caffeine will vary with length of brewing time and method of preparation.

Residue

The expectant mother should make certain that her food contains considerable residue such as is provided by fruit, especially raw; coarse vegetables, particularly uncooked; and whole-grain cereals and bread. This residue increases the bulk of the intestinal contents, stimulating peristalic action, thus helping to overcome the tendency toward constipation.

Summary

It has been seen that pregnancy is characterized by the need for increased amounts of all nutrients. For the woman who enters pregnancy in a state of good nutrition and is accustomed to eating a well-balanced diet, the change will not seem great. Indeed, her increased appetite will probably serve as an accurate gauge for increased intake. However, if her dietary habits have been poor, every effort must be made to encourage her to eat the proper food. Poor food habits are frequently of long standing and difficult to change, but the pregnant woman is often highly motivated to improve her diet to provide the best opportunities for her child's growth and development. For this reason, the nurse should consider pregnancy a good opportunity to influence the formation of good eating habits, which will carry beyond childbearing. Moreover, since it is usually the mother who selects and prepares food for the family, it is an opportunity to contribute to the nutritional health of the next generation.

POPULATIONS WITH SPECIAL NUTRITIONAL NEEDS

Adolescents

A great surge in physical, sexual, and physiologic development happens during adolescence. Growth occurs in virtually every skeletal and muscular dimension. If a young girl's nutrient stores are depleted by a poor diet and the increased demands of her own body for growth, then she will be ill prepared physically to sustain a pregnancy.

On the average, an adolescent girl does not achieve her full stature for approximately four years after menarche. If she becomes pregnant during this time, she is at increased biologic risk for pregnancy complications such as toxemia (pregnancy-induced hypertension), too much or too little weight gain, and anemia. At this age, she also is more likely to give birth by cesarean section since the pelvic girdle may not yet have reached its mature size.

Many teenagers have less than ideal eating habits. A large proportion of their caloric intake is often derived from "junk" foods such as potato chips, french fries, soft drinks, candy, and other sweets. Their diets are characteristically low in vegetables, milk, and milk products and are often deficient in calcium, iron, and vitamin C (ascorbic acid).

Dieting is a common preoccupation of adolescent girls. In an effort to "have a great figure," they often limit calories by skipping meals and/or adopting fad diets which may be deficient not only in needed calories but also in other nutrients essential for their growth. Many teenagers do not eat breakfast and thus may have nothing to eat for 16 to 18 hours from supper until lunch.

During pregnancy the teenager requires increases in nearly all nutrients, just as the older woman does. Specific amounts of nutrients are indicated in the table of Recommended Daily Allowances (RDA) (Table 10–1) and are discussed with respect to the adolescent in this chapter under each nutrient. The challenge of nutrition counseling for pregnant adolescents goes far beyond knowledge of RDAs, however. Eating habits, food likes and dislikes, peer pressures, and body image are all of equal—or even greater—importance. For some teens, informal group instruction structured as a rap session may be a more effective way of teaching. It should be remembered that the pregnant girl's mother is usually her primary food advisor. Very frequently, she prepares her daughter's meals throughout pregnancy and even beyond. Therefore, she should be included in any nutritional teaching.

Alcohol-Dependent Women

Alcohol interferes with the absorption and utilization of nutrients and with protein synthesis. Therefore, a woman who chronically abuses alcohol is likely to be malnourished. Even if she has stopped drinking just prior to conception, her stores of vitamins and proteins may be deficient. For this reason these women require special nutritional consideration in addition to the attention that should be paid to social and psychologic issues and the risk of fetal alcohol syndrome (see Chap. 11.)

The usual diet for pregnancy should be encouraged, taking into account the cost and availability of food. Dietary supplements may be indicated, depending on the severity of the alcoholism, the presence of secondary illness, weight loss or poor weight gain, evidence of intrauterine growth retardation, and the woman's eating habits.

Anemia is a common problem for these women, so particular attention should be given to encouraging foods high in iron and in instructing them about the most efficacious methods of taking iron supplements.

Obese Women

Obesity is not an uncommon condition for women of childbearing age. The reasons for being overweight and the issues of treating the problem successfully are multifaceted and highly complex. No attempt will be made to address these issues in this chapter. However, the maternity nurse should be aware of the major obstetric and nutritional concerns and be prepared to consult with appropriate professionals in nutrition, medicine, and nursing in order to assist the overweight pregnant woman in meeting her health needs and those of her fetus.

Women who are obese prior to conception are more likely to have pregnancies complicated by hypertension, hyperglycemia, and placental dysfunction. Their labors tend to be longer than average, and they have an increased incidence of postpartum hemorrhage. Their infants are more likely to be large for gestational age, and they have a higher incidence of neonatal asphyxia.[4] The asphyxia may be associated with the large size, the placental dysfunction, or with other nutritional and metabolic fators. In order to assist these women in achieving favorable maternal and perinatal outcomes, vigilant obstetric surveillance is required throughout gestation. Blood pressure, blood glucose, and placental function should be monitored carefully and attention given to the possibility of cephalopelvic disproportion early in labor.

There is a tendency among health care providers to advocate caloric restriction for obese women so there will be a net loss at the end of pregnancy. This probably is not advisable for several reasons: first, severe caloric restriction often results in insufficient intake of other essential nutrients; second, calories (energy) are needed for amino acid utilization; and third, in the absence of caloric intake, fat deposits are metabolized to provide energy needs. This latter phenomenon results in ketonuria, which has been associated with lower IQ scores in offspring when measured at four years of age.[5] For these reasons, the obese woman, like her thinner sister, should gain weight during pregnancy. However, her gain may be limited to the lower end of the recommended range of weight gain (approximately 20 lbs) since she does not require the deposition of additional fat stores (see Chap. 8, p. 161). Nutrition counseling should emphasize good eating habits and quality rather than quantity of foods.

[4] C. Calandra, D. A. Abell, and N. A. Beischer, Maternal obesity in pregnancy, *Obstet. Gynecol.,* 57:8–12, 1981.

[5] J. A. Church and H. W. Bernedes, Intelligence of children whose mothers had acetonuria during pregnancy, in *Perinatal Factors Affecting Human Development,* Pan American Health Organization, Scientific Publication No. 185. Washington, D. C., 1969, pp. 30–35.

Vegetarians

There is currently an increasing interest in vegetarianism. Although some persons follow a vegetarian diet as a result of their religious or moral beliefs, the most commonly cited reasons in the United States are related to health. Most vegetarians consume less refined sugar, fat, and cholesterol and more fiber than the average American. Such a diet is believed to be related to a lower incidence of cardiovascular disease, osteoporosis, diabetes mellitus, and some colon diseases. In addition, advocates of vegetarianism note that this diet avoids a number of environmental pollutants such as pesticides which are fat soluble and tend to accumulate in animal fat. A minority of persons may adopt this diet because it tends to be less expensive than one containing meat and animal products.

Vegetarians are classified into four basic types:

1. Lacto-ovovegetarians—those who eat vegetables and fruits supplemented with eggs and dairy products
2. Actovegetarians—those who supplement vegetables and fruits with dairy products but not eggs
3. Vegans or pure vegetarians—those who use no animal foods, eggs, or dairy products
4. Fruitarians—those who eat only fruits, nuts, honey, and olive oil

It is possible for women to follow any of these diets and still achieve adequate nutrition for both themselves and their fetuses, provided careful attention is given to eating a precise balance of food. It is easiest for lacto-ovovegetarians to achieve the goal of good nutrition and, as could be expected, most difficult for the fruitarian.

Calories

As for any pregnant woman, the diet must contain sufficient calories to support a weight gain of about 24 lb.

Vitamins

Many vitamins are contained in moderate amounts in plant sources and present little problem during pregnancy. However, very few plants contain vitamins B_{12} and D. Vegans who do not use eggs or dairy products should receive supplementation of these vitamins. In addition, because folic acid is readily destroyed in cooking, supplementation of this substance is also recommended. These needs can be met by taking a prenatal multivitamin which contains 400 mg folate, 5 mg vitamin B_{12}, and 10 mg vitamin D.

Minerals

Every pregnant woman should pay special attention to the consumption of iron and calcium. The gestational need for iron cannot be met by the average American diet and, as stated earlier, all women probably require iron supplementation during the latter two thirds of pregnancy. The increased need for calcium is readily met by drinking a quart of milk per day. If the woman does not use milk, a calcium supplement should be prescribed.

Protein

Meeting the increased protein needs of pregnancy is one of the biggest challenges for the vegetarian. In order to advise vegetarians about this aspect of their diet, it is necessary to understand the concepts of protein quality and complementarity.

There are 22 amino acids found in the human body. All but eight of these can be synthesized by the body. These eight must be consumed in the diet in specific proportions and are known as *essential* amino acids. Meat, fish, poultry, eggs, and dairy products contain all eight essential amino acids in the proper proportion and are said to be "complete" or high-quality proteins. As such, they can meet all the protein requirements by themselves. Proteins from plant sources are "incomplete" because they lack one or more of the essential amino acids, usually one of four: lysine, methionine, threonine, and tryptophan.

A food that is deficient in one amino acid may be combined in the same meal with another food deficient in a different amino acid to provide "complete" protein for that meal. For example, wheat which is deficient in lysine can be combined with a legume which is high in lysine but lacks methionine (a peanut-butter sandwich on whole-wheat bread). This is the concept of protein complementarity. Many cultures have traditional meatless meals that reflect an understanding of this concept. Examples include the Mexican corn tortilla with refried beans, Middle Eastern falafel (legume) with pita bread and sesame seeds, and the Italian pasta facoli (spaghetti and beans). It should be emphasized that these complementary protein foods must be eaten at the same meal in order to derive maximum benefit from the combination.

DIETARY MODIFICATIONS DURING LACTATION

The diet demands special consideration during lactation, just as it did during pregnancy, since the normal physiologic processes now are also altered and additional demands are placed on the body. Nutritional requirements are considerably increased above normal needs. Throughout the entire nursing period the mother's diet must be such that it will nourish her adequately and also aid in producing milk. The mother should be advised early in the postpartum period about the foods to include in an optimum diet. The physiologic costs of lactation in terms of many dietary needs are not completely clear, and utilization of certain foods may be altered during pregnancy and lactation. It appears, however, that nutritional requirements are increased.

Lactating women should receive substantially more calories, proteins, and calcium as well as modest increases in most other nutrients (Table 10–1). Milk production will not be good if there is any marked deficiency of protein or caloric intake. If the woman is able to sustain good milk production in the presence of nutritional deficiencies, she does so at a cost to herself.

Calories

Energy needs during lactation may be increased as much as 50 percent above the mother's normal requirements. Her diet must be sufficiently high in calories to meet the needs of her own body, to meet the caloric value of the milk secreted, which is 70 cal/100 ml, and to furnish the energy that is used in the actual production of milk. Thus, a mother who is secreting 850 ml of breast milk per day, the average amount secreted during established lactation, would need nearly 800 cal. In addition, she needs energy to produce milk. The caloric cost of lactation is uncertain. It has been estimated to be somewhere between 150 and 400 cal for production of 850 ml of breast milk. The additional caloric requirement is thus proportional to the actual amount of breast milk produced. When caloric requirements are not met, the mother must use her body stores to subsidize her caloric needs. The 1980 Recommended Daily Allowance of calories for the lactating woman is 500 cal above her usual nonpregnant intake (Table 10–1). During pregnancy 2 to 4 kg (5 to 10 lb) of fat was stored and is available to produce an additional 200 to 300 calories per day for about three months to assist in meeting the energy needs of lactation. For the mother who continues to breast-feed after three months, or for the woman who is underweight or feeding more than one infant, more than 500 calories may need to be added. Additionally, individual needs may require adjustment up or down, depending on how the woman is able to maintain her weight.

Protein

The estimated additional requirement for protein during lactation is based on the amount of milk excreted and on the amount of protein in the milk. Human milk averages 1.2 gm of protein per 100 ml. Assuming that the mother secretes an average of 850 ml (30 oz) of breast milk per day, with an upper limit of 1200 ml (42 oz), her daily output of protein may be as high as 15 gm per day. This means that the mother who is producing a large amount of breast milk needs to add to her own body's protein requirements an additional 15 gm of ideal protein each day. This allowance, based on a high milk secretion, should be ample for all mothers. However, to allow for variability in the quality of protein eaten, an additional 20 gm of protein per day is recommended for the period of lactation.

Although overall protein content of breast milk does not appear to be altered by deficient maternal diet, there is evidence that protein-deficient diets result in lowered amounts of lysine and methionine, two essential amino acids.[6] Thus, maternal protein deficiency may result in qualitatively poorer milk.

Calcium and Phosphorus

As in pregnancy, some physiologic adjustment that increases calcium uptake and calcium conservation also takes place during lactation. However, since calcium will be excreted in breast milk, an intake of dietary calcium above the mother's ordinary daily needs is important during lactation. The recommended calcium intake of the nursing mother is increased by 400 mg per day, which makes a recommended total intake of 1200 mg per day during lactation. One quart of milk per day will provide 1200 mg of calcium. Other foods in the daily diet will provide some additional calcium if needed.

Dietary phosphorus intake ordinarily equals or exceeds calcium intake. Phosphorus, therefore, is recommended in an amount equal to that of calcium. This increases the recommended allowance of phosphorus by 400 mg during lactation.

Other Minerals

Maternal sodium intake will influence directly the amount of sodium secreted in breast milk. On the other hand, maternal intake does not appear to affect the concentration in breast milk of iron, copper, or fluoride. The amount of iron in breast milk is fairly constant at 0.5 to 1.0 mg per day. For this reason, iron deficiency is not uncommon in breast-fed infants, particularly as the period of breast-feeding is lengthened. Iron supplementation of breast-fed infants thus is commonly recommended. Iron supplementation of the lactating woman also is common as a means of building up stores depleted by pregnancy, even though such supplementation does not affect milk levels.

[6] B. S. Lindblad and R. J. Rahimtoola, A pilot study of the quality of human milk in lower socio-economic groups in Karachi, Pakistan, *Acta Paediatr. Scand.*, 63:125, 1974.

Fat-Soluble Vitamins

Vitamins A and E are present in breast milk in appreciable amounts, thus suggesting a need for increased dietary intake (Table 10–1). The vitamin D requirement is uncertain and the breast milk content of vitamin D is low. Some authorities have recommended vitamin D supplementation for breast-fed infants, but it would seem that exposure to sunlight is almost universally practical and a preferred method.

Water-Soluble Vitamins

The recommended daily allowance for each of these vitamins is somewhat increased over nonpregnant, nonlactating levels. In addition, the amount of maternal intake is directly related to the amount secreted in the milk. Deficient maternal intake can produce deficiency diseases in the infant.

Fluids

A fluid intake up to 2500 or 3000 ml is important for adequate milk production. To facilitate adequate intake, it is a good plan to keep a pitcher or Thermos bottle of water on the bedside table and replenish it every four hours. Some mothers have experienced great thirst during nursing. Fluids during nursing relieve thirst, increase the amount of milk, and often stimulate the letdown of milk.

Restricted Foods

The mother may eat any food that agrees with her. The belief that certain substances from highly flavored vegetables such as onions, cabbage, turnips, and garlic are excreted through the milk to upset the infant's digestion is not given general credance. Some physicians believe that cabbage and members of the cabbage family have a tendency to give the infant colic. Others think that chocolate or certain berries may produce signs of allergy, such as rashes. Ordinarily, the mother may eat any kind of food she wishes unless she finds that her infant is disturbed by a particular one. Any food, of course, that causes her to have indigestion should be avoided.

Summary

Increase in the intake of all nutrients is necessary during lactation in order to maintain the maternal bodily needs and/or to supply appropriate levels of nutrients to the infant in breast milk. As during pregnancy, all of these increased needs may be met by increasing the quantity of a well-balanced diet. Should the quality of the diet be poor, nutritional counseling, not unlike that of pregnancy, is indicated. The lactating mother may have an additional difficulty in learning to schedule her time to allow herself opportunity for rest and adequate mealtimes.

NUTRITION DURING THE INTERCONCEPTIONAL PERIOD

The periods of pregnancy and lactation are short, albeit important, times compared to the lifetime of a woman. Attention to good nutrition should be an integral part of health care throughout the life cycle. The interval between pregnancies is especially important for the replenishing of stores depleted during pregnancy and lactation and for establishing optimum weight levels. It is appropriate that nutrition counseling be directed toward maintaining or improving the total family dietary habits.

Recently, considerable attention has been directed to the nutritional needs unique to women receiving hormonal therapy, specifically those women taking oral contraceptives. Most information to date is of a biochemical nature and its clinical implications are somewhat speculative. Tests indicating vitamin B deficiency are consistently reported in oral contraceptive users. It has been suggested that this may be a mechanism in the development of depression, and, although this information remains controversial, it is probably reasonable to consider B_6 deficiency as one possible cause of depression if a woman is taking oral contraceptives.

Other biochemical studies have suggested the need for increased folic acid, vitamins C, B_6, B_{12}, and certain trace elements for women taking oral contraceptives. On the other hand, requirements for iron, niacin, vitamin K, copper, and calcium may be diminished. It should be emphasized that the significance of these chemical findings is unclear at present; therefore, dietary alterations or supplementation should not be recommended until further investigations clarify the issues.

Because some women who use the intrauterine device for contraception have increased menstrual flow, it is advisable to follow hematocrit levels in this group of women. Dietary counseling should emphasize foods rich in iron, and iron supplementation even may be considered.

REFERENCES AND SUGGESTED READINGS

Borberg, C.; Gillmer, M. D. G.; Brunner, E. J.; Gunn, P. J.; Oakley, N. W., and Beard, R. W., Obesity in pregnancy: The effect of dietary advice, *Diabetes Care,* 3(3):476–81, 1980.

Brown, J. E.; Jacobson, H. N.; Askue, L. H., and Peck, M. G., Influence of pregnancy weight gain on the size of infants born to underweight woman. *Obstet. Gynecol.;* 57:13–17, 1981.

Calandra, C.; Abell, D. A.; and Beischer, N. A., Maternal obesity in pregnancy, *Obstet. Gynecol.,* 57:8–12, 1981.

Church, J. A., and Berendes, H. W., Intelligence of children whose mothers had acetonuria during pregnancy, in *Perinatal Factors Affecting Human Development,* Pan American Health Organization, Scientific Publication No. 185, Washington, D. C., 1969, pp. 30–35.

Committee on Maternal Nutrition, *Maternal Nutrition and the Course of Pregnancy: Summary Report,* Food and Nutrition Board, National Academy of Sciences, Washington, D. C., 1970.

Committe on Nutrition of the Mother and Preschool Child, *Oral Contraceptives and Nutrition—A Statement,* Food and Nutrition Board, National Academy of Sciences, Washington, D. C., 1975.

Hytten, F. E., and Leitch, I., *The Physiology of Human Pregnancy,* 2nd ed., Blackwell Scientific Publications, Oxford, 1971.

Metcoff, J.; Costiloe, J. P.; Crosby, W.; Bentle, L.; Seskachalam, D.; Sandstead, H. H.; Bodwell, C. E.; Weaver, F.; and McClain, P., Maternal nutrition and fetal outcome, *Am. J. Clin. Nutr.,* 34(Suppl.):708–21, 1981.

Naeye, R. L. Teenaged and preteenaged pregnancies: Consequences of the fetal-maternal competition for nutrients, *Pediatrics,* 67:146–150, 1981.

Pitkin, Roy, M., Nutritional support in obstetrics and gynecology, *Clin. Obstet. Gynecol.,* 19:489–513, 1976.

———, Assessment of nutritional status of mother, fetus and newborn, *Am. J. Clin. Nutr.,* 31(Suppl.):658–68, 1981

Worthington-Roberts, B.; Vermeersch, J.; and Williams, Sue R., *Nutrition in Pregnancy and Lactation,* 2nd ed., C. V. Mosby, St. Louis, 1981.

CHAPTER

11

Nursing Management of the Antepartal Client

DURING PREGNANCY WOMEN have an increased awareness of their bodies as they experience rapid contour changes and many new physical sensations. They also are likely to have an increased interest in health since they wish to provide the best possible environment for intrauterine growth and development. Their motivation to engage in sound health practices is typically high. These circumstances provide the nurse with an ideal opportunity to promote healthful self-care practices. Pregnant women are usually quite responsive to health education that helps them recognize normal bodily functions and increases their problem-solving skills to deal with deviations from normal.

This chapter will discuss some of the more common health practices with special recommendations for pregnancy. The so-called minor discomforts of pregnancy will be outlined. Emphasis will be placed on the nurse's role in facilitating the woman's self-care, which includes helping her to identify when she needs to seek consultation with a health care provider.

GENERAL HEALTH DURING PREGNANCY

Grooming and Hygiene

Pregnancy is a time of rapid and dramatic physical changes which require the woman to make continual adjustments in her self-image. With a little attention to herself, she can feel, as well as look, more feminine and attractive.

The excretory function of the skin is enhanced during pregnancy, resulting in increased perspiration. The skin and hair may become more oily, and more frequent bathing and shampooing may be necessary. Some women find it helpful to use a shampoo especially designed for oily hair and to adopt a hair style that is easy to manage.

Tub baths are permitted throughout pregnancy. During the latter weeks of gestation, however, the woman's physical clumsiness may make it more difficult to negotiate the climb in and out of the tub. At this time she may find it easier to shower, unless someone is available to help her out of the water. Baths tend to be quite relaxing and may be good therapy for tired muscles, backache, or insomnia. Bath oils, powders, and lotions are often a treat that makes a woman smell nice and feel special, and they need not be expensive.

If a chloasma or "mask of pregnancy" appears, the woman may wish to experiment with various makeup foundations if she finds it unattractive.

Clothing

Maternity fashions range from bathing suits to evening gowns. These clothes can be quite costly, but with a little care and effort the expectant mother can be well dressed on a very modest budget. Since maternity clothes almost never get worn out, friends or relatives of the same size are a good source of hand-me-downs. Garage sales and second-hand clothing stores are other inexpensive places to acquire a wardrobe. If the woman sews, she will find that maternity clothes are quick and easy to make. Since they require little fitting, even beginning seamstresses can produce very attractive garments.

It is wise to select fabrics that are washable. If the pregnancy occurs during warm weather, cotton or other absorbent materials are more comfortable. This is particularly true for undergarments.

Some women may find it desirable to wear a maternity girdle to support the enlarging uterus. This is particularly true of the woman who has flaccid abdominal musculature which gives poor natural support to the uterus. These women often get considerable relief from backaches and pressure symptoms when a girdle is worn since it lifts some of the weight of the heavy uterus from the blood vessels and ligaments. The girdle worn before pregnancy, regardless of how large, will not be satisfactory during pregnancy. It will become uncomfortable and may even be harmful, as it tends to push the uterus down into the pelvis, causing backache and cramps in the legs.

A brassiere that gives good support to the breasts is advisable. Most women will require a larger size during pregnancy to accommodate the normal growth of the breasts. A well-fitting bra should have wide, adjustable straps, some mechanism for expanding as chest circumference enlarges, and should support the nipple line about midway between the elbow and shoulder. All of the breast tissue should fit comfortably inside the bra cup. If the woman is planning to breast-feed she may wish to purchase a nursing bra which she can continue to use after the infant is born.

Any clothing that restricts circulation should be avoided, especially during pregnancy. As the woman gains weight, garments that fit properly before pregnancy may become too tight. Bras, panties, and knee socks are common offenders. Of course, garters should never be worn as they are especially apt to retard circulation, thus favoring development of varicosities and muscle cramps.

Shoes that are comfortable, provide firm foot support, and promote good posture and balance are advisable for everyone, including pregnant women. This does not mean that they must be unattractive or that frivolous shoes shouldn't be worn for some occasions. However, as the woman's center of gravity shifts owing to the increasing weight of the uterus, she will find it more difficult to maintain her balance in very high-heeled or platform-soled shoes.

Pregnancy is ordinarily a period of well-being for a woman. If she gives herself a little special care, she will increase her self-confidence in her appearance and will look happy and pretty.

Care of Breasts and Nipples

The importance of a well-fitting bra has already been mentioned. In addition, if the woman is planning to breast-feed, some preparation of the breasts and nipples during pregnancy is advisable.

Toughening the nipples for the abrasive and stretching action of sucking during breast-feeding has been given some consideration. Some authors have recommended the avoidance of soap on the nipples during pregnancy and lactation. This is felt to prevent drying and cracking by promoting the natural protective mechanisms of the body. Normally, dead cells form a protective covering for the nipples, while copious secretions of the sebaceous and sweat glands keep the skin pliable and maintain a normal acid condition. Frequent washing with soap tends to remove all these substances.

Ointments may inhibit evaporation of perspiration and cause the skin to become soft and tender, although lanolin is sometimes recommended.

Gentle rubbing of the woman's clothing is often an effective way to toughen the nipples. Either the mother may omit wearing her brassiere for a few hours each day, or if the brassiere has flaps, such as on a type used for nursing, the flaps may be left down for a few hours. Friction from drying with a rough towel is still another way to gradually toughen the nipples for nursing.

Some authorities have recommended manual expression of colostrum during the last month of pregnancy as a way of facilitating lactation. Milk then comes in earlier after birth, and the discomfort due to engorgement usually is avoided. Other writers, however, discourage this practice in the belief that the colostrum is wasted and the infant does not get the advantage of the immune substances it contains. More research is needed to determine if there is a unique advantage of colostrum over breast milk as well as to establish the efficacy of antepartum expression of colostrum.

Inverted nipples are a relative contraindication to breast-feeding because of the difficulties and frustration involved for many women. Much can be done to correct the inversion if it is recognized early in pregnancy. Rolling the nipple by grasping it between the thumb and finger and rolling very gently several times a day is often all the help that is needed. A Woolwich breast shield may be worn inside the bra. This is designed to exert pressure on the breast which will bring the nipple out. These shields are available from the La Leche League. Oral stimulation of the nipples by the woman's partner during sex play is another very effective treatment for inverted nipples.

Exercise

Exercise is beneficial to health as it improves circulation, enhances appetite and digestion of food, provides better bowel function, promotes restful sleep, and gives diversion from routine responsibilities. Walking is particularly recommended. Many physically active women continue to swim, jog, or play tennis well into their pregnancies. For the more sedentary woman, pregnancy may be a good time to embark upon a physical fitness program which will develop habits she can continue after childbirth. Many such programs are available through local YMCAs or even through do-it-yourself books. They are designed to increase flexibility, tone muscles, and improve cardiovascular conditioning.

Both the active and the sedentary woman should avoid fatigue and should stop exercising when she begins to feel tired. Moderation is the best watchword.

A change in balance with advancing pregnancy and the increased mobility of the pelvic joints may limit the pregnant woman's physical ability to continue some of her normal sports activities, at least in the latter weeks of pregnancy.

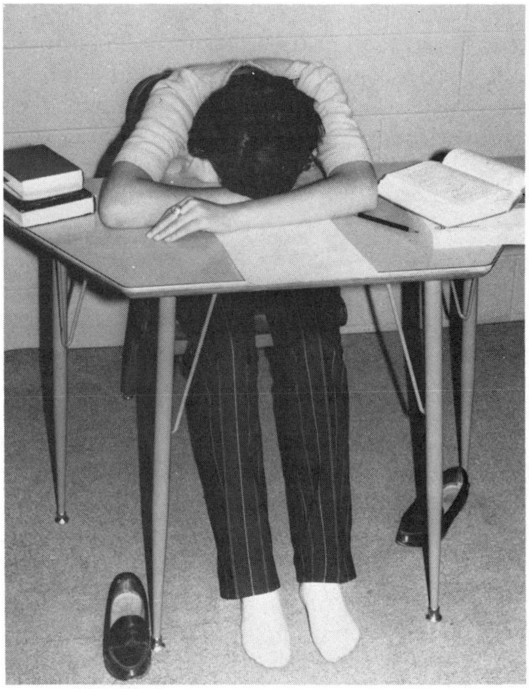

Figure 11–1. Relaxing at desk, with all muscles loose and limp, and feet flat on the floor.

Rest and Relaxation

Pregnant women tire easily, and every effort should be made to prevent undue fatigue. As the abdomen increases in size and weight, the body's center of gravity changes, and the pregnant woman is required to make a constant though unconscious effort to stand upright. Frequent rest periods are needed by all pregnant women, but are even more necessary for those with poor body alignment than for those who have good posture. Accordingly, the expectant mother may need rest frequently during the day, for 10 to 15 minutes at a time, in order to avoid needless fatigue. She should work and exercise in short periods, sitting or lying down if possible when tired. Many times some rest can be obtained by doing all work that can possibly be done in a sitting rather than a standing position.

If a woman is having trouble resting, it is often useful for the nurse to review a typical day with her in detail so they can plan together how to organize rest and work more efficiently. Sometimes the woman must adjust to less exacting standards of housekeeping in order to rest. Another woman may need help in setting limits for her preschool children to save herself steps. The woman who works outside her home may need suggestions for relaxation techniques and positions in order to get maximum benefit from her work breaks. (See Figure 11–1.)

Sitting can be fatiguing unless the hips are well back in the seat of a chair that gives adequate support to the back. The seat must not be so deep, however, that there is pressure under the knees and thus on the veins. The feet should rest on the floor or on a stool of suitable height, or a pillow. Sitting with the legs elevated on a stool, or pillow, will ensure rest as well as relieve a strain on varicosities and decrease swelling of the feet and legs (Fig. 11–2). For the position to be restful, the knees should be in slight flexion, and the footstool slightly lower than the chair to avoid pressure in the groins. Often a rocking chair, or a straight chair, with armrests

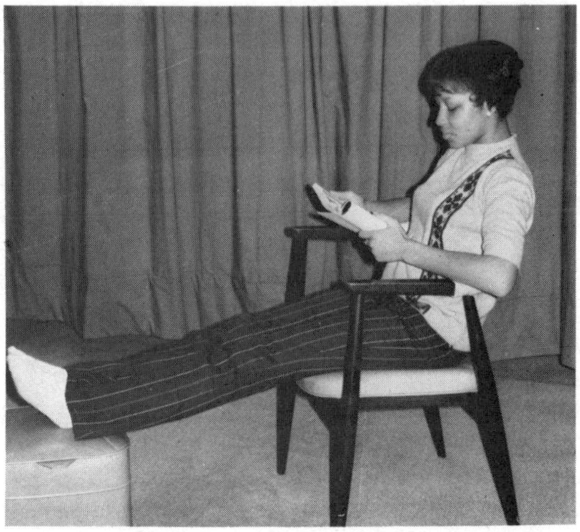

Figure 11–2. Relaxing in a chair with hips well back in the chair, adequate support to the back (not visible here), and legs elevated to relieve strain on varicosities and decrease swelling of feet.

and good back support, of a height that allows the feet to rest easily on the floor, is very comfortable for rest.

Fatigue often can be reduced by good posture and by taking care to avoid strain at work. Standing tall reduces stress. Changing position frequently is helpful. Stooping and lifting should be avoided whenever possible, but if they are necessary, the woman should bend at the hips or knees, keeping the back straight.

Since eight hours' sleep usually is considered necessary for the average person, the pregnant woman cannot expect to be comfortable with less. For good rest a comfortable position should be assumed, preferably on a bed with a firm mattress to prevent back strain.

In early pregnancy lying flat on the back with a pillow under the head and under the knees may be very comfortable. Clothing should be loose, and muscles should be allowed to become loose and limp. Slow abdominal breathing is conducive to relaxation and may help to induce sleep. Later in pregnancy when the abdomen enlarges, it usually becomes necessary for the mother to lie on her side with the hips partially rotated to allow the abdomen to rest on the bed. It may be necessary to use a pillow for support to the upper leg. All joints should be bent slightly to prevent muscle tenseness. With conscious effort, all of the skeletal muscles can be relaxed in this position.

Recreation is important to the expectant mother's pleasure and relaxation. It is advisable for her to continue most of her recreational activities during pregnancy, with limitations as necessary to avoid fatigue.

Sexuality

The desire for sexual expression may vary widely from one woman to the next and even from time to time for the same woman during pregnancy. There may be increased desire as the woman has a new awareness of her body and feels increasingly close to the man whose child she carries. At other times or in other women, this same body awareness may make intercourse repugnant to her. Still others have a fear of harming the baby.

Typically there is slight decrease in sexual tension during the first trimester because of fatigue and, perhaps, nausea. During the second trimester increasing pelvic congestion tends to heighten the woman's sexual desire; interest in sex may exceed that of her nonpregnant state. Again in the third trimester her interest in coitus declines as the fetus grows more demanding of her energy. In addition, her physical size makes positioning awkward. The penis thrusting against the "immovable object" of the fetal presenting part may be uncomfortable for both partners.

The man, too, varies in his sexual response to his pregnant partner. He may have diminishing sexual interest as pregnancy progresses because of the woman's swollen body and the fear of hurting her or the baby. Nurturant and protective feelings toward the woman may become dominant.

Couples should be aware that these changes in feelings are common. They are less likely to become confused and distressed by fluctuations in interest in sexual activity if they are able to anticipate it as a normal happening.

Adjustment to sexuality during pregnancy depends on the strength of the couple's total relationship, their maturity, culture, marital status, and feelings about this pregnancy. A couple with a stable, loving relationship who are able to communicate feelings to each other will adapt to each other more easily. They will be more apt to see sexual behavior as only one of many forms of intimacy.

Coital positions may need to be altered at various times throughout gestation to provide greater comfort. During the first trimester, breast tenderness may require avoiding direct pressure on the breasts, while in the third trimester the markedly enlarged uterus is clearly in the way of the traditional male-superior position. Many pregnant couples find the side-by-side, rear entry, or female-superior positions preferable. Coitus is necessarily gentler in these positions as well.

In the last trimester of pregnancy, the woman may experience a single orgasmic contraction lasting as long as a minute rather than the rhythmic, multiple contractions of the nonpregnant state. She also may have some cramps or a backache following orgasm resulting from the pelvic congestion. This is usually relieved by a back rub.

At the same time the woman's desire for coitus may be declining, she ordinarily has an increasing need for physical closeness and cuddling. Kissing, hugging, and caressing are important ways of expressing love and affection (Fig. 11–3).

There are no medically valid reasons for prohibiting sexual intercourse during a normal pregnancy. Certain complications or risk factors, however, may make restrictions necessary. These include threatened abortion, ruptured membranes, vaginal bleeding, and premature labor that has been stopped pharmacologically.

The Use of Drugs During Pregnancy

A single evening of television viewing is sufficient evidence that this is indeed a "drug culture." No human malady, however great or small, need be suffered if the drug commercials are to be believed. Pregnant women, no less than others, ingest a variety of drugs both prescribed and over-the-counter. For most of these drugs the effects on the fetus are unknown.

The dramatic tragedy of thalidomide-induced con-

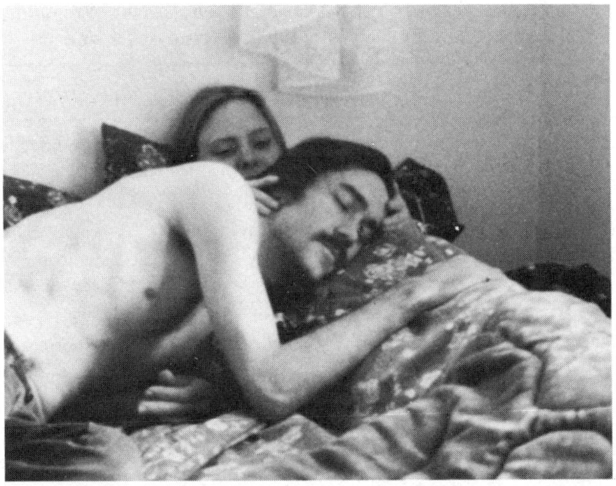

Figure 11–3. Intimacy is important for both expectant parents. During pregnancy changing physical contours as well as changes in libido may necessitate different expressions of affection.

genital anomalies raised the consciousness of the public as well as professionals to the risks inherent in medications taken during pregnancy. It is to be hoped that the result of this increased awareness will be a reluctance to prescribe or to take any but the most essential drugs during gestation.

Necessary Conditions for Drug Effects

In order for a drug to be teratogenic (cause damage to the developing fetus), the following conditions must be met:

1. The drug must cross the placenta and reach the fetus in concentrations sufficient to cause damage. It is generally believed that most drugs cross the placenta. The concentration achieved in the fetal bloodstream depends on a variety of factors. Probably, in most instances, there is an equilibration across the placenta so that the concentration in the fetus approximates that in the mother. In some cases the fetal concentration may be elevated because of the inability of the immature fetal liver to break down the drug or the immature fetal kidney to excrete it.

2. The drug must reach the fetus at a critical time for the development of a particular organ or structure. Different structures are vulnerable to damage at different times depending on when in embryonic or fetal life they are undergoing maximum differentiation (Fig. 11–4). In general, the first trimester is the period of greatest danger from malformation-inducing agents. Since the woman is unaware of her pregnancy for at least some part of this critical first trimester, there is a convincing argument for all women who are at risk to become pregnant to avoid taking drugs whenever possible.

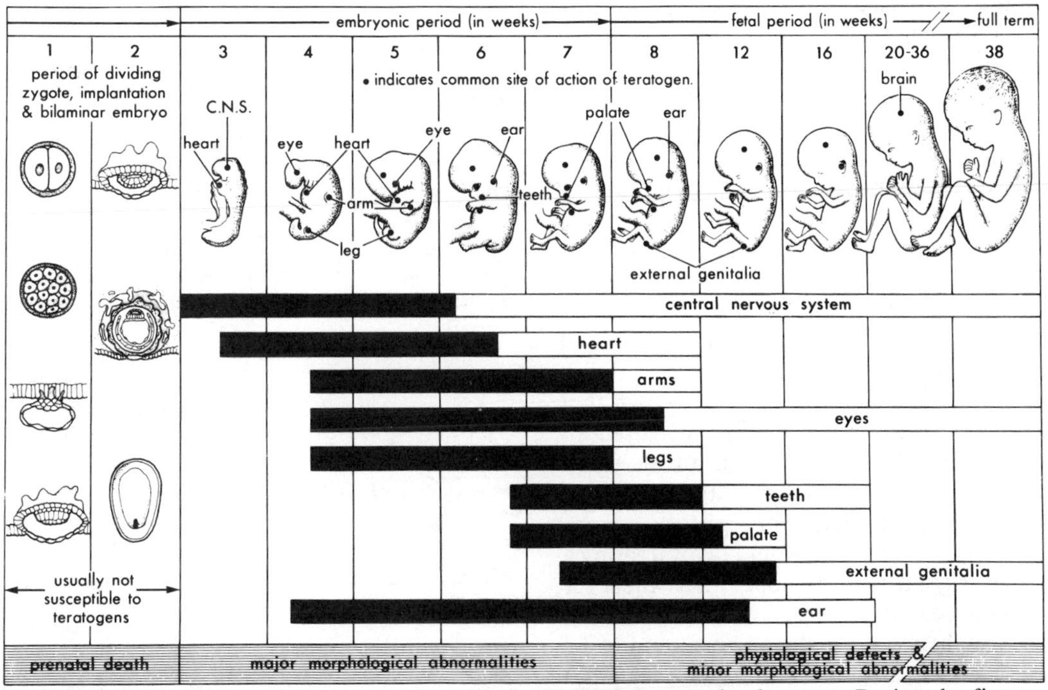

Figure 11–4. Schematic illustration of the sensitive or critical periods in human development. During the first two weeks of development, the embryo is usually not susceptible to teratogens. During these predifferentiation stages, a substance either damages all or most of the cells of the embryo, resulting in its death, or it damages only a few cells, allowing the embryo to recover without developing defects. Dark bars denote highly sensitive periods; white bars indicate stages that are less sensitive to teratogens. (Reproduced with permission from Keith L. Moore, *The Developing Human. Clinically Oriented Embryology,* 3rd ed., Philadelphia: Saunders, 1982.)

not have fetal monitoring in the absence of any risk indicators, or to choose early discharge within 8 to 24 hours after delivery. Such discussion should not replace consultation with the woman's physician, but it does provide valuable information at a time and location where the rooms and monitors can be seen and some of their mystique dispelled.

Expectant parents are taught that preparation-for-childbirth exercises are not designed to produce a painless childbirth, but rather to help them participate actively in the delivery of their infant. Preparation does not preclude use of analgesia, but it often reduces the amount necessary. Some women will not require medication. They are told that pain-relieving medication is available when it is indicated or desired. They are also taught that obstetric intervention, such as forceps delivery, may become necessary for delivery, and that the physician will make this decision according to the best interest of mother and fetus.

A growing trend in prenatal education is the inclusion of an increasing amount of information relative to parenting. Some groups are extending their classes into the postpartum period or are forming new groups of young parents to help them deal with the issues of childrearing.

In large families older children learn child care by practicing on their youngest siblings and the younger children practice on their nieces and nephews as their older siblings begin their own families. In the modern, smaller family such opportunities do not exist as often. When young couples become parents, their own mothers and other older women relatives are quite likely to be employed and unavailable to help with baby care and to act as role models. In addition, couples today tend to form isolated nuclear families which may be quite distant from the extended family, geographically as well as psychologically. Thus, the support structure as well as the sanctions of the kinship group are often missing. It is in an attempt to fill this gap that postpartum parent groups are being formed. The school system, too, in response to this need is increasing the sophistication and usefulness of the family life education courses being offered to young people.

The timing of classes during pregnancy depends to some extent on the length of the series of classes and their availability in the community as well as the couples' own schedule. Generally speaking, these classes should be arranged toward the end of the second trimester, which will permit completion by the thirty-sixth week of gestation. By this time the fetus is quite active, the woman looks pregnant, and is feeling well. She has adapted to her pregnancy and is now ready to consider preparation for the reality of labor and delivery and an infant. Whenever possible, the father should participate in the classes. He will gain needed information first hand and obtain the support necessary to facilitate the assumption of his new role. Some classes have one session for men only, so there is an opportunity to share feelings, doubts, and concerns without "feeling dumb" in front of the women.

RELAXATION TECHNIQUES, POSITIONS, AND EXERCISES

Physical preparation of the mother for childbirth through instruction in relaxation techniques, rest positions, and exercises is one of the objectives of parents' classes. This preparation is designed to help the pregnant woman minimize stress by improving her posture, developing an ability to relax and improve rest, practicing specific exercises for neuromuscular control and breathing response during labor, and learning methods useful in postpartum restoration of the body. Fathers are taught how to assist the woman with antepartum conditioning, with the practice of exercises, and about the techniques of coaching these exercises during labor. Since men, as well as women, are subject to stress and physical tension, it is to be supposed that the relaxation responses would be equally beneficial to them. (See Figure 11-10.)

The notion of deliberate physical conditioning for childbirth is a phenomenon of a technologic civilization where muscular activity is largely foreign to more sedentary occupations and birth is removed from the everyday experience.

Essentially each preparation-for-childbirth program stems from the Read or the Lamaze method, although there are variations in technique. However, all programs make the effort to erase previous negative impressions of pregnancy, labor, and delivery and plan to recondition the couple toward acceptance of a healthy positive attitude. Physical exercises to improve the woman's general well-being usually are included. Instruction in respiratory and relaxation techniques is designed to help

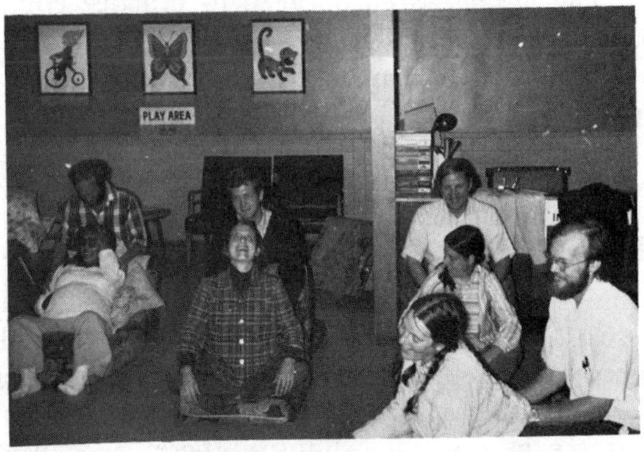

Figure 11-10. A group of expectant parents practicing relaxation and breathing exercises in preparation for labor and delivery.

the woman reduce her perception of pain arising from the uterine contractions and to participate actively in her labor and delivery.

The Read Method

The late Dr. Grantly Dick Read, a London obstetrician, originated the idea that pain during labor was caused by fear. He published his first book on the influence of fear on the course of labor in 1933 under the title *Natural Childbirth*. According to Dr. Read, women can be prepared for a natural physiologic labor unaccompanied by fear and tenseness when they learn to regard childbirth as a natural process. With education and preparation, the woman knows what to expect because she has learned the physiology of pregnancy, labor, and delivery, and she understands how to assist herself during the various phases of labor. By natural childbirth, Dr. Read meant labor and delivery uninhibited by physical, chemical, or psychologic factors and a labor that was not accompanied by great discomfort.

Dr. Read contended that to achieve natural childbirth the fear-tension-pain syndrome must be broken. This triad has considerable influence on the course of labor. Tension increases with fear, and tension may cause muscle spasms and increase pain. Tension not only interferes with cervical dilation, but also causes involuntary spasm of abdominal and back muscles, resulting in pain. With an understanding of labor and of the means of relaxation during labor, fear and apprehension are reduced, tension is lessened, and pain is decreased.

The Read method is sometimes called the psychophysical method of preparation. In this method, the mother is taught how to release muscle tension and how to relax all her muscles completely at her will. Slow abdominal breathing is practiced for use during contractions of much of the first stage of labor and is helpful in precluding painful spasms of the abdominal muscles. Rapid chest breathing is learned for use toward the end of labor if abdominal breathing becomes difficult at that time. The mother is encouraged to practice complete relaxation and abdominal breathing daily to achieve an increasingly greater ability to do so and to become so adept that it can be done at will and under stress.

The Lamaze Method

As the Read method of preparation for childbirth was becoming established, another method was devised, known as the psychoprophylactic or Lamaze method. Its author, Dr. Fernand Lamaze, accepted Dr. Read's theory that women often have been negatively conditioned to expect pain in childbirth; therefore, education to expunge previous negative impressions of childbirth is an important part of the program. Its major difference is in the method of preparation for labor. Lamaze joined Read's theory to the Russian psychoprophylactic system, based on pavlovian neurodynamics, using conditioned responses to uterine contractions.

The positive conditioning of the Lamaze method is accomplished through training in chest-breathing and relaxation techniques, which will become a specific response to uterine contractions, i.e., a conditioned reflex which prevents or diminishes the painful sensations arising from the contracting uterus. In this intensive training program the woman, who must be strongly motivated, is taught several specific levels of chest breathing, and she must learn with which kind of respiratory response, or level of chest breathing, she should react to the different phases of labor. Lamaze's chest-breathing method, as compared to Read's abdominal breathing, is considered easier and more comfortable throughout labor. The various levels of breathing and their use are described in detail in Chapter 20 and in Figure 20–4.

REFERENCES AND SUGGESTED READINGS

Becker, Constance, Comprehensive assessment of the healthy gravida, *JOGN Nurs.*, 11(6):375–78, 1982.

Campbell, Anne, and Worthington, E. L., Teaching expectant fathers how to be better childbirth coaches, *MCN*, 7 (1):28–32, 1982.

Daniels, M. B., and Manning, D., A clinic for pregnant teens, *Am. J. Nurs.*, 83(1):68–71, 1983.

Dzurec, Laura Cox, Childbirth education classes: Are they helpful? *MCN*, 6(5):329–32, 1981.

Grasso, Camille; Barden, Mary; Henry, Connie; and Vieau, Mary G., The Vietnamese American family—and Grandma makes three, *MCN*, 6(3):177–80, 1981.

Josten, LaVohn, Prenatal assessment guide for illuminating possible problems with parenting, *MCN*, 6(2):113–17, 1981.

Kim, M. J., and Moritz, D. A. (eds.), *Classification of Nursing Diagnosis: Proceedings of the Third and Fourth National Conferences*, McGraw-Hill, New York, 1982.

Lunney, Margaret, Nursing diagnosis: Refining the system, *Am. J. Nurs.*, 82(3):456–59, 1982.

Magee, J., The pelvic examination: A view from the other end of the table, *Ann. Intern. Med.*, 83:563–64, 1975.

Malasanos, L.; Barkasiska, V.; Moss, M.; and Slottenberg-Allen, K., *Health Assessment*, C. V. Mosby, St. Louis, 1981.

Martin, Bob J., and Reeb, Rene M., Oral health during pregnancy: A neglected nursing area, *MCN*, 7(6):391–92, 1982.

McKay, Susan R., Smoking during the childbearing year, *MCN*, 5(1):46–50, 1980.

Meleis, Afaf Ibrahim, and Sorrell, Lois, Arab American women and their birth experiences, *MCN*, 6(3):171–76, 1981.

Pritchard, J. A., and MacDonald, P. C., *Williams Obstetrics*, 16th ed., Appleton-Century-Crofts, New York, 1980.

Stephens, Cheryl J., The fetal alcohol syndrome. Cause for concern, *MCN*, 6(4):251–56, 1981.

CHAPTER

12

Psychosocial Adaptation of the Childbearing Family

DEFINITION OF FAMILY

Family-centered care is an underlying philosophy of this text. Repeatedly, the nurse-reader is exhorted to bear in mind that pregnancy and childbirth occur in the context of a family. Thus, it seems imperative to identify what is meant by a family.

Most people are clear about who and what constitutes their families. Yet to arrive at a universal definition that fits all families is very difficult since composition and functions vary considerably among modern families. An in-depth discussion of family structure and function is beyond the scope of this text. Suffice it to say that the American family has undergone significant changes during the past 50 years as a result of the changing social context in which it exists. Although the isolated nuclear family is still predominant, a variety of family structures are encountered. All of these families may be defined as *two or more people bound together by some form of ties and having some common goals.* The "ties" may be legal, as in marriage, affectional, or blood relationships. The goals may be economic, reproductive, affectional, and so on. Goals are closely associated with family functions. That is, one determines another. Some family scholars maintain that there are no longer any societal functions that are unique to the family. Other maintain that the family still serves to provide affection and understanding to its members and as the primary resource for the socialization of children.

Variant Family Forms

The *nuclear family* is the most common family structure encountered by the perinatal nurse. Over 80 percent of births occur in these families. Some authors differentiate between married couples who are expecting their first child and couples who already have one or more children, calling the former "beginning nuclear families." In any event, a nuclear family connotes a man and woman who are married to each other together with their children. The nuclear family is often referred to as a person's family of procreation, in contrast to the family of orientation which consists of his/her parents and siblings.

The *extended family* is made up of the larger kinship group to which the nuclear family belongs. It usually includes at least the parents and siblings of the couple and often grandparents, aunts, uncles, and cousins (Fig. 12-1).

Unmarried couples may live together in intimacy and

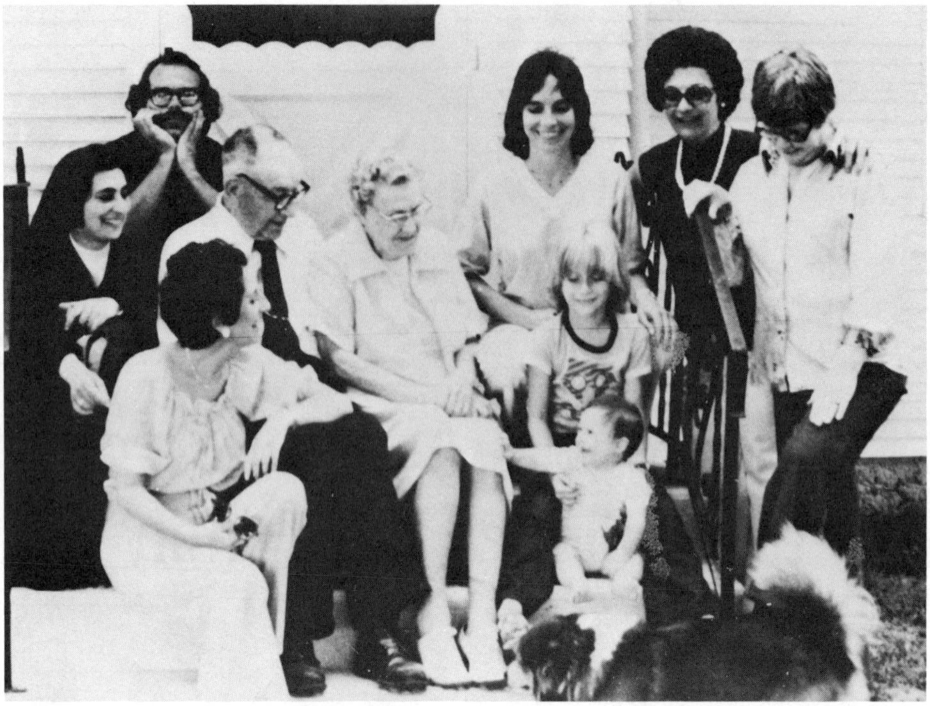

Figure 12–1. The extended family is an important source of support for the new parents. It provides role models, affection, and a sense of continuity over generations.

have children believing that the legal sanctions of marriage are unnecessary and inhibiting to their freedom to love each other. These couples present much the same situation to the nurse as the nuclear family. However, their relationship is likely to be a source of conflict with their extended family and thus may present issues of limited social support.

Single-parent families are increasingly common in the United States. In 1980, 18 percent of births were to unmarried women. It is estimated that about half of all children will spend some part of their first 18 years living in a single-parent household, either because their mother never married or as a result of death or divorce. Some of these pregnancies are accidental, some are planned. Single women who wish to have a child may purposefully become pregnant either by artificial insemination or by sexual intercourse. Parenthood is a long and often arduous job requiring much support. When giving care to a single parent, nurses should be particularly careful to assess the social support network of the woman as well as her ability to seek help, establish linkages, and utilize resources.

Lesbian couples are a variation of the unmarried-couple family style in which two women live together in sexual intimacy. The nurse may encounter these families in pediatric practice if they are caring for a child or children from previous heterosexual relationships. In addition, an increasing number of homosexual women are choosing to become pregnant, most frequently by artificial insemination.

Before providing care for any family, it is valuable for nurses to have a clear sense of their own families and of their values with respect to family life and reproduction. If secure with their own beliefs, they will be better able to intervene with families without making value judgments.

EFFECT OF PREGNANCY ON THE FAMILY

Change as a Characteristic of the Family

Transition and change are central to family experience. The family is in continual dynamic interaction among its members and with the community outside the family. Relationships within the family change, sometimes gradually, sometimes abruptly, as the members mature, as new members join, and some members leave. Interactions with the community also change, depending on the age and developmental stage of the family members, as well as many other circumstances such as health, employment, and family needs and interests. Some of the expected changes or transitions encountered by most, if not all, families are the birth of a child (children), departure of children from the parental home, aging, and death. In addition, all families face some unexpected situations such as divorce, illness, changes in economic circumstances, alcohol or drug use, school problems, violence, and so on.

Family Change Resulting from Pregnancy

Pregnancy normally results in significant family change as the result of anticipating and then realizing the addition of a new member. Although each family is affected in a slightly different way, the changes that most families can expect to some degree are described here.

Increased Number of Relationships

The addition of one new member increases the number of intrafamilial relationships geometrically. With a couple there are two relationships: his with her and hers with him. However, by adding one infant the number of relationships within the family increases to six, since each member has a relationship with two other members. The general formula for calculating the number of relationships in a family is

Number of members $\times$ $(n - 1)$

Thus, for a family of 4 there are $4 \times 3 = 12$ relationships.

Role Realignment

During pregnancy the couple begins to prepare for their new roles as parents. Not only must each individual acquire a sense of role function and a sense of self in that role, but he or she must reorder the sense of the partner to include the partner's new role. Thus, a woman pregnant for the first time not only has to acquire the mother role but has to begin to interact with her mate as a father as well as a husband, lover, and so on.

Social Networks

Changes in the couple's social network often occur during pregnancy and childrearing. New friends and acquaintances who share the experience of pregnancy and infants may be added. Some old acquaintances may have less and less in common and gradually drift apart. The family often seeks new contacts to help them cope with this transition such as childbirth education classes, parent support groups, and experienced parents from their extended families and acquaintances.

Sexual Relations

For many couples there is a period of heightened sexual enjoyment during at least part of pregnancy. For others there are diminished libido and discomfort with intercourse. Fear of injuring the fetus is a common inhibiting factor. In addition to the challenges of pregnancy, the early weeks after birth present additional barriers to sexual relationships with sleep interruptions, episiotomy discomfort, fatigue, and so on. Sex during pregnancy and post partum is discussed more fully in Chapters 11 and 24, respectively.

Time

During pregnancy couples notice a change in the way time is allocated as new activities are added. Antepartal health supervision visits usually require several hours each when travel and waiting time is considered. The couple may attend childbirth classes, spend time shopping for baby things and preparing the nursery. In addition, as the pregnancy progresses the woman may find that she needs to rest more frequently and cannot comfortably do work at her accustomed pace. After the birth of the infant, even more radical changes in the use of time occur.

Finances

Having a baby is expensive—even during pregnancy. In addition to the cost of antepartal care and hospitalization for delivery, there are expenditures for transportation to and from the clinic or physician's office, babysitters for other children, maternity clothing, prenatal vitamins and iron, and so on. Furthermore, many women are now in the labor force, and the loss or interruption of their incomes for part or all of pregnancy and early infancy may be a real economic hardship. Although these costs may seem to be self-evident, few couples are aware of them, and therefore do not plan for them in their budgets.[1]

Change as a Crisis

Families respond to change in highly individual ways. Some appear to take everything in stride with no appreciable shift in equilibrium, while other families may completely disintegrate in what objectively appear to be very similar circumstances. According to family crisis theory, an objectively defined *stressor event* may or may not result in a *crisis* for the family system depending on a number of family characteristics. These characteristics include:

1. *Vulnerability to Stress.* Families in which there is greater role flexibility seem more immune to stress and change since they can shift roles more readily

[1] J. E. Mulligan, "Hidden Costs of Pregnancy." Unpublished data, University of Wisconsin, Madison, School of Nursing.

to accommodate to changes. As an example, the Marches believed everyone should pitch in to accomplish whatever household tasks needed doing. As a result, both parents and the teenage son were reasonably adept at cooking, laundry, and cleaning. When Mrs. March was gone for 10 days to care for her aging mother, the rest of the family managed quite nicely. Vulnerability is also affected by the number of stressors. Stress is additive. A family may cope very well with a pregnancy. However, if the pregnancy occurs while the father is unemployed, a grandparent is critically ill, and an older child is having school problems, the pregnancy may be the proverbial straw on the camel's back.

2. *The Definition the Family Makes of the Event.* This is another way of saying "what is the family's point of view or perception of the event." If the family places a high value on children, that family will define even an unplanned pregnancy differently than another family with less regard for children. The 28-year-old married woman with reasonable economic security will likely view pregnancy differently than the 40-year-old woman who has a contraceptive failure or the 14-year-old girl who didn't know she could get pregnant the first time she had intercourse.

   Changes (events) that were anticipated are generally viewed more favorably and tolerated more readily than unexpected events. Those that are perceived to require relatively minor changes in the family system usually are regarded more favorably than those considered to cause major upheaval.

   In summary, an event is less likely to produce family crisis if it is considered by the family to be congruent with family values, if it requires a small amount of immediate change, and if it has been anticipated.

3. *Family Resources for Management.* Even events that the family defines as catastrophic may be dealt with fairly readily provided there are adequate resources.
   a. *Intrapersonal characteristics.* Individuals who are mature, imaginative, and possess good problem-solving skills are more capable of adapting to stress and change. In addition, if family members have generally good self-concepts and believe they are in control of their lives, they are less likely to view a situation as problematic.
   b. *Coping behaviors.* Coping is a process of maintaining the family system in a balance that facilitates unity and organization and encourages individual growth and development. It can reduce vulnerability to stress, strengthen resources, and change the social circumstances. According to McCubbin and his associates, coping behaviors simultaneously involve maintaining intrafamily communication and organization, promoting independence and self-esteem of each member, maintaining family cohesion, maintaining and developing social support, and attempting to control the impact of the stressor event on the family system.
   c. *Social support.* A major family resource is the extent to which they are a member of a community of mutual regard and support and the extent to which there exists a network of persons and services upon whom they can call for help. Support may take the form of emotional or moral support, assistance with tasks such as caring for children or giving a ride to the doctor's office, or material aid such as loans of money or baby clothing and equipment.
   d. *Financial resources.* Families with adequate incomes, health insurance, and so on generally manage easier than those less well-favored economically.

Nursing Intervention in Family Crisis

In assessing the family's response to pregnancy and the coming child, the nurse may use the family characteristics described above as a useful framework. In many families, short-term interventions can have a significant impact on family vulnerability, clarify the family's definition of the event, and increase their resources for management. Table 12–1 outlines some suggestions for nursing care. Significant family disruption will require longer term therapy and may be most appropriately treated by referral to a family counselor.

EFFECT OF PREGNANCY ON THE MOTHER

Pregnancy is a developmental event. This is self-evident from the point of view of the fetus. The entire gestational period is uniquely designed for the most dramatic and concentrated period of growth and development in human life. But for the pregnant woman, the mother, it is also a developmental and maturational period. It has been seen already that physiologically the changes are enormous. Virtually every organ and system undergoes substantial growth and development as well as functional modifications. In addition, it is a time of identity reformulation and reordering of interpersonal relationships. As her body changes in contour and appearance, she asks herself, "Who am I?"

Developmental Tasks

Although pregnancy is a biologically normal event, it is an exceptional one in the life of a woman and her family

Table 12–1. Outline of Suggested Nursing Actions Based on the Family Crisis Model*

Elements in the Family Crisis Model	*Suggested Nursing Activities*
VULNERABILITY TO STRESS	In initial interview, obtain information about other potential stressors such as unemployment, illness or recent death in family, career changes, marital problems.
DEFINITION FAMILY MAKES OF EVENT	Determine if pregnancy was planned. Ask what other family members have said about pregnancy. Provide opportunity for woman to express feelings. Explain most women and men are initially ambivalent about pregnancy.
FAMILY RESOURCES FOR MANAGEMENT	
Intrapersonal characteristics	Assess problem solving abilities of woman and family. Use anticipatory guidance and role play to enhance or develop skills.
Coping	Ask how woman and family have dealt with other experiences in the past. For example, in preparing for labor help woman think of what has been helpful in other situations when she has been in pain.
Social support	Determine kinship and friendship network. Determine how interpersonal resources are used. Provide information about support groups, neighborhood resources, etc.
Financial resources	Make appropriate referrals for public assistance programs such as WIC or Medicaid. Refer to community resources which may assist with baby clothes, etc.

*The practicing nurse will be able to add many other suggestions based on experience and individual family needs.

and, as such, requires a shift in the organization of values and roles. These characteristics have led several authors to describe pregnancy within the framework of crisis theory as a maturational or developmental crisis. This crisis acts as an impetus to a lengthy period of adaptation and reorganization, often necessitating the development of new coping mechanisms, acquisition of new knowledge and skills, and modification of interpersonal relationships.

How each woman works through the crisis of pregnancy will be determined largely by her own style as well as the culture in which she lives. There is, however, an increasing belief in the theory that her "work" can be described by certain developmental tasks common across cultures. Deutsch, Bibring, Caplan, Tanner, and Rubin have described various tasks or goals to be achieved by the woman during the nine months of her pregnancy. These tasks are briefly summarized as follows:

1. Acceptance of pregnancy as a symbiosis with the fetus and then moving toward acceptance of the infant as an individual distinct from herself in preparation for the physical separation of delivery.
2. Ensuring acceptance of the child she bears by her significant others.[2]

[2] Reva Rubin, Maternal tasks in pregnancy, *Matern. Child Nurs. J.*, 4:143–53, 1975.

3. Seeking safe passage for herself and her child through pregnancy, labor, and delivery.[3]
4. Adoption of the mother role.

Erik Erikson and other developmental theorists have postulated that each life stage has certain tasks that can be most efficiently accomplished given the age, social and psychologic development, and other parameters of that stage. They have suggested further that failure to master the developmental tasks of any given stage interferes with the ability to meet successfully the challenges of the stage to follow. In colloquial terms this can be stated as "you must crawl before you can walk."

The tasks of pregnancy can be regarded as a special case of Erikson's developmental stage theory. These tasks are the particular way in which a woman works out the stage of Generativity vs. Stagnation during that very circumscribed time defined by the conception and delivery of an infant. She works at the tasks simultaneously, weaving them all tapestry-fashion throughout gestation. One or the other of the tasks may assume dominance for an individual woman, and, for all women, there appears to be a shifting dominance of tasks from trimester to trimester as pregnancy progresses. The woman must achieve some resolution of each task for each of her pregnancies.

Trimester I

If a single word could be chosen to characterize the first trimester of pregnancy, it would be ambivalence. Regardless of how planned and how desired the pregnancy, the awareness of the fact that conception has indeed occurred causes the expectant mother to doubt the wisdom of her choice. Another time—any other time—might have been better. She realizes a certain loss of control over her body and, indeed, her whole destiny. If the option of abortion is set aside, the woman finds herself embarked upon a course from which there is no escape except through the trial of labor and birth. Following that, she is a mother forever. Added to that is her feeling of physical ambivalence. Her symptoms are primarily of absence of menstruation rather than the presence or addition of anything. She is tired, she may be nauseated. She is not ill, but she doesn't feel well either.

During this first trimester the woman seeks confirmation of her pregnancy and reassurance that she can bear a child. She wants—and needs—an expert opinion that what she believes is true, that she is healthy and that the pregnancy is "good." This is the goal of the first antepartum visit to the physician.

In addition to accepting herself as pregnant, the woman must ensure acceptance of her pregnancy by those who are important to her. This appears to be the most crucial of the tasks, since its successful accomplishment secures the support necessary for the woman as she becomes a mother. It seems to give her the energy for her other tasks, yet it differs from the other tasks in that it is bound to social interaction, whereas most of the remaining tasks are internal.

By around 16 weeks of gestation most women have resolved the ambivalence of rejecting/accepting and have incorporated the idea of self-as-pregnant-woman. This psychologic acceptance of pregnancy is analogous to physical implantation. If the blastocyst does not attach firmly to the uterine wall, development stops and the pregnancy is aborted. Similarly, if the pregnancy is not psychologically accepted, the development of attachment to the child stagnates and the mother-child relationship may be aborted.

Trimester II

As the second trimester begins, the physical changes that are occurring hasten the resolution of ambivalence. The woman has increasing energy, her nausea is gone, she begins to acquire a pregnant figure. She feels good and has a sense of well-being. Then quickening occurs. This event makes the woman acutely conscious of a presence within. She says she has felt Life. At first she regards the infant as part of herself. Gradually, throughout the rest of gestation, the infant becomes a reality that is within her but is not her. She must achieve this attitude in order to bear the idea of birth, physical separation. This shift in attitude is achieved in interaction with the fetus and in a rich fantasy life. She pokes her tummy to get the infant to poke back. She places her husband's hand on her belly so he, too, can feel. She describes the infant as sleeping or active. She attributes intention to him. "He just kicks at bedtime to keep me awake." She dreams and daydreams how he will be: boy or girl, blue eyes or brown, curly hair or bald, and, most of all, normal or abnormal.

As she begins increasingly to regard the infant as a reality apart from herself, the pregnant woman begins to consider her role as a mother. She must sort out for herself what being a mother means and what the cost/benefit balance is for her. This is closely wrapped up with the idea of self-identity—Who am I? The pregnant woman is assisted in her ability to rework old problems and come up with better solutions and a clearer identity by the characteristic shift in personality equilibrium which occurs as a phenomenon of pregnancy. This is most evident to the observer in the extraordinary openness and talkativeness of pregnant women. Thus, it appears pregnancy offers women a unique and valuable maturational opportunity.

Exploration of what motherhood is all about is accomplished primarily through the woman's relationship with her own mother. It is not unusual to find an in-

[3] *Ibid.*

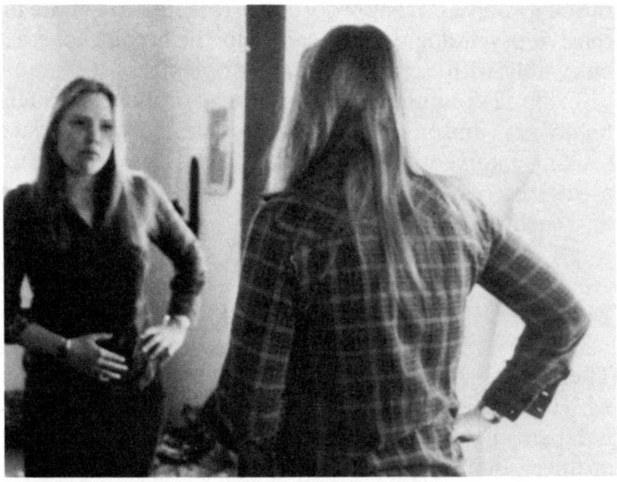

Figure 12–2. The woman's changing contours during pregnancy prompt a reexamination of self and body image.

crease in frequency of visits, letters, and telephone calls between a mother and her pregnant daughter. For women who have not had a close relationship with their mothers, there is often an attempt at reconciliation.

Because of the intense work of accepting the infant and adapting to her role change, the pregnant woman has a characteristic introversion and passivity. This change begins with the second trimester and gradually increases until around the seventh or eighth month (30 to 35 weeks). Her most essential reality is within. All her relationships and interests become reordered. Only those relationships and interests that are essential to her in this situation of being pregnant are compatible with her inner world.

The woman, as well as her family, is often confused by this change from her former outgoing, giving self. She now is often preoccupied and wishes to be given to rather than to give. She is increasingly dependent and looks for much love and attention, gifts of time and self to her. Fathers feel shut out from a world they cannot fully share or even understand. As with all creative work, every energy is directed inward as the woman struggles to make both a baby and a mother.

Pregnant women are notorious for their emotional lability. Partly from preoccupation, partly from hormonal changes, and partly from realization of the impact of pregnancy, the woman becomes increasingly sensitive and irritable. She is equally likely to laugh uproariously at something which no one else regards as funny and to burst into tears without knowing why.

During the second trimester the pregnant woman develops an interest in learning about herself and her baby. This is the time most women seek out prenatal classes, read books, and talk with other pregnant women. She is definitely pregnant but not yet close enough to labor for it to be an imminent threat, so it is a "safe" time to gather all the information that she can. When labor does become imminent, she will be armed with knowledge and skills to master it safely.

Trimester III

During the last weeks of pregnancy the expectant mother hastens to complete all the tasks. Physically she is now great and clumsy; she tires more easily, has difficulty adjusting to her new body boundaries, and is uncomfortable. She begins to be tired of pregnancy but is still hesitant about delivery. The fluttering of her infant within has become vigorous intrusive kicks. She has an increasing sense of vulnerability, exhibited by preoccupation with locks on the door, cautioning others to drive carefully, and avoiding running, bumping children. The physical discomforts and increasing burden of the pregnancy serve to instill a psychologic readiness for labor and delivery in spite of the threats.

As evidence that she has accepted the infant as separate from herself, she makes decisions about his care, how she will feed him, what his name will be. Acceptance of the infant by others in the family assumes crucial importance. There must be a place for him when he comes—a physical niche in the house and, more importantly, an emotional niche in the hearts of his family. Rejection of the child now is a rejection of the woman herself. She must have approval of the product she is preparing. To promote this, she spends much time with her children describing how it will be to have an infant in the family. She urges participation of her husband in name selection, nursery furnishings, and preparation for and participation in the labor and delivery itself.

As desperately as the woman wants her husband to want the baby, he wants the wife back he feels he has lost to the child. If they love each other enough and are open to sharing and communication of feelings, both will get their wishes and the child will come into a richer home.

The end of pregnancy comes at last. The woman has moved through 40 weeks of growing into motherhood. Through an intricate intertwining of physical changes and psychologic work she has accepted first the pregnant state and then the fact of a child. She has sought help to assure her own health and the intactness of her child and has prepared herself and her loved ones to accept a new family member. Finally she returns full circle to the ambivalence of the first trimester. She hates the pregnancy, wants the child, but fears birth. Her behavior in labor will appear as a telescoping of the emotions and behaviors of the entire pregnancy. It is as if she makes an intense summary of the whole process of baby-making so that she is ready to begin the next step in mothering. If the work has gone well, particularly if she has established a secure support system for herself and her child, she is most likely to have continued success as a woman and as a parent.

Implications for Therapeutic Intervention with Families

The implications of this framework of emotional change and maternal tasks for therapeutic intervention with families during childbearing are considerable. Three suggested applications will be discussed briefly here as illustrations.

1. *As an organizing framework for antepartum teaching*

The concept of maternal tasks could serve effectively as a guide for organizing classes for expectant parents. Not only content but also timing and methodology are suggested. For example, infant care activities and how-to's might well be appropriate for the third trimester when the woman clearly perceives the infant as an individual separate from herself. The same content is likely to be met with indifference earlier in pregnancy because it is not synchronous with the woman's own agenda at that time. In contrast, information about her own body and how it works would be more suitably approached early in gestation when her concerns for "safe passage" are principally self-centered.

2. *Anticipatory guidance in self-understanding*

Knowing that pregnancy is commonly greeted with marked ambivalence under the best of circumstances can do much to reduce the guilt of a woman who finds herself with these feelings. Similarly, if she can be helped to recognize and understand in herself the increasing dependency, mood swings, and other emotions as features of pregnancy that are as normal as increasing uterine size, then she will find her feelings less confusing and disturbing. An interesting observation is the conflicting effect of these emotions of pregnancy and the current feminist movement. Young women who think of themselves as independent, assertive, and "liberated," find the feelings of pregnancy incongruent with their self-image and may well need help to resolve this dissonance.

3. *Anticipatory guidance for significant others*

Persons who live with pregnant women often describe them as "different people" than when they are not pregnant. A man may be confused and/or threatened by his wife's changing sexual response, for example. If he is clued to expect that her sense of vulnerability and introversion as well as her physical contours may cause a loss of interest in conventional sexual expression, a potential area of conflict may be avoided. At the same time, the couple may be helped to explore alternate methods of expressing love and affection, and the woman's increased need for tenderness and attention can be pointed out. The pregnant woman's alarming tendency to cry for "no reason" and to laugh at jokes that are not funny can cause consternation for both partners, especially if their relationship was not securely developed prior to conception. Understanding that such mood swings and inappropriate effect stem from the intensive psychologic work can help them cope together enjoyably with "crazy pregnant women."

Table 12–2 summarizes the physical findings, frequent behaviors, and maternal tasks by trimester. Suggested nursing interventions are indicated as a guide. It must always be remembered that each woman, each family, and each pregnancy is unique.

EFFECT OF PREGNANCY ON THE FATHER

The father's biologic involvement with pregnancy ends with conception. His social and psychologic involvement is dependent in many ways upon his relationship with the mother. In the extreme situation where the father is unaware that conception had taken place and never sees the mother again, it is highly unlikely that he would experience any of the changes described below. Thus, the man's experience with pregnancy is intrinsically different from that of the woman; yet there are many similarities when the couple shares the pregnancy and plans together for parenthood.

Developmental Tasks

The literature about fathers in pregnancy and birth has mushroomed in the past 15 years as men have taken more active roles and American society has become more accepting of men having an interest in birth and babies. A number of authors have identified developmental tasks that appear to describe the work of a man preparing for fatherhood. These include:

1. Acceptance of the pregnancy and fetus and the reality of having a baby.[4]
2. Adoption of father role. This involves mourning the change of life-style, loss of some degree of personal freedom, and the need to share his partner's attention with an infant.[5] In addition, Brazelton[6] emphasizes that the man reevaluates his role as a provider for his family, his readiness for the responsibility of a dependent, and the requirement of being a role model for the child to learn about masculinity.
3. Nurturance and support of the woman during pregnancy, birth, and early infancy. The traditional stereotype of the All-American Man has not included many characteristics that could be

[4] L. Barnhill, C. Rubenstein, and D. Rocklin, From generation to generation: Fathers-to-be in transition, *The Family Coordinator,* 28(2):229–35, 1979. L. Obzrut, Expectant father's perception of fathering, *Am. J. Nurs.,* 76:1440–42, 1976.

[5] L. Barnhill *et al., op. cit.*

[6] T. B. Brazelton, The parent-infant attachment, *Clin. Obstet. Gynecol.,* 29:373–86, 1976.

Table 12-2. Summary of the Antepartum Period*

Weeks' Gestation	*Physical Signs and Symptoms*	*Characteristic Behaviors*	*Maternal Tasks—In Order of Usual Dominance*	*Suggested Interventions*
0–16	Amenorrhea Fatigue Nausea, vomiting Breast tenderness and growth Frequent urination	Ambivalence Seeks medical supervision and confirmation of pregnancy Tells selected close persons of pregnancy Mood swings from depression → euphoria	Acceptance of pregnancy Seeks acceptance of pregnancy by significant others Seeks safe passage—first for herself, then for her infant	Confirm pregnancy History and physical exam—risk assessment Diet history and instruction Help to talk out and resolve ambivalence Anticipatory guidance/teaching (include family) related to Drugs Radiation Embryology Individual signs and symptoms Reportable signs of possible complications Normality of her mood swings
16–30	Quickening "Pregnant figure" ↑ Energy Feeling of well-being Round ligament pain	Wears maternity clothes Tells the world Interested in learning about birth and babies—reads books, seeks out and questions friends and family, attends classes ↑ Talkativeness ↑ Dependency as time goes on Begins examining relationship with own mother	Acceptance of infant Seeks acceptance of infant by significant others Adoption of mother role Seeks safe passage but in more abstract, general way than in other trimesters	On-going assessment of maternal/fetal status FHR Fundal height Urine tests B/P Nutrition Give to woman—time, knowledge, pamphlets, etc. Anticipatory guidance/teaching (include family) related to Libido changes Mood swings Dependency Introversion Reportable signs of possible complications
30–40	Dependent edema Pressure in lower abdomen Frequent urination Round ligament pain Backache Insomnia Clumsiness Fatigue	↑ Introversion ↑ Dependency (craves attention and tenderness) May ↓ interest in genital sex Intensifies study of labor and delivery ↑ Vulnerability Prepares nursery—buys baby things Decides on feeding method	Safe passage for self and infant through labor and delivery Ensuring acceptance of infant by significant others Acceptance of infant as individual apart from herself Adoption of the mother role	Continue physical assessment at more frequent intervals Reassure—give ego support for attractiveness and self-worth Anticipatory guidance/teaching (include family) related to Signs and symptoms of labor Environmental modification for coming infant and to provide rest for mother Fulfilling maternal dependency needs Early infancy, especially developing parent/child attachment (help them verbalize mental picture of infant and concepts of selves as parents)

*It is well to remember that women and pregnancies differ, and, while an outline may serve as a useful overview and guide, the nurse should assess each client individually. Health care during pregnancy should be a cooperative endeavor between the clients and the professionals, with the client taking an active role in planning and decision-making.

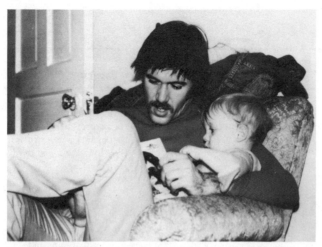

Figure 12-3. Many fathers are taking a more active role in all areas of child care than in prior generations.

described as gentle, tender, or nurturant. However, like all stereotypes, this one probably does not fit most men. Still, it is helpful for many men if the nurse provides some information about the typical emotional/psychologic responses of women to pregnancy, suggests ways he might be helpful, and supports and reinforces his efforts.

4. Adaptation to the physical changes in the woman. He must adjust to the differences in the way the woman's body looks, feels, and smells. This has implications for their sexual relationship, for his pride in her appearance, and, indirectly, for how the woman feels about her own body. This concrete evidence of the pregnancy helps him gain awareness of the fetus, particularly during the last trimester when he can see and feel fetal movement. To the extent that he is seen publicly with her, the pregnancy becomes known and social interactions become available to assist his role development. Unlike the woman, no one can recognize an expectant father on sight! He must tell people or be seen with a pregnant wife.

Fathers' Participation in Pregnancy and Birth

Some cultures provide for the ritual participation of the father in pregnancy and birth. Certain activities, chants, and behaviors are prescribed to allow the male to share in the revered mystery of birth, to ward off evil spirits, or for other societal reasons. Such ritual practices are known as couvade. American culture does not have a formally recognized couvade, although the term appears in the literature, often to describe a man's physical identification with the pregnancy through symptoms of nausea, bloating, toothache, and so on. Many health care professionals have a view of what men "should" do during pregnancy that is as rigid as the ritual couvade. From believing men were not interested in pregnancy—a woman's world—nurses now often assume all men to be vitally interested and totally involved. Attendance at childbirth classes and being present in the delivery room is assumed, and fathers who do not do so may be suspect. It is important to strike a middle ground that recognizes individual differences among fathers.

The degree of involvement chosen by a man is dependent upon his age and stage of development, his acceptance of the pregnancy, his own personal style, his relationship with his wife, and her expectations of him.

Katharyn Antle May (1980) has described a typology of detachment/involvement styles that men adopt during pregnancy. These styles allow for a wide range of personal investment as well as different expressions of involvement. These styles, as defined by May, are:

1. *The Observer Style:* men who see themselves as bystanders and report little emotional investment in the pregnancy. Although they may be delighted to be having a child, the pregnancy itself is something their wives do. They may be very supportive of her but do not enter into decisions about feeding method, choice of health care practitioner, and so on.
2. *The Expressive Style:* men who are intensely emotionally involved in the pregnancy. Their relationship with the woman is characterized by much mutuality as they try to share how it feels to be pregnant. These men often use the expression "*We* are pregnant."
3. *The Instrumental Style:* men who see themselves as caretakers or managers and emphasize tasks to be accomplished such as keeping clinic appointments and making purchases. The man with this style will attend childbirth classes and birth because it is part of his "job" rather than for the "experience" of doing so.

Although this typology of styles has yet to be tested with diverse populations of men, it does serve to illustrate the wide variety of participation the nurse may observe in fathers. It should be emphasized that there is no value attached to the various styles; that is, one is not better or more adaptive than another. The nurse should assess the congruity between the man's style and his wife's expectation of him. If there is incongruency, it may be helpful to facilitate communication between the couple to make their needs, wishes, and expectations known to each other.

Preparation of the Father for Labor and Birth

Most prenatal classes focus on the woman's experience in labor and birth and the father's role in helping her. It is also important to help the father anticipate what the experience will be like for him. He should give thought to how he might respond to seeing someone he loves in pain and how he will react to the various sights, sounds, and smells of the hospital and the labor and birth rooms. He should be aware ahead of time of the typical maternal behaviors during labor, of the amount of time required for various actions and phases of labor, and of the color and appearance of the infant at birth. This anticipatory guidance will help him cope more effectively when the actual event occurs.

EFFECT OF PREGNANCY ON SIBLINGS

The coming of another baby means the older child will have to share parents' time and space and that his/her position in the family will change. The child will gain the relationship with a sibling and a new status and position in the family as a big sister or big brother. Parents can help this transition to be a positive one for the child by making the coming of a new infant a family affair in which everyone can participate at his or her own level.

When to tell children about the coming baby depends to some extent on the age of the child as well as the parental preferences. Very young children who do not have a good concept of time may become impatient if told too early, whereas older children may guess from overheard conversations or maternal appearance if not told until later. A useful guideline for telling children is when the mother's body begins to change so that the early signs of pregnancy are noticeable.

Pregnancy offers a natural opportunity to discuss sexuality and reproduction with children. They are most often concerned about how the baby got inside Mommy, how its going to get out, and whether or not the birth will hurt Mommy. Care should be taken to answer children's questions but not to overexplain or provide more information than they are ready for. In explaining how the baby "gets out," it is desirable to describe both vaginal and cesarean births so children are prepared if a cesarean becomes necessary. This is especially important if the mother anticipates a cesarean birth. Libraries and bookstores have a number of good books both for parents and for children.

Children should be included in the preparation for the infant to the extent they are capable and interested. Some suggested ways for doing this include:

1. Accompanying mother to prenatal visit; hearing fetal heart tones
2. Calling grandparents to report progress of pregnancy
3. Doing breathing and relaxation exercises with mother
4. Shopping for baby things
5. Helping fix space for baby, put clothes in dresser, draw a picture for the baby's wall, and so on

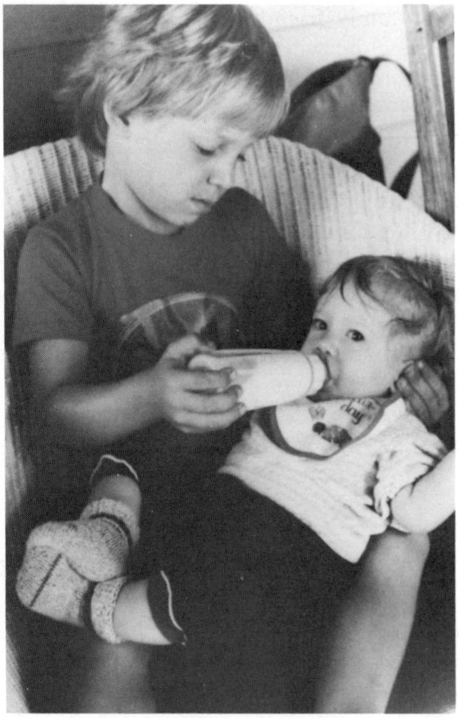

Figure 12–4. This young man enjoys the company of his sister and she doesn't seem to mind that he isn't the most expert at holding her.

6. Feeling fetal movement
7. Practicing baby care with dolls

Preparations that involve changes for the toddler or preschooler should begin well before the birth so there are not too many adjustments to be made at once. For instance, a move from crib to grown-up bed can occur several months before the baby comes so the baby doesn't appear to be taking away his or her bed.

Children enjoy hearing about their own birth and babyhood and looking at pictures of themselves as babies. This reinforces their importance in the family and helps them appreciate the advantages of being "big."

For young children the separation from mother during her hospitalization may be very difficult. Plans should be made early so the child knows just where he/she will be and who will take care of him/her. Some short experiences away from mother during pregnancy may be helpful preparation for some children. Older preschoolers or schoolagers benefit from a tour of the hospital to see where mother will be or pictures of hospitals to show people eating off trays and so on. It is usually possible to arrange for children to visit their mothers and new infants during their hospital stay.

Parents who are planning to have their children present for the labor and birth will need to make particular preparation for this. It is usually advisable to designate a relative or family friend as the support person for the child so the child will have someone to help him/her, answer questions, and so on when mother becomes preoccupied with labor and father is busy helping mother. Hospitals and birth centers that permit children's attendance at birth usually will have guidelines to help parents in this preparation.

Finally, it is good to talk with children about what new babies are like and what is involved in their care.

No matter how well prepared the child is, the parents can expect some behavioral changes to occur. Some children temporarily regress to less mature behavior, become more dependent or demanding, or misbehave in general. Parents need support to recognize this as normal and temporary and to guide their children patiently back to their previous "grown-up" behavior.

EFFECT OF PREGNANCY ON GRANDPARENTS

Becoming grandparents makes people realize the passing of time as they are now the "older generation." At the same time, it provides for many a sense of achievement as they see their own children grown and assuming adult roles. There is also a feeling of continuity as their family is carried on into the next generation.

Women whose daughters are pregnant tend to relive their own pregnancies and labors. They may recall with their husbands the joys, doubts, struggles, and victories of their earlier married life when they themselves were beginning families. The concerns women have for their daughters depend on individual and family values as well as their own pregnancy and childrearing experiences. They may be excited and supportive or very negative. One woman whose daughter had struggled successfully with a weight problem all during adolescence and young adulthood was very distressed to see the daughter's hard-won slim figure "balloon out" with pregnancy. Another remembered her two pregnancies as so miserable that she was hesitant to talk to her daughter for fear of frightening her.

Many women becoming grandmothers for the first time are employed full time outside the home. They may be concerned about fulfilling their roles as grandmothers as they reflect on the models set by their own mothers and grandmothers.

Grandparents want to offer help and advice to their children, and they may be among the best qualified to do so because of their years of living and parenting experience. However, their help may not always be well received by the young families who have ideas and values of their own. Depending on the age differences between parent and child, there may be a considerable generation gap during which new information, new technology, and new trends in childbearing and childrearing have come into fashion.

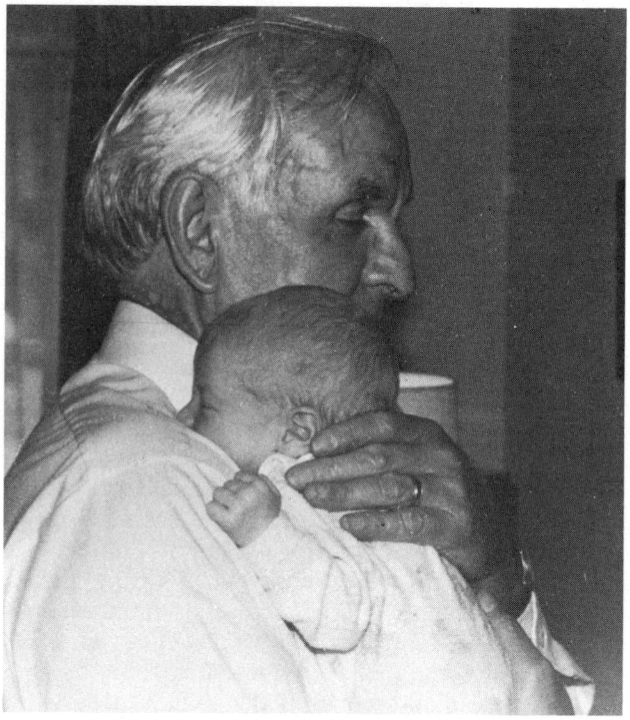

Figure 12–5. A grandfather's shoulder can be a very special place.

Although the nurse may rarely have the opportunity to speak with the parents of her pregnant clients, she can often help indirectly. The pregnant woman can be encouraged to discuss her mother's childbearing experiences with her and to talk with her about what would be helpful for her to do for the new family.

Children benefit from contact with the older generation as much as the reverse is true. New parents need the emotional, and sometimes material, support that is available from their extended families. Thus, intergenerational ties are well worth cultivating.

REFERENCES AND SUGGESTED READINGS

Barnhill, L.; Rubenstein, C., and Rocklin, D., From generation to generation: Fathers-to-be in transition, *The Family Coordinator,* 28(2):229–35, 1979.

Bibring, G. L., A study of the psychological process in pregnancy and of the earliest mother-child relationship, *Psychoanalytic Study of the Child,* 14:113–21, 1959.

Brazelton, T. B., The parent-infant attachment, *Clin. Obstet. Gynecol.,* 19:373–86, 1976.

Caplan, G., *An Approach to Community Mental Health,* Grune and Stratton, New York, 1961.

Cranley, M. S., Development of a tool to measure maternal-fetal attachment, *Nurs. Res.,* 30(5):281–84, 1981.

Cronenwett, Linda R. and Kunst-Wilson, William, Stress, social support and the transition to fatherhood, *Nurs. Res.,* 30(4):196–201, 1981.

Deutsch, Helene, *The Psychology of Women: Motherhood.* Bantam Books, New York, 1973.

Erikson, Erik, *Childhood and Society.* Basic Books, New York, 1956, Chapter 7.

Harding-Weaver, R., and Cranley, M. S., An exploration of paternal-fetal attachment behavior, *Nurs. Res.,*32(2):68–72, 1983.

May, Katharyn A., A typology of detachment/involvement styles adapted by first-time expectant fathers, *West. J. Nurs. Res.,* 2(2):445–53, 1980.

——, The father as observer, *MCN,* 7(5):319–22, 1982.

McCubbin, Hamilton I., *et al.,* Family stress and coping: A decade review, *Journal of Marriage and the Family,* 42(4):855–71, 1980.

Neugarten, B. L., and Weinstein, K. K., The changing American grandparent, *Journal of Marriage and the Family,* 26(2):199–204, 1964.

Obzrut, L., Expectant father's perception of fathering, *Am. J. Nurs.,* 76:1440–42, 1976.

Olson, Marjorie, L., Fitting grandparents into new families, *MCN,* 6(6):419–21, 1981.

Perez, P., Nurturing children who attend the birth of a sibling, *MCN* 4(4):215–17, 1979.

Robertson, J. T., Grandmotherhood: A study of role conceptions, *Journal of Marriage and the Family,* 39(1):165–74, 1977.

Rubin, Reva, Maternal tasks in pregnancy, *Matern. Child Nurs. J.,* 4:143–53, 1975.

Tanner, Leonide M., Developmental tasks of pregnancy, in Betty S. Bergersen *et al.* (eds.), *Current Concepts in Clinical Nursing,* Vol. 2, Mosby, St. Louis, 1969.

CHAPTER

13

Maternal and Fetal Assessment in High-Risk Pregnancy

IN SPITE OF the fact that pregnancy is a physiologic, not a pathologic, phenomenon, approximately 15 percent of pregnancies in the United States are at risk because of maternal and/or fetal factors. Chapter 9 discussed the personal, socioeconomic, and nutritional factors, as well as the medical reasons, why a pregnancy may be at risk. The importance of screening and early detection of women in these categories was emphasized. Watchfulness throughout pregnancy to ensure early recognition and treatment of abnormal conditions cannot be too insistently urged.

This chapter will discuss the antepartum care of women whose pregnancies are deemed at risk for any reason. Chapter 14 will discuss obstetric complications, and Chapter 15 will consider complications resulting from preexisting conditions.

GOALS OF HIGH-RISK ANTEPARTUM CARE

The goals for antepartum care of the high-risk pregnant woman are the same as those of all pregnant women. That is, to minimize maternal, fetal, and neonatal mortality and morbidity and to foster the optimal growth and development of both parents and child. The difference, from the nurses' perspective, is one of degree. For the woman whose pregnancy remains uncomplicated, little or no intervention is necessary in the traditional sense of illness care. These women and their families usually have sufficient resources to cope productively with childbearing and rely on health care professionals for validation of their well-being, early recognition of any deviations from normal, and instruction and supportive care, the amount depending largely upon the sensitivity of the caregiver. On the other hand, families experiencing a high-risk pregnancy have all the needs of low-risk families—perhaps doubled—plus the need for medical intervention to deal with the pathology. The entire period of the complicated pregnancy becomes very literally a period of intensive care. Indeed, the high-risk obstetric service may be named the Maternal Intensive Care Unit.

How can these goals be achieved? Without offering any easy formula for success, several important factors are discussed here briefly.

Factors in Goal Attainment

1. Consumer Education

Health care professionals at all levels should assume responsibility for increasing public awareness about what constitutes quality health care. Consumerism has had some beneficial effects on health care in general as people have insisted on stripping away the medical mystique and becoming partners, if not bosses, in their own health care. Professionals must be responsive to this and enter into dialogue so there can be mutual growth and mutual benefit.

2. Availability of Care

Financial barriers to care discriminate against those at highest risk for complicated pregnancy. Low socioeconomic status has the highest degree of correlation with such risk factors as poor nutrition, anemia, toxemia, premature and small-for-gestational age infants, and others. Geographic distribution of qualified personnel is an additional barrier to the availability of care. Because the percentage of women requiring high-risk care is small, a relatively large delivery base (about 15,000 per year) is required to support a perinatal center. Regionalization has been one attempt at making a concentration of skilled personnel and physical resources available within a reasonable distance of all women in the region.

3. Improved Quality of Antepartum Care for All Women

Appropriate screening, universally instituted, would detect deviations from normal very early and possibly prevent many high-risk pregnancies. Treatment of clients should meet individual needs. Increasing the accessibility to care will not have the desired effect unless the acceptability is also improved.

Personnel most qualified to deal with a given problem should be available to the client, and the clients should enter the health care system prior to conception. In this way, many genetic, nutritional, and other complications might be averted.

4. Appropriately Trained Personnel in Adequate Numbers

This includes perinatologists and neonatologists as well as clinical nurse specialists, midwives, home health aides, and others.

5. "Team"-Directed Care

Pregnancy offers opportunities for many different professionals to intervene in ways that positively influence the physical and mental health of whole families. This is especially true of the high-risk pregnancy where the needs are varied and may require highly specialized expertise. Such a team approach can be particularly effective when individual members are mature enough to set aside professional territoriality and work in colleagueship for *patient* care rather than medical care or nursing care or nutrition care.

Throughout this text, but especially in the area of high-risk pregnancy, little, if any, effort is made to distinguish between medical management and nursing care. It is believed that the complexity of the services required by families is so great that no one profession can reasonably expect to work alone. In any given situation, traditional professional roles may be reversed as in the case of E. C., a very young, frightened, and often hostile girl with chronic renal disease. One of the resident physicians was able to develop a warm, trusting relationship early in her pregnancy. Consequently, it was he who provided the major portion of teaching, supportive care, and general TLC (Tender Loving Care), while the nurse on the team worked with the senior physician to manage laboratory studies and other medical details.

6. Focus of Care

Professionals working with childbearing families have as their focus the pregnant woman as an individual who is a member of a family and a community. This is a departure from the traditional medical model which focuses on a pathology and how to cure it.

A FRAMEWORK FOR NURSING ASSESSMENT OF HIGH-RISK PREGNANCY

The dynamics of high-risk pregnancy are the closely interwoven relationships of four overlapping factors: the physiology of gestation, the pathology of the complication, the psychology of pregnancy, and the psychology of illness. It will become clear to the reader that there is much that is unknown about the interaction of these factors. Still, the careful consideration of such interactions can serve as a useful framework for determining the status of a particular woman and, to some extent, that of her family. Such an assessment is useful in establishing priorities of care, determining areas where women and families desire and/or need assistance, and describing outcome criteria that can be utilized to evaluate the effectiveness of the care given.

Physiology of Pregnancy

During gestation striking modifications in physiology occur to meet the demands of the developing fetus. Virtually all the woman's organ systems undergo some change, so that it is accurate to think of pregnancy as an alternate biologic state. Although there are certain commonalities, these changes tend to be individual for each woman and for each pregnancy, so that no two pregnancies are exactly alike, even if the same woman is experiencing them. Monitoring the extent and appropriateness of these physiologic changes is an essential part of all antepartum care—high- or low-risk.

Pathology of Complications

Whatever the complication of pregnancy, be it a preexisting chronic illness, an intercurrent acute infection, or an obstetric complication, there will be a specific pathology that affects selected organ systems and alters function. This alteration may be slight or it may be life-threatening. Because of the advances in medical science, many women are becoming pregnant who might not have survived to reproductive age or who might have been infertile in another era. For this reason it is not uncommon to see women with conditions about which the impact on pregnancy (and vice versa) is poorly understood. Conditions such as toxemia or diabetes mellitus have been widely studied and there are many empirical data in the literature to give the practitioner an idea of mortality and morbidity risks, preferred treatment protocols, and so on. Where such data do not exist, the practitioner needs a systematic method of determining potential risks to mother and fetus because of the complication. Analysis of the pathology as it affects or interferes with the ordinary physiology and management of pregnancy is one such method. The following three examples will illustrate the problem.

M. J. seeks care at the Maternal Intensive Care Clinic because of pregnancy complicated by mitral valve stenosis secondary to a childhood streptococcal infection. The nurse will recognize that both the increasing cardiac output and the increasing heart rate characteristic of normal pregnancy will likely produce negative effects in this woman. Furthermore, remembering the pattern of these increases, the nurse will be able to foresee that the woman's risks of pulmonary edema, cardiac failure, and other cardiac pathology will rise in a linear fashion from the third month of pregnancy until approximately the twenty-eighth week, then there will be a plateau-like interval until labor, when the risk is again increased. She also will know that the rapid hemodynamic changes that accompany parturition make the immediate postpartum period the time of greatest risk for congestive heart failure. Applying the old saw that forewarned is forearmed, the nurse can use this knowledge to plan with the woman and other team members for optimal safety at times of highest risk. In this situation the normal physiology of pregnancy adversely affects the preexisting pathology.

R. S. has had intestinal bypass surgery in order to effect weight loss. Although she had weighed in excess of 400 lb, at the time of her pregnancy she weighed 215 lb. Because of the loss of several feet of intestines, a significant amount of absorptive surface has been lost. In pregnancy one typically expects a weight gain of approximately 25 lb because of fetal growth as well as maternal tissue development. In order to ensure adequate nutrition to the fetus, careful consideration must be given to high-quality protein foods of high digestibility and in frequent small servings to facilitate maximum absorption. Needless to say, a woman for whom weight loss has been such a priority will need considerable support and instruction about her present need to gain weight.

B. L. has developed severe preeclampsia during the third trimester of her first pregnancy. Preeclampsia is characterized by generalized vasospasm, which interferes with the flow of blood to and from vital organs. Since oxygen and nutrients are carried to the placenta and thus to the fetus by the maternal bloodstream, it can be expected that intrauterine nutrition may suffer as a result of preeclampsia. Indeed, the nurse will understand that it is quite reasonable to expect the delivery of a small-for-gestational-age infant and should alert the neonatal team about this likelihood.

Psychology of Pregnancy

The characteristic emotional and developmental phenomena of pregnancy have been discussed in Chapter 12. It is widely recognized that these phenomena both influence, and are influenced by, the physiologic changes that are occurring simultaneously. At the simplest level, it is the physiology that first makes the woman aware of the fact of her pregnancy. In addition, endocrine changes have been suggested as factors in the mood swings of pregnancy among other processes. A passing knowledge of psychosomatics would indicate that the woman's attitude toward pregnancy and motherhood may intensify the nausea, vomiting, fatigue, and other physical irritations of gestation, or, conversely, it may minimize, or even eliminate, them as factors to be considered.

When intervening pathology threatens the life or well-being of the woman herself, or her child, there can be severe obstacles to the orderly progression of attachment and other maternal tasks. The woman's concept of herself as a woman and consequently as a mother may be clouded by an awareness of her "imperfection" in not having what she regards as a "normal pregnancy." Nurses and others in contact with high-risk pregnant women should be particularly sensitive to these feelings, and, whenever possible, intervene to help the woman and her family cope with these difficulties and prepare as well as possible to assume the parenting role. To this end it is usually helpful to spend some time each visit focusing on the "normal" aspects of her pregnancy and the positive findings regarding both herself and her infant. One woman, following a pregnancy cared for in the high-risk obstetric service of a university medical center, said that, although she was convinced she received the best care possible, "no one ever talked to me about having a little baby. I was so excited, but I felt the doctors and nurses only wanted to know about my liver studies."

Psychology of Illness

Society prescribes a specific sick role that allows a person to regress honorably to a position of increased passivity and dependency and to be temporarily excused from meeting some or all of his obligations. Pregnancy, too, is characterized by an increased passivity and dependency, during which the woman is very actively involved in self-reevaluation and in role and relationship adaptation. When these two events coincide, as they often do in a high-risk pregnancy, how do they enhance or inhibit each other?

Pregnancy is regarded as a healthy, usually happy, event. What happens when it is an unhealthy and an anxious time? In spite of ordinary fears for their own well-being and that of their children, most healthy women are hopeful and expect a healthy outcome for themselves and their infant. When the threat to life and health is a very real one because of complications, how can that hope be maintained without giving false hope? These are questions largely without answers that must be considered individually with each client family until some research is available that might give more general direction.

If the complicating condition is one that predates the pregnancy, it is useful to have some historical information. The age and developmental stage of the woman at the time of diagnosis, as well as the time elapsed since diagnosis, may give evidence of the degree of acceptance of the diagnosis. As an example, if a young woman becomes a juvenile diabetic during adolescence and the dietary restrictions become a weapon in her struggle for independence from her parents, one would not be surprised to find her in conflict with the nutritionist, whom she places in the role of controlling mother. Similarly, a woman who denies the reality of her diagnosis may place herself and/or her fetus in jeopardy by refusing to accept treatment. One young woman with Gaucher's disease felt well and expressed doubt concerning the accuracy of her diagnosis, although it had been made some five years previously and repeatedly confirmed. She felt if the diagnosis were accurate that she must have a very mild, and, therefore, quite harmless variety. She steadfastly refused genetic counseling and was persuaded by her husband to accept obstetric care at a perinatal center only to please him.

This brief look at the physiology, pathology, and psychology of pregnancy and its accompanying complications points out how closely they influence each other. To examine only some of these factors is to fail to recognize the woman as a whole person. It is only in attempting to assess the interaction of these elements as they relate to an individual that the nurse can form a picture of what it is like for this woman, this fetus, this family, to experience a high-risk pregnancy.

MONITORING MATERNAL WELL-BEING DURING HIGH-RISK PREGNANCY

Because of the unique relationship between mother and fetus, it is somewhat artificial to speak of monitoring maternal and fetal well-being separately. Throughout gestation the woman's nutrition and physical status as well as her emotional status are observed in order to promote her optimal health. The pathology that complicates the pregnancy is followed, using the tests and procedures appropriate to the individual pathology. For example, diabetics will have blood glucose values taken, renal function studies will be routine for those women with kidney disease, and so on. It is important to keep in mind when interpreting the results of these tests that normal values during pregnancy may be significantly different from normal values in the nonpregnant state. (See Appendix 3 for common laboratory values during pregnancy.)

Bed Rest

Bed rest is commonly prescribed for a variety of obstetric and medical complications of pregnancy. Among these are threatened abortion, renal disease, chronic hypertension, acute hypertensive disease of pregnancy, multiple gestation, placenta previa, and increased risk of preterm labor. The mechanism by which bed rest may benefit the pregnancy or, indeed, whether or not it is a benefit at all, has not been clearly documented. However, in all cases, the intended beneficiary of the bed rest is the developing fetus. It is believed that bed rest will enhance uteroplacental circulation, prevent or decrease uterine irritability, and overcome the effects of gravity, thus providing a more hospitable intrauterine environment and preventing an untimely birth.

The effects of prolonged bed rest on the pregnant woman include limiting her ability to carry out other responsibilities related to older children, household management, or work outside the home. In addition, such enforced inactivity may have an effect on the woman's mental and physical health. Depression, anxiety, and lowered self-esteem are not uncommon findings after several weeks of bed rest. Women may report physical symptoms of weakness, dizziness, and nausea.

Case Reports. Susan, a gravida 3, para 1, with a 3-year-old-son, was a class F diabetic with hypertension and renal disease. She chose pregnancy realizing the risks and the necessity for extreme bed rest. She was advised to rest in bed except for meals and bathroom activities from the twelfth week of gestation. By midpregnancy she was unable to attend clinic visits except by wheelchair since whenever she stood up, she became dizzy and fainted. For the last two months of pregnancy she wept frequently and worried greatly about what a "bad mother" she was since her son required care and supervision she could not provide.

Bed rest was prescribed for Linda, also a diabetic, at approximately 28 weeks' gestation as a result of increasing blood pressure. This required that she take a leave from her job as a bank teller. She had no other children and, as her friends were also career women, she was alone in the house all day. Her loneliness and lack of stimulation during the day caused her to place great demands on her husband to be "entertaining" (his word) in the evening, a challenge he felt he could not meet after a long day of physical labor as a roofing contractor. The last weeks of pregnancy were thus marked by considerable marital discord which was not totally resolved weeks after delivery.

Ellen, gravida 4, para 0, began bed rest at 26 weeks' gestation because of her twin pregnancy. This woman, after three weeks of bed rest, began to complain of weakness and nausea whenever she would be up to eat or shower. She worried that she would not have the strength to go through labor. She also reported feeling depressed and that it was increasingly difficult to concentrate. For example, she found that although during her first two weeks of bed rest she read extensively, later she could only attend to a book for 10 to 15 minutes at a time before losing interest. She also found she easily became disoriented about time since "all parts of the day are the same to me." She said, "When you just lie in bed all day and don't accomplish anything, make any contribution, it's hard to tell yourself that it's important enough just making these babies."

Nursing Interventions

When bed rest is prescribed, the nurse will need to set aside a period of time to help the woman plan for this radical change. It is very important that family members participate in this preparation, if that is at all possible. If they cannot be there in person, the nurse and/or the physician should take the responsibility for telephoning the husband or other significant adult in the household to discuss the implications of the prescribed bed rest.

The first step in helping the family plan is to make sure that everyone has the same understanding of the meaning of bed rest. Does this mean flat in bed 24 hours a day, or can the woman be up and about for meals and bathroom privileges? Some people may interpret bed rest as "just lazing around," avoiding any long or vigorous periods of activity but not necessarily being in bed. It is best to be as specific as possible.

There are a number of "hot tips" for coping with bed rest that families have found useful. The nurse can suggest these, as well as helping each family problem-solve for their unique situation.

Since social isolation is one of the major drawbacks of bed rest, thought should be given to minimizing this. The telephone should be within easy reach of the woman's resting place. Visits from friends and family members are perhaps the most helpful measure.

Varying the place of bed rest diminishes the monotony. Some time might be spent in the living room or even outside in warm weather. Dressing in different clothes for day and night helps maintain some time orientation. Continuing her own ritual of getting ready for bed in the evening will help combat the sleeplessness that may occur because the woman has been lying down all day. "Job lists" may structure older children's activities as well as being useful contributions to the family's work. Very young preschool children generally will require some child care assistance, but mothers can spend valuable time with them reading, doing puzzles, building with blocks, or anything she can participate in from a reclining position.

An exercise program will help prevent the physiologic complications of bed rest (orthostatic hypotension, increased cardiac work load, decreased respiratory effort, loss of appetite and constipation, increased risk of thrombus formation) as well as provide an activity to punctuate the day. A routine of about 15 minutes of muscle-toning exercises can be worked out in consultation with a physical therapist or exercise physiologist. If done at bedtime, this also may promote relaxation and sleep.

Hospitalization

It is not uncommon for periods of hospitalization to be required during the course of a high-risk pregnancy. Sometimes these may be quite extended periods. The diabetic woman may be admitted for diabetic control and teaching. A hypertensive woman or one with renal disease may require complete bed rest and almost continuous monitoring of kidney functions and fetal well-being. Third trimester hemorrhage may dictate hospitalization for other women.

Whatever the reason that precipitates admission to the hospital, this is likely to be a very stressful experience for the family. Her very presence in a hospital emphasizes the severity of the risk to mother and infant. In addition, the family is separated, and hospitals are universally uncomfortable places to take up residence.

Besides caring for the high-risk pregnancy, the team of caregivers must direct their attention in two other directions: facilitating the woman's adaptation to being an inpatient, and assisting the family to modify their lives to accomodate the absence of an important member. The accomplishment of one will help with the other. If the woman knows her children are safely cared for at home by grandma or a neighbor, she can rest somewhat easier. If her husband contrives to keep up with his job, manage the household, and still find time to visit her, her contentment will be greater. Conversely, if the family is comfortable in the understanding that both they and the woman are kept clearly informed regarding the plan of care, they will accept the inconveniences easier. If they also see that their wife or daughter or mother is treated with respect and her privacy is valued, a bad situation will be a bit better.

Opportunities for frequent visiting by family members, including children, should be available. If complete bed rest is not necessary, the use of passes to permit an afternoon or day away from the hospital should be considered. Every effort should be made to secure facilities on the antepartum unit where the couple can be alone. Separation due to the hospitalization can place a great strain on the relationship unless there is some opportunity to be together to discuss family matters, to be physically intimate, or even to have an argument in privacy.

Time passes slowly for these hospitalized women, especially if they feel well. It is a constant challenge to them and to the staff to provide occupation and diversion. Reading, needlework, television, and puzzles become tiresome after a while. It is often helpful if several antepartum women are able to share a room. In such situations they are very helpful to each other, and many close friendships develop.

METHODS OF MONITORING FETAL STATUS

The severity of maternal disease is reflected in the growth and development of the fetus. It is difficult, if not impossible, to think of a condition that places the mother at risk without affecting her fetus. Indeed, the fetus is usually the more vulnerable of the two. Thus, it is important to attempt to evaluate fetal well-being throughout complicated gestations.

Although at present the therapeutic repertoire for intrauterine intervention remains quite limited, it is often possible to forestall the more calamitous events. This is particularly true during the third trimester. At this time, careful observations of fetal status may permit delivery prior to damage from placental insufficiency. For the fetus whose intrauterine existence is made precarious by chronic hypertension or toxemia, the environment of a modern neonatal intensive care unit may be much more hospitable. On the other hand, determination of fetal lung maturity may prevent delivery of an infant too immature to adapt successfully to extrauterine life.

Physical Examinations

1. At each antepartum visit the height of the fundus is measured from the symphysis pubis to the upper rim of the fundus. This measurement gives an estimate of the growth of the fetus. Failure of the uterus to grow properly is suggestive of intrauterine growth retardation, while sudden increases in growth may indicate a multiple gestation or polyhydramnios.

2. In addition, the abdomen is palpated to determine uterine contour as well as presentation and position of the fetus. Unusual contours are indicative of anatomic abnormalities of the uterus and often predispose to breech or transverse presentations. Unusual presentation in a normal uterus may suggest an abnormally implanted placenta or fetal anomalies.

3. The woman should be questioned about fetal movement, how it varies over time and how it compares with her other pregnancies. Although fetal movement is quite variable and made even more so by the subjectivity of the reporting, a sudden change in movement bears further investigation. This is especially true if the change is one of decreased movement or of no movement.

4. Auscultation of the fetal heart rate with a standard fetoscope or doptone is an important diagnostic tool for several reasons. The time of initial auscultation with the fetoscope is corroborative evidence of gestational age. Periodic counting establishes the individual baseline for each fetus against which variations can be measured. Bradycardia (less than 100 beats per minute) is associated with congenital heart disease, and tachycardia (more than 180 beats per minute) is suggestive of maternal fever or thyrotoxicosis, or fetal hypoxia, or certain drugs that produce maternal tachycardia.

The presence of a normal fetal heart rate, however, has no predictive value, and the nurse should not be overly reassured by hearing a heartbeat in the face of other ominous signs. Absence of fetal heartbeat should be further evaluated by an ultrasound examination for cardiac pulsation before a diagnosis of intrauterine death is considered.

Amniocentesis

Amniocentesis consists of introducing a needle through the abdominal and uterine walls into the amniotic cavity in order to remove some fluid for examination (Fig. 13–1). Amniotic fluid may be analyzed for a wide variety of constituents. The most clinically applicable include chromosomes and metabolites for genetic diagnosis and/or counseling, bilirubin for monitoring Rh-sensitized fetuses, and surfactant for ascertaining fetal pulmonary maturity. These are discussed in greater detail below.

The Procedure

Prior to the procedure the woman and her family should have a careful explanation of the procedure itself, what information is being sought, and its importance to them and to the fetus. A step-by-step outline of what will be done and how it will feel permits the parents to visualize the event and anticipate their responses and ways of coping.

After changing into a hospital gown to protect her clothing, the woman is made as comfortable as possible on the examining table. The supine position during the procedure is often uncomfortable, particularly as gestation progresses and the uterus grows heavier. Especially during the third trimester, the woman may experience supine hypotension. This, accompanied by her natural anxiety, brings about dizziness, nausea, and occasionally vomiting. She may appear quite pale and feel clammy, although complaining of being too warm. A slight elevation of the head of the examining table or movement to a semilateral position often will prevent

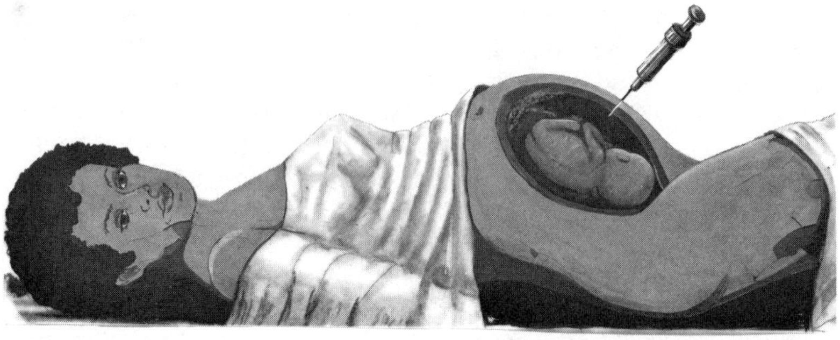

Figure 13–1. Cross section through a pregnant uterus showing the relationship of the amniocentesis needle to the fetus and placenta.

this troublesome situation. A cool cloth for her head or throat is often soothing and an emesis basin within easy reach is a wise precaution.

Next, mineral oil will be applied to her abdomen, and an ultrasound "picture" taken of the fetus to identify the location of the placenta, fetal anatomy, and a pool of amniotic fluid (Fig. 13–2). The abdomen is then prepped with an antiseptic solution, a local anesthetic infiltrated into the skin, and a long, small-gauge needle inserted into the identified pool of amniotic fluid. The necessary amount of fluid is withdrawn and sent for the appropriate laboratory analyses.

Women have described the pain of the procedure as being comparable to the sensation of having blood withdrawn from the arm. In addition, many describe a pulling sensation as the fluid is being aspirated.

When the amniocentesis is completed, the fetal heart tones should be auscultated to be sure there have been no immediate ill effects on the fetus. If the woman has been dizzy or nauseated, she usually will feel better if she rests on her side for a few minutes before leaving the examining room.

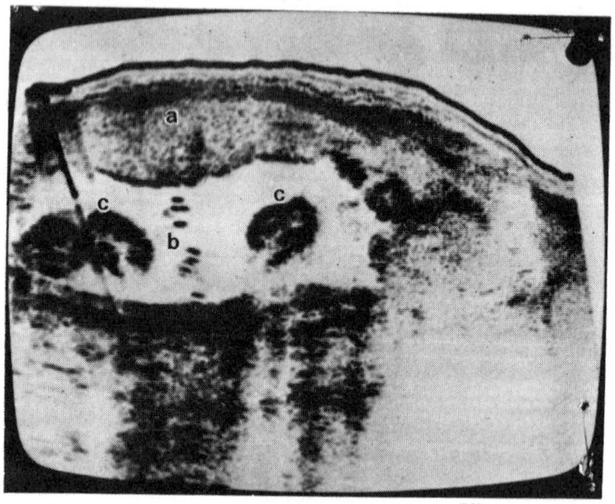

Figure 13–2. Sonogram performed prior to an amniocentesis to localize a safe pool of amniotic fluid removed from fetal vital parts and placenta. Note the marker which shows not only the location but also the depth of penetration required. Structures easily identified are *a*, placenta; *b*, umbilical cord; *c*, cross section through fetal limbs. (Courtesy of R. O. Friday, M.D., Department of Radiology, Madison General Hospital, Madison, Wisconsin.)

If blood is aspirated during the procedure, it should be analyzed at once to determine whether it is fetal or maternal blood. In the event it is fetal, close monitoring of fetal heart rate for 1 to 2 hours is a wise precaution.

Purposes of Amniocentesis

GENETIC DIAGNOSIS When amniocentesis is performed for genetic diagnosis, it is generally done as early as is practical, usually about 14 to 16 weeks' gestation. The fluid obtained may be chemically examined, cells floating in the fluid may be examined, or fibroblasts may be cultured from the cells and studied. This latter procedure requires from three to five weeks to obtain a sufficient amount of material for examination. Genetic disorders characterized by chromosomal abnormalities (trisomies, translocations, and others) and certain metabolic disorders can be diagnosed in this manner.

An additional tool for prenatal diagnosis of genetic defects is the determination of alpha-fetoprotein (AFP), a protein produced by the yolk sac and the fetal liver. This substance reaches its peak at about 14 to 16 weeks' gestation and then declines steadily throughout pregnancy. In the presence of open neural tube defects (anencephaly, spina bifida, meningomyelocele), the amount of AFP in amniotic fluid is increased eight times that of normal.

MONITORING OF RH-SENSITIZED FETUSES The monitoring of Rh-sensitized fetuses is discussed in Chapter 14, along with the subject of pregnancy complicated by isoimmune disease.

Maturity Studies

Prematurity is the leading cause of perinatal death. Whenever possible, it is desirable to determine prior to birth whether or not the fetus is capable of surviving in the extrauterine environment. Ideally, then, delivery would be postponed until such maturity is achieved. Unfortunately, the present state of the art does not always permit this. The more commonly used indicators of fetal maturity are discussed below.

LECITHIN/SPHINGOMYELIN RATIO (L/S) A surface-active phospholipid-protein substance known as surfactant normally lines the alveoli of the lungs. Surfactant is produced by the alveolar lining cells of adults and infants and is secreted onto the surface of the alveoli to form a lining film which lowers the surface tension in the alveoli. Surface tension is ordinarily quite high between any two moist surfaces and would therefore be a hindrance to alveolar expansion without the presence of surfactant. For effective respiratory function in the newborn, it is essential not only that the potential air spaces are developed but also that surfactant is being produced in sufficient quantities to prevent atelectasis and respiratory distress. (See Chapter 30.)

Lecithin is the major constituent of alveolar surfactant, and sphingomyelin is one of several related phospholipids which complete its makeup. These substances, produced in the fetal lung, are washed out into amniotic fluid by the respiratory-like movements of the fetal lung and chest and can be measured in amniotic fluid. The ratio of lecithin to sphingomyelin is determined to assess the degree of fetal lung development. The lungs have a developmental sequence that is, in part, independent of gestational age. The amount of lecithin at a given age varies among individual infants, some producing greater or lesser quantities than the average.

Lecithin is produced beginning at about 20 to 22 weeks' gestation and gradually increases throughout pregnancy, while the amount of sphingomyelin remains essentially the same. Until approximately the thirty-fifth week, a less stable form of lecithin is produced, a form more sensitive to acidosis, hypothermia, and other stress. Around 35 weeks there is a surge of the major surfactant lecithin, which is very stable and active. This explains in part why premature infants are more susceptible to respiratory distress syndrome.

At the time of the lecithin surge at 35 weeks, the amount of lecithin rises to more than two times that of sphingomyelin, and thereafter the ratio continues to rise. Thus, L/S ratio gives the best prediction for extrauterine survival, since adequate pulmonary function is of critical importance, and this ratio is a functional measurement of pulmonary alveolar stability. Although the values may differ from one laboratory to another, according to Gluck who did the initial work, when the lecithin to sphingomyelin ratio is greater than 2.0, the fetus is considered to have pulmonary maturity and to be unlikely to develop respiratory distress syndrome. Ratios in the 1.0 to 1.9 range indicate a possibility for the development of respiratory distress, while ratios less than 1 are associated with severe respiratory distress. If an infant with an immature L/S ratio must be delivered, the neonatal team must be alerted and plans made for immediate respiratory support therapy after birth.

Although research is inconclusive at this time, there is some evidence that several factors may act to enhance or delay surfactant production in addition to the infant's own individual pattern of development. Stress appears to be a factor that promotes earlier pulmonary maturation. Therefore, some conditions such as toxemia, narcotic addiction, intrauterine growth retardation, and premature rupture of the membranes have been associated with an early rise in L/S ratios.[1] Some investigators have suggested that mild diabetes mellitus retards surfactant production, but others have refuted this.

In 1968 Liggins observed that corticosteroid injection of fetal lambs improved the survival ratio when they were prematurely delivered. Since then he has demonstrated similar effects in humans.[2] Numerous studies are being conducted in an effort to substantiate the efficacy of this treatment. To date, the results indicate that betamethazone does enhance fetal lung development and reduce the incidence of respiratory distress syndrome if administered between 30 and 34 weeks' gestation. It appears to be more effective in female fetuses than in male and in black fetuses than in white ones. However, it must be remembered that RDS is not the only cause of morbidity and mortality in prematurely born infants. For this reason, a conservative management approach is usually adopted. Attempts are made to postpone delivery until a mature L/S is obtained, if this can be done safely for both mother and fetus. Repeat amniocentesis is done after a reasonable interval. Depending on the gestational age and the risks inherent in maintaining the pregnancy, this interval may be 3 to 4 days or it may be 1 to 2 weeks.

Approximately 5 ml of amniotic fluid is needed for the L/S ratio test, which requires 1 to 1½ hours to complete. If the test is not to be done for several hours after the fluid is obtained, it must be refrigerated, as the lecithin may deteriorate at room temperature. Bloody or meconium-stained fluid may give false results.

THE LUNG PROFILE Although it is very rare for an infant to develop respiratory distress syndrome (RDS) after having a mature L/S ratio (2.0), the false-positive rate is much higher. That is to say, a significant proportion of infants (46 percent in some studies) whose L/S ratios were immature (less than 2.0) do *not* subsequently develop RDS. This lack of specificity is troublesome when dealing with very high-risk pregnancies. For this

[1] Louis Gluck and Marie V. Kulovick, Lecithin/sphingomyelin ratios in amniotic fluid in normal and abnormal pregnancy, *Am. J. Obstet. Gynecol.*, 115:539–46, (Feb. 15) 1973.

[2] G. C. Liggins and R. N. Howie, A controlled trial of antepartum glucocorticoid treatment for prevention of the respiratory distress syndrome in premature infants, *Pediatrics*, 50:515, (Oct.) 1972.

reason, a more detailed examination of the components of surfactant is done in many centers. This examination, referred to as the "lung profile," includes the L/S ratio and the percentages of desaturated lecithin, phosphatidyl inositol (PI), and phosphatidyl glycerol (PG). The concentration of PI rises until about 35 to 36 weeks' gestation and then declines, while PG appears about the thirty-fifth week and rises sharply until term. The percentage of desaturated lecithin gradually increases throughout gestation from about 22 weeks. The measurement of these additional fractions of surfactant presents a more complete picture of lung development. It enhances the high accuracy of the positive (mature) L/S ratio. More important, knowing the levels of each fraction enables the physician to interpret low or intermediate levels of L/S ratios by noting the developmental level each has achieved. This permits some quantification of just how immature the lungs are and provides data with which to predict the best time to repeat the test in expectation of a mature reading. The lung profile also permits evaluation of some high-risk pregnancies. Delayed lung maturation characterized by L/S ratio greater than 2.0 with no PG has been reported in gestational diabetes.[3] Accelerated lung maturation (L/S ratio less than 2.0 with PG present) has also been noted. It appears that infants do not develop RDS when the PG level is at least 3 percent, irrespective of the L/S ratio (Kulovich, Hallman, and Gluck, 1979).

The lung profile has a distinct advantage when a bloody tap of fluid is obtained. PG is not present in blood and therefore will not inflate the values as may happen with the L/S ratio alone.

"FOAM" TEST ("Shake" Test, "Bubble" Test). The "foam" test, also called the "shake" test or "bubble" test, is a simple and rapid test for the presence of surfactant in amniotic fluid. Although it is useful as a screening test, it lacks the precision of the L/S ratio and is therefore not as useful for decision-making in complex high-risk situations. The test is performed by shaking a 1:2 dilution of 90 percent ethanol and amniotic fluid and observing the foam or bubbles that appear at the surface of the liquid. A complete ring of bubbles which remains for 15 minutes is considered a positive test and is correlated with mature lungs. A negative test is not interpretable and requires a specific L/S determination if immediate information is necessary.

AMNIOTIC FLUID CREATININE The concentration of the metabolic end product creatinine increases progressively in the amniotic fluid as the fetus approaches term. It is assumed that this rise is due to the fetal urine excretion, reflecting increasing muscle mass, as term approaches. Creatinine values of 2 mg per 100 ml of amniotic fluid appear to correlate closely with a pregnancy of 37 weeks' duration or more.

However, because this test is only an indirect measure of the vital pulmonary maturity and, for example, could be subject to variation in pregnancies complicated by intrauterine growth retardation, its greatest usefulness is in uncomplicated pregnancies. In situations where confirmation of maturity is desirable before scheduling a cesarean section or elective induction of labor, this test appears to be highly satisfactory. A maternal serum creatinine value should be obtained to ensure that the amniotic fluid level is not a reflection of maternal excess.

BILIRUBIN LEVEL IN AMNIOTIC FLUID A marked decrease in the normal amount of bilirubin in the amniotic fluid occurs as the fetus approaches term. The bilirubin virtually disappears in the last month of gestation. Using the optical deviation of 450 nm as an index, a fall in optical density in the last weeks of pregnancy is considered by many to be an assurance of fetal maturity. Exposure of the fluid to light at any time for more than a few seconds may invalidate this test.

CYTOLOGIC STUDIES OF CELLS IN AMNIOTIC FLUID Although the fetus desquamates cells throughout his intrauterine existence, the sebaceous glands become functional and shed cells rather late in gestation. The sebaceous cells are distinguishable from other shed cells by the presence of lipid globules. The percentage of these fat cells gives an indication of fetal age. The cells are recognized by the use of a Nile blue sulfate stain. In general, a lipid cell count of 20 percent or greater indicates 36 weeks' gestation or more. The test may be invalid if the amniotic fluid is contaminated with blood or meconium or if vernix caseosa particles are visible to the naked eye. The test, however, does help to distinguish the premature from the mature infant.

Laboratory Studies of Placental Function

Placental insufficiency is a significant factor in intrauterine growth retardation and in fetal death. Without an adequately functioning placenta sufficiently supplied by maternal circulation, the fetus cannot obtain enough nutrients and oxygen for health and growth. For this reason, measures of placental function are particularly good indicators of fetal well-being.

Estriol Excretion Studies

The measurement of estriol excretion in the maternal urine is particularly well suited to the purpose of estimating both placental function and fetal well-being. As discussed in Chapter 8, this hormone is produced by

[3] Marie V. Kulovick and Louis Gluck, The lung profile. II. Complicated pregnancy, *Am. J. Obstet. Gynecol.*, 135(1):64–70, 1979.

the joint activity of fetus and placenta and thus requires a certain level of health in both.

Estriol is excreted in the maternal urine in progressively increasing amounts throughout pregnancy. Although values may vary from one laboratory to another, the mean values are usually considered to be as follows: 1 mg per 24 hours at 20 weeks' gestation; 8 mg at 28 weeks; 12 mg at 32 weeks; 17 mg at 36 weeks; and 30 mg at term. There is a wide variation in the normal value for any individual in a given 24-hour period. This variation is usually the result of maternal factors such as the completeness of the 24-hour urine collection, amount of fluid intake, kidney dynamics, and the amount of bed rest. It is commonly accepted practice to perform a creatinine measurement on all specimens collected for estriol determination. Because creatinine levels remain fairly constant unless there is an unusual period of strenuous exercise, a creatinine level above 1.0 mg per 24 hr gives reasonable assurance of a complete specimen collection. (In situations where there is significant renal pathology, individual interpretations must be made.)

Because of the normally wide variations in estriol values mentioned above, it is important to keep two things in mind when making clinical interpretations. First, single values of estriol are meaningless by themselves unless they are in the extremely low range incompatible with fetal survival (usually less than 2 mg per 24 hr). Rather, the trend of values over time is more important, with consistently rising values being indicative of fetal well-being regardless of the absolute numbers. Second, in order for a decreasing value to be significant, there must be a 50 percent drop from the previous value. This information indicates the necessity for doing serial assays at least three times per week in order to be able to observe developing trends (Fig. 13-3). Daily urine collections are not unusual in situations of grave risk to the fetus.

Urine collections for estriol determination are usually begun at about 32 weeks' gestation and continued until term. This procedure is often one of the more annoying and stressful aspects of the medical regimen with which the woman is asked to comply. Every effort should be made to give careful instructions about the procedure and its importance and to provide supportive care as needed. Particular emphasis should be placed on the importance of collecting all urine for a 24-hour period. The usual procedure is to begin with the second voiding in the morning and end with the first voiding (inclusive) the following morning. The collection usually is made easier if the woman is provided with a container which fits under her toilet seat as well as a leakproof jar in which to store the urine until it is delivered to the laboratory. Refrigeration is not necessary.

The nurse should be aware that certain drugs may influence estriol values, usually causing them to be lowered. Among these drugs are methenamine (MAN-

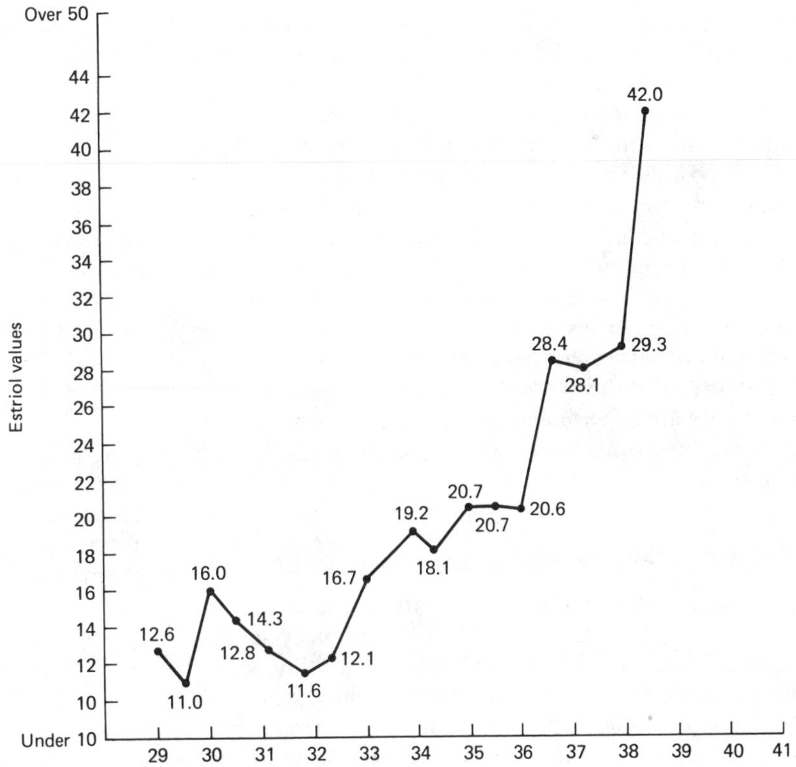

Figure 13-3. Graph of the actual urinary estriol values for a young woman who is a Class A diabetic. Notice that, although individual values may remain unchanged from the previous recording, or may even drop, the overall trend is a rise as gestation progresses.

DELAMINE), ampicillin, laxatives containing phenolphthalein, and corticosteroids. Furthermore, in pregnancies complicated by Rh isoimmunization or eclampsia, estriol values are not reliable indicators of fetal well-being.

Serum Estriol

In some centers the amount of estriol in maternal serum is measured rather than the urinary estriol. This has the advantage of a single withdrawal of blood in contrast to the 24-hour collection of urine. Values are interpreted in the same manner as for the urinary estriol.

Estriol-Creatinine Ratio

Still another way of monitoring the levels of estriol is to determine the ratio of estriol to creatinine, usually in the first morning urine sample. Since creatinine levels remain constant, the ratio will increase as the amount of estriol increases. Thus, the same guidelines for observing trends over time are applicable in evaluating the E/C ratio. An obvious advantage of this method is the avoidance of inconvenient 24-hour urine collections.

Human Chorionic Somatomammotropin (HCS)

Human chorionic somatomammotropin, also known as human placental lactogen (HPL), is a hormone produced by the placenta in increasing amounts throughout pregnancy. Like estriol, it has the potential of serving as an index of placental function and therefore of fetal well-being. It has the advantage of being a serum study which can be done weekly, thus avoiding the difficulties inherent in 24-hour urine collections. Present methods of assay, however, are expensive and not easily performed in most laboratories. With the development of more practical laboratory methodology, this test may become a useful adjunct to high-risk pregnancy management. It shows particular promise in the treatment of postdate pregnancies where it has been shown to be useful in predicting which postdate pregnancies involve a dysmature, and therefore at risk, fetus. However, normal values are so variable that interpretation is difficult at present and other tests should be considered together with the HPL.

Ultrasonic Echo Sounding or Sonor

Ultrasonic echo sounding (sonor) utilizes pulsed sound waves of very high-frequency, 1 to 10 million cycles per second. These sound waves are projected as tiny beams of energy from a transducer applied directly to the woman's abdomen. They echo, or reflect, from interfaces of tissues of different acoustical density. These echos are received by the same transducer that transmitted them, converted into electrical impulses, and displayed on an oscilloscope or television screen. In obstetric usage the most common method of display on the oscilloscope is the B-scan; that is, cross-sectional images of the patient are obtained by moving the transducer over the patient. More recent equipment permits this information to be displayed in eight to ten shades of gray (gray scale). A permanent record can be made of the television display by means of photography.[4] Real-time ultrasound is a dynamic imaging method that makes it possible to observe fetal movements.

Uses of Ultrasound

The uses of ultrasound in obstetric practice fall into two general categories: the assessment of the fetus at risk and the routine screening of all fetuses. The assessment of the fetus at risk includes gestational age assessment, detection of fetal abnormalities through visualizing fetal anatomy, location of amniotic fluid pools for amniocentesis, diagnosis of abnormal fetal presentations and abnormal implantations of the placenta, and identification of intrauterine growth retardation. Equipment and scanning procedures are being developed for use with large numbers of patients as a screening tool. A number of authorities recommend that all fetuses be scanned during the first half of pregnancy as a means of assessing gestational age, detecting twins or other multiple gestations, discovering missed abortions, hydatid moles and other nonviable pregnancies, and detecting fetal abnormalities. This routine early scanning is controversial and is yet to be widely accepted.

Gestational Age Assessment

An important use of ultrasound is the determination of gestational age. Crown-rump length is measured in the first trimester; later the biparietal diameter (BPD) of the fetal head is measured. These measurements are compared to a nomogram to determine gestational age (Fig. 13–4*A* and *B*).

Intrauterine Growth Retardation (IUGR)

Serial measurements of the biparietal diameter are used to monitor fetal growth and therefore to detect deviations from the normal growth curve. These measurements may be technically difficult to obtain in late pregnancy when the head is well down in the pelvis. In addition, they are subject to error because of the "brain-sparing" phenomenon. Intrauterine growth retardation tends to affect weight and length before head size. Thus, an infant may be quite small for gestational age and still

[4] Jay P. Sackler and Anthony M. Passalaqua, Diagnostic uses of ultrasound, *Postgrad. Med.*, 60:95–101 (Aug.), 1976.

Figure 13-4. *A*. Sonogram of pregnant uterus showing fetal head against a grid for measuring biparietal diameter. This BPD of 79 mm corresponds to a gestational age of approximately 30 weeks on the nomogram shown in *B*. Note the location of the placenta, which is the white area in the lower right-hand corner. (Courtesy of R. O. Friday, M.D., Department of Radiology, Madison General Hospital, Madison, Wisconsin.)

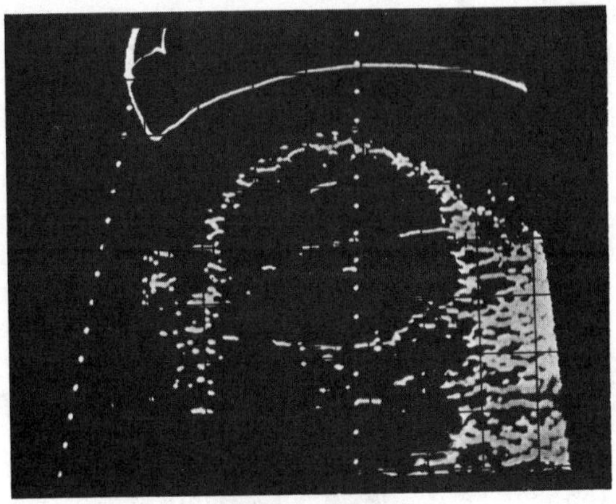

A

Figure 13-4. *B*. A graph showing the growth curve of the fetal biparietal diameter from 19 weeks till term. The three lines indicate the 5th, 25th, and 75th percentiles respectively.

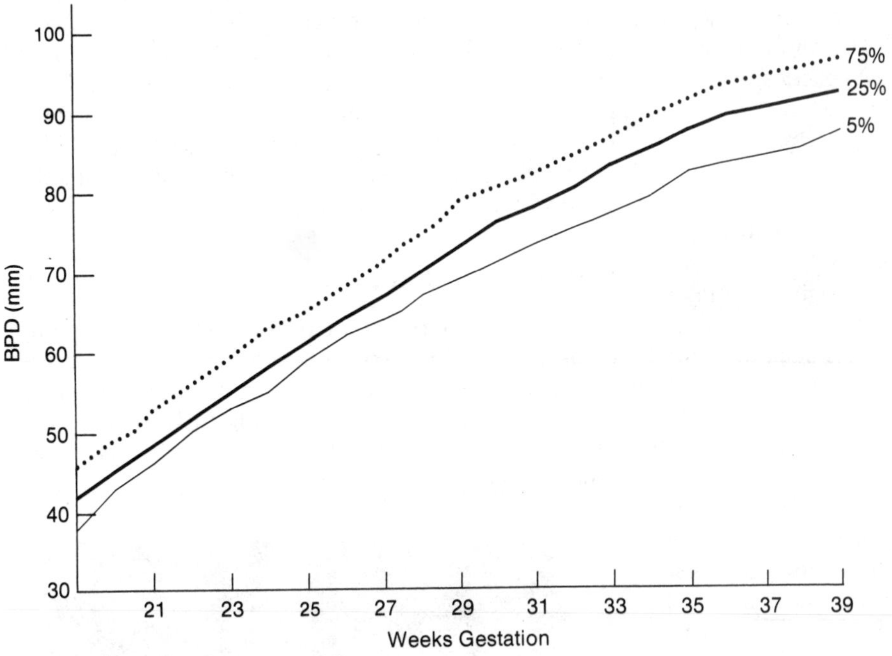

Name________________ Hospital # ________________

	Date	BPD	Wks Gestation Assigned
1st Scan			
2nd Scan			

1. Growth Percentile ________________
2. EDC ________________
   A. By Single Scan ________________
   B. By Menstrual Age ________________
   C. By Average of A & B ________________
   D. By GASA ________________
3. Delivery Date ________________

B

have a biparietal diameter within normal limits. This, however, does not mean the functional development of the brain will not suffer.

Because of the disadvantages of the biparietal diameter, research is being directed at other means of detecting intrauterine growth retardation. A variety of fetal dimensions are being studied. Among these are cross sections of the abdomen as a measure of liver size, one of the organs most diminished in size by IUGR, femoral length, and various combinations of measurements designed to estimate fetal weight.

Findings indicative of asymmetric growth retardation (normal head size, small weight, and/or length) are believed to be associated with placental insufficiency occurring late in gestation. Symmetrically small infants are more likely the result of a long-term, chronic insult, of abnormalities such as intrauterine infection or chromosomal disorders, or the infants are just genetically small.

Fetal Anatomy

Depending on the sophistication of the equipment and the skill of the operator, considerable information can be obtained about the fetus. Respiratory movements, cardiac activity, and blood flow through the major vessels can be observed, as can the emptying and filling of the bladder. Structural abnormalities such as spina bifida, abnormal limbs, and tumors can be detected.

Placental Evaluation

One of the most common uses of ultrasound is the localization of the placenta in situations where placenta previa is suspected. In these cases, ultrasound can either confirm or deny placenta previa as the cause of third trimester bleeding and therapeutic intervention can be planned accordingly (Fig. 14–3).

A recent advance is the classification of placentas based on their ultrasonic characteristics. Four grades of placenta (0–III) have been described which, in simplest terms, represent a continuum from immature to mature. These findings suggest yet another way that clinicians may be able to gather data for the assessment of the fetus.[5]

Safety of Ultrasound

All available data support the belief that intrauterine ultrasound at diagnostic doses produces no significant effects on the fetus or newborn. Follow-up studies demonstrate no ill effects up to one year after birth. Long-term follow-up studies are underway and should be followed to further evaluate the safety of this tool for perinatal care.

Patient Education

When a woman is to have an ultrasonic examination, certain explanations are necessary. First, she should be reassured that there are no known ill effects of the procedure either for herself or her infant. The procedure is a painless one, although the woman may become tired and uncomfortable from the hard examining table. An additional source of discomfort is the fact that the procedure is most successful if the woman has a full bladder. Finally, the woman should expect that a contact medium such as mineral oil will be applied to her abdomen to facilitate the examination (Fig. 13–5).

The opportunity to see their infant has a profound effect on most parents, particularly if real-time equipment is used and they can watch movement. A Polaroid picture should be given to the parents whenever possible. It is speculated that this experience of seeing their infant enhances the attachment process.

Monitoring Fetal Activity

Because the coordination of fetal movement requires complex neurologic control, fetal activity is an indirect indicator of central nervous system function and integrity. For this reason, the monitoring of fetal activity has been suggested as a reliable method for surveillance of fetal well-being.

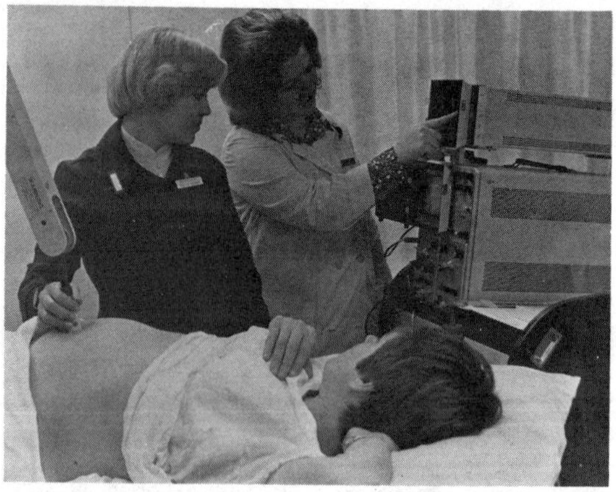

Figure 13–5. As the technician passes the ultrasound transducer over the abdomen a nurse explains to this mother that the upper screen is used to ensure that sound reception is adequate. The lower screen is where the biparietal picture will appear. (Copyright Sept./Oct., 1976, The American Journal of Nursing Company. Reproduced with permission from Karen G. Galloway, "Placental Evaluation Studies: The Procedures, Their Purposes, and the Nursing Care Involved," MCN, *Am. J. Maternal Child Nursing* 1(5):300–306 (Sept.–Oct.) 1976, p. 303.)

[5] P. A. Grannun and J. C. Hobbins, The placenta, *Radiol. Clin. North Am.* 20 (2):353–65, 1982.

Fetal movement has been documented on real-time ultrasound at 7 weeks' gestational age. Early movements appear jerky and uncoordinated. By 10 weeks, single limb movements are noticeable, and by 12 weeks, various combined movements of head, limbs, and torso occur. Gradually the movements become smoother and more coordinated. By 16 weeks, the fetus is large enough that the movements are perceptible to the mother. Mothers describe several kinds of movements: short but strong, probably representing single limb or body movements, usually referred to as "jabs" or "kicks"; longer, more complex, movements described as "rolling over, stretching"; very rapid movements which may or may not be rhythmic and are identified by the mother as "flutters" or "hiccoughs." Although research has failed to detect any consistent diurnal variation in the incidence and frequency of fetal activity, most women report greater activity in the evening when they are at rest. It has also been noted that women report most movement when lying down, less when sitting, and least when standing. This may be due to the attention the woman pays to the fetus, or it may be that the motion of being up and about is more soothing to the fetus. Other explanations could be speculated upon as well.

Monitoring of fetal activity can be done by real-time ultrasonography or by various electromechanical devices. However, the most practical method is maternal perception. The woman is instructed to lie on her left side and focus her attention on the fetus, counting each movement for a given period of time and to report at once if the number of fetal movements is less than some critical number per observation period. The length of the recommended observation period and the critical number of fetal movements vary among health care providers but a common schema is at least three movements in a one-hour observation period. Periods of fetal inactivity greater than one hour are not believed to represent physiologic rest periods and have been reported to be associated with increased fetal risk.[6]

Whenever a woman is requested to monitor movements of her fetus, the nurse should evaluate her ability to distinguish fetal movement from Braxton-Hicks contractions and other abdominal sensations. It is also important that the woman be able to explain why she is counting the movements and that she understands the charting instructions, the critical number of movements, and what to do if she detects decreased or absence of fetal activity.

If decreased activity is reported, further testing of fetal well-being using other assessment techniques is carried out.

[6] J. Patrick, K. Campbell, L. Carmichael *et al.*, Patterns of gross fetal body movements over 24-hour observation intervals during the last 10 weeks of pregnancy, *Am. J. Obstet. Gynecol.*, 142:363–71, 1982.

The Nonstress Test

The heart rate of the healthy fetus will accelerate in response to movement, just as an adult's heart rate increases with exertion and then returns to a baseline at rest. By monitoring the fetal heart rate in relation to fetal activity a reliable assessment of the fetal condition can be made.

The nonstress test is so named to distinguish it from the contraction stress test (CST) or oxytocin challenge test (OCT) which evaluates the fetal heart rate in response to the stress of uterine contractions. However, the nonstress test is actually an observation of the response of heart rate to the stress of activity. This test is indicated in any pregnancy where there is reason to suspect the fetus to be at risk for hypoxia or malnutrition.

Whenever possible, the woman and her family should be alerted to the possibility of the nonstress test well before it is needed. As with any procedure, they should be aware of the reasons for doing the test, the kind of information that will be obtained, how that information will be used, and what their role is in the procedure.

After the woman is comfortable in a semi-Fowler's position on a bed or in a recliner chair, the fetal heart rate transducer is secured firmly to her abdomen where it will pick up the fetal heart rate clearly. This is attached to a continuous fetal heart rate monitor which will print a tracing of the heart rate on a paper strip. The woman is asked to mark the tracing paper or signal to the nurse whenever she feels fetal movement. If no fetal movement occurs, rubbing or palpating the abdomen may stimulate activity. Some observers report increased fetal activity when maternal blood sugar is at its highest so it may be recommended that the mother eat a meal or snack just prior to the test. Because the fetal sleep-wake cycle is 20 to 40 minutes, the usual length of time for a nonstress test is about 40 minutes. The resulting fetal heart rate tracing is read, and the findings categorized as follows.

1. *Reactive.* A pattern characterized by an acceleration of the fetal heart rate in response to each of three to five movements occurring during any 20-minute segment of monitoring time. The increase in heart rate should be at least 15 to 20 beats per minute and last 20 sec. Figure 13–6 shows a tracing of a reactive nonstress test.
2. *Nonreactive.*—a pattern that lacks the characteristics described as reactive. A nonreactive test may occur when there is no acceleration of heart rate in response to movement or when the fetal activity is markedly decreased or absent. Either circumstance requires further investigation.

Nonstress tests are repeated at weekly intervals as long as they are reactive. A nonreactive test ordinarily will be

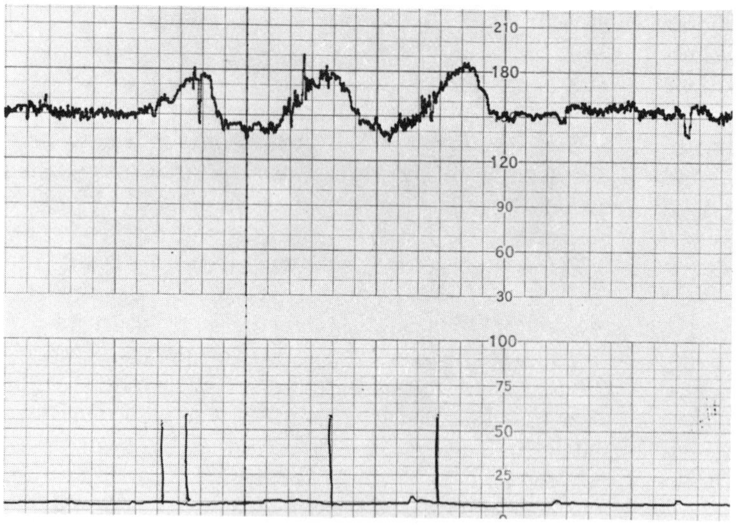

Figure 13–6. Fetal heart rate tracing illustrating a reactive non-stress test (NST). The vertical lines on the uterine activity graph represent fetal movement. Note that the fetal heart rate accelerates from a baseline of approximately 150 beats per minute in response to each period of fetal movement.

followed by an oxytocin challenge test (OCT) for a more precise evaluation of the fetal status.

Oxytocin Challenge Test (OCT)

The oxytocin challenge test involves the administration of intravenous oxytocin to stimulate uterine contractions while simultaneously monitoring uterine activity and fetal heart rate with an external monitor. It is well known that uterine contractions interfere with uteroplacental blood flow. In pregnancies where there is a diminished fetal-placental reserve, the fetus will become hypoxic during a contraction. This hypoxia will be reflected in the monitor tracing as a late deceleration. (For a detailed discussion of fetal heart rate patterns, see Chapter 19.)

If late decelerations occur in response to contractions, and they cannot be corrected by altering the maternal

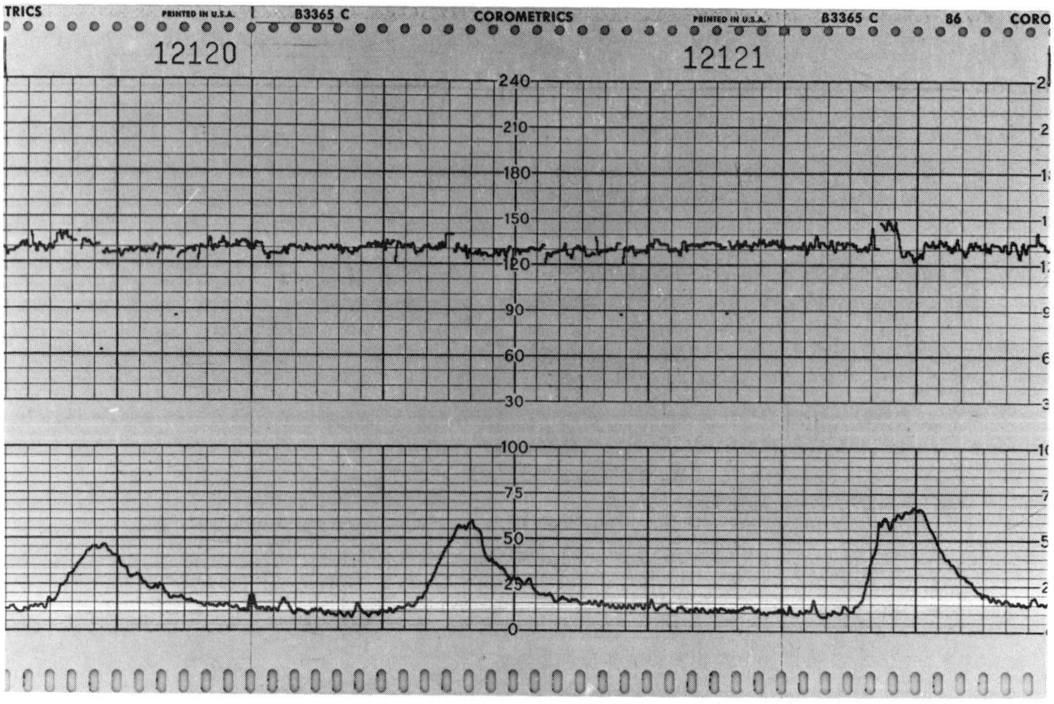

A

Figure 13–7. *A*. Fetal monitor tracing of a negative oxytocin challenge test (OCT). Note the regularity of the fetal heart rate at 140 beats per minute in the presence of good quality uterine contractions occurring every 3 minutes.

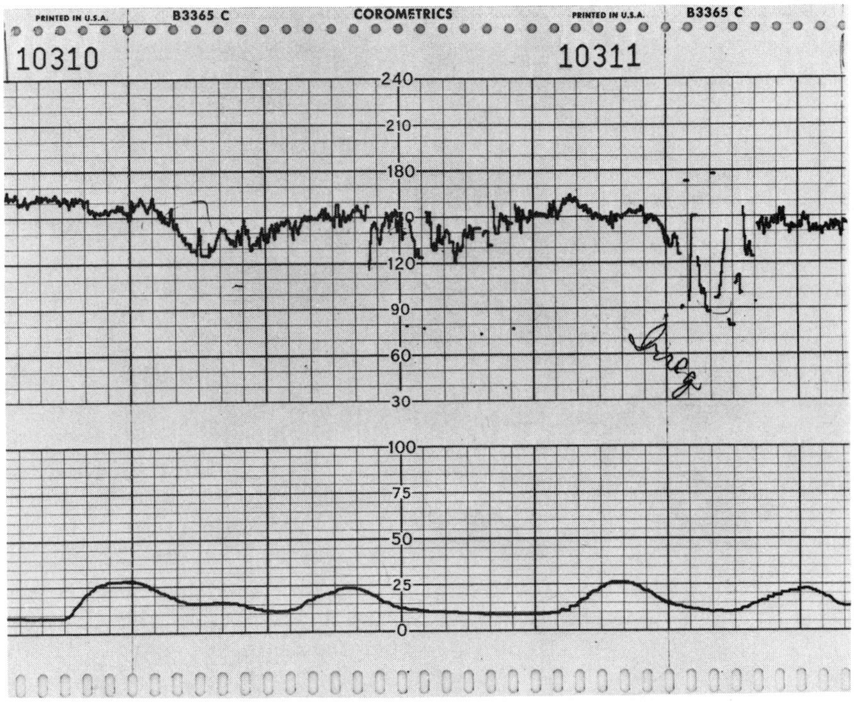

B

Figure 13–7. (Cont.) *B.* Fetal monitor tracing of a positive oxytocin challenge test (OCT). Late decelerations occur with each contraction, indicating a likelihood of placental insufficiency.

position, the OCT is said to be positive (Fig. 13–7). These fetuses are unlikely to tolerate labor and vaginal delivery and are at very high risk for intrauterine growth retardation, intrauterine asphyxia, and death. In the presence of a positive OCT and a mature L/S ratio, labor is induced and a cesarean section performed if warranted by continued late decelerations and fetal acidosis.

The OCT is said to be negative when no untoward changes occur in the fetal heart rate during contractions. The fetus who has a negative OCT is felt to be at no danger from the intrauterine environment for the ensuing week unless there is a change in maternal status. Should there be a change in maternal status, such as the development of toxemia, change in diabetic control, or dropping estriol values, the fetus should be reevaluated. Otherwise the test will be repeated on a weekly basis from about 32 to 34 weeks' gestation until delivery.

OCTs may be interpreted as inconclusive if clear-cut results cannot be obtained. Common causes for these results are insufficient or excessive uterine activity, poor recording of uterine activity because of obesity, edema, or polyhydramanios, and poor recording of fetal heart rate because of excessive fetal activity. Such tests should be repeated within 24 hr.

An OCT may be designated "suspicious" when occasional but inconsistent late decelerations occur. Such tests are usually repeated in 48 to 72 hr.

The woman having an oxytocin challenge test should plan to spend about a half day for this procedure. Although the test itself requires an average of about 90 min, it is not uncommon for up to three hours to be utilized. After changing into a gown, the woman assumes a semi-Fowler's position in bed, and the external microphone or ultrasound transducer is applied to record the fetal heart rate. A tocodynamometer is used to measure uterine activity (Fig. 13–8). After recording 15 to 30 min of baseline fetal heart rate, an intravenous infusion of oxytocin is begun by continuous infusion pump. Oxytocin is initially delivered at the rate of 0.5 mU/min with the rate being increased every 15 min until contractions of "good" quality occur at the rate of 3 in 10 min. The quality of the contractions is subjectively determined by the nurse doing the test. When the monitor tracing has been evaluated, the oxytocin is discontinued and the woman observed until contractions have stopped.

The amount of skilled professional time required for this test makes it quite costly as well as inconvenient for the woman and her family. In addition, there is a risk of initiating premature labor.

The time required for the OCT can be profitably used to develop sound nurse/client relationships, to do informal teaching, and to observe ways the woman and her family cope with the procedure. Many couples have found the oxytocin challenge test to be a useful "dress rehearsal" for labor and have used the opportunity to

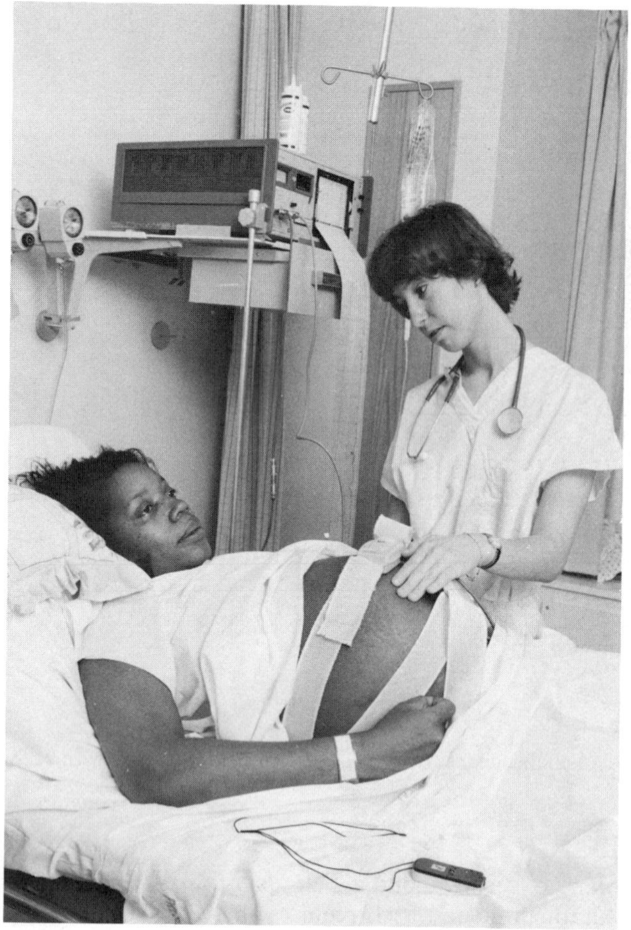

Figure 13-8. This woman is having an oxytocin challenge test (OCT). The tocodynamometer (on the left) and the transducer (on the right) are applied to the abdomen to monitor the uterine activity and the fetal heart rate, respectively. [Courtesy of The Presbyterian Hospital in the City of New York. Photo by Elizabeth Marshall.]

practice coaching and breathing techniques. They have learned to use the monitor to help them time contractions and breathing patterns. In addition, these periods of intense focusing on the movements and heart rate of their infant may facilitate the attachment process.

Biophysical Profile

No single test is conclusive in diagnosing the fetal condition. It is a standard practice to use multiple measures to assess health status in infants and adults. As the capability of fetal assessment increases, this principle is being applied more and more to these tiny patients.

Individually, fetal assessment tests are most reliable in identifying the healthy fetus. If the test is normal, the likelihood of the fetus being normal is extremely high. However, abnormal tests do not have the same predictive accuracy. They are said to have a high false-positive rate; that is, the tests frequently indicate an abnormality when, in fact, none exists. By combining a number of tests and using their composite results, the false-positive rate can be significantly decreased.

One combination of tests that is currently recommended is the nonstress test and the ultrasonic assessment of fetal breathing movements, total fetal movements, fetal tone, and qualitative amniotic fluid volume. Table 13-1 summarizes this profile which is obtained weekly or more often as indicated by the clinical situation.

It can be expected that the science of fetology and fetal medicine will grow more rapidly in the next decade. The perinatal nurse must be prepared to assist families in acquiring necessary information and in making informed choices about health care for themselves and their unborn. The nurse also shares with other health profes-

Table 13-1. Fetal Assessment Tests That Comprise One Example of a Fetal Biophysical Profile*

Test	*Results*	
	Normal	*Abnormal*
Nonstress test	Reactive—3-5 movements/20 min FHR ↑ 15-20 beats lasting 20 sec with each movement	Nonreactive—absence of movements and/or FHR accelerations as outlined in reactive results
Fetal body movements	Present—at least three discrete movements visualized on ultrasound in 30-min observation	Absent—two or less movements in 30 min
Fetal tone	Body in universal flexion. In 30 min, observe at least one extension of extremity or spine with return to flexion	Spine and/or extremities in partial-complete extension. Hands open
Fetal breathing	At least one episode breathing movements lasting at least 60 sec during 30-min observation	The absence of breathing movements meeting the criteria described for normal
Amniotic fluid	Fluid present throughout uterine cavity. At least one pocket of fluid greater than 1-cm diameter	Fluid absent in most of uterine cavity No pool of fluid as large as 1-cm diameter

*Table prepared with reference to F. A. Manning, L. D. Platt, and L. Sipas, Antepartum fetal evaluation: Development of a fetal biophysical profile, *Am. J. Obstet. Gynecol.*, 136(6):787-95, 1980.

sionals the responsibility for monitoring the cost-benefit issues of such technology.

REFERENCES AND SUGGESTED READINGS

Kulovick, Marie V., and Gluck, Louis, The lung profile. II. Complicated pregnancy, *Am. J. Obstet. Gynecol.*, 135(1):64–70, 1979.

Kulovick, Marie V.; Hallman, Mikko B.; and Gluck, Louis, The lung profile. I. Normal pregnancy, *Am. J. Obstet. Gynecol.* 135(1):57–63, 1979.

Lieber, Marilyn T., "Nonstress" antepartal monitoring, *MCN,* 5(5):335–39, 1980.

Neilson, J. P., and Hood, Valerie D., Ultrasound in obstetrics and gynecology. *Br. Med. Bull.*, 36(3):249–55, 1980.

Patrick, J.; Campbell, K.; Carmichael, L.; *et al.,* Patterns of gross fetal body movements over 24-hour observation intervals during the last 10 weeks of pregnancy. *Am. J. Obstet. Gynecol.*, 142:363–71, 1982.

Platt, Lawrence D., and Manning, Frank A., Fetal breathing movements: An update, *Clin. Perinatol.*, 7(2):423–33, 1980.

Rayburn, William F., Clinical implications from monitoring fetal activity, *Am. J. Obstet. Gynecol.*, 144(8): 967–79, 1982.

CHAPTER 14

Pregnancies at Risk: Obstetric Complications

SOME PREGNANCIES ARE high risk because of complications peculiar to pregnancy alone. These complications, which are the subject of this chapter, include:

1. Pernicious vomiting of pregnancy
2. Antepartum hemorrhagic conditions, in particular abortion, placenta previa, and abruptio placentae
3. Premature labor
4. Prolonged pregnancy
5. Isoimmune disease
6. Hypertensive disease of pregnancy; including toxemia
7. Polyhydramnios
8. Fetal death

PERNICIOUS VOMITING OF PREGNANCY

Pernicious vomiting of pregnancy, or *hyperemesis gravidarum,* may develop during the first three months of pregnancy.

Signs and Symptoms

In pernicious vomiting, the nausea and vomiting in the morning may persist for hours; it may occur later in the day, or even at night; or it may be so persistent that the woman will be unable to retain anything taken by mouth. There may be pain in the stomach, hiccups, and gastric pyrosis (heartburn). Thirst becomes severe. After food is no longer present in the stomach, the emesis is composed of mucus and bile. Considerable weight may be lost during this period.

Whenever vomiting is severe enough to produce nutritional deficiency or dehydration, it is considered hyperemesis. If untreated, further deterioration will occur with ketosis, jaundice, fever, and peripheral neuritis. Death may occur from hepatorenal failure.

Etiology

It is the general opinion that all vomiting of pregnancy is of an organic nature fundamentally. Since some degree of "morning sickness" occurs in about one half of all pregnant women, it is believed that all forms of vomiting in pregnancy are due to some factor commonly present in normal gestation. This factor is unidentified, but possible causes that are considered are a toxic element, or a maladjustment of maternal metabolism, or a change in gastric motility. Pernicious vomiting may develop when this factor becomes unusually active or when it is present to an extraordinary degree. Neuroses or psychologic disturbances resulting from all the adjustments that must be made to a pregnancy, however, may exert an important influence and may be superimposed on the underlying organic cause. An interrelation of the toxic or organic and the neurotic factors is generally acknowledged. The extent to which the woman reacts to the underlying cause is somewhat determined by her emotional stability and her mental reaction to the necessary adjustments during pregnancy.

Treatment and Nursing Care

In many instances pernicious vomiting is prevented by management of "morning sickness."

Drug therapy is often useful. A tranquilizer or sedative may be ordered. An antihistamine, antiemetic, and/or anticholinergic drug may give relief of nausea and vomiting if it is not too severe.

Vomiting often can be treated satisfactorily at home, but, if it remains persistent, hospitalization is advised. The goals of therapy are to counter starvation, correct fluid and electrolyte balance, prevent ketosis, and provide help for emotional distress or neurosis. Dehydration and starvation are treated by parenteral fluids, calories, and vitamins, and a gradual resumption of food. The rest, sedatives, and change of environment that can be given in the hospital may be beneficial in resolving emotional conflicts. Tact and understanding and reassurance are important aspects of care.

For the first 24 to 48 hours of hospitalization all food and fluids by mouth, including water and ice chips, are restricted in order to rest the gastrointestinal tract. As patients with pernicious vomiting usually have a bad taste and dry mouth, a refreshing mouthwash is offered frequently.

Carbohydrate, electrolytes, vitamins, and fluid are given parenterally during the first few days. From 2500 to 3000 ml of fluids are given daily.

An accurate record is kept of fluid intake, urinary output, and all emesis.

After this treatment for one to two days, small servings of solid foods—crackers, dry toast and jelly, dry cereal, baked or mashed potato—are given every two hours, or the solid food is alternated with liquid nourishment in small amounts, not more than 100 ml at one time. Hot tea, carbonated fluids, cold fruit juices, and crushed ice are usually easy to retain. Gradually more liquid is allowed so that the mother is taking as much as she desires up to one-half hour before and after the solid food. It is best not to mix the solid and liquid food for a few days. Some parenteral fluids may be necessary during these first few days, depending on the oral intake.

All foods should be served in very small amounts, attractively prepared, and either very hot or very cold. The dishes should be removed from the bedside as soon as the mother has finished eating. Anything that appeals to the mother, or for which she has a particular craving, may be given, although generally fats are restricted and carbohydrates are encouraged during the first few days. The diet is increased slowly to six small meals daily, this being followed by a gradual resumption of a regular diet.

If vomiting should recur after the patient has taken food, the treatment of nothing by mouth and parenteral fluids is repeated, and feedings are then again gradually resumed.

The mother usually recovers quickly with early and persistent treatment. A few continue to vomit to some extent throughout pregnancy. On rare occasions prolonged hospitalization with hyperalimentation may be required in order to maintain nutrition.

The impact of hyperemesis on the fetus is directly proportional to the severity of the disease. If it is promptly treated and corrected, the fetus should suffer no ill effects. If weight loss and dehydration are prolonged, fetal nutrition may be jeopardized. Maternal ketosis is thought to influence fetal brain development (Chapter 10, page 204).

ANTEPARTUM HEMORRHAGE

Hemorrhage is a life-threatening situation whenever it occurs. If it occurs during pregnancy, two lives are endangered: that of the mother and that of the fetus. As usual in high-risk pregnancies, it is the fetus who is more vulnerable. However, in spite of blood transfusions and modern surgical techniques, obstetric hemorrhage remains one of the three leading causes of maternal mortality.

Table 14–1 outlines the major sources of obstetric hemorrhage according to the period of gestation when they are most apt to occur. It should be remembered that there may be considerable overlapping among the groups.

Spontaneous Abortions

Termination of a pregnancy prior to viability (20 to 24 weeks' gestation) is known as an abortion. Abortions

Table 14–1. Important Sources of Hemorrhage During Pregnancy

Early to Midpregnancy	*Mid- to Late Pregnancy*	*Intrapartum and Postpartum*
Abortion	Placenta previa	Uterine atony
Extrauterine pregnancy	Marginal sinus	Retained placenta
Molar pregnancy	Vasa previa	Lacerations
Tumors of vulva, vagina, or cervix	Abruptio placentae	Uterine inversion

Table 14-3. Care of the Woman with Third-Trimester Hemorrhage

Patient Care Goals	*Nursing Interventions*
I. Determine extent of blood loss	1. Obtain history of onset, duration, amount of bleeding, and associated symptoms 2. Observe perineal pads for amount of bleeding 3. Monitor vital signs of mother and fetus (frequency is determined by severity of clinical symptoms)
II. Provide volume replacement	1. Insert intravenous conduit 2. Request type and cross-match for blood 3. Administer fluids and blood as prescribed 4. Monitor intake and output
III. Minimize chances for further bleeding	1. *NO* vaginal or rectal exams 2. Bed rest in position of comfort 3. Anticipate delivery by cesarean section
IV. Reduce anxiety	1. Keep woman and family advised of treatment plan 2. Share realistic hopes for maternal/fetal/neonatal outcome

Incompetent Cervix

A few women deliver premature infants because of a condition termed *incompetent cervix*. Termination of pregnancy owing to this complication usually occurs in the second trimester, too early for survival of the very immature infant.

Usually after the fourth month of pregnancy, the cervix dilates without the usual painful uterine contractions. The membranes later rupture, labor begins, and an immature fetus is delivered. The etiology of cervical incompetency is not known, but previous trauma to the cervix is a factor in some cases. It usually does not occur in primigravidas. (See Chap. 8, page 131.)

Treatment consists of reinforcing the cervix with a purse-string suture, which is usually placed about the cervix between the fourteenth and eighteenth weeks when the major risk of spontaneous loss is over. This procedure is done under general anesthesia and requires two to three days of hospitalization on the average. If contractions occur as a result of the uterine manipulation, tocolytic (labor-suppressing) medications are prescribed. The woman should be advised to expect some spotting from the cervical incision for several days but to immediately report any bright-red bleeding or bleeding that seems excessive to her. She should abstain from intercourse and douching until a follow-up visit is made to the physician two weeks postoperatively. She also should be alerted to the possibility of finding tiny pieces of suture on her perineal pad. These are from the absorbable suture used to close the cervical incision, *not* the suture placed to hold the cervix closed. This is not really a suture at all but a heavy mercelline band. When the cervical incision is well healed, the woman may return to her usual activities, including sexual intercourse.

Treatment is fairly successful in maintaining pregnancy. When the pregnancy reaches term, the suture may be removed to permit vaginal delivery, or in some cases the suture is left in place and the woman is delivered by cesarean section.

Premature Rupture of Membranes

Premature spontaneous rupture of the membranes occurs in 10 to 15 percent of all pregnancies. Not all of these result in premature birth, however. This terminology is somewhat misleading, since the word "premature" refers not to the duration of the pregnancy but to the fact that the bag of waters ruptures prior to the onset of labor. Obviously this can, and does, occur at term as well as before term.

When membranes rupture, it is essential to determine the gestational age of the fetus. If the pregnancy is at or near term (more than 37 weeks), labor should be induced and a delivery accomplished within 24 hours of the rupture. The risk of infection to both fetus and mother rises quite sharply after 18 to 24 hours of ruptured membranes, and neonates tolerate infection very poorly.

When the fetus is not mature, a more conservative approach is usually taken. Labor is not induced and may even be pharmacologically inhibited. Pregnancy may be allowed to continue until fetal maturity is established, unless symptoms of infection appear (elevated maternal temperature, foul-smelling vaginal discharge). It is even possible that a short period of ruptured membranes may enhance fetal lung maturation. It is suggested that stress stimulates the fetal adrenals to produce corticosteroids, which in turn induce the enzymes that produce surfactant.

Women should be carefully instructed to seek professional evaluation whenever they suspect that the membranes have ruptured, regardless of when in gestation this occurs. Diagnosis of ruptured membranes is discussed in Chapter 17.

Prevention of Premature Labor

Antepartum care which assists the woman in the maintenance of her own good health is an important factor in preventing premature labor and birth. Good nutrition, although not a prevention for premature labor, does favor the optimum growth and development of the fetus in a healthy mother and helps prevent a small-for-gestational-age infant.

Little is known that is specifically helpful in preventing premature labor. For some women at special risk, bed rest is recommended because it helps to improve uterine blood flow and, therefore, intrauterine nutrition. It also may decrease uterine irritability and the tendency to go into labor, although this is not clearly established.

Although the incidence of premature labor was not affected, one group has reported success in significantly reducing the incidence of premature birth through a program of education for both pregnant women and health care providers. All women were screened to determine their risk for premature labor, and all were instructed carefully in self-detection of early signs of labor. Those who were judged to be high risk were followed weekly in a special clinic. Intensive staff training was directed toward early and aggressive management of all preterm labor. Using this program they were able to reduce the rate of preterm birth during the first year to 2.4 percent from 6.5 percent.[3]

Suppression of Premature Labor

From very early in pregnancy women should be aware of the importance of reporting immediately any contractions that increase in frequency and intensity. Pharmacologic means of stopping premature labor are increasing in effectiveness and availability. These drugs are most useful in early labor. Postponing objective evaluation of the contractions because "it's too early for labor" can result in being too late for most effective use of the drugs.

Women who have been determined to be in premature labor may be candidates for pharmacologic inhibition of labor, provided the fetus is alive but immature, and there are no maternal or fetal indications for terminating the pregnancy. Such indications could include, among other factors, bleeding from placenta previa or abruptio placentae, intrauterine infection, erythroblastosis fetalis, severe preeclampsia or placental insufficiency. In addition, cervical dilation should not be greater than 4 cm, and some authors believe that the membranes should be intact. (See Table 14-4).

The drugs commonly used for suppression of labor include ethyl alcohol and the beta-adrenergic agents, such as ritodrine. Alcohol blocks the secretion of oxytocin by the maternal pituitary and also crosses the placenta to block secretion of fetal neurohormones. The beta-adrenergic drugs make myometrial cells less sensitive to oxytocin and prostaglandins. Both drugs are thought to increase uterine blood flow.

Alcohol

Alcohol is no longer recommended for use as a labor suppressant except in extraordinary circumstances. In the unlikely event that it is prescribed, it should be administered intravenously as a 10 percent solution in dextrose and water. The goal is to achieve a blood level of 0.12 to 0.16 percent. This is approximately the level that results from three good drinks at a cocktail party (0.10 percent is defined as legal intoxication by most states for driving purposes). Side effects include those of intoxication from oral intake of alcohol and are often quite distressing to the woman and her family. This factor, together with the anxiety precipitated by the threatened loss of their infant, demands a high degree of skill and sensitivity on the part of the nurses and physicians giving care. Labor may be successfully delayed three or more days in up to 66 percent of clients, depending on patient selection. Alcohol is generally unsuccessful if the membranes are ruptured or if the cervical dilation is greater than 4 cm. When treatment is unsuccessful, attention must be given to the fetus/neonate whose blood alcohol level will approximately equal that of the mother. Personnel expert in neonatal resuscitation should be present at delivery as ventilatory assistance may be necessary owing to prematurity and/or respiratory depression resulting from the alcohol.

Table 14-4. Criteria for Selecting Patients for Pharmacologic Inhibition of Premature Labor

Presence of "true" labor
Gestational age between 20 and 37 weeks
Immature fetal pulmonary development
Cervical dilation less than 5 cm
No contraindications to continuing pregnancy—For example:
- Intrauterine infection
- Severe vaginal bleeding
- Severe preeclampsia
- Placental insufficiency
- Erythroblastosis fetalis
- Fetal death

[3] M. A. Herron; M. Katz; and R. K. Creasy, Evaluation of a preterm birth prevention program: Preliminary report, *Obstetrics and Gynecology,* 59(4):452–456, 1982.

Ritodrine

The beta-adrenergic-receptor stimulators relax myometrial cells by a complex mechanism which is outlined in Figure 14–6. In addition, all of these agents have varying effects on the beta receptors of other organs. $Beta_1$ receptors increase heart rate and cardiac contraction force and are responsible for lipolysis and relaxation of intestinal muscle. $Beta_2$ receptors mediate glycogenolysis and relax the smooth muscle of arterioles, bronchi, and the uterus. All drug actions other than uterine relaxation are considered side effects when the purpose is inhibition of labor. The various members of this drug family vary widely in the number and severity of side effects, but all increase maternal heart rate and produce some peripheral vasodilation. The most important implication of this is its effect on uteroplacental blood flow. Ritodrine hydrochloride (YUTOPAR) is the only one of the beta-adrenergic agents currently approved by the Food and Drug Administration (FDA) for use in premature labor. Research is progressing on others in an effort to perfect a drug that acts only on the $beta_2$ receptors of the myometrium without affecting the heart, blood vessels, and other organs.

Ritodrine is administered intravenously to women who meet the criteria outlined in Table 14–4. An additional criterion for this drug is that the mother is free from cardiac disorders, especially those associated with arrhythmias and from hyperthyroidism. Ritodrine may precipitate arrhythmias or heart failure in these women.

While receiving the intravenous infusion, the woman should lie in a left lateral position to optimize uteroplacental blood flow. Fetal heart rate is monitored continuously, together with uterine activity. Maternal heart rate and blood pressure should be taken and recorded at 15-minute intervals. Serum electrolytes and blood glucose levels should be evaluated, particularly if ritodrine infusion is prolonged. Initially, 50 to 100 mcg of ritodrine per minute are infused. This dosage is increased in increments of 50 mcg every 10 minutes until uterine activity ceases. It is recommended that the intravenous infusion of 150 to 350 mcg per minute be maintained for 12 to 24 hours after contractions stop. One half hour before the intravenous infusion is discontinued, an oral dose of 10 mg of ritodrine is given, followed by 10 mg every 2 hours for 24 hours. The woman is then instructed to take 10 to 20 mg every 4 to 6 hours until term or until fetal maturity can be documented. The incidence of side effects of ritodrine is summarized in Table 14–5.

Care of women in premature labor is most appropriately carried out in a perinatal center where personnel have the training, expertise, and equipment to make maximum use of the latest research drugs and techniques. Furthermore, should attempts at arresting labor fail, the infant will be delivered where a neonatal intensive care unit will give him the best chance for survival. Delivery in the center also avoids the separation of parents and infant, which occurs when only the infant is transported to the intensive care nursery after being born in a community hospital.

Management of Premature Labor

When it is not possible or desirable to arrest premature labor, then the management must be directed at pro-

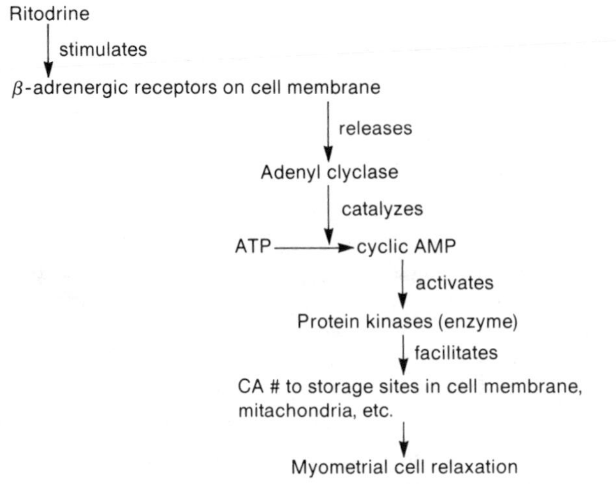

Figure 14–6. Schematic representation of mechanisms by which ritodrine and other beta-adrenergic-receptor stimulators bring about uterine relaxation and thus stop labor. (Source: Tom P. Barden, "The effect of drugs on uterine contractility," in E. J. Quilligan and N. Kretchmer (eds.), *Fetal and Maternal Medicine,* New York: Wiley, 1980.

Table 14–5. Incidence of Side Effects of Ritodrine Hydrochloride (YUTOPAR).*

	Incidence (percent)	
Side Effect	*Oral*	*Intravenous*
Increased maternal heart rate	80	80–100
Increased fetal heart rate	—	80–100
Increased maternal systolic pressure	—	80–100
Decreased maternal diastolic pressure	—	80–100
Irregular maternal heart rate	10–15	33
Chest pain or tightness	—	1–2
Anxiety	—	5–6
Emotional upset	—	5–6
Jitteriness	5–8	5–6
Nervousness	—	5–6
Restlessness	—	5–6
Headache	—	10–15
Nausea and vomiting	5–8	10–15
Reddened skin	—	10–15
Skin rash	3–4	Rare
Trembling	10–15	10–15

*Source: *1983 U.S.P. Dispensing Information,* United States Pharmacopeial Convention, Rockville, Md., 1982.

viding an optimal environment for the labor and delivery of a premature infant. The objectives of care for a woman in premature labor include the following:

1. To assist the woman through labor in such a way that she is able to maintain ego integration
2. To maximize fetal oxygenation
3. To provide support to enable the woman to conduct her labor with minimal analgesia/anesthesia

The woman in premature labor comes to the laboring experience without the readiness for parturition which characterizes the woman at term. She has not completed the tasks of pregnancy. She is physically and psychologically unready for her infant. The crib and room are not even prepared. In a very real sense, she is a premature mother. In addition, she carries a burden of guilt which may be quite awesome. She fears the loss of her child so, as in all grieving, she asks herself what she did wrong. Her husband, too, will likely feel he should have taken better care of her, not had sexual intercourse, or whatever he imagines may have contributed.

These feelings are a normal part of the grief of parents in premature labor. They should be encouraged to express these feelings and concerns and helped to understand that they are usual and normal feelings. On the other hand, they should be given factual information so they can come to realize, at least intellectually, that they did not do something "wrong," that they are not inferior persons.

Fear of losing the child is another real factor. Rubin has described one of the tasks of pregnancy as "securing safe passage for herself and her child."[4] This has certainly not been accomplished as yet by those women in premature labor. A significant manifestation of this fear may be the denial of reality. Some women do not accept labor itself and may put off seeking medical attention, thinking it can't be labor because "it is not time yet." Or, accepting labor, they deny the seriousness of the situation. Much can be done to put this fear into proper perspective and help the parents focus on reality by keeping them well informed of the progress of labor, the fetal status, the plan of care, and the expectations of the professionals caring for them. If it is at all possible during labor, a member of the neonatal team who will be caring for their infant should be introduced to the parents. Depending on the stage of labor and the woman's discomfort, the neonatal nurse or physician can briefly explain what immediate care the infant will be likely to receive, and that the parents will be able to come into the nursery to see, touch, and care for their infant as soon as they wish.

The second objective of care is to maximize fetal oxygenation. The premature is more vulnerable to the stress of labor that is a term fetus. Continuous fetal heart rate monitoring is indicated to constantly assess fetal response to contractions. Blood from fetal scalp samples may be analyzed for blood gases and pH, if indicated by the occurrence of significant fetal heart rate abnormalities.

Women should not labor in a supine position regardless of gestational age because of the risk of the vena caval syndrome. This condition, caused by the compression of the vena cava by the pregnant uterus, results in diminished placental perfusion and, potentially, fetal hypoxia. The left lateral position seems to favor the best placental perfusion, but either side or sitting up is suitable if the woman is comfortable. Women in normal labor often prefer to be out of bed moving about or sitting in a chair.

Maternal hyperventilation should be particularly avoided as it can cause a maternal alkalosis. This, in turn, may decrease the release of oxygen to the fetus, resulting in fetal hypoxia and acidosis. Hyperventilation may be brought on by severe anxiety, or it may be the result of improperly performed childbirth breathing techniques. The mother and her coach should be reminded of the importance of the deep, "cleansing breath" at the beginning and end of each contraction and of the necessity to use a normal breathing pattern between contractions. If the mother's fingertips begin to tingle (an early symptom of hyperventilation), it may be helpful for her to breathe in and out into a small paper bag. This will increase the carbon dioxide content of the inspired air.

At the time of delivery the mother should be on her back for the shortest time possible. Some authorities recommend the Sims position for delivery, but this is not usually acceptable in the United States. An episiotomy generally is performed to lessen the risk to the infant of intracranial hemorrhage. For the same reason, outlet forceps may be used to shorten the second stage of labor and reduce the pressure on the fetal head. Someone skilled in neonatal assessment and resuscitation should be in attendance to receive the infant.

The third goal of care is to keep analgesia and anesthesia at a minimum to avoid respiratory depression in the neonate. To do this, expert care and support of the laboring woman are essential. The woman relies on the nurse to help her maintain contact with time and reality and to help her control her own body in order to retain dignity. To meet these expectations appropriately, the nurse must be continuously available to the woman and her family in order to establish and maintain a therapeutic relationship.

Finally, the small premature infant may deliver through an incompletely dilated cervix. For this reason, the nurse should be especially sensitive to maternal behavior that signals the approach of second stage of labor.

[4] Reva Rubin, The maternal tasks of pregnancy, *Matern. Child Nurs. J.*, 4:143–53, (Fall) 1975.

PROLONGED PREGNANCY

A pregnancy that extends beyond 42-weeks duration is designated *postterm* or *postdate*. The reasons for prolonged gestation are unknown, although perhaps as many as 10 percent of all pregnancies fall into this category.[5]

Effects of postterm pregnancies on the mother are primarily psychosocial in nature. For many weeks she has focused on a time for delivery, only to have that time come and go without an infant being born. In an effort to make appropriate judgments about her care, physicians and nurses cross-examine her in detail about the accuracy of her menstrual dates and other events until she may question what she really knows. If tests or interventions are instituted, her anxiety about her infant and herself will rise markedly. Nursing care should be directed toward helping the woman utilize family and social support systems, providing information and reassurance about fetal assessment, and acting as a sounding board for her fatigue and frustration with "still being pregnant."

Fetal effects of prolonged gestation are quite variable. Some fetuses will continue to grow, which may lead to dystocia and birth injury because of their large size. Others fail to grow as gestation continues and indeed may even lose weight due to malnutrition. These latter infants, termed *dysmature* or *postmature,* are typically scrawny with long nails, abundant scalp hair, loose, desquamated skin, and a characteristic worried expression on their faces. Dysmaturity is correlated with increased incidence of placental lesions, increased perinatal death, and neonatal morbidity.

With the present methods of fetal/placental assessment, it is not possible to identify which prolonged pregnancies will compromise the fetus until placental insufficiency is fairly advanced. For this reason postterm women should be evaluated for induction of labor. If menstrual dates and other determinants of gestational age are reasonably accurate and the cervix is favorable, an oxytocin induction should be undertaken.

When gestational age is in question or the cervix unfavorable, pregnancy may be continued under very close supervision. Gestational age should be verified and fetal well-being assessed by means of serial estriol determinations and non-stress tests or oxytocin challenge tests.

During labor the fetus should be continuously monitored by electronic means as he is at high risk of hypoxia. Particular attention should be paid during the second stage of labor as bearing-down efforts may further compromise placentofetal respiratory reserves. Additional nursing measures include maintaining maternal position for maximal uteroplacental blood flow and providing supportive care to minimize the use of analgesia and anesthesia.

Personnel skilled in resuscitation should be present at delivery. Some authors recommend delaying clamping of the cord to permit an increased blood supply to counteract hypovolemia and dehydration, two threats to the dysmature neonate.[6] Special neonatal care of these infants is discussed in Chapter 29.

Dysmature babies tend to score lower than term babies on the Brazelton interaction and motor scores and are often described as "difficult" by their mothers.[7] These infant characteristics have the potential for initiating a vicious cycle of parent-infant interaction, which could result in inappropriate infant stimulation, neglect, or even abuse. Nursing care should emphasize helping parents recognize their baby's cues and provide appropriate stimulation to enhance his growth and development. Close follow-up should be assured at least through the first year of life.

ISOIMMUNE DISEASE

Isoimmune disease is primarily a disorder of the fetus and neonate, caused by maternal sensitization to fetal red cell antigens and subsequent transfer of the resulting antibodies to the fetus. This occurs when the fetus possesses a red blood cell antigen, inherited from the father, that is absent in the mother.

Although the fetal circulatory system is entirely separate from the mother's and the blood of mother and fetus does not mix, it is possible for fetal blood cells to pass through the placenta into the maternal circulation. When these blood cells are incompatible with the mother's blood, she may produce antibodies to them. These antibodies, in turn, can pass through the placenta into the fetal circulation and destroy fetal red blood cells, sometimes to a severe degree. This condition is known as hemolytic disease of the newborn or erythroblastosis fetalis.

One of 150 births is marked by detectable hemolytic disease of the newborn. The most severe form of the disease is the result of an incompatability of the Rh, or Rhesus, blood groups. This will be discussed in some detail in the following pages.

An incompatibility may also occur between the ABO blood groups of the mother and fetus. This usually re-

[5] Jack A. Pritchard and Paul C. MacDonald, *Williams Obstetrics,* 16th ed., Appleton-Century-Crofts, New York, 1980, p. 949.

[6] Helmuth Vorherr, Placental insufficiency in relation to postterm pregnancy and fetal postmaturity, *Am. J. Obstet. Gynecol.,* 123:67–103, (Sept.) 1975.

[7] Tiffany M. Field *et al.,* Developmental effects of prolonged pregnancy and the postmaturity syndrome, *J. Pediatr.,* 90:836–39, (May) 1977.

sults when there is a type-O mother and a type-A fetus, although it has been known to occur with a type-B fetus. Type-O blood, of course, contains both anti-A and anti-B serum antibodies. This is the most common cause of hemolytic disease, but it is usually mild. It differs from Rh isoimmunization in several important ways: (1) it can occur as readily in a first pregnancy as in a subsequent one, (2) it does not necessarily increase in severity with each subsequent gestation, (3) it does not require intrauterine therapy. Additionally, incompatibility of ABO blood types may protect against Rh immunization. For example, if the fetal red cells are type A, Rh(+) and the mother is type O, Rh(−), the anti-A in the mother's serum will destroy any fetal cells entering maternal circulation before they can stimulate an immune response to the Rh antigen.

About 2 percent of isoimmune disease is caused by other, rare blood groups. Those most often implicated are the Kell, Kidd, Duffy, and MN factors. These antigens, besides being quite rare, are rather weak and do not usually produce severe disease. Sensitization to these antigens is often the result of a previous blood transfusion.

Isoimmune Disease Caused by Rh Incompatibility

Isoimmune disease due to Rh incompatibility occurs when Rh antigens enter the blood of an Rh-negative mother and she produces anti-Rh antibodies. These maternal antibodies readily cross the placenta into the fetal circulation. If the fetus is Rh-positive, the antibodies attach to the erythrocytes and cause hemolysis. The antibodies are harmless to the mother herself, since the Rh antigen is absent from her cells, and they are harmless to an Rh-negative fetus.

The hemolytic process may begin early in pregnancy and be so intense as to cause death *in utero* from profound anemia. It may begin later and be mild enough to permit birth of a normal-appearing liveborn infant in whom hemolysis continues to a variable, sometimes only mild, degree. To compensate for loss of cells, the hemolytic process is accompanied by an overdevelopment of erythropoietic tissue in bone marrow, liver, and spleen. Anemia and jaundice occur as a result of erythrocyte destruction, and there are many nucleated red blood cells in the circulating blood owing to the hyperactivity of blood-forming tissue.

The Rh Factor

The Rh factor, which is a cause of incompatibility between maternal and fetal blood, is really an antigenic system. It was first observed in 1939 by Levine and Stetson.[8] They reported an antibody present in the blood of a woman who had delivered an erythroblastotic, stillborn infant. Her serum agglutinated not only the infant's blood but also her husband's blood.

One year later Landsteiner and Weiner published the results of their work with Rhesus monkeys. They had immunized rabbits with Rhesus red blood cells and found that the resulting rabbit serum agglutinated not only Rhesus cells but also the cells of 85 percent of the human population. In other words 85 percent of humans had this antigen on their red cells; 15 percent did not. Those persons possessing the antigen were designated Rh-positive; those lacking the antigen were designated Rh-negative. It was soon discovered that this newly named Rh antigen was the same substance responsible for the fetal death in Levine and Stetson's case report and, indeed, for many of the maternal-fetal blood incompatibilities.

The Rh blood groups vary in their proportions depending on the population under discussion, just as other blood groups do. On the average, about 15 percent of the caucasian population is Rh-negative. There are fewer Rh-negative persons in the Negro race (about 8 percent) and fewer still among Orientals (1 to 2 percent).

The Genetics of the Rh Factor

It became evident very soon after Landsteiner and Weiner's discovery that the Rh factor is, in fact, a very complex gene locus. Geneticists are in disagreement about whether there is a single locus with multiple alleles or three very closely linked loci. The clinical relevance is not affected by this technical point, however.

There are five major Rh antigens: *C, c, D, E, e.* The genetic alternative to *D* is designated *d,* although it does not appear to be antigenic. The gene or genes carrying the Rh antigens are, like all genes, located on chromosomes, which are always in pairs—one of which has been derived from the mother and one from the father. An individual then receives one chromosome from his mother carrying a *C* or *c* and a *D* or *d* and an *E* or *e.* He likewise receives one chromosome from his father carrying a *C* or *c* and a *D* or *d* and an *E* or *e.* A single chromosome does not carry both a *C* and *c,* a *D* and *d* or an *E* and *e;* it must be either a large-letter or a small-letter gene. Large letters symbolize the dominant Rh-positive genes, while small letters symbolize the recessive Rh-negative genes.

It can be seen that there are a large number of possible combinations of genes. A person may be *CDE/CDE, cde/cde, CDe/cde, cDe/cDE* and so on and on. The genotype, or the kind of Rh genes carried by an individual's chromosomes, is determined by laboratory tests using antisera specific to the various antigens.

The *D* is the most strongly antigenic and as such is responsible for most of the fetal-maternal pathology related to the Rh factor. For this reason, in clinical terminology, Rh-positive means literally *D*-positive and

[8] P. Levine and R. E. Stetson, An unusual case of intragroup agglutination, *JAMA,* 113:126–27, 1939.

Rh-negative means *D*-negative or *d*. The Rh-positive individual may have two *D* genes, designated as *DD,* in which case he is homozygous. Or, he may have one *D* and one *d,* designated *Dd,* and he is then heterozygous. Because the Rh-positive trait is dominant, the presence of only one *D* makes a person Rh-positive. If both genes are *d,* the individual is *dd,* designated Rh-negative.

In addition to the major Rh antigens, a number of variants of *C* and *D* are known. Of these only the *D* appears to be clinically significant. This variant, designated D^u, reacts weakly or not at all with anti-*D* serum and may give a false Rh-negative classification. For this reason, antiserum specific to the D^u should always be used to double-check red cells thought to be *D*-negative.

Persons who are Rh-negative (i.e., lacking the *D* antigen) can be stimulated to form antibodies that will destroy Rh-positive (*D*-positive) red cells. This stimulation occurs when an Rh-negative person is transfused with Rh-positive blood or when red cells of an Rh(+) fetus enter the circulation of an RH(−) mother. Once antibody formation, or sensitization, has occurred, any further contacts with the antigen will result in a hemolytic reaction. Therefore, if Rh-positive fetal blood cells pass through the placenta into an Rh-negative maternal circulation, antibodies are produced to the fetal red cell antigens. The antibodies then pass back from the mother's blood into fetal circulation, where they hemolyze fetal red cells (see Fig. 14–7).

How does an Rh-negative woman become pregnant with an Rh-positive fetus? The woman must possess only Rh-negative genes, since that is a recessive trait. Therefore, it is clear that the fetus must have inherited an Rh-positive gene from the father. The mating of an Rh-negative female with an Rh-positive male occurs about 12 times in 100, but not all of the offspring are affected with isoimmune disease. Some of them may themselves be Rh-negative. A review of the genetics will explain how this happens. If the father is homozygous (*DD*), all of his children will be Rh-positive regardless of the mother's blood type. [Remember, *D* or (+) is dominant.] However, if he is heterozygous (*Dd*), a mating with an Rh-negative woman (*dd*) would result (on the average) in half of his children being Rh-positive (*Dd*) and half Rh-negative (*dd*) (see Fig. 14–8 for a diagram).

Firstborns of Rh-neg.–Rh-pos. matings are seldom

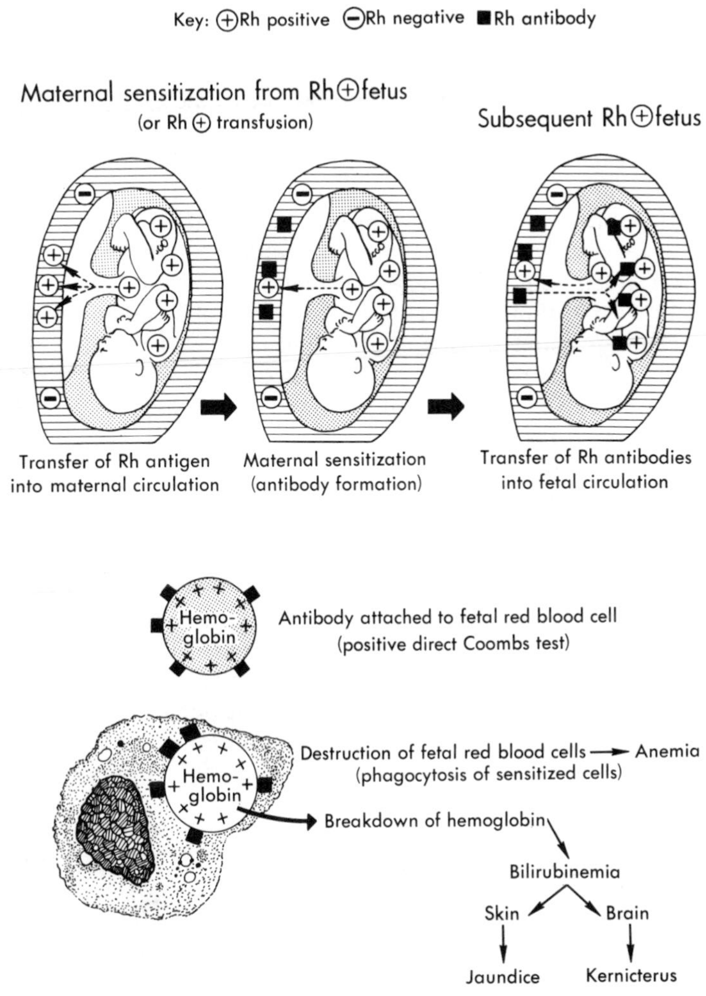

Figure 14–7. Erythroblastosis fetalis. [Adapted by permission from *Erythroblastosis Fetalis*, Ross Clinical Education Aid No. 9. Ross Laboratories, Columbus, Ohio, 1962.]

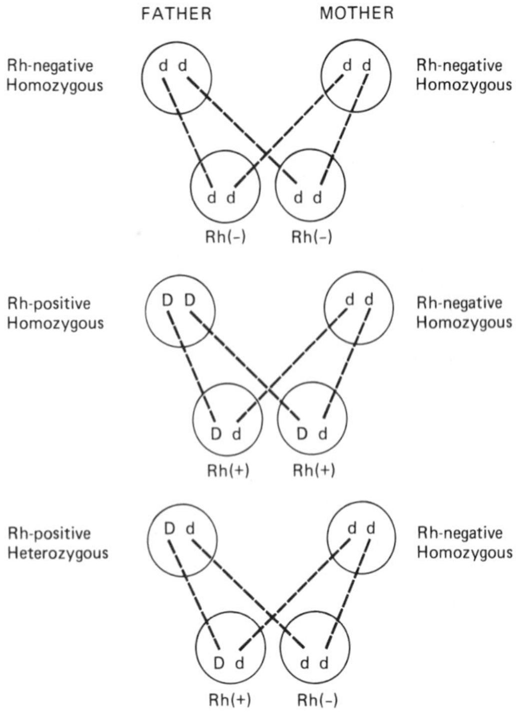

Figure 14–8. Illustration of inheritance of the Rh genes *D* and *d*. The *C* and *c* and *E* and *e* genes are inherited in the same manner.

sensitized. It is believed that the most likely time for fetal cells to escape into maternal circulation is near or at the time of placental separation. This does not allow time for antibody formation to occur and to affect the fetus before birth. First children may be affected if the mother was previously sensitized by a transfusion or by an abortion which went undiagnosed. Practitioners performing elective abortions are not always knowledgeable or conscientious about the use of RhoGam (see below), and some Rh-negative women are sensitized in this way.

Fetal antigens are not always able to pass through the placenta into the maternal circulation. If they do pass through to the mother, they may be rapidly hemolyzed and unable to stimulate antibody formation, as occurs when there is a coexistent ABO incompatibility. Or the mother may not produce any antibodies to them for reasons that are not completely understood.

On the average, about 15 percent of the offspring of Rh-negative females and Rh-positive males will be affected by isoimmune disease if no prophylactic treatment is employed. Once a woman has developed a concentration of antibodies sufficient to cause hemolytic disease in an infant, each subsequent Rh-positive infant is likely to have increasingly severe disease.

Antepartum Diagnosis and Management

Detection and treatment of Rh isoimmunization begin early in pregnancy at the first antepartum visit. At this time the ABO and Rh blood groups should be documented and an antibody screen performed. If the woman is Rh-negative and has no history of a preceding affected infant, it is useful to determine the father's Rh type. If he is negative, the fetus also will be negative and no disease will occur.

If the woman is found to be Rh-positive with no antibodies, a normal pregnancy and delivery are probable, at least with respect to isoimmune factors. However, it is wise to repeat the antibody screen at 28 weeks' gestation to rule out the possibility of difficulty from any of the rare blood antigens.

If the mother is Rh-negative and the antibody screen is negative, rescreening is done at 24, 28, and 34 weeks' gestation to detect any sensitization that develops during pregnancy. In addition, she will be evaluated to receive RhoGam in the postpartum period (see below).

If the mother is Rh-negative and antibodies are found with an indirect antiglobulin (Coombs) test, titration is made to determine the degree to which they are present. Subsequent monthly titrations will reveal whether the titer rises or remains the same. If the titer remains at or below a *critical* level (usually defined as 1:8) on repeated determinations throughout gestation, the pregnancy usually will be delivered at term with no further treatment.

Detection of an antibody titer above the *critical* level indicates significant sensitization and requires evaluation by means of amniocentesis. Unfortunately, the level of the titer does not correlate well with the severity of the fetal disease. A more precise estimate of the degree of fetal illness is obtained by analyzing amniotic fluid samples for bilirubin content. Normally, the amount of bilirubin in amniotic fluid declines steadily throughout gestation until it virtually disappears in the last month. If maternal antibodies are destroying fetal red cells, excessive bibirubin will be excreted as an end product of hemolysis by the fetal skin and kidneys. Thus, the more severe the hemolysis, the greater the amount of bilirubin in amniotic fluid.

Amniotic fluid is obtained by amniocentesis as described in Chapter 13. Care must be taken to place the fluid immediately in a light-excluding container, as exposure to light for more than a few seconds will cause deterioration of the bilirubin and may give a falsely low value. The optical density of the fluid is analyzed in a spectrophotometer, which measures the light absorption. Normal amniotic fluid, when plotted on a logarithmic scale, will describe a straight line from about 350 to 700 nm, but when bilirubin is present, a bulge appears in the graph at about 450 nm. The extent of this bulge can be measured and plotted against gestational age to gauge the severity of the hemolytic process.

When the optical density (OD) falls within zone I of the Liley graph (see Fig. 14–9), the fetus is only mildly affected, if affected at all, and may be suspected of being

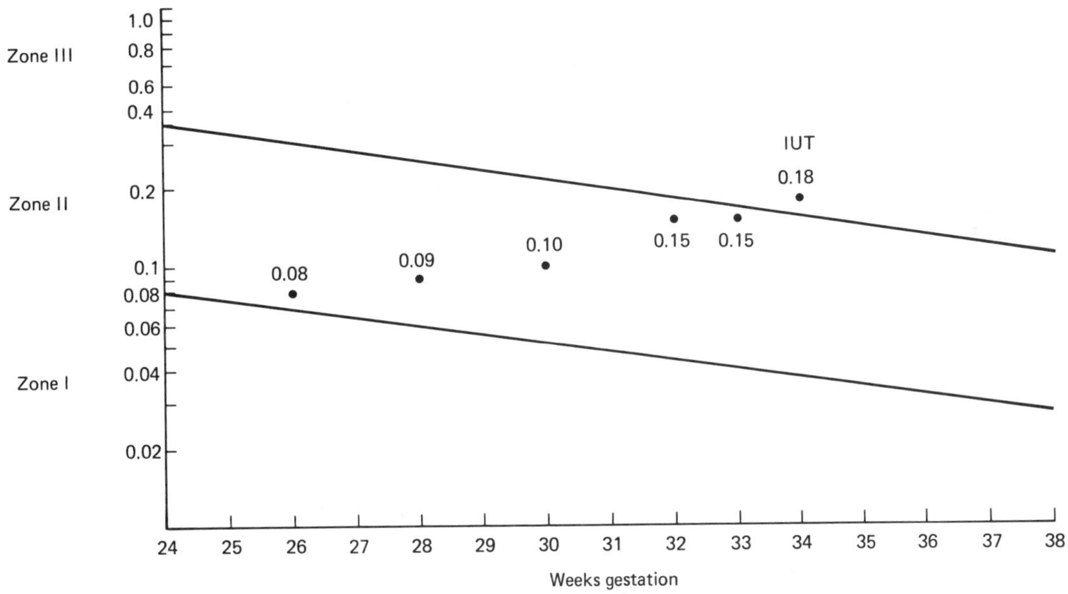

Figure 14–9. A Liley graph showing the optical density for a 29-year-old Rh(−), GIV, PII. Her first child was unaffected; the second was an Rh(−) child; the third pregnancy terminated in a spontaneous abortion at 14 weeks' gestation. At the initial antepartum visit at 12 weeks' gestation in the present pregnancy the antibody titer was 1:128. Amniocenteses were begun at 26 weeks gestation and continued biweekly and then weekly. At 34 weeks, with an optical density in zone III and a fetal L/S ratio of only 1.8, an intrauterine transfusion was performed. At 36 weeks a 2450-gm male infant with an L/S of 3.6 was delivered vaginally following an oxytocin induction. The infant did well, requiring a single exchange transfusion and phototherapy for hyperbilirubinemia. His parents took him home on the tenth day of life.

Rh-negative. Zone II indicates a moderate degree of disease. If serial ODs follow the normal downward trend, the pregnancy is usually allowed to continue until 35 to 37 weeks' gestation, when labor is induced following confirmation of fetal lung maturity. A reading in zone III is indicative of a severely affected fetus, and immediate treatment must be undertaken to avoid permanent disability or death. If the fetus is mature, delivery is effected at once. When the fetus is not mature, intrauterine transfusion is undertaken.

Since 1963, intrauterine transfusions have been done on fetuses that would not otherwise be able to survive *in utero* until sufficiently mature to be born. Recently the use of ultrasonography to direct the placement of the transfusing catheter has markedly improved the safety of this procedure. After the insertion of the catheter into the peritoneal cavity of the fetus, a volume of type O, Rh(−) packed red cells commensurate with the fetal weight is infused. These cells, absorbed into fetal circulation, improve fetal anemia and oxygenation. Since these cells are Rh-negative, they are not hemolyzed. The transfusions may be repeated at approximately two-week intervals until fetal lung maturity is achieved and delivery can be effected.

Figure 14–10 outlines the steps in diagnosis and management of isoimmunization in pregnancy as described above.

The major threat to the life of the fetus and newborn in hemolytic disease is anemia. Preparations should be made for immediate delivery room transfusion of the neonate whenever the birth of a severely affected infant is anticipated. Postnatally, hemolysis continues for varying lengths of time and, if untreated, may result in kernicterus, deposition of bilirubin in brain tissue. This irreversible condition may cause profound mental retardation. *In utero* bilirubin is cleared by the placenta and the maternal liver and thus represents no threat to the fetus. For a discussion of the care of neonates with hemolytic disease, refer to Chapter 30.

Prevention of Rh Isoimmunization

Much progress has been made in the prevention of Rh disease with the availability of anti-D immunoglobulin (RhoGam).

The likelihood of maternal infusion with fetal red cells is highest around the time of delivery when placental separation takes place. Normally these fetal antigens would stimulate an active immunity (antibodies) in the mother. However, if a high concentration of anti-D gamma-globulin can be administered, a passive immunity will result. The injected anti-D will destroy the antigenic fetal cells before they have the opportunity to stimulate active production of antibodies by the mother (Fig. 14–11).

Since it is not known how long a time period is re-

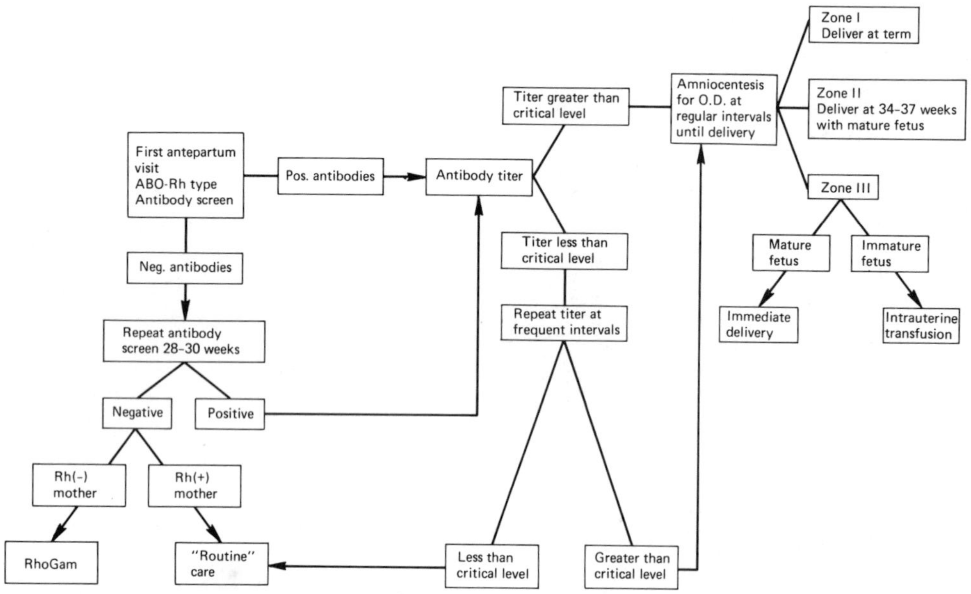

Figure 14–10. Path diagram outlining the management of isoimmunization during pregnancy.

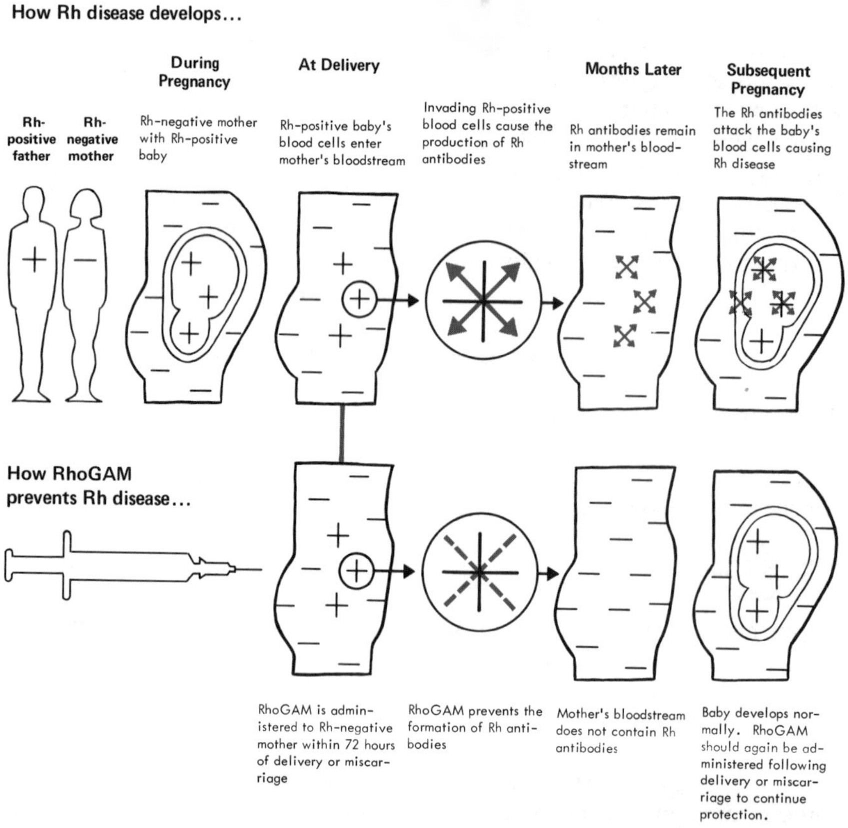

Figure 14–11. How Rh disease develops. How RhoGAM prevents Rh disease. [Reproduced with permission from Ortho Diagnostics, Raritan, N.J., 1968.]

quired for the formation of antibodies, it is recommended that RhoGam be given to the mother within the first 72 hours post partum. A dose of 300 mg of the preparation is injected intramuscularly after observing the following precautions:

1. Delivery has occurred within the past 72 hours
2. Mother is D(−), $D^u(-)$
3. Mother is *not* sensitized (negative Coombs test to D or D^u)
4. Infant is D(+) (or abortus of unknown blood type)
5. Infant is Coombs negative to D or D^u
6. Individual RhoGam dose has been cross-matched with maternal red cells and is compatible

Each pregnancy should be followed carefully with antibody screening and RhoGam given after each birth whether full-term or premature.

Sensitization also can occur as a result of spontaneous or induced abortions, ectopic pregnancies and amniocentesis involving piercing of the placenta. For pregnancies terminated prior to 12 weeks' gestation and for prophylaxis after amniocentesis, MICRhoGAM may be given. This consists of 50 mg of Rh-immune globulin and will protect against fetal-maternal hemorrhages of 4 to 5 ml. It has the added advantage of not requiring cross-matching. When the mini dose is administered following a genetics amniocentesis at 16 weeks' gestation, a second dose is recommended to be given at 28 weeks' gestation.

It should be emphasized that RhoGam cannot reverse or decrease sensitization once it has occurred. In addition, it is only effective against the D antigen, which is the one most commonly responsible for isoimmune disease. Sensitization can occur, however, to other of the Rh antigens or to other blood factors.

HYPERTENSION

Hypertension is one of the most serious, and, at the same time, most common complications of pregnancy, occurring in approximately 7 percent of all gestations. It accounts for 15 to 20 percent of maternal mortality, as well as contributing significantly to perinatal morbidity and mortality.

The hypertensive states of pregnancy have been classified by the American College of Obstetricians and Gynecologists into three major categories: (1) pregnancy-induced hypertension (preeclampsia and eclampsia), (2) chronic hypertension antedating pregnancy, and (3) chronic hypertension with superimposed toxemia. It should be emphasized, however, the differentiation of these disorders is often very difficult. Frequently diagnosis is only possible retrospectively, and then it may be somewhat arbitrary, since the criteria tend to be neither precise nor mutually exclusive.

The proportion of the various categories of hypertensive disease varies somewhat according to the characteristics of a given obstetric population. In general, preeclampsia accounts for between 80 and 90 percent of all hypertension in pregnancy. However, since chronic hypertension is more common in black women than caucasian women, this percentage would be likely to change if the population were largely black. Similarly, both preeclampsia and eclampsia are primarily diseases of primigravidas, so a very young population composed mainly of women in their first pregnancies, such as might be found in some housing developments or university communities, would tend to have a larger proportion of toxemias.

Pregnancy-Induced Hypertension

Pregnancy-induced hypertension or toxemia is a disease of the last half of gestation characterized by hypertension, edema, and proteinuria. It has been described for as long as written records have been kept. Its occurrence has been attributed to evil spirits, bad humors, and, more recently, to sodium intake and weight gain during pregnancy. Therapy has varied with the theories of etiology and the sophistication of the art and science of medicine. Aligning the woman's body with the magnetic poles of the earth was once a popular treatment, as were various herbs and incantations and, perhaps, even "eye of newt; toe of frog."[9]

The cause of toxemia remains unknown today, although much has been learned about the underlying pathology. Research into etiology and physiologic mechanisms is hampered by the lack of suitable laboratory animals, since no species apart from humans is susceptible to this disease.

It is known that functioning trophoblastic tissue is necessary for the occurrence of toxemia, although apparently the presence of the fetus is not necessary, since women with hydatid moles have a markedly increased incidence of the disease. Other predisposing factors include age (very young and very old gravidas), parity (classically a disease of nulliparas), multiple gestations, diabetes mellitus, and chronic hypertension. In addition, the incidence of all toxemia, but especially eclampsia, is significantly higher in less favored socioeconomic circumstances. This has caused speculation that a nutritional basis may exist for the disease. Frequency as well as quality of antepartum care no doubt plays a significant role as well, particularly with regard to eclampsia. Recently, evidence has been presented to indicate that the occurrence of preeclampsia may be determined by a single recessive gene.[10] The familial nature of this disease has long been recognized by nurses.

[9] William Shakespeare, *Macbeth,* Act III, Scene i.

[10] L. C., Chesley, Hypertension in pregnancy: Definitions, familial factor, and remote prognosis, *Kidney International,* 18:234–40, 1980.

Numerous hypotheses regarding the cause of toxemia have been advanced only to be discarded. One current hypothesis is that of reduced uteroplacental blood flow. A number of investigators have been able to induce hypertension in pregnant dogs or sheep by ligating the uterine arteries and thus producing uterine ischemia. Uterine blood flow is known to be reduced in chronic hypertension and some diabetes mellitus, two of the predisposing factors. Also there is anatomic confirmation that the diameter of the uterine arteries is greater in multigravidas than in primigravidas. It is not decided, however, whether the uterine ischemia is actually the first cause of the toxemia or whether it is the result of some other factor, as yet unknown. Another popular hypothesis suggests that "something" produces an increased vascular sensitivity, accounting for vasospasm which causes uterine ischemia.

It is postulated that the ischemic placenta undergoes premature aging and may develop infarcts and other degenerative changes. Catabolic end products from this process are released into the maternal bloodstream, where they bring about a mild disseminated intravascular coagulation. This is aggravated by the hemoconcentration characteristic of the more severe forms of toxemia.

Regardless of where these changes occur in the cause-effect cycle, there is agreement that the most basic underlying pathologic change is that of *generalized vasospasm*. If this vasospasm is kept in mind, all of the clinical symptoms of the disease may be explained, as well as the majority of therapeutic interventions.

Symptoms

Toxemia should be thought of as a single disease which exists on a continuum of severity ranging from mild preeclampsia through severe preeclampsia to eclampsia. Patients, however, do not necessarily progress through the disease in this sequence. The woman may present initially with very severe preeclampsia or, less commonly, eclampsia. Mild preeclampsia may progress rapidly to eclampsia or may remain quite stable with only minimum therapy. For this reason, an extraordinary degree of vigilance is required in order to control the disease effectively.

The cardinal signs of preeclampsia are three: hypertension, edema, and proteinuria. The presence of hypertension together with either edema or proteinuria or both is diagnostic of this condition.

Hypertension is defined as a blood pressure of 140/90 or a rise in systolic pressure of 30 mm Hg or more and a rise in diastolic pressure of 15 mm Hg or more over baseline values. The elevation over the individual's own baseline is the more valuable criterion, since many women of reproductive age may have normally low readings, especially in the midtrimester. It is also valuable in detecting preeclampsia when it is superimposed on chronic hypertension. The blood pressure elevation should be noted on two separate occasions taken six hours apart in order to establish a definitive diagnosis. Since this, however, is not a practical procedure in most outpatient settings, treatment usually is begun without meeting this strict criterion.

Blood pressure readings of 160/100 mm Hg are indicative of severe preeclampsia. Systolic readings over 200 usually are associated with an underlying chronic hypertension. Patients with systolic pressures over 200 are at significant risk for cerebrovascular accidents and require vigorous medical therapy.

Edema is the least precise of the clinical parameters of preeclampsia, though it is often the first one to be detected. Edema of the lower extremities is almost a universal finding in pregnancy because of the mechanical obstruction of veins by the heavy uterus as well as changes in venous pressure. For this reason, edema of the face and hands is given greater significance. A sudden increase in weight (greater than 500 gm or 1 lb per week) without any other explanation is suspicious of developing edema. The woman may complain of a sudden tightness of her rings or of edema present upon rising in the morning. Facial edema may not be apparent to the woman or her family unless the onset is quite sudden. But the nurse who only sees her at weekly intervals may immediately notice a change in her appearance since the last visit.

Proteinuria is indicative of the extent of glomerular damage due to the toxemia and usually appears later than other symptoms. In order to be considered diagnostic, values greater than 1 gm/liter (or 1+ on a standard dip stick) must be detected. Whenever a possibility of preeclampsia exists, care should be taken to obtain a clean-voided urine specimen for analysis. Vaginal discharge, characteristic of late pregnancy, readily contaminates the urine specimen and may give a falsely high reading. Twenty-four-hour urine assays are more reliable than a single voiding. Protein values over 500 mg/24 hours are diagnostic of preeclampsia. As preeclampsia becomes severe, urine may be highly concentrated, scant in amount, and contain casts, red and white blood cells, and epithelial cells. Oliguria is a grave prognostic sign.

While mild preeclampsia is characterized by edema and/or proteinuria together with hypertension, as the disease progresses and the vasospasm becomes more severe, other signs and symptoms begin to appear. There is increasing central nervous system irritability as evidenced by headaches, dizziness, visual disturbances, and hyperreflexia. Fundoscopic changes may be seen as a result of the vasospasm and perhaps also because of central nervous system alterations. These changes include retinal edema, arteriolar constriction or spasm, and hemorrhages. Rarely, retinal detachment may occur due to extreme retinal edema. Reattachment is usually spontaneous after delivery and resolution of the disease process. Epigastric pain is a late and ominous symptom. The pain is generally felt to be due to hepatic capsular stretching resulting from edema and/or hemorrhages.

The occurrence of a convulsion or coma, in addition to the symptoms of preeclampsia, is diagnostic of eclampsia. This constitutes one of the gravest complications in obstetrics. Maternal mortality may be as high as 10 percent, while perinatal mortality approaches 25 percent.

All the symptoms enumerated for preeclampsia become more severe with eclampsia. Severe edema distorts the woman's features until she may be unrecognizable. Oliguria or even anuria is noted, and proteinuria varies from a few grams per liter to 30 to 40 gm/liter. Blood pressure averages 180/110 mm Hg, although it may be much higher.

Convulsions, both tonic and clonic, occur in eclampsia. At first all muscles go into a state of tonic contraction; then they alternately contract and relax. The convulsions are sometimes preceded by an aura, but often are so entirely unheralded that they occur while the patient is asleep. They ordinarily begin with a twitching of the eyelids or facial muscles. The eyes are wide open and staring, and the pupils are usually dilated. Next the whole body becomes rigid, and then alternate contraction and relaxation of all muscles begin. The twitchings proceed from the muscles about the nose and mouth to those of the neck and arms, and so on, until the entire body is in spasm. The patient's face is usually cyanotic and badly distorted, with the mouth being drawn to one side. She clenches her fists, rolls her head from side to side, and tosses violently about the bed. She is totally unconscious and insensible to light, and during the seizure respirations cease. Her head is frequently bent backward. Her neck forms a continuous curve with her stiffened, arched back. Another distressing feature is the protruding tongue and the frothy saliva, which may be blood stained if the patient bites her tongue. Finally, muscular movements become milder, and then the patient lies motionless. After a long, deep breath, respiratory movements are resumed.

Convulsive attacks vary greatly in their intensity and duration. There may be only a few twitches, lasting 10 to 15 seconds, or violent convulsions lasting as long as two minutes. Their number and severity increase with the seriousness of the patient's condition.

The patient lapses into a coma after a convulsion. This also varies in length and profundity, her condition during the intervals being very suggestive of the probable outcome of the disease. Some patients have no recollection of the seizures and may even fail to remember anything that happened within several hours, or even days, before the attack.

During the acute stage the respirations are, as a rule, labored and noisy, and cyanosis may be present. The temperature is often normal or rises to 38.3° C (101° F). It may go as high as 39.4° C (103° F) or 40° C (104° F), in severe cases, and this is a serious prognostic sign.

When eclampsia develops during late pregnancy, labor may begin and the baby be born spontaneously, or the fetus may die, after which the condition begins to improve and the stillborn infant is delivered later.

When eclampsia occurs in labor, contractions usually increase in force and frequency, thus hastening delivery, after which the condition begins to improve. Death or expulsion of the fetus is usually followed by improvement within 12 to 24 hours (coma may continue a few hours or a day) and by ultimate recovery, provided adequate treatment is continued and the condition has not become critical before delivery or death of the baby.

In postpartum eclampsia the convulsions occur soon after delivery—almost always within the first 24 hours.

The most frequent causes of death in eclampsia are congestive heart failure, cerebrovascular accidents, and complications of obstetric operations. Improved antepartum care as well as better methods of treatment for both preeclampsia and eclampsia have led to a significant decrease in maternal and perinatal mortality.

Prevention

Eclampsia is considered to be a preventable disease in almost every circumstance. A woman who assumes responsibility for her own health care, seeks antepartum consultation, and recognizes changes in her body needing evaluation will be diagnosed and treated before eclampsia occurs. Preeclampsia, treated knowledgeably, can almost always be controlled so it does not progress to convulsions. Professionals caring for pregnant women have a serious responsibility not only to recognize and treat early symptoms but also to instruct their clients in what signs and symptoms to report immediately. Every effort should be made to develop a relationship where the woman, though not overly dependent, feels free to call with questions at any time. In this way she is unlikely to delay reporting symptoms because she doesn't "want to bother you."

Preeclampsia is not preventable at present. Although good antepartum care has markedly reduced the mortality and morbidity caused by the more severe forms, there is no evidence that any feature of even the best antepartum care has reduced the overall incidence of preeclampsia.

In the recent past, several measures widely prescribed to prevent preeclampsia have been proven to be of no value and, in fact, potentially harmful. Restriction of dietary salt and caloric intake as well as the use of diuretics have been shown to be detrimental. Severe electrolyte imbalance can result from limited sodium intake, particularly if combined with the use of thiazide diu-

Table 14–6. Nursing Management of Inpatients with Toxemia

Patient Care Goals	*Nursing Interventions*
I. Decrease central nervous system irritability	1. Modify environment to ensure rest and quiet a. Eliminate noise, bright lights, other harsh stimuli b. Minimize number of personnel giving care c. Initiate painful and/or intrusive procedures after sedation d. Promote comfort at bed rest 2. Explain all plans and procedures simply and briefly 3. Administer sedative drugs as prescribed 4. Be alert to changing clinical status a. Assess knee-jerk reflexes b. Determine subjective symptoms (irritability, headache, blurred vision, epigastric pain) c. Keep emergency support materials readily available (e.g., O_2, suction, airway, $MgSO_4$, sedatives)
II. Control blood pressure	1. Measure and record B/P (frequency is determined by severity of clinical symptoms) 2. Have B/P taken by the same person using the same cuff whenever possible 3. Administer antihypertensive drugs as prescribed (usually when diastolic pressure exceeds 110 mm Hg)
III. Promote diuresis	1. Encourage continuous bed rest in left lateral position 2. Monitor renal function a. Dip-stick exam for urine protein b. Collect 24-hour specimen for protein and creatinine clearance 3. Monitor effects of therapy a. Record accurate intake and output (minimum output: 20 ml/hr) b. Weigh daily at same time using same scale
IV. Monitor fetal well-being	1. Auscultate and record FHR 2. Instruct and support during amniocentesis 3. Collect 24-hour urine specimen for estriol determination 4. Perform FAD and/or OCT 5. Reassure parents realistically, based on available data
V. Deliver the infant	1. Review parents' knowledge of labor and delivery 2. Give instructions about induction of labor and electronic fetal heart rate monitoring 3. Introduce parents to intrapartum nurse prior to onset of labor 4. Introduce parents to appropriate neonatal staff

retics. In fact, there is growing evidence that increased salt intake may be necessary to maintain the positive sodium balance of a normal pregnancy. This is usually accomplished by advising the woman to salt her food to taste, since she will doubtless be increasing her overall food intake.

Weight control is likewise of no value in preventing preeclampsia. As discussed in Chapter 10, inadequate weight gain is associated with an increased incidence of small-for-gestational-age infants.

Diuretics have failed to demonstrate any reduction in the incidence of preeclampsia in double-blind studies. Rather, they have been associated with severe maternal electrolyte imbalance, fetal and neonatal hyponatremia, and neonatal thrombocytopenia. By reducing the effective intravascular volume, diuretics may actually promote vasospasm, thus further reducing uterine blood flow. Furthermore, when given prophylactically throughout pregnancy they may mask the development of early signs of impending toxemia.

Although a cause-effect relationship between nutrition and toxemia has not been proven, there is some reason to believe that a good diet, high in protein, may be helpful. Periods of rest, preferably with the woman lying on her side, may enhance uterine blood flow. Certainly these two precautions are beneficial enough to the woman's general health and well-being that no harm can be done in emphasizing them, even without proof they will prevent toxemia.

Since early detection of the beginning symptoms of preeclampsia is so beneficial, it would presumably be even more beneficial to detect those women who are going to develop preeclampsia before clinical symptoms appear. In 1974, Gant and his associates found that women between 28 and 32 weeks' gestation, who later developed toxemia, demonstrated an increased sensitivity to the pressor effects of angiotensin II. In addition, he found that these same women demonstrated a rise in diastolic blood pressure of at least 20 mm Hg when turned from a lateral to a supine position. Initial reports indicated that more than 93 percent of the women who showed the rise in diastolic pressure subsequently developed toxemia.[11] Subsequent studies have failed to replicate this high percentage, and the clinical value of this observation is unconfirmed. Continued research is needed to develop means of detecting which women will develop preeclampsia before symptoms appear, as well as means for differentiating pregnancy-induced hypertension from other hypertensive disorders.

Treatment

The only cure for toxemia is delivery of the pregnancy. Therefore, if delivery is undesirable because of the immaturity of the fetus, efforts are directed at controlling the symptoms to insure both maternal and fetal safety until delivery can be reasonably undertaken. The extent and vigor of medical intervention depend on the severity of the disease at any given time. Constant reevaluation and modification of the plan of care is usually necessary.

The most usual situation is for a woman who has been receiving regular antepartum supervision to present in the third trimester at a regular appointment with some generalized edema and a slight elevation in blood pressure. Proteinuria may or may not be present. A diagnosis of mild preeclampsia is made. The woman is advised to maintain bed rest, notify the nurse or physician of any subjective change in status, and return to the office or clinic in three to four days. A mild sedative (usually sodium phenobarbital) may be prescribed to make bed rest more palatable as well as for its anticonvulsive effects. Bed rest, especially on the left side, facilitates venous return, promotes diuresis, and enhances uterine blood flow. Public health nurse consultation may be sought to monitor blood pressure at home. A case summary will illustrate this care.

M. W., a 19-year-old primigravida, presented in the physician's office at 37 weeks' gestation with a blood pressure of 138/90 (previous readings were 100–110/70), 2+ to 3+ edema of feet, legs, and hands, and a trace of protein on the urine dip stick. She had gained 2½ lb since her last visit ten days earlier. The diagnosis of preeclampsia and its implications were carefully discussed with M. W., and she was advised to go on bed rest at home and return to the office in four days. She was encouraged to lie on her left side as much as possible and to get up only to go to the bathroom or to eat. When M. W. returned to the office four days later, she still had some dependent edema, but her blood pressure was 112/76, her urine contained no protein, and she had lost 1800 gm (4 lb) from diuresis. This woman was followed closely until 39 weeks' gestation when she went into labor spontaneously and delivered a 3150-gm (6 lb 15 oz) girl. Except for continued edema and slight elevation of blood pressure to 130/90 during labor, there were no further clinical manifestations of preeclampsia.

For this woman bed rest was a reasonable request, which she was readily able to carry out. She had previously resigned from her job, had no other children, and lived with her husband who was able to rearrange his work commitments to allow time for him to be very nurturant toward his wife.

In contrast, consider the following case.

V. L., a 22-year-old gravida three, para one, lived in a mobile home eight miles from town and nearly three miles from her nearest neighbor. Her husband, a long-distance truck driver, was away from home 11 out of every 14 days. During this time V. L. was alone with her three-year-old daughter. Bed rest in these circumstances would be virtually impossible unless the nurse used tact and resourcefulness to help this family problem-solve. In this case daytime child care and help with grocery shopping were arranged through a local church and a home health aide visited every other day. Later, the husband was able to negotiate with his company for some short-distance drives for several weeks of the pregnancy. At 38 weeks a 2700-gm (6 lb) boy was delivered following induction of labor.

When bed rest at home does not improve the symptoms, or when the presenting symptoms are more severe, hospitalization is necessary. The goals of therapy are to decrease central nervous system irritability, control the blood pressure, promote diuresis, monitor fetal well-being and, ultimately, to deliver the infant.

The newly admitted woman is placed on bed rest, and environmental stimuli are kept to a minimum. Loud talking, bright lights, and unnecessary traffic in and out of her room are to be avoided. Reflexes are checked at frequent intervals for hyperactivity, and the presence of clonus is noted. Sodium phenobarbital or some other mild sedative or tranquilizer is usually prescribed. Careful explanation of all procedures as well as the overall plan of care will further alleviate the woman's anxiety.

Renal function is evaluated by means of creatinine clearance tests and 24-hour urine protein determinations. A strict intake and output record is kept to detect any changes in volume of urine. Weight obtained at the same time each day indicates the extent of diuresis.

An amniocentesis usually is done to determine fetal lung maturity. Twenty-four-hour urinary estriol is measured as an indicator of fetal/placental function, and/or an oxytocin challenge test (OCT) or fetal activity determination (FAD) may be done. If the fetus is near term and has a mature L/S ratio, labor usually will be induced after the maternal symptoms have been controlled for 12 to 24 hours. If preeclampsia is severe, delivery may be necessary before optimal fetal maturity for both maternal and fetal welfare.

The woman who does not respond to bed rest and sedation with lowered blood pressure and diuresis must be treated more aggressively. The usual therapy is magnesium sulfate, administered either intramuscularly

[11] Norman F. Gant *et al.*, A clinical test useful for predicting the development of acute hypertension in pregnancy, *Am. J. Obstet. Gynecol.*, 120:1–7, (Sept. 1) 1974.

or intravenously. This drug is an effective anticonvulsant as it decreases central nervous system irritability by acting directly on the central nervous system as well as at the myoneural junction. A secondary effect is the lowering of blood pressure owing to vasodilation. Patients receiving magnesium sulfate by either route should have an intravenous conduit in place, receive nothing by mouth, and have an indwelling catheter in the bladder to permit hourly assessment of urinary output.

When magnesium sulfate is given intramuscularly, the initial dose is usually 10 gm (20 ml of a 50 percent solution). It is divided so that 10 ml are given into each buttock; 1 ml of a 1 percent local anesthetic agent is usually added to each 10 ml of magnesium sulfate solution to reduce the discomfort of the injection. If the patient is still hyperactive in four to six hours and if urinary output is satisfactory, magnesium sulfate may be repeated in a 5-gm dose.

Intramuscular administration of magnesium sulfate should be deep into the gluteal muscle, preferably into the ventrogluteal area. It is advisable to discard the needle used to draw the solution from the ampul and to attach another sterile dry needle to the syringe for administration of the drug. In this way it is possible to avoid any irritant solution on the outside of the needle. As injection of the medication is made, the needle may be moved about to obtain a wider dispersion of the drug. The area of administration should be massaged and a dry, warm pack applied.

Intravenous administration of this drug is more common. It avoids the painful intramuscular injection, but also has the added safety of a more predictable action, which is more readily controlled. In contrast, medication injected intramuscularly may have quite variable absorption rates and, once injected, cannot be retrieved. A frequent dose schedule for intravenous magnesium sulfate is a "loading" dose of 4 gm followed by the continuous infusion of 1 to 2 gm per hour. Magnesium blood levels are often used to determine the rate of flow.

Regardless of the route of administration, certain clinical criteria must be met prior to the administration of any subsequent doses. These criteria are (1) respirations greater than 12 per minute, (2) urinary output at least 30 ml per hour, and (3) presence of the knee-jerk reflex.

Magnesium sulfate is eliminated from the body chiefly by the kidneys, and if the urinary output is low, it may be retained in the blood until a high, dangerous concentration is reached. This may depress respirations and cardiac action. The patient must be watched for respiratory depression. It is believed that this depression does not occur until after the knee-jerk reflex disappears.

A further safeguard against magnesium overdose, as well as a means of assuring doses sufficient to prevent convulsions, is the monitoring of maternal magnesium blood levels. Magnesium equilibrates fairly readily across the placenta so the fetal blood level reflects that of the mother, and the neonate may have respiratory depression if born with high magnesium blood levels. Maternal blood levels of 4 to 6 mg per 100 ml are usually sufficient therapeutically and do not cause neonatal depression at birth.

An intravenous calcium preparation, 10 percent calcium gluconate, is an immediate antidote to magnesium sulfate. It should always be available at the patient's bedside in case of respiratory or cardiac arrest. (See Table 14–7).

Occasionally magnesium sulfate alone is not sufficient to reduce central nervous system irritability and sodium phenobarbital is given as well. Smaller doses of the barbiturate are necessary when used together with magnesium sulfate. Barbiturate should be avoided in labor, since there is no available antagonist.

An antihypertensive drug is sometimes required to lower blood pressure. When the diastolic pressure cannot be reduced below 110 mm Hg with magnesium sulfate alone, a drug such as hydralazine (APRESOLINE) may be given. This drug has the advantage of dilating peripheral vessels, and thus does not diminish uterine blood flow. Care should be taken to maintain the diastolic pressure no lower than 90 mm Hg in order to maintain placental perfusion.

As soon as the maternal condition is stabilized and fetal maturity is established, induction of labor is begun with continuous oxytocin infusion as described in Chapter 22. The magnesium sulfate is continued through labor. In preeclampsia the uterus is highly responsive to oxytocin, and vaginal delivery can almost always be achieved. Continuous fetal heart rate monitoring should be employed to assess the fetal response to labor.

In the unfortunate event that the disease progresses to eclampsia, immediate efforts are directed toward control of convulsions, stabilization of blood pressure, and maintenance of renal function. Usually four to six hours are sufficient to control the symptoms and stabilize the patient. Delivery should then be accomplished with dispatch.

The intracranial pressure is frequently raised in patients wtih eclampsia, and they are therefore very irritable, so that any stimulation may start a convulsion.

Table 14–7. Precautions for Women Receiving Magnesium Sulfate

1. Continuous nursing attendance
2. Intravenous conduit in place
3. Foley catheter connected to drainage
4. $MgSO_4$ given *only* when:
    - Respirations > 12 per minute
    - Urine output > 20 ml per hour
    - Knee-jerk reflexes clearly present
5. Calcium gluconate available at bedside

To this end, there are innumerable details to be considered. Every effort is made to keep the patient as quiet and free from stimuli as possible. A quiet, darkened room is important. Every act must be performed as quietly as possible. The nurse should walk lightly and guard against kicking or striking the bed. Talking should be in low tones, doors should be opened and closed quietly, and papers should not be rustled or furniture scraped. Since any manipulation may excite a convulsion, the patient should not be disturbed more than is absolutely necessary. Only the care essential for treatment and for observation should be given.

Constant nursing care is necessary, and the patient must never be left alone for even a second. She must be carefully observed for any change in condition and especially for twitchings, cyanosis, and excessive mucus. Someone must be present to prevent the patient from injuring herself during convulsions and to remove mucus from the respiratory passage as it collects.

Restraint during convulsions should be as mild as possible, since resistance increases the patient's excitement while her need is to be quieted, but she must be protected against falling out of bed and against injuring her tongue. During a convulsion there is great danger of the patient's biting her tongue unless something is placed between her teeth at the very onset to prevent their closing on the tongue. A small roll of bandage, a clean cloth tightly rolled, several tongue depressors wrapped with gauze or a piece of thick rubber tubing may be used and must be at the bedside, available for immediate use. Hard wooden mouth gags are not satisfactory because of the danger of bruising or cutting the mucous membranes or even breaking a tooth.

Careful watching and proper positioning are necessary to keep the patient from aspirating excessive pulmonary secretions and vomitus. The comatose patient, or one who is vomiting, is usually turned on her side and the foot of the bed elevated to favor drainage of secretions from the air passages. Suction may be necessary to remove mucus. The pulmonary secretions may be greatly increased. Fluids should never be given orally, for fear of aspiration.

The blood pressure, urinary output, temperature, pulse, and respirations are checked at least every hour and more frequently if clinical condition warrants. A decrease in the urinary output or a rise in any one of the other signs is considered unfavorable. An indwelling catheter is usually inserted so that the urinary output can be carefully watched. It should be at least 30 ml per hour. The fetal heart tones are checked at regular intervals. Labor frequently begins after eclampsia develops; if not, labor should be induced as soon as the patient's condition is stable. Examinations, however, are kept to a minimum.

Sedatives are administered, sometimes in fairly large doses. The respirations must be closely observed. Magnesium sulfate is used to lower blood pressure and control convulsions.

A 5 to 10 percent dextrose in Ringer's lactate solution may be used to provide fluids, electrolytes, and caloric intake and to overcome acidosis. From 2500 to 3000 ml total fluids are usually given in a 24-hour period. Output must be closely monitored to avoid circulatory overload.

As in the case of preeclampsia, induction of labor is by oxytocin infusion. Cesarean section usually will not be done except for obstetric indications or fetal distress.

Regardless of the severity of the antepartum toxemia, the woman remains at risk for convulsions for at least 24 hours post partum. For this reason vigilant care and medical treatment are continued until diuresis occurs and definite improvement in all symptoms is noted.

Prognosis

In general, the prognosis for preeclamptic patients is good when treatment is prompt. If improvement is not evident with bed rest and medical treatment, delivery of the baby is effective. Recovery is usually quite prompt after delivery, with disappearance of all signs of toxemia in 10 to 14 days (Fig. 14–12). In some patients hyperten-

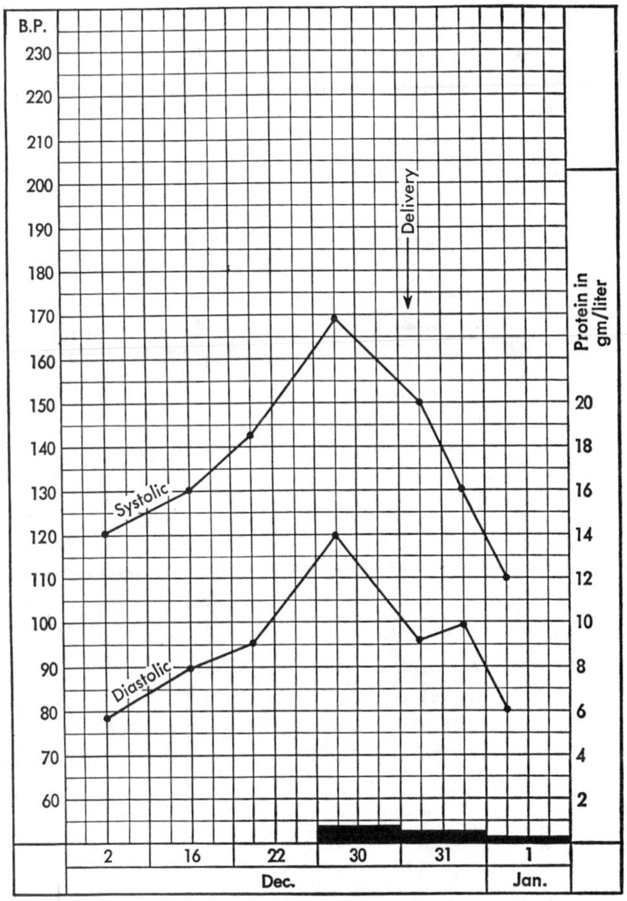

Figure 14–12. Fall in blood pressure and decrease in protein are rapid after delivery of a woman with severe preeclampsia.

sion persists, but it is thought that most such patients have underlying chronic hypertension. There may be a recurrence of toxemia, at least to a mild degree, in subsequent pregnancies.

The final outcome of eclampsia depends on many factors. The prognosis is more favorable after delivery, especially when the urinary output increases. When signs and symptoms increase, the outlook is unfavorable. The patient may die due to pulmonary edema, cardiac failure, or pneumonia due to aspiration of mucus, blood, and fluid, which may be drawn into the lungs by the deep, stertorous breathing. Exemplary nursing care can virtually prevent this latter complication.

When recovery begins, it is comparatively rapid. In 24 to 48 hours the urinary output may be as high as 4 to 6 liters per day. An increase in the urinary output is the first sign of improvement. Edema disappears in four to five days, and as the woman loses all this fluid, there is a marked difference in her appearance. The patient soon begins to feel well unless she has developed aspiration pneumonia or other infection. The weight decreases rapidly, the blood pressure drops to normal in about two weeks, the protein and casts disappear from the urine in about a week. All symptoms subside in two to four weeks.

In preeclampsia the primary risk to the fetus is intrauterine growth retardation, resulting from poor placental perfusion. In addition, premature delivery may be necessary because of the severity of maternal disease as well as the increasing risks to the fetus of remaining in an environment of malnutrition. Intrauterine death may occur as a result of placental insufficiency, eclamptic convulsions, or abruptio placentae. The neonatal risks are chiefly those of the small-for-gestational-age infant and/or the premature infant. Overall perinatal mortality in toxemia is estimated to be approximately 25 percent, with eclampsia accounting for most of this.

Prior to postpartum discharge from the hospital, the nurse should sit down with the woman (and her family if she desires) and review the course of events, answering any questions she might have. Implications for follow-up health care, contraception, and future pregnancies also should be discussed.

If the woman is not normotensive by four to six weeks post partum, chronic hypertension is suspected and further medical evaluation is indicated. The use of oral contraceptives is contraindicated in hypertensive women, so alternate forms of contraception should be considered until confirmation of normal blood pressure readings. If the woman is a primigravida, the chances are good that she will not have toxemia in future pregnancies. If, however, there is a predisposing factor, such as diabetes mellitus, which will still be present during subsequent gestations, she should take particular care to alert physicians to her risk at the time of any future antepartum care.

Chronic Hypertensive Disease

Hypertensive disease, also termed essential hypertension or hypertensive vascular disease, is not peculiar to pregnancy but is frequently first recognized in pregnancy. It presents some of the same symptoms as toxemia, and pregnancy may be an aggravating factor. The patient with essential hypertension often develops a superimposed preeclampsia or acute toxemia. Hypertensive disease in pregnancy is seen most frequently among pregnant women in the older age group, in multigravidas, and in obese women. It appears that the greater incidence of hypertension during pregnancy in women over 30 years of age is the result of preexisting or latent hypertension, which predisposes to development of blood pressure elevation during pregnancy. When the tendency to develop hypertension in later years exists in any woman, she is more likely to develop an increase in her blood pressure during pregnancy.

Signs and Symptoms

Evidence of this disease is variable. Frequently the only sign of chronic hypertensive disease in pregnancy is hypertension before the twenty-fourth week of gestation. In many of these women a persistently elevated blood pressure and possibly slight changes in the retinal blood vessels are the only evidences of the disease throughout pregnancy. Signs are typically present from the onset of pregnancy, unlike in patients with acute toxemia. These women usually feel well with the possible exception of having headaches. A small percentage of patients have a more advanced disease and show varying degrees of cardiac, renal, and/or retinal damage. Blood pressure readings may vary from slight elevation to levels of 300/160 mm Hg and are frequently normal during midtrimester. Marked narrowing and tortuosity of the retinal blood vessels and retinal exudates and hemorrhages may be present if the disease is severe, especially if the kidneys are involved. Proteinuria and edema are ordinarily not present, as in an acute toxemia, unless there is severe renal involvement.

About 25 percent of patients with chronic hypertensive disease in pregnancy develop a superimposed preeclampsia. This is apt to occur earlier than preeclampsia ordinarily appears and is likely to be a more severe form. This development may be manifested by a sudden exacerbation of previous signs, sudden weight gain, edema, protein in the urine, and retinal hemorrhages and exudates. Fetal growth retardation is frequently seen and is a major risk.

Diagnosis

It may be difficult to differentiate between hypertensive disease and preeclampsia unless it is definitely known that the woman had hypertension before her pregnancy. Examination of the eyegrounds may show hemorrhages and exudates which are not always present in preeclampsia. The response of the blood pressure, weight, urinary output, and protein output while the patient is under treatment of bed rest and dietary control may be of value in diagnosis.

Sometimes chronic hypertensive disease cannot be differentiated from preeclampsia until some time after delivery. The differential diagnosis can usually be made during the puerperium since in preeclampsia the blood pressure usually falls rapidly to normal, the weight decreases rapidly, and the casts and protein disappear from the urine in from two to four weeks. In chronic hypertension, although the blood pressure falls somewhat and protein, if present, decreases as the condition improves, by the end of the puerperium the blood pressure is still elevated, and casts and protein may be present in the urine (Fig. 14–13).

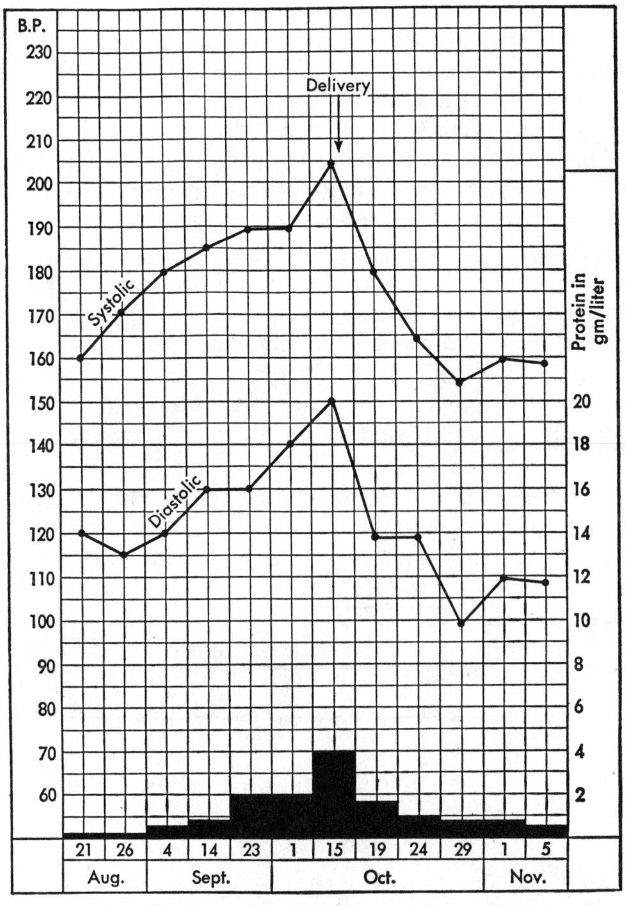

Figure 14–13. Persistence of high blood pressure and protein after delivery of a woman with severe chronic hypertensive renal disease, who additionally had a superimposed preeclampsia during the last month of gestation. Compare this with Figure 14-12 which shows rapid recovery from severe preeclampsia following delivery.

Treatment and Nursing Care

Observations of blood pressure, weight gain, and proteinuria are important. Hypertensive disease cannot be prevented through antepartum care, but evidence of disease can be recognized early and proper treatment instituted to minimize its effects and decrease the major risks of preeclampsia and intrauterine growth retardation.

Patients with mild hypertensive disease frequently need only careful evaluation of their cardiovascular status, close observation during pregnancy, and instructions to report untoward symptoms early. Considerable rest and limitation of activity are very important. A common recommendation is for the woman to rest four hours per day in addition to her nighttime sleep. The four hours need not be at a single time, but a rest period should not be less than one hour. If this regimen is not sufficient to keep her normotensive, more extensive bed rest, up to 24 hours a day, may be recommended. Rarely, antihypertensive drugs are required. In this event and/or if a superimposed toxemia develops, hospitalization and intensive care are required.

Careful assessment of fetal growth and evaluation of placental function are important.

Hospital treatment and nursing care are approximately the same as for preeclampsia: rest in bed, a high-protein diet, adequate fluids, and close observation of the patient's general condition.

To discover any change in condition, the weight is checked frequently, sometimes daily, the blood pressure is taken once or more daily, and an accurate record of the fluid intake and output is kept. The urine is examined for protein. Headache, dizziness, and/or visual disturbance should be noted and reported to the physician immediately.

Kidney-function tests and examinations of the cardiovascular system are often made. The results of such findings, the severity of symptoms, and the response of treatment determine subsequent care.

Prognosis

If hypertensive disease is mild and if preeclampsia is not superimposed, the pregnancy usually continues without hazard. Severe hypertension, cardiac or renal involvement, advanced retinal changes, and a superimposed preeclampsia may endanger the mother and may be associated with death of the fetus. Many physicians believe that pregnancy is contraindicated and may recommend that it be terminated in the small number of patients who have a severe form of the disease. If a superimposed acute toxemia develops, there is a high incidence of fetal death *in utero* and an increased incidence of abruptio placentae. When such a condition does not respond to intensive treatment, the physician may recommend early delivery of the baby. These patients are likely to have a recurrence of an acute toxemia in subsequent pregnancies.

HYDRAMNIOS

Hydramnios (sometimes referred to as polyhydramnios) is the presence of an excessive amount of amniotic fluid. The normal amount of fluid near term is between 500 and 1000 ml, or slightly more. An amount of over 2000 ml is considered excessive. Between 2000 and 3000 ml of amniotic fluid is relatively common; much larger amounts may develop but occur infrequently. Any amount over 3000 ml is considered clinically significant.

The cause of hydramnios is not clear. It is known to occur frequently in association with fetal malformations and in pregnancies complicated by diabetes and severe erythroblastosis. Amniotic fluid may be increased in amount in twin pregnancies and sometimes in the toxemias of pregnancy. The increase to an excessive amount of fluid is usually gradual, but in rare cases is occurs suddenly.

Diagnosis of hydramnios usually is made through clinical observation, since it is difficult to estimate or measure the amount with accuracy. The uterus enlarges more than expected for the period of gestation. Palpation of the fetal small parts, hearing of the fetal heart tones, and ballottement of the fetus may be difficult. Ultrasound examination permits a more quantitative estimate of the amount of amniotic fluid.

Symptoms caused by hydramnios result from the pressure of the enlarged uterus on adjacent organs and are related to the degree of distention. Pressure against the diaphragm may cause distress. Edema of the lower extremities occurs frequently. Generalized abdominal discomfort may develop. However, maternal discomfort may be only slight, since the increase in fluid is usually very gradual. Labor tends to begin prematurely. The uterine muscle may become atonic due to excessive stretching.

Occasionally, maternal symptoms of shortness of breath are severe as a result of hydramnios. Amniocentesis unfortunately affords only a very short period of relief and in women in the latter weeks of pregnancy may be associated with premature labor. This usually precludes amniocentesis as a useful procedure for relief of hydramnios unless labor and delivery are desired. However, some practitioners have had favorable results in chronic hydramnios with removing 500 to 700 ml of fluid every three to four days to allow the fetus to reach maturity.

FETAL DEATH

Fetal death late in pregnancy usually is recognized by the mother through the absence of fetal movements. It is a subjective, but a significant sign, and warrants further investigation. The mother may suspect that movement has ceased when the fetus actually is healthy but becomes less active as he nears term. On the other hand, even when fetal movements have ceased, the mother may believe she feels movement, and it is difficult for her to accept any other fact. Death of a fetus, or suspected death, causes the mother much concern over carrying the dead fetus and a great deal of worry over what she may or may not have done to cause its death. She needs a great deal of reassurance that she could not have avoided the death, and both parents will need much immediate emotional support and, later, guidance in future pregnancies.

Fetal life must be assumed until diagnosis proves that death has occurred. Sometimes this diagnosis is difficult and takes considerable time. Some diagnostic methods will obviously depend upon the period of gestation.

In the early months of pregnancy, failure of uterine growth over a period of several weeks is significant. Negative pregnancy tests point to fetal death, but sometimes a pregnancy test may remain positive for several weeks because the placenta may continue to produce chorionic gonadotropic hormone for a few weeks after fetal death.

Later in pregnancy, absence of fetal heart tones is strong evidence of fetal death but not infallible. Urinary estriol becomes very low (less than 2 mg per 24 hours) and is a very useful confirmatory test. X-ray shows overlapping of skull bones several days after death. Ultrasound findings include characteristic echoes from the head and thorax, as well as evidence of overlapping skull bones. Amniotic fluid may be analyzed for the presence of creatinine phosphokinase (CPK), which is markedly elevated in fetal death after 48 to 72 hours. The uterus fails to grow and may even become smaller.

In many women labor will begin spontaneously within a few weeks after fetal death, but induction of labor usually is carried out when the diagnosis is definitely confirmed. Prolonged retention of a dead fetus presents some danger of fibrinogenopenia in the mother, and it is psychologically disturbing to her.

A dead fetus usually shows maceration and peeling of the skin at birth, and the amniotic fluid is small in amount and meconium-stained or reddish in color.

REFERENCES AND SUGGESTED READINGS

Aure, B. Intrauterine transfusions: The nurse's role with expectant parents, *Nurs. Clin. North Am.,* 8:817–826, 1972.

Fost, N., Chudwin, D., and Wikler, D., The limited moral significance of "fetal viability", *Hastings Center Report,* 10:10–13, 1980.

Gant, Norman F. *et al.,* A clinical test useful for predicting the development of acute hypertension in pregnancy, *Am. J. Obstet. Gynecol.,* 120:1–7, (Sept 1) 1974.

Hypertension in pregnancy—Continuing education credit feature, *Am. J. Nurs.*, 82(5):791–822, 1982.

Penticuff, J. H., Psychologic implications in high-risk pregnancy, *Nurs. Clin. North Am.*, 17(1):69–78, 1982.

Pizer, H. and Palinski, C. O., *Coping with a Miscarriage,* Mosby, St. Louis, 1980.

Quilligan, E. J. and Kretchmer, N. (eds.), *Fetal and Maternal Medicine,* Wiley, New York, 1980.

Wein, S. G., The unspoken needs of families during high-risk pregnancies, *Am. J. Nurs.*, 81:2047–53, 1981.

Wetzel, S. K., Are we ignoring the needs of the woman with a spontaneous abortion? *MCN,* 7(4):258–59, 1982.

CHAPTER

15

Pregnancies at Risk: Preexisting Health Problems

BOTH THE PREGNANT woman and her fetus may be at risk because of the existence of a chronic organic disease in the mother or because of an acute illness occurring during gestation. These illnesses are likely to result in a suboptimum intrauterine environment, which places the fetus at a disadvantage for normal growth and development from the very beginning of life. At the same time the normal physiologic adjustments of pregnancy may severely stress maternal organs already impaired by a chronic illness.

Ideally, women who are at risk for complications should be identified prior to pregnancy. Counseling at this time will enable them to make more informed decisions about childbearing, as well as provide time to correct remedial conditions and stabilize others so that each woman begins pregnancy in her optimal state of health. Women (and their families) whose pregnancies are concurrent with a chronic disorder should expect that medical supervision will be more intense, office visits will be more frequent, more diagnostic studies will be done, antepartum hospitalization may be necessary, and the cost will be much greater both in dollars and in stress. On the other hand, they can also expect a generally favorable outcome for both mother and infant, provided they are given access to the quality of care that is possible today in perinatal intensive care settings.

INFECTIONS IN PREGNANCY

Since no special privileges of immunity are conferred with conception, pregnant women are susceptible to any infectious agents that can affect the general population. Sexually transmitted organisms as well as others may cause disease in the mother and adversely affect the health of the unborn child. A disturbing characteristic of many of these infections is that, while the maternal disease may be very mild, or perhaps even asymptomatic, severe developmental anomalies and even death may occur in the embryo/fetus. (See Table 15–1.)

Vaginal Infections

Although not unique to pregnancy, vaginal infections often are exacerbated during this time due to the altered vaginal environment. The two most common infections are *Trichomonas vaginalis* and candidiasis.

Table 15–1. Infections in Pregnancy

Infection	*Causative Organism*	*Mode of Transmission*	*Maternal Symptoms*	*Fetal/Neonatal Effects*
Toxoplasmosis	*Toxoplasma gondii*	Maternal: raw meat, cat feces Fetal: transplacental	Asymptomatic or headache, malaise, low-grade fever	IUGR,* microcephaly, hydrocephaly, chorioretinitis, hepatosplenomegaly; death frequent; if lives, MR* and developmental lag
Rubella	Rubella virus	Maternal: pharyngeal secretions Fetal: transplacental	Pharyngeal inflammation, lymphadenopathy, macular rash	Cataracts, hemolytic anemia, congenital heart defects, MR, deafness
Cytomegalic inclusion disease	Cytomegalovirus	Maternal: most body fluids, sexual intercourse Fetal: transplacental, contact with infected birth canal	Asymptomatic or, rarely, mild mononucleosis-like symptoms	IUGR, microcephaly, MR, deafness, congenital heart defects
Herpes genitalis	Herpesvirus hominis, type II	Maternal: sexual intercourse Fetal: contact with infected birth canal, less often transplacental	Painful vesicles in genital area	Mild: few skin lesions, recovery likely Severe; viremia, CNS involvement, high mortality rate
Streptococcus	Beta-hemolytic streptococcus, group B	Maternal: ascending genital tract organisms Fetal: ascending through ruptured membrane, contact with infected birth canal	Amnionitis, puerperal sepsis	Septicemia, meningitis, mortality high
Syphilis	*Treponema pallidum*	Maternal: sexual intercourse Fetal: transplacental	Vary with stage of infection; may be asymptomatic, chancre, rash, etc.	Midtrimester abortion, congenital syphilis (septicemia, skin lesions, anemia, jaundice, periostitis)
Gonorrhea	*Neisseria gonorrhoeae*	Maternal: sexual intercourse Fetal: contact with infected birth canal	Often asymptomatic, urethritis, cervicitis, pelvic inflammatory disease	Ophthalmia neonatorum
Chickenpox	Varicella virus	Maternal: airborne viruses Fetal: transplacental	Characteristic skin lesions, high fever	Congenital varicella, rare but mortality is high
Mumps	Mumps virus (myxovirus group)	Maternal: airborne viruses Fetal: transplacental	Parotitis, fever	Spontaneous abortion, premature birth, stillbirth; congenital anomalies

*IUGR, intrauterine growth retardation; MR, mental retardation.

Trichomonas vaginitis (Trichomoniasis)

This common vaginal infection is caused by the *Trichomonas vaginalis,* an actively motile, flagellate protozoan. It is sexually transmitted and may produce a profuse, irritating, foamy secretion, yellowish green in color, and of an unpleasant odor. This discharge is very irritating to the vagina and the external genitalia and causes intense itching. Diagnosis is made by the "hanging drop" method, that is, a microscopic examination of vaginal discharge suspended in a drop of normal saline. The protozoa can be seen swimming about in the suspension.

The specific cure for trichomoniasis is the drug metronidazole (FLAGYL). This may be prescribed as a single 2-gm dose, as two 1-gm doses to be taken in a single day, or as a seven-day course of 250 mg to be taken three times a day. The obvious convenience of the single dose makes it preferable in the nonpregnant woman. However, during pregnancy, the seven-day course should be prescribed because it results in lower fetal blood levels. The drug should be avoided during the first trimester, and some believe its use in the second and third trimester should be restricted to those women who do not respond to palliative treatment. During lactation the single-dose regimen is recommended with interruption of breast-feeding until 24 to 48 hours after treatment is completed. Breast milk should be expressed and discarded during this time and a formula given to the infant.

PATIENT EDUCATION The nurse should advise the woman of several factors that will enhance the treatment plan. First, because this is a sexually transmitted infection, the sexual partner should be treated simultaneously. The single-dose method is preferred. It is advisable to use a condom during intercourse until symptoms have resolved. All alcoholic beverages are to be avoided during and for 48 hours after taking this medication as the combination may cause an accumulation of acetaldehyde, resulting in severe gastrointestinal side effects. The importance of taking the full course of therapy at evenly spaced times should be emphasized. The medication may be taken with food to minimize gastrointestinal irritation.

Candidiasis

Yeast infection, caused by *Candida (Monilia) albicans,* also often flares up during pregnancy because the increased glycogen content of the vaginal epithelium is conducive to its growth. It produces a profuse white, watery, curdy discharge which is very irritating to the vagina and external genitalia.

Candidiasis is usually treated either with nystatin or with miconazole, both of which are antifungal medications usually administered as vaginal suppositories. Nystatin may be preferable during the first trimester as small amounts of miconazole are absorbed systemically.

PATIENT EDUCATION Although symptomatic relief is obtained in 48 to 72 hours, it is essential that the full course of therapy be carried out. The use of minipads protects clothing from vaginal drainage resulting from the suppositories and increases the woman's comfort. The nurse may review general hygiene measures and the use of cotton rather than nylon underpants to minimize reinfection risks. Because candidiasis is often associated with other conditions, the nurse should investigate the possibility of diabetes mellitus as well as the recent or current use of broad-spectrum antibiotics, steroids, or oral contraceptives. When labor ensues before the candidiasis has been cured, the nurse should be alert for the development of thrush in the newborn.

DOUCHING The presence or absence of symptoms will often determine whether treatment is given for vaginal discharge. Sometimes douches seem indicated for excessive vaginal secretion and are prescribed by the physician. Several important precautions are necessary when douching during pregnancy to prevent high fluid pressure and possible entry of air or fluid into the uterus. Hand bulb syringes should never be used. The douche bag should be held no higher than 2 ft above the level of the hips, and the douche nozzle should not be inserted more than 3 in. These are safe precautions in douching at any time, but should be particularly observed during pregnancy.

The TORCH Complex

The letters in TORCH stand for toxoplasmosis, other agents, rubella, cytomegalovirus, and herpes virus. The "other agents" most commonly refers to group B beta-hemolytic streptococcus as well as syphilis and gonorrhea.

Toxoplasmosis

Toxoplasmosis is caused by the protozoa, *Toxoplasma gondii.* It is transmitted through the ingestion of raw or undercooked meat as well as in the feces of cats. Women should be cautioned to cook meat thoroughly, particularly pork, which never should be eaten rare. House cats that do not kill and eat the raw meat of small rodents are probably not a threat. If the woman has concerns because of her cat, she may have someone else handle the kitty litter and pay particular attention to good hand washing and other hygienic practices.

Toxoplasmosis in the adult is frequently asymptomatic. If symptoms do occur, they are mild and nonspecific, consisting of malaise, headache, myalgia, low-grade fever, and occasionally a macular rash. The organism readily crosses the placenta causing congenital infection. The infected infants exhibit a variety of serious conditions, including intrauterine growth retardation, microcephaly, hydrocephaly, chorioretinitis, jaundice, and fever. They rarely live more than a few days. Less severe infections may not be diagnosed until later in infancy when the child may present with mental retardation, seizures, chorioretinitis, or developmental lag.

Because it is generally asymptomatic in the adult, detection during pregnancy usually is possible only through screening. A serologic test for the detection of antibodies may be done. At the present time such screening is not recommended as a routine for all pregnant women. Women at particular risk because of dietary habits or who have special concern arising from their pets may be screened.

Should an active toxoplasmosis occur during pregnancy, treatment may be considered. The drug of choice is pyrimethamine, a folic acid antagonist, which is not without its own risks for the developing fetus. For this reason there must be a definitve diagnosis of infection as well as a careful consideration of the risks of the teratogenic effects of the drug versus the risks of damage to the fetus from the infection.

Beta-hemolytic Streptococcus

Group B beta-hemolytic streptococcus is currently attracting notice as a factor in both neonatal and puerperal infections. It has been associated with urinary tract infections, septic abortions, stillbirth, and serious neonatal disease. It is estimated that it constitutes part of the normal flora of the genital tract in about 15 percent of the women of childbearing age. The fetus may become infected by organisms ascending through ruptured membranes or from passage through an infected birth canal.

This infection can be devastating in the neonate as it often runs a fulminate course ending in fatal streptococcal meningitis. Because of this, many practitioners routinely culture the cervix and vagina of women presenting with premature labor or ruptured membranes. Early identification of group B streptococcus may permit antibiotic therapy in the neonate before the infection is overwhelming.

Efforts to eliminate the organism in the mother by prenatal screening and antibiotic therapy have not proved practical. Success requires treating the woman's sexual partner as well as herself, and even then recolonization is frequent.

Rubella

Rubella, or German measles, is a mild virus infection in children and adults that can produce a severe malformation syndrome in the fetus.

The virus is spread person to person in pharyngeal secretions. Symptoms include pharyngeal inflammation, lymphadenopathy, and a macular rash, which typically begins on the face and spreads to the trunk. It is not uncommon for the disease to be subclinical and go unnoticed by those affected.

Transplacental transmission results in infection of the fetus. The severity of its effect depends on the developmental stage of the fetus at the time of infection. The first trimester with its rapid organogenesis is the most sensitive period, and infection during this time may result in congenital anomalies in the form of cataracts, hemolytic anemia, congenital heart defects, mental retardation, and deafness. Approximately one fourth of fetuses exposed during the first trimester will be born with this multiple malformation syndrome. Even when the infant does not appear affected, he or she can shed live viruses for many months after birth. Precautions should be observed in the newborn nursery to protect employees who may be pregnant or at risk to become pregnant.

The percentage of women of childbearing age who have no serologic evidence of previous rubella infection has been reduced from 25 to 10 percent with the introduction of the vaccine. Since the vaccine consists of attenuated live viruses, it should never be given to pregnant women, as the attenuated viruses cross the placenta in the same way as the wild variety and at least theoretically, can produce the same results. Before children are immunized, their mothers should be ascertained either to be already immune themselves or at no risk to become pregnant during the ensuing two months. Pregnant women who have no serologic evidence of past infection should receive the vaccine early in the postpartum period when adequate protection against pregnancy in the next two months has been assured.

Cytomegalovirus

Cytomegalovirus (CMV) is a member of the herpesvirus group of which five are known to infect humans. Besides CMV these include the varicella/zoster virus (responsible for chickenpox/shingles), the Epstein-Barr virus, herpes simplex virus type I (cold sores), and herpes simplex virus type II.

Cytomegaloviruses are ubiquitous agents, and it has been estimated that nearly 100 percent of the population are affected in some parts of the world. The incidence tends to be lower in more favored economic environments where sanitation standards are higher. The infection is rarely symptomatic, although a mononucleosis-like syndrome has been described in young adults. Viruses are shed for as long as several years in saliva and urine. It has also been cultured from semen and from cervical smears, indicating that there may be a venereal transmission.

The significance of this virus in pregnancy lies in its ability to cause fetal infection. Although studies are difficult to do because of the typical absence of any symptoms of maternal infection, it is felt that the most critical time is during the second month of gestation. Infants are affected in much the same way as in rubella infection. They are small for gestational age, microcephalic, and mentally and developmentally retarded. Deafness and congenital heart defects also have been observed. When maternal infection occurs in the last trimester, infants have been known to become infected during passage through the birth canal. These infants shed viruses but do not exhibit clinical symptoms.

At present there is no way known to prevent infection or to treat the congenital disease. Tragically, most diagnoses are made retrospectively after the birth of an infant with multiple malformations.

Herpes Simplex

Herpes simplex virus, type II, is one of the antigenic types of herpesvirus hominis. It was previously thought to cause disease below the diaphragm (herpes genitalis), in contrast with type I which produces disease above the diaphragm, most notably the "cold sore," herpes labialis. However, it is now known that both types can be found anywhere on the body, and both are capable of producing severe disease in the newborn.

Herpes is a sexually transmitted infection, characterized by exquisitely painful vesicles surrounded by an erythematous area which progress to shallow ulcers, pustules, and crusts, with healing occurring spontaneously in about 10 days to 3 weeks. These occur on the cervix, vaginal wall, and vulva and may extend to the buttocks and thighs. The initial infection may be accompanied by symptoms of systemic illness, presumably caused by a transient viremia.

The virus may then enter a latent phase and be harbored by the individual indefinitely, giving rise to recurrent infections when the virus is activated. Numerous modes of therapy have been attempted, but all have been unrewarding. Symptomatic treatment in the form of sitz baths, wet compresses, lotions, and analgesics can provide some relief from the discomfort.

The maternal infection may be transmitted to the fetus and neonate. The usual mode of transmission is through contact with cervical and vaginal vesicles on the way through the birth canal, although a few cases of transplacental transmission have been documented. The neonates at greatest risk are those whose mothers had an onset of a primary herpes infection shortly before delivery. If the virus is present at birth, it is estimated that 40 per cent of vaginally delivered neonates will be infected. More than one-half of the infected infants die, and one-half of the survivors have permanent neurologic or visual damage. For this reason, a cesarean section is generally recommended for the woman with active herpes lesions. Should premature rupture of the membrane occur, cesarean section should be performed prior to four hours' elapsed time since rupture, or as soon as possible, in order to prevent ascending infection.

Syphilis

Syphilis in a pregnant woman is a serious condition meriting prompt and efficient treatment. Once the leading cause of fetal and neonatal mortality and morbidity, it is now an entirely preventable disease. Yet the incidence of congenital syphilis is increasing as a reflection of increased incidence of parental syphilis, as well as a tragic commentary on the inadequacy of antepartum care.

The first, and absolutely indispensable, step toward efficient treatment of syphilis in pregnancy is a diagnostic test. In all but eight states prenatal serologic test is required by law. Even without the force of law, omission of such an examination from antepartum care would be indefensible.

The serologic screening test should be done early in gestation in order to permit treatment of the mother prior to the sixteenth week of gestation. The *Treponema pallidum* spirochetes cannot penetrate the early placenta but may begin to do so any time after the fourth month.

Positive serologic tests identified after the sixteenth week should nevertheless prompt treatment for the mother's health, as well as for the transplacental treatment of the fetus. All cases of syphilis should be reported to public health officials in order that all contacts can be identified and treated.

Penicillin is used as treatment in all stages of syphilis. It is a safe, effective treatment that quickly eliminates the infectiousness of the disease, prevents later complications, and effectively prevents congenital syphilis. It is easier to administer than the drugs formerly used, rarely has serious toxic effects, and does not require a long period of treatment. Adequate penicillin levels usually are maintained for about two weeks. Even though the mother does not have a negative serology by the time she delivers, a nonsyphilitic baby can be expected if she has shown a favorable response to treatment by monthly quantitative blood tests. Several months may elapse following treatment before a negative maternal blood test is obtained. A rapid drop in titer is expected after treatment of early syphilis. Even a small drop is considered a favorable response in late or latent syphilis, in which the decline may be quite delayed and very gradual. Retreatment is indicated in cases not showing the normally expected response.

Gonorrhea

Gonorrhea, once considered conquered by penicillin, is reaching epidemic proportions in the United States. In 1982 there were nearly one million reported cases in this country.[1] The enormous increase in the incidence of this disease is felt to be due to the high percentage of infected individuals who are asymptomatic (70 to 82 percent) and to increasing antibiotic resistance. There has been a 30-fold increase in the amount of medication needed for cure between 1950 and 1977. In February, 1976, a penicillin-resistant, beta-lactamase-producing gonococcus was isolated.[2]

Diagnosis of gonorrhea is made by culturing the *Neisseria gonorrhoeae* from the endocervical canal. Routine screening cultures are currently recommended at the first antepartum visit, with repeat cultures at 36 weeks' gestation for those women at high risk for reinfection.

Although the majority of cases are asymptomatic, the vaginal discharge from an infection may become profuse and purulent. It may cause great discomfort from irrita-

[1] U.S. Dept. Health, Education and Welfare, Public Health Service, Center for Disease Control, *Morbidity and Mortality Weekly Report* 32 (1), 1983.

[2] Michael R. Spence, Genital infections in pregnancy, *Med. Clin. North Am.*, 61:139–51, (Jan.) 1977.

tion and itching of the vulva, or even excoriation of the mucous membrane, and sometimes abscesses of the vulvovaginal glands. The chief danger to the mother in an untreated gonorrheal infection is that, after delivery, the organisms may travel from the lower genital tract to the uterine cavity and the fallopian tubes. There they cause inflammation, or possibly a general postpartum infection. Sterility may be one of the results of an untreated gonorrheal infection.

The greatest danger to the infant is infection of the eyes during passage through the birth canal. This is the reason for the special care given to the eyes of the neonate immediately after birth (see Chapter 21).

The treatment of choice is intramuscular aqueous procaine penicillin G, 4.8 million units. Probenecid, 1 gm, is frequently administered concomitantly to maintain high serum levels by blocking renal tubular secretion of the penicillin.

Tuberculosis

Although the pregnant woman with tuberculosis must receive special care, routine roentgenograms as a part of antepartum care, to detect early lesions, currently are not often advised. If infection is found, both the infection and the pregnancy need ideal management. It appears that pregnancy does not exert an adverse effect on tuberculosis, but the progress of the disease must be halted. To promote resolution and healing, the mother receives the care she would ordinarily have for a tuberculous infection without a superimposed pregnancy. This treatment remains essentially unchanged during pregnancy. Long-term planning is essential for adequate rest and supervision. Suitable arrangements must be made for the care of the infant since the mother will be unable to care for her child until her disease is arrested.

To reduce the physical strain of labor, a low forceps delivery usually is considered advisable for shortening the second stage. Excessive sedation and inhalation anesthesia are avoided, insofar as possible, to prevent suppression of the cough reflex. During delivery and the postpartum period, good drainage of secretions is maintained to prevent accumulation in the bronchi. The mother is not allowed to nurse her infant because of the danger to the infant from exposure to the disease and also the added strain this would place on her.

With adequate long-continued care, the tuberculous patient usually may be carried safely through pregnancy without ill effects.

Tuberculosis is rarely transmitted to the fetus, and there seems to be no predisposition to the disease. The infant may be infected easily by his mother after birth from droplet contact. Accordingly, he/she is not allowed to nurse, and the mother should not care for the child in any way. BCG vaccination of the infant may be considered, but this does not decrease the need for preventive measures against infection of the infant.

If a woman becomes pregnant after a tuberculosis infection has responded well to treatment, but while the lesion is still somewhat unstable, she is given all possible safeguards during pregnancy, labor, and the puerperium. Hospitalization during a part of the pregnancy and for a longer than usual period during the puerperium is advisable.

Pregnancy is usually safe without danger of recurrence of tuberculosis when a period of two years has elapsed after the lesions have been well controlled. Safety increases with time since this allows for more effective healing.

Urinary Tract Infections

During pregnancy alterations occur in the collecting systems of the urinary tract that favor the development of infection. These alterations, evident as early as the tenth gestational week, consist primarily of a dilation and hypokinesis of the kidney pelves and ureters. The result of these anatomic changes is a relatively static column of urine in the upper collecting system which facilitates the ascending migration of organisms to the kidney itself. Therefore, bacteriuria is more likely to result in pyelonephritis in the pregnant woman than in the nonpregnant woman. In fact, pregnant women with untreated bacteriuria have a 30 percent incidence of acute pyelonephritis.[3]

Whether or not pregnant women have an increased susceptibility to bacteriuria per se has not been established conclusively. The pathogenesis of bacteriuria and bladder infections is the same regardless of the gravid state. That is, organisms migrate from the rectum to the urethra and thus to the bladder. This migration may be facilitated by careless perineal wiping and sexual intercourse. Whether the vaginal environment or other factors are more favorable to this migration of organisms during pregnancy is not known. It is known from epidemiologic studies that 3 to 7 percent of pregnant women have bacteriuria and that this is frequently asymptomatic. If untreated, about one third of these women will develop acute pyelonephritis because of the static column of urine which provides a pathway from the infected bladder to the kidney.

Urinary tract infections, principally pyelonephritis, are associated with an increased incidence of premature labor and thus pose a potential hazard to the fetus. It does not appear that the mother is at increased risk for chronic renal disease because of acute pyelonephritis in

[3] H. G. Dixon and H. A. Brant, The significance of bacteriuria in pregnancy, *Lancet*, i:19–20, (Jan.) 1967.

pregnancy, unless there are abnormalities leading to repeated infections that antedate the pregnancy.

Because bacteriuria is apt to progress to an acute pyelonephritis and because it is so frequently asymptomatic, routine screening for this disorder should be an integral part of antepartum care. There are a number of inexpensive, commercially available, screening cultures that can be done easily by the nurse or physician in the office/clinic setting. Positive findings on such a screening test should be followed by a conventional urine culture in the clinical laboratory. The woman should be carefully instructed and assisted, if necessary, in the collection of a midstream specimen following careful cleansing of the vulva with a nonbacteriostatic soap. If the urine cannot be plated for culture immediately, it should be refrigerated to prevent bacterial multiplication prior to plating. Findings of 100,000 bacteria per ml of urine indicate infection and require treatment for the eradication of the bacteriuria.

Treatment

Antibiotics of choice for bacteriuria are those that achieve high urinary, as opposed to high serum, concentrations. Sulfisoxazole (GANTRISIN, AZO GANTRISIN) and nitrofurantoin (FURADANTIN) are commonly used drugs. In addition, the woman should be instructed in ways to enhance the natural body defenses against infection. She can do this best by increasing her fluid intake and spending several periods each day in the left lateral position to increase blood flow to the kidneys.

Women who have had positive urine cultures should be recultured upon completion of the course of drug therapy. Cultures should be repeated each month for the remainder of gestation and again at six weeks post partum, since recurrence is common. Successful treatment of bacteriuria can decrease the incidence of acute pyelonephritis from 30 percent to less than 5 percent. Failure to eradicate the bacteriuria or persistent recurrence is indication for a complete urologic evaluation after the anatomic changes of pregnancy have been reversed (six weeks post partum).

Should pyelonephritis occur, the woman will typically complain of sudden paroxysms of pain in the region of the kidney in addition to the usual symptoms of a bladder infection (frequent micturition, urgency, burning on urination). The kidneys may be swollen and very tender to palpation and the woman may have a fever and sometimes chills. A catheterized urine specimen will contain bacteria and pus and possibly protein.

Bed rest and increased fluid intake are begun. A urine culture is done to identify the causative agent in order that an organism-specific antibiotic may be prescribed. After the specimen is obtained for culture, a broad-spectrum antibiotic is begun, pending results of the culture which takes 24 hours to grow. Prompt treatment is essential to prevent fibrosis of tissue which may result from the inflammation.

CHRONIC RENAL FAILURE

Women with chronic renal failure for whatever reason typically have impaired fertility. However, should conception occur, a successful pregnancy is possible.

The gravest threat to both mother and fetus is uncontrolled hypertension. This accelerates the progress of renal insufficiency and causes intrauterine malnutrition and its attendant risks.

Proteinuria is markedly increased during pregnancy in these women. However, this is most likely a result of increased glomerular filtration rate and not an indication of progression of the underlying disease.[4]

Very careful management throughout gestation by a multidisciplinary team which includes a nephrologist will be essential. In addition to the immediate stresses of the pregnancy, the family will likely need some support and counseling related to childrearing because of the nature of the mother's chronic disease and her life-span expectations.

THYROID DISEASE

Modifications in thyroid structure and function in pregnancy are discussed on page 141. To summarize, there are an elevated T_4 and T_3 because of an increase in thyroxine-binding capacity. However, the free T_4 and T_3 remain unchanged from the nonpregnant state, resulting in normal peripheral thyroid activity (Fig. 15-1). Hyperplasia of the gland is a common physiologic finding during pregnancy.

Hypothyroidism

It is a popular, though undocumented, notion that hypothyroid women have reduced fertility. Whether or not their ability to conceive is affected, they are much less likely to carry the pregnancy successfully to term. There is an increased incidence of all forms of fetal wastage as well as premature labor and the birth of infants who are severely handicapped both physically and mentally.

Thyroid hormone crosses the placenta with some difficulty and probably not in its intact form but as either an inorganic iodide or some as yet undefined organic iodide. It is evident from the above discussion, however, that passage is essential for normal fetal growth and development, especially prior to the time when the fetus

[4] B. S. Strauch and J. P. Hayslett, Kidney disease and pregnancy, *Br. Med. J.*, 4:578–82, (Apr.) 1974.

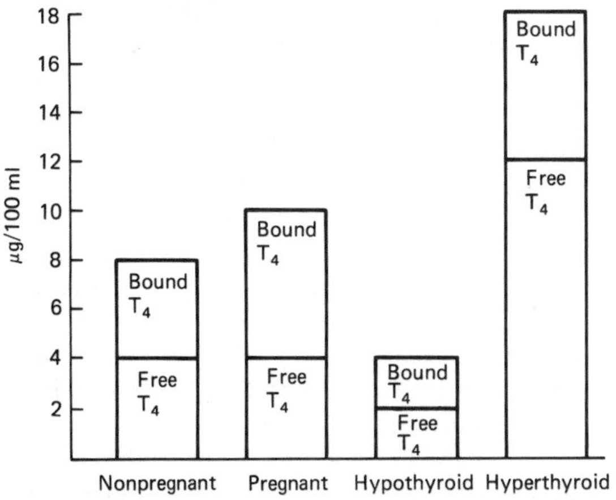

Figure 15-1. Comparison of thyroid hormone levels in nonpregnant and pregnant women with the levels typical of hypo- and hyperthyroidism. Note that the amount of free, and thus active, thyroxine remains unchanged in pregnancy, although the total amount increases due to the action of estrogen which enhances protein-binding capacity.

is capable of synthesizing his own thyroxine (approximately 12 weeks' gestation). Maternal hypothyroidism therefore requires full thyroid replacement in the form of exogenous hormone.

Hypothyroidism is only rarely diagnosed during pregnancy. A fairly common situation arises, however, when a young woman who is already taking thyroid extract seeks antepartum care. Not infrequently, the thryoid extract was prescribed without adequate documentation of hypothroidism because of adolescent complaints of obesity, fatigue, and/or menstrual disorders. Even though the majority of these women will probably be euthyroid, it is wise to continue the therapy until delivery, since normal thyroid function will be depressed for several weeks following the discontinuation of exogenous therapy. Even transient periods of hypothyroidism may threaten the outcome of the pregnancy.

Hyperthyroidism

The incidence of thyrotoxicosis in pregnancy is approximately 0.2 percent or 1 in every 500 pregnancies.[5] Diagnosis during pregnancy is difficult because many of the symptoms of normal pregnancy are similar to those of hyperthyroidism.

The appropriate treatment during pregnancy is medical rather than surgical and consists of the administration of antithyroid drug in dosages sufficient to maintain the patient as very slightly hyperthyroid. Since both propylthiouracil (PTU) and methimazole (TAPAZOLE) readily cross the placenta, fetal thyroid is protected by keeping the mother in the slightly hyperthyroid range. This goal is achieved by monitoring the T_4 and the free thyroxine index (FTI) at frequent intervals (every 2 to 3 weeks) and adjusting the drug dosage to maintain the T_4 at 1.4 times the upper limit of normal for the laboratory, and the FTI at or near the upper limits of normal.

The woman should be advised about the importance of taking the prescribed drug regularly in order to maintain relatively stable blood levels. She and her family usually will benefit from a discussion of the personality changes (emotional lability and irritability) that result from the disease process. Understanding that these are a result of the hyperthyroidism and will improve with therapy may lessen the impact. At the same time these are also typical emotional responses to pregnancy, so it is also important to provide the usual counseling about maternal emotions and development.

Infants born to mothers who have received antithyroid therapy should be monitored closely during the newborn period for evidence of hypothyroidism. Neonatal hypothyroidism due to *in utero* exposure to PTU or methimazole is transient, responds favorably to treatment, and has rarely been associated with long-term effects on growth and development.

CARDIOVASCULAR DISEASE

Rheumatic heart disease and congenital heart defects are the most common cardiac complications of pregnancy, since these are the heart conditions most likely to affect women of childbearing age. Of these, mitral stenosis is by far the most common lesion. Although the particular pathology may dictate some specific therapy, some general principles of management pertain to all pregnant women with heart disease.

Activity and Rest

Pregnancy places significant demands on the cardiovascular system of healthy women (Chapter 8, pages 143–50). As normal gestation advances, there is a progressive decline in cardiac reserve and an increasing tendency toward tachycardia with even mild exertion. This is particularly evident during the third trimester. In a study of women with asymptomatic or only mildly symptomatic heart disease, it was found that cardiac output failed to increase during pregnancy to the expected normal levels. The increased incidence of prematurity and low-birth-weight babies in women with

[5] K. R. Niswander, R. Gordon, and H. W. Berendes, *The Women and Their Pregnancies,* W. B. Saunders, Philadelphia, 1972.

Table 15-2. Physiologic Alterations in Pregnancy That Stress Cardiovascular Function

1. 20–25% increase in O_2 requirements
2. 25% increase in cardiac output
3. 50% increase in plasma volume
4. Weight gain due to
   a. Increased maternal and fetal body bulk
   b. Salt and water retention
5. Sudden hemodynamic changes at delivery
   a. Splanchnic vessel engorgement
   b. Sudden decrease in intraabdominal pressure

heart disease is further evidence that the heart cannot always meet the demands of the growing fetus.[6]

The physiologic alterations that may place increased stress on cardiovascular functioning during pregnancy are summarized in Table 15-2.

For these reasons, limitations of activity with frequent rest periods seem a wise precaution for the pregnant woman with heart disease. The extent of these limitations will depend primarily on the severity of the cardiac disease. The American Heart Association classifies persons with heart disease into four functional categories, depending on their symptoms in response to activity. Those who are asymptomatic with exertion are termed class I; those who are symptomatic with strenuous activity are class II. Class III contains those who are symptomatic with ordinary activities of daily living, and class IV is reserved for those who are symptomatic with even very mild activity. Clearly the woman who fits into class I will require fewer restrictions during pregnancy than those in more severe classes.

As early as possible in gestation, the family should sit down with the nurse and attempt to work out a systematic plan for the woman to rest and reduce her work load. Such planning cannot be limited to establishing a schedule of nap times. Discussions of task reassignment may evoke strong feelings of what is "proper" for various family members to do. The woman may feel so guilty about the unfinished tasks that, even though she is lying down for the prescribed time, she does not rest. Providing for the care and safety of small children in the home may necessitate obtaining help from neighbors, extended family members, day care centers, or others.

For some women prolonged hospitalization may be necessary, although the benefits of such a step should be weighed carefully against the stresses of a disrupted family and the discomforts of being in a hospital. Frequently, a well-planned rest and activity schedule at home is more beneficial, particularly if household help and public health nursing are available.

When the woman is not lying down, she should wear pressure-graded elastic stockings to prevent pooling of blood in the lower extremities and promote venous return to the heart. These stockings should always be applied before arising from a period of rest in the lateral position.

Fear and worry are additional sources of stress on the heart. Although no one is likely to go through a nine-month period totally free from anxiety—especially not the nine months of a high-risk pregnancy—expert nursing care can reduce this stress. Factual information about the interrelationships of pregnancy and heart disease should be available to the family in a form they can understand. All planning should be done with the woman and her family as active participants. The nurse should strive to enhance the family's ability to support each other, as well as providing support herself.

Nutrition and Fluids

The importance of nutrition during pregnancy has been emphasized repeatedly. For the woman with heart disease this is especially important, since she and her fetus are already faced with factors that predispose to intrauterine malnutrition.

Because of her restricted activity, there may be a need for fewer calories for the cardiac patient. Avoiding excessive weight gain is quite important because of the increased cardiovascular hazards resulting from obesity. A diet containing 80 to 100 gm of protein and enough calories to sustain an even progressive weight gain of 15 to 20 lb is usually recommended. Consultation with a nutritionist is important. If weight gain is low, urine may be checked for ketonuria.

Fluid and sodium restriction are contraindicated during pregnancy. Diuretics are unnecessary unless cardiac disease is severe and the risk of decompensation and pulmonary edema is high. Diuretics other than thiazides are usually selected, and careful attention must be paid to electrolyte balance.

Intrapartum Care

Generally, a vaginal delivery at term provides the safest intrapartum experience for the woman with heart disease.

Every effort is made to reduce strain and facilitate circulatory activity—a useful goal for any laboring woman. The left lateral position is preferable, and constant nursing attendance should be available to provide support. Continuous fetal heart rate monitoring is indicated, and the mother's ECG may be monitored as well.

Pain relief is important because of the added cardiac work produced by pain. Analgesics should be used judiciously, keeping in mind the fetal effects of the drug. Conduction anesthesia in the form of epidural or caudal is frequently recommended. Care should be taken that

[6] Kent Ueland, M. J. Novy, and J. Metcalfe, Hemodynamic responses of patients with heart disease to pregnancy and exercise, *Am. J. Obstet. Gynecol.*, 113:47–59, (May) 1972.

the woman is well hydrated to minimize the danger of cardiovascular side effects from the anesthesia.

Delivery is usually by low forceps extraction to avoid the strain of maternal bearing-down efforts.

Postpartum Care

Dramatic hemodynamic changes occur in the mother at the time of delivery and separation of the placenta. For this reason, the immediate postpartum period probably constitutes the period of greatest risk for the cardiac patient. Careful and frequent monitoring of maternal vital signs in a recovery room setting is crucial during this time. Immediate cardiac consultation should be available should symptoms of congestive heart failure or other complications arise.

Early ambulation should be encouraged to prevent venous thrombosis. As in the antepartum period, elastic stockings should be worn to prevent pooling in the large dilated veins of the lower extremities.

Both parents should have immediate and continued access to their newborn. The nurse, however, should be sensitive to signs of fatigue in the mother and help her set limits for herself to conserve energy. Decisions about infant feeding should be considered very seriously in the light of the mother's capacity for activity. Breast-feeding may place too great a strain on her heart. In addition to the physiologic demands of lactation, the mother would be less able to delegate infant care to the father and others if she were breast-feeding.

Discharge planning should include a consideration of the mother's ability to undertake the care of her infant and resume her daily activities and will necessarily involve the family.

DIABETES MELLITUS

Before the availability of commercially prepared insulin in 1921, diabetes and pregnancy rarely occurred together. Few juvenile diabetics lived to reproductive age, and those who did were frequently sterile. In the rare instances where pregnancy did occur, the maternal and perinatal mortality was enormous. Currently, after more than 60 years' experience with insulin, maternal mortality has been virtually eliminated, but perinatal mortality remains as high as 10 to 20 percent. This is well above the 2 to 3 percent perinatal mortality for the general population.

Team Approach to Care

Diabetes is a highly complex disease that affects multiple body systems. There remains much about it that is poorly understood. The physiologic and psychologic interactions with pregnancy are many and, perhaps, even less well understood. Perhaps more than any other high-risk pregnancy, this situation calls for the expertise of many highly specialized disciplines working as a team with the client. No single professional has the skill and knowledge to meet all the needs of these families experiencing a diabetic pregnancy. For these reasons, it is strongly recommended that care for pregnant diabetic patients be concentrated in regional perinatal centers where the necessary human as well as technical resources for expert individualized care can be made available.

By combining the expertise of nurses, physician specialists, nutritionists, and social workers, a number of perinatal centers have achieved perinatal mortality rates approaching those of the "normal" population. Such an approach requires close cooperation and communication among all members of the health team and, perhaps most important, an active involvement of the pregnant women and their families in all aspects of care.

Effects of Diabetes on Pregnancy

The potential impact of diabetes on pregnancy is very impressive. This impact, however, can be significantly lowered by maintaining good maternal diabetic control throughout the antepartum and intrapartum periods. The frequency and severity of complications are also influenced by the duration and severity of the diabetes.

Dr. Priscilla White has classified diabetes in pregnancy according to the age at onset and duration of the disease as well as the extent of diabetic complications.[7] (Table 15-3).

It is possible for a woman to be classified in one category and, at a later time, require reclassification because of progression of her diabetes and/or elapsed time. Generally speaking, the further down the alphabet the woman is classified the greater the risk to her fetus.

The incidence of toxemia is markedly increased in diabetics. Whereas approximately 7 percent of all pregnancies are complicated by toxemia, 25 to 50 percent of diabetic pregnancies are affected, depending on the diet, quality of antepartum care, diabetic control, and diabetic complications. Polyhydramnios affects as many as 25 percent of diabetic pregnancies, and vaginal and urinary tract infections are very common.

All forms of fetal wastage are increased in the diabetic woman, particularly third-trimester intrauterine death. The fetus is extremely vulnerable to maternal ketoacidosis as well as to the placental insufficiency which may accompany more severe diabetes.

Infants of diabetic mothers are classically thought of as large for gestational age. Maternal hyperglycemia results in fetal hyperglycemia. This, in turn, causes increased fetal islet cell stimulation and subsequent high

[7] Priscilla White, Pregnancy and diabetes, Medical aspects, *Med. Clin. North Am.*, 49:1015-24, (July) 1965.

Table 15-3. Classification of Diabetes in Pregnancy

Class A —	Pregnant women whose blood sugar is abnormally elevated only during pregnancy. Dietary regulation is adequate for control and no insulin is required. Fetal survival is high.
Class B —	Pregnant women whose diabetes is of less than 10 years duration, whose disease began at age 20 or older, and who have no vascular involvement.
Class C —	Pregnant women whose diabetes began between age 10 and age 19, whose disease has lasted 10–19 years.
Class D —	Pregnant women whose diabetes has lasted 20 years or more, whose disease began before age 10, and who may have vascular involvement and benign retinopathy.
Class E —	Pregnant women in whom calcification of the pelvic arteries has been demonstrated on x-ray. (This classification is not employed in current practice.)
Class F —	Pregnant women whose diabetes has caused nephropathy (proteinuria, azotemia).
Class R —	Pregnant women whose diabetes has caused proliferative retinitis (changes in the retina of the eye causing progressive loss of sight).

Source: Based on information from Priscilla White, Pregnancy and diabetes, medical aspects, *Med. Clin. North Am.* 49:1019 (July) 1965.

insulin levels. This fetal insulin, needed to metabolize the large glucose loads that cross the placenta from maternal circulation, acts as a growth factor, causing increased deposition of glycogen, fat, and probably protein. Thus, these infants are both longer and heavier than the norm for their gestational age. However, macrosomia is not invariably present in infants of diabetic mothers. Women in White's classifications D through R are more likely to deliver infants who are small for gestational age because of insufficient placental perfusion.

Congenital malformations occur in 5 to 10 percent of diabetic pregnancies. While the precise reason for this risk is not clear, it is supposed to be a result of some intrauterine environmental factor (e.g., hypo- or hyperglycemia) rather than of a genetic, inherited factor. Evidence for this is found in studies that reveal no increased risk for anomalies when the father, rather than the mother, is a diabetic. The most common malformations are congenital heart defects, neurologic defects, small left colon syndrome, and caudal regression syndrome. The latter syndrome, unique to infants of diabetic mothers, is characterized by imperfect development from the waist down and may be associated with cleft lip and palate, congenital heart defects, and upper limb abnormalities.

Complications that may be anticipated in the neonatal period include respiratory distress syndrome, hypoglycemia, hyperbilirubinemia, and hypocalcemia.

Inheritance of Diabetes

Parents often ask about the likelihood of their child having diabetes. The mode of inheritance of diabetes is a matter of some controversy among geneticists. A likely hypothesis is that it is a multifactorial condition. That is, a number of genes are responsible for the trait (polygenic rather than monogenic), and environmental or nongenetic factors contribute to its expression. It is generally believed to be inherited as an autosomal recessive with reduced penetrance, but whether the disease itself, a predisposition to the disease, or still another characteristic is inherited has not been clarified. Congenital diabetes is virtually unknown. The stronger the family history, however, the greater the likelihood of the child manifesting the disease at some time in his life. The older he/she gets, the greater the risks. For example, if only the child's mother is diabetic, the child's chances of having diabetes by age 25 is 8 percent, but the chances of being diabetic by age 85 increase to 25 percent.[8] Absolute risk values or percentages contain much guesswork. In general, however, infants of diabetic mothers are about 22 times as likely to become diabetic at some time in their lives than are individuals in the general population.[9] It is important to note that good health practices, especially good nutrition and maintenance of optimal body weight, can reduce the risk significantly.

Effects of Pregnancy on Diabetes

A thorough knowledge of the normal alterations in carbohydrate metabolism during pregnancy is essential to the understanding of the effects of gestation on diabetes and, in fact, to the understanding of medical management. The reader is referred to Chapter 8, pages 162–66, for a review of these changes (Fig. 15-2).

During the first half of pregnancy the major factor having an impact on carbohydrate metabolism is the fetal need for glucose and amino acids. It is believed that the fetus, like the brain, can utilize only glucose for energy needs. Glucose is transported rapidly across the placenta by facilitated diffusion, effectively lowering maternal blood glucose. The active transport of amino acids to the fetus also reduces the amount of "raw materials" available to the maternal liver for gluconeogenesis. The net result of all this is a tendency toward hypoglycemia. If, in addition, the woman is bothered by decreased appetite or nausea and vomiting of pregnancy, the blood glucose levels may fall dangerously low. As blood glucose levels fall, fat is broken down into fatty acids to serve as an auxiliary fuel source. These fatty acids cross the placenta to the fetus, where they are potentially hazardous to neurologic development.

In view of the above discussion, it is apparent that the

[8] J. M. Darlow, Charles Smith, and L. J. P. Duncan, A statistical and genetical study of diabetes. III. Empiric risks to relatives, *Ann. Hum. Genet.*, 37:157–73, (July) 1973.

[9] David Rimoin, Inheritance in diabetes mellitus, *Med. Clin. North Am.*, 55:807–18, (July) 1971.

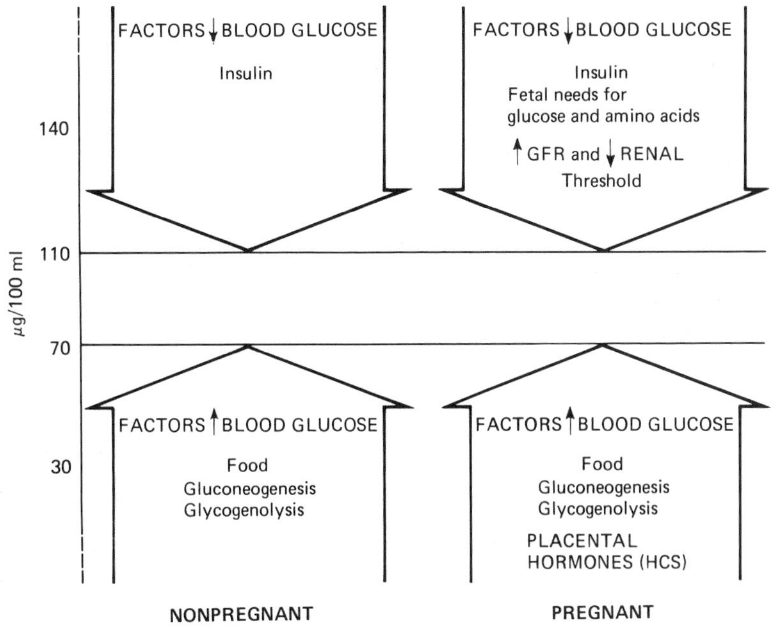

Figure 15–2. Factors which operate to maintain appropriate blood glucose levels in nonpregnant and pregnant women. Although new factors are added during pregnancy, the net result for the healthy woman is normoglycemia.

diabetic pregnant woman will need to increase her carbohydrate intake during the first half of gestation, and she also may need to decrease her insulin dosage. Care should be taken throughout pregnancy to distinguish between ketoacidosis that results from inadequate insulin dosage and that caused by starvation or inadequate carbohydrate intake. The treatment for the first is more insulin, while the treatment for the second is more carbohydrate.

The increasing supply of placental hormones, principally human chorionic somatomammotropin (HCS), has caused the second half of pregnancy to be characterized as diabetogenic. A woman with a predisposition to diabetes may display glucose intolerance and/or clinical diabetes at this time. Her pancreatic activity is adequate to meet normal needs, but she has no reserve capacity to increase insulin production to compensate for the insulin antagonism of HCS (Fig. 15–3). The insulin-dependent diabetic can accommodate to this challenge of pregnancy only by increasing her dose of exogenous insulin. Very careful control of blood glucose levels is necessary to prevent ketoacidosis, which is a common cause of intrauterine death.

An additional factor operating during pregnancy is the change in renal function characterized by an increased glomerular filtration rate without a commensurate increase in tubular reabsorption. As a result, glucosuria is not well correlated with blood glucose. Therefore, urine tests cannot serve as determinants of appropriate insulin dosage.

The influence of pregnancy on long-term complications of diabetes has not been conclusively demonstrated. It is known that the better the diabetic control, the less likelihood there is for nephropathy, retinopathy,

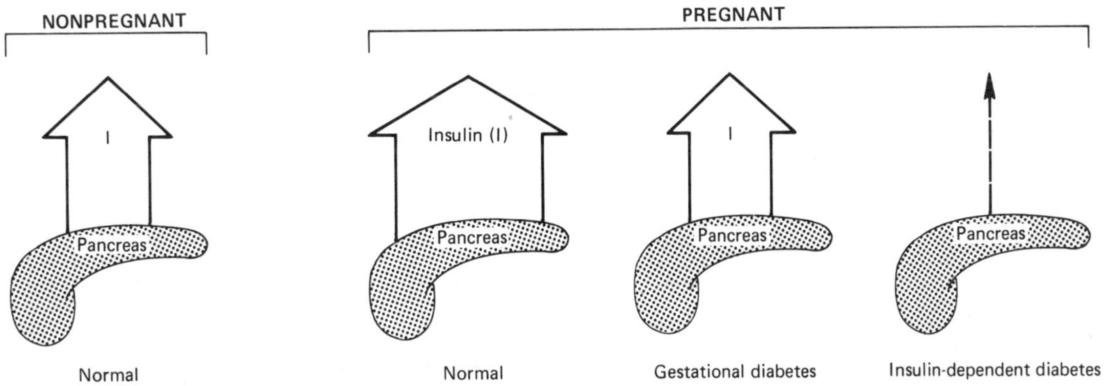

Figure 15–3. Diagrammatic representation of the way in which the pancreas compensates during pregnancy for the insulin antagonist effects of the placental hormones (principally HCS). Notice the pancreas of the gestational diabetic, although producing insulin, does not increase its output of this substance during pregnancy. The pancreas of the insulin-dependent diabetic produces no insulin for all intents and purposes.

and other complications to occur. Since pregnancy is a period of time when blood glucose levels may be particularly difficult to control, it is at least theoretically possible that pregnancy contributes indirectly to the progression of diabetes. Conversely, many women are more rigidly controlled during pregnancy than at any other time because of the fetal intolerance to hyperglycemia as well as to wide fluctuations in blood glucose. Furthermore, women are frequently motivated to become better informed about their disease during this time and thus, perhaps, improve their health practices for future living.

Diabetic Screening

The first step toward improving pregnancy outcome in diabetic pregnancies is an efficient screening program for early diagnosis. As discussed in Chapter 9, a blood glucose determination should be a part of routine antepartum care for all women. Typically, this is done at about 28 weeks' gestation when the placental hormones are beginning to exert their greatest influence. However, early screening in the first trimester is indicated for any woman whose history suggests she may be at particular risk. Factors in the history that prompt earlier screening include family history of diabetes, previous large-for-gestation-age infant (birth weight over 4000 gm), previous unexplained stillbirth, neonatal death, or congenital anomalies, recurrent infections (especially candidial vaginitis and urinary tract infections), obesity, and glycosuria.

Prior to the screening blood glucose, the woman's dietary pattern should be reviewed. If she is eating less than 200 to 250 gm of carbohydrate per day, she should be instructed in a diet that will provide this intake for three days before the screening test. Failure to do this may result in a false-positive test, since the pancreas will be unable to respond appropriately to the sudden, unaccustomed carbohydrate challenge.

When the two-hour postprandial blood test is used for screening, blood glucose values of 140 mg/100 ml of plasma (or 120 mg/100 ml of whole blood) or less are considered normal. An ordinary meal containing 100 gm of carbohydrate provides a more physiologic test than the commercially prepared glucose drinks, although the drinks have the advantage of convenience. The motivation of the client as well as her ability to follow directions should be assessed as a means of selecting the appropriate test methods.

Fasting blood glucose or the glucose tolerance test also may be used for screening. The same precautions of three days of high carbohydrate intake should be observed as for the postprandial test. Fasting blood glucose levels of 110 mg/100 ml of plasma or less are considered to be within the normal range. In evaluating the glucose tolerance test in pregnancy, it is important to remember that the fasting value will be lower than in nonpregnant individuals, but that the two- and three-hour values are normally higher. Norms for each individual laboratory should be consulted.

Gestational Diabetes

Gestational diabetes is an abnormal glucose tolerance during pregnancy with a return to normal after delivery. Women who manifest this disorder are variously described as prediabetics, subclinical diabetics, or potential diabetics. They are individuals who do not have the capacity to increase insulin production sufficiently to compensate for the diabetogenic effects of the placental hormones. Maternal and fetal complications are increased significantly. Although dietary control is usually sufficient without exogenous insulin and there is a return to normal glucose tolerance post partum, these women are at increased risk to develop diabetes later in life. This is especially true if they do not maintain a normal body weight.

The impact of a diagnosis of gestational diabetes on the woman and her family is likely to be crisis-provoking. The necessity for adopting a dietary regimen, the added threats to the pregnancy, and the long-term implications of a difficult chronic disease may be, at least temporarily, overwhelming. Careful instruction and frequent contacts with supportive professionals can do much to facilitate the mobilization of the family's coping behaviors.

The gestational diabetic woman requires the same close supervision as the insulin-dependent diabetic. Evidence of placental insufficiency and possible jeopardy to the fetus must be carefully checked. Even when the diabetes is very mild, the hazard of placental insufficiency increases toward term gestation. Pregnancy should not be permitted to continue postterm.

During the postpartum period the woman should obtain appropriate nutritional consultation for weight control and receive instructions about health maintenance to prevent or detect later development of overt diabetes.

Insulin-Dependent Diabetes

Initial clinical assessment of the insulin-dependent diabetic pregnant woman should include a thorough discussion of her experience with diabetes, her knowledge of the disease, and her own methods of managing her disease. Such discussions can provide valuable information about the individuality of the woman, her coping patterns, and probable needs and responses.

One of the primary goals of diabetic management in the nonpregnant individual is to foster independence in the client so that she can competently adjust her own glucose-insulin balance to meet the needs of daily living and minor illnesses. Some of this independence must necessarily be relinguished during pregnancy because of the necessity for closely monitoring maternal and fetal well-being.

It is therefore crucial to a satisfactory working relationship between client and professional that the woman be encouraged to assume as much autonomy in her care as she desires and is capable of achieving. An openness in communication will foster mutual trust which can only benefit the client and her developing fetus.

Preconception Control

The incidence of major congenital malformations in infants of diabetic mothers has remained unchanged in spite of the many advances in knowledge and scrupulous application of optimal standards of care. It is believed that these malformations occur as a result of an inhospitable intrauterine environment occurring during the first few critical weeks of embryonic life. During much or all of this time, the woman may be unaware of her pregnancy, yet already she is changing physiologically. Changes in estrogen and progesterone levels, as well as early pregnancy symptoms, may produce significant changes in diabetic control, resulting in hypo- and/or hyperglycemia. In addition, many women achieve a pregnancy without optimal control of their blood glucose. Thus, conception and embryonic development may take place under inadequate conditions.

The ideal situation is for the woman who has insulin-dependent diabetes to seek consultation with the health care team prior to conception. At that time, she and her partner can find out what the risks are and what management of a diabetic pregnancy will involve. If they elect to attempt conception, they should plan to do so only after optimal control of the woman's diabetes has been achieved. Typically, the woman is counseled about nutrition after a review of her current dietary plan, and her diabetic control is evaluated by means of blood glucose determinations. The length of time required for preconception control depends on the kind of control and health habits the woman already has. Usually, when she has been normoglycemic for one month, she is advised to discontinue contraceptive measures and attempt to conceive. Needless to say, she is well advised to return for antepartal care as soon as she becomes pregnant. Some women may be seen as early as three to four weeks' gestation, having just missed their first menstrual period. Although it remains to be seen whether such an approach will effect a reduction in congenital malformations, it appears to offer the best opportunity now known for healthy growth and development.

Antepartum Care

Over and above the usual goals for all antepartum care, there are two major objectives for care of the insulin-dependent diabetic. These are (1) to maintain careful diabetic control, and (2) to evaluate placental function and fetal well-being.

Diabetic control is achieved through the balance of dietary intake and insulin as determined by periodic blood glucose determinations. Diet should be reviewed in consultation with a nutritionist who will assist the woman to define a dietary pattern compatible with her cultural and personal food preferences, life-style, and economic status. Caloric intake should be sufficient to permit a weight gain of approximately 25 lb. This will vary according to activity level and other factors, but, in general, a diet of 1800 to 2200 calories is satisfactory. The diet should contain 80 to 100 gm of protein and carbohydrate equivalent to 40 to 45 percent of the calories. In order to avoid the wide fluctuations in blood glucose, the carbohydrate content should be evenly distributed throughout the day. Regularity in both the timing and the content of meals and snacks is very important in order to avoid insulin reactions. The diet may require frequent alterations in response to symptoms of pregnancy such as nausea, heartburn, and pressure of the uterus on the stomach. A bedtime snack is desirable to reduce the risks of the overnight fast.

It is often helpful to both client and nutritionist if the woman keeps a diet diary of all foods and beverages and the time she eats them. Reviewing this diary may assist the nutritionist to diagnose problem areas, and it is also an excellent means of teaching meal planning, calorie counting, and food values.

Insulin dosage is adjusted on the basis of blood glucose levels obtained at frequent intervals throughout gestation. Biweekly or even weekly blood tests are not uncommon. Practitioners differ in their approach to blood glucose collections. Some use a profile of three two-hour postprandial samples on a single day, others use fasting blood samples, and others may use a combination. The therapeutic goal is to maintain the fasting level below 120 mg/100 ml and/or the postprandial level below 150 mg/100 ml. The usual insulin prescription to achieve this goal is a combination of an intermediate or long-acting insulin with multiple doses of regular insulin at meal time. It is to be expected that the insulin requirements will gradually increase throughout gestation, especially during the second half. It is usual for the insulin dosage to increase 70 to 100 percent over prepregnancy amounts.[10] It is important to emphasize that urine tests are not reliable indicators for modifying insulin dosage during pregnancy.

The availability of reliable and portable reflectance colorimeters for the home measurement of blood glucose has made it possible for pregnant women to take

[10] Philip Felig, Diabetes mellitus, in *Medical Complications During Pregnancy, (2nd ed.)* edited by Gerard N. Burrow and Thomas F. Ferris, W. B. Saunders, Philadelphia, 1982.

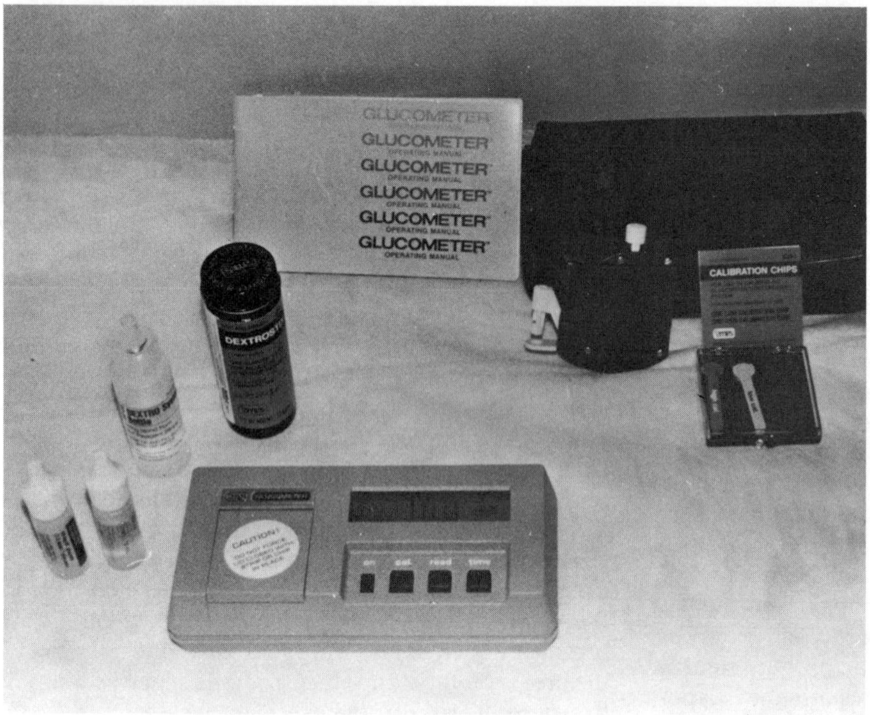

A

Figure 15–4. *A*. One kind of reflectance colorimeter for use by the patient for measuring her blood glucose level at home. *B*. A finger puncture is made with a stylet. *C*. Blood is applied to the reagent strip. *D*. After waiting exactly 60 seconds, the blood is rinsed with a stream of water. *E*. The reagent strip is inserted into the reflectance meter, the appropriate controls punched and the blood glucose level appears as a digital readout in the small black window at the upper right of the machine.

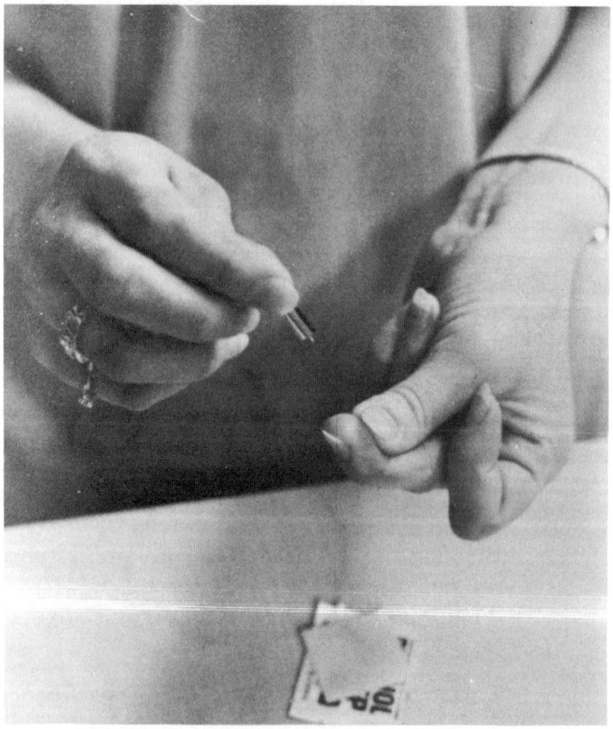

B

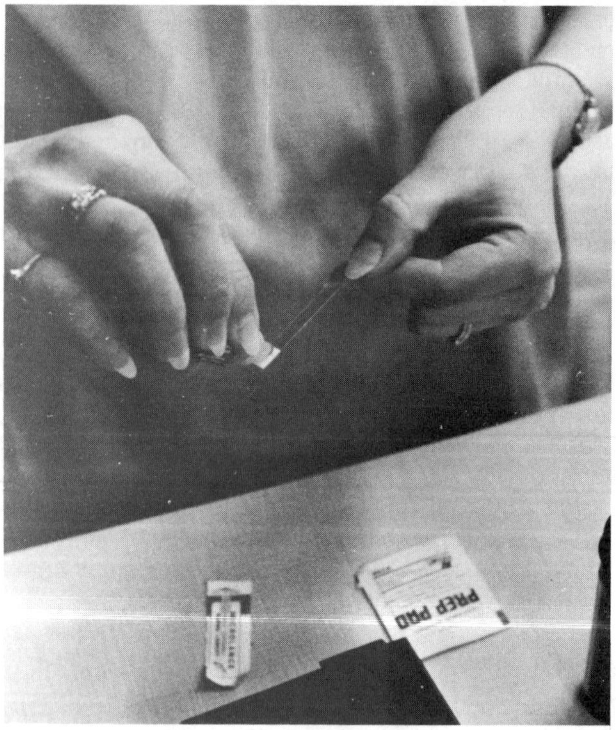

C

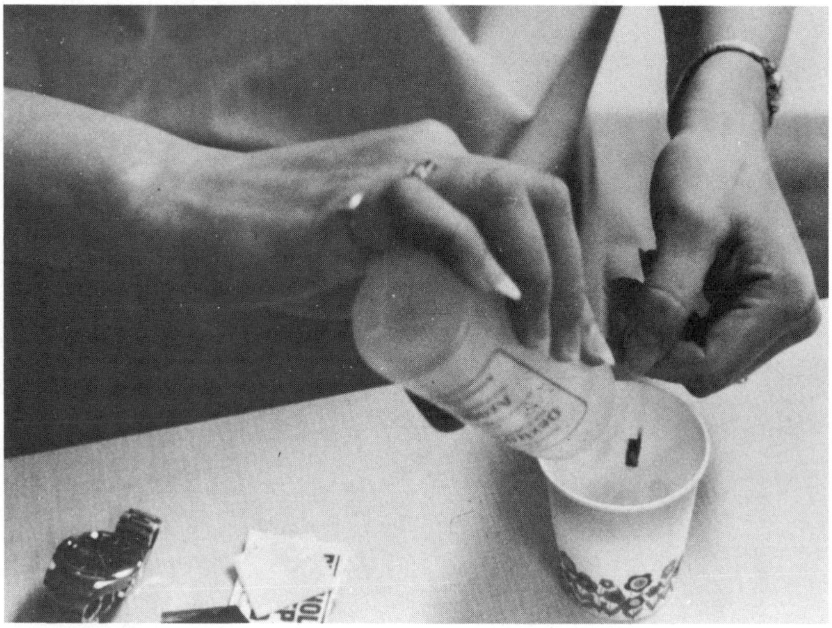

D

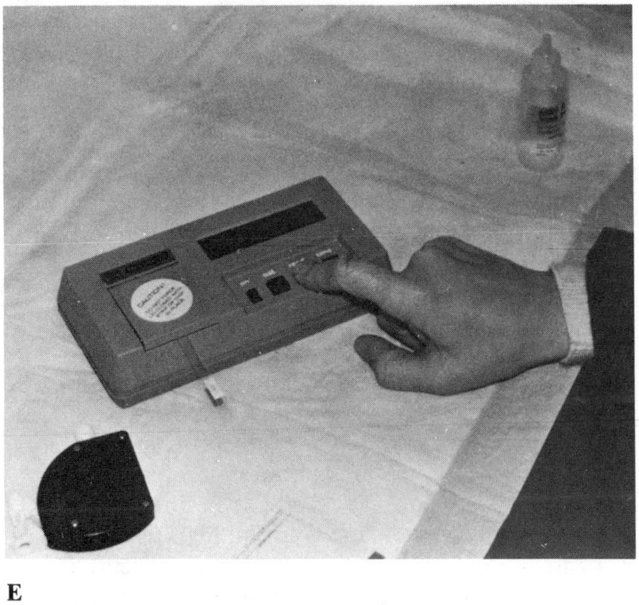

E

a more active role in their own health care and to achieve a more precise control of their blood glucose levels (Fig. 15-4). In addition, many centers are testing the use of insulin infusors and insulin pumps in an effort to achieve a more physiologic distribution of insulin throughout the day (Fig. 15-5). Nurses should familiarize themselves with the current practices in their communities as this is a dynamic and rapidly changing field of practice.

Assessment of Fetal Well-Being

As the third trimester begins, evaluation of fetal/placental function becomes paramount. An important cause of intrauterine fetal death is placental dysfunction. Early recognition of signs of impending failure permits lifesaving intervention. Maternal insulin requirements provide a crude indication of placental function, since insulin is inactivated by the placental hormones. Failure to require increasing insulin doses or, more ominously, a sudden drop in insulin requirements should cast suspicion on the efficiency of the placenta.

Twenty-four-hour urinary estriol determinations or estriol-creatinine ratios are evaluated two to three times per week, beginning at approximately 32 weeks' gestation. Weekly nonstress tests (NST) and/or oxytocin challenge tests (OCT) are also started at about 32 to 34 weeks' gestation. Any test results indicative of placental insufficiency should suggest the need for prompt assessment of fetal maturity and possible delivery. See Chapter 13, for a discussion of these tests.

Management of the diabetic pregnancy can almost always be accomplished in an ambulatory setting. Periodic hospitalization, however, may be necessary for the woman who is in poor diabetic control, who has ketonuria, or who demonstrates evidence of placental insufficiency. In addition, a brief period of hospitalization may be the most efficient means of conducting a concentrated program of health education.

Intrapartum Care

Historically, it has been good obstetric practice to perform cesarean sections routinely on all diabetic women at 35 to 37 weeks' gestation. Since the incidence of intrauterine fetal death was known to be highest during the last three to four weeks of gestation, this practice was a reasonable preventive approach. Cesarean section was

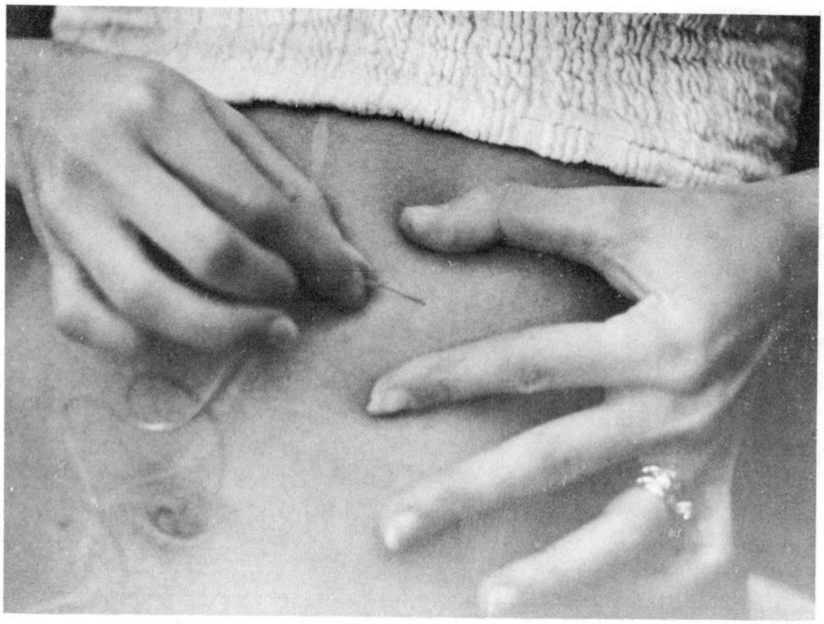

A

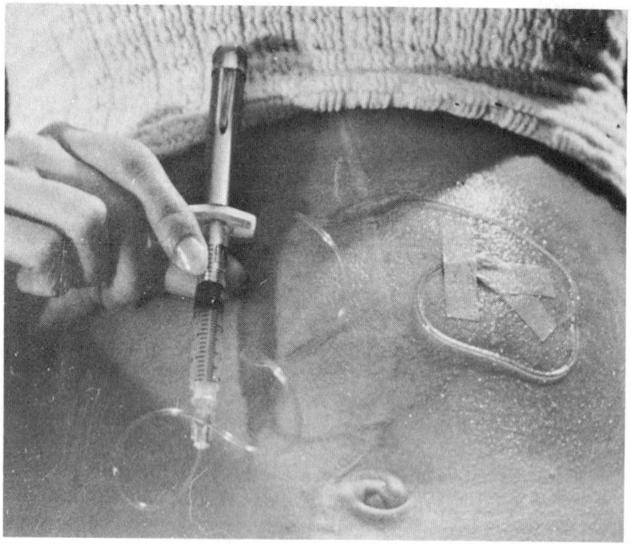

B

Figure 15–5. *A*. Woman is shown inserting a needle subcutaneously into her abdomen. *B*. Shows needle taped in place and attached to the insulin infusor by a short length of polyethylene tubing. Note the clip on the infusor which can be used to attach it to the woman's belt or other piece of clothing.

preferred over vaginal delivery because, even if the condition of the cervix permitted induction at this early time, the fetus tolerated labor poorly and often succumbed during the intrapartum period.

Currently several factors are changing this practice. The ability to closely monitor placental function and to assess fetal response to labor by continuous fetal heart rate records and scalp capillary blood gases permits both the longer continuation of pregnancy and the potential for safe conduct through labor. In addition, the development of reliable biochemical tests for fetal lung maturity allows the timing of delivery when adequate neonatal pulmonary function is more assured. As long as there is adequacy of placental function, as evidenced by rising urinary estriol values and reactive non-stress tests, many centers are allowing the pregnancy to continue until near term to give the fetus the benefit of intrauterine growth. Near term, personal and obstetric readiness for labor are increased and induction of labor is facilitated.

During labor, or in preparation for cesarean section, maternal blood glucose levels are maintained by the intravenous infusion of glucose or other sugars and regular insulin. There is an attempt in some centers to maintain maternal glycemia under 100 mg/100 ml for several hours prior to delivery. This appears to reduce the risk of neonatal hypoglycemia by providing the fetus an intrauterine period of "withdrawal" from the high glucose loads previously available from the mother.

For the diabetic woman, as for all high-risk pregnant women, laboring is a highly mechanized event. It requires extraordinary skill and sensitivity on the part of the nurse to integrate all of the data from patients and machines and make sound judgments about care. Even greater expertise is needed to permit the laboring woman to maintain her self-esteem and to control her labor and birth in ways that are safe and acceptable to her and to the father. If possible the couple should be attended during labor by physicians and nurses whom they have known through pregnancy. The father or another supportive person should be present throughout labor and delivery. As soon as initial assessment has been made of the infant at birth to ensure adequate respirations, the parents should be offered their infant to see, touch, and hold. Unless there are either maternal or neonatal complications, the mother may initiate breast-feeding during the first one to two hours of life. Emphasis during a high-risk labor must always be on the family—never on the gadgetry.

Postpartum Care

Endocrine and metabolic changes occur precipitously with the termination of pregnancy. The contrainsulin effects are abruptly stopped, and insulin requirements are markedly decreased for the first few days post partum. Regular insulin is usually given on a sliding scale, depending on the amount of glycosuria, for two to three days before intermediate or long-acting insulin is prescribed. It typically requires three to six months for the insulin requirements to return to their prepregnant level.

The diabetes may be quite brittle for a time after delivery, and the nurse must observe the patient closely for signs of insulin reaction, hyperglycemia, and acidosis. The tendency toward postpartum infections is increased in the diabetic, and even mild infections can severely compromise diabetic control.

The stress of diabetic reregulation, the possibility of an infant who requires special observation and care, as well as the usual anxieties and discomforts of involution may combine to delay comfortable mother-infant contact. Mothers need help to understand and accept themselves if there is not an immediate flood of maternal feeling. Parental attachment can be facilitated by flexible, family-centered policies that permit free access of parents to their infants.

Nutrition consultation should be obtained prior to discharge from the hospital. Emphasis will be on nutritional requirements for lactation, if that is appropriate, and on caloric intake to achieve optimal weight.

Referral to community health agencies, if not initiated antepartally, should be accomplished at the time of discharge. Telephone follow-up within two or three days of going home is quite helpful for all mothers, but especially for those who have had a high-risk pregnancy. For some women the postpartum period is a time of considerable letdown after the intense, almost constant, attention they received during the final weeks of their pregnancy. A period of weaning from the intensive care team members may be necessary.

Observation and special care of the infant of a diabetic mother are discussed in Chapter 30.

AGE AS A RISK FACTOR IN PREGNANCY

Women in their early twenties have been described as the most biologically fit for reproduction. But is there an optimum age socially or psychologically or developmentally for a person to become a parent? This is a question that awaits discussion and investigation. For the present, it can only be said that women at either extreme of the reproductive life span are at increased risk for both medical and social/psychologic complications of childbearing.

Adolescence

Pregnancy during adolescence received considerable attention in the middle and late 1970s from virtually every facet of society. Birth rates have increased steadily in the under-16 age group while declining in all other age groups. Such pregnancies, generally beginning outside of marriage, place significant stress on the young women involved, their families, and society as a whole.

The girl, not yet a woman, still developmentally occupied with her own physical and psychologic growth, is thrust into a role for which she is ill prepared. She needs very special nutritional care to ensure proper growth for her child, as well as for her own continued physical growth. Because of her physiologic immaturity, nutritional status, and frequent reluctance to seek early antepartum care, she is at increased risk for toxemia, premature labor, low-birthweight infant, and operative delivery.

All too frequently, teenage pregnancy means the interruption of education, which may substantially alter the girl's future life chances. Premarital conceptions are highly correlated with marital disruptions, as approximately three out of four teenage marriages end in divorce. If the girl does not choose to marry, she must make other very difficult decisions related to her future and that of her child. More and more single women are not relinquishing their infants for adoption but are choosing to raise them alone. This has implications for the support services, financial as well as social, needed to help these mothers.

Although services for unwed mothers are rather widely available, little or no attention has been paid to the unwed father. What are his needs for counseling, for education? What are his rights with regard to his unborn child? Social and health agencies and the courts are beginning to address these issues, but there is much yet to be done.

Even more neglected are the parents of these adolescents. Professionals waste little time and no sympathy on these parents who are doubly in crisis. The quality of their parenting is called into question by the out-of-wedlock pregnancy. They hurt for themselves and they hurt for their child, whom they love. In addition, they must deal with the loss of their grandchild if adoption is elected or with adjustment to their new relationship to their daughter as a single parent.

Many references are available that deal more comprehensively with individual aspects of care for the adolescent pregnant girl. The reader is referred to these for assistance in individualizing nursing care for this vulnerable segment of the childbearing population.

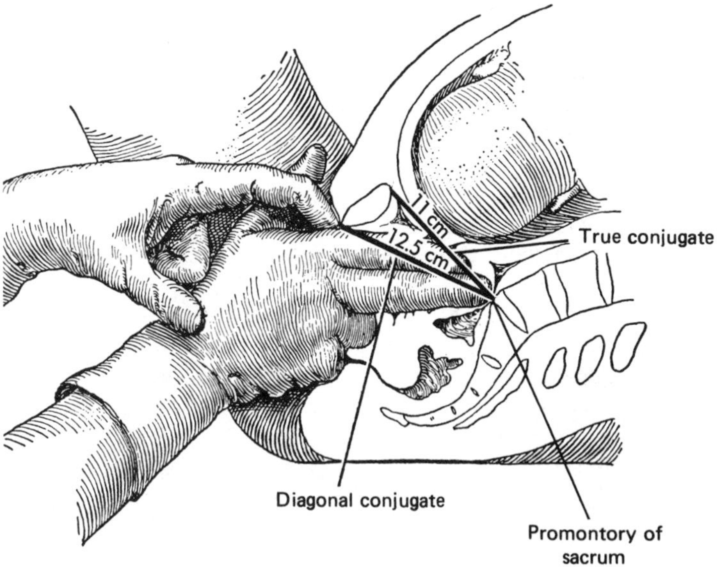

Figure 16–7. Diagram showing method of measuring the diagonal conjugate in order to estimate the length of the true conjugate.

promontory of the sacrum (Fig. 16–7). The point at which the lower margin of the symphysis pubis rests on the forefinger is then marked by the nail of the index finger of the other hand, and the fingers in the vagina are withdrawn. The nail of the index finger, which is used as the marker, is held firmly in place until the distance between it and the tip of the second finger (the finger that touched the sacral promontory) is measured. This distance is the length of the diagonal conjugate, which normally measures 12.5 cm. The diameter of the true conjugate is then estimated by subtracting 1.5 to 2.5 cm from the measurement of the diagonal conjugate (Table 16–1).

It may be difficult to reach the promontory of the sacrum during the early months of pregnancy because of tightness of the vaginal tissues and rigidity of the perineum. Measurement of the diagonal conjugate therefore is sometimes deferred until the middle part of pregnancy, when these tissues stretch more easily. Measurement of the diagonal conjugate may be somewhat uncomfortable for the patient and requires reassurance by the physician and the nurse.

Table 16–1. Average Measurements of Diameters of the Female Pelvis

Diameter	*Average Length in Centimeters**
Inlet measurements	
True conjugate	11
Obstetric conjugate	10.6
Diagonal conjugate	12.5
Transverse	13
Oblique (right and left)	12.75
Midpelvic measurements	
Anteroposterior	11.5
Interspinous (transverse)	10.5
Outlet measurements	
Anteroposterior	11.5
Intertuberous (transverse)	11
Posterior sagittal	7.5

*All measurements represent average figures.

MIDPELVIC MEASUREMENTS There is no satisfactory manual or instrumental method of measuring the midpelvis; measurements can be obtained only by x-ray. However, an approximate but useful estimate of the space in the midpelvis may be obtained by vaginal examination. The ischial spines, which project into the region of the midpelvis (Fig. 16–4), are felt readily during a vaginal (or rectal) examination. Although the distance between these spines cannot be measured clinically, their bluntness or prominence can be estimated. The slope of the side walls of the pelvis, the curve of the sacrum, and the width of the sacrosciatic notch also can be palpated during vaginal examination.

A midpelvic contraction may be suspected if the ischial spines are prominent, if the side walls of the pelvis converge, or if the sacrosciatic notch feels narrow. A contraction of the midpelvis also may be suspected when the intertuberous measurement (transverse diameter of the outlet) is 8.5 cm or less, because the distance between the ischial spines is usually small whenever the space between the ischial tuberosities is decreased.

PELVIC OUTLET MEASUREMENTS Measurements of the pelvic outlet also are made with the patient in the lithotomy position. In addition to measurements being made, the coccyx is examined for mobility at this time, and the general contour of the pelvic outlet is ascertained. The shape of the subpubic arch is outlined by palpation of the bony sides of the outlet from the symphysis pubis down to the ischial tuberosities. When the thumbs of each hand are placed along the descending portion of the pubic bone on each side of the pelvis, the angle at which these bones come together can be observed. Information about the width of the pubic arch is very valuable in making an estimate of the adequacy of the outlet and hence, indirectly, of the midpelvis. A narrow arch, which is typical of a male pelvis, is almost always associated with other characteristics of a masculine-type pelvis.

In addition to estimation of the width of the pubic arch, distances between points also are measured. The distance between the inner, lower aspect of the ischial tuberosities, the intertuberous diameter, which is the most important measurement of the outlet, is measured with a pelvimeter (Fig. 16-8) or with the examiner's hand. When the examiner uses the hand to make this measurement, three or four knuckles of one hand are pressed between the ischial tuberosities and the distance across the portion of the hand that fits into this space is measured. The average measurement between the ischial tuberosities is 11 cm.

The posterior sagittal diameter, a distance that has special importance when the intertuberous diameter is short, is obtained by measuring, with a pelvimeter, the distance from the midpoint between the ischial tuberosities to the tip of the sacrum. This distance is normally an average of 7.5 cm in length.

X-Ray Pelvimetry

X-ray technique may be used to measure the diameters of the pelvis that cannot be measured clinically and at the same time to recheck measurements that have been obtained with the pelvimeter and the hand. If the x-ray is taken late in pregnancy or during labor, it not only aids in determining pelvic size and shape, but also provides valuable information about the relationship of the fetus (presentation, position, and station) to the maternal pelvis (Figs. 16-9 and 16-10).

X-ray examinations are a valuable diagnostic aid in pregnancy, but because they increase, albeit slightly, the radiation exposure on *two* individuals, they are used only when clinical examination indicates that additional information is essential. Although diagnostic x-rays have some slight effect on any exposed body cells

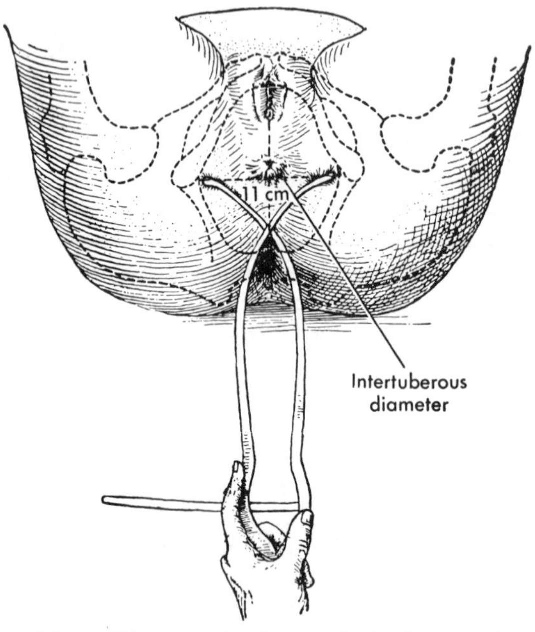

Figure 16-8. Diagram showing method of measuring the transverse diameter of the outlet (intertuberous diameter).

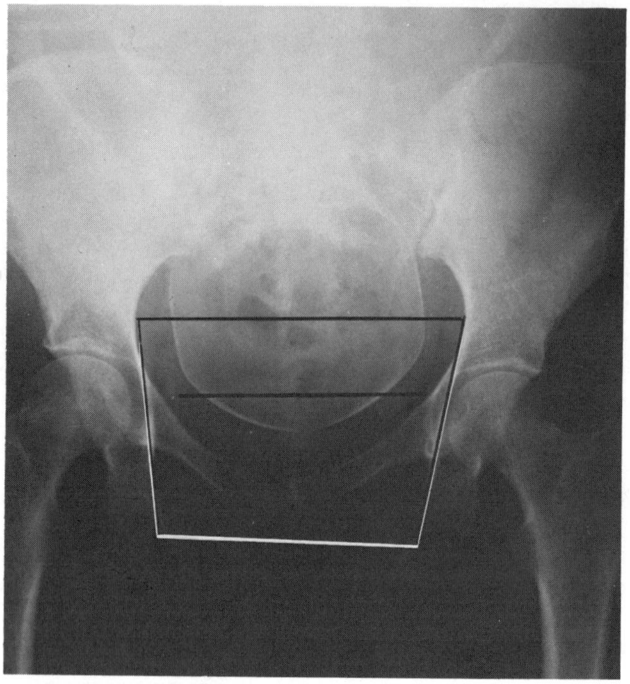

Figure 16-9. Anteroposterior view of a roentgenogram of a pelvis taken to determine the size of the pelvis, its general architecture, and the relationship of the size of the fetal head to the size of the pelvis. This x-ray was taken on a primigravida in labor whose measurements by clinical pelvimetry seemed to be within normal limits, but in whom the fetal head apparently was not engaging.

The horizontal dark lines on the film designate the diameters measured. The uppermost horizontal line indicates the transverse diameter of the inlet, which measured 12.2 cm. The center horizontal line runs between the ischial spines and measures the transverse diameter of the midpelvis; this measured 10.1 cm. The lowermost horizontal line lies between the ischial tuberosities and thus measures the transverse diameter of the pelvic outlet; this was found to be 10.2 cm. (After the distances had been measured on the film, a correction factor was applied to make adjustment for magnification and other technical considerations.)

This x-ray shows the presentation to be cephalic with the occiput anterior. The back lies anteriorly and slightly to the right. The fetal head is small compared to the size of the pelvis.

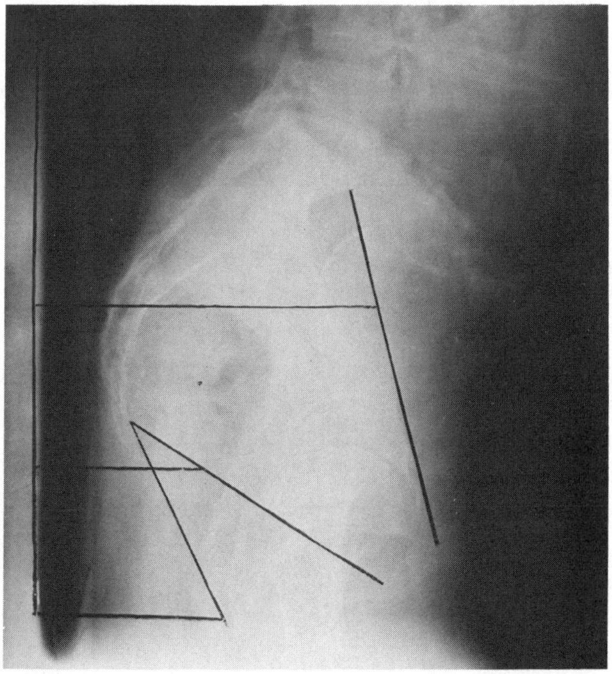

Figure 16–10. Lateral view roentgenogram of the pelvis shown in Figure 16–9. This x-ray was taken with the patient in an upright position and shows that the fetal head is engaged just within the pelvis. The oblique dark lines designate the diameters measured. The anterior line is the AP diameter of the pelvic inlet which measured 13.1 cm; the center line indicates the AP diameter of the midpelvis which measured 10.7 cm; and the posterior line shows the posterior sagittal diameter which measured 7.8 cm. (These measurements are the readings after application of the correction factor.)

The conclusion that was drawn from the x-rays shown in Figures 16–9 and 16–10 was that the pelvic diameters are adequate for the size of the baby and that there is no apparent reason for difficulty in delivery due to disproportion between the fetal head and the bony pelvis.

(somatic effect), the major concern in their use during pregnancy is the effect on reproductive cells (genetic effect). The genetic effect of radiation on reproductive cells may be cumulative from the time of conception through the reproductive years. Deleterious or harmful mutations may be produced which are then passed on to the next generation. Pelvic x-rays are in the gonadal region, and when taken during pregnancy they involve two persons, a mother in the reproductive years and a very young individual, the fetus. The gonads of both the mother and the fetus are exposed to a certain amount of radiation; in addition, the fetus receives radiation to other parts of his body.

To keep radiation exposure to a minimum, the physician will carefully evaluate the need for an x-ray and then take all precautions possible in the technique and method of taking the films, precautions that keep the exposure as low as possible. Whenever justifiable, an x-ray examination is postponed until after onset of labor. The fetus is then well beyond the period during which the x-ray may have a deleterious effect on his somatic development. Also, the x-ray serves several purposes; it provides information about fetal size, maturity, position, and development, in addition to size of pelvis.

X-ray pelvimetry, if necessary, ordinarily is done only as indicated sometime during the course of labor. It becomes imperative in conditions such as suspected disproportion between the fetal head and the pelvis, abnormal presentation and position, suspected abnormal fetal development, and prolonged or arrested labor. In the hope that x-ray pelvimetry may prove unnecessary, physicians await labor before obtaining films on a woman with a pelvis of questionable size. For example, descent of the fetal head with the beginning of labor might terminate fears regarding the adequacy of the pelvic inlet.

Whenever a patient in labor must have an x-ray, it is highly desirable that a nurse accompany her to the x-ray room. The patient and her husband are often worried and frightened, and the reassurance of a nurse is of great comfort to them. The mother is usually uncomfortable from her labor, which sometimes has continued for hours, and both parents will be concerned over its outcome and the safety of mother and child. The nurse can help to interpret the purpose of the x-rays and the general overall procedure in taking the films. The nurse also can be of considerable assistance in helping the patient move into the proper positions for the films (views from several positions may be necessary) and should remain in the room, close to the patient, until all is in readiness for taking the films. In most instances the patient can be left alone during the short interval required for taking the x-ray, and, if possible, the nurse should leave the room because she/he too must keep total radiation dosage to a minimum. If the occasional patient requires assistance from the nurse in maintaining a position, or for some other reason, lead-lined aprons are available for the nurse's protection. The nurse must observe labor carefully while the patient is in the x-ray department and while en route and must be prepared to notify the physician immediately at the appearance of signs of imminent delivery or threatened uterine rupture and also be prepared to handle other emergencies.

THE FETAL HEAD

The fetal head is the most important part of the body from the standpoint of passage through the birth canal. The head is the largest and least malleable part of the body; it is also the part that ordinarily passes through the birth canal first. The process of labor is essentially a series of adaptations of the size, shape, and position of the fetal skull to the size and shape of the maternal pelvis—an adaptation of the "passenger" to the "passage." Since the pelvis is quite rigid and inflexible, adjustment must be made by the fetal head, which is moldable because of incomplete ossification and bone fusion at this age. If the head passes through the pelvis safely, the rest of the delivery usually will be accomplished with comparative ease, unless the fetus is excessive in size. A marked disproportion between the diameters of the head and the pelvis, or limited moldability of the head, constitutes a serious complication, which will be described later as a complication of labor (Chapter 22).

Bones of the Skull

The fetal skull is proportionately larger than other parts of the body; the face forms a relatively small part of the head. The major portion of the head, the dome or vaultlike structure, which forms the top, sides, and back of the head, is made up of separate and as yet ununited bones—two *frontal,* two *parietal,* two *temporal,* and one *occipital* bone. The bones are separate structures with membranous tissues between their margins. The membranous tissues between the bones are called *sutures,* and the irregular membranous areas at the intersection of two or more sutures are called *fontanels.*

Sutures and Fontanels

The sutures are named and situated as follows: the *frontal* lies between the two frontal bones; the *sagittal* extends anteroposteriorly between the parietal bones; the *coronal* lies between the frontal bones and the anterior margin of the parietals; while the *lambdoidal* suture separates the posterior margins of the parietals from the upper margin of the occipital bone (Fig. 16–11). These sutures can be palpated on vaginal, and sometimes rectal, examination.

There are two fontanels of obstetric significance. The *anterior,* or *large, fontanel,* also called the *bregma,* is located at the meeting of the coronal suture from each side, the sagittal suture, and the frontal suture (Fig. 16–11). It is diamond- or lozenge-shaped, is about 3 cm in diameter, and is usually not obliterated during labor. The *posterior,* or *small, fontanel* is a triangular space at the intersection of the sagittal suture and the lambdoidal sutures (Fig. 16–11). This space may be obliterated as the surrounding bony margins approach each other during labor.

The sutures and fontanels are of great diagnostic value during labor because some can be outlined during a rectal or vaginal examination after the cervix has thinned and dilated. Correct recognition of these sutures and fontanels will determine the fetal position. The fontanels are differentiated from one another by their size and also by the number of suture lines that enter the space.

Areas of the Skull

The skull is divided into four areas that are designated the occiput, the vertex, the bregma, and the sinciput (brow). The *occiput* is the region behind the small fontanel and is named from the bone that forms it; the *vertex* lies between the two fontanels and extends on each side of the head to the protuberances of the parietal bones; the *bregma* is the area of the large fontanel; and the *sinciput* (brow) is the area in front of the large fontanel and is formed by the frontal bone (Fig. 16–11). Terms used to describe presentation and position of a fetus indicate the relationship that exists between an area of the fetal skull and an area of the maternal pelvis.

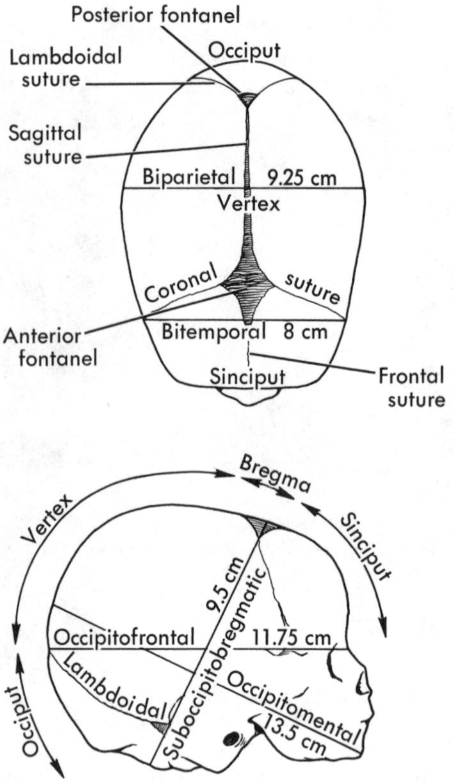

Figure 16–11. Top and size views of fetal skull, giving average length of important diameters.

Diameters and Circumferences

Information about the normal shape and average size of a newborn's head is important from the standpoint of the relationship between the measurements of the head and the measurements of the bony canal through which the head will pass during birth. The diameters that are usually described and their normal size are as follows (Fig. 16–11):

1. The *occipitofrontal diameter* (abbreviation, OF), measured from the bridge of the nose to the occipital protuberance, is 11.75 to 12 cm.
2. The *biparietal diameter* (BP) is the greatest transverse diameter, being the distance between the parietal protuberances, and measures 9.25 cm.
3. The *bitemporal diameter* (BT) is the greatest

distance between the temporal bones and measures 8 cm.

4. The *occipitomental diameter* (OM) is the longest diameter. It extends from the point of the chin to the most prominent part of the occiput and measures 13.5 cm.
5. The *suboccipitobregmatic diameter* (SOB), measured from the undersurface of the occiput, where it joins the neck, to the center of the anterior fontanel, is 9.5 cm.

The *greatest circumference* of the fetal head is at the plane of the occipitofrontal diameter and measures 34.5 cm (13.8 in.). The *smallest circumference* is at the plane of the suboccipitobregmatic diameter and measures 32 cm (12.8 in.). With a normally flexed fetal head, this is the circumference that must traverse the birth canal. Until the fetus weighs approximately 4500 gm (10 lb), the circumference of the head is greater than the body circumference at the shoulders. The size of the shoulders is therefore not likely to present a problem during delivery unless the fetus has developed to excessive size and the circumference at the shoulders has become greater than the circumference of the head. Even then, the size of the shoulders may not cause difficulty if their firmness does not interfere with a certain amount of compression in their passage through the pelvis.

The measurements given above, like all of those which it is possible to give, only represent averages taken from a large number of term infants. Individual variations will be found among normal infants. For example, the size of the infant is affected by race. Black infants average a smaller size than those of the white race. As might be expected, the size of the parents is likely to be reflected in the size of their infants; parents of large stature tend to have large infants.

Molding

The fact that the skull is made up of separate bones, with soft membranous spaces interposed between them, permits its being compressed and changed in shape to a considerable extent as it passes through the birth canal. In this process, called molding, opposing margins of bones meet, or overlap to such a degree that the shape of the head changes and certain diameters are appreciably diminished (Fig. 26–7*A*, Chapter 26). Such change permits passage of the fetal head through a relatively narrow canal. Moldability varies greatly, however, and the difference in the degree of compressibility of heads of approximately the same size may determine the difference between an easy and a difficult birth, or even the impossibility of passage through the birth canal. A newborn's head may be so distorted and elongated by the molding process that its abnormal appearance gives the parents great concern; the nurse can be quite confident, however, in giving them assurance that the head will assume its normal outline in a few days.

FETOPELVIC RELATIONSHIPS

Knowledge of the exact relationship of the fetal position to the maternal pelvis is important in management of labor and delivery. Examinations are made during the latter part of pregnancy to determine this relationship and to estimate the fetal size. Further examinations are made at the onset of labor to confirm previous findings or discover changes and, at intervals during labor, to ascertain that the fetal progress through the birth canal is satisfactory. The fetal position in relation to the maternal pelvis is described as lie, presentation, and position of the fetus. This relationship is determined by abdominal palpation and rectal and vaginal examination, and sometimes by x-ray.

During the latter months of pregnancy the fetus is curved and folded upon itself into an ovoid mass which corresponds to the shape of the uterine cavity. In this position it occupies the smallest possible space. The relationship of the various parts of the fetal body to one another, the posture assumed *in utero,* is called the fetal *attitude.* The usual intrauterine posture, or characteristic attitude, is with the back flexed; the head bent forward, with the chin close to the chest; arms crossed on the chest; thighs flexed on the abdomen; and knees bent. The umbilical cord lies in the space between the upper and lower extremities. With a few exceptions, the long axis of the fetus is parallel to the long axis of the mother, and most frequently the head is downward (Fig. 16–12). Although the fetus moves about and changes its position during the early part of pregnancy, it is less likely to alter

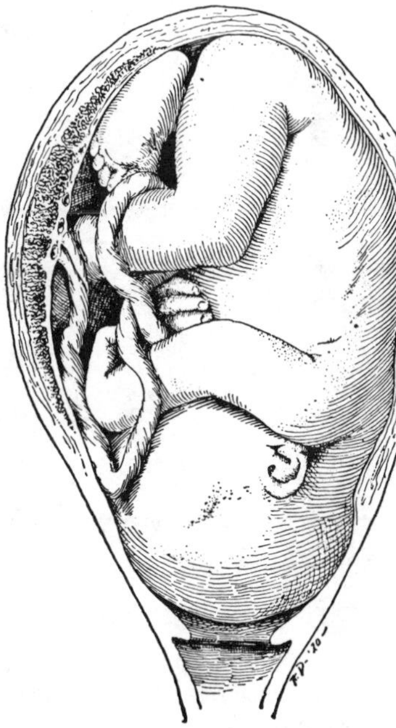

Figure 16–12. Most common attitude of fetus in uterine cavity at term.

its relation to the maternal body during the tenth lunar month and quite unlikely to do so after the onset of labor. Before present methods of determining fetal intrauterine position, it was believed that the fetus stood upright in the uterus until toward the end of pregnancy and then somersaulted to the position it occupied just before birth (Fig. 16–13).

Lie of the Fetus

Lie is the term employed to indicate the relationship of the longitudinal axis of the fetus to the longitudinal axis of the mother. The lie may be either longitudinal or transverse. In a *longitudinal lie,* the long axis of the fetal body is parallel to the long axis of the maternal body. In the *transverse lie,* the longitudinal axis of the fetal body is at right angles to the longitudinal axis of the maternal body.

Presenting Part and Presentation

The terms "presenting part" and "presentation" are used to designate the part of the fetal body that lies closest to, or has entered, the true pelvis. The part of the body that is lowermost is called the *presenting part.*

The *presentation* of the fetus is named after the presenting part and is therefore a phrase used to describe the fetus in terms of its lowermost part. In longitudinal lies the head or the breech (buttocks) will be the lowermost portion of the fetus and thus the presenting part. When the head is lowermost (presenting part), it is termed a *cephalic* presentation (Fig. 16–14*A*), and when the breech is downward (presenting part), it is called *breech* presentation (Fig. 16–14*B*). In transverse lie the shoulder is usually closest to the pelvic inlet (presenting part), and it is termed a *shoulder* presentation (Fig. 16–15). Well over 99 percent of all lies are longitudinal. A transverse lie is a serious obstetric complication.

Cephalic presentations are further divided into two main types, vertex and face presentation, and two transitory types, sincipital and brow presentation. These terms define more specifically the area of the fetal head that becomes the presenting part. The degree of flexion that the fetal head assumes in relation to his own body determines the area of the head that will be lowermost.

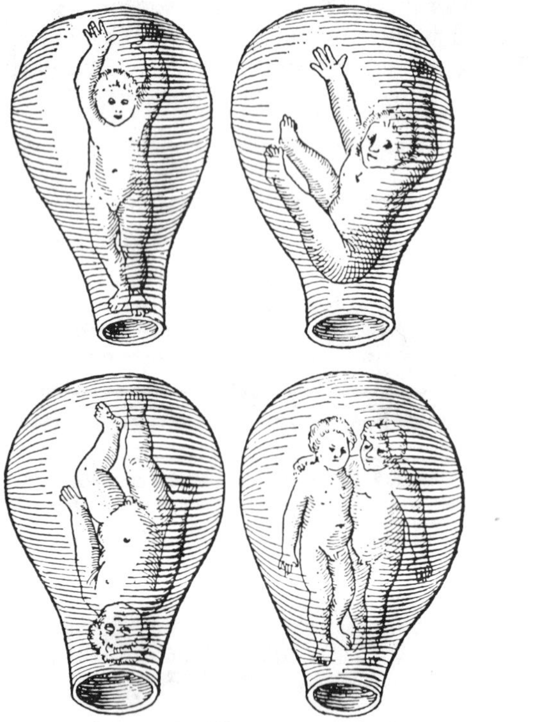

Figure 16–13. Illustrations from the first textbook on obstetrics, Roesslin's "Rosengarten," 1513, showing a former concept of fetal positions *in utero*.

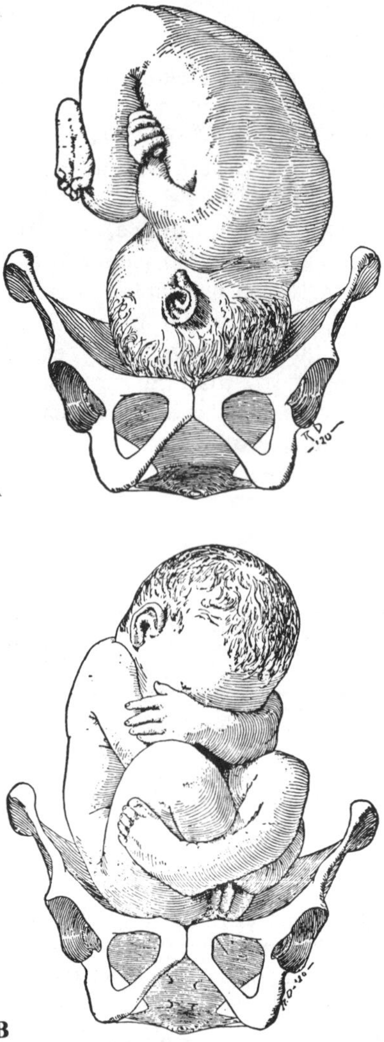

A

B

Figure 16–14. *A*. Attitude of fetus in vertex presentation. *B*. Attitude of fetus in complete or full breech presentation.

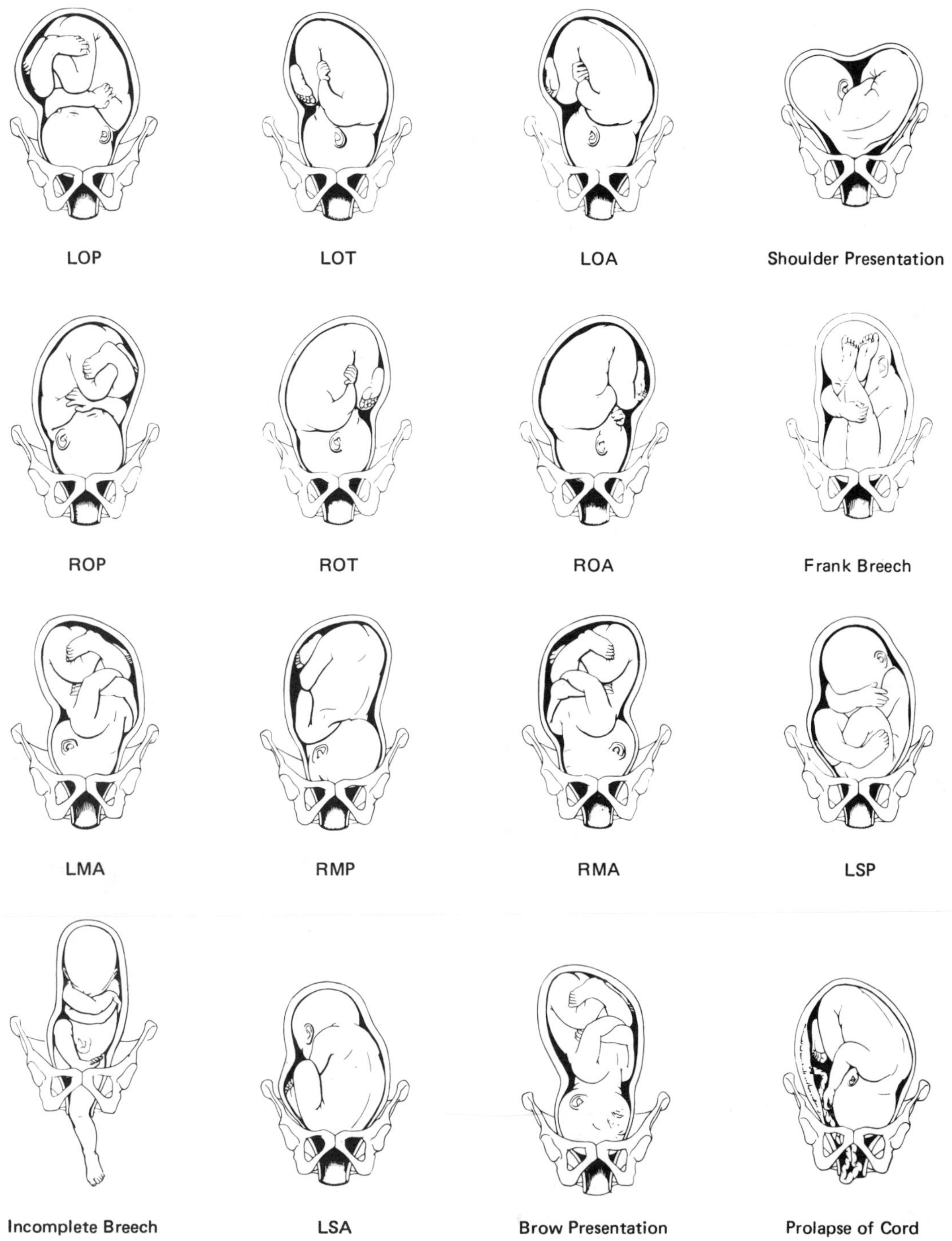

Figure 16–15. Categories of presentation. (Reprinted with permission from Obstetrical Presentation and Position, Ross Clinical Education Aid #18, Ross Laboratories, Columbus, Ohio.)

The posture usually assumed is one in which the head is sharply flexed with the chin near the chest; the vertex is then lowermost in the pelvis, making a *vertex presentation* (Fig. 16–14*A*). Occasionally the head is sharply extended with the occiput nearly touching the back and the face lowermost; this is called a *face presentation* (Fig. 16–15).

The fetal head may assume a position intermediate between sharp flexion and sharp extension; when it is partly flexed, the large fontanel is the lowermost part making a *bregma* or a *sincipital presentation;* and when it is partly extended, the brow becomes the presenting part, making a *brow presentation* (Fig. 16–15). Sincipital and brow presentations are usually transient; the head either flexes or extends more completely as labor progresses, and the presentation changes to vertex or face, the vertex being far more common. Cephalic presentation occurs in over 96 percent of longitudinal lies; the ratio of vertex presentation to face is over 300 to 1.

Breech presentations also are described in several varieties according to the position of the fetal lower extremities in relation to its body. The fetal legs may be in the position that they characteristically assume *in utero* with the thighs flexed on the abdomen and the legs flexed on the thighs (squatting position); the buttocks and the feet then present, and the term *complete breech* or *full breech presentation* is used (Fig. 16–14*B*). Often the legs are extended so that they lie against the anterior trunk with the feet touching the face; in this position only the buttocks present, and the term *frank breech presentation* is applied (Fig. 16–15). In another variety, *incomplete breech presentation,* one or both feet or knees have prolapsed so that they are lower than the buttocks and become the presenting part (Fig. 16–15). When only one foot presents, the other leg assumes the position that it would take in either a complete or frank breech presentation. An incomplete breech presentation may be of two types, a *footling presentation,* either *single* or *double,* or a *knee presentation.* Breech presentation occurs in about 3.5 percent of deliveries, and the frank breech is the most frequent.

Presentation does not become fully established until the presenting part has entered the pelvic inlet, and it therefore may change during the latter part of pregnancy, most frequently changing from breech to cephalic. The possibility of change lessens, however, as the end of pregnancy approaches.

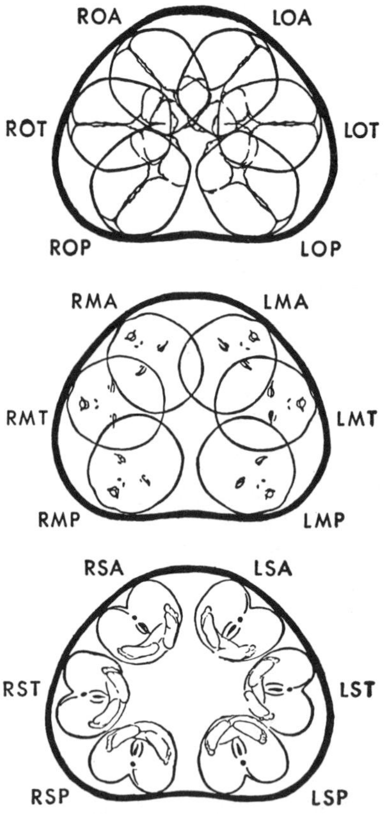

Figure 16–16. Diagrams showing the six possible positions of a vertex presentation, a face presentation, and a breech presentation as seen when looking at the pelvis from below.

Position

After the lie and presentation of the fetus have been established by the examiner, the relationship of the presenting part to the maternal pelvis is defined more specifically. This is done by stating the *position* of the fetus. The term "position," as used here, means the relation that an arbitrarily chosen point on the presenting part of the fetus bears to a specific part of the maternal pelvis. The arbitrary points designated for describing the fetal position are the occiput in a vertex presentation, the chin (mentum) in a face presentation, the sacrum in all varieties of breech presentations, and the scapula in a shoulder presentation. For purposes of stating quite precisely the relationship of the arbitrarily chosen point (occiput, chin, or sacrum) to the maternal pelvis, the pelvis is divided into six segments—an anterior, transverse, and posterior segment on the right side, and an anterior, transverse, and posterior segment on the left side. The occiput, the chin, or the sacrum may occupy any one of these six segments, thus making it possible to describe six positions for each presentation (Fig. 16–16).

When the fetus is so positioned in the uterus that the head is lowermost and flexed, with the chin resting on the chest, the vertex is the presenting part, and the occiput is the arbitrarily chosen point. If the occiput is found to be lying in the left anterior segment of the maternal pelvis, the position is occiput left anterior. However, in general usage, the right or left side is usually specified first when position is stated, and the position described above is called a left occiput anterior instead of an occiput left anterior.

Positions usually are expressed in abbreviations, determined by the first letter of each word; the left occiput anterior position therefore is usually stated as an LOA position. When the occiput is turned *directly* toward the maternal left side, neither to the front nor the back, the position is a left occiput transverse, or LOT, and when it lies in the left posterior segment of the pelvis, the position is left occiput posterior, or LOP. As there are three corresponding segments on the right side of the pelvis, anterior, transverse, and posterior, there are six possible positions for the fetus to occupy in the vertex presentation (Figs. 16–15 and 16–16). The names and abbreviations of these positions are shown in Table 16–2. Similarly, there is a possibility of six face positions (Fig. 16–16) and six breech positions (Fig. 16–16). When

Table 16-2. Categories of Lie, Presentation, and Position of the Fetus *in Utero*

Lie	*Presentation*		*Position and Abbreviation*			
Longitudinal	Cephalic	Vertex	Left occiput anterior	LOA	Right occiput anterior	ROA
			Left occiput transverse	LOT	Right occiput transverse	ROT
			Left occiput posterior	LOP	Right occiput posterior	ROP
		Face	Left mentum anterior	LMA	Right mentum anterior	RMA
			Left mentum transverse	LMT	Right mentum transverse	RMT
			Left mentum posterior	LMP	Right mentum posterior	RMP
		Sincipital	....			
		Brow	....			
	Breech	Complete (full) breech	Left sacrum anterior	LSA	Right sacrum anterior	RSA
		Frank breech	Left sacrum transverse	LST	Right sacrum transverse	RST
		Incomplete breech	Left sacrum posterior	LSP	Right sacrum posterior	RSP
		Footling Single Double				
		Knee				
Transverse	Shoulder		Left scapula anterior	LScA	Right scapula anterior	RScA
			Left scapula posterior	LScP	Right scapula posterior	RScP

the chin (mentum) rests in the left anterior segment of the maternal pelvis, the position is left mentum anterior, or LMA. When the breech presents and the sacrum is in that relation, the position is left sacrum anterior, or LSA (Figs. 16-15 and 16-16).

In a shoulder presentation (transverse lie) there are only four positions, since the shoulder is either anterior or posterior on the right or the left side of the maternal pelvis (Fig. 16-15). The scapula (of the presenting shoulder) usually is chosen as the point of direction; sometimes the acromion process is chosen.

The fetal position may change frequently before engagement of the presenting part. The back may be toward one side of the maternal body on one day and toward the other side on another day. After the presenting part becomes engaged in the pelvis, positional changes are in a narrower range, taking place from one segment to another on the same side of the pelvis.

Internal rotation of the head (in the pelvis), one of the movements in the mechanism of labor, described on pages 345–46, brings about a change in position whereby the anteroposterior diameter of the head comes to lie in the anteroposterior diameter of the pelvic outlet; this change is necessary for the head to emerge from the pelvis. The rotation is usually such that the occiput comes to lie directly behind the symphysis pubis; the position is then described as *direct occiput anterior, direct OA*. Sometimes the head turns so that the occiput lies in the hollow of the sacrum, this is known as *direct occiput posterior, direct OP*.

Some positions are more common than others at the onset of labor. Since a vertex presentation occurs in the majority of cases, the occiput position is most common. The head enters the pelvis with the occiput in a transverse position more frequently than in an anterior or posterior position and is directed toward the left side of the maternal pelvis more frequently than toward the right side.

ENGAGEMENT AND STATION

Engagement of the Presenting Part

Engagement means that the presenting part of the fetus has descended into the pelvis to the level where its widest diameter has passed through the pelvic inlet. In cephalic presentation the widest diameter is the biparietal, and in breech presentation it is the intertrochanteric. Engagement of the head thus means that the fetus has descended into the pelvis to a level where the biparietal plane (the greatest transverse diameter) of the head has passed through the pelvic inlet. Engagment of the head is evidence that the pelvic inlet is large enough to accommodate the fetal head. Engagement does not provide information about the relationship between the size of the head and the remainder of the pelvic canal (the midpelvis and the pelvic outlet).

Engagement may be gradual or quite sudden. In the majority of women in their first pregnancy, engagement takes place before the onset of labor; many times it occurs somewhere around two weeks before labor begins and at times even earlier. In women who have previously had children, engagement generally does not take place until the onset of labor. The fetus does not sink into the pelvis as readily as in a first pregnancy because the multigravida is likely to have more relaxed abdominal muscles and there is less downward pressure on the fetus.

In certain abnormalities, or in disproportion between the fetal head and the maternal pelvis, engagement of the head may not take place until after labor is well established, or possibly not at all. An unengaged head at the beginning of labor in a primigravida is not necessarily indicative of disproportion between the fetal head and the maternal pelvis, but close observation for such a possibility is considered essential.

Engagement is ascertained by abdominal palpation and by vaginal or rectal examination. From abdominal examination, engagement is determined by palpation of the presenting part of the fetus for the degree of its descent into the pelvis. In vertex presentation, this is ascertained from the part of the fetal head that can be felt when the examiner's hands are placed on each side of the lower abdomen and the fingers are pushed downward toward the pelvis. If the lower part of the head can be palpated with the fingers, it is not engaged; if it cannot be felt, it is probably engaged.

On vaginal or rectal examination, engagement is determined by the relationship of the lowermost part of the presenting part of the fetus to the level of the ischial spines. In vertex presentation, the head is engaged when its lowest part is at or below the level of the ischial spines, unless it is markedly elongated due to molding of the bones or swelling of the scalp. If unusual elongation is suspected, an x-ray ordinarily is indicated to establish the relationship between the fetal head and the pelvis.

In breech presentation, engagement of the breech has taken place when the bitrochanteric diameter has passed through the inlet of the pelvis. The breech is less likely to engage prior to the onset of labor than is the fetal head, but descent of the breech ordinarily progresses well during active labor. Estimation of degree of descent is likely to be more difficult in breech than in vertex presentation. X-ray facilitates diagnosis when there is doubt. Since the breech is smaller than the head, its engagement does not have the same significance concerning size of the pelvic inlet as does engagement of the head. Descent of the breech in the pelvis is important to the progress of labor.

Station of the Presenting Part

The station of the presenting part is the degree to which it has descended into the pelvis. A method of describing station is to state the distance (in centimeters) between the lowermost level of the presenting part and the level of the ischial spines. The most dependent area of the presenting part may be at the level of the spines or above them or below them.

The relationship between the presenting part and the ischial spines is determined by vaginal or rectal examination; the soft rectovaginal wall readily permits palpation through it on rectal examination. In the examination, the most dependent portion of the presenting part (usually the top of the fetal head) is located first; next the side walls of the pelvis are palpated to find the ischial spines, and an imaginary line is drawn between them; then the vertical distance (up or down) between this imaginary line and the most dependent portion of the presenting part is estimated in centimeters.

The station (degree of descent) is stated in numerical terms. The line between the ischial spines is called a zero station, any distance above the line is called a minus station, and any distance below the line is called a plus station. When the lowest level of the presenting part is on the level of the line between the ischial spines, the presenting part is said to be at zero station (or at the spines); when it is above the line, it is said to be at −1 (1 cm above), −2 (2 cm above), or −3 (3 cm above) station; and when it is below the line, it is described as at +1 (1 cm below), +2 (2 cm below), or +3 (3 cm below) station (Fig. 16–17).

Certain general terms, other than numbers, may be used to describe degree of engagement. A presenting part that is not engaged is said to be *high;* it may be further described as floating or as fixed in the inlet. Both of these stations can be determined by abdominal palpation. When palpation reveals the presenting part to be freely movable above the pelvic inlet, it is described as *floating;* when it is entering the pelvis, as *dipping* or entering; and when it is no longer movable, but not yet low enough to be engaged, it is described as *fixed in the inlet.* When the head has descended to the place where the biparietal plane has passed through the pelvic inlet, the term *engaged* is used, and when the presenting part is well below the level of the ischial spines, it is said to be *low.* If the presenting part is sufficiently low to push on the pelvic floor, the degree of descent may be described by the term *on the pelvic floor,* and when it has de-

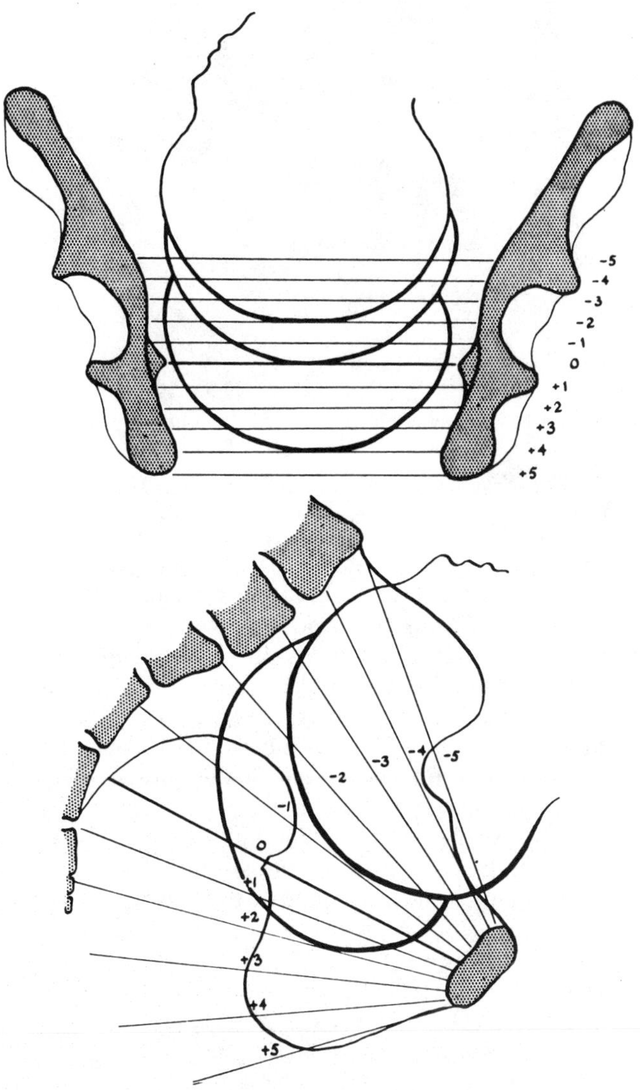

Figure 16–17. Station of the fetal head. Representation of the designations of fetal station, anteroposterior (top) and lateral (bottom) aspects, as the relation of the forward leading edge of the fetal presenting part to the plane of the ischial spines (*station 0*), in centimeters above (minus values) and below (plus values) this reference plane. While parallel in the anteroposterior view, the planes diverge in the lateral view (wider posteriorly than anteriorly) as they follow the curvilinear pelvic architecture. In the anteroposterior view, fetal heads are shown at station −2 (dipping), 0 (engaged), and +4 (on pelvic floor); in lateral view, −1 and +2. (Reproduced with permission from Emanuel A. Friedman. *Labor: Clinical Evaluation and Management*, 2nd ed. New York: Appleton-Century-Crofts, 1978.)

Table 16–3. Correlation of Terms Used to Describe Descent of the Presenting Part into the Pelvis

Broad Terms	*Specific Terms*	*Station*
Presenting part high	Floating	−4
	Dipping	−3
		−2
	Fixed, but not engaged	−1
	Engaged	Ischial spine > -0- < Ischial spine
		+1
Presenting part low		+2
	On the pelvic floor	+3
	Bulging of the perineum	+4

scended so far that it distends the perineum, the term *bulging of the perineum* is used. This last usually occurs only toward the end of labor (Table 16–3).

Accurate information about the degree to which the presenting part has descended at the beginning of labor, and about the rate of descent during labor, is necessary in evaluation of progress of labor. Descent may occur prior to labor, during dilation of the cervix (first stage of labor), during the second stage of labor, or, gradually, at all these times; this is explained more completely in Chapter 17. Degree of descent is determined each time the woman is examined during the latter part of pregnancy and during labor.

DIAGNOSIS OF PRESENTATION AND POSITION

Presentation and position of the baby are ascertained by means of abdominal palpation, vaginal examination, and x-ray.

Abdominal Palpation

Palpation of the fetal body through the maternal abdominal wall is ordinarily possible during the latter months of pregnancy because the uterine and abdominal muscles are so stretched and thinned that the various parts of the fetal body can be felt through them. Abdominal palpation is the most useful method of making a diagnosis of presentation and position in the latter part of pregnancy; it also can be used for the same purpose during labor, if it is performed in the intervals between uterine contractions. Palpation is sometimes difficult with hydramnios, and it may be impossible in very obese women. Abdominal palpation is also used to obtain other important information. It is one means of determining the distance to which the presenting part has descended into the pelvis. If the head has not descended, it may be possible to detect disproportion between the fetal head and the pelvic inlet by ascertaining whether or not the head overrides the symphysis pubis when it is pressed toward the inlet. Palpation is also used to make a rough estimate of the fetal size.

Abdominal palpation is a method that is readily available to the nurse for determination of presentation and position. During this examination the client should lie flat on her back with her knees slightly flexed. The bladder should be empty for comfort and for ease of palpation. Successful results require that pressure be applied to the abdomen with firmness and evenness, but this must be done gently. Cold hands, or quick, jabbing motions with the fingers, will usually stimulate the muscles lying beneath them to contract, thus somewhat obscuring the outline of the fetus. Such movements are also uncomfortable for the woman, whereas firm, even pressure, started gently, with warm hands, ordinarily does not cause discomfort. Abdominal palpation should be performed in a systematic manner. One such system, described below, consists of four maneuvers, often called the maneuvers of Leopold.

Before beginning the maneuvers of Leopold, the general contour of the uterus should be observed and outlined, to determine if the fetal body is parallel or transverse to the maternal body. As noted above, the fetal body is usually parallel to the maternal body, and the presentation is either cephalic or breech. With this much information, the examinations described below are made to ascertain presentation and position more exactly.

First Maneuver (Figs. 16–18 and 16–22)

The purpose of the first maneuver is to determine what is in the fundus; this is usually either the breech or the head. Facing the client the nurse gently applies the entire tactile surface of the fingers of both hands to the upper part of the abdomen, on opposite sides and somewhat curved around the fundus of the uterus. The outline of the pole of the fetus that occupies the fundus may be palpated. If the head is uppermost, it will be felt as a hard, round object which is movable, or *ballottable,* between the two hands, and if it is the breech, it will be felt as a softer, less movable, less regularly shaped body.

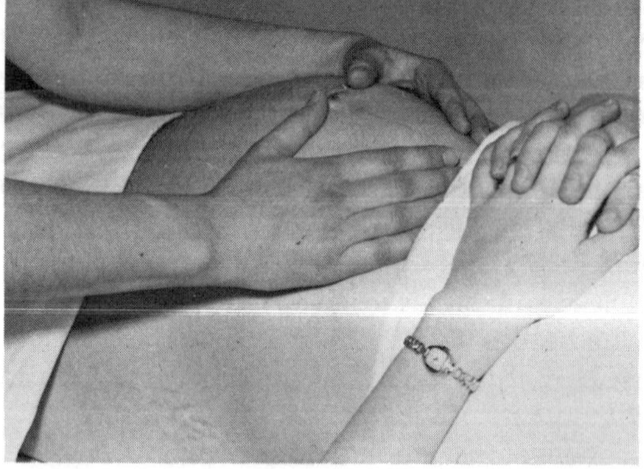

Figure 16–18. First maneuver in abdominal palpation to discover position of fetus.

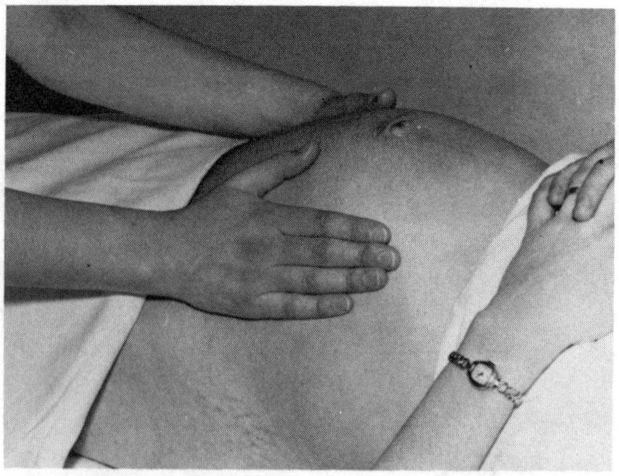

Figure 16–19. Second maneuver in abdominal palpation.

Second Maneuver (Figs. 16–19 and 16–22)

Having determined whether the breech or the head is in the fundus, the next step is to locate the fetal back and small parts in their relation to the right and left side of the mother. This is accomplished, while still facing the woman, by sliding the hands down to a slightly lower position on the sides of the abdomen. Firm, even pressure is made with the entire palmar surface of both hands. The back is felt as a smooth, hard surface under the palm and fingers of one hand, and it offers a resistance that prevents the hand from being pressed in as deeply as the hand on the opposite side. The small parts (hands, feet, elbows, knees) are felt as irregular knobs or lumps under the hand on the side opposite from the back.

As the same time that the fetal back is palpated, the nurse should note whether it is in the anterior or lateral portion of the right or left side of the abdomen. This information will be valuable in determining the relationship of the presenting part to the anterior, transverse, or posterior segment of the maternal pelvis.

Third Maneuver (Figs. 16–20 and 16–22)

The third maneuver confirms the impression gained by the first maneuver as to which fetal pole is directed toward the pelvis and also indicates whether the presenting part is floating or has entered the pelvis. The thumb and fingers of one hand are spread as widely as possible, applied to the abdomen just above the symphysis pubis, and then brought together to grasp the part of the fetus that lies between them.

Either head or breech may be identified; the head gives the sensation of a hard, round mass at the lower fetal pole. If engaged, the presenting part may be difficult to palpate because it has descended so deeply into the pelvis. If the lower pole is movable, engagement has not occurred; if the lower pole is fixed, it may be engaged or merely entering the pelvic inlet.

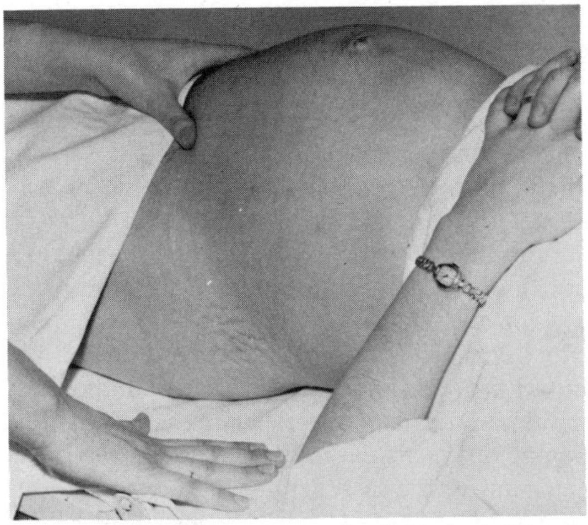

Figure 16–20. Third maneuver in abdominal palpation.

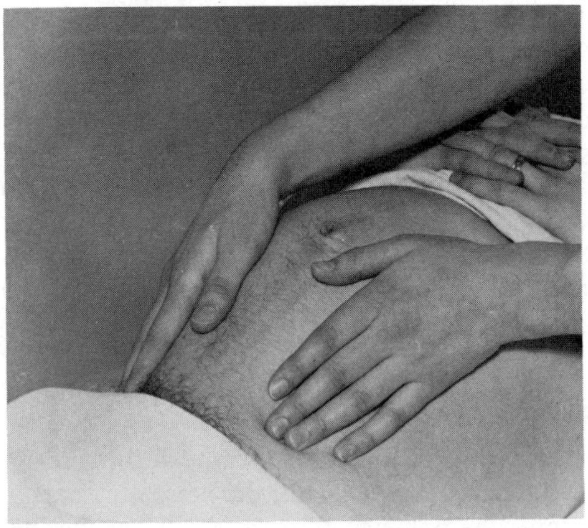

Figure 16–21. Fourth maneuver in abdominal palpation.

Fourth Maneuver (Figs. 16–21 and 16–22)

The fourth maneuver is of particular value after the presenting part has become engaged. The nurse faces the woman's feet and places the tips of the fingers of each hand on each side of the midline of the lower abdomen. Deep pressure is then made in a downward and slightly inward direction—toward the pelvic inlet—with somewhat of a gliding motion that moves the skin on the lower abdomen downward along with the fingers. With the head presenting, the fingers on one side may be arrested in their downward progress by the cephalic prominence, the most marked protrusion of the fetal head, while the fingers on the other side may descend farther. A cephalic prominence felt on the same side as the small parts is the brow; this gives evidence that the head is

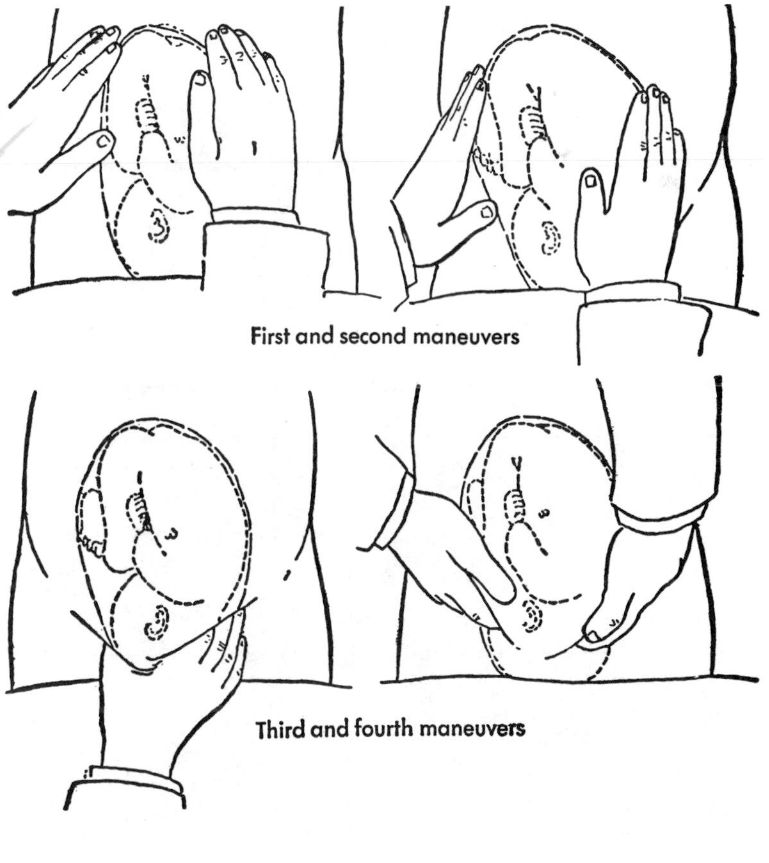

Figure 16–22. Diagram showing relation of examiner's hands to fetus in the four maneuvers in abdominal palpation.

flexed, that the vertex is lowermost in the pelvis, thus that the presentation is vertex. A cephalic prominence on the same side as the fetal back is the occiput; the head is then extended and the face is downward, making a face presentation.

The fourth maneuver helps to determine how far the presenting part has descended into the pelvis. When the cephalic prominence is readily palpable, the head is not engaged. After engagement, it becomes quite difficult to feel the cephalic prominence.

Vaginal Examination

When a vaginal examination is done during pregnancy, while the cervix is still closed, the presenting part of the fetus must be palpated through the lower uterine segment. This makes identification of landmarks difficult and the findings concerning presentation and position may add little to those obtained by abdominal palpation. However, from vaginal examination, information concerning the station of the presenting part, the softness and length of the cervix, and the pelvic configuration can be ascertained.

During labor, when the cervix has thinned and dilated, a vaginal examination provides valuable information about presentation, position, and station of the fetus, as well as information about cervical effacement and dilation. The presenting part is palpated more easily through a dilated cervix and landmarks often can be differentiated. In a vertex presentation, a diagnosis of position is made by feeling the sutures and fontanels of the fetal head and determining from them which segment of the pelvis is occupied by the occiput. In a face presentation, the features of the face are differentiated; and in a breech presentation, the buttocks and the sacrum are palpated for their placement in the pelvis. Fairly accurate determinations can often be made by rectal examination, but when there is a question of cephalopelvic relationship or of an abnormal presentation, or when there is doubt about the findings of a rectal examination, a vaginal examination is essential. Findings on vaginal examination are usually more reliable than those on rectal examination, since the cervix and the fetal landmarks are palpated directly rather than through several layers of maternal tissue. In general, rectal examinations are now obsolete and are ordinarily replaced by vaginal examinations. Details of performing a vaginal examination, one that nurses frequently make, are presented in Chapter 20.

X-Ray

Presentation, position, and station of the fetus can be visualized by an abdominal x-ray. This method of diagnosis is sometimes used when abdominal palpation of the fetus is difficult or impossible for some reason (for example, obesity) or when the information gained by vaginal examination during labor is uncertain (Figs. 16–23 and 16–24). X-ray is often used to gain additional information when the fetus is found to be in a markedly

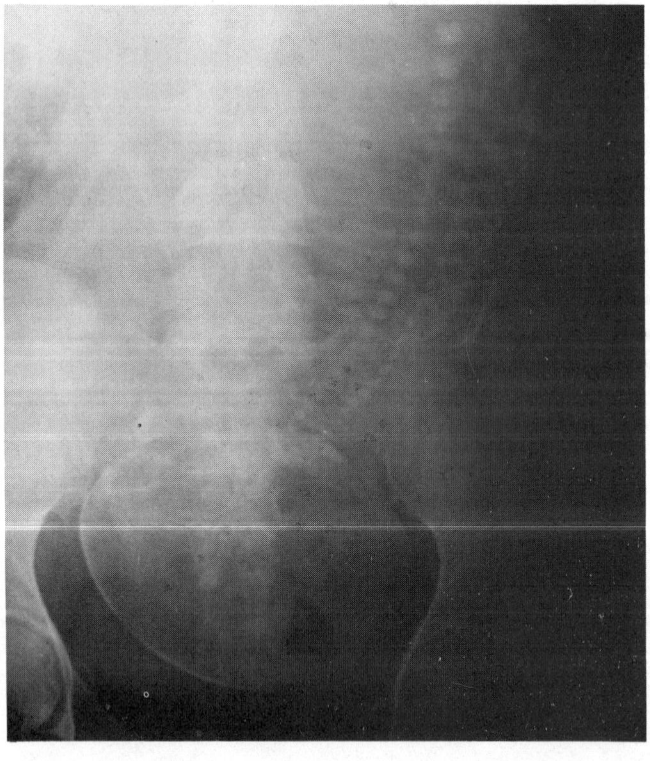

Figure 16–23. An x-ray taken on a woman who was believed to be close to term. It had previously been determined that a cesarean section was indicated, but since the gestational age was not definitely known and palpation of the abdomen was difficult, a roentgenogram seemed indicated to determine fetal size and position.

The x-ray shows a single well-developed fetal skeleton with the head presenting at the inlet and with the back lying to the left and anteriorly. The fetal size and skeletal development correspond to those of the last month of gestation. There is no evidence of fetal skeletal abnormalities.

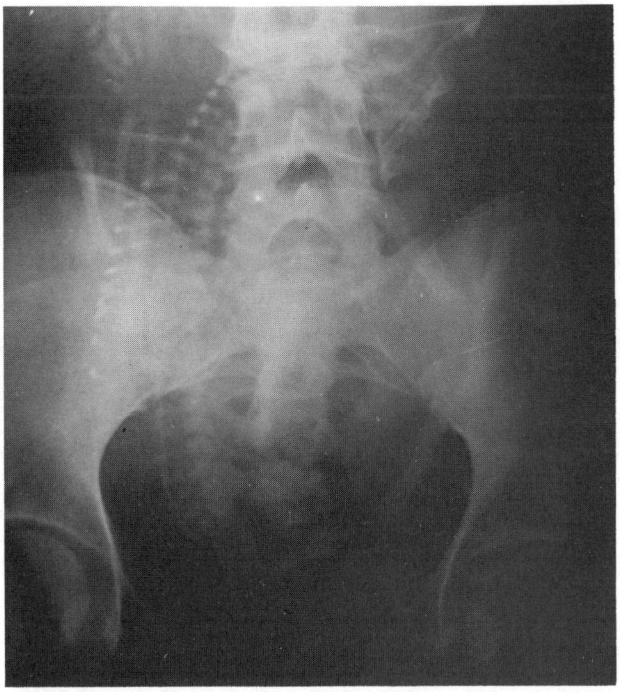

Figure 16–24. This roentgenogram shows a well-developed fetus in a frank breech presentation with the sacrum to the right and anterior.

abnormal position. When x-ray pelvimetry is required to determine whether disproportion exists between the maternal pelvis and the fetal head, fetal presentation, position, and station can also be determined from the pelvimetry films. An x-ray is of value in making an accurate diagnosis when there is a question of multiple pregnancy; it is an aid in estimating the size and development of the fetus; and it may show the existence of fetal abnormalities.

AUSCULTATION OF THE FETAL HEART

The fetal heart is auscultated when abdominal palpation is done, and preceding and following other examinations. The fetal heart is heard through a stethoscope placed against the mother's abdomen (Fig. 16–25).

The sounds of the heartbeat are usually transmitted through the convex surface of the fetus that lies closest to the uterine wall; in vertex and breech presentations this is the back, and in face presentation it is the thorax. The area of the mother's abdomen in which the fetal heart is heard best depends on the position of the baby and the degree of descent into the pelvis. In cephalic presentations the heart usually is heard best below the umbilicus; this may be very low, close to the pelvic region, if the head is deeply engaged. In breech presentation the heart usually is heard best at, or above, the level of the umbilicus. When the occiput occupies the anterior segment of the maternal pelvis, the fetal heart generally is heard best near the midline of the maternal abdomen; when the occiput is in the transverse segment of the pelvis, the heart is heard farther toward the maternal side; and when in the posterior segment, the heartbeat is heard far toward the maternal back. Location of the maximal fetal heart sound sometimes reinforces the findings of presentation and position by palpation.

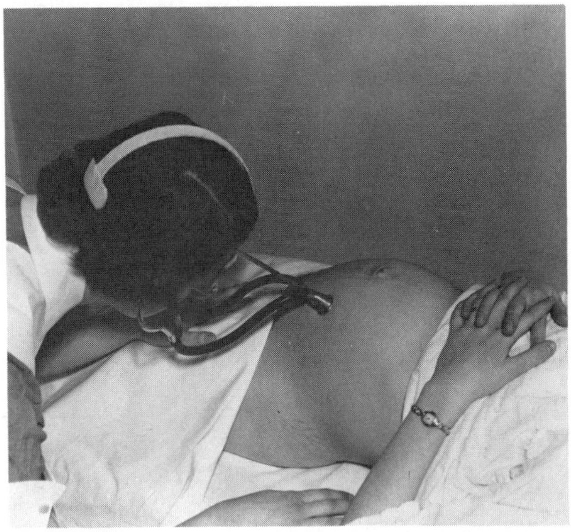

Figure 16–25. Auscultation of the fetal heart.

REFERENCES AND SUGGESTED READINGS

Friedman, Emanuel A., *Labor: Clinical Evaluation and Management,* 2nd ed., Appleton-Century-Crofts, New York, 1978.

Iffy, Leslie, and Kaminetzky, Harold A. (eds.), *Principles and Practice of Obstetrics and Perinatology,* Vol. II. John Wiley, New York, 1981.

Oxorn, Harry, *Oxorn-Foote Human Labor and Birth,* 4th ed., Appleton-Century-Crofts, New York, 1980.

Pritchard, Jack A., and MacDonald, Paul C., *Williams Obstetrics,* 16th ed., Appleton-Century-Crofts, New York, 1980.

Verralls, Sylvia, *Anatomy and Physiology Applied to Obstetrics,* 2nd ed., Pitman Medical Limited, Turbridge Wells, Kent, 1980, Chapters 2 and 13.

CHAPTER

17

The Clinical Course and Mechanism of Labor and Delivery

Revised by Sue A. Frazier, R.N., M.S.N.

THE PROCESSES that lead to progressive effacement and dilation of the cervix and the descent of the presenting part, with eventual expulsion of the fetus and the other products of conception, is known as *labor*. The actual birth of the infant is called the *delivery*. Ordinarily labor occurs near the end of the tenth lunar month, at which time pregnancy is said to be *at term*.

At term the pregnant uterus is a thin-walled, muscular sac containing the mature fetus, the placenta to which the fetus is connected by the umbilical cord, and the amniotic fluid, which surrounds the fetus. The fetus and fluid are contained in the sac formed by the amniotic and chorionic membranes. The average fetus at term is about 50.8 cm (20 in.) long and weighs about 3400 gm (7½ lb).

Somewhere near term, contractions of the uterine muscle become forceful enough to expel the products of conception, the series of processes being called labor. Sometimes pregnancy ends prior to term; when this occurs *after* the fetus has reached the period of viability (about the twenty-sixth week of pregnancy), but *before* the end of the thirty-sixth week of gestation), the term *premature labor* is used. From the end of the thirty-sixth week to term the fetus and hence the labor may be considered as term.

The course of labor is dependent on many variables, each differing not only from one woman to another, but also in successive labors of the same woman. A typical course of labor may be outlined as described below, with the understanding that any given labor may differ markedly from this prototype.

At the onset of labor the uterine contractions are weak and infrequent, being anywhere from 10 to 30 minutes apart. As labor progresses, the contractions become more forceful and more frequent until the interval between them is approximately 2 to 3 minutes. These involuntary uterine contractions dilate the cervix until it is large enough to permit the fetus to pass through; then with the aid of voluntary contractions of the abdominal muscles, the uterine contractions move the fetus down through the birth canal. Finally the placenta is separated from the uterine wall and expelled.

The three factors—powers, passenger, and passage—concerned with the process by which the fetus is born have been discussed previously. The passage, the passenger, and their interrelationship have been described in Chapter 16. The present chapter will describe in detail the powers—those forces that move the passenger through the passage—as well as the mechanism by which such passage takes place.

LABOR

Cause of Labor

The cause of the onset of labor is not definitely known. Many theories have been advanced to explain why the muscular contractions, which have occurred painlessly and without expulsive force throughout pregnancy, finally become effective at approximately the end of the tenth lunar month of pregnancy. It is also not known why some labors occur before and others after the expected date.

Labor appears to be the result of a combination of factors, which include fetal control, steroid hormone changes, production of prostaglandins, oxytocin stimulation, and uterine muscle changes. It appears that all these factors play some role, and that labor is the result of a combination of interrelated physiologic changes, particularly endocrine changes, but all factors are not necessarily essential at any one time.

From evidence to date, it is thought that at some appropriate time, determined by the fetus, the fetal pituitary gland secretes increasing amounts of ACTH and oxytocin. Fetal ACTH is believed to stimulate the adrenal to increased activity, and fetal oxytocin is thought to cross the placenta and add to the action of maternal oxytocin. Evidence of the influence of the fetal endocrine system is not certain, but is inferred from observations of prolonged pregnancies associated with fetal pituitary and adrenal abnormalities.

ACTH and possibly fetal prolactin stimulate the fetal adrenal to secrete increasing amounts of cortisol, which precipitates a series of events that initiate labor and also promote fetal lung maturation.

Steroid hormone changes that take place near the end of pregnancy include a decrease in progesterone production (progesterone withdrawal), which allows increased uterine muscle excitability, and an increase in estrogen production, which enhances rhythmic uterine contractions and their responsiveness to oxytocin. These changes in production of steroids by the placenta appear to be the result of increased fetal adrenal gland activity—utilization of progesterone and increased production of estrogen precursors.

Prostaglandins, which stimulate uterine contractions, increase significantly in amniotic fluid during labor and may thus have a considerable influence on the initiation of labor.

The myometrium becomes more excitable and contractile with increasing volume as pregnancy progresses, and it is known that the uterus becomes more responsive to oxytocin with advancing pregnancy. Although definite evidence is lacking, it is assumed that oxytocin plays a role in the initiation of labor.

Although the exact processes are obviously not known, changes in endocrine relationships appear to stimulate the onset of labor. Some of these changes begin to appear several weeks before labor begins.

Stages of Labor

The process of labor is divided into three periods or stages:

First stage or stage of dilation—begins with the onset of regular contractions and ends with complete dilation of the cervix.

Second stage or stage of expulsion—begins with complete dilation of the cervix and ends with complete delivery of the fetus.

Third stage or placental stage—begins immediately after the fetus is born and ends when the placenta is delivered.

The Forces of Labor

The forces of labor are muscular contractions, primarily of the uterine muscle and secondarily of the abdominal muscles. Uterine muscle contractions effect all the changes during the first stage of labor, which lead to complete effacement and dilation of the cervix. The secondary force of abdominal muscle contractions is effective only after the cervix has been completely dilated and at that time is ordinarily added to the primary force.

Duration of Labor

The duration of normal labor may vary from an extremely short time, comprising only a few contractions, up to approximately 24 hours. Although there is wide variation, the average length of first labors is approximately 12½ hours. This is an average figure; some primiparous labors will be considerably shorter and some much longer. When the 12½ hours are divided according to the duration of each stage, the length may be as follows: first stage, 11 hours; second stage, 70 minutes; and third stage, 10 minutes. Subsequent labors average about 8 hours in length, with a first stage of a little over 7 hours, a second stage of 30 minutes, and a third stage of 10 minutes.

The duration of labor depends in part on the effectiveness of the powers—the strength and frequency of the uterine contractions—and also in part on the amount of resistance that must be overcome as the fetus accommodates to the bony pelvis while the soft tissues stretch to permit passage of the fetus. The longer labor in primigravidas as compared with multigravidas is due chiefly to the greater resistance offered by the cervix, by the soft parts of the vagina and pelvic floor, and by the perineum.

Premonitory Signs of Labor

Sometimes labor seems to start suddenly, but often signs of its approach appear several hours, a day, or even a week or more before its actual onset. In general, these signs are lightening, false labor pains, changes in the cervix, show, and rupture of the membranes. The woman herself can be aware of all of these signs with the exception of changes in the cervix, which may be noted by the nurse or physician when a sterile vaginal examination is done. Lightening and sporadic false labor pains may occur at any time during the last weeks of pregnancy, and the nearness of labor cannot be closely judged from these signs. The appearance of bloody show and rupture of the membranes are better evidence of imminent labor. In some instances the woman is not aware of any premonitory signs of labor; in other instances she has noticed most, or all, of the signs.

Lightening

Lightening is the descent of the uterus downward and forward, which takes place when the presenting part descends into the pelvis far enough to become fixed, and often deep enough to become engaged. With descent of the uterus, the top of the fundus settles to the level that it had reached at about the eighth month of pregnancy, and the lower part of the abdomen becomes more prominent. As with engagement, lightening may come about gradually or quite suddenly, and it is more common in women with good abdominal muscle tone. Primigravidas are much more likely to experience lightening than multigravidas.

The woman is aware of the occurrence of lightening, which she often speaks of as "dropping" of the baby, through a lowering of her waistline and through relief of pressure in the upper abdomen but increased pressure in the pelvic region. She usually breathes more comfortably after this change in abdominal contour, but, at the same time, may have cramps in her legs, more difficulty walking, frequent micturition, and pressure in the rectum.

The time at which lightening takes place may vary from a few weeks to a few days before the onset of labor. In multigravidas lightening may not occur before labor. Lightening is a sign of approaching labor, but because of the variable time of its appearance, it is not very useful in predicting the onset of labor. As a rule, lightening is evidence that the fetal head will not be too large for the pelvic inlet.

False Labor Pains

Contractions that may be more or less regular and may become quite uncomfortable, but that subside without effecting dilation of the cervix, are termed *false labor*. This occurs more often in the multigravida than in the primigravida. In false labor, the painless uterine contractions, called *Braxton-Hicks contractions,* which may have been present throughout pregnancy, become painful, similar to true labor contractions. These moderately painful contractions often occur at night and then subside toward morning.

The appearance of false labor pains usually indicates that true labor is imminent, but sometimes false labor contractions recur for days before true labor begins, and they may even recur intermittently for three to four weeks before the onset of labor. It is difficult to distinguish false labor from true labor, and the woman may enter the hospital thinking that she is in labor.

This is a disappointing experience for her. Sometimes a woman is admitted to the hospital for a second or even a third time in false instead of true labor. She will need considerable assurance that false labor is not uncommon and that she does not need to be apologetic for being unable to distinguish false from true labor contractions.

False labor may be suspected when the contractions occur irregularly, when they do not appear with increasing frequency, and when their intensity does not increase. The discomfort from false labor contractions is usually located in the abdomen instead of beginning in the back, as with true labor contractions, and it is generally not intensified, and may be lessened, with activity. *The major differentiating feature is that the cervix does not change appreciably in thickness and does not dilate during false labor, while in true labor the cervix becomes progressively thinner and dilation takes place.*

Changes in the Cervix

As labor approaches, the cervix, which during pregnancy has been long, relatively firm, and closed, usually becomes softer and shorter and sometimes slightly dilated. It may have become very short, almost completely obliterated, by the time labor begins, and the diameter of the external os may have increased in size to a measurement of 1 to 2 cm.

Show

A tenacious mucoid vaginal discharge may appear shortly before the onset of labor. This may be pinkish in color or it may be slightly blood streaked. The discharge is known as the *show* or *bloody show,* or it may be termed *expulsion of the mucous plug*. This mucus, secreted by the cervical glands, has accumulated in the cervical canal during pregnancy, where it served to close the opening leading to the uterine cavity. As the cervix shortens and the canal enlarges toward the end of pregnancy or at the onset of labor, the mucous plug is expelled from the canal and discharged from the vagina. Sometimes some of the superficial mucosa of the cervical canal is expelled with the mucous plug. The slight oozing that accompanies this separation results in the blood streaking.

Labor ordinarily begins 24 to 48 hours after the mucous plug or show appears. However, the mucous plug may not be observed until the onset of labor, and

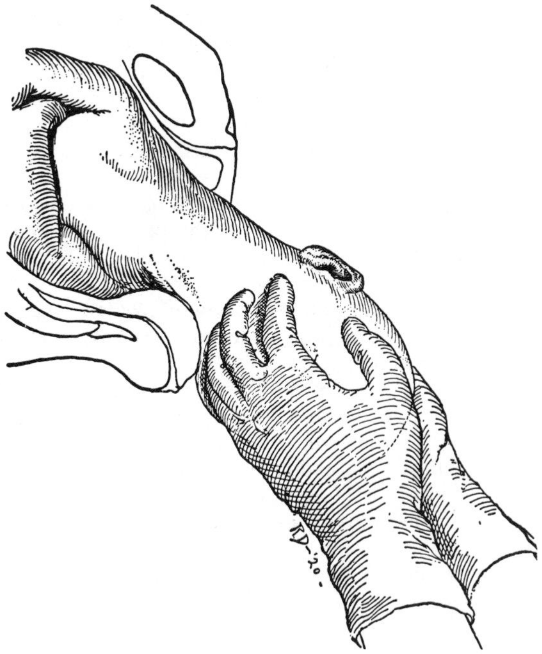

Figure 17-9. *Gentle* downward traction is sometimes made to impinge the anterior shoulder under the symphysis pubis.

position, rotate to the anteroposterior position, with one shoulder near the symphysis pubis and the other shoulder resting on the perineum (Fig. 17-9). As the shoulders rotate internally, the head, which is on the outside, rotates externally.

EXPULSION *Delivery of the shoulders* takes place quickly after external rotation of the head. Almost immediately the anterior shoulder becomes fixed under the symphysis pubis; very soon the posterior shoulder is delivered over the perineum by pivoting upward; and promptly thereafter the anterior shoulder follows (Figs. 17-9 and 17-10). Sometimes the anterior shoulder delivers first. After the shoulders are delivered, *expulsion of the rest of the body* is rapid. A definite mechanism is not necessary for birth of the rest of the baby, which is smaller than the head and shoulders, but

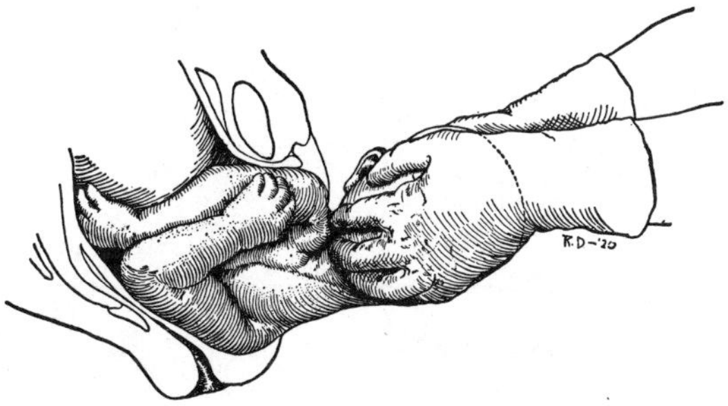

Figure 17-10. Lifting the head during delivery of posterior shoulder.

the body follows the upward curve of the lower part of the birth canal.

Pattern of Descent of Fetus

As with the pattern of cervical dilation, the pattern of descent of the presenting part of the fetus may be divided into a latent phase and an active phase, with a slow beginning of active phase, and a later phase of maximum slope (Fig. 17-5). Until cervical dilation enters the phase of maximum slope, there is essentially no downward movement of the presenting part of the fetus from its station at the onset of labor. After such a latent phase, descent slowly begins its active phase during the phase of maximum slope of cervical dilation.

Descent reaches its maximum slope at the same time that the dilation curve begins the deceleration phase. Thus, when dilation of the cervix is nearly complete, the presenting part begins its descent through the pelvis in a fairly rapid, progressive manner. The phase of deceleration of labor is thus a combination of progressive cervical dilation, although somewhat slower, and beginning of rapid descent.

Descent of the presenting part of the fetus continues its steady downward movement to the end of the second stage of labor, normally proceeding in an uninterrupted linear descent until it reaches the perineum and thereafter is delivered from the birth canal. In continuing its steady downward movement the presenting part adjusts to the pelvis according to the cardinal movements of the mechanism of labor.

The slope of descent, without complicating factors, averages 1.6 cm/hour in primigravidas and is normally greater than 1.0 cm/hour. In multigravidas it averages 5.4 cm/hour and is normally greater than 2.1 cm/hour.

As noted previously, these events comprise the pelvic functional division of labor.

Evaluation of the Labor Pattern

To determine if labor is progressing satisfactorily and within the wide variation that is possible in normal labors, it is very helpful to examine the progress of each woman in labor according to the normal curves of dilation and descent. Figure 17-5 shows the cervical dilation and the descent curves as they interrelate in a normal labor.

Labor curves can be constructed easily for each woman in labor, using a graph as shown in Figure 17-11. As the progress of labor is recorded, a pattern of progress of cervical dilation and progress of descent of the presenting part evolves. From observation of these patterns a fairly objective evaluation of the progress of labor can be made. If abnormal patterns in any of the

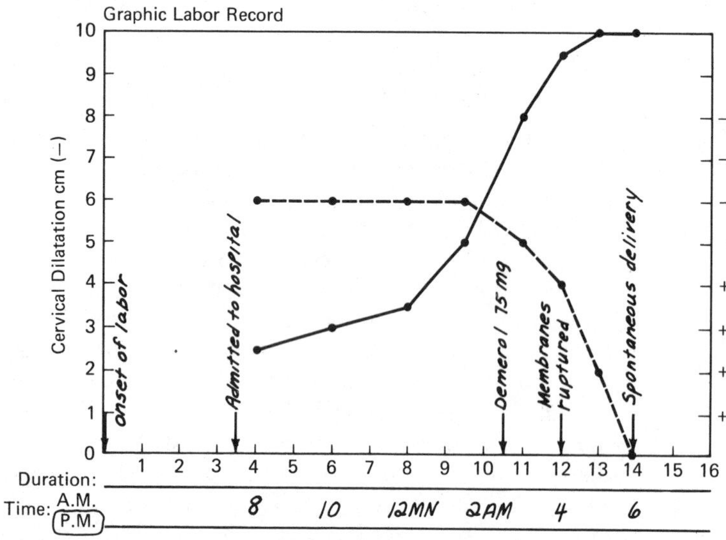

Figure 17–11. Representative graphic labor record showing cervical dilation and descent patterns as they evolved, taken from a patient's hospital chart. [Reprinted with permission from Emanuel A. Friedman, "Patterns of Labor as Indicators of Risk," *Clin. Obstet. Gynecol.* 16:172–173 (Mar.) 1973, p. 175.]

Using a square-ruled graph paper, the hours of labor are written across the paper horizontally, numbers are written along the left side in ascending order to represent centimeters of cervical dilation, and numbers are written along the right side in descending order to denote station of the presenting part.

The onset of labor is recorded as the time of onset of regular uterine contractions as perceived by the woman herself. Each examination for cervical dilation and station of presenting part is recorded on the appropriate line along with the time of the examination. As each recording is joined to the previous notation, a pattern of cervical dilation and descent of the presenting part evolves.

phases of labor develop, they can be recognized early and managed as described in Chapter 22.

Third Stage (Placental Stage)

The third stage of labor, called the placental stage because the placenta is delivered during this period, is made up of two phases—the phase of placental separation and the phase of placental expulsion.

At the beginning of the third stage, the uterus, which contracted down as its contents were diminishing during the birth of the fetus, is a firm mass above a collapsed lower uterine segment and is quite freely movable in the abdominal cavity. Its walls are considerably thicker than they were earlier in labor, and it has so decreased in size that the top of the fundus lies slightly below the umbilicus. Its cavity now contains only the placenta and the fetal membranes.

Placental Separation

Contractions of the uterine muscle continue at 3- to 4-minute intervals as in the first and second stages, but with minimal or no discomfort; they can be felt by an examiner palpating the uterus through the abdominal wall. On palpation of the uterus one may note a perceptible change in shape with contraction and relaxation. While the placenta is attached, the uterus assumes a globular shape during a contraction and a flattened (discoid) shape during relaxation; after the placenta is separated, its shape is globular also during relaxation. A persistent globular shape is therefore a sign of placental separation.

With the sudden decrease in the overall size of the uterus as the infant is born, there is a corresponding decrease in the surface area at the site of placental attachment. With this decrease in size, the placenta becomes considerably thicker, but being a noncontractile organ, it cannot completely accommodate itself to the decreased area of its place of attachment. It begins to fold up and is literally squeezed off the uterine wall. Separation usually takes place in the first few minutes of the third stage; it may occur as soon as the infant is born or may take place during the next few contractions of the uterine muscle.

Placental separation takes place in the spongy layer of the decidua, and a portion of the decidua is expelled with the placenta. Detachment usually begins at the center of the placenta, but sometimes it starts at its edges (Fig. 17–12). Some bleeding accompanies separation. When detachment begins at the center of the placenta and pro-

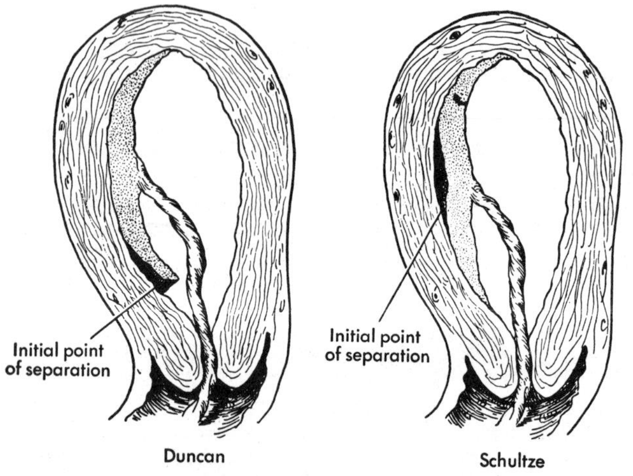

Figure 17–12. Diagrams showing the Duncan and Schultze mechanisms of placental separation and extrusion.

gresses to its margins, blood collects in the space behind the placenta and generally does not appear until the placenta is expelled. When separation starts at the edges, there may be a continuous trickling of blood throughout the third stage.

The fetal membranes and the decidua vera are also unable to accommodate to the decreased uterine size; they become thicker, but cannot completely adjust themselves, and their separation begins. Separation of the membranes is completed by traction of the placenta. As the placenta slides out of the uterus, the membranes, which are continuous with it, are dragged along and are peeled from the inner surface of the uterus.

Placental Expulsion

After the placenta is separated, the continuing uterine contractions push it out of the upper cavity into the relaxed lower uterine segment or into the upper portion of the vagina. As it slides into the lower segment, it fills this cavity, which has been collapsed, and pushes the fundus upward. After expulsion of the placenta from the upper segment, the uterine muscle contracts firmly and the cavity of the fundus becomes very small. Uterine contractions do not effect further expulsion of the placenta. It lies in the lower uterine segment or the vagina as a foreign body until additional pressure is applied to it, either by abdominal muscle contractions, as in the second stage of labor, or by manual means. The physician may facilitate placental expulsion by exerting downward pressure on the uterus.

The placenta can be delivered by bearing-down efforts of the mother, which increase intraabdominal pressure, but this method may take considerable time or may be impossible if the mother is under the influence of analgesia or anesthesia. Its expulsion from the lower uterine segment or the vagina therefore is usually completed manually. To some extent, the length of the third stage varies according to the time that elapses before effort is made to express the placenta. When the physician expresses the placenta, he places his hand over the fundus of the uterus and makes downward pressure on it; the uterus in turn places pressure on the placenta and pushes it out of the vagina. The fetal membranes, because of their attachment to the placenta, follow immediately.

Signs of Placental Separation and Expulsion from the Upper Uterine Segment

Four signs generally make their appearance when the placenta has separated and dropped into the lower uterine segment. The uterus changes from a discoid to a *globular shape* when the placenta separates; this shape *persists* during relaxation as well as during contraction. There is usually *bleeding from the vagina* with separation; this may come with a gush if the placenta has separated from its center first, or it may appear as a continuous trickling when separation begins at the edges. As the placenta sinks into the lower uterine segment or into the vagina, the *fundus rises* up to or above the umbilicus, and the *umbilical cord,* which is protruding from the vagina, becomes *limp* and *advances* several inches.

Mechanism of Extrusion of the Placenta

As the placenta is delivered, it appears at the vaginal outlet with either the fetal or the maternal surface foremost. In the most common method, known as the *Schultze mechanism,* the placenta becomes inverted on itself, and the glistening fetal surface appears at the vaginal outlet first. There is ordinarily little bleeding before the placenta is extruded; blood from the placental site collects behind the placenta and follows immediately after its expulsion (Fig. 17–12). Less frequently, the placenta descends sideways and presents at the vaginal outlet with its roughened maternal surface; this is called the *Duncan mechanism.* It is usually accompanied by slight but continuous bleeding during the third stage (Fig. 17–12).

Contraction of Uterine Muscle Following Third Stage

The uterus continues contracting as separation and expulsion of the placenta take place. It becomes a solid mass of muscle that lies below the level of the umbilicus; its walls are thick and lie so close to each other that they practically obliterate the cavity (Figs. 17–13 and 17–14). The tightly contracted muscle fibers constrict the large blood vessels that were opened up at the placental site with separation of the placenta, and they control bleeding by acting as ligatures. Inadequate muscle contraction results in excessive bleeding (described under the heading "Postpartum Hemorrhage" in Chapter 25).

A certain amount of bleeding takes place from the placental site during the third stage of labor even when muscle contraction is excellent; the amount varies from 50 to 200 ml (1.7 to 7 oz). In addition, there is some bleeding from an episiotomy. The total amount of blood lost in the third stage is often from 200 to 300 ml (7 to 10 oz).

The necessary continuous observation of the mother during the first hour or longer after delivery for excessive bleeding and for systemic reactions to the stress of labor is described on pages 427–30. After the completion of labor, which is an exhausting experience, the mother is in great need of rest. Unless labor has been short, she is very tired physically and, in addition, has been under considerable emotional strain. At the same time, however, she is promptly wide awake, exhilarated by the birth of the infant and the feeling of relief that the labor

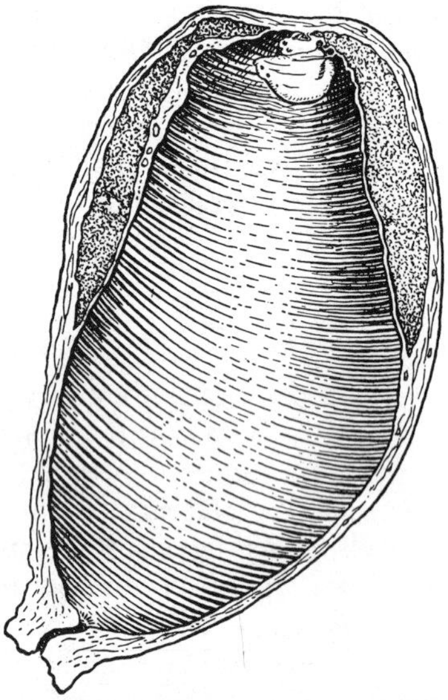

Figure 17–13. Longitudinal section through uterus showing thinness of uterine wall before expulsion of fetus, contrasting sharply with thickened wall in Figure 17–14—twin placentas are still adherent in upper segment. [Drawing of photograph of specimen in the obstetrical laboratory, Johns Hopkins Hospital.]

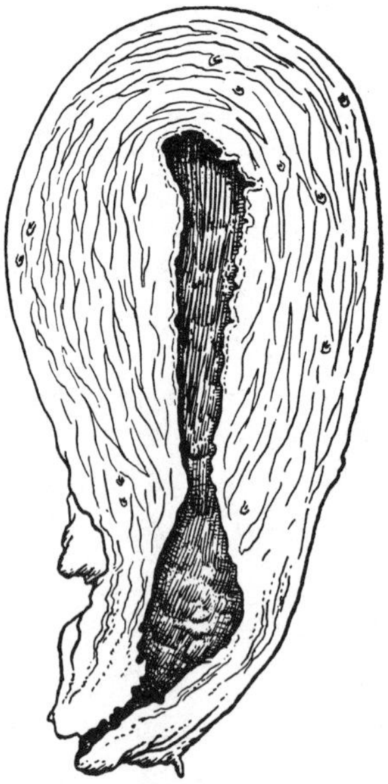

Figure 17–14. Longitudinal section through uterus, immediately after delivery, showing marked thickening of wall as a result of muscular contraction. [Drawing of photograph of specimen in the obstetrical laboratory, Johns Hopkins Hospital.]

is finished, and she is not immediately aware of her exhaustion.

The mother also has a great need to see and hold her infant immediately after birth. She should be given this opportunity just as soon as possible so that mother and child can begin to form a close attachment to each other in this first very early period after birth.

After seeing and holding her infant and visiting with her husband, she may be ready for rest and sleep.

REFERENCES AND SUGGESTED READINGS

Caldeyro-Barcia, Roberto, The influence of maternal position on time of spontaneous rupture of membranes, progress in labor, and fetal head compression. *Birth Fam. J.,* 6(1):7–15, 1979.

Friedman, Emanuel, *Labor: Clinical evaluation and management* (2nd ed.) Appleton-Century-Crofts, New York, 1978.

Liggins, Graham C., New concept of what triggers labor. *Contemp. Ob/Gyn,* 19:131–141 (May) 1982.

Miller, Frank C. Monitoring uterine activity. *Contemp. Ob/Gyn,* 13:35–39, (June) 1979.

Oxorn, Harry, and Foote, William, *Human labor and birth* (4th ed.). Appleton-Century-Crofts, New York, 1980.

Pritchard, Jack A., and McDonald, Paul, *Williams obstetrics* (16th ed.). Appleton-Century Crofts, New York, 1980.

Roberts, Joyce; Malasanos, Lois; and Mendez-Bauer, Carlos, Maternal positions in labor: Analysis in relation to comfort and efficiency. In Regina Lederman and Beverly Raff (eds.), *Perinatal parental behavior.* Liss, New York, 1981. (*Birth Defects: Original Article Series,* 17(6), 97–128, 1981.)

Sosa, Roberto A., and Cupoli, J. Michael, The birthing process: The effects on the parents, In Robert A. Knuppel (Guest ed.), *Clin. Perinatol.* 8:197–210, (Feb.) 1981.

CHAPTER

18

Pain Management During Labor and Delivery

Revised by Sue A. Frazier, R.N., M.S.N.

PAIN MANAGEMENT DURING labor and delivery is of primary concern to the laboring woman, her significant others, and the clinical staff caring for them. Individualizing the patient's care mandates a knowledge of the multiplicity of factors that contribute to her pain and discomfort. Although the physiologic stressors inherent to uterine contractions and the resultant resistance of the lower segment, cervix, and pelvic floor musculature are a given, any one woman's perception of and response to those stressors will depend on her unique prepregnancy and pregnancy history. Thus, a comprehensive, personal profile of the patient prior to the onset of labor can be particularly helpful in anticipatory pain management. Such a profile should include the patient's cultural background, her assessment of pain experiences, responses, self-management, as well as her concerns about labor pain. In addition, a nursing assessment as to the patient's attitude and acceptance of the pregnancy should be included. As this profile develops over the course of the pregnancy, the question of "desired" pain management can be raised and a variety of strategies can be explored. All too often, discussions and decisions regarding pain management are left until the woman is in active labor when all of her energies are invested in the immediacy of the event.

NONPHARMACEUTICAL PAIN MANAGEMENT

Somatopsychic methods used to relieve the pain and discomforts of labor and delivery are those methods taught in education-for-childbirth programs. Although these various programs may have marked theoretical differences, they all prepare women for labor and delivery by helping them understand the physical and emotional aspects of the experience and by teaching controlled relaxation techniques. The prepared woman is less distressed by the pain of labor than the one who is unprepared. She is better able to cope with the discomfort of labor than the woman who is fearful and anxious, and she is less fearful of the various phenomena of labor because she knows what to anticipate. (Education for Childbirth is discussed more fully in Chapter 11.)

Preparation for childbirth does not preclude use of analgesia and anesthesia. The need for medication is minimized, however, when the woman is trained how to respond to contractions and when she has support and guidance in her efforts from an interested and skilled person.

Emotional support during labor also can help alleviate discomfort in women unprepared for labor. Often they can be assisted with proper breathing during contrac-

Concern has been expressed that early mother-infant relationships may be adversely affected by depressant drugs and especially that this effect may come at a critical imprinting time. A depressed infant, and sometimes a depressed mother, may not be able to respond appropriately to carry out normal mother-infant interactions. The infant's responsiveness to the mother's voice, to her efforts to alert him or to soothe him, and his response to attempts to feed him may be impeded.

FACTORS DETERMINING CHOICE OF ANESTHESIA

Many factors are considered in selecting anesthesia for an individual client. No one method is preferable. Among factors considered are existing complications of pregnancy, such as antepartum bleeding, toxemias, diabetes, or heart disease; presentation and position of the fetus, such as breech; maturity of the fetus; the time the patient last ate; the availability of an anesthesiologist; the mother's desire to participate in the delivery; and the mother's wishes, if possible. Although it is not always desirable for the patient to determine the type of anesthesia, her objection to a particular method is an important consideration. When not contraindicated, regional anesthesia may be chosen over inhalation because of the mother's desire to be awake and to participate as much as possible in the birth and the desire of both parents for the father to participate in the labor and delivery experience.

Although aspiration of vomitus by the mother is more likely to occur with inhalation anesthesia than with other kinds, inhalation may be the method of choice in some cases. Among reasons for its use is the relaxation that it will provide for a delivery in which good relaxation is necessary. It may be more quickly administered than conduction anesthesia when the need for immediate delivery arises. The duration and depth of inhalation anesthesia are easily controlled. With the relatively light amount of anesthesia required for many deliveries, the inhalation method may present little or no problem of fetal depression, although the threat of maternal aspiration is always present.

Regional anesthesia reduces danger of maternal aspiration of food and fluid and, when used for analgesia during labor, eliminates use of narcotic drugs. However, regional anesthesia is sometimes contraindicated. It is not used in cases of obstetric hemorrhage because of the hypotension that often accompanies conduction anesthesia. Spine deformities in the woman are another contraindication to its use. It has also been advised that paracervical block should be contraindicated in prematurity, in the presence of preexisting fetal distress, and in the presence of uteroplacental insufficiency.

REFERENCES AND SUGGESTED READINGS

Bonica, John J., *Principles and Practice of Obstetric Analgesia and Anesthesia,* Vol. I., Davis, Philadelphia, 1967.

Brackbill, Y.; Kane, J.; Manniello, R. L.; and Abramson, D., Obstetric premedication and infant outcome, *Am. J. Obstet. Gynecol.,* 118:377–85, (Feb. 1) 1974.

Caton, Donald, Obstetric anesthesia and concepts of placental transport: A historical review of the nineteenth century, *Anesthesiology,* 46:132–37, (Feb.) 1977.

Fishburne, John I. Jr., Local anesthetics in obstetrics, *Contemp. Ob/Gyn.,* 6:101–105, (Oct.) 1975; 7:15, (Feb.) 1976.

Grad, Rae Krohn, and Woodside, Jack, Obstetrical analgesics and anesthesia, *Am. J. Nurs.,* 77:242–245, (Feb.) 1977.

Joyce, Thomas H., III (Guest ed.) Symposium on obstetric anesthesia and analgesia, *Clin. Perinatol.,* 9:3–135, 191–225, (Feb.) 1982.

Nicolls, Evaline, *et al.,* Epidural anesthesia for women in labor, *Am. J. Nurs.,* 81:1826–30, (Oct.) 1981.

Pohodich, Jane, *Selected Drugs Used During Labor and Delivery: Effects on the Fetus and Neonate,* A staff development program in perinatal nursing care, Series 3: Intrapartal Care: Module 1. March of Dimes Birth Defects Foundation, White Plains, N.Y., 1980, p. 24.

Ralston, David H., and Shnider, Sol M., The fetal and neonatal effects of regional anesthesia in obstetrics, *Anesthesiology,* 48:34–64, (Jan.) 1978.

Roberts, Joyce, Factors influencing distress from pain during labor, *MCN,* 8:62–66, (Jan.-Feb.) 1983.

Vadurro, Judith Farrell, and Butts, Priscilla, Reducing anxiety and pain of childbirth through hypnosis, *Am. J. Nurs.,* 82:620–23, (Apr.) 1982.

Warren, Thomas M., and Ostheimer, Gerard W., A guide to complications of paracervical block, *Contemp. Ob/Gyn.,* 20:69–89, (July) 1982.

Zurawski, Glenn F., and Shnider, Sol M., How anesthetic drugs affect neonatal neurobehavior, *Contemp. Ob/Gyn.,* 17:179–89, (June) 1981.

CHAPTER

19

Nursing Management of Fetal Responses to Labor

ASSESSMENT OF THE FETUS

THE SECOND INTRAPARTUM client, the fetus, is more difficult to assess than the laboring woman. Most of the usual means of physical examination are unavailable to the nurse, since the fetus cannot be directly inspected, palpated, or manipulated.

The stress of uterine contractions poses a potential threat to every fetus. Fortunately, the vast majority are healthy and possess sufficient reserve to withstand labor with no ill effects. For the benefit of the few who cannot readily tolerate labor, however, the nurse must maintain a high index of suspicion and carefully assess each fetus throughout the intrapartum period.

Because the chances of fetal distress are greater in high-risk pregnancies, the first step in fetal assessment is careful attention to the maternal history and the antepartum course of events. This is accomplished on admission to the labor suite by interview with the mother and review of the antepartum record (see page 383). Additional information about fetal presentation and position as well as a very crude estimate of fetal size can be obtained by palpation of the maternal abdomen (Leopold's maneuvers). Vaginal examinations give further evidence of presentation, position, and station of the presenting part. Other studies of a chemical or electronic nature may have been done during pregnancy or may be done during labor. Studies such as L/S ratio and ultrasound scans are discussed in Chapter 13.

Although all clinical data must be considered in relationship to the total situation, the single most informative parameter of fetal well-being during labor is the fetal heart rate. For this reason, observation of the fetal heart rate is an important responsibility of the nurse caring for a woman and fetus in labor. The rate must be counted often and recorded each time it is counted. It is essential that the nurse recognize abnormalities in rate so that prompt medical consultation may be obtained when necessary.

PATTERNS OF FETAL HEART RATE

The normal range of fetal heart rate (FHR) is 120 to 160 beats per minute. Although the rate differs in different fetuses, it usually remains constant within a small variation of less than 10 beats per minute in an individual fetus. If the heart rate has been carefully noted throughout gestation, the antepartal rate should provide a reasonably reliable baseline against which to compare the intrapartum values.

The uterine contractions of labor cause a transient reduction or arrest in maternal blood flow through the placenta. A healthy fetus will have enough oxygen reserve to sustain him during this time, and no change in baseline heart rate will occur. In addition, the contractions compress the fetal head and body, and circulation through the umbilical cord can be occluded during a contraction if the cord is in a position where it receives pressure. The fetus may respond to these stresses of labor with a momentary slowing of the heart during some of the contractions, but then it quickly resumes the baseline rate. *Brief* arrests in maternal blood flow through the placenta and *short* periods of pressure do not appear to affect the fetus adversely, especially if the interval between contractions permits a complete recovery.

Abnormalities in the pregnancy; strong, long, very frequent contractions; or failure of the uterus to relax completely between contractions are likely to interfere with adequate fetal-maternal exchange in the placenta. Under such conditions the reduction in exchange of oxygen and carbon dioxide between fetal and maternal blood results in fetal hypoxia, hypercapnia, and metabolic disturbances, resulting in acidosis, all of which cause fetal distress. The fetus responds to distress with adaptive reactions in his circulatory system and his heart rate in an attempt to protect his vital organs and to restore his placental exchange to normal. Reactions to inadequate exchange manifest themselves in changes in normal FHR patterns. These changes may be manifested as alterations in the baseline rate or as periodic changes occurring in relation to uterine contractions.

Baseline Fetal Heart Rate

Baseline fetal heart rate is defined as the heart rate when the woman is not in labor or the rate between periodic changes during labor. In the absence of periodic changes (i.e., in normal labor), it is simply the level of the heart rate in beats per minute. Any rise or drop in baseline which persists for more than 10 minutes is regarded as a change to a new baseline.

The baseline FHR above 160 beats per minute is designated as *tachycardia* and is frequently associated with fetal immaturity and/or maternal fever. Tachycardia is often the first response of the fetus to hypoxia and, as such, should be regarded as an early sign of fetal distress until proven otherwise.

A baseline FHR below 120 beats per minute is designated as *bradycardia*. Persistent bradycardia may be associated with congenital heart anomalies or, when accompanied by periodic changes in FHR, fetal distress and neonatal depression.

In addition to determining the level of the baseline FHR, which can be accomplished readily using a fetoscope, continuous FHR monitors permit an evaluation of the *variability* in the baseline. The level of the baseline, as well as the various periodic changes that may occur, is determined by a physiologic control mechanism which consists of interacting cardioaccelerator and cardiodecelerator reflexes. This interaction is dynamic rather than static, as the reflexes respond to each other and to other physiologic stimuli. As these accelerator and decelerator reflexes attempt to achieve balance, momentary fluctuations occur about the FHR baseline. These beat-to-beat fluctuations are considered to be a sign of a well-developed and well-functioning neurologic system.

Baseline variability is of two types: short term and long term. Short-term variability is the interval between successive heartbeats or beat-to-beat variability. The magnitude of this variability is about 2 to 3 beats per minute. Long-term variability refers to cyclic fluctuations over time and are of an average magnitude of 5 to 20 beats per minute. Figures 19–1 and 19–2 illustrates these two types of variability.

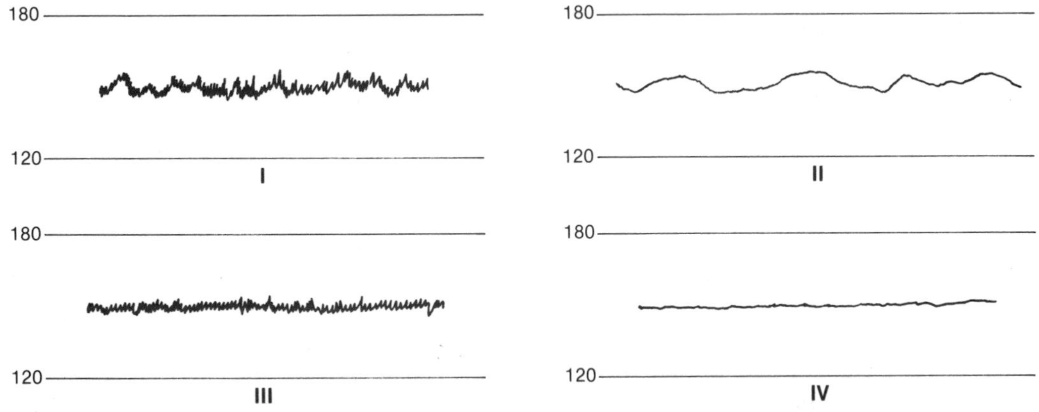

Figure 19–1. Fetal heart rate variability. I. Both long-term and short-term variability is illustrated. II. Long-term with no short-term variability. III. Short term with no long-term variability. IV. Neither short-term nor long-term variability.

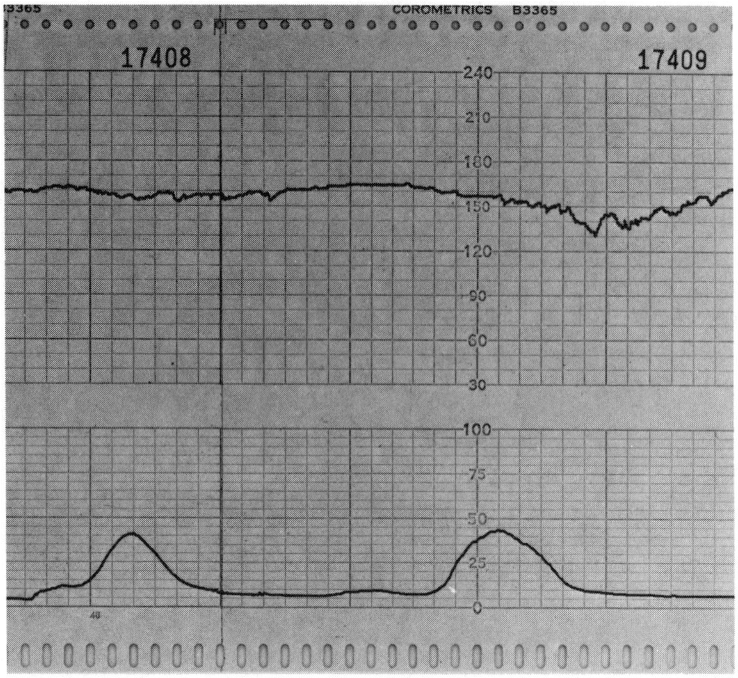

Figure 19–2. Fetal monitor tracing showing loss of short-term variability in the baseline fetal heart rate. Compare this almost smooth baseline with that seen on the tracing in Figure 19–15. A *late deceleration* can be seen in conjunction with the second uterine contraction.

Changes in baseline variability are believed to reflect changes in central nervous system status. Maternal medications such as narcotics, tranquilizers, magnesium sulfate, or other central nervous system depressants will temporarily reduce or eliminate baseline variability. In the absence of maternal medication, loss of baseline variability must be regarded as an ominous sign of fetal hypoxia and acidosis. Short-term variability is lost fairly early in a hypoxic episode with long-term changes occurring later. The presence of a uniform long-term variability without any short-term variability is known as a *sinusoidal pattern* of variability. It is an exceedingly rare finding and is thought to be associated with severe tissue hypoxia such as might be encountered with anemic fetuses suffering from erythroblastosis.

Periodic Fetal Heart Rate Changes

Periodic changes in fetal heart rate occur in relation to uterine contractions. These alterations may be either accelerations or, more commonly, decelerations. They are transitory departures from the baseline level followed by return to the baseline after a short interval. Accelerations may occur in association with contractions as the fetus attempts to compensate for the temporarily decreased placental blood flow, or they may occur as a response to fetal activity. (See discussion of NST, Chapter 13.) Tactile stimulation of the fetus during vaginal examinations or by the contracting myometrium during contractions also may produce FHR accelerations. Accelerations that recur with each contraction may result from isolated compression of the umbilical vein and may precede the development of variable decelerations. Accelerations of 10 to 50 beats per minute occurring late in the contraction cycle and accompanied by loss of beat-to-beat variability are ominous signs of fetal distress and frequently evolve into late decelerations.

Decelerations are classified according to the *shape* of the deceleration curve. Some decelerations are of uniform shape and reflect the shape of the uterine contraction curve, while others are of variable shape and have little or no correlation with the shape of the uterine contraction. FHR deceleration patterns may be further classified according to the *time relationship* between the onset of the uterine contraction and onset of the deceleration.

The classification according to the time relationship is as follows.

Early Deceleration

Early deceleration has its onset early in the contraction cycle, reaches its lowest point at the time of the acme (peak) of the contraction, and has generally returned to the baseline by the end of the contraction. The degree of deceleration is usually proportional to the amplitude (intensity) of the contraction, although the heart rate rarely falls below 110 to 115 beats per minute (Fig. 19–4).

Early decelerations are thought to be caused mainly by compression of the fetal head, which results in increased intracranial pressure and decreased cerebral blood flow. The resulting local hypoxia stimulates the vagus nerve and produces a transient rise in vagal tone,which slows the heart rate (Fig. 19–3). Early decelerations occur only

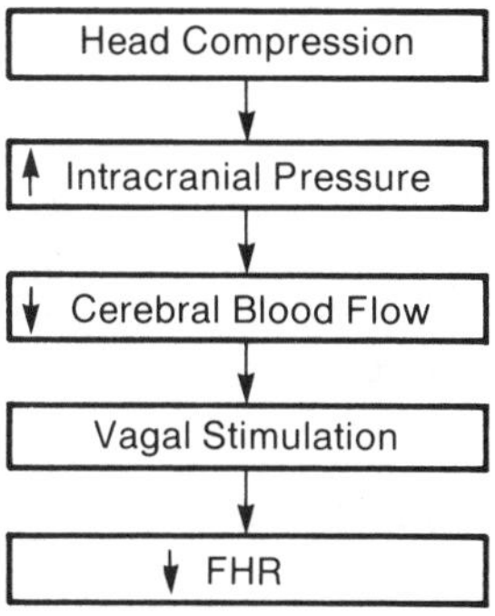

Figure 19-3. Mechanism of early deceleration of fetal heart rate.

in vertex presentations and are most common between 4 and 6 cm cervical dilation. They occur more frequently when the membranes are ruptured.

Even though cerebral hypoxia is one feature of the pathophysiology of early decelerations, these episodes are brief and appear to be well tolerated by the fetus. They are considered innocuous and are not associated with neonatal depression. Their clinical significance results from the need to differentiate them from late decelerations, which are similar in shape but occur at a different time in the contraction cycle and represent fetal distress.

Late Deceleration

The late deceleration, like the early deceleration, is of uniform shape. Unlike the early deceleration, it has its onset later in the contraction cycle, reaches its lowest point well after the acme of the contraction, and may not begin recovery until after the contraction has subsided (Fig. 19-4).

Late decelerations are a sign of fetal hypoxia resulting from a reduction in maternal blood flow through the intervillous space during a contraction. There is a lag between the height of the contraction and the late deceleration, reflecting the fact that intervillous blood flow and, consequently, oxygen transfer to the fetus decreases as the contraction becomes more severe. In addition, some oxygen continues to be available to the fetus from oxyhemoglobin. In consequence, there is a lag in the fall in fetal Po_2 below a critical level.

Any condition in which there is a reduction in fetal-maternal exchange in the placenta is likely to result in

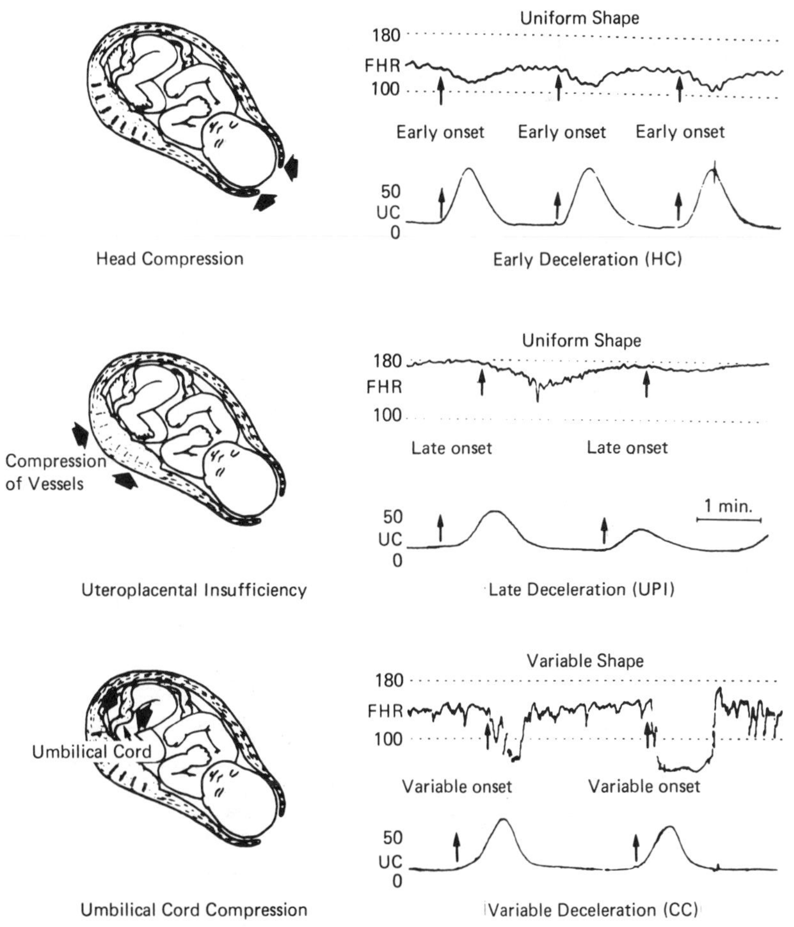

Figure 19-4. The three periodic fetal heart rate patterns.

The early deceleration pattern is thought to be due to fetal head compression. It is of uniform shape, reflects the shape of the associated intrauterine pressure curve, and has its onset early in the contracting phase of the uterus. Hence, it has been labeled "early deceleration." HC = head compression, UC = uterine contraction.

The late deceleration pattern is thought to be due to acute uteroplacental insufficiency as the result of decreased intervillous space blood flow during uterine contractions. It is also of uniform shape and reflects the shape of the associated intrauterine pressure curve. In this case, however, in contradistinction to the uniform FHR early deceleration pattern (above), its onset occurs late in the contracting phase of the uterus. Hence, it has been labeled "late deceleration." This FHR deceleration pattern is considered indicative of uteroplacental insufficiency. UPI = uteroplacental insufficiency.

The variable deceleration pattern is thought to be due to umbilical cord occlusion. It is of variable shape, does not reflect the shape of the associated intrauterine pressure curve, and its onset occurs at a variable time during the contracting phase of the uterus. CC = cord compression. (Reproduced with permission from Edward H. G. Hon, *An Introduction to Fetal Heart Rate Monitoring*. North Haven, Conn.: Corometrics Medical Systems, Inc., 1973.)

should be advised of this and their approval secured prior to assembling the equipment. Except in emergency situations, a brief lesson on monitors should be given, allowing the couple opportunity to closely examine the equipment. This is particularly important when a fetal electrode is to be applied. No parent relishes the idea of having a piece of steel screwed into her infant's head! However, when they have seen the electrode and been reassured that it only penetrates the skin about 1 mm, they probably will be much more comfortable.

Once the monitor is in place and operating, many parents are fascinated by seeing the tracing of their fetus' heart. If the husband is coaching his wife in breathing and relaxation, he will find the uterine contraction tracing very helpful in knowing when to cue her for the cleansing breath at the beginning and end of a contraction.

All labor room personnel must carefully train themselves never to enter a labor room and look first at the monitor tracing before acknowledging the presence of the woman. Certainly the worst offense is to enter, check the tracing, and leave, as if no patient were there at all. The laboring woman and her fetus must remain the central focus with the monitor only one adjunct to quality care.

Finally, it should be noted that the monitor tracings are only as useful as the expertise of the human practitioners makes them. Unless there are skilled nurses and physicians available to interpret the FHR patterns and take appropriate action, monitors are of no value.

TREATMENT OF FETAL DISTRESS

Early recognition of an abnormal fetal heart rate pattern often permits treatment before the condition of the fetus becomes serious. Some measures can be instituted readily, and they frequently modify or eliminate the cause of the distress. Among such actions are change in maternal position, correction of maternal hypotension, decrease in uterine activity when an oxytocic is used for stimulation of labor, and administration of oxygen to the mother.

A summary of interventions appropriate for various FHR findings is contained in Table 19-2.

Maternal Position Change

Change of maternal position may have the effect of correcting one of several different possible causes of interference with good circulation to the fetus or to the placenta. A change of position may relieve pressure on the umbilical cord during uterine contractions, and a change from a supine to a side position may remove pressure of the uterus from the large blood vessels in the abdomen.

The *umbilical cord may be in a position where it becomes compressed* between the fetus and the uterine wall or the maternal pelvis during contractions. Interference with good circulation through the umbilical cord is likely to result in a fetal heart rate pattern

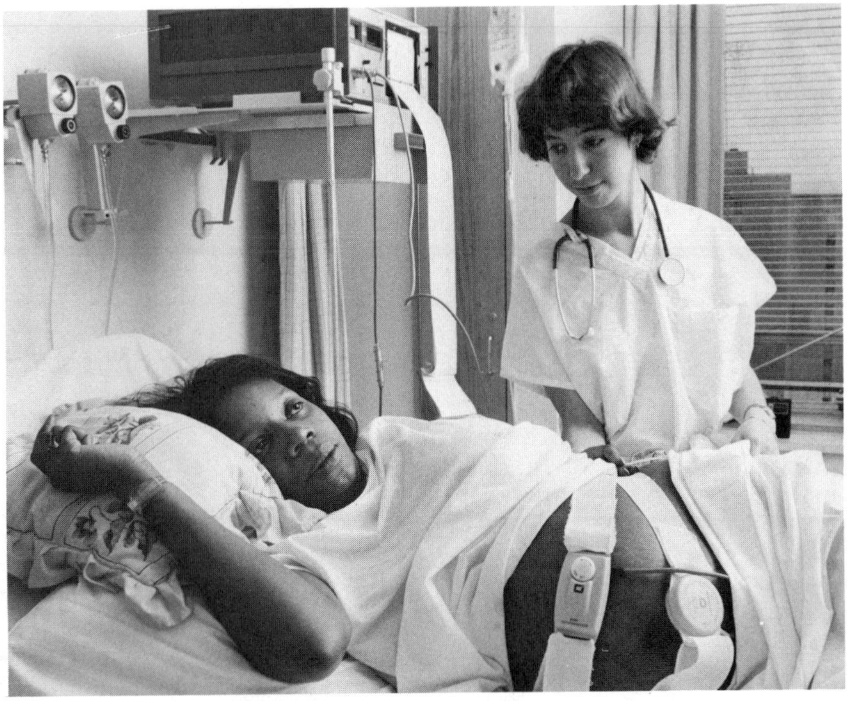

Figure 19-16. This woman in labor is being monitored using an external continuous fetal heart rate monitor. The tocodynamometer (L belt) records uterine activity while the Doppler unit (R belt) monitors the fetal heart beat. The woman is turned toward her side to provide for optimal circulation to the uterus and placenta. [Courtesy of The Presbyterian Hospital in the City of New York. Photo by Elizabeth Marshall.]

Table 19–2. Summary of FHR Patterns, Their Underlying Pathophysiology, and Suggested Interventions

FHR Pattern	*Characteristics*	*Underlying Pathophysiology*	*Therapeutic Intervention*
BASELINE CHANGES			
Tachycardia	Baseline over 160 bpm or a rise of 10% of previous baseline	Mild fetal hypoxia Maternal fever Maternal tachycardia Fetal neurologic immaturity	Monitor maternal vital signs Change maternal position Continue to watch closely
Bradycardia	Baseline under 120 bpm or a drop of 10% of previous baseline	Congenital heart abnormalities Fetal distress (when accompanied by periodic changes)	Inform neonatal personnel Change maternal position Administer oxygen to mother Prepare for immediate delivery
Loss of variability	Smooth baseline as recorded by *internal* fetal monitor	Maternal medication Fetal acidosis (especially if accompanied by late decelerations) Fetal neurologic immaturity	Note time and dose of medication on record See "late decelerations" below
PERIODIC CHANGES			
Early deceleration	Uniform shaped dip Onset, maximal fall, and recovery coincides with onset, peak, and end of contraction	Head compression	Distinguish from late deceleration Observe mother for progress in labor as these are usually indicative of cervical dilatation of 4–6 cm or more
Late deceleration	Uniform shaped dip Onset coincides with peak of contraction with recovery occurring at the end or after the end of the contraction	Uteroplacental insufficiency	Correct underlying cause; e.g.; Supine hypotension—change maternal position Conduction anesthesia—elevate legs, increase hydration with IV fluids, apply elastic stockings or leg wraps Uterine hyperactivity—reduce or discontinue dosage of oxytocin Left lateral position during labor Administer oxygen to mother Fetal scalp sampling Be prepared for operative delivery if fetal condition warrants
Variable deceleration	Variably shaped dip Usually shaped like a V or a squared U May occur any time during contraction cycle May be nonrepetitive	Cord compression	Change maternal position If severe, lasting more than one minute—attempt upward displacement of presenting part; help mother into knee-chest or Trendelenburg position; prepare for immediate delivery if pattern does not improve Administer oxygen to mother

associated with distress. Decelerations in fetal heart rate due to umbilical cord compression may occur at variable times in relation to the associated uterine contractions. Sometimes the decelerations begin early in a contraction and sometimes later, and they may be of variable duration. Very frequently a change in the mother's position will redistribute pressure points and modify or alleviate pressure on the umbilical cord during contractions.

A pregnant woman at or near term may develop hypotension while lying in the supine position. While the woman is on her back, the heavy uterus may press on the inferior vena cava and interfere with venous return to the heart. The impaired venous return results in reduced cardiac output and consequently a fall in arterial pressure. As a result, exchange of oxygen and carbon dioxide between maternal and fetal blood is reduced and the fetus is likely to begin to show signs of distress.

Hypotension resulting from pressure on the inferior

vena cava usually can be remedied by having the mother change to a side position. Although it may not be readily determined if a mother's supine position is the cause of distress to either mother or fetus, a change to a side position is advocated if signs of difficulty appear. Previous occurrence of a hypotensive syndrome in a mother during the latter part of her pregnancy suggests that it is not advisable for her to lie on her back at any time during labor. Actually a side position is recommended for all women in labor.

It may not be possible at first to determine the cause of an abnormal fetal heart rate pattern. Initially, however, it is important to change the mother's position as soon as an abnormal fetal heart rate pattern appears. Change in maternal position ordinarily can be carried out easily and it usually can be instituted immediately.

Correction of Maternal Hypotension

Maternal hypotension interferes with good perfusion of blood through the placenta and may result in reduced exchange of blood gases and other materials between maternal and fetal blood. Restoration of good maternal arterial pressure is essential to increasing the blood flow through the intervillous space and consequently adequate transfer of materials across the membranes.

Corrective measures for hypotension include elevation of the legs and rapid administration of intravenous fluids. A side position corrects the supine hypotensive syndrome. When spinal anesthesia is used, careful observation of blood pressure and readiness to combat hypotension are important to the fetus as well as the mother. The nurse should not wait for the physician to arrive to carry out corrective measures for hypotension. She should quickly change the mother's position, elevate the foot of the bed, and begin administration of intravenous fluids.

Control of Uterine Contractions

Strong uterine activity virtually stops blood flow through the intervillous space, at least during the peak of the contractions. If the contractions are long, there may be considerable impairment in transfer of oxygen and carbon dioxide across the placenta. When the contractions are also frequent, the relaxation intervals between them may be too short for the fetus to be able to recover adequately from the previous impairment of transfer of blood gases. The length of these intervals of relaxation is significant since fresh oxygenated blood is circulated through the intervillous space to meet the needs of the fetus during these intervals.

Stimulation of uterine muscle contractions with an oxytocic is the leading cause of strong, long, frequent contractions. Occasionally unusually strong contractions develop in a spontaneous labor.

Abnormally strong, frequent contractions accompanying oxytocin stimulation can ordinarily be avoided. Careful regulation of the amount of the medication usually will keep the contractions within physiologic limits. If contractions become abnormal, the nurse should immediately decrease or terminate the oxytocin. A decrease in length and frequency of contractions usually will provide sufficient time for fresh blood to circulate through the intervillous space in the interval between the stresses of contractions. This will permit adequate transfer of oxygen and carbon dioxide between mother and fetus.

Administration of Oxygen

Administration of oxygen to the mother will increase the maternal blood oxygen tension, often increase transfer of oxygen to the fetus, and may help to keep the oxygen tension of the fetal blood above a critical level. Administration of oxygen to the mother when the fetus is distressed has often been found to reduce the incidence of late deceleration. Oxygen may be used effectively for a sudden episode of fetal difficulty, while preparation is made for other treatments.

Administration of Glucose

Partial asphyxia causes rapid mobilization of glucose, and if the fetus does not receive an adequate amount of glucose from his mother, his own glycogen stores may become depleted. Since glucose readily passes across the placenta from mother to fetus, administration of intravenous glucose to the mother will assure that she is not becoming hypoglycemic and that glucose will be readily available to the fetus as it is needed.

FETAL BLOOD ANALYSIS

Examination of blood taken from the fetal scalp may serve as an important additional factor in the evaluation of the fetus and in making a decision whether or not operative delivery is indicated. Almost any disturbance that affects the fetus can result in acidosis. Since the range of pH in which body cells can function in a normal manner is very small, a fall in the pH of the fetal blood poses a serious risk. When facilities are available to carry out the procedure, analysis of fetal blood for acid-base balance may be used to obtain valuable information about the reactions of the fetus to the stresses of labor. Analyses of blood aid in identifying fetuses with intrauterine asphyxia and also those who have clinical signs of distress but no evidence of acidosis. Such analyses may be helpful in determining when immediate delivery is indicated.

The presence of late decelerations with normal

variability is the usual indication for scalp sampling. Most practitioners also reserve this procedure for situations where labor is progressing well, and delivery can be anticipated to occur in approximately 1 hour or less. Serial samples are obtained every 15 to 30 minutes as long as the pattern of late decelerations continues and the patient has not delivered. An operative delivery may be avoided as long as the pH remains above 7.25. A downward trend between 7.25 and 7.20 or any one finding below 7.20 is an indication for immediate delivery by the most expeditious means, often cesarean section.

This procedure allows the physician to differentiate between late decelerations caused by reflex changes and those that are associated with acidosis and are thus more dangerous. In the first instance, it is safe to continue labor and vaginal delivery as long as the pH remains normal; in the second instance, it is necessary to deliver the fetus as soon as possible. In settings where the obstetric and laboratory expertise are not available for fast and efficient fetal scalp sampling, it is customary to perform cesarean sections for fetal distress whenever late decelerations are observed and delivery is not imminent.

A sample of fetal blood for analysis is obtained by collection of a few drops of capillary blood from the fetal scalp. An instrument for making a very small incision in the skin of the scalp is inserted through the cervical canal after the membranes are ruptured. A few minims of blood are collected from the small scalp puncture wound into a heparinized capillary tube. The puncture site usually bleeds very little. The pH of the blood is immediately determined. The blood may be analyzed for changes in Pco_2 and base excess or deficit, as well as for level of pH.

Fetal scalp blood may also be used to type and crossmatch the Rh-sensitized infant for immediate extrauterine exchange transfusion.

DELIVERY OF THE INFANT

An abnormal fetal heart rate pattern may develop as a result of a combination of causes. The presence of one complication may exaggerate the effects of another. As an example, severe uterine contractions may contribute to the effects of decreased blood flow through the placenta from another cause, such as maternal hypotension or decreased functional capacity of the placenta.

Corrective measures for fetal distress will be effective in a large number of patients. If the fetus has not been affected severely, his condition may return to normal when the cause of his distress is removed. If an abnormal fetal heart rate pattern persists after institution of therapeutic measures, it is likely that the physician will make the decision that labor should be terminated by operative delivery.

PASSAGE OF MECONIUM

Passage of meconium *in utero* may be a sign of fetal distress. The bowel shows increased peristalsis during hypoxia, and its contents are likely to be expelled. The fetus may expel meconium during any period of distress, either during the latter part of pregnancy or during labor. As meconium escapes from the bowel, it mixes with the amniotic fluid, giving the fluid a yellowish-green or dark-green color. The discolored fluid is described as *meconium-stained amniotic fluid.*

Meconium-stained amniotic fluid can be recognized through intact membranes, if the fluid is observed through an amnioscope, introduced through the cervix. Amnioscopic examinations may be carried out in some circumstances during pregnancy if the fetus is likely to be at risk. However, under most circumstances, passage of meconium is not observed until the membranes rupture and the amniotic fluid begins to drain. The meconium may appear as a thick, tarry material draining from the vagina, or it may be well mixed with the amniotic fluid. The color of the fluid is likely to be dark when the meconium staining is of recent origin; it becomes more yellow than green if the meconium was passed several days or weeks earlier.

Meconium-stained fluid should be considered a sign of previous fetal hypoxia and a warning signal that the condition of the fetus may worsen. Its appearance should be immediately reported to the physician. The fetus should be carefully protected against undue stress and closely observed during the remainder of labor. Excessive fetal movements are occasionally noted in association with meconium passage and are considered further evidence of fetal difficulty.

Meconium is expelled under normal as well as abnormal circumstances when the breech is the presenting part. Uterine contractions apply considerable pressure on the baby's abdomen, and meconium is easily forced out of the bowel by this pressure. Although fetal hypoxia may be present, passage of meconium during labor when the breech is presenting is not a clue to the fetus' condition; other observations must be relied on for evidence of fetal distress.

The presence of meconium-stained amniotic fluid should be reported to the nursery staff as soon as it is noted and arrangements made for pediatric attendance at delivery. In addition to the risk of a depressed or asphyxiated neonate, meconium aspiration is a serious threat to the infant (see Chapter 30).

REFERENCES AND SUGGESTED READINGS

Banta, H. D., and Thacker, S. B. Costs and benefits of electronic fetal monitoring: A review of the literature. DHEW Publication # (PHS) 79-3245, 1979.

Freeman, Roger K., and Garite, Thomas J., *Fetal Heart Rate Monitoring,* Williams & Wilkins, Baltimore, 1981.

Haverkamp, A. D.; Orleans, M.; Langendoerfer, S.; McFee, J.; Murphy, J.; and Thompson, H. A controlled trial of the differential effects of intrapartum fetal monitoring. *American Journal of Obstetrics and Gynecology,* 134:399–412, 1979.

Langerdoerfer, S., *et al.* Pediatric follow-up of a randomized controlled trial of intrapartum fetal monitoring techniques. *Journal of Pediatrics,* 97:103–107, 1980.

McDonough, Marilyn; Sheriff, Dee; and Zimmel, Patricia, Parents' responses to fetal monitoring, *MCN* 6:32-34, 1981.

Paul, Richard H., Fetal distress, in E. J. Quilligan and N. Kretchmer (eds.), *Fetal and Maternal Medicine,* Wiley, New York, 1980.

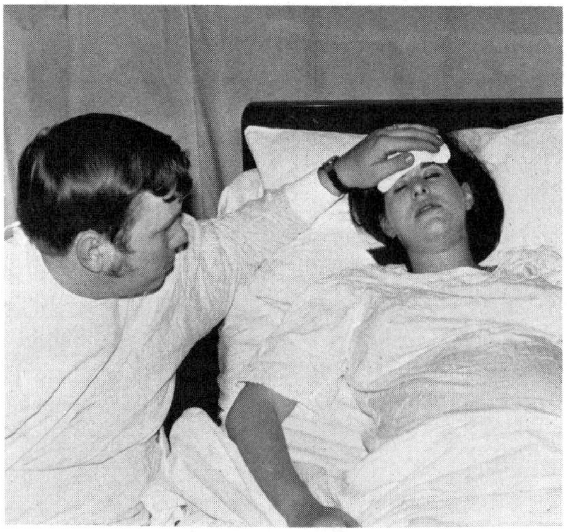

Figure 20–5. The husband is encouraging and coaching his wife during labor, and is providing physical comfort. The mother appears to be giving full concentration to slow, even, pant breathing and to relaxation of the muscles that are not involved in labor.

begins to wane, she decelerates the pace of her breathing. It is helpful to the mother if her husband or another person tells her when 15, 30, and 45 seconds have passed (Fig. 20–6). Intense concentration and active participation with each contraction take a great deal of effort, especially if the contractions come in close succession. The mother may begin to feel tired and become discouraged, and needs encouragement to continue in her efforts. It is helpful to the mother to have someone check her for muscle release as well as for breathing techniques. It is important that her breathing remain shallow and superficial to avoid hyperventilation.

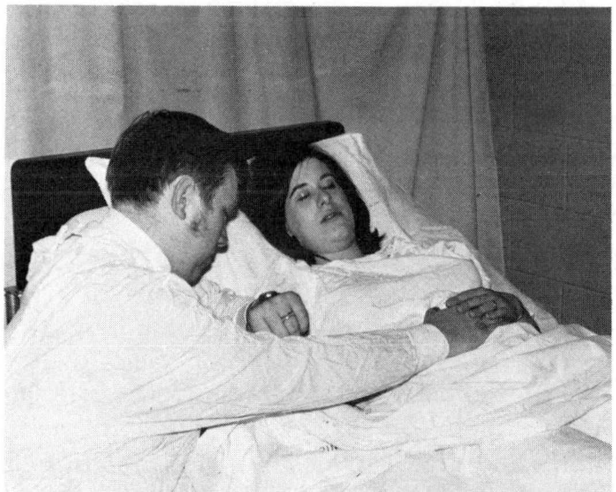

Figure 20–6. The mother accelerates her rapid, but light shallow chest breathing toward and over the peak of her contraction and then decelerates the pace of her breathing when her contraction begins to wane. Her husband is assisting her in determining when the peak of the contraction has passed and is also checking her for muscle release. Note that the mother's left hand appears relaxed.

During the transition phase of labor the mother may change to a rapid, light, pant-blow breathing. She blows her breath out forcefully at intervals while doing shallow panting during each contraction. This is the most difficult phase of her labor. The mother may feel irritable and she may be uncomfortable from leg cramps, nausea, chills, and perspiration. She may feel a vague sense of loss of control. She needs encouragement and reminders that she will soon be ready to push with her contractions. Complete relaxation between contractions is very important at this time. Concentration on breathing and relaxation will be most effective if distractions are kept to a minimum.

Hyperventilation may become a problem with rapid breathing if the breathing is not shallow enough or if panting is prolonged. Hyperventilation increases the loss of carbon dioxide and leads to a respiratory alkalosis and the appearance of symptoms. The mother may feel tingling and numbness in her hands and feet and may develop carpopedal spasms. Possible adverse effects of maternal alkalosis on the fetus are being investigated.

The effects of hyperventilation can be overcome by having the mother slow the rate of her breathing and hold her breath for a few moments or rebreathe air in a paper bag. The prepared mother ordinarily will keep her breathing sufficiently shallow, and she has usually been instructed in management if she notes symptoms of hyperventilation. She may overanticipate, however, the necessity for rapid breathing and need reminders to slow the rate of breathing if it becomes very rapid, or a suggestion to keep her breathing very shallow. When an untrained mother breathes with hyperventilation, she is likely to become distressed by both the symptoms and her lack of understanding of their cause. She needs explanation to relieve her concern and needs instructions in proper breathing. Since some trained mothers have difficulty in using rapid shallow breathing effectively and some become fatigued with the method, changes in respiratory techniques, with substitution of a slower breathing for the very rapid breaths, have been made in some education-for-childbirth classes.

Most methods of preparation for childbirth recommend that the mother take a deep breath in and out at the start of each contraction, before beginning the series of shallower breaths used during the contraction. They also recommend that she take a deep inhalation at the end of a contraction and then let her breath out slowly and relax as with a sigh. The deep inhalation and slow exhalation used at the beginning and the end of each contraction are often called a complete breath or a cleansing breath. The slow, deep breath provides for a good exchange of oxygen and carbon dioxide before and after the shallower breathing that is done during the contraction. It also may be useful in overcoming hyperventilation. In addition, a complete or cleansing breath at the end of a contraction helps the mother to define for herself that the contraction has ended and it provides a good beginning for the relaxation between contractions.

Mothers prepared by the Lamaze method may use light rhythmic massage (effleurage) over the lower abdomen in conjunction with their controlled breathing. This may be done by the mother herself or by her husband or the nurse. The massage is used as an aid in relaxing the abdominal muscles during contractions.

The need for analgesia is minimized when the mother has been prepared for labor and when she has the support of a skilled person. However, its use need not be eliminated during either the first or second stage of labor. The mother should know that she may ask for pain relief if she feels she needs it, or medication may be offered when the person caring for her observes signs suggesting the need for analgesia. Use of medication for pain relief and for relaxation does not mean failure in carrying out a preparation-for-childbirth program.

Some women are not prepared for labor. The unprepared mother is likely to be very anxious and tense and will need a great deal of support, assistance with relaxation, and detailed explanation of what is taking place as labor proceeds. She will, however, respond to the reassurance of a calm, sympathetic, and understanding nurse and often can be given considerable assistance with relaxation by instructions and suggestions that seem indicated at the moment. Instructions and frequent reminders to breathe slowly and deeply during each contraction will be very helpful to her. When she is concentrating on slow, deep breathing, she is less likely to tense other muscles in her body than when she takes short, quick breaths or holds her breath at intervals.

Administration of Drugs

Drugs that have a tranquilizing effect are often used during labor to relieve anxiety and apprehension, and analgesic drugs are frequently administered to reduce pain. These drugs are another means of reducing the discomfort of labor. They are described more completely in Chapter 18. The time of administration, the kind of drug used, and the dosage are determined by the physician, but the observations of the nurse caring for the client will be useful in the decision. The nurse informs the physician of the mother's request for pain relief and of her own observations of the mother's reactions to labor.

Since all drugs given to the mother affect the fetus as well, a general dictum is that the less medication given during labor the better. It should also be remembered, however, that an anxious mother in severe pain who is having difficulty coping with contractions may also distress her fetus. Increased maternal epinephrine produced in response to anxiety, can reduce uterine blood flow; therefore, the progress of labor actually may be impeded by severe anxiety. A carefully chosen analgesic and/or tranquilizer, when coupled with appropriate nursing support, is often sufficient to enable the woman to relax, get some rest, and regain control of her labor.

In general, intravenous administration of analgesics is desirable, providing faster relief at lower dosages. This also permits greater accuracy in predicting effects on the fetus, since it is not necessary to account for variability in the rate of muscular absorption. The administration should be timed to permit a sufficient interval for the placenta to clear the drug from fetal circulation prior to delivery. In general an analgesic should be given about 2 hours prior to the anticipated time of birth.

After administration of a drug, it is important that the nurse provide an environment conducive to relaxation. The mother is made as comfortable as possible for a period of rest by suggesting that she attempt to void, changing bed linen if needed, and assisting her into the most comfortable position. The fetal heart is auscultated before the drug is administered, and the mother's pulse, respiration, and blood pressure are checked. The mother is usually informed that she is being given medication for rest and is urged to relax as much as possible in order to obtain maximum benefit from the drug. The room should be quiet and its temperature adjusted to the mother's comfort; most mothers wish to have the room quite cool.

After administration of a drug, the nurse must monitor the mother and fetus carefully. The mother is watched for respiratory depression. Careful observation of strength and frequency of contractions is necessary; labor may be slowed or it may progress rapidly. It may be difficult to decide from the mother's reactions when the second stage is reached, and close observation for signs of progress in labor is important. If a drug that causes excitement is given, the mother must be watched every moment to prevent her from injuring herself. The fetal heart tones are checked frequently. If continuous electronic fetal heart rate monitoring is being employed the nurse should note the time and dose of the medication on the monitor read out sheet as well as in the woman's hospital record. A diminished base line variability is commonly seen for a period of time after the drug is given.

Discomfort from Pressure

Pressure of the fetal head on pelvic structures—nerves, ligaments, and organs—may cause discomfort, sometimes severe, in the lower back, the pelvis, and the legs.

Low backache, over the lumbosacral region, may be experienced with each contraction, or it may be continuously present, with exacerbation during contractions. In some labors, pain in the lower back causes more discomfort throughout labor than the abdominal pain that accompanies each uterine contraction. Massage of the lower back with the palm of a hand, in the form of firm back rubbing, mainly pressure, may give relief. This massage may be done by the support person or by the nurse (Fig. 20-7). A small pillow placed under the lumbar region, if the mother is on her back, may give some comfort.

Cramps in the legs, especially if the fetal head is low in the pelvis, may be a source of discomfort in labor. These cramps usually cause excruciating pain and require immediate attention; they may return at frequent intervals. Relief is obtained by elevating and extending the leg, making pressure on the knee to keep the leg straight, flexing the foot, and forcibly pushing the forefoot as far as possible toward the knee (Fig. 20-8). Stepping on the foot and walking about relieve muscle cramps if the mother is able to be up.

Pressure on the rectum, if the baby's head has descended low in the pelvis, is another source of discomfort, sometimes through a considerable part of labor. This pressure may prompt the mother to ask for the bedpan frequently, only to find that she cannot use it. Use of the bedpan often and unnecessarily is tiring; its frequent use may be reduced if the nurse gives the mother an adequate explanation for this constant feeling of a desire to empty her bowel. Since pressure on the rectum is often a sign of imminent delivery, especially if it appears late in labor, the nurse must assure herself of the stage to which labor has progressed when the mother complains of this pressure.

Occasionally, when the head is deeply engaged, there is so much *pressure low in the pelvis* that the mother has a certain amount of *involuntary bearing down* with contractions before dilation of the cervix is complete. Such effort usually cannot be controlled, but the mother should be advised against any voluntary effort to bear down during the first stage. Voluntary effort at this time does not hasten labor, uses energy unnecessarily, and may possibly cause edema of the cervix and small cervical tears. Pant-blow breathing during contractions may reduce the urge to push down.

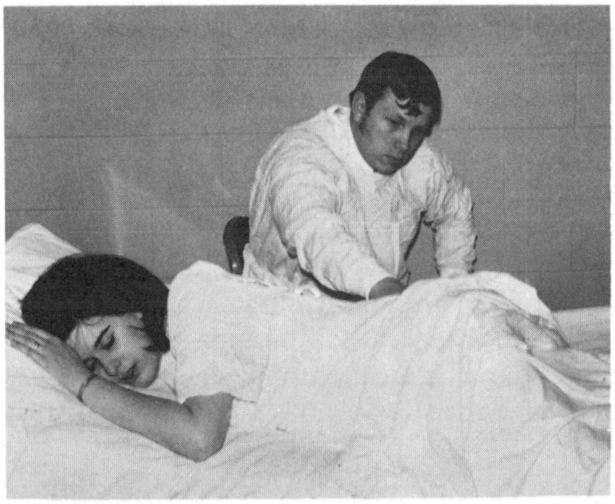

Figure 20-7. This woman's husband is putting very hard pressure over her lumbosacral area during contractions to provide relief from back pain.

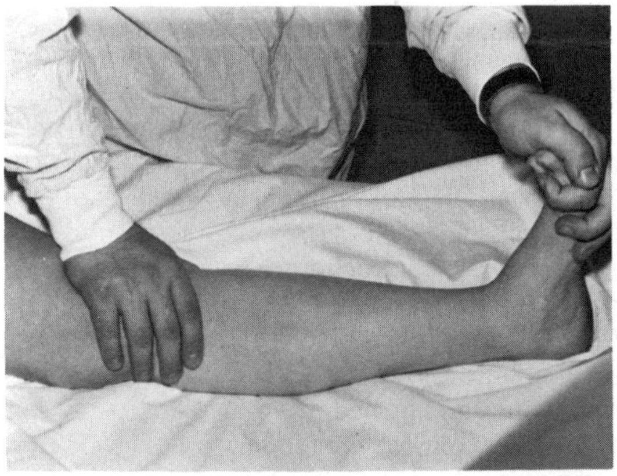

Figure 20-8. A leg cramp may be relieved by counterpressure on the foot. The leg is kept straight by pressure on the knee and the foot is flexed by forcibly pushing the forefoot toward the knee.

ASSESSMENT OF MATERNAL PHYSICAL RESPONSE

Important functions of the nurse caring for a woman in labor are (1) careful observation of the mother and the fetus in order to assess their reactions to the stress of labor, and to detect early signs of complications that may affect their welfare, and (2) close observation of the progress of labor.

Temperature

The mother's temperature is taken every 4 hours unless prolonged labor or fever indicates that more frequent observation, along with other vital signs, is desirable. Normal labor has relatively little effect on the mother's temperature, and it should be expected to remain within normal limits. A rise to 37.6° C (99.6° F), or above, should be reported to the physician and is an indication for frequent checking.

Pulse and Respiration

The mother's pulse and respiration change relatively little during normal labor, except possibly during a contraction. The pulse and respiration are observed every hour; any increase is reported to the physician and indicates the need for more frequent observation. A pulse rate of 100 beats per minute is generally considered the upper limit of normal.

Blood Pressure

The mother's blood pressure is checked on admission to the hospital and every hour thereafter, unless more frequent observation is indicated by elevation prior to or at the time of admission, or by the presence of other signs of preeclampsia. It is best to obtain the blood pressure reading between contractions because there may be an increase from 5 to 10 mm Hg during a contraction.

Frequent checking of blood pressure, as often as every 15 to 30 minutes, may be necessary if it is elevated. The doctor should be notified of an increase to 140 mm Hg systolic and 90 diastolic, or sooner if the blood pressure was low on admission and appears to be steadily rising. Although the urinary output should be carefully recorded at all times, it must be particularly noted when the blood pressure is elevated.

Intake and Output

The importance of close observation of fluid intake and urinary output has been described on page 388.

Headache

A headache during labor may be an indication that toxemia is developing. The blood pressure should be checked if a headache develops and both observations reported to the physician.

Vaginal Bleeding

Bleeding from the vagina, other than bloody show, however slight, necessitates immediate report to the physician. Vaginal bleeding usually can be distinguished from bloody show by the character of the drainage. The show is a mucoid material containing a small amount of blood, whereas bleeding which is due to other causes appears as a trickle, or as a gush of bright-red blood not mixed with mucus. At times it is difficult to determine the difference between bloody show and vaginal bleeding. If the nurse has any questions, she must bring it to the physician's attention.

Other Observations

The nurse must be alert to many other signs of impending danger and report all abnormal behavior so that treatment can be instituted early. Among some of the other signs that may indicate development of complications are dizziness, visual disturbances, frequent vomiting, epigastric pain, abnormally long and hard contractions or rigidity of the uterus, extreme sensitivity of the lower abdomen or constant abdominal pain, and undue restlessness.

ASSESSMENT OF THE PROGRESS OF LABOR

Observation of Uterine Contractions

The *frequency, duration,* and *strength of the uterine contractions* should be carefully observed by the nurse. The woman and her support person may be asked to help time the contractions for short intervals, and they frequently do so without request. Their observations are very useful, but the nurse must make her own evaluation of contractions at frequent intervals. The mother's and the nurse's evaluation of contractions are not always in complete agreement. The mother may not feel discomfort at the beginning and at the end of the contraction, and its actual duration may be longer than the period of her discomfort; or she may continue to have discomfort, due to pressure, after the contraction has ended and therefore believe that it lasted longer than it actually did. An estimate of the strength of the contraction by the mother's reaction also may not be completely reliable because of the differences in reaction by different women to contractions of approximately the same intensity.

To make her own observations of uterine contractions, the nurse places her hand lightly on the mother's abdomen, over the fundus of the uterus, and gently palpates with her fingers changes in uterine muscle tone. With experience she can learn to detect the beginning of a muscle contraction, feel its maximum firmness when the uterus seems to "stand up" and become hard, and perceive when the muscle is again relaxed. The nurse should stay with the mother long enough at any one time to observe several contractions in order to note the general pattern. It is important for her to ascertain that the uterine muscle relaxes completely in the intervals between the contractions.

The *length of the contraction* is the time interval between the first sensation of tightening of the muscle and its subsequent complete relaxation—this may differ from the time during which the mother feels discomfort. The *frequency of the contractions* is the time interval from the beginning of one contraction to the beginning of the next; it is not the time that elapses between the end of one contraction and the beginning of the following one (Table 20-1). The *strength of the contractions* can be estimated by the firmness of the uterine muscle. A weak contraction is one in which the uterine muscle becomes firm, but not hard; the contraction also is generally short, around 30 seconds' duration. A moderate contraction is usually longer, around 45 seconds' duration, and the uterine muscle becomes moderately firm. A strong contraction generally lasts around 60 seconds, and the uterus becomes very hard. During a hard contraction the examining fingers cannot indent the uterus, whereas some indentation is possible with weaker contractions.

Table 20-1. A Record of the Length and Interval Between Uterine Contractions.*

Interval	*Beginning of Contraction*	*Duration of Contraction*
	7:12	50 seconds
3 min.	7:15	60 "
4 min.	7:19	60 "
4 min.	7:23	50 "
3 min.	7:26	50 "
3 min.	7:29	50 "
4 min.	7:33	60 "

*The frequency with which contractions occur is timed from the beginning of one contraction to the beginning of the next. When contractions are timed at various intervals during labor, a chart similar to the above may be kept at the woman's bedside. The frequency and length of the contractions are recorded for short periods of time. This aids the nurse in accurately recording her observations of the contractions on the woman's record. This chart shows that the woman had contractions of 50 to 60 seconds' duration occurring every three to four minutes.

Palpation of the abdomen for evaluation of uterine contractions must be done gently and with a minimum amount of manipulation. The examining hand need not be moved about on the abdomen from one area to another, and frequent efforts to indent the uterus are not necessary. The mother's abdomen is often very tender and manipulation adds to her discomfort.

Among the many factors that affect the progress of labor, the force of the uterine contractions exerts an important influence. Labor can be expected to progress steadily, and sometimes rapidly, when the uterine contractions are strong, last approximately 60 seconds, and recur at three- to four-minute intervals, unless the resistance of the soft tissues is great or the relationship of the fetus to the mother's pelvis makes passage difficult.

Uterine contractions also may be continuously monitored by a tocodynamometer or by an intrauterine catheter as described in Chapter 19.

Examinations to Determine Progress of Labor

Abdominal Palpation

At an early examination of the mother after the beginning of labor, the abdomen is palpated, according to the description on pages 329–32 for diagnosis of presentation, position, and engagement of fetus. Abdominal examination may be repeated later in labor for further observation of position of the fetus and for descent of the presenting part, and the findings of the examination may be correlated with those obtained by rectal or vaginal examination. Abdominal examination must be made between contractions.

Vaginal Examination

Vaginal examinations are frequently employed methods of determining the progress of labor. Progress is ascertained by palpation of the cervix for degree of effacement and dilation and of the fetal presenting part for station and position. The examination is made when the mother is admitted to the hospital in labor and is repeated at intervals during labor, perhaps only once but often several times.

To some extent, the progress of labor can be followed by the other observations enumerated in this section on "Assessment of Progress of Labor." Vaginal examination is used to confirm the judgment that labor is progressing, concluded from other signs, and is performed whenever necessary to determine more definitely the amount of progress that has been made. The frequency of examinations varies considerably in individual situations and is somewhat determined by the reliance that can be placed on other signs of progress. Since the examinations are not entirely without danger of infection to the birth canal and are also disturbing to the woman, they are not repeated more often than seems essential.

When a vaginal examination is to be performed, the nurse should explain the procedure, assist the mother to a position on her back, ask her to flex her knees, and drape her in such a manner that she will be covered, but with the perineal area exposed. The nurse provides a sterile glove and lubricant and remains with the mother during the examination to provide support and to encourage her to relax her muscles during the examination when it is being done by the physician (Fig. 20-9).

For some examinations, such as questionable cephalopelvic disproportion, abnormal presentation, questionable placenta previa, and further evaluation of the pelvis, a lithotomy position is used during the vaginal

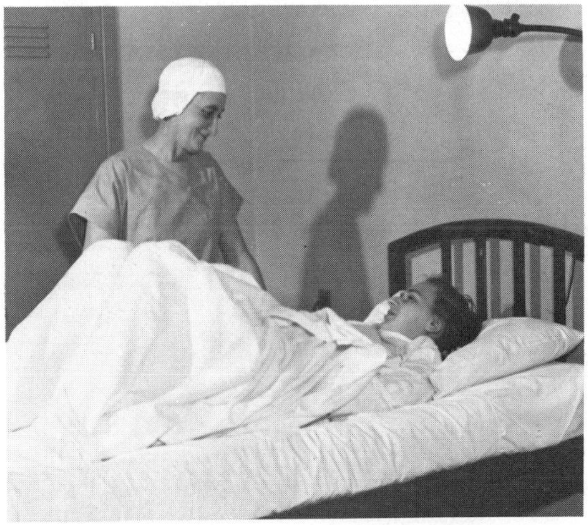

Figure 20-9. Woman covered with a cotton blanket awaiting an examination to determine progress of cervical effacement and dilation and station and position of the fetus. The drape can be removed as much as necessary to expose the perineal area sufficiently for the examination. The nurse is available to coach the mother with the appropriate breathing and relaxation techniques during a physician's examination.

examination. Because such examinations cannot be done satisfactorily with the woman on her bed, she is placed on an examining table or the delivery table where better positioning and better preparation can be done.

VAGINAL EXAMINATION BY THE NURSE The nurse herself often performs vaginal examinations. Such findings, added to the nurse's other observations, increase her information concerning the progress of labor. To become skillful in using vaginal examinations as a means of determining progress, the nurse must have many opportunities to perform the examination and at first needs assistance in interpreting the findings.

To proceed with a vaginal examination, two fingers of a gloved hand are lubricated and introduced into the vagina. The cervix, the presenting part, and the ischial spines are palpated directly for the following information; the consistency, effacement, and dilation of the cervix, the station of the presenting part, and the position of the fetus (Fig. 20-10).

During palpation of the cervix, its opening is felt as a depression with a surrounding circular ridge. The *amount of cervical dilation* is determined by palpating this depression and estimating its diameter in centimeters (Fig. 20-10). The *amount of cervical effacement* is determined by palpation of the thickness of the ridge around the depression (Fig. 17-3). See Chapter 17 for a more complete description of cervical effacement and dilation. The *consistency of the cervix* is also noted at this time; a cervix that is soft usually thins and dilates faster than one that is still firm. Sometimes *information about the integrity of the membranes* is obtained during this examination. If the membranes are intact, they are sometimes felt bulging through the cervical opening, especially during a contraction; if the membranes are ruptured, amniotic fluid may drain out of the vagina during a contraction.

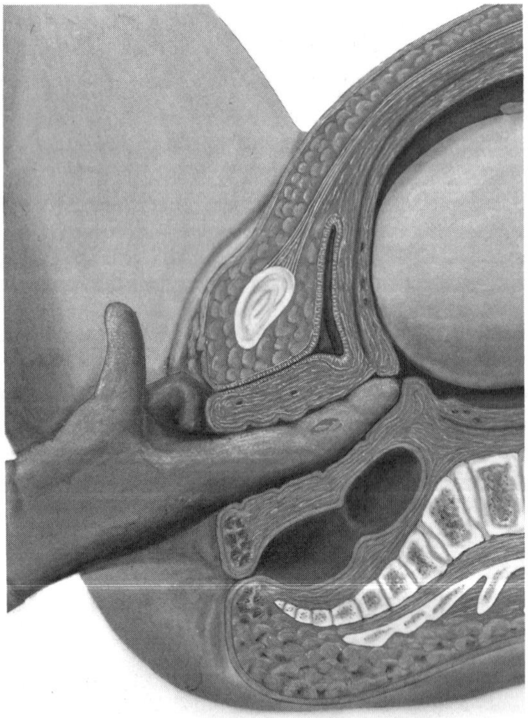

Figure 20-10. Diagram showing method of asertaining cervical effacement and dilation, station of the fetal head, and position of the fetus by means of a vaginal examination. The examining finger palpates the cervix, the fetal head, and the ischial spines.

The *station,* or degree of descent, is ascertained by touching the fetal head, feeling for the ischial spines on the side walls of the pelvis, and correlating the level of the head to the level of the ischial spines. The stations of the head are described on page 328 and in Table 16-3 on page 329.

It may be possible to determine the *position of the fetus* on vaginal examination if the cervix is quite well dilated. When the vertex is presenting, the sagittal suture usually can be felt through the cervical opening, and if dilation is advanced, the suture can sometimes be followed to a fontanel. By feeling some portion of the landmarks of the fetal head it may be possible to determine the placement of the occiput. Correlation of the direction of the sagittal suture with the findings of an abdominal examination may be helpful in diagnosing the position. The positions assumed by the fetal head are described on page 326 and its sutures and fontanels on page 322.

Overlapping of sutures owing to marked molding of the head may interfere with differentiation of landmarks. Sometimes the soft tissues of the fetal head become very edematous during labor, making palpation of the underlying structures difficult or impossible.

The nurse must be aware of contraindications to a vaginal examination, which include *vaginal bleeding, however slight,* and abnormal findings upon abdominal palpation, such as a transverse presentation.

Vaginal examinations may be made either during or between contractions. An examination made between contractions reveals the amount of cervical dilation and effacement and descent of the head when the cervix and the head are not under pressure of a contraction. An examination performed during a contraction shows the maximum amount of thinning and stretching of the cervix and descent of the head under the influence of a contraction. There may be some recession in cervical effacement and dilation after each contraction, but the cervix does not completely return to its state before the contraction began. Each contraction makes some change; toward the end of labor this change may be rapid.

Signs of the Transition Phase

The appearance of the transition phase is evidence that the first stage will soon be completed. This phase may be recognized by changes in the mother's behavior and by an increase in the intensity of contractions and an increase in pressure in the pelvis made by the presenting part. The contractions become intense and frequent and are sometimes so close together that they seem almost continuous. Pressure on the rectum increases and cramps in the legs and buttocks may begin or become more marked. The back and abdomen often become sore to touch. This discomfort may be so marked that the mother requests the nurse not to touch her abdomen to palpate uterine contractions, and when palpation is necessary, it must be done very lightly. The mother may have nausea and sometimes emesis at this time.

The mother's entire mien grows more serious during the transition phase. Relaxation becomes more difficult, and she may have trembling of her legs which she may find difficult or impossible to control. The mother may feel irritable at this time, and she may become restless. Signs of amnesia to varying degrees also may appear.

Signs of Approach or Onset of Second Stage

Rupture of the Membranes

The membranes may break at any time before or during labor, but when rupture occurs after the mother has been in labor for several hours, it may be an indication that the cervix is completely dilated. The station and position of the presenting part may change when the membranes rupture, and there is some possibility of prolapse of the umbilical cord with the gush of fluid, if the presenting part is still high in the pelvis at the time of rupture (Fig. 22-3, page 440). The nurse should instruct the mother to notify her at once if she feels a sudden gush of fluid from the vagina. The amount of fluid that escapes will depend on the point of rupture and the position of the presenting part; it may vary from a small amount that soaks only a portion of the pad under the mother to a quantity that completely saturates the lower bedding. After rupture has occurred, some fluid will escape with each contraction. Rupture of the membranes should be reported to the physician promptly. The fetal heart should be checked immediately for rate and rhythm, and a vaginal examination is usually made at once to determine the condition of the cervix and the station and position of the presenting part. The color of the amniotic fluid is observed, and evidence of staining with meconium reported to the physician.

Increase in Bloody Show

Increasing bloody show, resulting from tiny lacerations in the cervix, is a good indication that labor is progressing well and that the cervix is steadily dilating. There may be considerable increase in bloody show toward the end of the first stage. This bloody mucoid discharge must be distinguished from bright-red blood, which is abnormal during labor.

Nausea and Vomiting

Sudden appearance of nausea and vomiting, if it has not been present throughout labor, is often a sign that the first stage has ended. The nurse also must realize that complications such as toxemia may first present this way.

Pressure on the Rectum

At the end of the first stage of labor the mother usually has an almost continuous desire to empty her bowels, because of pressure made on the rectum by the presenting part as it descends more deeply into the pelvis. This descent frequently takes place when the cervix becomes completely dilated, and if pressure has not been present in early labor and then rather suddenly appears, it may be a sign that the second stage has been reached. In addition to rectal pressure, cramps in the buttocks, thighs, and legs also may begin.

Involuntary Bearing Down

When the mother begins to bear down involuntarily with contractions, the second stage of labor probably has begun. Whenever there is bearing down, the perineum must be inspected for bulging at the height of the contraction.

Deep Grunting Sounds

Deep grunting sounds during contractions, in contrast to earlier utterances of a sharp and complaining nature, often signify that the second stage has begun. The grunting sound may appear very suddenly and may be so distinct from earlier sounds that this sign of second-stage labor is unmistakable, at least to the experienced obstetric nurse.

The Mother's Feeling That She Is Ready to Deliver

When the mother, especially the multigravida, says that her "baby is coming" she is usually correct, regardless of the findings of a recent vaginal examination, even if it was performed only a few minutes earlier. Such a remark must not be ignored. Although a very recent examination revealed little cervical dilation, it is important to realize that the cervix can dilate very rapidly, and the mother's observation demands further investigation.

Bulging of the Perineum

Bulging of the perineum is always a sign that delivery is imminent.

Close observation of the mother is necessary to allow adequate time to prepare for delivery. If the mother is to be taken to a separate delivery room for birth, the time at which she is moved will depend on how soon the birth of the baby is anticipated. The intensity of uterine contractions, the station and position of the presenting part, and previous progress are considered in making this judgment.

The primigravida usually is taken to the delivery room when the cervix has become completely dilated, if the head is low and in an anterior position. If the head has not descended to the perineal floor or has not rotated anteriorly, the mother may remain in her bed in the labor room during the early part of the second stage of labor. She is encouraged to bear down with contractions and is observed closely for advancement of the presenting part.

The multigravida, who ordinarily completes the latter part of the first stage of labor and all of the second stage quite rapidly, is often taken to the delivery room when the cervix is 7 to 8 cm dilated. If her progress is rapid, there may not be adequate time for complete preparation if it is not begun before the second stage. On the other hand, if there is reason to expect that delivery of the multigravida will be delayed, preparation for the birth may not be started before complete dilation of the cervix has been reached.

The nurse caring for the mother in active labor must be alert to the possibility of rapidly changing conditions. When a multigravida who is having strong contractions suddenly shows signs of second-stage labor, rapid delivery can usually be anticipated. If the mother's membranes rupture, if she feels sudden pressure on her rectum, and if she begins to have involuntary bearing down, the nurse must notify the physician immediately and quickly prepare for delivery. The nurse also must appreciate that in some instances conditions are favorable in the primigravida for rapid completion of the latter part of the first stage and of the entire second stage of labor. In such case, labor in the primigravida may be quite similar to that of a multigravida.

It is usually preferable for the woman to give birth in the same room in which she has labored. This provides greater comfort for her and avoids the annoying interruption of her concentration which occurs with a move. It can also permit a more orderly preparation of equipment by the staff.

SECOND STAGE (STAGE OF DESCENT AND BIRTH)

The second stage of labor is shorter and more intense than the first stage. The uterine contractions are stronger, more frequent, and more expulsive, and the fetus steadily descends through the birth canal. The mother must be attended at all times by someone who is capable of recognizing any change in condition. Vigilance in observing the progress of labor, and in watching both mother and fetus for signs of complications, is of extreme importance.

Care of the Mother

Most of the care that was given in the first stage of labor is continued during the second stage. Close observation of the progress of labor, and observation for unfavorable signs are of extreme importance. The mother needs continuing emotional support, she may need coaching in making the best use of expulsive efforts to deliver the baby, and she needs relief from discomfort insofar as possible. She needs a person capable of giving expert care with her at all times.

Amniotomy (Artificial Rupture of the Membranes)

If the fetal membranes do not rupture spontaneously at complete dilation of the cervix, they are ruptured artificially at the beginning of the second stage since they may now retard progress of labor. Under conditions favorable for the onset of labor and with the presenting part low in the pelvis, an amniotomy may be performed before labor begins, being used as a method of induction of labor. At other times, the membranes are ruptured at varying times during the first stage of labor, either after labor is established or after cervical dilation is progressing well.

In performing the amniotomy, precautions are taken to prevent contamination of the vagina, and close observation is made of its effects on the labor and the fetus. The mother's vulva is washed with an antiseptic solution. The physician prepares his or her hands and puts on sterile gloves. A sterile forceps, frequently an Allis clamp, or a sharp hook, is introduced into the vagina to rupture the membranes, which are usually quite tense. The break is made between uterine contractions. Sometimes only the forceps is introduced into the vagina to grasp the membranes and break them; at other times the physician performs a vaginal examination and inserts the instrument while two fingers of one hand are in the vagina touching the membranes. The physician may hold the fingers in the vagina while some of the amniotic fluid drains out and then note the change that may take place in the position of the presenting part. As following spontaneous rupture, the rate of the fetal heart is observed and recorded immediately following artificial rupture of the membranes, and the color and characteristics of the fluid are observed and recorded.

Pushing with Uterine Contractions

During the second stage the force of intraabdominal pressure is added to intrauterine pressure to move the fetus through the birth canal. This force is exerted through bearing-down efforts at the time that the uterine muscle is contracting. Bearing down is discouraged before the cervix is completely dilated, but is advised as soon as the second stage begins.

Bearing down is reflex and spontaneous during the second stage, and as labor advances it becomes a very strong impulse. Occasionally a woman does not use this reflex advantageously during the early part of the second stage, and coaching is helpful. The nurse is often the person who explains to the woman what she should do and gives her encouragement. Mothers who have attended preparation-for-childbirth classes have had instructions in pushing; they need support in their efforts.

Good breathing technique, contraction of abdominal muscles, and relaxation of the perineum are important for effective pushing. As the contraction begins, the woman is encouraged to use quick, shallow breathing as she feels the contraction build. The urge to bear down will cause her to involuntarily hold her breath and push toward the area of greatest pressure, the vagina. Ordinarily she will return to rapid, shallow breathing briefly, then bear down again. She may repeat this pattern several times depending on the length of the contraction. Her urge to push will likely vary from one contraction to another. The practice of exhorting the woman to hold her breath and bear down using a Valsalva manuever for as long as she possibly can is not physiologic and may actually be harmful as well as less effective.

The effect of bearing down is increased if the woman is in a good position for pushing. The position, which appears to be most favorable, is one in which her back is rounded, chin on chest and her knees are bent and drawn up. Some women may assume this position on their sides, or they may prefer kneeling or squatting. However, the majority of women will choose a semi-sitting position similar to that shown in Figure 20–11.

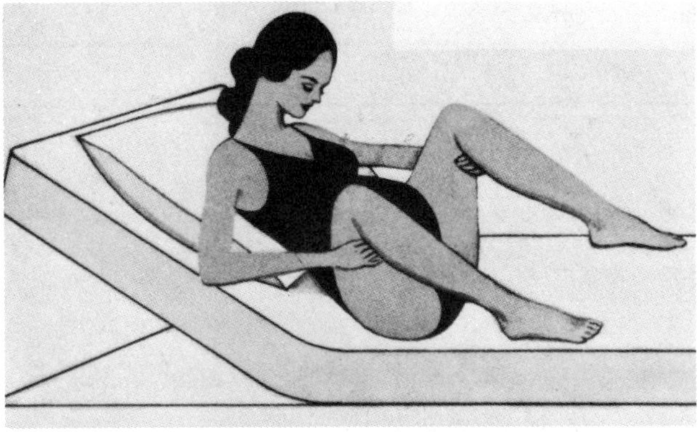

Figure 20–11. Pushing position. The position and breathing in this illustration have been practiced during pregnancy, but without actual pushing, as is done during the second stage of labor. The stretch afforded by the pushing position, without simultaneous use of the breathing pattern, may give a mother some relief from middle backache during the antepartum period if she wishes to use it for that purpose. (Reproduced with permission from Maternity Center Association, *Preparation for Childbearing*. 4th ed. rev. New York: Maternity Center Association, 1982, p. 34.)

This position takes advantage of the assistance of gravity in aiding the descent of the fetus. In addition it is similar to the position used in bearing down to evacuate the bowels and, as such, is familiar. The arms and legs should be flexed and relaxed.

The mother is urged to relax as much as possible between contractions. When the contraction is over, the mother should let out her breath, lean back, take a deep breath and sigh it out, and try to relax all over. Every minute between contractions should be used for rest.

Although the contractions of the second stage are very strong, the mother usually feels less discomfort than she

Table 20–2. Summary of Observations and Nursing Care During Labor

Phase of Labor	*Mechanisms of Labor*	*Responses of Patient*	*Nursing Interventions*
FIRST STAGE			
LATENT PHASE			
0–2 or 3 cm	Cervical effacement Slow dilation (duration: primigravida—8 hr; multigravida—3 to 5 hr)	Surge of energy and excitement Talkative, outgoing Easily distracted from contractions Anxiety is low and promotes learning	Orient to hospital environment and personnel Assess history and physical status Assess attitudes, past experiences, expectations Teach about labor Practice breathing and relaxation techniques
2–3–4 cm	Effacement completed Slight acceleration of rate of dilation	Becomes quieter; settles into rhythm of contractions Breathes with contractions May grimace, squeeze hands	Teaching still appropriate but should be specific to immediate needs Reemphasize relaxation; purpose of contractions

(*Continued*)

Table 20–2. (Cont.)

Phase of Labor	*Mechanisms of Labor*	*Responses of Patient*	*Nursing Interventions*
		Less easily distracted but still interested in surroundings	Monitor physical status: Vital signs including FHR Voiding Amount and character of vaginal discharge Warmth and comfort Oral hygiene
ACTIVE PHASE			
5–6–7 cm	Period of most rapid dilation Dilation for primigravida should be at least 1.2 cm/hr; for multigravida at least 1.5 cm/hr	Serious, talks only in short sentences or phrases; cries out in pain Focused on self and her pain Restless, tossing body about during contractions Regression and increasing dependency Own resources may not be adequate to cope with contractions	Anticipate needs: Sponge face Keep bed clean and dry Care for dry, cracked mouth Check bladder for fullness Stay at bedside working through each contraction with patient; praise woman's efforts, point out progress Reinforce supportive efforts of the father Use touch to soothe, relax, comfort Check FHR q 15 min, B/P q 30 min Observe for hyperventilation May need analgesia to enhance coping
8–9–10 cm	Slight deceleration in rate of dilation around 8–9 cm Descent of presenting part	Maximum concentration needed to cope with contractions May be nonverbal except for moans, single words, cries for help Nausea, occasional vomiting Legs shake uncontrollably Back pain and perineal pressure often continuous; can't distinguish beginning and end of contractions	Continue physical and supportive care as above Use palpation or uterine contraction monitor to help patient define contractions and rest periods Observe perineum for bulging
SECOND STAGE	Expulsion of fetus	Becomes exhausted by great physical effort May be amnesic between contractions May become aggressive: hitting, scratching, vulgar language Panic that she will rip apart	Direct pushing efforts with father for each contraction Provide comfort measures and facilitate rest between contractions: Cool cloth to face Keep perineum clean and dry Environment quiet Encourage efforts; point out progress Explain preparations being made for delivery Check FHR with each contraction Help with panting for delivery of head and shoulders
THIRD STAGE	Expulsion of placenta	Relief, fatigue, euphoria Cries with relief and joy Talkative Focused on infant and husband; keenly aware of people and things in environment	Congratulate Initiate contact with infant Coach in relaxation for delivery of placenta and perineal repair

did during the latter part of the first stage. With bearing down, she generally feels that she is accomplishing something and making progress in the delivery of her infant. She should be given assurance that she is doing well and that her efforts are advancing the infant.

As the second stage progresses, the father is able to see first the bulging of the perineum and then the top of the infant's head as it comes further down the birth canal with each contraction. This visible sign of progress is not only encouraging and exciting for him but enables him to effectively urge the mother on through the last few difficult moments of labor.

The birth of the infant and immediate postdelivery care of mother and infant are discussed in Chapter 21.

Table 20-2 gives a summary of the physiologic and psychologic changes during labor and appropriate nursing interventions for each stage and phase of labor.

REFERENCES AND SUGGESTED READINGS

Barnett, M. M., Infant outcome in relation to second stage labor pushing method, *Birth,* 9(4):221-229, 1982.

Brown, C., Therapeutic effects of bathing during labor, *J. Nurse Midwifery,* 24:13-16, 1982.

Howe, C. L., Physiologic and psychosocial assessment in labor, *Nurs. Clin. North Am.,* 17(1):49-56, 1982.

Lederman, R. P., Lederman, E., Work, B. A., and McCann, D. S., Relationship of psychological factors in pregnancy to progress of labor, *Nurs. Res.,* 28(2):94-97, 1979.

Maloni, Judith A., The birthing room: Some insights into parents' experiences, *MCN* 5(5):320-25, 1980.

McKay, S., Second stage labor. Has tradition replaced safety? *Am. J. Nurs.,* 81(5):1016-1019, 1981.

Mercer, R. T., Hackley, K. C., and Bostrom, A. G., Relationship of psychosocial and perinatal variables to perception of childbirth, *Nurs. Res.,* 32(4):202-207, 1983.

Penny, K. S., Postpartum perception of touch received during labor. *Res. Nurs. Health,* 2:9-16, 1979.

Roberts, Joyce, Alternative positions for childbirth—Part I: First stage of labor, *J. Nurse Midwifery,* 25(4):11-18, 1980.

——Alternative positions for childbirth—Part II: The second stage of labor, *J. Nurse Midwifery,* 25(5):13-19, 1980.

Sosa, R. A., and Cupoli, J. M. The birthing process: The effects on the parents. *Clin. Perinatol.,* 8(1):197-210, 1981.

Sosa, Roberto; Kennell, John; Klaus, Marshall; Robertson, Steven; and Urrutia, Juan, The effect of a supportive companion on perinatal problems, length of labor, and mother-infant interaction, *N. Engl. J. Med.,* 303(11):597-600, 1980.

CHAPTER

21

Nursing Management During Delivery

CARE OF THE MOTHER and fetus during the first stage of labor has been described in Chapter 20. This chapter deals with the actual delivery of the infant (second stage of labor), delivery of the placenta (third stage of labor), and the immediate care of both mother and newborn after the birth (fourth stage of labor).

The second and third stages of labor may take place in the same room as the first stage, or the woman may be moved to another room known as the birth room or delivery room. The place of birth may depend in part on the preference of the woman and in part on the normalcy of labor and expectations for a normal birth.

When a delivery room is used, the woman is transferred from her bed to the delivery table during either the latter part of the first stage or the early part of the second stage of labor, depending on her parity and progress of labor. Final preparation for delivery may be made immediately after this transfer, or after a variable period of bearing down with contractions, depending on the imminence of the birth. Efforts are made to allow sufficient time, thus avoiding hasty or inadequate preparation, and yet not to complete the preparation too far in advance of the actual delivery. When preparation is made too early, the mother's legs may be in stirrups an undue length of time; this may lead to muscle soreness, sluggish leg circulation, and venous thrombosis. Early preparation also leaves sterile supplies uncovered for a long time, which increases danger of contamination.

It is desirable for the same nurse who cared for the mother during labor also to care for her during delivery. This nurse will be a familiar person in a strange environment, and communication between the nurse and the parents will probably have been well established. If the father will be with his wife during delivery, it is also desirable that he accompany her to the delivery room at the time this transfer is made.

THE DELIVERY ROOM

All or a considerable part of the second stage of labor, and also all of the third stage, may be conducted in the delivery room. Maintenance of aseptic technique to prevent infection in both mother and newborn is crucial. An adequate amount of equipment for the management of complicated as well as normal births, for administration of anesthesia, and for meeting all emergencies is equally important.

Prevention of Infection

The woman in labor is very susceptible to infection brought to her from without. Personnel in the delivery room must be dressed in clean uniforms that have not been worn outside the labor and delivery room area. A cap must be worn to keep loose hair from falling on the sterile field and a mask to prevent droplet infection from the mouth and nose. Both mouth and nose must be well covered, and the mask must be changed at least every hour, and preferably every one-half hour, but a mask will not be sufficient protection if any of the attendants has a bacterial respiratory infection. No one with an infection of any type should attend the woman in labor. Only personnel directly concerned with the delivery should be permitted in the delivery room, and then only when in proper operating room attire. The delivery room is used only for obstetric clients. Frequent hand washing is important. A soap or detergent that contains hexachlorophene (G-11) or another bacteriostatic agent usually is preferred to other soaps.

Everything that touches the perineal region or that is used directly for the delivery—gloves, gowns, instruments, draping sheets, towels, and gauze—must be sterile. Preparation of the hands, gowning, and gloving of persons who directly assist with the delivery is similar to preparation for assisting with an operation.

Equipment

Much of the equipment in the delivery room is similar to that of the operating room; some is different because of the special purpose for which the delivery room is used.

Gloves, gowns, drapes, and many of the instruments and suture equipment are similar to those of an operating room. Some equipment, such as obstetric forceps, is special for the purpose of delivery.

The delivery table usually consists of two adjoining sections that can be separated easily; it is equipped with stirrups and with hand grips; and it is adjustable to various heights and positions. The mother is often put in the lithotomy position, with her legs in stirrups, for the delivery, and the lower half of the table is rolled under the main section for easier access to the perineal area.

Anesthesia machines and anesthetic agents and supplies are the same as those used in the operating room.

Equipment must be available for adequate care of the newborn. This includes a heated crib or incubator and warmed blanket, an umbilical cord clamp, identification material, silver nitrate solution, penicillin, or tetracycline for the eyes, and aspiration, oxygen, and intubation equipment in case the infant needs resuscitation.

Equipment and supplies for administration of intravenous fluids, for blood transfusion, and for drugs that may be necessary to meet an emergency must be available. Other essential equipment consists of suction devices for both mother and newborn and an oxygen supply for both. Emergency call lights or signals and facilities for adequate lighting and for adequate temperature control are important. Mechanical devices must be checked frequently for proper function.

Since most deliveries are normal and only a small amount of supplies are used, much of the equipment mentioned above will be used infrequently. It is prepared to be available and in readiness for the less common complicated deliveries and the emergencies that may arise.

NURSING ASSESSMENT

Observations of the Mother

Frequency of making observations and the vigilance in watching for changes must be increased during the second stage because of the increased rapidity and stress of labor. The uterine contractions are observed closely. The monitor is watched carefully, or the abdomen is palpated for frequency, duration, and strength of contractions, and also to ascertain that the uterine muscle relaxes well between contractions. The abdominal contour during contractions is observed to make certain that the uterus is contracting evenly.

The perineum is inspected during bearing down for bulging or for appearance of the presenting part, and also for abnormal vaginal discharge, such as bleeding and expulsion of meconium. Before the fetal head can be seen at the vaginal outlet, or its advance noted by bulging, the stage of its descent is sometimes ascertained by palpating through the perineum, the fingers of a gloved hand pressing upward on one side of the vulva.

The mother's vital signs, with the exception of temperature, are checked frequently. The pulse and blood pressure are taken every 5 to 10 minutes.

Muscle cramps in the legs may be a source of discomfort and will need immediate attention (see Fig. 20–8, page 395). The uncomfortable feeling of perspiration on the face may be relieved by wiping the face frequently and by applying a cool, moist cloth to the forehead. Discomfort caused by dryness of the mouth and lips may be relieved by moistening the lips with a wet cloth.

Observations of the Fetus

The reactions of the fetus must be very carefully observed throughout the second stage of labor. As in the first stage, this is done by close observation of the monitor or by auscultation of the fetal heart and by watching for expulsion of meconium. Fetal distress may be brought about by an interference with its oxygen supply. Heart rate pattern is watched very carefully and checked every five minutes, or following each contraction, during the entire second stage, until the fetus is born.

Oxygen administered to the mother may satisfactorily treat the fetus if signs of hypoxia appear and thereby prevent respiratory depression at birth. This treatment may be beneficial when the fetus is deprived of an adequate oxygen supply from such causes as a low concentration of oxygen with an anesthetic agent, obstruction in the maternal respiratory tract, respiratory depression due to drugs, a failing maternal circulatory system, placental separation, or pressure on the umbilical cord during contractions. With signs of fetal hypoxia, high concentration of oxygen may be administered to the mother between, as well as during, contractions while awaiting spontaneous delivery, or while preparation is being made for an operative delivery.

PUSHING WITH CONTRACTIONS

Pushing with contractions, as described on page 400, is continued throughout the second stage of labor. Pushing on the delivery table is facilitated by a semipropped position, with back curved and head forward. The mother's head and shoulders can be supported by raising the head of the delivery table or with extra pillows. If her legs are not in stirrups, she can flex her thighs toward her abdomen and grasp her thighs or her legs just below the knees while she pushes.

The father usually supports the mother's back as she pushes and coaches her in breathing and in relaxation between contractions.

PREPARATION FOR DELIVERY

Traditionally the lithotomy position has been used for delivery and the mother's legs are put in stirrups when the delivery is imminent. Sometimes the mother is delivered with her knees bent and her feet resting on the foot end of the delivery table. Many physicians prefer the lithotomy position for easier access to the perineal area and for readiness in the event that an operative delivery becomes necessary as an emergency measure. A side-lying (Sims') position also may be used if the woman prefers and labor is normal. Squatting and kneeling positions also are used occasionally. In the usual, uncomplicated birth, the woman may be left to assume any position she prefers.

When the lithotomy position is used, care must be taken to prevent a strain on the ligaments of the pelvis during positioning of the legs in stirrups. They must not be separated too widely, and one leg should not be placed higher than the other. It is important that both legs are elevated together and placed into the stirrups at the same time. The legs or thighs should not be permitted to press against the bars holding the stirrups. The legs are strapped to the stirrups immediately after being placed there, to avoid the danger of the mother's moving a leg out of the stirrup. They must never be unstrapped after the delivery until the very moment that they are to be put down on the table, since the mother may be partly under the influence of an anesthetic and unexpectedly move her legs. When the legs are taken out of the stirrups, they must be moved gently and both should be lowered to the bed at the same time. Such movement will lessen ligament and muscle strain and prevent any sudden change in circulation and blood pressure.

The perineal region is regarded as the field of a major surgical operation and is prepared accordingly. Preparation consists of thorough washing of the skin of the lower abdomen, inner aspect of the thighs, vulva, and anal region to make it as clean as possible. During preparation, precautions are taken to avoid bringing bacteria to the mother and also carrying bacteria from her own skin to the vagina and thus permitting entry to the uterine cavity. All materials used for this preparation are sterile, and the nurse wears cap and mask and sterile gloves.

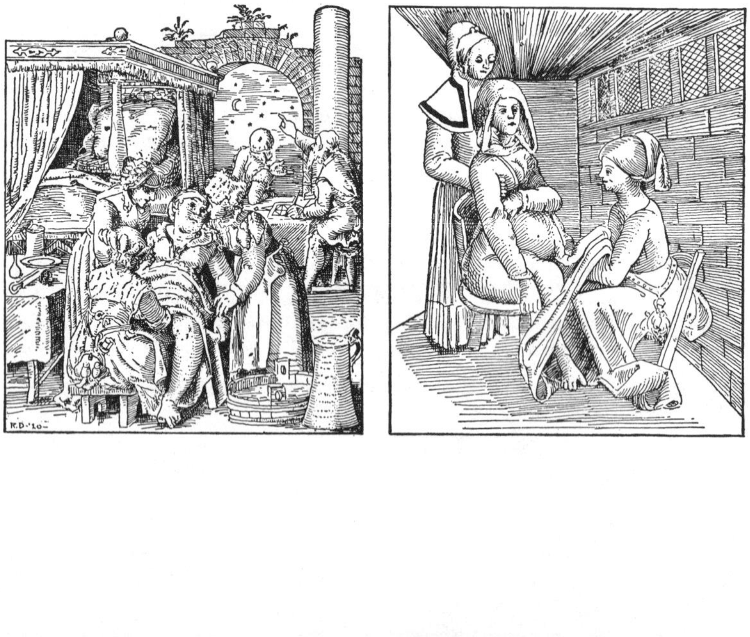

Figure 21-1. Old prints illustrating early ideas of suitable methods of making examinations and conducting deliveries, furnishing contrast with present-day methods. Concern seems to be divided between the patient and the signs of the zodiac in the picture at left.

A fairly typical method of preparation for delivery, or sterile vaginal examination, is as follows. The mother's legs are positioned in stirrups, and she is covered with a sheet according to the extent of area to be prepared. The mother should be protected from embarrassment of unnecessary exposure at all times during labor. The field which is to be prepared for examination or delivery must be uncovered, and a certain amount of exposure is unavoidable, but there are many ways in which the nurse may show consideration for the mother and she will appreciate this effort.

The lower half of the delivery table should not be removed until everything is in readiness for skin preparation and draping. The mother should never be left alone for a moment without careful observation of the perineum after the lower portion of the table has been removed.

The nurse washes her hands and arms using soap or detergent containing a bactericidal agent, puts on a pair of sterile gloves, and then prepares the skin. Firm, even movements are made for washing the perineal region, using soap or detergent containing an appropriate bactericidal agent. These movements are repeated a sufficient number of times to clean the skin well, removing all blood and mucus. Each sponge is used only once, being discarded after approaching the anal region, or after stroking away from the vaginal opening in any direction. Washing is done from the center outward to avoid carrying material from surrounding areas to the vaginal outlet. The vaginal orifice is covered with a dry cotton ball while the surrounding skin area is prepared, to prevent solutions from entering the vagina. After the perineal area is washed, it is rinsed with sterile water, and other antiseptic solutions may then be poured over or sprayed on the skin. If fluid is poured over the vulvar region, it is not allowed to run into the vagina from the surrounding skin.

After skin preparation, as much of the prepared area as possible may be covered with sterile drapes. The gloves used for preparation are considered contaminated. A sterile gown and a fresh pair of sterile gloves should be put on before sterile linen and other supplies are handled. Sterile leggings are placed over the mother's legs and as deeply into the groin as possible, and sterile sheets are placed under her buttocks and over her abdomen. Commercially packaged sterile drapes of a waterproof paper, which are disposable after use, are ordinarily used.

Since skin can only be cleaned, not sterilized, care is taken to avoid touching the vulva and surrounding skin insofar as possible during examination and delivery. Special precautions are taken against touching the anal region with sterile gloved hands. Whenever draping sheets or towels become wet from amniotic fluid and blood, they must be considered contaminated from the skin underneath; wet drapes are therefore not touched, and if possible they are replaced with dry ones. Instruments, towels, and sponges that are ordinarily used for a normal delivery are arranged on a table that has been covered with a sterile draping sheet.

An area on which the infant may be placed, for immediate care after birth, is arranged. For this, a warmed incubator or crib may be covered with a sterile sheet. Sufficient padding with sterile blankets or towels over the area where the infant will be placed is provided to protect him and to keep the area under him sterile. The newborn's skin is wet, and inadequate layers of draping sheet will become moist throughout and unsterile from the table underneath.

While the above preparations are being made, the physician or midwife prepares the hands and arms as for surgery and puts on a sterile gown and gloves for the delivery. If a local anesthetic or a pudendal block is planned, an anesthetic drug is injected into the vulvar and perineal tissues after the preparation and draping. If the mother has not recently emptied her bladder she may be catheterized at this time. The perineum is kept clean while awaiting the birth of the fetus by sponging in a downward direction, with cotton balls soaked in an antiseptic solution. Amniotic fluid and bloody mucus may drain from the vagina. Also particles of fecal material are sometimes expelled while the mother is bearing down, because of the pressure that is exerted on her rectum by the fetal head.

BIRTH OF THE FETUS

Delivery of the Fetal Head

The physician or midwife controls delivery of the fetal head to prevent its rapid and forceful expulsion at the height of a contraction. Uncontrolled, forceful extrusion of the head may result in a deep tear in the perineal tissues and may also be injurious to the infant because of a sudden change of pressure on the head. Sometimes, when the perineum has offered considerable resistance to the head, the resistance is suddenly overcome; one contraction may then force the head out of the vagina. If the head is not yet well extended, force against the perineal body instead of upward toward the vaginal opening increases the possibility of a deep perineal tear. Delivery of the head is therefore controlled so that it emerges from the birth canal slowly and in good extension. The head is often delivered between contractions, the time at which control is easiest.

To control delivery, a hand is placed on the fetal head, after it begins to distend the perineum and separate the labia, and held in such a position as to be able to control its progress if this becomes necessary. While placing pressure on the occiput, upward pressure may also be applied on the brow through the perineum, a method

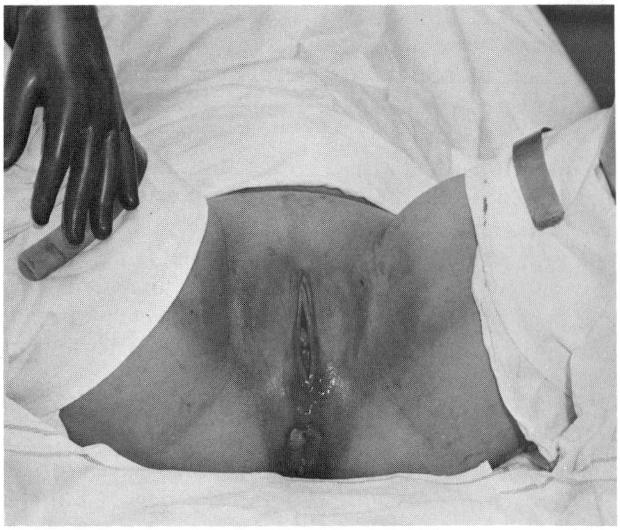

Figure 21–2. The baby's head is appearing at the vulva at the height of a contraction; separation of the labia is beginning.

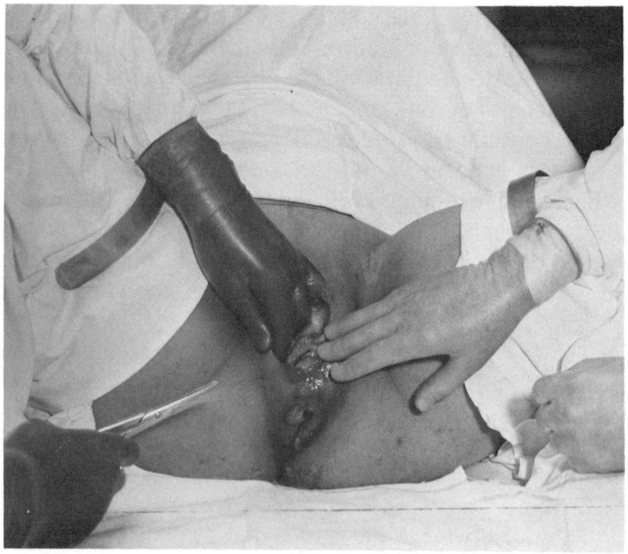

Figure 21–4. Preparation for an episiotomy during a contraction. Note that the perineum has become quite thin and that the anus has begun to distend.

termed *Ritgen's maneuver.* For this maneuver, the fingers are covered with sterile toweling and, after the head has descended far enough to distend the vulva with its parietal bosses, the fingers of one hand are placed directly behind the anal region, or directly before it in a modified procedure, and upward pressure is exerted through the perineum while the other hand is held in readiness to restrain progress of the head should the vulvar resistance be overcome suddenly.

With restraint on the occiput, and sometimes upward pressure on the fetal chin, delivery of the head is slow and controlled in a manner favoring extension (see Figs. 21–2, 21–3, 21–4, and 21–5 for appearance, advance, and birth of head during normal delivery).

The mother may be asked to pant during the last few contractions before the birth of the head, after crowning occurs, so that bearing down, which is involuntary, and the resultant intraabdominal pressure will be considerably reduced, preventing rapid advancement of the head. The head then may be allowed to advance slowly during a uterine contraction, or the physician may deliver it after the contraction has ceased. For delivery between contractions a certain amount of pressure is necessary. This pressure may be applied from above by asking the mother to bear down, this time without a

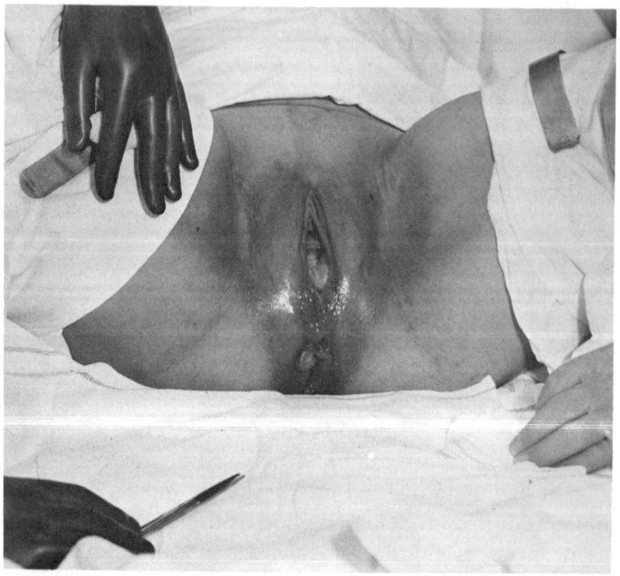

Figure 21–3. Advance of the head is indicated by distention of the vulva and perineum.

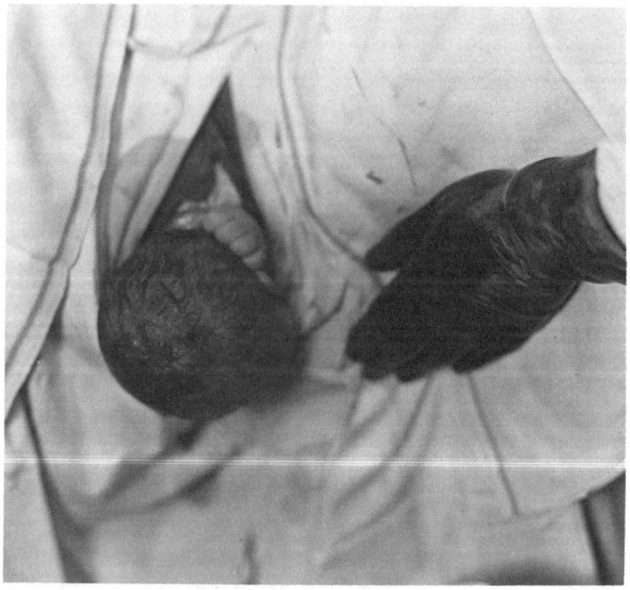

Figure 21–5. The head has been born, and external rotation toward the right has taken place. In this delivery a hand has prolapsed alongside the head; this is not ordinarily the case.

simultaneous uterine contraction; or an assistant may exert a small amount of pressure on the uterine fundus.

Episiotomy (Perineal Incision) and Perineal Laceration

Lacerations are occasionally prevented, and often limited in extent, by skillful delivery of the infant, but in spite of the most careful efforts, tears of some degree will occur in most primigravidas and in many multigravidas unless an episiotomy (incision of the perineum) is done. A laceration may be no larger than a nick in the vaginal mucous membrane, it may extend down into the perineal body to any degree, or it may extend entirely through the perineal body and through the rectal sphincter. Perineal lacerations are very likely to occur when the perineal tissues are rigid and do not stretch well, or when they are friable; when the infant is delivered rapidly; when the infant is large; when a small pelvic outlet does not permit the head to fit closely against the symphysis pubis; and when delivery takes place from an abnormal presentation or position. Lacerations are usually described as being of first, second, or third degree, according to their extent.

A *first-degree laceration* is one that extends only through the fourchet, the vaginal mucous membrane, and the skin at the anterior margin of the perineum, without involving any of the muscles.

A *second-degree laceration* is one that involves the muscles of the perineal body. It extends down into the perineal body to varying degrees, sometimes to the rectal sphincter, but not through it. Such a tear usually extends upward into the vagina on one or both sides, making a triangular injury.

A *third-degree laceration* extends entirely through the perineal body and through the rectal sphincter and sometimes up the anterior wall of the rectum. This variety is often called a *complete tear,* in contradistinction to those of first and second degree, which are incomplete. A third-degree tear occurs infrequently. When the laceration extends up the anterior wall of the rectum, the term *fourth-degree laceration* is sometimes used to designate the extent of involvement.

Sometimes *lacerations* occur in the *labia* or *around the urethra.* These may be only slight abrasions, or they may be deep enough to bleed freely.

Episiotomy (Perineotomy)

An episiotomy, which is an incision through the perineal body, is very frequently performed, shortly before the fetal head is born, to facilitate delivery by enlarging the vaginal orifice. The major purposes of an episiotomy are (1) to spare the muscles of the perineal floor from undue stretching and bruising, and (2) to prevent prolonged pressure of the fetal head against the perineum. An episiotomy also will prevent the frequently unavoidable tears of the perineum, and substitute repair of a clean-cut incision for an irregular tear. It is especially useful in cases of rigid perineum, when rapid delivery is necessary, when laceration seems inevitable, when presentation and position of the fetus are abnormal, and when the infant is premature.

An episiotomy incision starts at the posterior margin of the vaginal opening and either may be made directly in the midline down to the sphincter ani muscle, called a *midline* or *median episiotomy,* or made at a 45-degree angle to either side, termed a *mediolateral episiotomy.* A blunt-pointed scissors is used to make the incision, which is ordinarily performed at the height of a contraction, while the perineum is stretched (Fig. 21–4). For the comfort of the mother, analgesia ordinarily is used when the incision is made. Analgesia may be obtained from a regional anesthetic previously administered or from a local infiltration of the perineum. The episiotomy is usually performed when the fetal head is low enough to distend the perineum and apply some pressure to the incision. Generally it is done before undue stretching has occurred, but not so early as to allow for excessive blood loss while awaiting the birth of the infant.

The decision as to whether to make a midline or a mediolateral incision will depend on a number of factors. The midline incision is easy to repair, heals well, and probably heals with less discomfort to the mother than the mediolateral, but there is danger of extension through the sphincter muscle if further tearing occurs. Extension of a mediolateral episiotomy does not injure the sphincter muscles, therefore it may be employed when the infant is large or when the presentation or position is unusual. Many physicians favor the midline incision in most cases, preferring to incise the sphincter ani if a laceration appears imminent.

Palpation for Umbilical Cord Around the Fetal Neck

Immediately after birth of the head, the physician palpates around the neck to determine whether or not loops of umbilical cord surround it. At times one or more loops of cord do encircle the fetus' neck, and they may be so tight that the vessels become constricted. If these coils of cord are fairly loose, they may be slipped over the head, but if they are tight the cord is clamped and cut immediately.

Delivery of the Shoulders and Body

The fetus' shoulders appear at the vulva as soon as external rotation of the head has taken place, and they usually are born spontaneously. However, it may be necessary to hold the infant's head between the two hands and make gentle downward traction to guide the anterior shoulder under the symphysis pubis, then lift the head upward to deliver the posterior shoulder, and downward

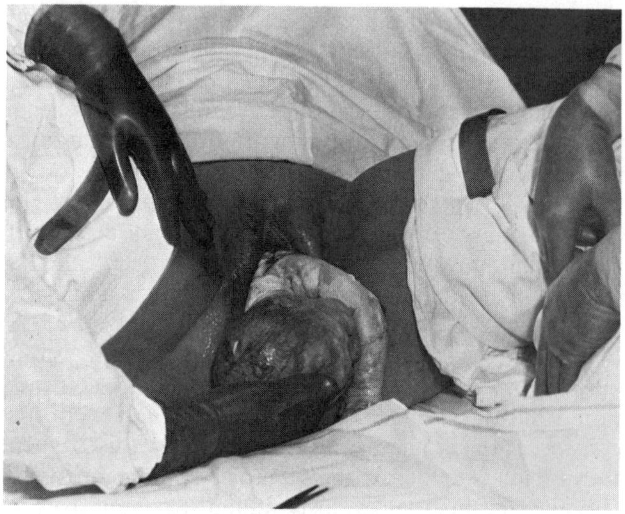

Figure 21-6. The anterior shoulder has been delivered. Birth of the rest of the body follows quickly.

again to deliver the anterior shoulder (Figs. 21-6, and 17-9 and 17-10 on page 347). At times it is found to be easier to deliver the anterior shoulder first. After delivery of the shoulders, the rest of the body usually follows easily.

Manipulations to deliver the shoulders and body must be gentle to avoid injury to the brachial plexus or the clavicle or the nerves of the arm. Any necessary traction is made moderately and only in the direction of the long axis of the fetus to avoid bending the neck on the body, which may result in excessive stretching of the brachial plexus. The fingers are not placed in the axillae to aid delivery, since this may put undue pressure on the nerves of the arms.

If force is necessary for delivery of the shoulders or for extrusion of the body, it is applied from above, by bearing-down efforts of the mother, or by suprapubic pressure made by an assistant.

As soon as the body is delivered the infant is held head downward for postural drainage of secretions and to decrease the risk of lung water syndrome (Fig. 21-7). The infant then is usually placed on the mother's abdomen for the parents to see and touch. Simultaneously the infant is dried off and covered to prevent chilling. The cord is clamped and cut, and the newborn may be moved to a warmed incubator for further care or left next to the mother's warm body well covered (Fig. 21-8).

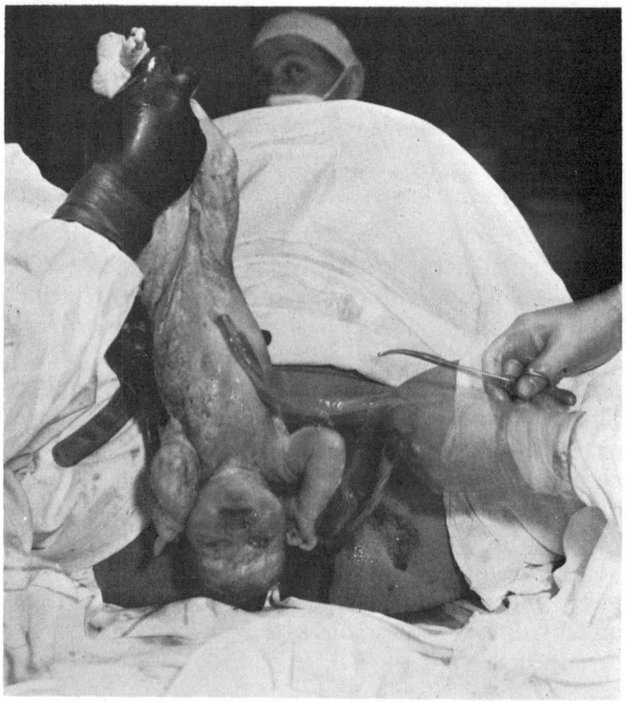

Figure 21-7. The infant is held with his head dependent for postural drainage of lung water and secretions in the respiratory tract. The physician is ready to clamp and cut the umbilical cord after respirations are initiated, unless need for immediate resuscitation is apparent. The baby will probably be placed on a level with the mother's body (the placenta) before the cord is clamped.

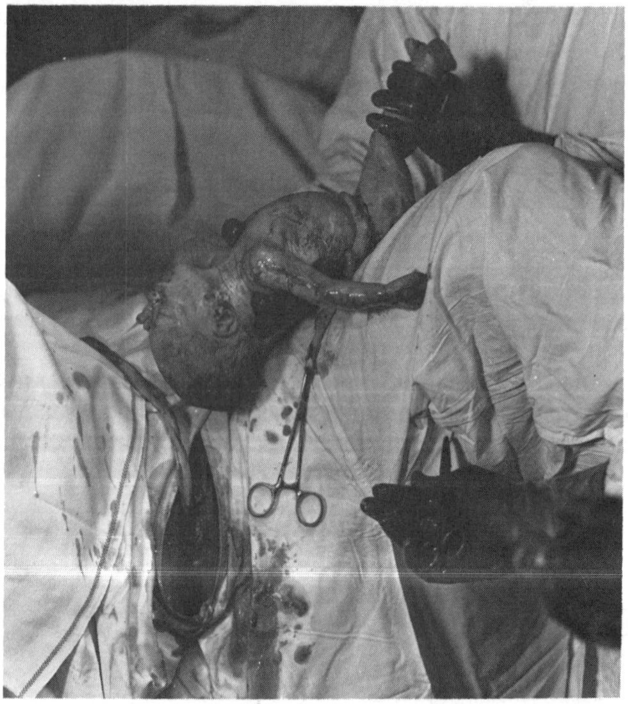

Figure 21-8. The umbilical cord has been severed, and the baby is shown to his parents and then, moved to an incubator for further care.

IMMEDIATE CARE OF THE NEWBORN

Establishing Respirations

The newborn requires prompt attention to ascertain that respirations begin at once, or to give aid that will assist in establishing adequate respirations. The lungs must immediately take over the respiratory function of the placenta, which, until birth, has served as the organ through which gas exchange has taken place.

Respirations are established within one minute after birth in most normal infants; many take their first breath within a few seconds and often cry vigorously as soon as they are born. A strong cry shortly after birth is evidence that the respiratory system has begun functioning well. Some infants, however, have a delay in onset of respirations, or they make respiratory movements shortly after birth but do not sustain these. With these infants resuscitative efforts must be taken immediately to prevent asphyxia, which progresses rapidly if untreated, and which may result in damage to brain cells or in death of the infant. Resuscitation should be done by the most experienced health team member present. Each nurse should be skilled in the techniques and should take prompt positive action if the physician is not immediately available.

Clearing the Air Passages

Fluid and mucus, and sometimes blood, meconium, and vernix, may be present in the newborn's mouth, nose, and pharynx at birth; it is of the utmost importance that this material is not aspirated with the first inspiration. A newborn who has not become asphyxiated during a normal labor and birth process will probably not aspirate with inspiration. An asphyxiated infant is likely to aspirate the secretions that are present in the mouth and oropharynx when the first breath is taken. Equipment that should be immediately available to clear the infant's respiratory tract is shown in Figure 21-9.

To permit secretions to drain by gravity from the pharynx, postural drainage should be instituted immediately after birth. The newborn is held in a position with the head dependent and the neck extended, before the first breath is taken, if possible, so that foreign material is not drawn into the trachea and lungs (Fig. 21-7). Sometimes an infant gasps before the body is completely delivered and before he can be held head down, but postural drainage is instituted as quickly as possible.

Some physicians use a rubber bulb syringe to remove excess mucus from the mouth and nose as soon as the fetal head is delivered, or they wait until immediately after delivery of the entire body, or they use suction at both times, after birth of the head and again after delivery of the body (Fig. 21-10). When suction is used, the mouth is aspirated first, since stimulation of the nose may cause the infant to gasp and aspirate secretions from the mouth. The initial suction of the mouth with the bulb syringe may induce coughing and gagging and facilitate the infant's own efforts to clear fluid and mucus.

Suction on a catheter also may be used to aspirate the

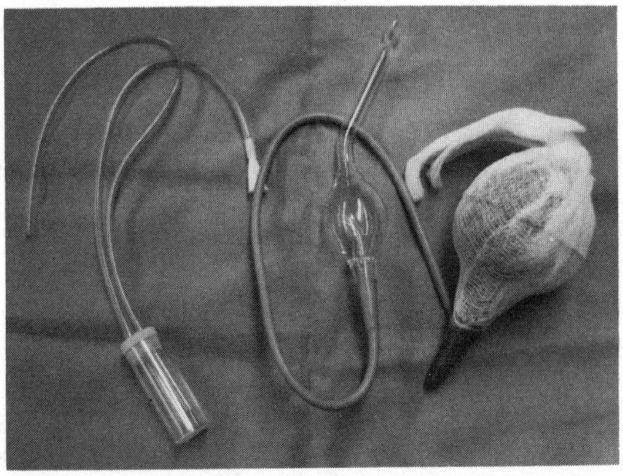

Figure 21-9. Equipment that may be used to remove secretions from the baby's mouth, nose, and throat.

Right, soft rubber bulb syringe. A piece of gauge placed around the syringe prevents slipping when it is handled with rubber gloves.

Middle, a soft rubber catheter, size no. 12 or 14 French, attached to a glass mucous trap.

Left, a plastic catheter with mucous trap. The mucous trap may be used to send the mucus to the laboratory for culture. The unit is disposable.

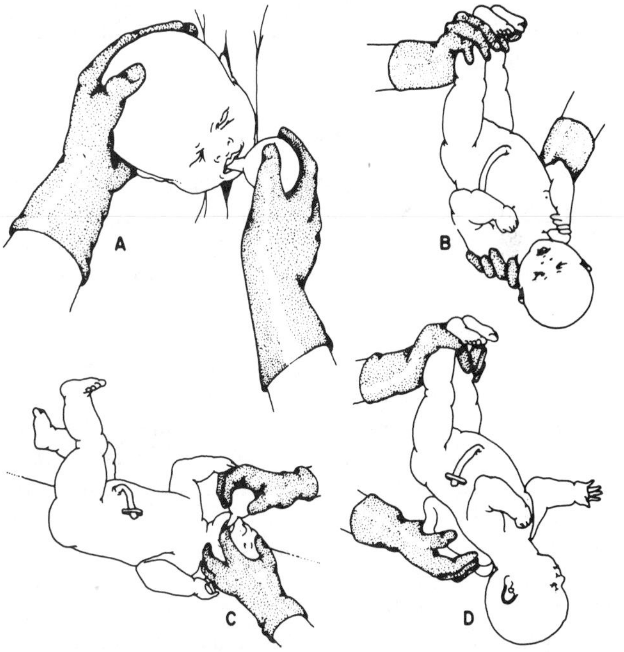

Figure 21-10. Vaginal delivery. *A*. suctioning a nasopharynx and oropharynx with bulb syringe, following delivery of the infant's head; *B*. the umbilical cord is clamped and cut; *C*. the infant is placed in a 20° head-down position and suctioned with a bulb syringe; *D*. the infant is thoroughly dried. (Reproduced with permission from G. W. Ostheimer, "Resuscitation of the Newborn," in M. D., Lough et al. (eds.): *Newborn Respiratory Care*. Chicago: Year Book Medical Publishers, Inc., 1979.)

mouth, pharynx, and nose. A disposable polyvinyl catheter attached to mechanical suction or to a DeLee mucous trap on which the operator makes suction (Fig. 21-9) may be used. The catheter may be more effective than the bulb syringe because it reaches farther down into the throat.

For further suctioning, the newborn is provided with warmth and put in the supine position with head lowered. To permit the infant's airway to extend and straighten, the head is slightly extended by placing a hand or a pad under the shoulders to elevate them. The infant's jaw is brought forward to lift the tongue from the posterior pharynx. The suction catheter is placed as far back as possible into the infant's throat, and suction is made on the mouthpiece of the mucous trap. The position of the catheter is changed frequently. The nose may also be aspirated.

Suctioning must be gentle to prevent injury to mucous membranes, and all should be brief—less than a minute is recommended. Unless suctioning is brief, the infant may hold his breath and develop laryngeal spasm during stimulation of the pharynx. Prolonged suction also may cause severe bradycardia and cardiac arrhythmia, complications that may result from vagal stimulation and lack of adequate oxygen.

Gastric suction also is done sometimes, but it is ordinarily delayed until respirations are established. Early gastric suction also may cause bradycardia and cardiac arrhythmia.

Maintaining Body Temperature

The infant is born into a room many degrees cooler than his body, and he will begin to lose body heat immediately. From the moment of birth the newborn must be kept warm to minimize the metabolic demands that are produced when heat production is increased to maintain the body temperature. A sterile blanket should be in readiness to cover the baby at birth. The infant should be quickly dried with a warm towel to reduce heat loss from evaporation of amniotic fluid from the body. The wet blanket should be replaced by a warm dry one. When the blanket is prewarmed, the newborn does not need to warm it with his own body heat.

To provide warm surroundings the newborn then should immediately be placed in a delivery room incubator warmed to 97 to 98° F (36.1 to 36.7° C) or preferably one with an overhead radiant heater. A radiant heater over the incubator will provide warmth while the infant is receiving care. If a source of radiant heat is not available, blankets around the infant will reduce radiation of heat from the infant's body to the cold tables and walls of the delivery room. If inhalation anesthesia is used, it is essential that any source of radiant heat or lamp is either properly grounded or is used outside the delivery room.

Immediate Appraisal of the Newborn

Appraisal of the neonate should begin the moment the infant is born. The newborn should be carefully observed for the time of the first gasp, the first cry, and the beginning of sustained respirations, and a record made. The nurse usually has the responsibility of making these observations. Many infants take their first gasp and begin crying within seconds after birth. It is therefore important to note the time of birth on a clock with a second hand so that the time of the first gasp, first cry, and sustained respirations can be recorded in the exact number of seconds that they appear following birth.

Most hospitals use a scoring system, devised by Dr. Virginia Apgar in 1952, for making a clinical evaluation of the newborn's condition at 1 minute after birth and again at 5 minutes and perhaps at 10 minutes.

The Apgar Scoring System

In the Apgar scoring method five vital signs—heart rate, respiratory effort, muscle tone, reflex irritability, and color—are observed at exactly 1 minute after complete birth of the infant, irrespective of delivery of the placenta. Each sign is evaluated according to the degree to which it is present and is given a score of 0, 1, or 2 (Table 21-1). The five scores, one given to each of the five signs, are added together for a total score. It has a possibility of ranging from 0 to 10. An infant in excellent condition could receive the maximum score of 10, and one in poor condition would receive a very low total score, possibly even 0.

All signs do not have equal importance, and they are not individually independent. Color is the least important sign and the first to change, and the heartbeat is the most important and the last to be absent. When all signs are not present, they disappear in the following order: color, respirations, muscle tone, reflex irritability, heartbeat.

Scoring is done by one of the persons in the delivery room who observes the infant during the first minute after birth. The nurse may be requested to make the observations and scoring; she may want confirmation from another person until she has had experience. Two observers, however, do not necessarily obtain the same total score, but variations should not be wide. Scoring does not interfere with other care and can be done while the newborn is receiving other necessary attention.

Scoring has been found to be easiest when a decision is made quickly, between 55 and 60 seconds after birth of the infant. For this reason, careful timing of birth on a clock with a second hand is important. The person doing the scoring may find it helpful to make a quick survey of the newborn's general appearance and decide in which order to observe the signs. If the infant cried immediately at birth, the observer may wish to check the respira-

Table 21-1. Apgar Scoring System*

Sign	*0*	*1*	*2*
Heart rate	Not detectable	Slow (below 100)	Over 100
Respiratory effort	Absent	Slow, irregular	Good, crying
Muscle tone	Flaccid	Some flexion of extremities	Active motion
Reflex irritability			
1. Response to slap on sole of foot	No response	Grimace	Cry
2. Response to catheter in nostril (tested after oropharynx is clear)	No response	Grimace	Cough or sneeze
Color	Blue, pale	Body pink, extremities blue	Completely pink

*Scoring chart arranged according to information from Dr. Virginia Apgar.

tions and color first. If the infant seems mildly depressed and respirations are absent at this time, the last three signs to disappear—muscle tone, reflex irritability, and heartbeat—can quickly be checked. If the newborn seems severely depressed, concentration on the last two signs to disappear—heartbeat and reflex irritability—is important.

HEART RATE The heart rate is the most important sign. It may be checked by observing pulsation in the umbilical cord at its juncture with the abdominal wall, by feeling the pulsation in the cord, or by auscultation of the heart with a stethoscope. A heart rate under 100 beats per minute is a sign of serious asphyxia and indicates resuscitation is necessary. If bradycardia is present, the other signs will be absent or present in only a minimal degree. If the heart rate increases during resuscitation, the prognosis is generally good; failure to increase during ventilation is a grave sign or an indication of ineffective resuscitation efforts.

RESPIRATORY EFFORT Respiratory effort is the second important sign. The vigorous infant should have respirations well established within 1 minute. The newborn usually cries lustily at birth and continues to breathe well. The infant whose breathing is shallow, slow, and irregular and who has only a weak cry is considered to be having some difficulty. Apnea requires early treatment.

MUSCLE TONE Muscle tone is scored according to the amount of flexion of the extremities and their resistance to extension. A term infant with excellent muscle tone keeps the arms and legs flexed, resists efforts to extend them, and has good movement of all extremities. If tone is only moderate, the infant appears sleepy, is not active, and does not keep the extremities flexed consistently. Poor muscle tone indicates that the infant has a low blood and tissue pH and is asphyxiated. An infant without tone is very limp and unresponsive.

REFLEX IRRITABILITY The reflex irritability sign is often tested by a slap on the sole of the infant's foot. The vigorous infant responds to this stimulation with a cry. If the response is not good, the infant will only grimace, and if he is quite depressed, he will not respond.

As an alternative method, reflex response may be tested by placing the tip of the catheter that was used to clear the pharynx of mucus just inside the nose. This method is not easily used before the infant has been moved to a table away from the field of delivery and may therefore not be the method of choice when clamping of the umbilical cord is delayed. A vigorous infant responds with a cough or sneeze when the catheter is placed just inside the nose. The less vigorous one responds with only a grimace, and the depressed infant does not respond. Lack of response indicates that the nervous system is depressed.

COLOR Color is the least important sign. Most infants, even when vigorous, do not become completely pink in 1 minute. All infants have some cyanosis at birth, and 1 to 3 minutes usually elapse, even in the healthy infant before the entire body is pink. Vigorous infants that receive a score of 2 for all other signs may therefore have only a score of 1 for color, because their extremities may still be blue at 1 minute after birth. For this reason, even the infant in excellent condition often has a score of less than 10. If the infant's entire body is blue or pale at the end of 1 minute the score for color is 0.

GROUPING ACCORDING TO SCORE The infant may be placed into one of three broad clinical groups according to the score he receives. Vigorous infants score from 7 to 10. These infants usually cry within a few seconds after birth. They generally do not require treatment. Infants in the depressed group score 4, 5, or 6, and may require some resuscitative measures to improve their condition. They have good heart rate and reflex irritability, but do not make satisfactory respiratory effort, their color is cyanotic, and their muscle tone may not be good. Infants in the severely depressed group score from 0 through 3; these infants require immediate resuscitation.

RESUSCITATION OF THE NEWBORN

The infant who does not breath at birth will have a rapid (1) decrease in blood Po_2 (decrease in concentration of oxygen in the blood), (2) rise in blood Pco_2 (in carbon dioxide concentration in the blood), and (3) fall in pH of blood and tissues. The Po_2 falls to a very low level, approaching zero, in 1 minute. Carbon dioxide continues to accumulate and the Pco_2 can rise to a very high level in 3 to 4 minutes. When adequate oxygen is not available, glucose is incompletely metabolized to lactic acid instead of being completely metabolized to carbon dioxide and water. Liberation of this lactic acid into the bloodstream and the accumulation of carbon dioxide results in a rapid fall in pH. Acidosis and lack of oxygen interfere with the normal function of body cells, and both must be corrected early. Unless resuscitative measures are instituted quickly, the infant's heartbeat will decrease in rate and heart action will soon stop.

If the infant does not breathe almost immediately after birth, ventilation of the lungs must be started at once to prevent or reverse sharp changes in physiologic condition. Ventilation of the lungs is used to reoxygenate the blood, remove carbon dioxide, and raise the pH by removal of carbon dioxide and restoration of complete glucose metabolism. Most infants who do not breathe within 1 minute after birth need only a few inflations of the lungs to initiate spontaneous breathing. A severely depressed infant may need ventilation for minutes or even hours. Ventilation is continued until the infant has sustained respirations.

The condition of the infant at birth is related to the degree of hypoxia or asphyxia before birth. An infant who has not suffered hypoxia, caused by antepartum complications or the labor and delivery process, is likely to require very little assistance or none with breathing. Infants with a severe depression, usually caused by asphyxia prior to birth, require that resuscitation be started immediately, without waiting to ascertain the 1-minute Apgar score. The heart should immediately be auscultated for evidence of its action; poor muscle tone indicates a serious condition. The longer ventilation of the lungs is delayed, the longer is the delay before spontaneous breathing will begin. Anesthetic agents administered to the mother may increase the infant's difficulty in spontaneous breathing. Cooling of the infant increases the rapidity of fall in pH. Cooling along with asphyxia can produce an almost irreversible condition within a few minutes.

Resuscitative measures include first making certain that the airway is clear, administration of oxygen, intermittent positive pressure ventilation to expand the lungs, and occasionally infusion of a base to help restore the pH of the infant's blood. Methods of resuscitation are described below. In general, resuscitation should begin with the measures that are the least vigorous, and, if those are not effective, move to the more aggressive ones.

If the infant is breathing, but not with regularity, suction of the mouth and oropharynx and administration of oxygen may be sufficient treatment to improve respiratory function. Sometimes sensory stimulation, such as rubbing the infant's back or a quick slap to the soles of the feet, and oxygen flow with a mask against the face may stimulate respiration. If these measures are not quickly effective, or if the infant is not breathing, suction and positive pressure ventilation with a bag and mask or tracheal intubation as well as administration of oxygen become necessary. If the infant is obviously unresponsive at birth, no time can be lost in ventilation of the lungs. Table 21-2 summarizes suggested care for establishment of adequate respiratory function according to the infant's Apgar score.

Very important to resuscitation is to anticipate a problem and to be ready for it. Personnel and equipment for resuscitation must be ready at all times, so that the infant can be given aid immediately, even when difficulty is not expected. Someone in the delivery room should always be assigned to be responsible for assisting the infant in case he has difficulty breathing.

Clearing the Air Passages and Provision of Warmth

Clearing the air passages and providing warmth are essential to all infants and surely cannot be omitted in care of the newborn with respiratory difficulty. This has been discussed under "Resuscitation" above. The need for clearing of the air passages before attempting ventilation is rather obvious, but the need for warmth is just as great.

Maintenance of body temperature is critical because cooling causes increased consumption of oxygen and

Table 21-2. Summary of Suggested Care of Infants Immediately After Birth to Assist in Establishment of Adequate Respiratory Function

Apgar	*Action to Be Taken*
9–10	Dry infant's skin and protect against heat loss. Observe closely and check Apgar at 5 min to assure that condition remains good.
7–8	Dry skin. Protect against heat loss. Suction mouth and nose for mucus if indicated. Give oxygen (warmed and humidified if possible) by mask if color is dusky. Stimulate to cry. Observe closely and check Apgar in 5 min for improving condition.
4, 5, 6	Dry skin and place in heat-gaining environment. Give oxygen with mask—use bag-and-mask ventilation if not breathing well. Suction upper airway. Stimulate to cry. Expect prompt improvement—if not, continue with bag-and-mask ventilation and oxygen.
1, 2, 3	Provide warmth, preferably radiant heater. Use oxygen bag and mask immediately. Check to make sure lungs are being ventilated. Suction mucus from airway. Use laryngoscope and tracheal intubation tube if there is reason to suspect obstruction. Stimulate infant to take deep breaths and to cry. Expect improving condition. If no improvement by 5 min, consider need for correction of acidosis, correction of hypovolemia, glucose infusion.

glucose, both of which are essential for the energy that the brain and other cells need, and cooling quickly leads to acidosis and acid-base disturbance. The newborn with respiratory difficulty may not have enough oxygen available to meet the even greater metabolic demands that are created by the stress of chilling.

An infant in need of resuscitation sometimes cannot be as carefully protected as recommended, but every effort must be made to keep him warm. Whenever possible, resuscitative procedures should be carried out under a radiant heater. When this cannot be done the infant should be covered with warm blankets as much as circumstances permit.

Sensory Stimulation

If the airway is clear, a mildly to moderately depressed infant often can be stimulated to take deep breaths, and to cry, by rubbing the back, flicking the soles of the feet or flicking a finger against the heels several times. This method already may have been used to check reflex response, but may be repeated for stimulation. More vigorous methods, such as forcibly spanking the buttocks, slapping the back, or compressing the chest, are ineffective, waste valuable time, and may be injurious.

Oxygen

As a first measure, oxygen administered by a mask held next to the infant's face will increase the oxygen inspired during the first breaths. Increased oxygen to the brain may improve respirations. The infant's respirations, tone, reflexes, and heart rate are closely observed while oxygen is administered. If the infant does not breathe adequately within a minute or two or if the heart rate drops or does not improve if already low within 15 to 30 seconds with administration of oxygen, other treatment is usually started to prevent increasing asphyxia.

Ventilation

Mask-and-Bag Inflation

A mask and anesthesia bag may be used to administer oxygen in 100 percent concentration. The mask is held snugly over the infant's face, the head is tilted back slightly, the chin is held up and forward, and oxygen is administered by intermittent pressure on the bag (Figs. 21-11 and 21-12). Ventilation is begun with a light squeeze on the bag and thereafter the squeeze is regulated according to chest movements. Careful observation for amount of chest expansion is essential. It may be necessary to apply increasing pressure on the bag at first and then to decrease pressure when the lungs open. Ventilation is carried out at 55 to 60 times per minute. An oropharyngeal airway may be put in place prior to ventilation to hold the tongue away from the posterior pharynx so that it does not obstruct the airway. It is im-

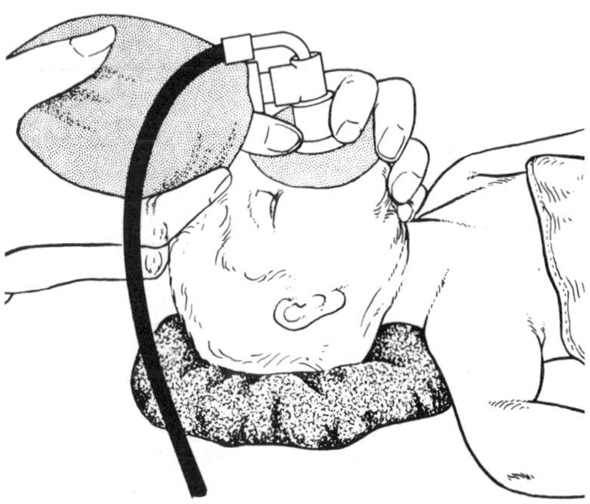

Figure 21-11. Artificial ventilation of the newborn with bag and mask. (Reproduced with permission from *Guidelines for Perinatal Care* by the American Academy of Pediatrics, Evanston, IL and The American College of Obstetricians and Gynecologists, Chicago, 1983.)

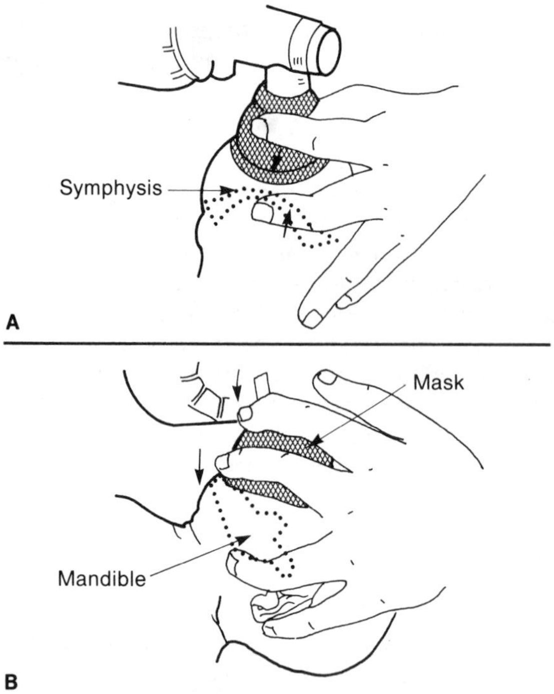

Figure 21–12. This illustration shows in greater detail the method of holding the bag and mask when it is used for inflating the lungs. The mask is applied firmly to the face, and counterpressure is exerted. (*A*) with the middle finger against the symphysis menti, or (*B*) with the ring finger behind the angle of the mandible. (Reproduced with permission from Kenneth R. Niswander, *Obstetric and Gynecologic Disorders: A Practitioner's Guide*, Medical Examination Publishing Co., Flushing, N.Y., 1975.)

portant to know the capabilities of the resuscitation bag used, as some, especially self-inflating ones, will only deliver 40 percent oxygen and may not deliver any without compression. Oxygen may pass into the infant's stomach and gentle pressure on the infant's abdomen may be necessary to deflate the stomach. If bag-and-mask ventilation continues more than 5 minutes, a nasogastric tube should be passed to provide for stomach decompression.

With effective ventilation the infant's chest should soon aerate well, the color should improve rapidly, and the heart rate should quickly reach a normal rate.

Direct Laryngoscopy and Tracheal Intubation

If the infant does not quickly improve with the use of mask and bag and oxygen, a laryngoscope is introduced to visualize the larynx, suction is used to clear the larynx and trachea, and a tube is inserted into the trachea to be used for inflation of the lungs. For the severely depressed infant (Apgar score 0, 1, 2, or 3), the laryngoscope ordinarily is used immediately, without first using the methods described above.

A pencil-handle laryngoscope with a premature blade is used to visualize the larynx. For its insertion the infant is placed on his back on a firm surface; the head is positioned over a towel so that it will be extended, with the chin pointing slightly upward; and the infant's head is kept in a straight line with his body. After insertion of the laryngoscope, suction may be made with a catheter to remove mucus, blood, meconium, or vernix (Fig. 21–13), or an endotracheal tube may be inserted and suction made through it. The laryngoscope is removed and the endotracheal tube is left in place until respirations are established.

Clearing the trachea may be sufficient to stimulate respirations, which is evident when the infant makes a gasping sound. If respirations do not begin, the lungs are inflated through the endotracheal tube by one of several methods, until the infant gasps and breathes.

Artificial respiration may be given by breathing into the endotracheal tube a few times, using short breaths that cause the infant's chest to rise gently. Air from the room may be used before each breath into the tube or a tube from which oxygen is flowing freely may be placed into the operator's mouth to increase the amount of oxygen delivered to the infant. Intermittent pressure on an anesthesia bag, attached to the endotracheal tube with an adaptor, may be used to inflate the lungs and deliver oxygen, or a respirator may be used to deliver oxygen, under controlled pressure, into the endotracheal tube.

Use of Respirator

A positive pressure respirator may be used for artificial ventilation if ventilatory support is still needed after the initial resuscitative efforts. The infant is likely to be transferred to the intensive-care nursery for this care. The respirator is set for the desired resuscitative pressure. Pressures of 15 to 20 cm of water are usually

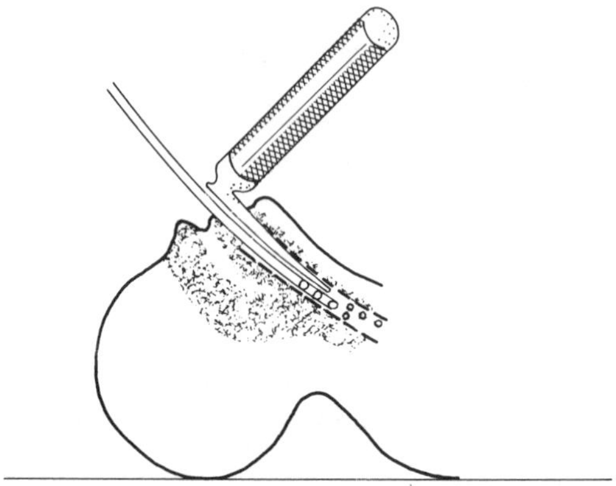

Figure 21–13. Meconium and mucus in the respiratory tract can be removed by quick, brief suction through a laryngoscope.

safe when carefully applied, but brief pressures as high as 30 cm or more water pressure may be necessary at first to expand the alveoli. Oxygen is administered by controlled intermittent pressure. The lungs deflate between each application of pressure by their elastic recoil. The intermittent positive pressure thus inflates the lungs, supplies oxygen, and removes carbon dioxide.

Inflation, by any method, is used for the shortest time and with the lowest pressure that is effective. A few inflations may be sufficient, or repetition for several minutes or occasionally several hours may be necessary before spontaneous respirations are well established. Required pressures and tidal volumes change rapidly during the first minutes of ventilation. Use of a method or machine that permits easy adjustment to the necessary change is important. Movements of the chest are observed during inflation. If the stomach rises, the tracheal tube is in the esophagus; its position must be changed. The endotracheal tube is removed when respirations are well established, usually after the infant has taken several spontaneous breaths. Sometimes it must be kept in place for a longer period until there is assurance that respirations are sustained.

Mouth-to-Mouth Inflation

Mouth-to-mouth breathing may be used instead of a bag and mask if equipment is not immediately available. Equipment is not necessary for mouth-to-mouth breathing, and it is therefore a method always available in an emergency.

To do mouth-to-mouth breathing, the infant is placed on his back on a firm surface, and the operator places his mouth directly over the infant's mouth and nose or over two or three layers of clean gauze first put over the infant's face, if gauze is readily available. The infant's nose and mouth must be covered with the operator's mouth, or if the nose is not covered, it must be held closed so that air will not come out through it. The infant's head should be tilted back slightly and the lower jaw should be pushed forward so that the chin juts out; this lifts the tongue and raises it from the posterior pharynx, where it may obstruct the air passage. Air is breathed into the infant at a rate of 35 to 40 times per minute. The breaths into the infant must be gentle so that the lungs are not injured. The breaths should be no more vigorous than the person's normal breathing; only the air in the mouth, not the lungs, is used. The operator should look for chest expansion; a small amount of chest movement is sufficient to indicate that the procedure is being performed vigorously enough.

While carrying out mouth-to-mouth breathing, the individual should take in a breath of room air before each breath into the infant or, if oxygen is available, take in a breath of oxygen from a tube attached to the oxygen supply; this increases the amount of oxygen that is delivered to the infant. Room air or oxygen will dilute the carbon dioxide present in the operator's mouth at the end of his own expiration. A depressed infant already has acidosis; additional carbon dioxide may increase it and therefore should be limited as much as possible.

Since air breathed into the infant's mouth and nose may enter either the lungs or stomach, the individual's hand should put slight pressure over the infant's epigastrium to prevent the stomach from being filled with air. The elastic recoil of the infant's lungs will usually deflate them, but expiration will be favored by slight pressure on the infant's chest.

Mouth-to-mouth breathing is sometimes disapproved of because of danger of infection. Its ready availability however, and its effectiveness may make it the best procedure in certain instances. Antibiotics may be administered after use of this method if signs of sepsis appear or if a WBC indicates possible infection.

External Cardiac Massage

Closed chest cardiac massage is initiated when a heart rate is not detectable and does not return with three or four insufflations. With cardiac massage the heart is manually compressed and artificial circulation is maintained. As the heart is compressed between the chest wall and the vertebral column blood is forced into the arteries. Relaxation of pressure allows the heart to fill with venous blood. When combined with proper ventilation, manual heart compression is often able to maintain sufficient blood pressure to keep the heart and brain adequately oxygenated until the heart can begin beating by itself (Fig. 21-14).

To perform external cardiac massage the infant's sternum is rhythmically compressed at the rate of 100 to 120 times per minute while artificial ventilation is also given. The infant is placed in the supine position on a firm surface. The index and middle fingers of the operator's hand are pressed sharply against the *middle* third of the infant's sternum to a depth of 1/2 to 3/4 inch at the rate of 100 to 120 times per minute. The heartbeat is coordinated with the ventilation at a ratio of 3 cardiac massages to 1 ventilation—3 heartbeats, pause for 1 ventilation, 3 heartbeats, pause for 1 ventilation, and so on. The two procedures should not be performed simultaneously because the pressure applied during cardiac massage may injure a lung that has just been inflated. The pressure for cardiac massage is best applied against the middle third of the sternum, since pressure against the lower third is less effective and limits movement of the liver. The peripheral pulses are monitored for evidence of adequate perfusion of the peripheral vessels.

An alternate method of cardiac massage is for the operator to place his hands around the infant's chest with the fingertips to the infant's back and the thumbs touching over the sternum. The middle third of the ster-

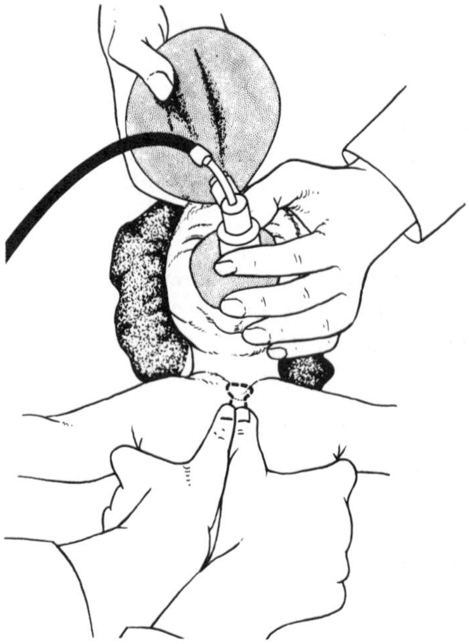

Figure 21-14. Administering external cardiac massage. The fingers of both hands support the infant's back while both thumbs apply pressure on the middle of the sternum, which should be compressed about two thirds of the distance to the spine at a rate of 100 to 120 times per minute. (Reproduced with permission from *Guidelines for Perinatal Care* by the American Academy of Pediatrics, Evanston, IL and The American College of Obstetricians and Gynecologists, Chicago, 1983.)

num is compressed vigorously with the thumbs. This technique is more applicable if the infant should for some reason be kept in the lateral position. The two-finger technique, however, has the advantage of being carried out successfully with one hand, leaving the other free to palpate the temporal or femoral pulses.

Ventilation must be maintained during the time that compression of the heart is carried out. Cardiac compression and ventilation are continued until a regular heartbeat is discerned. Massage is stopped briefly every 30 seconds for observation of signs of spontaneous heartbeat. As soon as a rhythmic beat can readily be heard, massage is discontinued.

Use of Epinephrine

Epinephrine may be used in conjunction with cardiac compression to stimulate the heart if other methods fail to produce a cardiovascular response. It may be administered intracardiac or intravenously. Care must be used in preparing the minute dose of 0.05 to 0.1 mg from the concentrated standard solution. A standard epinephrine ampul (1:1000) contains 1 mg/ml or 1000 μg. This 1-ml ampul is diluted to 10 ml with saline or 5 percent glucose, making a 1:10,000 dilution. A dosage of 0.1 ml/kg of a 1:10,000 solution may be ordered. If a more dilute solution is desired, 9 ml of the 1:10,000 solution are discarded and the remaining 1 ml is again diluted to 10 ml, making a 1:100,000 dilution.

Administration of a Base

If asphyxia is severe, intravenous infusion of a base may help to restore the blood pH. With asphyxia the pulmonary arterioles constrict, resistance to blood flow is high, and less blood reaches the alveolar cells. Also, the ductus arteriosus does not close or it opens again, permitting blood to be shunted past the lungs. The pulmonary arterioles and the ductus arteriosus are sensitive to blood Po_2 and pH. Ventilation of the lungs will supply oxygen and if the blood Po_2 can be raised in this way, the pulmonary arterioles will respond with reduced resistance. However, dilation of the pulmonary arterioles is also dependent upon a blood pH above the level of 7.2.

In severe asphyxia the blood pH is low and must be raised for good lung response to oxygenation. Removal of carbon dioxide by ventilation will improve the pH somewhat, but when the pH is very low and response to assisted ventilation is poor, administration of a base may be important in treatment. Initially sodium bicarbonate may be given intravenously over a two- to five-minute period into one of the vessels of the umbilical cord to raise the pH to a level at which the lungs will respond by arteriolar dilation to take up the oxygen that is being administered by ventilation. Initial dose of sodium bicarbonate is 2 to 4 mEq/kg diluted two to five times with water for injection. Dilution of the base before injection is essential. After the initial injection, the base may be continued by slow intravenous drip.

Since sodium bicarbonate breaks down to carbon dioxide, good ventilation is essential when sodium bicarbonate is used. Ventilation is also very useful in reducing acidosis by removal of carbon dioxide from the body. The importance of adequate ventilation is stressed in the following:

Marked Metabolic Acidosis

A pH less than 7.05 and a base deficit of 15 mEq/liter or more should be corrected by infusing 0.5 M[1] $NaHCO_3$ at a rate of 1 mEq/kg/minute or slower for a dose calculated by the formula

$$\text{mEq} = 0.3 \times \text{weight (kg)} \times \text{base deficit in mEq/liter.}$$

No bicarbonate should be infused unless ventilation is being assisted effectively and $Paco_2$ *is nearly normal or low.* The ability of this buffer to raise pH depends upon the ability of the lungs to eliminate the CO_2 produced by the buffering process ($H^+ + NaHCO_3 \rightarrow Na^+ + H_2CO_3 \rightarrow H_2O + CO_2$).[2]

[1] $NaHCO_3$ is most commonly available as a 1.0 M solution. This should be diluted 1:1 with sterile distilled water, not 5% or 10% dextrose, to halve the osmolarity.

[2] Gordon B. Avery, *Neonatology,* 2nd ed., Lippincott, Philadelphia, 1981, p. 192.

Administration of Glucose

Intravenous glucose, 5 or 10 percent, will provide a source of energy for the infant whose stores may quickly be depleted. The glucose is important to assure that the infant's metabolic requirements, which are likely to be increased with this stress, will be adequately met. Glucose administration is begun as soon as other emergency measures permit.

Drugs

The use of drugs in addition to the resuscitative measures described above is very limited. If the infant's depression is believed to be caused by a narcotic administered to the mother during labor, a *narcotic antagonist,* such as naloxone (NARCAN), may be administered after the air passages have been cleared and the lungs have been ventilated. This drug reduces the respiratory depression and other side effects of morphine and its derivatives, but has no effect in lessening depression caused by other drugs, such as barbiturates, or by anesthetics.

NARCAN may be administered intramuscularly or by injection into the umbilical vein. If the infant's circulation is satisfactory, the effect from intramuscular injection becomes apparent in a few minutes.

Narcotic antagonists, such as nalorphine (NALLINE) or levallorphan (LORFAN) or naloxone (NARCAN), may be administered to the mother 5 to 15 minutes prior to delivery, if depression of the infant from a drug administered to the mother is anticipated. Since a narcotic antagonist is a depressant of itself, the infant must be closely observed for such effect after its administration. NARCAN is the drug of preference for the newborn and therefore for the mother, because it does not depress respiration or cause sedation and would not do harm by such action if the infant's depression was not narcotic-induced.

Stimulants

Most stimulants, including such drugs as alphalobeline, pentylenetetrazol (METRAZOL), and nikethamide (CORAMINE), are considered potentially dangerous to a depressed infant. In the infant, the margin between therapeutic dose and toxic dose of stimulants is often very narrow. Such drugs are only considered on rare occasions. Use of epinephrine has been discussed.

Evaluation of Circulatory Status

An infant with asphyxia may have hypovolemia and hypotension. If the infant has a low circulating blood volume, he will have inadequate perfusion of some organs and will develop shock. The infant is likely to appear pale and "shocky." Poor capillary filling may be noted when an area of skin is blanched by firm pressure and return of color is slow. The extremities may be cold and the pulses may be weak, especially the radial and posterior tibial pulses. Other early signs are a low arterial or central venous pressure, and metabolic acidosis. Blood pressure should be monitored frequently on an asphyxiated infant by Doppler or from the umbilical artery if the vessel must be entered. Tachycardia may or may not be present. Anemia may or may not be present initially but will appear later.

When shock is present, treatment must be started early. For initial blood volume expansion, albumin, 1 gm/kg of body weight, diluted 1:4, with dextrose 5 percent in water or physiologic saline, may be used. After this the infant's response is evaluated and a determination of further therapy is made. For severe hypovolemia and for infants with severe asphyxia, administration of plasma or whole blood may be indicated for circulatory support. Some of the initial effects of the sodium bicarbonate administered for acidosis may result from its effect as a volume expander as well as from the correction of pH.

Subsequent Observations

An Apgar score should be done on all infants at 5 minutes after birth, but such evaluation of an infant who required resuscitation is absolutely essential. An infant with a low score at 1 minute after birth should soon have a higher score if he responds well to resuscitation. If the infant's score has not reached 8 at 5 minutes of age, another scoring is indicated at 10 minutes and perhaps more frequently.

For any infant who received a high Apgar score at 1 minute of age, a second scoring at 5 minutes is also indicated. An infant with a high score at 1 minute usually does not drop to a lower one, but he also needs further close observation because the condition may change rapidly, especially if obstructing material is obstructing the trachea, or if the infant is under the influence of drugs administered to the mother.

It is important to make an accurate record of the time of each Apgar score on an infant. Scoring at specific times assures regular observation of an infant during the early period of life and greatly increases the likelihood of identifying an infant in distress. All other behavior of the infant must be closely observed and described. Respiratory effort, movement of the chest, rate of respirations, heart rate, and color are valuable observations. Frequency and lustiness of cry, whether spontaneous or stimulated, should be recorded. Muscle tone and activity must be closely observed, since an infant with poor tone, who lies in a flaccid position, may require treatment for acidosis.

Continuous close observation in the nursery is mandatory for any infant who has required resuscitation or who has become chilled.

Care of the Umbilical Cord

The umbilical cord is compressed a few inches from the baby's abdominal wall with two hemostatic clamps and cut between the clamps. The placental end of the cord is placed on the mother's abdomen until the placenta is expressed, to prevent its contamination from contact with the mother's anal region (Fig. 21-8). The clamp is left on the placental end of the cord until the placenta is expelled, because of the possibility of another infant in the uterus and the danger of serious blood loss from that infant through the open cord.

The umbilical cord may be clamped immediately after the newborn's birth, or clamping may be postponed for a few minutes, until pulsation in the umbilical cord ceases. A short delay in clamping of the cord permits the amount of blood which flows between the placenta and the infant to stabilize. Blood is pushed from the infant to the placenta as he passes through the birth canal, flows back quickly and overcompensates, and then some returns to the placenta and begins to stabilize. Holding the infant at the level of the perineum permits good equalization of the blood between infant and placenta. Delay in clamping of the cord until the respirations are established also provides a reservoir for the lung fluid which is quickly removed from the infant's lungs by his circulatory system. Clamping of the cord may be necessary early when the umbilical cord is snugly around the infant's neck and when resuscitation must be instituted immediately. It may be desirable when the mother is deeply anesthetized to avoid further anesthesia to the infant, or when complications, such as hemolytic disease, are anticipated. The time of clamping is determined for the individual infant.

The umbilical cord stump is ligated close to the infant's abdomen with a small plastic or metal clamp or a cord tie, and the hemostat is removed. Several kinds of umbilical cord clamps are available. They ordinarily are left on the cord for 12 to 24 hours and removed when the umbilical cord vessels are crushed and thrombosed.

If a ligature of bobbin is used to ligate the cord, it must be strong and heavy enough to be noncutting. It is tied tightly, in a square knot that will not slip and permit bleeding, about an inch from the infant's abdominal wall. If the ligature is applied slowly and at interrupted intervals, the Wharton's jelly in the cord is squeezed out from under the ligature, and the blood vessels will be constricted better than with one rapid pull on the tie. When the Wharton's jelly is not squeezed out, it may escape later and the cord will then retract, leaving the tie loose, with subsequent bleeding. It is considered a safe precaution to bend the cord back on itself and tie it a second time with the same ligature, as the danger of hemorrhage from a loosely tied cord is serious.

The blood vessels are clearly visible at the ends of the moist, freshly cut umbilical cord. The two arteries can be seen as two small vessels of equal size and the umbilical vein as a larger vessel. Examination for the number of vessels in the umbilical cord and a record of the findings are recommended. Infants with only one umbilical artery are reported to have a higher incidence of congenital anomalies, especially renal and gastrointestinal. A finding of only two umbilical vessels serves as an alert for a search for other anomalies in the infant.

A dressing is not applied to the umbilical cord stump, but it and the surrounding area must be kept clean to prevent infection. Precautions consist of careful hand washing prior to care, keeping moisture around the cord to a minimum, and application of 60 percent alcohol or other antiseptic several times a day (see Chapter 27).

Care of the Eyes

The infant's eyes may become infected during birth if gonococci are present in the birth canal, but proper care of the eyes at birth will prevent almost all cases of ophthalmia neonatorum. A germicide properly dropped into the eyes soon after birth will kill any organisms that are present.

The Credé method, named for and made famous by the Viennese obstetrician who introduced it in 1881, was to drop from a glass rod a single drop of nitrate of silver, 2 percent, into each eye immediately after birth. The routine use of this prophylaxis reduced the occurrence of ophthalmia in Credé's clinics from 10 to 1 percent among the newborns. Later the strength of silver nitrate was reduced to 1 percent and was made mandatory in many countries.

Since penicillin is highly gonococcocidal, its use has often been recommended as a prophylactic agent against ophthalmia neonatorum, and it has been used as a preventive treatment. Its efficiency is good, but it, as well as silver nitrate, has certain disadvantages. Penicillin sensitivity, although rare, may occur, and there is the possibility of infection with an antibiotic-resistant strain of gonococcus. Some physicians, therefore, do not wish to abandon the silver nitrate treatment.

A prophylactic treatment against ophthalmia neonatorum is required by law or regulation in most states in this country; in a number of them the silver nitrate method is specified. Others permit the use of tetracycline or erythromycin ophthalmic ointment.

Before instillation of drops or ointment into the eyes, the outer surface of each eyelid is wiped from the nose outward with a sterile cotton ball moistened with sterile water to remove mucus, blood, and vernix.

For instillation of silver nitrate, wax ampuls containing a 1 percent solution are supplied by state health departments. This is an important safety factor since danger of accidental use of a stronger solution is eliminated. The ampuls are hermetically sealed, so that the solution does not deteriorate rapidly, as does a more exposed solution in a dropper bottle. They should be protected, however, from exposure to light. They also eliminate danger of evaporation and subsequent increase in concentration of solution. Each ampul contains sufficient solution for treatment of one infant. To use the ampul, one end is pierced with a sterile pin, allowing the solution to be squeezed out one drop at a time.

For instillation of silver nitrate, the lower lid is pulled downward as far as possible and 2 drops of a 1 percent solution of silver nitrate are placed into the conjunctival sac (Fig. 21-15). After the lid is released, the solution will spread over the entire conjunctiva. Care must be taken not to drop the medication directly on the cornea, where it may cause trauma and injury. Excess solution that squeezes out of the eye when the lids are closed should be wiped off. If it is not removed, it causes a brown or black discoloration of the skin around the eyes that must wear off and that concerns the parents until it disappears.

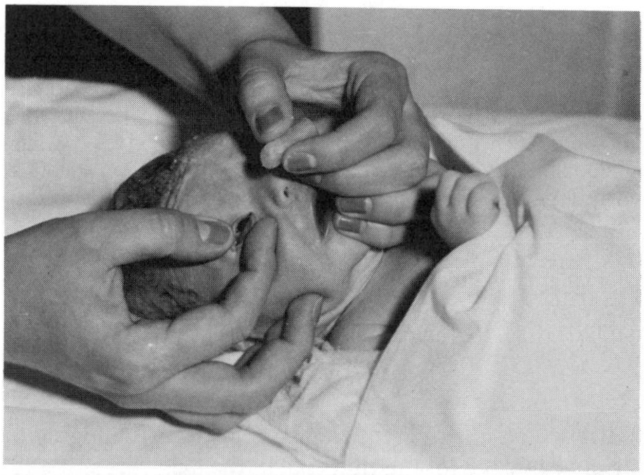

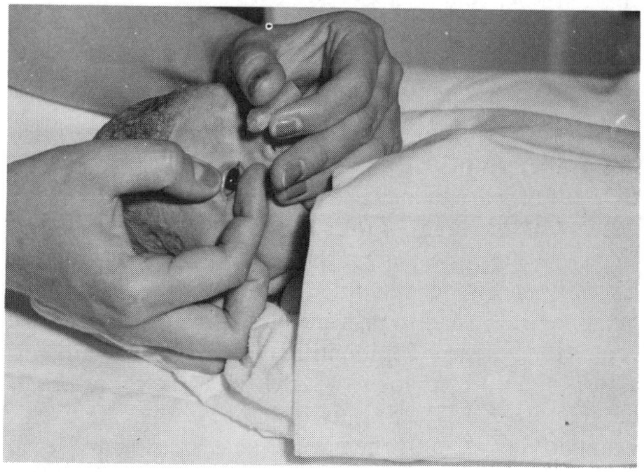

Figure 21-15. Placing drops of a 1 percent silver nitrate solution into the conjunctival sac for prevention of ophthalmia neonatorum.

Top: The eyelids are not sufficiently separated, and there is danger of dropping the medication directly on the cornea, where it may cause trauma and injury.

Bottom: The eyelids have been separated sufficiently to permit placing the medication on the lower eyelid or into the conjunctival sac.

The silver drops may be left *in situ* without further treatment, or the eyes may be irrigated 1 to 2 minutes after the instillation, using warm *sterile* water or warm physiologic salt solution and a soft bulb syringe. The irrigation will wash out excess silver nitrate and form a precipitate with the remainder when saline is used. Care must be taken that the silver nitrate is not washed out of the eyes so soon after instillation that it does not have time to be effective.

When an antibiotic is used as a prophylactic agent against ophthalmia neonatorum, it is usually instilled into the eyes as drops or as an ophthalmic ointment. To prevent antibiotic solution or ointment from becoming inactive, it must be kept refrigerated and not used beyond the expiration date.

Prophylactic treatment of the eyes has traditionally been carried out as soon as possible after birth and before the infant leaves the delivery room. From studies of mother-infant bonding it becomes advisable to postpone this treatment for about an hour or two so as not to interfere with the infant's quiet and alert eye contact with his mother. Such contact between mother and child seems to trigger important maternal attachment responses to her infant during the very special period following birth.

Eye treatment is best postponed to early care of the newborn in the nursery, when the same procedure that has been described above may be carried out after the mother has had initial contact with her infant.

Identification

Every newborn must be properly identified *before the infant and the mother are transferred from the delivery room.* Identification bands with identical numbers for both infant's and mother's wrists or bands fastened to the infant's wrist and ankle are frequently used (Fig. 21-16). Minimum identifying information on the bands includes the infant's sex and surname, the mother's given name, and the date and time of birth. Other identifying information such as the name of the physician also may be added. The nurse preparing the identification bands should have another person check the information with her as additional certainty against error.

The identification band is checked each time the infant is taken to the mother or moved from the bassinet for any reason. The mother is shown the identification and is instructed to check it each time the infant is brought to her. The infant is discharged without removal of identification unless he is wearing two identical

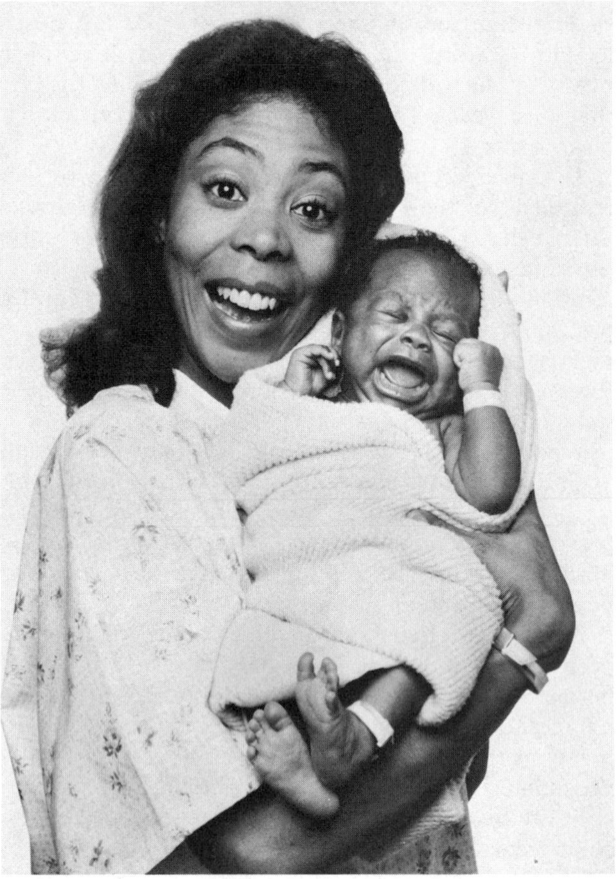

A

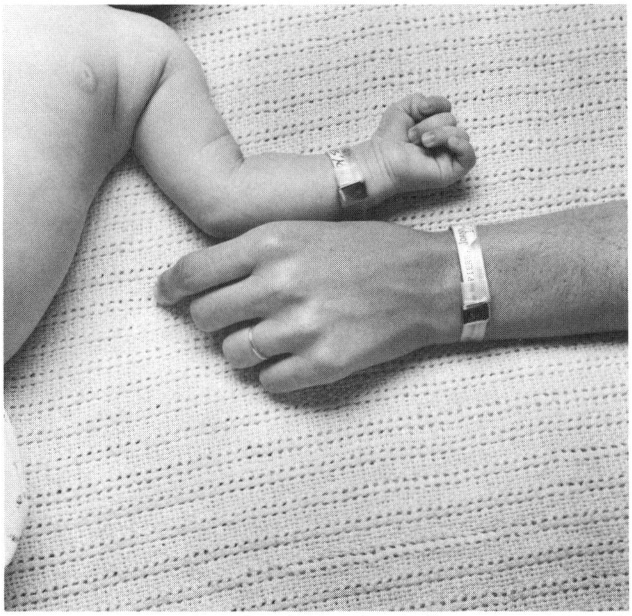

B

Figure 21–16. Correlated Mother/Baby Ident-A-Band® bracelets, available from Hollister Incorporated. With this newborn identification system three joined bands bearing identical numbers and inserts for recording of other identical identifying information can easily be separated and applied to mother and infant before either leaves the birth room. *A*. Mother and infant shown with a band around mother's wrist and identical bands around infant's wrist and ankle. *B*. Shows the wrist bands in greater detail. (Photographs courtesy of Hollister Incorporated.)

bands, in which case one is removed and attached to the infant's record.

A footprint, which is a permanent means of identification, should also be made and filed with the hospital records (Fig. 21–17). In some states footprinting is mandatory. The footprint does not replace other more readily observable methods of identification, but is used as a supplemental means in case doubt arises concerning an infant's identity. This is especially important after the infant leaves the hospital. The print is made on a form that contains other identifying data, similar to that on the identification band, and also the mother's fingerprint.

If taken carefully, a footprint is positive identification, because the arrangement of the ridges on the fingers, toes, palms, and soles is unique to each individual. These ridges are present at birth; they begin forming in the fetus about the fourth month; and they do not change during the individual's lifetime.

The footprint should be made in the delivery room whenever possible. A print of the mother's finger, on the same record as the infant's footprint, is also made at this time. In some hospitals an infant's palmprint or fingerprint is taken instead of a footprint; these are somewhat more difficult to make.

Ridges in an infant's skin are fine, and the footprint must be made with great care to be legible. Smudging of prints or heavy inking that fills in the skin ridges makes the print illegible and useless.

To make a print of the infant's foot, the nurse should study the instructions for the particular material to be used. Instructions that apply to all methods are as follows. The infant's foot is wiped clean and dry, and lint is brushed off. A thin film of printer's ink is applied to the foot, care being taken that the ink is not so heavy that it fills the ridges of the skin. The foot is then pressed firmly on the paper on which the print is to be recorded. Excessive pressure is avoided, and both paper and foot must be held firmly to prevent smudging. The ball of the foot is the best area for identification of ridge detail, and efforts should be made to get this area as clear as possible (Fig. 21–17). The print is examined immediately with a magnifying glass. If the nurse is able to recognize some ridge detail, the print can be considered legible; if not, it must be redone.

The American Academy of Pediatrics and the American College of Obstetricians and Gynecologists make the following statement regarding footprinting for neonate identification:

> Footprinting and fingerprinting has in the past been recommended for purposes of neonate identification. Techniques

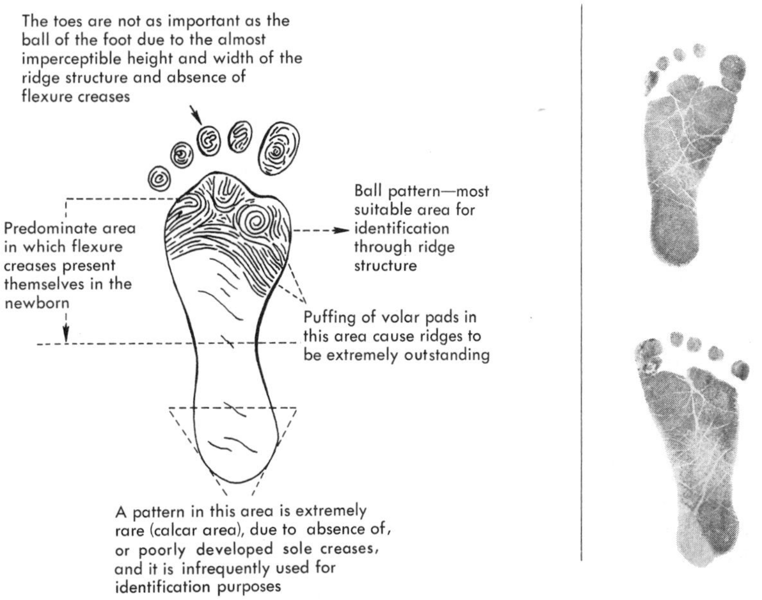
The toes are not as important as the ball of the foot due to the almost imperceptible height and width of the ridge structure and absence of flexure creases
Ball pattern—most suitable area for identification through ridge structure
Predominate area in which flexure creases present themselves in the newborn
Puffing of volar pads in this area cause ridges to be extremely outstanding
A pattern in this area is extremely rare (calcar area), due to absence of, or poorly developed sole creases, and it is infrequently used for identification purposes

Figure 21-17. Footprint identification pointers. (Reprinted with permission from Footprinting Pointers and Procedures. Bureau of Maternal and Child Health, New York State Department of Health, Albany, N.Y.)

such as sophisticated blood typing are now available and appear to be more reliable. If utilized, dermatoglyphics should be done carefully. Individual hospitals may want to continue with footprinting and fingerprinting, but universal use of this practice is no longer recommended.[3]

Inspection for Abnormalities

Before the newborn is taken from the delivery room, physician and nurse inspect the infant for abnormalities, especially those that may not be apparent immediately, such as supernumerary digits, clubfoot, hypospadias, imperforate anus, and birthmarks. They again observe the infant's color and general behavior to determine if special attention is required, such as incubator care or oxygen.

Protection from Chilling, Trauma, and Infection

Warmth, gentle handling, and cleanliness are imperative throughout the entire regimen of an infant's care. Until birth the fetus' existence was completely dependent on the mother, but immediately after birth independent functions of respiration and changes in circulation must be established. The infant must also begin existence in surroundings that are very different from the protective and unchanging environment of the mother's body.

One of the most immediate environmental changes for the infant is temperature. The delivery room is many degrees cooler than the very warm habitat from which he has just emerged. Body warmth is a valuable aid in helping to establish normal functions, so every effort is taken to prevent undue cooling.

To protect the infant against infection, all equipment used for care is sterilized, if it can withstand sterilization, or is kept as clean as possible. It is important that persons caring for the infant wash their hands before giving care.

The infant is protected from trauma by gentle handling during all care, especially removal of mucus, stimulation of respirations, and treatment of the eyes.

Baptism

The Roman Catholic Church teaches that baptism is necessary for salvation. Parents who are Roman Catholic wish to have their infant baptized if it is in danger of death. If time permits, a priest should be called to administer baptism. If there is not sufficient time, the nurse or the physician should perform the baptism. Baptism is conferred by pouring ordinary water on the child's forehead while saying the words: "I baptize you in the name of the Father and of the Son and of the Holy Spirit." It is necessary for validity that the person performing the baptism have the intention of doing what the Roman Catholic Church wishes. The Church teaches that every fetus and embryo should be baptized if possible.

Most Protestants observe infant baptism. Those who practice this rite usually desire to have their infant baptized if his condition is serious. The physician or nurse should, therefore, consult with the parents to determine their wishes regarding their child's baptism, and arrange to call a minister of their faith. If time does not permit calling a minister, an emergency baptism may be per-

[3] American Academy of Pediatrics and American College of Obstetricians and Gynecologists, Guidelines for Perinatal Care, American Academy of Pediatrics, Evanston, IL, and American College of Obstetricians and Gynecologists, Washington, D.C., 1983.

formed by anyone else. If times does not permit for consulting with the parents regarding their infant's baptism, the physician or nurse should baptize the infant, since many Protestant parents consider this rite very important and desire to have it done. The baptism is administered by pouring water, usually with the palm of the hand, over the child's head, and at the same time saying the words: "I baptize thee (or you) in the name of the Father and of the Son and of the Holy Ghost." If time permits, the Lord's Prayer and/or Apostles' Creed may also be spoken; however, these are not essential to the rite of baptism.

Early Contact of Newborn with Mother

Every effort must be made to permit the mother to see and touch her newborn as soon as possible after birth, especially if the infant is well, alert, and responsive. A sensitive period in mother- and father-infant attachment in the early minutes and hours of life make early mother-infant contact important to later development.

Facilitating the mother's opportunity to touch and explore her infant should be at her pace. She may wish only a very short period of contact at first because of fatigue and preoccupation with other events. A short time, or perhaps a longer time, later she will wish to have more contact, or she may wish to hold the infant for a longer time from the beginning (Fig. 21-18). It is important for persons caring for the mother to avoid comments that may inhibit her own expression of what she wishes to do and how she feels. It is not helpful to the mother who says she is disappointed that she did not have a boy to remind her that she should be happy to have a healthy infant regardless of sex. A better response would be, "Boys are nice, but sometimes things don't come out as we hoped." One should not add to this, "but girls are just fine." When the father is in the delivery room he also has the opportunity to have early contact with his infant (Fig. 21-19).

There ordinarily does not need to be concern over the infant becoming chilled while he is with the mother. As the mother holds the child in her arms she provides some body warmth. The mother's later contact with her infant in the recovery room can be a warmer room and sometimes a portable warmer can be used.

The opportunity for early parent-infant contact as parents wish it, without needing to conform to hospital practices, is an important reason why they choose home birth or birth at an alternative birth center.

THIRD STAGE (PLACENTAL STAGE)

The third stage of labor and the hour immediately following delivery of the placenta are, at times, hazardous to the mother. This period requires careful management because of the great danger of hemorrhage.

Delivery of the Placenta

Immediately after the birth of the infant, the uterus is palpated for placental separation. The uterus can readily be felt through the mother's abdominal wall. The nurse may place a hand on the mother's abdomen and gently

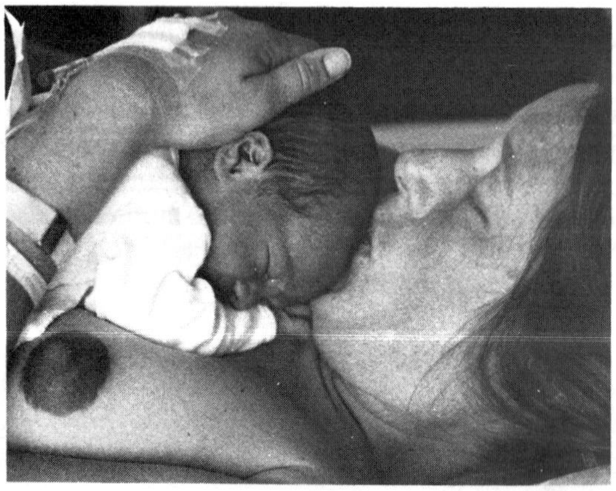

Figure 21-18. Mother cuddling her baby a few minutes after birth. The intravenous infusion is firmly anchored so that it does not inhibit maternal-infant interaction. (Photograph courtesy of Dr. and Mrs. Daniel Wikler.)

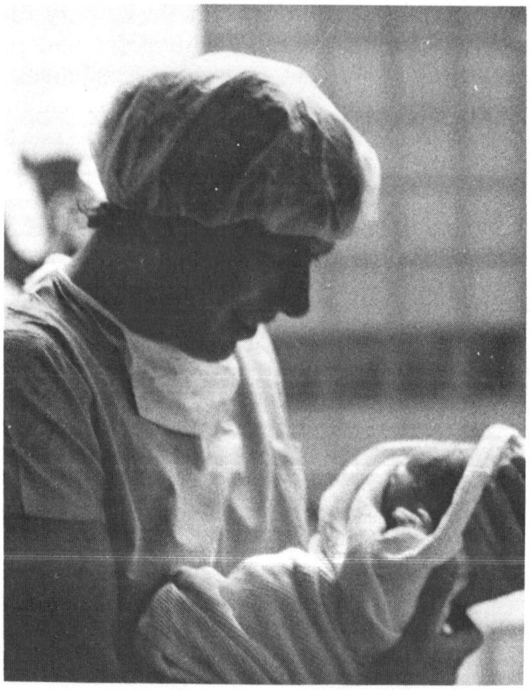

Figure 21-19. The father takes his turn inspecting his newly born infant in the delivery room. He is wearing a scrub suit for his participation in the birth. (Photograph courtesy of Dr. and Mrs. Daniel Wikler.)

palpate the fundus, noting its consistency, and its height in relation to the level of the mother's umbilicus.

Since the placenta may descend very quickly into the lower uterine segment or into the vagina, the nurse also watches for and reports the signs of this occurrence—a rise in the abdomen of the uterine fundus, an increase in the amount of umbilical cord protruding from the vagina, and a trickling or a spurt of blood from the vagina. The nurse palpates the uterus for the above signs, watching very carefully that the uterus does not relax and enlarge (balloon out) from bleeding into the uterine cavity.

After the placenta has separated, pressure is exerted on it from above to effect its delivery. The physician or nurse-midwife first ascertains that the uterus is firmly contracted; massage may be used to stimulate contraction of the muscle, and then firm but gentle, steady, downward pressure is exerted on the fundus in the direction of the pelvic inlet (Fig. 21-20). In this manner pressure is exerted on the placenta with the fundus. The umbilical cord may be used to guide the placenta out of the vagina, but traction on it is avoided. Sometimes the mother is asked to apply the pressure by bearing down, but such efforts are frequently not practicable at this time. In either case, the uterus must be firm before pressure is applied to avoid inversion of the uterus, which involves prolapse of the uterine fundus, through the cervix, into the vagina. This is a grave obstetric accident.

The physician holds the hand or a basin just below the vaginal outlet to receive the placenta and supports it close to the vulva to prevent sudden tension on the membranes and possible tearing of the membranes before their separation from the uterine wall is complete (Fig. 21-20). The membranes are then slowly peeled from the inner surface of the uterus by gentle traction. They are extracted by pulling the placenta gradually away from the vulva, or by turning the placenta over several times to twist the membranes, or by alternately grasping them with a forceps and applying gentle traction (Fig. 21-21). The latter method is especially useful if the membranes have torn away from the placenta.

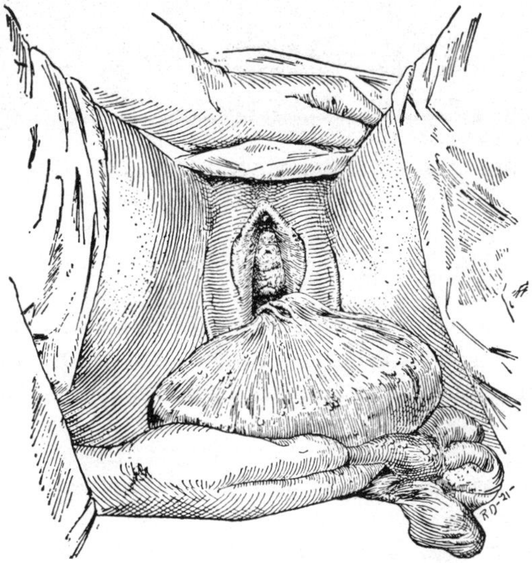
Figure 21-20. Delivery of the placenta.

The placenta and membranes are examined immediately to see if the cotyledons of the placenta fit together and if the membranes are complete. If fragments of either break off and remain in the uterus, they prevent its firm contraction and thus may be a cause of postpartum hemorrhage. It is to prevent tearing that only gentle pressure and traction are used in expressing the placenta and withdrawing the membranes. The use of force is more likely to leave small particles adherent to the uterine wall. After inspection, the placenta is placed in a receptacle for disposal. Sometimes a laboratory examination of the placenta is ordered. In addition to inspection of the placenta, some physicians routinely palpate the inside of the uterus to assess for complete placenta delivery.

If a placental fragment has remained in the uterus, although small and causing no immediate bleeding, it is manually removed at once because of the possibility of causing bleeding at a later time. Occasionally separation of the placenta is delayed, or spontaneous separation does not take place, or the placenta separates, but is retained in the uterus. Several attempts at simple expression may be necessary before the placenta is expelled, with intervals of waiting and careful observation for bleeding between such efforts. Manual removal becomes necessary when the placenta does not separate or when it cannot be expressed following its separation (see page 451).

With delivery of the placenta, there is a gush of the blood that collected behind it during its separation. The amount varies considerably, frequently between 50 and 200 ml. The amount of blood behind the placenta is, to a large extent, determined by how firmly the uterine muscle fibers contracted as the placenta separated and also by the length of time that elapsed between its separation and its expulsion. The bleeding usually subsides quickly. The blood vessels, which are as large as a lead pencil, are closed by involuntary contractions of the network of uterine muscle fibers in which they are enmeshed, and which are sometimes referred to as "living ligatures." If the bleeding continues, contraction of the muscle fibers is stimulated by massage and by oxytocic drugs.

The uterus should be a firm, hard mass after delivery of the placenta and should remain so; this is evidence of strong muscle contraction. For a variable period of time a hand is kept on the mother's abdomen to palpate the fundus continuously to ascertain that it remains firmly contracted and, if relaxation occurs, to detect this immediately. As soon as relaxation of the muscle is

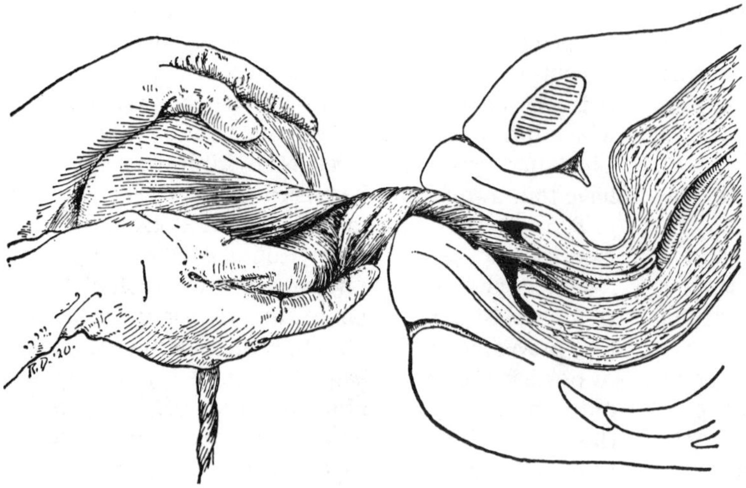

Figure 21–21. Twisting the membranes while withdrawing them from the uterus.

discerned, the uterus is firmly grasped through the abdominal wall and massaged gently until the muscle contracts. If the uterus has not spontaneously risen upward in the abdomen following the pressure that was placed on it to expel the placenta, it may be necessary to pull it up before it can be grasped for massage. The uterus is freely movable at this time and usually can be moved upward if the fingers of both hands are placed against the lower abdominal wall, just above the pubic bones, and pressed inward and upward so that they make pressure against the lower part of the uterus and lift it up.

Oxytocic Drugs

Drugs with an oxytocic[4] action are often given after delivery of the placenta to stimulate contraction of uterine muscle fibers; they are sometimes given during or immediately after delivery of the infant's body. The drugs used for this purpose are an oxytocic alkaloid of ergot, natural or synthetic, and the oxytocic principle of the posterior pituitary hormone in synthetic form.

Ergonovine maleate is the principal oxytocic alkaloid of ergot, a fungus that grows on rye and other grains. A term frequently used as a synonym for ergonovine is ERGOTRATE, a trade name for the drug. Ergonovine is a powerful stimulant to uterine muscle contraction and exerts an effect that may last for hours. The contraction of the uterine muscle is sustained after administration of the drug and is a valuable aid in control of postpartum bleeding.

Ergonovine may be administered orally or parenterally. It is prepared in tablet form in doses of 0.2 mg ($^1/_{320}$ gr) for oral administration and in 1-ml ampuls containing 0.2 mg ($^1/_{320}$ gr) dissolved in water for injection intramuscularly or intravenously. The usual amount of ergonovine administered at one time by any route is 0.2 mg. The uterine muscle contracts quickly, within a very few minutes after an intramuscular injection, and even within 5 to 10 minutes after oral administration, since the drug is readily absorbed from the gastrointestinal tract. The oral route of administration is used after the mother is permitted to take fluids. Ergonovine is generally contraindicated in women who have hypertension, particularly when it is caused by toxemia. The nurse should check the blood pressure before she gives this drug.

A synthetic derivative of ergonovine, methylergonovine maleate (METHERGINE), is often used in place of ergonovine. It is also prepared in 0.2-mg ($^1/_{320}$ gr) doses and may also be administered by either the oral or parenteral routes.

Ergot preparations are being used less and less as a routine postpartum medication. Intravenous administration of a 0.2-mg dose (1-ml ampul) as a rapid injection is inadvisable. It may cause severe hypertension due to serious cerebral vasospasm.

Oxytocin, the oxytocic principle of the posterior pituitary hormone, also produces marked contractions of the uterine muscle. Unlike the long-sustained contraction produced by ergonovine, these contractions last for only 5 to 10 minutes, after which there are intermittent periods of muscle relaxation. The periods of rhythmic contractions of the uterine muscle are very strong, however.

Posterior pituitary extract contains two hormones, oxytocin (PITOCIN), with strong oxytocic properties, and vasopressin (PITRESSIN), with marked vasopressor and antidiuretic properties. The pressor and antidiuretic principle is undesirable because hypertension and water retention are common problems in pregnancy; for this reason the oxytocic principle alone is administered in preference to the entire posterior pituitary extract. Oxytocin is produced synthetically, and the synthetic hor-

[4] Oxytocic means rapid parturition. An oxytocic is an agent that promotes the rapidity of labor.

mone (PITOCIN or SYNTOCINON) is now used in place of the natural hormone.

Oxytocin is prepared in an aqueous solution for injection containing 10 USP units in 1 ml of solution; it is available in 0.5- and 1-ml ampuls and is administered intramuscularly or intravenously; it has no value by the oral route. When given intramuscularly after delivery, the usual dosage is 10 units. Oxytocin is not administered in such a large dose in a single intravenous injection. When it is given intravenously, 10 or more units are diluted in 500 to 1000 ml of 5 percent dextrose in Ringer's lactate or in water, and it is administered as an intravenous infusion, since a large single dose intravenously may produce a profound hypotension. In addition to postpartum administration, intravenous infusion of oxytocin is used for induction of labor, but it then is administered with extreme caution (more dilute, very slowly) because of danger of violent uterine contractions (see pages 442–44).

When oxytocics are administered intramuscularly following delivery, they are often given most easily into the deltoid muscle because the position of the mother and draping sheets interfere with using other areas. It is important to use a needle at least 2.5 cm (1 in.) in length in order to reach the muscular tissue of the arm. The area should be thoroughly massaged for quick absorption.

The time of administration of an oxytocic drug in relation to delivery of the infant or delivery of the placenta varies with the preference of the physician. Some physicians give an oxytocic at the time the infant's body is being delivered or immediately thereafter (before the end of the third stage of labor), and sometimes repeat an oxytocic at the end of the third stage; others object to the administration of any oxytocics before delivery of the placenta. When an oxytocic is used during or immediately after the birth of the infant, it is done in an effort to deliver the placenta quickly and thereby reduce blood loss. The incidence of retained placenta and its manual removal is higher when oxytocic drugs are administered before its delivery than when they are withheld until the end of the third stage.

The nurse who is responsible for preparing the drugs, and probably for their administration, must have a clear understanding of which oxytocic the physician wants given and of when the drug is to be administered. In general it seems advisable to wait with administration of an oxytocic until after delivery of the placenta.

If the uterine muscle does not contract well after the administration of an oxytocic drug, an intravenous infusion of oxytocin is commonly started.

Repair of the Perineum

An episiotomy or a laceration is repaired either in the interval between the delivery of the newborn and expulsion of the placenta or after delivery of the placenta. Some physicians prefer to wait until the end of the third stage of labor before the repair is begun in order to deliver the placenta as soon as it has separated and also to avoid placing tension on the repaired area if exploration of the uterus is necessary. Bleeding from the wound is kept to a minimum by placing pressure against the edges of the wound with sterile gauze until it can be sutured. Other physicians prefer to do the repair while waiting for the placenta to separate. It may be necessary to interrupt the repair temporarily to deliver the placenta when its separation has taken place.

Regardless of when the repair is done, the physician, an assistant, or frequently the nurse, must palpate the uterus for size and consistency during the time that the physician is doing the repair. If the placenta is not delivered, observation is made for signs of placental separation and its expulsion into the lower uterine segment and for evidence of any enlargement of the uterus from bleeding into the cavity. If the placenta has been delivered, observation is made to ascertain that the uterus remains firmly contracted. When the nurse is responsible for making the observations, she informs the physician immediately of changes in uterine size and consistency.

The cervix is frequently inspected for lacerations and is repaired if indicated. Cervical inspection is made before the perineum is repaired. Additional information on cervical lacerations is given on page 451.

In the repair of an episiotomy or a laceration, the structures of the perineum—vaginal mucosa, levator ani muscle, facisa, and skin—are anatomically approximated. Chromic catgut sutures varying in size from no. 00 to no. 0000 are frequently used; these are put in place with a round needle with either a taper or a cutting edge. Anesthesia, usually regional or local, is used during the repair. If regional anesthesia was used for delivery, it is frequently still effective.

If a tear has been sustained around the urethra, the repair is made with thin, nontraumatic needles and fine catgut, size 000 or smaller, since the tissue in this area is thin and tears easily. Following this repair, an indwelling catheter may be placed into the bladder for a day or two to prevent trauma or tension on the sutured area, which may accompany a catheterization should the mother be unable to void.

FOURTH STAGE OF LABOR (IMMEDIATE POSTPARTUM PERIOD)

Although the puerperium is considered to begin following delivery of the placenta, the immediate postpartum period is so closely associated with the process of labor that it is included with the care of the patient in labor. The mother is still in the delivery room at the beginning of this immediate postpartum period, and when moved from the delivery room she needs continuous observation for a variable period of time, to prevent complications that may result from labor and delivery.

Labor is ordinarily divided into three stages, as previously described, but from time to time the immediate postpartum period has been referred to as a fourth stage of labor.

The duration of the fourth stage of labor is variable. It has long been customary to consider the first hour post partum as a special period during which the mother needs continuous observation. This one hour of close observation is sufficient for most mothers, but often the events of labor and delivery make one hour an inadequate time for recovery from labor. The immediate postpartum period, or "fourth stage of labor," should therefore be considered as that interim of time after delivery of the placenta that is necessary to assure that the mother is reacting satisfactorily to the stress of birth, that the uterus is remaining firmly contracted, and that vaginal bleeding is not excessive.

After delivery and repair of the episiotomy, the vulva is cleaned of blood with sterile cotton balls; the thighs and buttocks are dried; a sterile pad is applied to the perineum or placed under the buttocks; and the mother is moved to a clean bed. The mother is usually tired and often cold at the conclusion of labor and she may have a shaking chill. The reason for the chill is not known. It may be in part a nervous reaction or in part may be due to vasomotor changes. Although this chill is not serious, the mother is nonetheless uncomfortable and should be warmly covered. A warmed, cotton blanket usually adds to the comfort of all women immediately following delivery.

Many hospitals have a postpartum recovery room to which the mother is moved following delivery, for close observation until there is assurance that immediate complications are not likely to develop. Recovery room care includes observation of vital signs, of contraction of the uterus, and of the amount of vaginal bleeding.

The mother's vital signs are checked immediately after delivery and at least every 15 minutes during the immediate postpartum period; deviations from a normal range require more frequent checking, sometimes every 5 minutes. A marked rise or fall in blood pressure and/or pulse rate are reported immediately to the physician. A toxemia of pregnancy may cause the blood pressure to rise immediately post partum, even when it has not been unduly elevated during labor. Blood loss during delivery may result in rising pulse and respiratory rate and a lowering of blood pressure. Response to drugs may affect the vital signs. Existing cardiac or respiratory disease may influence vital signs. Headache, dizziness, and persistent nausea and vomiting are also reported.

To detect early uterine muscle relaxation, the nurse places a hand on the mother's abdomen to palpate the fundus every 10 to 15 minutes for at least one hour after delivery, and longer if indicated by previously existing conditions. During this period, sometimes referred to as "the placental hour," the consistency, the size, and the height of the uterus are observed (Fig. 21–22). As long as the uterus is felt as a firm, round mass below the umbilicus, its irregularly arranged muscle fibers are contracted around the blood vessels and will prevent excessive blood loss. If the fundus feels soft and boggy, its muscle fibers are relaxed, constrictions are accordingly somewhat released from the open vessels, and serious bleeding may occur unless these fibers are stimulated to contract again. The uterine muscle may suddenly relax and a severe hemorrhage may occur very quickly.

Observation of the size and height of the fundus as

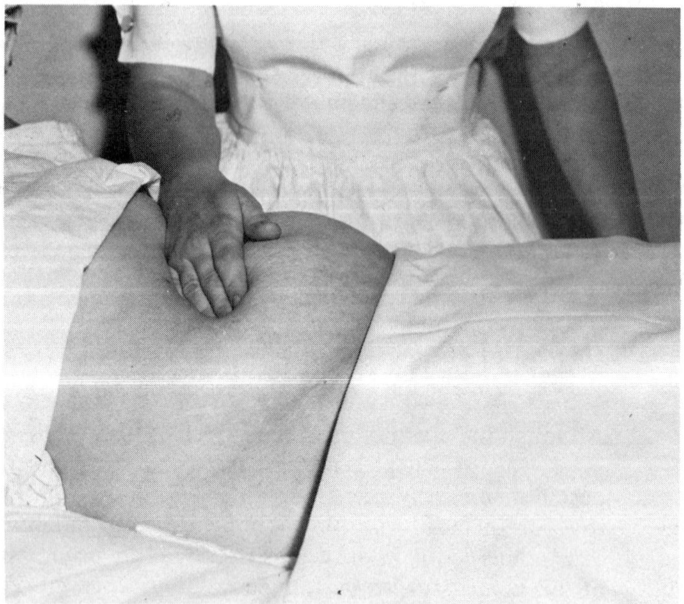

Figure 21–22. The nurse palpates the fundus very frequently after delivery of the placenta to observe the consistency, size, and height of the uterus. This is an essential safeguard against hemorrhage due to uterine muscle relaxation.

well as its consistency is essential, because blood can be retained in the uterus with the muscle fairly well contracted around the blood clot. Consistency of the muscle may then be misleading, but an enlarged uterus high in the abdomen, above the umbilicus, will be indicative of excessive bleeding within the uterus.

If the uterus relaxes or rises in the abdomen, it should be grasped through the abdominal wall and massaged vigorously until it contracts. The fundus should be grasped by the entire hand, with the thumb curved across the anterior surface and the fingers directed deep into the abdomen, behind it, or it may be held between the two hands—one to give support and the other to massage (Fig. 21-23). Rubbing the top of the fundus with the fingers is usually not sufficient stimulation. Massage is discontinued as soon as the uterus has contracted, but vigilance in observation for further relaxation is essential. The physician is notified of departures from normal uterine consistency and size.

Palpation and gentle massage of the uterus, just sufficient to expel clots from the vagina if present, may be carried out every 15 minutes or so for the first hour or two, but vigorous massage should not be used unless the uterus relaxes. Massage may cause uterine muscle fatigue; this fatigue then predisposes to relaxation. Unnecessary massage makes the mother uncomfortable, the uterus being sensitive to manipulation after delivery.

If there has been no relaxation of the uterine muscle during the first hour after delivery of the placenta, there is usually no great danger of hemorrhage. The mother may then be made comfortable in any position she desires and left to rest, but the nurse must still return frequently to check on the consistency of the uterus and the amount of vaginal bleeding.

The mother should be taught how and where to palpate her uterus, what it should feel like when firmly contracted, and how to massage it. She can then assist in making observations.

The perineal pad must be inspected frequently to discover excessive external bleeding. Although the uterus remains firm and is probably not a source of excessive blood loss, bleeding may originate from the cervix or vaginal wall and appear on the perineal pad. Saturation of more than one or two perineal pads with blood during the first hour is considered excessive. A small continuous dribble of blood from the vagina can soon become a serious blood loss and it must be observed as closely as larger gushes. It is also important to look for pooling of blood under the buttocks. Such evidence of bleeding may be missed unless the nurse frequently examines the pad under the woman's hips.

Intravenous fluids begun during labor or delivery are likely to be continued for a variable period of time in the recovery room. Sometimes oxytocin has been added to the intravenous fluids to aid in uterine muscle contractions.

The mother usually has great thirst following delivery, due to restriction of fluids in the later part of labor and loss of fluid in the effort that is exerted during labor and delivery. Unless nausea is present, she will wish to have large amounts of water to drink. Ordinarily fluids are not contraindicated, and, unless there is a reason for withholding them, the nurse should give the mother cold water, or other liquids, as soon as she wishes and in the quantity she desires. Many women are extremely hungry after the birth and may enjoy a snack.

The mother may be exhausted and tense after delivery. She may have generalized discomfort and perineal pain. To ensure rest and relaxation, she may wish to have an analgesic drug when she returns from the delivery room. If the mother is then made as comfortable as possible by a change of perineal pads, proper amount of covering,

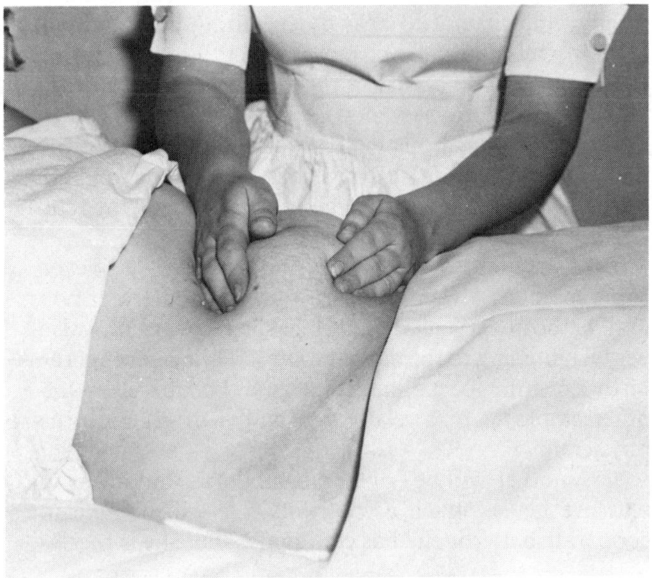

Figure 21-23. Grasping the uterus through the abdominal wall and massaging vigorously to stimulate contraction of the muscle.

comfortable position, and a quiet, well-ventilated room she will be able to rest.

Many mothers expect to sleep immediately, but may find that sleep is not possible for several hours and sometimes not for 8 to 12 hours, because of the physical and nervous exhaustion and the excitement that follows the birth of the infant. The nurse should explain this to the mother and advise her that if sleep is not possible, she should try to lie quietly and get as much rest as she can.

The mother remains in the recovery room from one to several hours, being moved to the postpartum unit when the fundus remains firm, vaginal bleeding is not excessive, and vital signs are stable.

Mother and infant are often moved from the delivery room together, unless this is contraindicated by the condition of either, frequently with the mother holding the infant in her arms. The father accompanies them from the delivery room. The infant may remain with the mother for a time, depending upon physical condition and provisions for keeping him warm, or the infant may be taken to the nursery where he is weighed, wrapped in warm blankets, and placed in a warmed bassinet. Depending upon the alertness of the infant and the mother, the infant may be taken back to the parents for another get-acquainted visit while the mother is in the recovery room.

EMERGENCY DELIVERY BY THE NURSE

It sometimes happens that labor progresses with unexpected rapidity, and the nurse is confronted with the emergency of being alone with the mother during part or all of the delivery.

When the fetus is making such rapid descent that the nurse expects it may be born before the physician's arrival, she may be able to slow labor somewhat by instructing the mother to open her mouth, breathe deeply, and try not to bear down during contractions. Such instructions must be repeated continuously during each contraction because of the mother's almost uncontrollable desire to bear down. Exerting force to delay birth is very dangerous from the standpoint of injuring the fetus and causing it to have marked hypoxia, and the nurse is *never* justified in forcibly holding back the fetal head.

The nurse must not leave the mother alone—not even for a moment—when delivery is imminent. The infant may be born very suddenly while she is away. It is also very frightening to the mother to be left alone, even if the birth does not occur immediately. Someone else—another employee or a relative—usually can summon the physician.

The mother will be frightened, and it is important to reassure her as much as possible. She will be able to cooperate better if she has confidence that she is receiving adequate care until the physician arrives. Calmness of the nurse is essential to the mother's reassurance.

To assist with the delivery, the nurse should put on a pair of sterile rubber gloves or cover her hand with a sterile towel, whichever is more easily available, and apply moderate pressure to the fetal head as it is advancing with contractions, not with the intent of retarding delivery, but to prevent a rapid, unassisted birth. It is rapid distention of the perineum that causes lacerations; also sudden expulsion of the fetal head at the height of a contraction may cause injury to the brain. As the scalp appears at the introitus, the nurse should apply pressure to the head during contractions to prevent its sudden expulsion and to keep it well extended by pressing it up toward the symphysis pubis so that the perineum is not unduly and rapidly stretched. The head should be allowed to progress a little farther with each contraction. After the brow is visible, pressure is gradually released and the head allowed to emerge, or the mother may be asked to bear down between contractions to deliver the head between, rather than with, the force of uterine contractions.

The nurse should remember that there is no need for haste in delivery of the head, since a slow delivery is less dangerous to both the mother and the fetus than rapid expulsion. If the membranes have not ruptured when the head is born, they must be broken immediately to minimize aspiration of fluid. Blood and mucus should quickly be wiped from the infant's mouth and nose when the head is delivered. After the head is born, it drops down toward the mother's rectum, and external rotation takes place.

The shoulders usually will be born spontaneously with the next contraction, or the mother may be asked to bear down to deliver them. Occasionally the shoulders are not delivered in a reasonable time and some assistance is given. To assist in delivery of the shoulders, the infant's head may be held between both hands, and with a gentle downward motion the anterior shoulder can be brought under the symphysis pubis, and then with a gentle upward motion the posterior shoulder may be delivered. The rest of the body follows easily. All manipulation must be very gentle to prevent injury to the infant's neck or arms.

The infant should immediately be held with the head dependent; additional mucus and fluid should be cleared from the air passages. Respirations and cry are usually spontaneous in this type of delivery, but if the infant does not breathe immediately, he should be stimulated by flicking the soles of the feet.

After delivery of the infant, the nurse's hand should be placed on the mother's abdomen to palpate the uterus for size and consistency and to make certain that she is not bleeding. If the uterus remains firm, there is no necessity for delivering the placenta before the physician's arrival. If it appears necessary to deliver the placenta, the nurse should make certain that the fundus is firm and then ask the mother to bear down to expel it from the vagina. If the mother's efforts do not deliver the placenta, the nurse may make gentle downward pressure on the fundus with her hand on the mother's abdomen. The nurse should support the placenta on her hand as it is expelled. After delivery of the placenta, the uterus must remain firm; it should be carefully observed and massaged when necessary. If massage is not successful in producing uterine contractions and bleeding persists, the nurse should use additional treatment measures if available. Administration of oxytocin, 10 IU intramuscularly, stimulates muscle contraction, and use of appropriate intravenous fluids, such as dextrose 5 percent in Ringer's lactate solution, helps to maintain an adequate blood volume. It is advisable whenever possible for the nurse to have prior clarification of actions she may take in emergency situations.

There is no reason for haste to cut and tie the umbilical cord even if the placenta is separated soon after the infant is born. Bleeding does not occur through the surface of the placenta. An intact umbilical cord prohibits moving the infant any distance, but if he is well covered, he will be sufficiently warm until there is time to give him further attention. After the breathing is well established, the infant does not need other care immediately; the nurse can attend to matters that may be more urgent. When sterile equipment can be obtained, the umbilical cord is wiped with an antiseptic solution and clamped and cut under conditions that are as clean as possible.

When the nurse must manage an emergency delivery until the physician arrives, she will need to do whatever is necessary to protect mother and infant, but she should not do more than the emergency demands, allowing delivery to proceed normally insofar as possible and with minimal assistance.

Precipitate Delivery

Sometimes delivery has taken place before the physician or nurse arrives. Such an unassisted delivery is termed a *precipitate delivery*. Immediate attention must be given to the newborn to prevent aspiration of fluid in his attempts to breathe as he lies in the amniotic fluid that escapes after delivery. The infant must be picked up immediately and held head-dependent for postural drainage. There will be no time for hand washing otherwise recommended prior to handling an infant. As soon as the infant's breathing is established, the mother is observed for evidence of excessive uterine bleeding, and care of mother and infant is continued as outlined above.

Delivery Outside the Hospital

In the event of an emergency delivery in a home or elsewhere outside the hospital, the cleanest area possible should be selected for the birth of the infant. When delivery is imminent, the mother should remove clothing that may interfere with the birth. If possible, something should be put under the mother's hips for protection—a clean towel or cloth or plastic or newspaper if available.

The person who will assist at the delivery should wash the hands thoroughly, preferably under running water, if circumstances permit. If in addition, an antiseptic agent such as alcohol or pHisoHex is available, it may be applied to the hands and allowed to dry. The mother must be cautioned against touching the vaginal opening. As a reminder to keep her hands away from the perineal area, she may be instructed to clasp her hands over her chest, or to grasp her knees.

After the birth and establishment of respirations, the infant may be placed on the mother's abdomen, on the side, with the head down. Such a position promotes drainage of mucus. The mother's body will provide warmth and, in addition, the infant should be dried and covered to reduce loss of body heat.

If mother and infant are to be transported to a hospital immediately, the placenta may be delivered through the mother's bearing-down efforts or it may remain in the lower uterine segment or vagina and be delivered later. It is important for the nurse to keep the uterus firm to prevent excessive bleeding.

Under unusual circumstances, when the mother cannot receive medical care for some hours, the umbilical cord may be cut and clamped after urgent matters have been given attention. Tape or narrow strips of white cloth and scissors may be boiled for this purpose. If possible, the cord should be cleaned before it is cut, especially if an antiseptic such as alcohol is available. Since there is danger of infection through the open end of an umbilical cord if it is cared for with unclean equipment, it is best to leave the cord intact until much later if there is assurance that better facilities will then be available.

The infant must be kept warm by being wrapped in blankets and being placed in the mother's arms. If there is mucus, postural drainage can be instituted by positioning the infant with the head toward one side. Unless contraindicated by either the infant's or mother's condition, the infant may be put to breast. As soon as the placenta has been delivered, sucking at the breast stimulates the uterine muscle to contract.

If there is any possibility of separation of mother and infant, as in a disaster, identification of the infant by some means is very important.

REFERENCES AND SUGGESTED READINGS

American Academy of Pediatrics and American College of Obstetricians and Gynecologists, *Guidelines for Perinatal Care,* American Academy of Pediatrics, Evanston, IL, and the American College of Obstetricians and Gynecologists, Washington, D.C., 1983.

Boggs, Thomas R., Avoiding morbidity during the first 60 minutes of life, *Contemp. Ob/Gyn.,* 15:47–65, (May) 1980.

Cogan, Rosemary, Pain and hyperventilation with fast panting, slow panting, and "He" breathing during labor. *Birth Fam. J.,* 4:59–64, (Summer) 1977.

Friedman, Emanuel A., *Labor: Clinical Evaluation and Management,* 2nd ed., Appleton-Century-Crofts, New York, 1978.

Huprich, Patricia A., Assisting the couple through Lamaze labor and delivery, *MCN,* 2:245–53, (July–Aug.) 1977.

Iffy, Leslie, and Kaminetzky, Harold A. (eds.). *Principles and Practice of Obstetrics and Perinatology,* Vol. II, John Wiley, New York, 1981.

Jennings, Betty, Emergency delivery: How to attend one safely, *MCN,* 4:148–53, (May–June) 1979.

Klaus, Marshall H., and Kennell, John H., *Parent-Infant Bonding,* 2nd ed., C. V. Mosby, St. Louis, 1982, Chap. 2.

Landry, Karen E., and Kilpatrick, Darla M., Why shave a mother before she gives birth? *MCN,* 2:189–90, (May–June) 1977.

Lum, Sister Barbara; Batzel, Ruth Lortz; and Barnett, Elouise, Reappraising newborn eye care, *Am. J. Nurs.,* 80:1602–03, (Sept.) 1980.

McKay, Susan R., Second stage labor—Has tradition replaced safety? *Am. J. Nurs.,* 81:1016–19, (May) 1981.

Ostheimer, Gerard W., Resuscitating the depressed neonate, *Contemp. Ob/Gyn.,* 15:27–36 and 41, (Apr.) 1980.

Oxorn, Harry, *Oxorn-Foote Human Labor and Birth,* 4th ed., Appleton-Century-Crofts, New York, 1978.

Phillips, Celeste R., The essence of birth without violence, *MCN,* 1:162–63, (May–June) 1976.

Pritchard, Jack A., and MacDonald, Paul C., *Williams Obstetrics,* 16th ed., Appleton-Century-Crofts, New York, 1980.

Scanlon, John W., Fast action for the distressed newborn, *Contemp. Ob/Gyn.,* 18:151–60, (July) 1981.

CHAPTER

22

Complications of Labor; Obstetric Operations

Revised by Sue A. Frazier, R.N., M.S.N.

LABOR AND DELIVERY do not always proceed in the normal manner described in Chapter 17. Abnormalities may develop in any of the three stages.

A difficult labor is termed *dystocia*. This is a slow or complicated labor and/or delivery that may result from any condition that interferes with the normal mechanical processes and clinical progression of labor. Included among such aberrations are faulty cervical effacement and dilation, failure of fetal descent, abnormal uterine muscle action, uncommon fetal presentations and positions, and pelvic contractions. Less frequent are excessive size of the fetus, certain fetal abnormalities, poor abdominal muscle contractions, abnormalities of the pelvic organs, and overdistention of the uterus from such conditions as multiple pregnancy or hydramnios, which decrease the efficiency of uterine contractions.

Sometimes labor with associated abnormalities, although prolonged, terminates in a spontaneous delivery. At other times, operative interventions are necessary.

ABNORMAL LABOR PATTERNS AND UTERINE MUSCLE ACTION

Prolonged or Arrested Labor

In the past, labor was considered prolonged when it continued for more than 24 hours after the onset of regular uterine contractions. Such a definition is very broad, has only a single criterion, does not define the time at which a problem arises, and may include women who actually have a normal labor pattern in all but the latent phase. A current method of defining abnormal labor and recognizing one that is prolonged is to compare each phase of the labor to an established normal labor curve.

Many problems arise when labor is prolonged. The incidence of perinatal morbidity and mortality is increased. The woman is vulnerable to intrauterine infection and to postpartum hemorrhage; she becomes fatigued and exhausted and may become dehydrated. Intravenous fluids can supply minimum fluid requirements, but the woman does not receive adequate food or rest during a long labor. The fetus is subjected to prolonged stress from uterine contractions, and there is increased likelihood of infection in the fetus, with intact as well as with ruptured membranes.

A graphic analysis of each labor will help the professional to recognize undue prolongation of labor in any of its phases, so that appropriate treatment can be given early. It is advisable to record the time and the findings of each observation of cervical dilation and station of the presenting part on a Friedman graph as shown in Figure 17-11. The professional can then compare the particular labor curve with a normal curve to evaluate the labor in progress and appraise its normalcy or deviation in one or more of the specific dilational or descent phases.

Labor may be prolonged or arrested in any one of the cervical dilational phases of labor or in the fetal descent pattern (Figs. 22-1 and 22-2). Six specific dysfunctional labor patterns may be defined; these are described below. Each pattern is an independent entity, which may appear individually or in combination with any of the other patterns in a given labor.

Prolonged Latent Phase of Cervical Dilation

The latent phase of cervical dilation is ordinarily considered prolonged when it exceeds 20 hours in the primigravida and 14 hours in the multigravida. A prolonged latent phase has often been called primary dysfunctional labor. The acceleration phase also may be prolonged and can be considered along with a long latent phase, since it is often affected by the same causative factors (Fig. 22-1).

Among the causes of prolonged latent phase of labor are false labor, a long, firm cervix which is not prepared by the softening and shortening that usually occur prior to onset of labor which thus must be accomplished during the latent phase, dysfunction of uterine contractions, and excessive sedation early in labor.

When the latent or acceleration phases of labor are prolonged, the patient becomes very tired before active labor begins. A period of rest for the exhausted patient, as well as for the uterine muscle, is often beneficial. Medication for pain is administered in sufficient dosage to give relief, good rest, and sleep if possible. During or after a period of rest most labors advance into the active phase with a normal pattern and subsequently are followed by vaginal delivery. Some women awaken not in labor, indicating that they were in false labor. In a small number of cases the labor pattern may remain unchanged. If oxytocin stimulation of uterine contractions is not contraindicated, it may be used when progress of labor does not improve after therapeutic rest.

The prognosis for a prolonged latent phase is usually good for vaginal delivery and the fetus is usually not at risk.

Prolonged Active Phase of Cervical Dilation

The active cervical dilation phase is considered prolonged if cervical dilation during the phase of maximum slope does not progress at 1.2 cm or more per hour in a primigravida or 1.5 cm or more per hour in a multigravida (Fig. 22-1).

Prolonged Descent of the Presenting Part

The descent phase of labor, which reaches its maximum slope toward the end of the first stage of labor (concurrent with the deceleration phase of cervical dilation), is prolonged when the slope of descent does not progress at at least 1 cm per hour in primigravidas and 2 cm per hour in multigravidas (Fig. 22–2).

Discussion of Prolonged Active Phase and Prolonged Descent

Prolonged active phase dilation and prolonged descent are considered together here because of certain similarities. The cause is often not known, although cephalopelvic disproportion is present in about one-third of these cases. Sometimes malposition of the fetus, excessive sedation of the mother, and early conduction anesthesia slow the labor.

To determine the possible cause of a long active phase

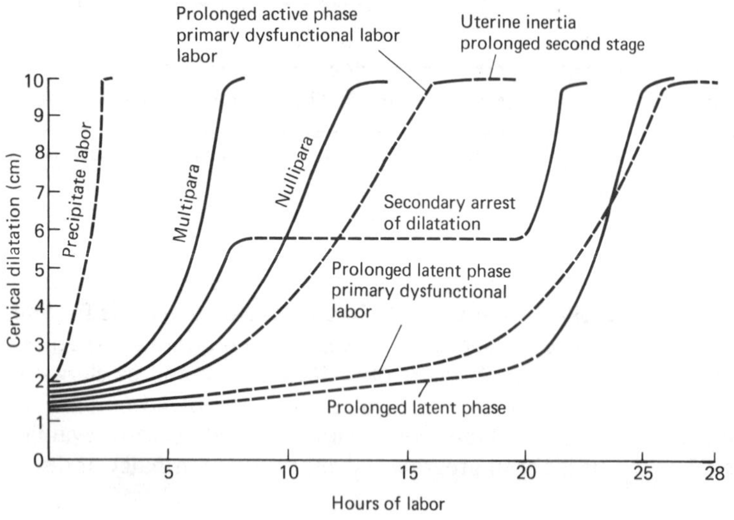

Figure 22–1. Normal and abnormal labor curves as diagrammed in the time relationship of cervical dilation and progression of first and second stages of labor. The duration of labor and its pattern is different in primigravidas and multiparas. The multiparas have definite advantages through previous labor experience: they display better coordinated and stronger uterine activity, faster cervical dilation, and an easier and more rapid expulsion of the fetus through the birth canal. The net result is a shorter duration of labor by an average of 4–8 hours as compared to primigravidas. In precipitate labor the first and second stage may be very short and inseparable; in these cases the child may be born within a few minutes by a few uterine contractions.

Prolonged or arrested labor patterns in the cervical dilational phases of labor are prolonged latent phase, prolonged active phase, prolonged deceleration phase, and secondary arrest of dilation. (Reproduced with permission from Nicholas S. Assali (ed.), Maternal Disorders. Volume I in *Pathophysiology of Gestation.* New York: Academic Press, 1972, p. 191.)

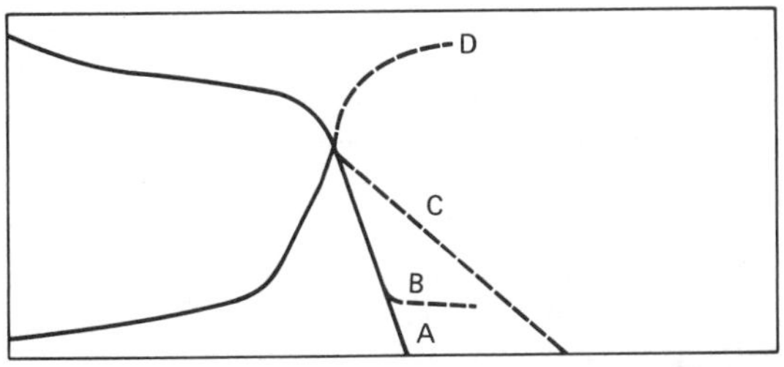

Figure 22-2. Abnormal patterns of descent of the presenting part during labor according to Friedman's graphic labor patterns. *A.* Normal descent pattern. *B.* Arrest of descent. *C.* Prolonged descent. *D.* Prolonged deceleration. Prolonged deceleration, a part of the cervical dilation pattern, is shown with abnormal descent pattern because of its close relationship to abnormal progress of the presenting part through the pelvis.

of cervical dilation or a prolonged descent phase, and the appropriate treatment, the mother's pelvis and the fetal position are reexamined. A sterile vaginal examination is done to ascertain the condition of the cervix, to determine the presentation and position of the fetus, and to reevaluate the size and configuration of the pelvis. X-ray pelvimetry may be done to measure the pelvis accurately, determine the exact fetal position, and evaluate the cephalopelvic relationship.

If a cephalopelvic disproportion exists, a cesarean section is done to deliver the infant. If neither disproportion between the fetus and the woman's pelvis nor fetal malposition is detected, physical and emotional supportive measures are indicated, and conservative management is recommended. Dilation and descent may proceed slowly, followed by vaginal delivery, or if labor continues without progress, a cesarean section may yet become necessary.

Intravenous fluids are used during a prolonged labor to prevent dehydration, provide glucose, and maintain a good electrolyte balance. Sedation and analgesia rarely inhibit normal progress of the active phase of dilation as is so often evident in the latent phase, but with abnormally slow progress, sedation can diminish advancement even more.

Sometimes during the course of a long labor, an amniotomy may be done with the anticipation of improving contractions. An amniotomy is carefully considered since it may not prove helpful, and it may lead to complications arising from premature rupture of the membranes.

Stimulation of contractions with oxytocin by intravenous drip may be used if there are no contraindications. Oxytocin is not used if it cannot be anticipated that the fetus will pass through the birth canal easily, or if the uterus is overdistended. Oxytocin may be administered for a few hours, discontinued for a period of rest, and then resumed. The procedure for oxytocin infusions is described later in this chapter.

Risk to mother and fetus from the delivery following prolonged active phase of the dilation or prolonged descent of presenting part is not significantly increased if management is conservative, if labor progress continues, and if delivery is spontaneous or by low forceps. Difficult forceps delivery increases risk to the fetus considerably. Prolonged labor, however, does increase the risk of infection to mother and fetus.

Prolonged Deceleration Phase of Dilation

The deceleration phase of dilation is prolonged when it exceeds 3 hours in a primigravida and 1 hour in a multigravida. Although the deceleration phase is a part of the cervical dilation pattern, a prolongation of this phase is closely related to abnormal descent of the presenting part through the pelvis. It is an arrest pattern.

Secondary Arrest of Dilation

An arrest in dilation during the phase of maximum slope is diagnosed by documenting that there has been no progress in cervical dilation for over a period of 2 hours or longer (Fig. 22-1).

Arrest of Descent

Arrest of descent is diagnosed when there is an arrest in the descent pattern, usually in the second stage, for at least 1 hour (Fig. 22-2).

Discussion of Prolonged Deceleration, Secondary Arrest, and Arrest of Descent

Cephalopelvic disproportion must be suspected in prolonged deceleration, secondary arrest, and arrest of descent. A pattern of arrest is often the first sign of disproportion and constitutes a warning. Other associated factors in arrest are fetal malpositions, excessive sedation, and conduction anesthesia in conjunction with other inhibitory factors. Evaluation for cephalopelvic disproportion and fetal position is essential whenever an arrest pattern develops.

If disproportion is not evident, continuation of labor is usually permitted. Therapeutic rest may be indicated for the woman who is becoming exhausted. Later, if there are no contraindications, stimulation with oxytocin may be instituted. Most women will respond to this stimulation with progress in dilation and descent. Occasionally progress is not good or fetal distress occurs, and a cesarean section will still be indicated.

If cephalopelvic disproportion is discovered, termination of labor by cesarean section as soon as possible is indicated.

Risk to the fetus is considerably increased with arrest patterns and therefore requires early diagnosis and careful management.

Table 22-1 summarizes the various abnormal labor patterns.

Table 22-1. Summary of the Pattern of Abnormal Labor*

Pattern	*Diagnostic Criterion*
I. Disorder of Preparatory Division of Labor†	
Prolonged latent phase	
Nulliparas	Latent phase duration of 20 hr or more
Multiparas	Latent phase duration of 14 hr or more
II. Disorders of Dilational Division of Labor†	
Protracted active-phase dilation	
Nulliparas	Maximum slope of dilation of 1.2 cm/hr or less
Multiparas	Maximum slope of dilation of 1.5 cm/hr or less
Protracted descent	
Nulliparas	Maximum slope of descent of 1.0 cm/hr or less
Multiparas	Maximum slope of descent of 2.0 cm/hr or less
III. Disorders of Pelvic Division of Labor†	
Prolonged deceleration phase	
Nulliparas	Deceleration phase duration of 3 hr or more
Multiparas	Deceleration phase duration of 1 hr or more
Secondary arrest of dilation	Cessation of active-phase progression for 2 hr or more
Arrest of descent	Cessation of descent progression for 1 hr or more
Failure of descent	Lack of expected descent during deceleration phase and second stage
IV. Precipitate Labor Disorders	
Precipitate dilation	
Nulliparas	Maximum slope of dilation of 5 cm/hr or more
Multiparas	Maximum slope of dilation of 10 cm/hr or more
Precipitate descent	
Nulliparas	Maximum slope of descent of 5 cm/hr or more
Multiparas	Maximum slope of descent of 10 cm/hr or more

*From Emanuel A. Friedman, *Labor: Clinical Evaluation and Management*, 2nd ed., Appleton-Century-Croft, New York, 1978, p. 63.

†I. Preparatory division includes latent and acceleration phases of cervical dilation. II. Dilational division encompasses the phase of maximum slope of dilation. III. Pelvic division includes both the deceleration phase of cervical dilation and second stage of labor concurrent with the maximum fetal descent slope.

Nursing Care

Nursing care of a mother during prolonged labor includes providing physical comfort, giving reassurance, and making observation of untoward effects. The mother often becomes anxious, discouraged, and frequently irritable, especially when she is tired. She needs much encouragement and is often less anxious when someone is with her. Constant nursing care by a calm, reassuring person should be provided if the mother wishes it. Reduction of tension may increase effectiveness of contractions. Frequent baths, back rubs, fresh linen, and changes of position are refreshing and add to the mother's general comfort. If she may be out of bed, a shower and fresh bed linen often help her to relax and rest more comfortably. When an analgesic is given, provision for good ventilation and a quiet environment promotes rest.

The mother is observed for signs of exhaustion, dehydration, and acidosis. Her vital signs are checked frequently. The fetal heart is closely observed. Deviations from normal are reported to the physician immediately.

When the uterus has not contracted well in the first or second stage of labor, a similar action can be expected in the third stage. It is necessary to watch for ineffective uterine contraction after delivery and be ready to give treatment if bleeding becomes excessive.

Precipitate Labor and Delivery

In contrast to the prolonged labor, an abnormally rapid, intense labor in which cervical dilation occurs quickly and descent of the presenting part is rapid is termed a precipitate labor. This should be distinguished from a "precipitate delivery" which usually refers to a rapid delivery over an unprepared and unsterile field.

In precipitate labor the uterine contractions are unusually strong and frequent, and in addition there may be little resistance from the maternal soft parts. The uterine contractions cause the cervix to dilate very rapidly and also move the fetus through the birth canal very quickly. Often the abdominal muscles also contract very strongly and thus assist in rapid delivery.

Precipitate labor has been defined as a labor of 2 to 4 hours in duration. The rate of cervical dilation in the active phase is greater than 5 cm per hour in primigravidas and greater than 10 cm per hour in multigravidas (Fig. 22-1).

Precipitate labor may be injurious to both mother and fetus. Trauma to both may be a serious problem, and hypoxia of the fetus may occur because of the rapidly occurring uterine contractions.

For precipitate delivery the fetal head should be controlled and guided over the perineum to prevent traumatic damage to the fetal head and the mother's perineum. No attempt, however, should be made to delay the delivery forcibly (See Table 22-1).

Abnormal Uterine Action

Abnormal uterine muscle contractions may be characterized as hypotonic or hypertonic.

Hypotonicity

Hypotonic contractions are short, irregular, infrequent, and often without much discomfort, with one or more of the following features in evidence: less than 15 mm Hg intrauterine pressure, duration of less than 40 seconds, and more than 3 minutes between contractions. The contractions may occur farther and farther apart and become very irregular. The uterus is easily indented even at the acme of the contraction, and the contractions are ineffective in promoting progress of labor.

Hypotonic contractions are most likely to occur in the active phase of dilation or in the second stage, usually after labor has been in progress for awhile; then labor is slowed or arrested. Hypotonic contractions may be a protection against labor continuing with strong contractions when there is some degree of cephalopelvic disproportion or an abnormality of fetal position. Other causes of hypotonic contractions are uterine overdistention and persistent OP position of the fetal head toward the end of labor.

Evaluation of the pelvis, the fetal position, and the relationship of the fetal head to the pelvis is made when hypotonic labor develops to rule out abnormalities. If none is found, the hypotonic labor usually is treated successfully by stimulation of the contractions with oxytocin, sometimes interspersed with periods of rest.

Hypertonicity

Hypertonic contractions occur frequently and are cramplike; they are regular, strong, and painful, but ineffectual in producing anything more than minor progress in the labor. In hypertonic dysfunction the uterine muscle usually maintains a greater than normal tonus, but the contractions themselves are of poor quality.

Duration of the contractions varies from 50 seconds back to 10 seconds and up to 70 seconds, their intensity varies from 20 to 40 mm Hg, and their frequency varies from 2 to 3 to 5 minutes. The contractions are erratic in all respects. They are clinically more painful than palpation of the uterus would indicate, and they can quickly cause maternal exhaustion. They are also likely to lead to early fetal distress because of inadequate relaxation between contractions.

Hypertonic contractions are most likely to occur in the latent phase of labor. As with hypotonic labor, hypertonic contractions may develop with cephalopelvic disproportion or abnormal fetal position. It is important to look for such underlying problems.

The initial treatment of hypertonicity usually consists of rest by stopping the abnormal contractions and the pain with morphine. The pain appears to aggravate the dysfunction and should be relieved. The medication is not likely to have adverse effects on the fetus because there is time for it to be eliminated before labor ends. If there is no underlying obstructive problem, normal labor often ensures after a period of good rest.

Occasionally the hypertonic uterine contractions do not convert to normal after rest. At that time, contractions may be stimulated with oxytocin in the hope that they will become normal; however, the drug must be administered with even greater caution—considerably smaller dosage—than normally used in stimulation of labor. The woman must be carefully observed for any evidence of tetanic contractions. The fetus must be monitored assiduously for signs of distress.

With either type of abnormal uterine contraction, hypotonic or hypertonic, a cesarean section will be performed if abnormalities in pelvic size or fetal position are discovered, if labor does not change and progress normally, or if fetal distress develops.

Tetanic Contractions

A patient has a tetanic contraction of the uterus when it stays contracted continuously more than 90 seconds, instead of relaxing at regular intervals. This condition usually occurs with overstimulation of the uterus with an oxytocin, or it may be found in prolonged labor, due to a mechanical obstruction to advancement of the fetus. These contractions are very painful. There is danger of asphyxia of the fetus due to interference with placental circulation and rupture of the uterus. Oxytocin, if being given, is promptly discontinued. An obstructed labor is ended as soon as it can be accomplished safely.

Pathologic Retraction Ring or Bandl's Ring

Normally there is a physiologic retraction ring between the upper and lower uterine segments during labor. In an obstructed labor this may become more pronounced and thus pathologic. An excessive amount of thinning of the lower uterine segment develops, and the upper segment becomes thicker and more tightly contracted than normal. The retraction ring rises to, or nearly to, the level of the umbilicus. It can be seen as a depression across the abdomen. There may be intense pain above the symphysis pubis. There is considerable danger of rupture of the uterus when a pathologic retraction ring develops. A cesarean section is done because the obstruction does not permit descent of the fetus.

Ruptured Uterus

A ruptured uterus is a splitting of the uterine wall at some point that has become thinned or weakened and is unable to stand the strain of further stretching or the force of uterine contractions. It is accompanied by an extrusion of all or a part of the uterine contents into the abdominal cavity. Spontaneous rupture of a normal uterus is a rare accident, and usually occurs only in obstructed labors and with improper use of oxytocin. A multiparous, aging uterus is more prone to rupture than that of a primigravida. Even a slightly obstructed labor, possibly due to a large baby, may be serious in a woman who has had many children. Rupture of the uterus at the site of a scar from a previous cesarean section sometimes occurs because of a weakened wall.

In obstructed labors the lower uterine segment becomes thinner and thinner as the contractions pull the retraction ring higher. Finally the lower segment becomes tetanic, the contraction ring becomes very prominent, and the pulse becomes rapid. A patient in whom there is some possibility of obstructed labor must be carefully observed for ballooning out of the lower uterine segment or rising up of a retraction ring. These signs and pain above the symphysis pubis are premonitory signs of rupture of the uterus. If they appear, prompt termination of labor is necessary.

A common sign of rupture is sudden and acute abdominal pain during a contraction, which the patient describes as being unlike anything she has ever felt and as though "something had given way" inside of her. With complete rupture there is immediate cessation of labor pains because the torn uterus no longer contracts. Bleeding takes place internally, and sometimes also through the vagina. The patient soon shows signs of shock. Her face becomes pale and drawn and covered with perspiration; her pulse is weak and rapid; she appears exhausted and may complain of chilly sensations and air hunger. On abdominal palpation the contracted uterus, partly or entirely empty, may be felt as a hard mass alongside the fetus. In some cases there is an incomplete rupture. Blood loss is then slower and signs of shock may be delayed.

Pain and abdominal tenderness are usually present with rupture, incomplete as well as complete. These signs should lead to the suspicion that rupture may have occurred. It may be possible to institute treatment before shock develops. First a laparotomy is done to remove the fetus, usually followed by a hysterectomy. Occasionally the laceration in the uterus is sutured, but it may be subject to rupture in a subsequent pregnancy. Blood transfusions are given to overcome shock and to replace the blood loss. Antibiotics are administered to prevent infection, to which the traumatized tissues are very susceptible.

A ruptured uterus is a grave accident. The fetus usually dies owing to placental separation. The maternal mortality rate is high. Early diagnosis, immediate treatment, blood transfusions, and antibiotics should improve maternal prognosis.

ABNORMAL PRESENTATION, POSITION, AND DEVELOPMENT OF THE FETUS

Variation in labor, with prolongation in the active phase of dilation or in descent of the presenting part or frequently in both, is likely when the fetal position is one of the less common varieties. Excessive size of the fetus influences labor. Occasionally an abnormal development of the fetus complicates labor and delivery.

Occiput Posterior Position

Labor is usually prolonged when the vertex presents with the occiput in the posterior portion of the pelvis, the occiput posterior position. The mechanism of labor is the same as that described for vertex presentation (Chapter 17) except that the occiput must rotate a longer distance to reach the symphysis pubis. When the occiput is in the anterior portion of the mother's pelvis, it rotates only 45 degrees to reach the symphysis pubis, while the distance is 135 degrees from the posterior position (Fig. 17-8). Internal rotation of an occiput posterior occasionally takes place as the head is descending, but often not until the vertex reaches the pelvic floor. The longer distance of rotation prolongs the second stage of labor.

In some cases the occiput rotates to a posterior position so that it lies directly over the sacrum instead of under the symphysis pubis. This is termed a *direct occiput posterior position*. During delivery from this position the part of the head near the large fontanel fixes itself under the symphysis pubis, and the head becomes more and more flexed until the occiput slips over the perineum. Spontaneous delivery occurs in many instances, but the second stage may be prolonged. An episiotomy is more likely and is apt to be made deeper than with the direct occiput anterior position since a larger diameter of the head distends the vulva during delivery.

In a small number of cases, the occiput does not rotate, a condition termed *persistent occiput posterior*. In others, rotation is incomplete with the head arrested when it reaches the transverse position. This is designated a *deep transverse arrest*.

With enough time, complete rotation of the head and spontaneous delivery often take place from an occiput posterior position. If the head is arrested and little or no progress is made, rotation may be completed manually or with the aid of forceps. Then forceps is used to deliver the head. The head may be delivered as a direct occiput posterior, or it may be rotated to an anterior position for delivery, provided this can be accomplished quite readily.

Breech Presentation

Breech presentation may alter the normal course of labor and complicate delivery. Labor and delivery in breech presentation are described later in this chapter.

Face Presentation

In a face (mentum) presentation the head is in extension as it descends into the pelvis instead of the usual position of flexion. Here the occiput points toward the back, and the face enters the pelvis first (Fig. 16-15). Diagnosis by palpation is sometimes difficult, and an x-ray may be necessary to establish it. X-ray pelvimetry is important to evaluate the pelvic size, a common influence on the method of delivery. Face presentations are rare, but perinatal mortality and morbidity rate are increased in this abnormal presentation.

Spontaneous delivery cannot occur unless the chin rotates anteriorly so that it lies under the symphysis pubis. This rotation may not occur until late in labor. When the chin lies anteriorly, the neck can slip around the short symphysis pubis without difficulty. If the chin lies posteriorly, the neck is too short to allow the chin to travel the relatively long distance along the anterior surface of the sacrum. Delivery is impossible without a change in position, unless the fetus is small enough to allow the shoulders to enter the pelvis also. When the chin lies posteriorly, spontaneous rotation to the anterior position often takes place after the face reaches the pelvic floor. If this does not occur, a cesarean section is performed. A cesarean section is considered preferable whenever any condition indicates that a vaginal delivery will be difficult or traumatic.

During delivery of the head, after the chin has rotated anteriorly, the mouth appears at the vaginal opening, the chin stems against the symphysis pubis, and the head flexes so that the nose, eyes, brow, and finally the occiput slip over the perineum. The face usually becomes edematous due to effusion of serum under the skin during labor, and the skull becomes markedly molded.

Transverse Lie

In a transverse lie the longitudinal axis of the fetus lies at right angles to the longitudinal axis of the mother, and a shoulder is usually over the pelvic inlet. This is called a shoulder presentation (Fig. 16-15). Delivery is impossible in this position unless the fetus is very small. If labor progresses with the fetus presenting transversely, the shoulder usually becomes wedged in the pelvis and the arm frequently prolapses into the vagina. If hard uterine contractions continue, a thinning and even rupture of the lower uterine segment may occur. Fortunately a transverse presentation occurs in only a small percentage of all cases.

Spontaneous version to a longitudinal presentation occasionally occurs after onset of labor; otherwise, a cesarean section is done.

In a primigravida a transverse lie is suggestive of a pelvic contraction. If x-ray pelvimetry shows a contracted pelvis, a cesarean section is performed before onset of labor. If the pelvis is of normal size, the cesarean section may be delayed until the onset of labor on the chance that the lie may change.

A transverse lie is frequently associated with placenta previa. This complication will determine the time at which a cesarean section is performed.

Excessive Size of Fetus

The relationship between the size of the fetus and the size of the pelvis is one determining factor between an easy and a difficult delivery. A slight disproportion may delay progress, and a greater one make delivery through the birth canal difficult or impossible. The fetal head must always accommodate to the mother's pelvis. With some degree of cephalopelvic disproportion, considerable molding of the head may be necessary, and this may prolong labor.

When a fetus develops to excessive size, the chance of a prolonged or difficult labor increases. The head is not only larger, but also less moldable, than that of an average-sized fetus. With average pelvic measurements, the fetal size usually presents no problem until the fetus reaches a weight of 4500 gm (10 lb). After the fetus reaches a size of 4500 gm, the size of the shoulder girdle also may complicate delivery. The circumference at the shoulders may then be greater than the circumference of the head, and they may not compress easily due to firmness.

Occasionally malformations of the fetus resulting in an enlargement of a part of the body may make delivery difficult.

PROLAPSE OF THE UMBILICAL CORD

The umbilical cord may prolapse into the cervical canal alongside the presenting part (occult prolapse) or through the cervix into the vagina and occasionally may protrude from the vagina. This complication can occur when the presenting part of the fetus does not fit firmly against the pelvic inlet (Fig. 22-3). It occurs most frequently when the membranes rupture while the presenting part is still above the pelvic inlet or with abnormal presentations, such as a footling breech. The condition is often first suspected by the nurse because of notation of a slowed fetal heart rate due to cord compression.

Prolapse of the cord endangers the life of the fetus through interference with its circulation; diagnosis is made by palpation of the umbilical cord below or alongside the presenting part on vaginal examination, or seeing the cord outside the vagina. The diagnosis of prolapsed cord demands immediate intervention directed at relieving or minimizing cord compression. This is done by quickly placing the patient in a knee-chest or exaggerated Trendelenburg position. If this positional change is insufficient to relieve the compression, the attending clinician should manually elevate the presenting part off the cord. Under no circumstance should the cord itself be directly manipulated. If a physician is not immediately available, the nurse must take the corrective action and direct others to notify the physician and make the necessary preparations for the delivery of the fetus.

When an umbilical cord has prolapsed, the fetus is delivered as quickly as possible. Time is very important. If the cervix is already completely dilated, immediate delivery through the birth canal may be possible. If the cervix is not completely dilated or if vaginal delivery would be delayed because of the possibility of some disproportion, a cesarean section is performed as quickly as possible. Haste in preparation for the cesarean birth is of utmost importance. During this preparation the physician may keep the fetal presenting part up from the umbilical cord by pressure applied to it from below through the vagina. Oxygen is given to the mother. The FHR is checked continuously.

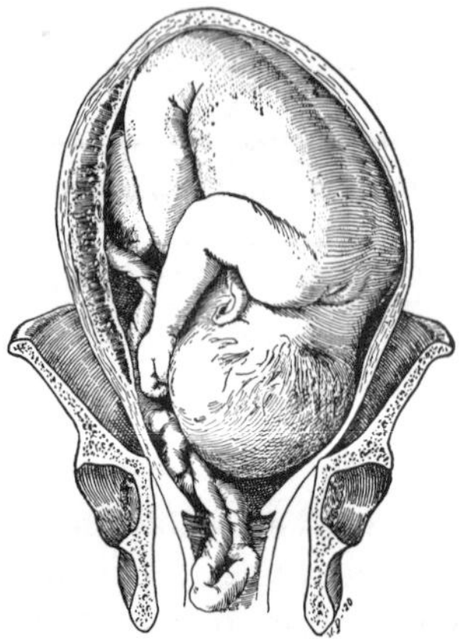

Figure 22-3. Showing how a prolapsed cord may be pressed between the fetal head and the pelvic bones, resulting in interference with circulation between the fetus and the placenta.

DYSTOCIA CAUSED BY PELVIC CONTRACTION

The size and configuration of the bony birth canal influence the progress of labor. Shortening of one or more of the pelvic diameters or variations in the shape of a pelvis of normal size alter the normal mechanism of labor to some degree. Labor may then be prolonged in the first stage by slow cervical dilation and in the second stage by the longer time required for molding of the fetal head, or delivery through the birth canal may be impossible.

The size and moldability of the fetal head may determine if delivery through a pelvis with some degree of contraction is possible. The outcome depends on the size of the pelvis in relation to the size of the fetus. For this reason, in two women with pelves of the same size and shape one will have a spontaneous delivery and the other require a cesarean section. The former has a relatively small fetus which can pass through her pelvis; the second woman's fetus is too large, or the head is not sufficiently moldable, for passage through the pelvis.

In some cases the pelvic measurements taken during the antepartum period determine a significant pelvic contraction and suggest that delivery should be by the abdominal route. A cesarean birth is then planned before the onset of labor.

Pelvic contractions are usually classified into four groups: inlet contraction, midpelvic contraction, outlet contraction, and combinations of inlet, midpelvic, and outlet contractions. As the fetal head passes through the birth canal, it may be arrested at any one of the divisions of the pelvis.

Inlet Contraction

If contraction at the pelvic inlet is pronounced, a cesarean birth is planned in advance. If the contraction is mild or borderline, the decision may rest on the relationship of the size of the fetal head to the size of the pelvis at the time of labor.

Engagement of the fetal head is evidence that the pelvic inlet is large enough to accommodate it. Before engagement, evidence of disproportion sometimes can be determined by grasping the head through the abdominal wall, pressing it toward the inlet, and checking for overriding of the head over the symphysis pubis. An x-ray with the patient in a standing position gives information on the relationship between the size of the fetal head and the size of the pelvis. Taken during labor it often demonstrates whether the head is engaging.

A *trial of labor* may be given in cases of borderline inlet contraction. The patient is allowed to have labor for several hours to determine if an uncomplicated vaginal delivery can be anticipated. Engagement may take place after labor is well established. If labor does not progress satisfactory with engagement of the head during a few hours of fairly strong contractions of about 50 mm Hg intrauterine pressure, 50 seconds' duration, occurring approximately every 3 minutes, a cesarean is done.

Midpelvic Contraction

Midpelvic contraction usually prolongs labor. The uterine contractions must push the fetal head through an area that is shortened more than normal, and this takes time. After the biparietal diameter has passed the midpelvic area and the head is on the perineum, delivery may progress rapidly and spontaneously, or forceps may be used to complete it. Midpelvic contraction may cause a transverse arrest of the head.

Outlet Contraction

When the pelvic outlet is contracted, the pubic arch is narrowed. The fetal head does not fit closely to the pubic arch and cannot emerge from the birth canal directly under the symphysis pubis. The head must occupy more of the posterior part of the outlet (the posterior triangle) as it emerges from the birth canal. The degree to which a contracted outlet causes dystocia depends on the posterior sagittal diameter as well as on the intertuberous measurement. When both measurements are decreased, dystocia is most likely to result.

Midpelvic contraction often accompanies outlet contraction and may add to or be the major cause of dystocia. In midpelvic contraction as in outlet contraction the head occupies the posterior portion of the pelvis in its passage. In the midpelvis the uterosacral ligaments, which partly form its posterior circumference, are often pliable enough to permit passage through a pelvis contracted between the ischial spines. At the outlet the apex of the posterior triangle is located at the tip of the sacrum, but there are no bony sides, and the perineum will distend to permit room for passage in most cases. Because of a certain degree of pliability of soft tissue at both the midpelvis and the pelvic outlet, narrowing in these areas does not present the absolute barrier to the fetus' passage that narrowing at the pelvic inlet may present. The pelvic inlet is a bony ring that is incapable of expansion, as compared with some degree of flexibility of the midpelvis and the outlet.

Pelvic outlet contraction increases the necessity for forceps deliveries. Since the occiput cannot emerge directly under the symphysis pubis, the perineum is consequently distended more than in delivery through a normal-sized outlet. A deep episiotomy is usually necessary to facilitate delivery and may be made in a mediolateral direction to prevent tearing through the anal sphincter.

INDUCTION AND AUGMENTATION OF LABOR

Today it is not uncommon for labor to be induced (artificially initiated). This is done either in the presence of obstetric or medical risk conditions such as premature rupture of the membranes, hypertensive disorders, diabetes, or any other condition associated with placental insufficiency or as an elective procedure. In the latter instance, the decision may be based on the patient's past obstetric history of very rapid labors or a woman's personal circumstances, such as living a long distance from a health care facility.

Regardless of the reason for inducing labor certain conditions are necessary for a successful induction. The cervix should show some of the changes that normally take place shortly before labor. It should be soft and partly effaced, and the canal should be open sufficiently to admit one finger. The fetal head should be fixed in the pelvis.

Induction of labor is contraindicated when there are contraindications to spontaneous labor. This would include previous cesarean birth and known cephalopelvic disproportion. Certain complications such as an abnormal fetal presentation and overdistention of the uterus require especially close supervision by the obstetrician if stimulation of uterine contractions is to be carried out. Some cases of antepartum bleeding are contraindications to induction of labor.

Two methods are used commonly for induction of labor. One is to administer a very dilute solution of oxytocin intravenously. The other method is artificial rupture of the membranes. Either of these procedures may be used separately or may be used together. A warm enema may be given before an induction is started, not only to clean the bowel, but also for its stimulating effect on the uterus.

The methods used to induce labor may also be used to augment or stimulate a labor that is not progressing well. As noted in the discussion of prolonged labor, certain conditions must be met before augmentation begins.

Amniotomy

An amniotomy or artificial rupture of the membranes must be carried out in the hospital. During a vaginal examination the physician loosens the membranes from their uterine attachment in the region of the cervix with a finger inserted through the cervix. Then he nicks the membranes with a sterile amniotomy hook, allowing amniotic fluid to escape. When the membranes are artificially ruptured to induce labor, the procedure may be carried out before oxytocin is started, or after labor is in progress with the use of oxytocin. Sometimes no further immediate treatment is given after rupture of the membranes, with the anticipation that this method alone will cause onset of labor in a few hours. Membranes are not ruptured if there is risk of prolapsed cord. The fetal heart is checked immediately after an amniotomy and closely observed thereafter.

When an amniotomy is done, a time limit is set—a commitment to deliver the fetus within 24 hours or preferably less. This presents a problem if labor does not begin and may necessitate delivery by cesarean section. Early amniotomy therefore is reserved for those women who are very likely to go into labor or who must be delivered for medical reasons even if labor does not occur.

Prior to the amniotomy the procedure should be explained to the woman so that she understands how it will feel and how it will affect her labor. Whenever possible, she should participate in the decision.

Another procedure that may be used to initiate the onset of labor is the stripping or loosening of the membranes from the lower uterine segment during a vaginal examination. This is frequently done in the physician's office, prior to hospital admission. If successful, labor may begin within a day or two.

Use of Oxytocin

When oxytocin is used to induce or augment labor, it is usually administered by intravenous drip in a very dilute solution. From 5 to 10 units of oxytocin (PITOCIN or SYNTOCINON) are added to 1000 ml of appropriate intravenous solution. Sometimes a lesser amount of oxytocin is used, giving a more dilute solution and making control of administration easier. The intravenous bottle must be well labeled with the name of the drug, the amount added, and the date and time of addition of the drug. The dosage of oxytocin administered from the mixture can be calculated from the amount of drug added to the amount of intravenous solution. Oxytocin 10 IU equals 10,000 milliunits (mU). When 10 IU (10,000 mU) of the drug are added to 1000 ml of fluid each milliliter of the mixture contains 10 mU of oxytocin. The oxytocin dosage used during induction of labor is spoken of as number of milliunits given per minute. The amount of oxytocin administered per minute is regulated by the number of milliliters of solution given per minute.

Administration of oxytocin is the responsibility of the physician. Oxytocin is a dangerous drug when used before delivery, and the nurse must not take full responsibility for giving it. A nurse skilled in care of labor patients and well informed about the implications of the use of oxytocin for stimulation of labor usually collaborates with the physician in monitoring maternal and fetal responses and making sure that the woman is never left alone.

Oxytocin induction may be administered by a very slow intravenous drip, with careful regulation of the number of drops per minute, or by use of a continuous infusion pump (Fig. 22-4). An infusion pump is highly preferable to the drip method, since it gives assurance of a constant rate. The fluctuations in rate that are permitted by the drip method may be especially dangerous when the uterus is very responsive to the drug.

When the oxytocin infusion is first started, it is given very slowly to test the patient's sensitivity to the drug. Then the flow may be gradually increased at 15- to 30-minute intervals to obtain the desired response in strength and frequency of uterine contractions. A professional palpates the uterus continuously while the flow is regulated. The induction is started with no more than 1 or 2 mU of oxytocin per minute or possibly only 0.5 mU. As the rate of flow is increased, it is also done slowly. Five to 10 mU per minute are often enough to stimulate good contractions; sometimes the dosage is increased somewhat more. As labor progresses, the flow may again be decreased, or the oxytocin may be discontinued when labor is well established. One method of changing dosage of oxytocin is to double the dose each time it is increased, going from 1 mU to 2 mU, then to 4 mU, and then to 8 mU. In decreasing the dosage it may be halved with each change, unless there is indication for immediately stopping the medication.

The rate of oxytocin administration is regulated according to the response of the uterine muscle. It is given at a rate that will produce effective uterine contractions of about 50 mm Hg pressure, lasting 40 to 50 seconds, occurring about every 3 minutes. Contractions should not occur more than every 2 minutes, since there must be time for adequate relaxation between contractions to avoid fetal distress. Contractions should not be greater than 60 to 70 mm Hg pressure; sometimes even less than 50 mm Hg will bring about cervical dilation. Contractions should not be longer than 60 seconds' duration; a longer contraction comes close to what might be considered tetanic.

When oxytocin is used for inducing or augmenting labor, the uterus may be very sensitive and responsive to the drug. Only a small dose of the drug may be necessary to produce effective contractions. Therefore a two-

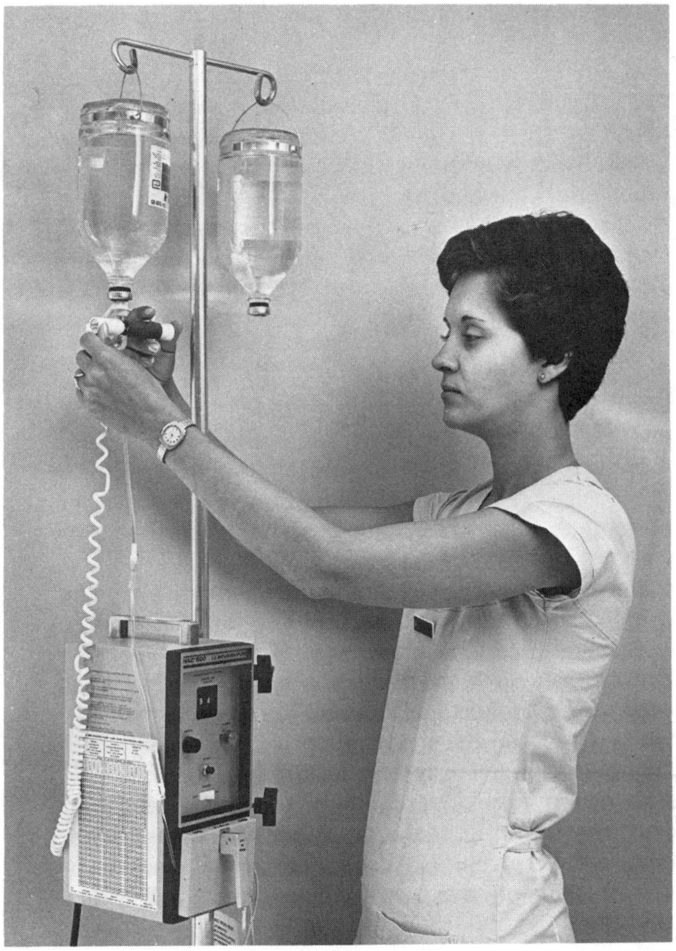

Figure 22–4. A continuous intravenous infusion pump, a precision instrument, which may be set at variable speeds to deliver exact volumes of fluid intravenously. An exact dose of oxytocin can be given within an exact time interval. It is apparent that calculations for various settings of the dial for delivery of different amounts of oxytocin as milliunits per minute have been attached to the machine.

bottle or piggy-back setup is recommended for oxytocin administration. This makes it possible to discontinue and restart the oxytocin drip readily without removing the intravenous needle. The intravenous solution without medication is given while the oxytocin solution is clamped off (Fig. 22–4).

Uterine contractions begin almost immediately after an oxytocin drip is started, but these early contractions are not true labor contractions. Later the contractions become more efficient contractions. Sometimes an induction is unsuccessful. If true labor does not start after several hours, or sometimes as long as 8 to 10 hours, the induction is discontinued. It may be restarted the following day. In some cases, such as the presence of diabetes or toxemia, when early delivery is indicated, an induction may be started before the cervix is well effaced. If unsuccessful, it may be repeated on several successive days to soften and efface the cervix and finally induce labor.

Careful observation of uterine contractions during oxytocin administration is absolutely essential. Tetanic contractions can develop. Severe and prolonged contractions could result in uterine rupture, premature separation of the placenta, and fetal hypoxia. When any danger signs appear, the oxytocin should be discontinued immediately. A hemostat should be at the patient's bedside for quick clamping of the intravenous tubing.

Although the nurse does not take the major responsibility for oxytocin administration, she usually assists with observation of the patient. The uterus is observed carefully for frequency and duration of contractions and for relaxation between contractions. The fetal heart is checked approximately every 15 minutes or more frequently if indicated. A change in rate or rhythm is reported immediately. The mother's blood pressure and pulse are checked every 15 minutes or oftener. Either a rise or fall in blood pressure or a rapid pulse is reported at once. Progression of labor and any unusual physical phenomena must be observed closely. When the drip method is used, the rate of flow of the oxytocin solution is watched carefully by counting the number of drops per minute at frequent intervals. Although the flow has been carefully regulated, it may accidentally increase in speed when the patient moves her arm or if the clamp on the tubing loosens.

If continuous electronic fetal heart rate monitoring and intrauterine pressure recording equipment are available, they are used to check uterine response to oxytocin. Careful and continuous clinical evaluation of uterine muscle response and fetal reaction to induction may be satisfactory with an uncomplicated pregnancy. Clinical evaluation is necessary for all patients when monitoring equipment is not available, but use of continuous electronic monitoring is highly desirable for all high-risk pregnancies.

When an oxytocin infusion has been used to induce labor, it may be slowed or discontinued during delivery and restarted after the placenta is expelled. It is then administered more rapidly than prior to delivery. Given after delivery, oxytocin aids in control of postpartum bleeding through stimulating the uterine muscle to contract.

Intramuscular injection, another method by which the drug is effective, should *not* be used for induction or augmentation of labor since the drug cannot be removed in case of an untoward reaction, and its effect continues until it is completely absorbed. Administration of oxytocin by the intravenous route is safer than any other method. Intravenously the dosage can be carefully regulated and promptly discontinued. The effect of the drug does not linger because oxytocin is rapidly inactivated and excreted. For these reasons, intravenous administration of oxytocin should replace all other methods.

Other Uterine Stimulants

Alkaloids of ergot are not used for induction of labor. They create contractions of a hypertonic or sustained nature or of an inappropriate frequency and do not permit adequate relaxation of the uterine muscle.

There is a growing interest in the use of prostaglandins (PGF_2 or $PGF_{2\alpha}$) for the induction of labor. Currently, PGF_2 is being used more for therapeutic abortions (see Chapter 14) than for inducing labor. The major drawbacks when it is administered orally or intravenously are the side effects. The problems of nausea, vomiting, diarrhea, and abdominal cramps make it unpleasant and unacceptable to the patient. As a result, attention is now being given to the local (cervical) application of prostaglandin. Because of its action on connective tissue, PGF_2 is proving to be an effective cervical priming agent. This "topical" approach would appear to hold much clinical promise.

Summary

In summary, careful monitoring is absolutely essential during induction or augmentation of labor. The physician or a properly instructed substitute must be with the patient constantly, and the physician must be immediately available to deal with any emergency that may arise. Inappropriate uterine muscle stimulation, which results in contractions more frequent than every 2 minutes and of very intense strength, or uterine tetany, leads to fetal hypoxia and may also endanger the mother.

OBSTETRIC OPERATIONS

Forceps Delivery

The obstetric forceps is an instrument used to extract the fetal head in certain conditions where progress is arrested and which may result in dangers, immediate or remote, to the mother and/or fetus. The forceps is a valuable instrument in obstetrics. Before its invention the only operative method of delivering a live fetus was by version and extraction, and in these cases the fetal death rate was high. Prior to the advent of forceps, the obstetric instruments in use were designed for the destruction of the baby *in utero*. Use of forceps may be hazardous, however, and this method of delivery is carried out only when all conditions for proper application are fulfilled (Fig. 22-5).

There are two groups of indications for use of forceps: those relating to the condition of the fetus and those relating to the mother. Indications for their use in the interests of the fetus are signs of fetal distress, as manifested by a change in the rate or rhythm of the fetal heartbeat. Fetal hypoxia may have many causes, including analgesia or anesthesia, premature separation of the placenta, pressure on the umbilical cord, and prolonged pressure of the head on the pelvic floor. Proper use of forceps is believed to reduce incidence of intracranial bleeding in the fetus, resulting from a long, hard labor.

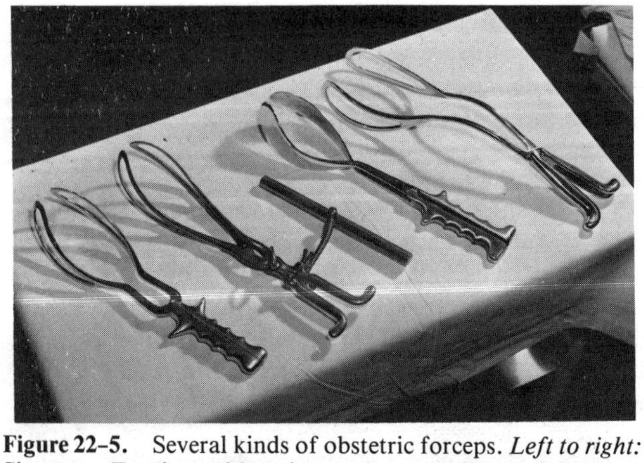

Figure 22-5. Several kinds of obstetric forceps. *Left to right:* Simpson; Tarnier, with axis traction attachment; McLean-Tucker; Piper, for delivery of the aftercoming head in breech extraction.

The most frequent indication for the use of forceps is poor progress of the fetal head through the birth canal. This slow progress may be due to poor contractions of the uterine and abdominal muscles, great resistance of the perineal muscles, or failure of the head to rotate. Other maternal indications are severe toxemia, heart disease, pulmonary disease, and exhaustion. Low forceps delivery in these conditions alleviates some of the exertion of the second stage of labor.

Forceps applications are usually designated as *low* or *mid-*, corresponding to the level to which the head has descended into the pelvis when the forceps is applied.

Low forceps operation is application of the blades after the fetal skull has reached the perineal floor, has rotated so that the sagittal suture is anteroposterior, and the head has become visible. This type of forceps delivery is relatively easy and is attended by little danger to mother or fetus (Figs. 22–6, 22–7 and 22–8).

Midforceps operation is application of the blades after the lowermost part of the skull is at or below the level or the ischial spines, but has not descended or rotated sufficiently to meet the criteria for low forceps. A midforceps delivery is more difficult and more serious than a low forceps delivery.

Many forceps operations are *elective low forceps*. The procedure is elective as distinguished from indicated when the physician elects to use forceps to deliver the fetus when immediate delivery is not absolutely necessary. In these cases spontaneous delivery could be expected to take place in approximately 15 minutes. The forceps is used to relieve the mother of the strain of the last part of the second stage of labor and to relieve the cerebral tissues of the fetus from pressure against the perineum. The criteria for a low forceps must be met. Only gentle traction is necessary, and the delivery is performed easily and with safety.

Unless there are indications for immediate delivery, a forceps delivery is usually not performed until the mother has been in second-stage labor for a variable period of time. Uterine contractions and bearing-down efforts will usually advance the head and perhaps rotate it, making a forceps delivery less complicated. The forceps is applied after the head has advanced satisfactorily for easy delivery, or when progress slows considerably or ceases.

All operative deliveries are potentially dangerous, but the danger is reduced to a minimum with proper indications and technique. A forceps delivery is often essential to prevent or minimize danger to mother and/or fetus.

Breech Extraction

Labor is usually longer in breech presentation than in vertex presentation. The membranes frequently rupture early, and the breech does not make a good dilating wedge. The incidence of prolapse of the umbilical cord is higher than in a vertex presentation, and the fetal heart must be observed frequently throughout labor. If continuous electronic fetal heart monitoring equipment is available, it is used.

Meconium is often expelled during labor, due to downward pressure of the contracting uterus on the fetus, but this does not have the same significance that it does in a head presentation. If the membranes are ruptured, meconium is seen draining from the vagina. Bed rest and constant watchfulness throughout labor are important.

If the presentation is a footling, one or both feet may prolapse through the vagina as labor progresses. This does not necessarily mean that birth is imminent. The patient is often not ready for delivery when the feet appear. They may prolapse when the cervix has dilated suf-

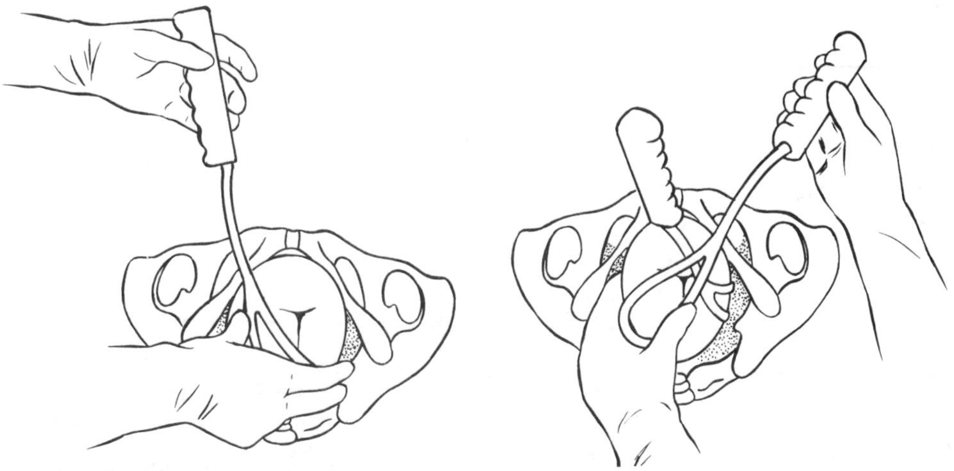

Figure 22–6. Low forceps extraction showing application of blades. [Reproduced with permission from J. Robert Willson; Elsie Reid Carrington; and William J. Ledger, *Obstetrics and Gynecology,* 7th ed. St. Louis: Mosby, 1983.]

CHAPTER

23

Nursing Management of the Postpartum Family: Physiologic Responses

THE PUERPERIUM[1] IS the interval from the end of labor until the return of the maternal physiology to its non-pregnant state approximately six weeks later. This time is also termed the postpartum[2] period.

The puerperium may be thought of as being composed of two distinct periods. During the first two to five days after birth, the majority of women in the United States remain in a hospital or maternity home. This may be described as the lying-in period, a rather gracious term which connotes the pace of a less technologic era. During the remaining longer period, the woman gradually resumes her former activities as she and her family work to integrate the new infant into the life of their household.

This is a dynamic and challenging time for the woman and for the family. Remarkable physiologic changes occur very rapidly in the woman's body. Both parents become acquainted with their new infant and learn many new skills and attitudes necessary for infant care. In some sense they become reacquainted with each other after the dramatic experiences of pregnancy and childbirth. Relationships with their other children and with the extended family must be adjusted and renewed. The pattern of day-to-day living changes in response to the sleeping and waking cycles of the infant. It is a time of much joy and fun and family closeness. But it is also a time of lost sleep, frustration, irritability, and feeling isolated from previous activities, interests, and friends.

This chapter and the one following will introduce the basic concepts necessary for the nurse to begin working with families during the puerperium. Emphasis will be on activities that maintain and enhance maternal health and, in Chapter 24, on teaching and anticipatory guidance of parents to facilitate their development as parents and as decision-makers for their own and their child's health.

PHYSICAL ASPECTS OF MATERNAL CARE

Throughout the puerperium, but especially during the first week, the mother's body undergoes a number of

[1] From *puer*, child, and *parere*, to bring forth.

[2] From *post*, after, and *partum*, bearing.

rapid changes. Although these are most marked in the pelvic organs and the breasts, the alterations that occurred in all the physiologic systems during gestation are reversed. Changes in the breasts are progressive, if the mother nurses her infant, preparing them for lactation. All other changes are retrogressive. The retrogressive genital changes are termed *involution*.

The alterations producing all these changes are normal, physiologic processes. However, because of the rapidity with which they happen, they may be disturbing to the woman unless she understands what is happening to her body. Furthermore, deviations from normal can occur and are most effectively treated if detected early. Consequently, women need information and teaching about the expected physical changes, but they also need systematic physical assessment to monitor the progression of involution.

During the time the mother is in the hospital, a physical assessment should be made daily. This provides the ideal setting for teaching and/or reinforcing good health practices. If the mother is discharged very soon after delivery or if she does not deliver in the hospital, arrangements may be made for visitation by a public health nurse. In addition, women can learn to observe their own uterine involution and to determine which subjective symptoms ought to be investigated with a health professional. This implies, however, that a significant amount of health education has taken place prior to the birth.

Postpartum Physical Assessment

The purpose of the postpartum physical assessment is to gather data about involutional changes, the mother's awareness of these changes, and her need for nursing care and teaching. An outline is given below. Following the outline is a discussion of the underlying physiology, health teaching, and nursing care pertinent to each area of assessment. The mother should be requested to empty her bladder immediately preceding the physical assessment.

1. *General Observations*
   Throughout the examination the nurse should keenly observe the mother's posture in bed, the ease (or lack of it) with which she moves about, her facial expressions, and her affect. These signs are clues to her energy level, her mood, and her general feeling of wellness or illness.
2. *Vital signs*
   These may be monitored at the time of the physical assessment or at some other time during the day that is routine for the agency. Late afternoon around 4 o'clock is a common time for daily vital signs since diurnal variations cause most people's temperature to be at its highest for the 24 hours during this period.
3. *Breasts*
   Both breasts are palpated, beginning in the axillae and moving toward the nipples, including all four quadrants. The degree of filling and/or engorgement is determined by the consistency of the breasts as well as the presence of milk and the subjective reports of the mother. The nipples are inspected for cracks.
4. *Abdomen*
   Palpation will detect any areas of unusual tenderness as well as the presence of flatulence. Should there be any reason to question intestinal motility (history of general anesthesia, abdominal distention, constipation, etc.), a stethoscope may be used to auscultate bowel sounds.
   A. *Uterus*
      The size of the uterus may be determined readily by palpating it through the soft, stretched muscles of the abdomen. The flat of the hand is placed at the level of the umbilicus and slowly moved downward while gently pressing on the abdomen until the top of the fundus is felt as a firm, globular mass. The height of the fundus is reported in relation to the umbilicus. For example, it is said to be at the level of the umbilicus, two fingerbreadths below the umbilicus, and so on.
   B. *Bladder*
      A full bladder may be palpated and often observed visually because of the flaccid condition of the abdominal muscles. It is particularly important to assess bladder distention during the first 24 to 48 hours post partum, when the urge to void may be dulled.
5. *Perineum*
   A. Episiotomy
   B. Hemorrhoids
6. *Lochia*
   Color, odor, and amount of vaginal discharge are noted.
7. *Lower extremities*
   Both legs should be viewed simultaneously for discrepancies in size and color. A check is made for Homan's sign.

Anatomic Changes and Nursing Implications

Care of the mother during the immediate postpartum period, the first few hours after delivery, is described in Chapter 21, Nursing Management During Delivery. During this immediate postpartum care, the vital signs, the contractility of the uterus, and the amount of vaginal bleeding are closely observed. When the fundus remains firm, vaginal bleeding is not excessive, and vital signs are stable, the recovery room care is discontinued. These observations, however, must be continued frequently during the next 12 to 24 hours. In addition, other aspects of physical care assume importance once the first critical postpartum hours are passed.

The Vital Signs

The *temperature* may rise to 38° C (100.4° F) shortly after a long labor, but it should return to normal within 24 hours. For various causes, some unexplained, the temperature may be slightly above normal at times during the first few days of the puerperium, without the patient seeming to be ill. A temperature of 38° C (100.4° F) is the upper limit of normality, and the patient is considered to have a morbid temperature if it reaches that point on any two days after the first 24 hours, providing the temperature is checked at least four times daily. (See Chapter 25, pages 486–89). The most frequent sites of infection are the uterus, breasts, urinary tract, and respiratory tract. Fever occurring on the same day that the breasts become engorged cannot be attributed to normal breast engorgement. Engorgement does not cause an elevation in temperature except in very rare instances of extreme engorgement when the temperature may be elevated for a few hours. However, if the temperature has been normal for several days or a week and then very suddenly rises to 38.3° C (101° F) or more, a breast infection is often the cause.

The normal *pulse rate* may be slow during the early puerperium, being about 60 to 70 beats a minute or occasionally as low as 50 beats. This is referred to as puerperal bradycardia. It is thought that this is caused by decreased strain on the heart after the birth of the infant and the reduction of the vascular bed with the contraction of the uterus. In 7 to 10 days the rate is usually back to normal. In some cases there may be an increase in the pulse rate, usually following a long, hard labor or a large blood loss at delivery. A tachycardia over 100 beats per minute warrants further investigation and medical consultation, since it may be an early sign of infection, hemorrhage, or pulmonary embolism.

All the vital signs (temperature, pulse, respiration, and blood pressure) are checked three to four times during the first 24 hours after birth. Thereafter, if all are stable, temperature, pulse, and respiration may be monitored daily. The blood pressure is not taken regularly after the first 24 hours unless it has been elevated before, during, or shortly after delivery. In that event it is measured every two to four hours, or more frequently if indicated, until it remains at a normal level for the patient. (See Chapter 14, page 287.)

Breasts

The anatomy and physiology of the lactating breasts, as well as the care of the breasts and nipples of the nursing mother, are discussed in Chapter 28, "Infant Nutrition."

For nonnursing mothers, breast care is directed at suppressing lactation and giving symptomatic relief to any discomfort that may occur.

The anterior pituitary gland produces and releases the lactogenic hormone prolactin almost immediately after delivery. This stimulates secretion of milk in the breasts. As they fill, they become tense and engorged. If the breasts are not emptied, milk secretion is not continued, since the pressure of milk accumulation inhibits further secretion. This process may cause considerable discomfort to the woman until the breasts soften, a process that takes approximately 36 to 48 hours.

Lactation may be suppressed pharmacologically by the administration of estrogens and/or androgens to inhibit the production of lactogenic hormone. In addition, estrogens are believed to render breast tissue refractory to stimulation by prolactin. Although quite effective in preventing the discomfort of engorgement, these drugs are not without hazard. A 1977 ruling of the Federal Food and Drug Administration requires that women be advised of the risks inherent in taking estrogens for any reason. Because of the relatively large doses required to suppress lactation, some feel the risks of coagulopathy outweigh the advantages of suppressing lactation, particularly since the treatment is not always entirely successful.

Another medication frequently prescribed to suppress lactation is Bromocriptine (PARLODEL). This drug inhibits the release of prolactin from the anterior pituitary thus restoring ovarian function and preventing lactation. The usual prescription is 2.5 mg twice a day for 14 to 21 days. A decrease in blood pressure is a frequent side effect of this drug and some women will experience dizziness or lightheadedness, especially when getting up from a sitting or lying position. The concurrent use of oral contraceptives and Bromocriptine is contraindicated.

Whether or not the mother receives medication to suppress lactation, some milk will be present in the breasts for varying lengths of time. The mother may observe some slight leaking of milk from the breasts, particularly during a warm shower, when she is cuddling her infant, or when she is sexually aroused. This may continue for several weeks.

If the breasts become uncomfortable from engorgement, symptomatic care is given until resolution occurs in about 24 to 48 hours. Wearing a proper fitting, supportive bra is important for relief from discomfort from the weight of the breasts. Application of ice bags may contribute to comfort, although some women find application of heat to be more soothing. A mild analgesic such as aspirin or acetaminophen may be given for pain relief as necessary. The breast pump should not be used to remove some of the milk from the breasts, since this will only stimulate further milk production.

Occasionally a mother may decide to breast-feed after

lactation-suppressing medication has already been administered. She should be reassured that regular sucking and emptying of the breasts by her infant will be adequate stimulation to milk production, and, that, with a little patience, an adequate milk supply and successful nursing will ensue. Mothers of sick and/or premature newborns have successfully begun breast-feeding several weeks after birth. Needless to say, such women must be strongly motivated and require support from significant others as well as health professionals.

While performing a postpartum breast examination, the nurse should evaluate the mother's knowledge and practice of breast self-examination (BSE) and review this with her as necessary.

The Abdomen

Because of the prolonged distention of the abdominal wall by the pregnant uterus and the possible rupture of the elastic fibers of the skin, the abdomen is soft and flabby. Sometimes the abdominal wall is so stretched that the rectus muscles separate in the midline. In that condition, known as *diastasis recti,* part of the abdominal wall is formed simply by skin, subcutaneous fat, fascia, and peritoneum. Restoration of the muscle tone requires two to three months and is greatly dependent on the physical constitution of the individual, the number of pregnancies, and the kind and amount of physical exercise.

Many women, especially primiparas, are surprised and disappointed that their flabby abdominal muscles make them look as if they were still pregnant. After the last fatiguing weeks of pregnancy, they are anxious to be slim and trim again. An empathetic remark, made at the time of examining the abdomen, will often encourage a woman to ventilate her feelings about how she looks. She can be reassured that this is a temporary situation and that she can speed the return of good muscle tone by doing some postpartum exercises.

The plan for exercising is determined by the type of labor and delivery the mother had and by her energy level and interest. Early exercises are light, require little exertion, and may be begun on the first or second postpartum day. More strenuous exercises are begun later. As at any other time, exercise must be taken with moderation and judgment, started slowly, and increased gradually according to individual tolerance.

Numerous booklets describing exercise regimen are available from pharmaceutical and formula companies as well as other sources. Many communities have organized exercise groups, especially for new mothers, conducted by the YMCA, parent education groups, or other organizations. Several representative exercises are described below.

DEEP ABDOMINAL BREATHING The mother is instructed to breathe deeply four or five times and on each exhalation to contract her abdominal wall. This may be done two or three times daily.

HEAD RAISING This exercise is done while lying flat on the back, without a pillow, and with the arms at the sides. The head is raised from the flat position trying to touch the chin to the chest while at the same time contracting the abdominal muscles. Raising the head is repeated several times; the exercise is done several times daily.

STRETCHING FROM HEAD TO TOE This exercise is done while lying flat with the arms extended above the head. This tenses both back and abdominal muscles and is useful for postural correction. Similarly, standing tall will improve posture.

LOWER BACK EXERCISE The mother lies on her back with her knees bent and feet flat on the bed or floor. Keeping one knee up, the other leg is slowly lowered to the floor while pressing the lower spine against the bed or floor. The secret to correct performance of this exercise is keeping the spine absolutely flat against the bed or floor.

All of the above exercises may be begun as soon as desired after delivery. In addition to increasing muscle tone, they are excellent for relieving backache and tension at the end of the day. As such they may be helpful to the new mother as a means of relaxation for rest and sleep during the first several months post partum.

KEGAL EXERCISE This is an isometric exercise for strengthening the muscles of the pelvic floor. It is advisable for women to develop a habit of doing this exercise during the antepartum period to minimize loss of tone in these muscles during pregnancy. It can be done at any time in any place and will reduce congestion and discomfort in the perineal area, increase the ability to control the muscles at the openings of the urethra, vagina, and rectum, and improve support to the pelvic organs. It consists of gradually tightening the muscles around the vagina and perineum and then, just as gradually, relaxing them. A good way to practice this in the beginning, in order to know how it is supposed to feel when done correctly, is to stop the flow of urine by contracting the perineal muscles. This exercise should be done many times a day, whenever the woman thinks of it.

LATER EXERCISES Rather strenuous abdominal exercises consist of leg raising and sitting up from a recumbent position. These are illustrated and described in Figures 23–1 and 23–2. In the leg-raising exercise it is recommended that only one leg be raised at one time and then only to about a 45-degree angle. Raising the leg to a 90-degree angle or raising both legs at one time may place too great a strain on the back. Similarly, bringing

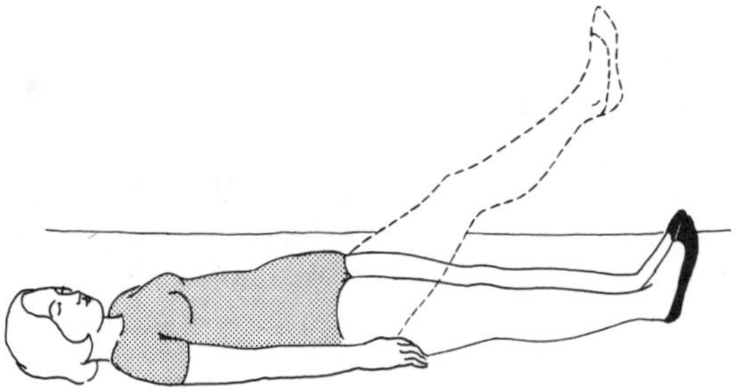

Figure 23–1. Strengthening the abdominal muscles by raising and lowering the legs. While lying on her back, the woman raises her right leg to approximately a 45-degree angle without bending the knee or raising the head and then lets it down slowly. Next the left leg is raised and lowered in the same way. Right and left legs are alternately raised and lowered as the exercise is continued.

A variation of a leg exercise is to bend the right knee and draw the thigh up over the abdomen and then straighten the leg and lower it. Next the left leg is drawn up and lowered in the same way. Right and left legs are alternately raised and lowered.

In either of these exercises each leg is raised and lowered only once or twice at first. Later the number of times is increased.

the body to an erect position in the sitting-up exercise may be too strenuous. Lifting the shoulders and upper back from the floor is often as much exertion as is advisable. Complete sit-ups should be done with the knees slightly bent to prevent strain on the muscles of the back and concentrate the effort in the abdominal muscles.

As these exercises require much effort, they must be increased very gradually. Each may be done only once or twice at first and slowly increased to several times twice a day. They should not be carried to the point of fatigue. These exercises are continued for several months. The results will depend on the amount of stretching during pregnancy, the ability of the muscles to regain their tone, and the degree to which the exercises are carried out.

Uterus

Remarkable retrogressive changes take place in the uterus during the puerperium. Immediately after delivery the uterine muscle is contracted so that the walls of the uterus are very thick, its cavity is flattened, and it forms a solid mass of tissue. The inner surface, where the placenta was attached, is raw and bleeding. After delivery the uterus is about the size of an infant's head and weighs about 1000 gm (2.2 lb). On palpation through the abdominal wall the top of the fundus can be felt at or slightly below the level of the umbilicus.

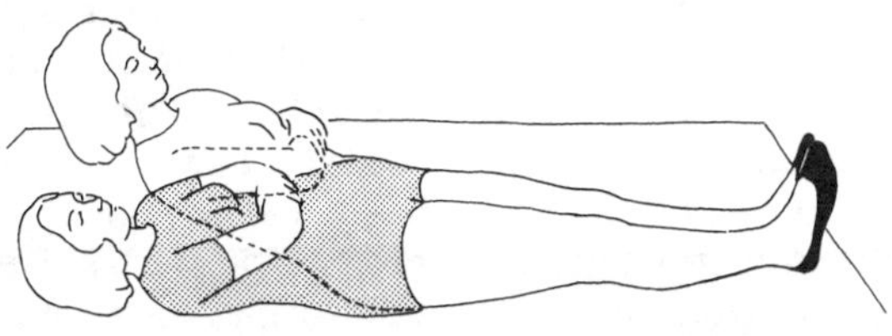

Figure 23–2. Strengthening the abdominal muscles by raising the upper part of the body. This exercise is started while lying on the back, without a pillow, and crossing the arms on the chest. The head and shoulders are raised just enough to clear the floor at first and gradually raised a little farther. Crossing the legs at the ankles may facilitate raising up from the recumbent position.

The uterus remains about the same size for two days and then decreases so rapidly in size that by the tenth day it usually cannot be palpated above the symphysis pubis. Its weight is decreased to about 500 gm (1 lb) at the end of one week. At the end of six to eight weeks the uterus has descended into the pelvic cavity and resumed approximately its original position and size, as well as its former weight of 60 gm (2 oz).

Uterine involution is accomplished by a process of *autolysis* or self-digestion. The muscle cells become much smaller. The protein material in the uterine walls is broken down into simpler components, which are absorbed and cast off, largely through the urine. This greatly increases the nitrogen content of the urine for several days. The change and absorption of uterine tissues are similar to the resolution that takes place in a consolidated lung in pneumonia.

There is evidently a close relation between the functioning of the breasts and of the uterus during the puerperium. Involution usually progresses more rapidly in women who nurse their babies than in those who do not.

The decidua, which remained in the uterus after the placenta and membranes separated, becomes differentiated into two layers within two or three days. The outer layer is cast off in the discharge from the uterus, and the inner layer, which contains the bases of the glands and a small amount of connective tissue, remains to regenerate new endometrium. The entire endometrium is regenerated in three weeks, with the exception of that over the placental area, which is not completely restored for six to seven weeks. The blood vessels of the placental area become either compressed or thrombosed after delivery of the placenta. It is believed that the large vessels present in the uterus during pregnancy then become obliterated and that new, smaller vessels develop.

Progress of uterine involution may be judged by the size and consistency of the uterus and the character, amount, and odor of the lochia. In describing the consistency of the uterus the terms "soft and boggy" or "firm and round" are often used. The size of the uterus is determined by its height and is measured by the number of fingerbreadths the top of the fundus lies above or below the umbilicus. Immediately after delivery the top of the fundus is often several fingerbreadths below the umbilicus. It rises to near the level of the umbilicus within several hours and remains there for a day or two and then descends into the pelvis and decreases in size (Fig. 23–3). The height of the fundus

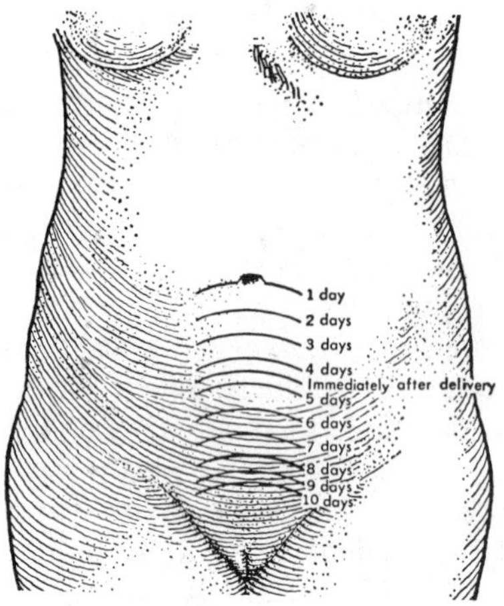

Figure 23–3. Approximate height of the fundus on each of the first 10 days after delivery.

should be measured when the bladder has been emptied recently, because the stretched uterine ligaments permit it to be moved about easily, and a distended bladder may push it up or to one side.

The normal rate of descent of the fundus cannot be stated exactly because of the great variations within normal limits in different individuals, but usually it is not palpable above the symphysis pubis after the tenth day. A daily record of the height of the fundus in the individual patient gives evidence of her rate of progress in involution. The nurse measures and records its height and consistency each day as part of the routine postpartum assessment.

If the uterus is involuting well, the lochia gradually decreases in amount and changes from rubra to serosa within a few days and then changes to lochia alba on approximately the tenth day. The amount and color of the lochia are recorded daily.

If the uterus remains soft and large and the mother continues to have a large amount of bright-red lochia, both signs of subinvolution, ergonovine in a 0.2-mg ($^1/_{320}$-gr) dose may be given every 4 hours for 24 hours or three or four times a day for one or two days. Bright-red vaginal bleeding or expulsion of blood clots may be caused by retention of a small piece of placenta or some of the fetal membranes. Involution is usually more rapid when the infant nurses because nursing stimulates uterine contractions.

Afterpains, caused by alternate contraction and relaxation of the uterine muscle, occur in about 75 percent of multiparas. They may be severe and often become worse while the mother is nursing her infant because of stimulation of the uterus. They usually do not last more than 48 hours. The primipara ordinarily does not have afterpains unless her uterus has been distended more than normal. If afterpains persist for much longer than 48 hours or if they are severe in the primipara, the possibility of retention of secundines (fragments of placenta or membranes) or blood clots is considered. The pains are aggravated by administration of ergonovine.

Relief of discomfort from afterpains is obtained by pain-relieving drugs. Analgesics commonly given are propoxyphene hydrochloride (DARVON), 32 to 65 mg, alone or concurrently with aspirin, or a combination of codeine, 30 to 60 mg (1/2 to 1 gr), and either aspirin, 0.30 to 0.60 gm (5 to 10 gr) or acetaminophen, 325 to 650 mg.

Women often accept afterpains as a discomfort that may be expected after delivery, and they may not inform the nurse of pain. To ensure that the mother is relieved of this discomfort, it is advisable that the nurse tell the multipara that she may have afterpains and that pain medication is available. Breast-feeding mothers may be hesitant to take medications that will be transferred to their infants in the breast milk. They should know that analgesics in the ordinarily prescribed doses are not harmful to the infant. Being tense and in pain, however, may have an adverse effect on the let-down mechanism, thus inhibiting optimal nursing. Pain medication taken 15 to 20 minutes prior to a feeding often will greatly enhance the mother's comfort and enjoyment of her infant.

Cervix, Vagina, Perineum

The cervix, vagina, and perineum, which have become stretched and swollen during delivery, gradually regain their tone during the puerperium. The cervix and lower uterine segment form a flabby, collapsed, hollow tube immediately after delivery and contract slowly. The cervical canal will admit the hand immediately after delivery, two fingers for a few days thereafter, and only one finger at the end of a week.

Small lacerations sustained by the cervix during labor heal during the puerperium, but it does not return to its exact predelivery state. The external os, instead of being a smooth round opening, now usually becomes a slightly irregular transverse slit.

Changes in the vagina occur slowly, and it does not return entirely to its original state. It gradually diminishes in size, and the rugae begin to reappear in three weeks. The hymenal ring is replaced by numerous ragged edges of tissue known as *carunculae myrtiformes.* The external genitalia, which have been somewhat distended during pregnancy, become smaller and more flabby. The stretched uterine ligaments become shorter as they recover their tone and regain their former state. Until the ligaments, the pelvic floor, and the abdominal wall are restored to normal tonicity, the uterus is not adequately supported and therefore may be displaced easily. The Kegal exercises described above are important for the rapid restoration of muscle tone of the perineal structures.

Bladder

Immediately after delivery the bladder is edematous and hyperemic. There may be some submucosal extravasation of blood, particularly in the bladder trigone. Some swelling and bruising are apt to be seen around the urethral meatus as a result of the trauma of delivery. In addition, the bladder has an increased capacity together with a decreased sensitivity to pressure. The renal pelvis and ureters are still dilated as during pregnancy.

Because of the above anatomic variations, there is a tendency for women to have some difficulty voiding during the immediate postpartum period. This tendency is aggravated by the general perineal swelling and tenderness of this period. Women who have had conduction anesthesia have particular difficulty because of the temporary interruption of neural function. Some women, although able to void, cannot completely empty their bladders, leaving residual urine after each voiding. In either case (inability to void or residual urine) the woman is at high risk for urinary tract infection because of the stasis of urine and the traumatized bladder tissues. It is, therefore, of utmost importance that the bladder distention be avoided, by catheterization if all else fails.

Assessment of urinary function is the first step in giving care. Reports of voiding should be elicited from the woman. It is also wise to measure the amount of urine the first several times the woman voids after delivery to determine whether or not a sufficient volume is being eliminated. It is not unusual for 300 to 500 ml of urine to be eliminated at one time because of the diuresis that occurs during the first couple of days post partum. The abdominal contour should be observed to help determine the presence of a distended bladder. It can be seen as a mass distending the lower abdomen, or it may be palpated above the symphysis pubis. (Figure 20–3, page 388, shows a distended bladder in an undelivered woman.) As the bladder fills, it pushes the uterus up higher in the abdomen and/or toward one side. Thus, detecting the fundus away from the midline or higher than normally expected should be reason to strongly suspect a full bladder.

If at all possible, bladder distention should be prevented by urging the mother to attempt to void within two to three hours after delivery. Almost all women are able to be up to the bathroom or at least to a bedside commode by this time. Bedpans should be used only as a last resort, since many women find it difficult or even impossible to urinate in a horizontal position. Since the temporary dulling of sensation in the bladder may prevent the mother from having an urge to void, she may need to be reminded to try urinating at intervals during the first 12 to 24 hours. Before resorting to catheterization the nurse should exhaust all other methods of encouraging voiding such as pouring warm water over the vulva. Sitting in a sitz bath of warm water is often helpful, especially if the woman is still having difficulty after 24 hours. Applying light pressure or massage just over the symphysis pubis compensates for the lack of abdominal muscle tone and is also useful in preventing residual urine by promoting a more thorough emptying of the bladder.

On the rare occasions when catheterization is necessary, strict asepsis and extreme gentleness are important. Catheterization of a postpartum patient may be difficult. The labia must be gently separated to prevent pulling on the perineal sutures, which causes the mother considerable pain, and yet separated far enough to visualize the meatus, which is frequently difficult to find owing to small lacerations and edema of the tissues of this area. A good light must be directed on the area. The cotton balls used for washing the area around the meatus should be squeezed dry enough to prevent the cleaning solution from running into the vaginal orifice, since this may be a source of contamination to the birth canal. There is danger of carrying lochia into the bladder, since it usually flows freely. A cotton ball placed over the vaginal orifice immediately after cleaning the area around the meatus helps to keep the vaginal secretions from spreading upward.

There is some controversy about whether or not an indwelling catheter should be inserted when a postpartum patient is unable to void or has residual urine. Some practitioners believe this allows the bladder to rest completely and eliminates the possibility of frequent catheterizations. Others believe that there is no more danger of cystitis from frequent catheterizations than from an indwelling catheter and that the muscle may regain its tone more quickly if the bladder fills and is emptied with some regularity. Conclusive research data are lacking to support either position. Any catheterization significantly increases the risk of urinary tract infections. Because of this, prophylactic antibiotics may be prescribed for these women. Fortunately, early ambulation, as well as improved antepartum and intrapartum care, has made this problem less common. Alert nursing care can further reduce the incidence by the skillful use of preventive measures.

For most women urinary function continues normally after delivery. There is a significantly increased urinary output for the first five to seven days owing to the elimination of the extra tissue fluids and intravascular volume accumulated during pregnancy. Gradually the renal pelves and ureters regain their tone and by four to six weeks after delivery the urinary tract has resumed its nonpregnant state.

Perineum

The vulva and perineum are bruised and tender for several days following delivery. In addition, most women have perineal sutures used in repair of the episiotomy or occasional lacerations.

Perineal care is given to keep the area clean and dry, to

eliminate odor, to promote healing, and to contribute to the woman's comfort. It is the same whether or not there are sutures.

In the past, perineal care was a highly ritualized procedure utilizing a large array of equipment and cleansing solutions and occupying many hours of nursing time. Now, however, it is realized that ordinary washing and careful attention to the usual measures of good hygiene are satisfactory. Because women are out of bed and active quite soon after delivery, the nurse's major responsibility is to teach and reinforce the mother's own hygiene practices.

Even if sutures are not present, the perineum should be regarded as an open wound because it is the uterine cavity itself which must be protected from infection. Therefore the principles of hand washing and cleansing from front to back should be strongly emphasized. Washcloths, sponges, or other materials that have come in contact with the anal area should be discarded and never used again around the vaginal and urethral openings. Perineal pads should be applied snug enough to avoid sliding back and forth, possibly transferring organisms from anus to vagina. A clean pad should be used each time the woman goes to the bathroom.

Perineal care should be given by the nurse whenever the mother's energy levels or illness indicate the need for such care. The mother is placed on a bedpan and the vulva, perineum, and groin are washed with soap and water, taking particular care to wash from front to back and to avoid any tension on the sutures. Warm water is then poured over the area to thoroughly remove the soap. After drying, a clean perineal pad usually is applied.

Self-care usually is done while showering or while sitting on the toilet. An extra washcloth should be provided the mother specifically for perineal cleansing. A very common and practical piece of equipment is a small plastic squeeze bottle. The mother fills it with warm tap water and uses it to rinse off the perineum after each voiding or defecation. In addition to washing off the lochia, it removes urine which may sting the sutures, and the warmth is soothing to the tender episiotomy. The perineum should be blotted dry with toilet tissue, again from front to back.

Perineal sutures cause some mothers considerable discomfort, occasionally for as long as seven or eight days. Others report only mild discomfort for the first few hours.

Ice applied to the perineum immediately after delivery reduces the amount of edema that occurs and thus prevents some of this discomfort. Women who have had a long second stage of labor, required unusual obstetric manipulations, or have extensive episiotomies and/or lacerations are particular candidates for this type of care. A rubber glove partially filled with crushed ice is an ideal size to fit next to the sutures.

After the initial recovery period, heat to the perineum gives some relief of discomfort. Dry heat from a heat lamp may be applied for 20 to 30 minutes two or three times a day. Perineal care should be given shortly before using the heat lamp to avoid drying lochia on the sutures and skin edges of the episiotomy repair. Sitz baths may be taken several times a day as a means of applying moist heat.

Analgesic ointments or sprays also may provide some relief. The ointments have the additional property of helping to keep the sutures soft and pliable, which prevents a drawing sensation. It is convenient to apply the ointment to a soft tissue which is then placed next to the sutures and held in position by the perineal pad.

If the mother experiences pain while sitting, she may be somewhat relieved by sitting on a large plastic air ring, which is inflated with just enough air to relieve pressure on the perineal area. If the perineum causes the mother much discomfort, analgesic medication may be necessary during the first few days.

Complaints of severe or persistent perineal pain should prompt immediate investigation, since it may be a symptom of a hematoma or other abnormality (Chapter 25, page 486).

Hemorrhoids, which may have developed (or, if present, become enlarged) during pregnancy, may become more edematous with the straining of the second stage of labor. They are sometimes very painful for a few days post partum, but gradually decrease in size and cause less discomfort as circulation improves.

The mother is kept as comfortable as possible from hemorrhoidal pain by one of several kinds of treatment. Among these are application of either heat or cold in the form of a heat lamp, warm moist pack, sitz bath, or ice compress; witch hazel compresses; analgesic ointment or spray; and rectal suppositories. Witch hazel compresses are analgesic and soothing. Applied for 20 to 30 minutes several times a day they often give considerable pain relief. Small flannel pads saturated with a solution of witch hazel 50 percent, glycerin 10 percent, and water, commercially available as TUCKS, may be used next to the perineal pad. They are placed in contact with the hemorrhoids and are changed as often as they become soiled.

If hemorrhoids were present before pregnancy, they usually subside to previous size during the puerperium. If they were not present before pregnancy, they will probably disappear completely.

Lochia

There is a vaginal discharge after delivery, termed *lochia.* It consists of uterine and vaginal secretions, blood, and the uterine lining that is cast off during the puerperium. During the first few days this discharge is bright red, consisting to a large extent of blood, and is termed *lochia rubra*. As the color gradually fades after two or three days and becomes pinker and more serous, the discharge is called *lochia serosa*. After about the tenth day, if involution is normal, the discharge is whitish or yellowish and is designated *lochia alba*. The normal characteristic odor of lochia is fleshy and resembles menstrual blood. A foul odor is suggestive of infection.

The total amount of the lochial discharge is from 150 to 400 ml. Nursing mothers bleed less totally, but may bleed more during first nursings. Under normal conditions the discharge is profuse at first, gradually diminishing until it entirely disappears by the end of the puerperium. A small amount of blood may be retained during the first day or two and expelled later as clots, without serious significance, and the discharge may be more blood-tinged after the patient becomes active. However, if the lochia is persistently blood-tinged, it may be an indication that the uterus is not involuting well or that a piece of placental tissue has been retained.

A woman should not be alarmed by a sudden gush of blood and clots upon first rising in the morning or after a long nap. While she is recumbent, lochia is apt to pool in the vagina and lower uterine segment for sudden release when she stands up. She generally can expect a slight increase in the amount of lochia when she first goes home from the hospital and increases her activity.

The duration of postpartum bleeding varies with individual women and with whether they are nursing or not. In general, a discharge sufficient to require the use of perineal pads persists for four to six weeks. If desired, tampons may be used after about three weeks or when sufficient perineal healing has occurred to make insertion comfortable. The Institute of Medicine recommends refraining from the use of tampons for several weeks post partum and suggests all women, especially adolescents, avoid the use of high absorbency ("super-plus") tampons to lessen their risk of toxic shock syndrome.[3]

Blood

A significant leukocytosis is present during and just after labor. A white cell count of 20,000 to 30,000/mm is not uncommon during labor, probably as a result of the physical exertion of this period. The blood count gradually returns to normal during the first postpartum week. During this time the white blood count is not as reliable an indicator of the presence of infection as it is at other times.

During the first postpartum week the increased plasma and red cell volumes gradually accumulated during pregnancy are reduced. This results in fluctuations in the laboratory values for hemoglobin, hematocrit, and red cell count. As a general rule of thumb, values that drop much below the level present just before labor are indicative of extraordinary blood loss and anemia.

For at least the first week following delivery, the pregnancy-induced increase in coagulation factors remains present. This places susceptible women at risk to develop thrombophlebitis and suggests the importance of exercising utmost care in preventive treatment (Chapter 25, page 489).

Lower Extremities

Because of the risk of thrombophlebitis (see above), examination of the legs should be a part of the daily physical assessment of all postpartum women. The legs are observed for redness and skin temperature and palpated for tenderness. Edema, which can result from venous occlusion, may be best detected by observing both legs simultaneously, since it is very rare for both legs to be affected. The presence of vascular inflammation often will be indicated by pain in the calf of the leg in response to the application of gentle pressure to dorsiflex the foot. Such an occurrence is known as Homan's sign.

Ambulation is important to prevent postpartum cardiovascular complications. A program of early and progressive activity should be instituted even for women who have had cesarean sections. Indeed, since surgery further increases the risk of thrombophlebitis, ambulation is especially important for these women. Healthy women who have had an uncomplicated pregnancy and vaginal delivery are able and usually wish to be up shortly after delivery.

Additional Aspects of Postpartum Physical Care

Rest and Sleep

Fatigue commonly accompanies the postpartum period. The last weeks of pregnancy are physically as well as emotionally tiring and labor is often exhausting. Added to this is the energy expenditure required to adjust to the new responsibilities of motherhood.

Providing mothers with adequate sleep and intervals of uninterrupted rest and relaxation is a goal that challenges the most skillful of nurses. Physical discomforts, including perineal tenderness, engorgement, and afterpains may prevent rest. Unaccustomed noises in the hospital, a strange bed, or a restless roommate are further difficulties. In addition, hospital schedules, infant needs, physician and nursing visits, telephone calls, family and friends may all interrupt the most carefully planned nap. Yet this rest is essential for the mental as well as the physical health of the mother. Coping with the challenges and joys of a new infant in the family can be almost impossible for a tired mother.

[3] Use of "super-plus" tampons discouraged, *Science*, 216:1300, 18 June 1982.

Postpartum women rarely have the energy to assert themselves to demand time for their own needs. Therefore, the nurse has a serious obligation to modify the environment to promote rest and to act as a patient advocate. It is very rare that any hospital personnel must ignore a "Do Not Disturb" sign on a mother's door. Vital signs can be taken a half hour later; routine chest x-rays can be scheduled at the convenience of the mother rather than the radiology department. Even most medications can be given a half hour earlier or later. As long as the mother remains in the hospital, she can take advantage of returning her infant to the nursery for supervision and care while she naps. However, since infants sleep much of their first few days of extrauterine life, most mothers are able to rest with their infants asleep in the crib beside them.

Most hospitals place some restrictions on visitors to the maternity unit in order to protect the mother's time for rest as well as to limit the potential sources of infection. Such restrictions should of course never apply to fathers who need to have free access to their wives and infants. Equally important is the need to provide a visiting time for other children in the family. Multiparas frequently express great loneliness for their older children and the children, particularly preschoolers, should have the opportunity to maintain contact with their mothers and to meet their new sisters and brothers. As long as reasonable precautions are taken to screen visiting children for infectious diseases, there appears to be no increased risk of infection from their presence on the maternity unit.

Since visiting hours are intended for the protection of the patient, it is necessary to modify them whenever individual or family needs are not met by the routine policy. A common example is the single mother who may wish her mother, sister, or boyfriend to have the unlimited visiting hours designated for fathers.

Nutrition and Elimination

An occasional mother will experience nausea or even vomiting immediately after delivery. Most mothers, however, are extremely hungry and thirsty after the physical exertion of labor. Maternity units should be equipped with facilities to provide a light lunch for mothers regardless of the hour of their delivery. Fathers who have done the work of labor support also are usually ready for a snack. Increased appetite and thirst usually persist for the first two or three days post partum.

There is a decided change in weight during delivery and the early puerperium. An initial loss of approximately 5 to 6 kg (11 to 13 lb) occurs with expulsion of the uterine contents. An additional loss of 2 to 2-1/2 kg (4-1/2 to 5-1/2 lb) takes place early in the puerperium. This in large part is caused by elimination of the normally increased fluid in the tissues during pregnancy. Even women who were not particularly aware of dependent edema during pregnancy are amazed to see how skinny their feet and ankles appear several days after delivery. Usually a woman will return to approximately her nonpregnant weight by the end of the sixth to eighth week.

The principles of nutrition for the lactating woman are discussed in Chapter 10.

Concern about the ability to have a bowel movement is relatively common in the puerperium, although it appears to concern physicians more than it does mothers. The sudden loss of intraabdominal pressures, relaxation of abdominal muscles, and the intestinal sluggishness acquired during pregnancy all contribute to the tendency toward constipation. In addition, mothers often fear they will tear their stitches or that a bowel movement will be extremely painful. Most women will not have difficulty if they eat a well-balanced diet with adequate fruits and vegetables and get a reasonable amount of exercise. The urge to defecate should be acted upon promptly. Gentle bearing down serves to relax the anal sphincter and make defecation more comfortable. Stool softeners are often prescribed for several days after delivery.

If a bowel movement does not occur by the third or fourth postpartum day or if the mother is distended and uncomfortable, a suppository or enema may be given. A rectal tube will often relieve distention.

When hemorrhoids are present or a fourth-degree laceration has occurred, suppositories and/or enemas are frequently necessary and the passage of stool may cause severe discomfort. An analgesic given at the time of the suppository or 15 or 20 minutes prior to the enema will usually be helpful, and a sitz bath immediately after defecating is soothing.

Bathing and Grooming

There is frequently profuse perspiration, especially at night, during the first few days post partum which may add to increased thirst. This gradually subsides and becomes normal by the end of a week. The perspiration sometimes has a strong odor. There may be an appreciable amount of desquamation of the skin.

Opportunity for a sponge bath should be provided as soon as practical after delivery, since the mother will probably feel sticky and sweaty after the work of labor. A few minutes taken to freshen up and brush her hair can make her feel like a new woman.

Mothers may take showers as soon as they feel able after delivery. It is wise for someone to be close by the first time a shower is taken, since even women who have been up and about may become lightheaded or faint in the warm shower.

Tub baths should be delayed for about a week until the cervix has closed as a precaution against infection. Sitz baths, which involve sitting in 2 to 3 inches of clean, warm to hot water, are exceptions.

Most women feel very feminine during the early postpartum period and enjoy shampooing and arranging their hair, manicuring their nails, and dressing up in pretty nightgowns.

Continued Health Supervision

Before leaving the hospital the mother should be instructed about making an appointment for a postpartum follow-up visit to her physician. The first medical postpartum checkup after discharge usually is made in approximately six weeks, at about the time the pelvic organs have returned to their normal condition. It includes examination of the breasts and pelvic examination to determine the condition of the perineum, uterus, cervix, and support to the rectum and the bladder. Blood pressure, weight, urinalysis, and sometimes a complete blood count are also included. Attention also is given to the mother's emotional adjustments.

A slight abnormality detected at the six-week examination usually can be corrected with little difficulty, but if it persists it may result in a more serious problem. If subinvolution, inadequate perineal healing, or uterine displacement is found, treatment can be started. If the cervix is red and eroded, a cauterization may be necessary. All cervical lesions receive careful treatment to prevent predisposition to gynecologic problems later.

The six-week examination completes the postpartum period, and it is also the beginning of a new period of health supervision. A pelvic examination usually is repeated after six months and one year. Adequate postpartum care over a period of a year may prevent or cure conditions that would otherwise cause trouble in later years.

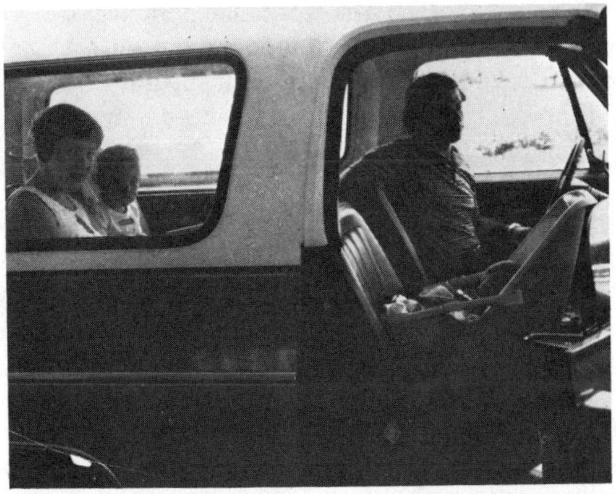

Figure 23-4. Family leaving the hospital for home after the birth of their baby. Notice this mother's way of meeting her two-year-old's needs by sharing the back seat with him while baby sister rides up front with daddy.

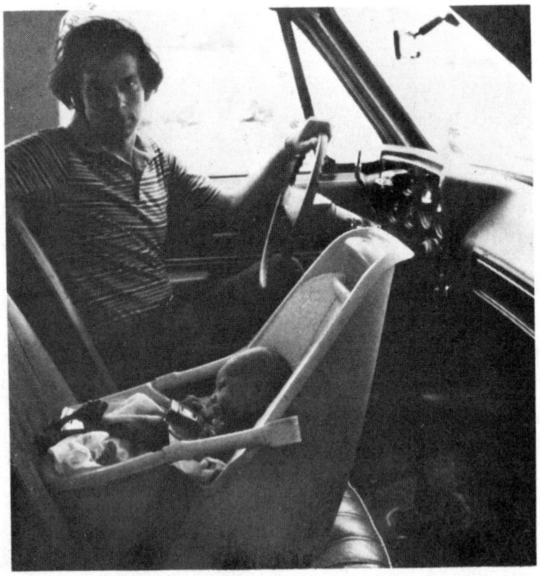

Figure 23-5. Baby snuggled safely in her car seat for the trip home from the hospital.

The first health supervision visit for the infant generally is made at about one month of age. It will include a physical examination and a discussion of infant care and behavior.

If a visiting nurse service is available to the mother, she is referred for a follow-up visit for herself and her infant if she desires. When a referral is not made, the mother is told of the visiting nurse service and how to secure this service should she need assistance.

REFERENCES AND SUGGESTED READINGS

Avery, M. D., Fournier, L. C., Jones, P. L., Sipovic, C. P., An early postpartum hospital discharge program: Implementation and evaluation, *JOGN Nursing,* 11(4):233–235, 1982.

Cibulka, N. J., Toxic shock syndrome and other tampon related risks, *JOGN Nursing,* 12(2):94–99, 1983.

McKenzie, C. A., Canaday, M. E., Carroll, E., Comprehensive care during the postpartum period, *Nursing Clinics of North America,* 17(1):23–48, 1982.

Meserve, Y., Management of postpartum breast engorgement in nonbreast feeding women by mechanical extraction of milk, *Journal of Nurse Midwifery,* 27(5):3–8, 1982.

Mynick, A., Instituting a postpartum self-medication program. *MCN,* 6:422–424, 1981.

Strelnick, E. G., Postpartum care: An opportunity to reinforce breast self-examination. *MCN,* 7:249–252, 1982.

Woolery, L. F., Self care for the obstetrical patient. A nursing framework, *JOGN Nursing,* 12(1):33–37, 1983.

CHAPTER

24

Nursing Management of the Postpartum Family: Psychosocial Responses

THE PSYCHOSOCIAL AND developmental events that occur as a part of the puerperium are perhaps even more dramatic than the physiologic events. Certainly they have a more lasting effect on the individuals and families involved.

THE FOURTH TRIMESTER

Although the puerperium is defined physiologically as the first six weeks after delivery, it is somewhat more accurate to think of the psychosocial and developmental adjustments as occupying the entire three- to four-month period following birth. Some authors have termed this the "fourth trimester." During this time the woman makes gradual adjustments from being pregnant to being nonpregnant and a mother. The infant continues to grow and makes the initial adaptations to family life, behaviorally as well as physically. The entire family responds to new expectations, responsibilities, and routines.

Because of her biologic involvement in childbearing and her subsequent physical interdependence with her infant during lactation, a woman experiences this period in a unique way. The experience is modified for each woman by the number of children she has had, her own childhood and parenting, experiences during pregnancy, the strength of her relationship with her child's father, her own self-concept, and many other things. Yet, there is some common pattern. This pattern should be familiar to nurses so it can be used as a framework for assessment, just as physical and laboratory values are used to assess physiologic homeostasis.

RESPONSES TO BIRTH

In some respects the change that occurs at delivery is an abrupt one; at one moment there is a pregnant woman and a fetus and at the next moment there is a mother and child. Yet the woman may not feel any more a mother than she did before labor just as a person doesn't suddenly feel married as soon as "I do" is said or suddenly feel educated because a diploma has been granted. Much has gone before to prepare her for this event, and much will follow. Although no longer pregnant, her body is still not what it was before pregnancy. Her uterus still fills much of the abdominal cavity and she still looks pregnant. Her physical state reflects in many ways how she feels. She is in transition; no longer pregnant but not quite feeling herself again and not really feeling like a mother (though she may not know how one feels when "feeling like a mother").

At the moment of birth there is an immediate relief of pain and most women experience a tremendous sense of peace and excitement. Joy is great because both mother and infant have survived the long-awaited and dreaded labor. Usually there is an eagerness to see and touch the infant and a desire to be close to a significant other to share the joy of the moment. During the first hour after delivery, women who have had relatively unmedicated labors tend to be quite talkative. They frequently review the recent events of labor. If the opportunity is presented, they will usually inspect and cuddle their infant and may begin breast-feeding. They may join the father in making telephone calls to announce the birth to their parents and friends.

Within a few hours after birth, the physical exertion of labor as well as the excitement brings on fatigue, and, if she is comfortable and the environment quiet, the woman may sleep soundly for several hours. It has been suggested that failure to obtain this sleep results in a delay of the restorative processes of the puerperium and a sleep hunger which persists for several days.[1]

DEVELOPMENTAL TASKS

During the first five to seven days, postpartum women are confronted with various tasks which they will continue to work out during the whole of the fourth trimester and perhaps, for some women and for some tasks, even beyond. These tasks include:

1. Achieving some closure or resolution of pregnancy, labor, and delivery
2. Reconciling the real infant with one of antepartal fantasy
3. Continuing the acquaintance-attachment to the infant
4. Replenishing physical and psychic energy
5. Learning infant care skills
6. Reestablishing family life and relationships to include the new infant member

[1] Reva Rubin, Puerperal change, *Nurs. Outlook,* 9:754, (Dec.) 1961.

TAKING-IN PHASE

The first few days post partum are characterized by a passivity and dependency not unlike the last trimester of pregnancy. Reva Rubin has very aptly described this time as the "taking-in" phase of the puerperium.[2] Women do indeed take in food, attention, and physical care with obvious enjoyment. They absorb every detail of their infant and their surroundings. It is as if they must fill themselves up after the draining experience of labor before they can give to the very dependent infant. Elements of this need for attention and nurturance continue throughout the puerperium, probably throughout parenthood. The literature on child abuse strongly suggests that mothers without supportive significant others are at risk for maladaptive parenting. The same is very likely true for fathers, although in the United States there are usually more opportunities for men to receive ego support from outside the family, especially during the first year of parenthood.

TAKING-HOLD PHASE

Gradually the woman moves from a state of predominant dependence to one of predominant independence. The timing of this transition depends on the individual woman as well as her experiences. Women whose pregnancy was medically complicated, whose labor was unusually long, or who had cesarean sections or other operative procedures generally have increased dependency needs over a longer period of time. Multiparas, women whose general health is good, and who view their pregnancies as positive experiences tend to move more quickly toward independence. On the average this occurs about two to three days post partum and coincides with an increase in physical well-being. By this time the muscular soreness from the work of labor is gone, bladder and bowel function are usually reestablished, engorgement of the breasts is subsiding, fatigue is less overwhelming, and, in general, physical restoration is well underway. After a couple of days' acquaintance the infant is beginning to be somewhat familiar, and women begin to plan for going home from the hospital, for resuming their responsibilities. Rubin terms this the "taking-hold" phase.

The observant nurse will easily detect the behavior changes that herald entry into this phase. The mother who has been still dozing when breakfast was served is suddenly showered and dressed with makeup on, waiting for her tray. Lists of tasks to be done and things to be

[2] *Ibid.*

purchased are made out for husbands, mothers, and babysitters. She writes birth announcements and takes a more active role in caring for her infant. Whereas earlier she was comfortable just being instructed, she now is eager to try doing things herself. She has increased confidence in her own opinions of how things should be done. As she begins to plan for the near future she is ready for discussions of public health nurse referrals, household help, other children's response to the infant, contraception, and other pertinent topics.

NURSING MANAGEMENT

Nursing care priorities should reflect an awareness of where a woman fits along the continuum of dependency to independency. During the taking-in or dependent phase, physical comfort measures should have prominence in the care plan. A back rub, a bed bath, or even a pillow-fluffing can help satisfy needs much deeper than skin care. At this time, too, a woman has an almost compulsive need to talk about her labor and delivery. To anyone who will listen she will give a detailed account of how she knew she was in labor, what her doctor said, how she behaved. She must fit all the pieces together and reconcile them with her expectations for herself. It is most helpful if the nurse who was with her during labor can help her talk out the experience, preferably with the father who was there also. In this way situations that were confusing during the stress of labor can be clarified, questions can be answered, and situations and events verified. Each member of the couple can be reassured of the "goodness" of his or her performance. This is also a valuable means of collecting data about which nursing care measures were helpful or not helpful to the couple, thus enabling the nurse to constantly improve her practice.

During the taking-in phase the mother needs ample opportunity to spend time with her infant. She may use this time to feed, to examine, or simply to watch her infant as he sleeps near her. The nurse can facilitate the acquaintance process by doing a physical examination of the infant in the mother's room, explaining all of the findings, and by pointing out those behaviors and characteristics of the infant that are unique. Although she enjoys her infant, a mother is more inclined at this time to send him to the nursery while she naps or to request a nurse to manage the soiled diapers. Later, as her independence increases, she is more likely to change the diapers herself or at least to ask for help to do so.

The mother's progression toward independence does not mean she no longer needs nursing care, merely that the kind of care is somewhat different. As she assumes responsibility for her own care and that of her infant she needs more guidance and teaching and more positive reinforcement that she is doing things right. She still needs rest, but because of her anxiety about doing everything herself, she may have a tendency to overextend herself. Now she needs help to plan for rest periods and to set limits for herself.

The taking-hold phase is often a time of rapid mood swings. As the woman begins to assume more and more of her responsibilities, they are occasionally overwhelming and periods of depression are not uncommon. In addition there is a natural letdown after the attention in pregnancy and the excitement of labor and delivery. The sudden shift in hormone balance, fatigue, physical discomfort, and lack of experience in caring for infants may further add to her feelings of depression. It is often reassuring for the mother to know that virtually all women experience some depression post partum. It is so common, in fact, that it has been termed the "baby blues." Talking about her feelings with her husband, with other women, or with the nurse may be very helpful. It also will be helpful if she receives positive feedback that she is doing well. If the infant goes to sleep when she soothes him, if the nurse praises the way she handles the infant, if her husband says she's a good mother, then her self-esteem will increase and her depression more likely will be mild and transient.

Effects of Early Discharge

In current maternity practice many women are leaving the hospital before achieving some stability in the taking-hold phase; some may be discharged within a few hours after delivery, and almost all are at home by the fourth or fifth postpartum day. This means that a substantial proportion of women are no longer in contact with the health care system at the time of their greatest readiness to learn about themselves and their infants. Nurses working in traditional postpartum settings must seek ways to resolve this situation. The use of printed instruction sheets and booklets which the mother can keep with her for reference may be useful. Referral to public health nursing services is helpful in areas where this is available. A few hospitals have established outreach services whereby hospital-employed nurses make home visits. Family or pediatric nurse practitioners may establish contact with the woman in the hospital or even prior to delivery and then provide the necessary nursing care from the time of discharge. It can be expected that a variety of patterns of care will emerge in the near future as nurses strive to meet the health needs, as well as the illness needs, of childbearing families.

Yet to be answered in research is the question of the influence of early discharge (24 hours or less after delivery), or even home delivery, on the rate at which a woman moves through the taking-in and taking-hold phases. It may be that this progression will be more rapid if the woman is in familiar surroundings with people she knows and loves. At the present time, however, it seems safe to expect every woman to have some period of increased physical and emotional dependency after giving birth. This has important implications for counseling families, helping them plan for the birth of their infants and for household help and support systems during the first week of the puerperium.

THE GROWTH OF PARENTING

The process by which an infant becomes attached to his caretaker has been carefully explored and described by Bowlby, Spitz, Ainsworth, and others during the past thirty years. It was not until 1970, however, that systematic efforts were begun to study this process from the maternal perspective.[3] The earlier research made clear that separation from and failure to form an attachment to a primary caregiver resulted in significant disturbances in the child's motor, mental, and affective development. The mother's failure to attach to her infant appears to have equally devastating effects on her offspring.

The mother-child relationship is an interactive one. That is to say, it is two-sided, with each member of the dyad responding to behaviors of the other in such a way that she in turn evokes a response. For example, the mother talks to her infant causing him to turn his head and look at her. The visual contact in turn evokes positive feelings in the mother toward her infant. This relationship begins during gestation as the mother works out the tasks of pregnancy in response to her own bodily changes, her kinesthetic awareness of her fetus, and the role defined for her by the culture in which she lives. If she does not accept her pregnancy as a positive event, if she does not respond to fetal movement with a growing awareness of the infant as an individual apart from herself, then the attachment process is likely to go awry at an early stage. The survival of the human infant in primitive society required that the mother be sufficiently attached to him to care for him from the moment of birth. Obviously, surrogate mothers and formula feedings no longer make this necessary for the continuation of the species. Nonetheless, most modern mothers are probably positively inclined toward their newborns when they see them for the first time.

Fathers also most likely begin to form an attachment to their infants during gestation as they anticipate parenthood with the mother. This attachment is apt to be stronger the more involved they are in sharing the experiences of pregnancy. Men who watch and feel fetal movement, attend Lamaze classes, and place a high value on children are more likely to be actively involved with their newborns.

Even though a certain attachment to the fetus develops during pregnancy, the emergence of the infant at birth adds an entirely new dimension to the relationship. It is somewhat analogous to being acquainted with someone only through correspondence and then meeting him in person. Now there is an individual that can be seen, touched, and heard, and who can respond in a variety of ways to the surroundings. This individual may be quite unlike the mental image of the letterwriter—and of the fetus. Time is required to decide if the reality is as acceptable as the fantasy.

All mothers tend to follow a similar pattern in getting acquainted with their infants. First there is an exploration and identification of the infant. Then, gradually, she claims him irreversibly as her own. This process may occur very quickly or it may require several days to weeks. Table 24–1 summarizes some of the factors that influence this process.

During the exploration and identification phase the mother can be expected to do certain things with her baby. These behaviors are briefly described below.

Table 24–1. Factors Influencing Maternal-Infant Attachment

Personal Characteristics
Relationship with her own parents
Previous experiences with infants
Cultural and/or ethnic background
Age and developmental level
Antepartal Factors
Planned conception
Acceptance of pregnancy as a positive event
Support of family and friends
Health during pregnancy
Attachment to fetus
Intrapartal Factors
Amount of active participation in labor and delivery
Amount of analgesia/anesthesia
Type of delivery (vaginal or cesarean)
Presence of support person(s)
Postpartal Factors
Health and responsivity of infant
Health of mother
Time of initial contact between mother and infant
Opportunity for continued contact and care of infant
Support of significant others
Skill of professionals in providing instruction, consultation, and support

[3] Clifford R. Barnett, P. Herbert Leiderman, Rose Grobstein, and Marshall Klaus, Neonatal separation: The maternal side of interactional deprivation, *Pediatrics,* 45:197–205, (Feb.) 1970.

Touch

The progression of maternal touch has been described by Rubin[4] and verified by numerous other observers. The mother begins touching her infant by stroking the extremities and the outline of the head with her fingertips, then gradually moving toward caressing him with the entire surface of her hand. At the same time she will usually touch and observe, first at arm's length, on her lap, or held slightly away from her body. Finally she will enfold the infant close to her body with both arms.

Eye-to-Eye Contact

This appears to be an extremely important component of the acquaintance process. Again and again mothers will be observed assuming an *en face* position with their babies. In this position where the two faces are in the same vertical plane each can look into the other's eyes. Mothers interpret their infant's gaze as having many positive intentions and spend much time coaxing their infants to look at them. It is very common on the postpartum unit to hear such comments as "Open your eyes. I know you're in there," "You're really looking me over," "Come on, look at mommy," and to her husband, "She opened both her eyes and looked right at me." (See Fig. 24–1.)

As the mother looks at and touches her infant she will begin to attribute to him characteristics that establish the infant as both unique and a member of the family. That is, she will begin to regard her infant as special and distinctly different from all others. Yet she will identify things about him that tie him to their family. Thus she will say the infant looks like her older brother or has her daddy's nose or a temper like Uncle Harry.

If a name was chosen during pregnancy, the mother will gradually "try it out" on her child. Sometimes she will decide it doesn't fit and a new name will be chosen. If a name has not been agreed upon prior to birth, sometimes the naming itself can be symbol of claiming the infant as her own.

It should be noted that the attachment process is closely related to the progress of the mother from taking-in to taking-hold. An integral part of what she is taking in is the infant. As the bond with the infant is strengthened and she "feels more like a mother," she begins to assume more responsibility for infant care. She has claimed him as her own and so she begins to take care of him.

Nursing Care to Promote Parent-Infant Attachment

Hospital routines designed primarily for the efficiency and convenience of physicians and nurses have done a great disservice to families for many years. Parents have been separated from each other during labor and birth and for much of the lying-in period. Infants were traditionally sequestered away in nurseries to be seen by their mothers only for feeding and by their fathers only through a window. Changes are occurring, however, and it is hoped that parents will now be able to be together whenever they choose and will have free access to their infants at all times. Consumer input into health care practices has been a valuable force in bringing about the much-needed changes in the care available to childbearing families. Many skilled professionals are now working in a variety of sensitive and imaginative ways to provide both the warmth and security of a family environment and the safety of modern medical technology.

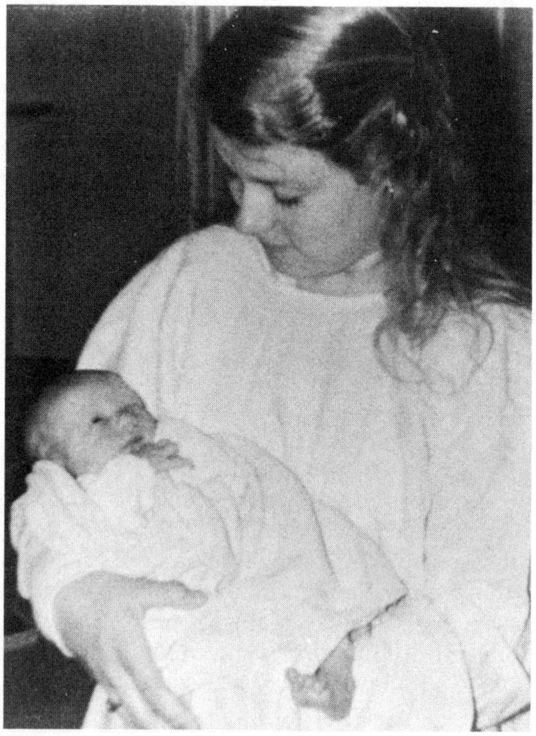

Figure 24–1. This young woman and her baby are beginning the acquaintance process. Notice the eye contact.

Promotion of healthy parent-infant relationships begins during antepartum care, or even long before. It continues during labor and delivery, when the woman is reassured by the presence of a significant other and a supportive professional. Efforts to enhance the self-esteem of the laboring woman will leave her better prepared to devote the necessary energy to her infant.

Preferably the mother is awake during delivery and both she and the father are participating actively in the birth of their child. In any event, it is important that both parents have the opportunity to see and touch their infant as soon as possible after birth. In animals, there exists a critical or sensitive period for maternal attachment. This is a short period of time, usually less than an hour, immediately following birth, during which the

[4] Reva Rubin, Maternal touch, *Nurs. Outlook,* 11:828–31, (Nov.) 1963.

mother animal must have contact with her offspring or she will abandon it. Obviously, adult humans, with their ability to reason, remember, and imagine are not apt to abandon their infants if they do not have contact with them in the first hour of life. Nevertheless there is some evidence that an initial period of separation contributes to maladaptive parenting in individuals who are at risk because of other factors.[5,6] Equally important is the fact that physiologically and psychologically both infant and mother are optimally disposed to begin attachment within the first hour after birth. Therefore, since only extremely rare circumstances necessitate separation, it should be avoided in order to facilitate the development of the parent-infant bond.

Immediately after birth and for about one hour thereafter the infant is in a quiet alert state. (See Chapter 26, page 531). During this time his eyes are open and he looks around. This is the ideal time for the parents to begin eye-to-eye contact. For this reason, it is recommended that the instillation of silver nitrate drops be postponed until after the parents have spent some time with their infant. While he remains in this first period of reactivity, the infant will often suck well at the breast. This provides him with valuable colostrum and provides the mother with the satisfaction of being a success at her first breast-feeding attempt. In addition, the sucking stimulates oxytocin production in the mother which promotes uterine contraction and minimizes bleeding. Early stimulation of the breast also may prevent, or at least minimize, engorgement.

When the nurse takes the infant to the parents for the first time, it is usually wise to spend a few minutes with them inspecting the infant together. The nurse should unwrap the infant and point out the physical characteristics of the newborn which could concern parents who have not had experience with such a young infant. Molding of the head, for example, can look very alarming to the unfamiliar observer. Parents often have questions about the appearance of the genitalia and the umbilical cord. By pointing out forceps marks, caput succedaneum, or fetal electrode marks, as well as the normal variations in the newborn's appearance, parents are reassured that the nurse is aware of these things and judges them to be normal (Fig. 24–2).

After checking over their infant with the nurse, most parents appreciate some privacy to be alone with each other and with their infant.

Throughout the hospitalization both parents should have free access to their infant. Hospital policies should enable the mother to keep her child with her as much as she wishes and yet be comfortable sending him back to the nursery if she feels the need for a break. It is important to remember that each mother and father will proceed at his or her own pace in developing a relationship with the infant. The nurse should provide support and opportunity for attachment to occur but should not push.

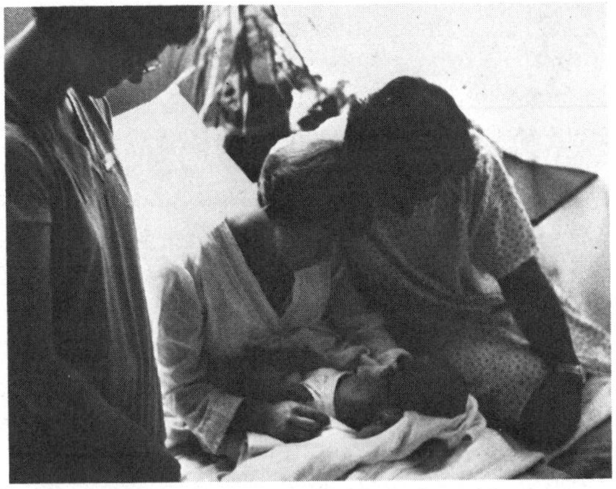

Figure 24–2. Nurse examining baby with parents.

There are a number of ways the nurse can encourage attachment as she cares for the postpartum family. Several suggestions are as follows:

1. Write the infant's first name on the crib identification card and use it when talking to or about him.
2. Serve as a role model for the parents. If they see a nurse cuddling and rocking an infant in the nursery or talking to him or stroking him to quiet him, they will recognize that these are important ways of caring for an infant. The nurse, however, should be cautious not to appear so expert in her handling of the infant that the parent feels she/he can never do as well.
3. Point out the infant's behaviors and help parents to interpret them. For example, some infants prefer to be held up on the shoulder so they can look around, others like to be cradled in the arms. Some infants are able to console themselves quite readily and are content to look around and "entertain" themselves. Snug swaddling comforts some infants and puts them right to sleep; others fight the confining blankets. Most infants stir and make noises or even cry out briefly in their sleep and then settle themselves again several times before finally waking up all the way for feeding. Learning to wait for the "real" waking up saves the frustration of trying to feed a drowsy infant.
4. Problem-solve with the parents about meeting infants' needs. For example, interpreting the meaning of an infant's cry is one of the major concerns of most new parents. Talking together about ways they can distinguish among cries of hunger, discomfort, anger, illness, or just self-expression allows parents to check the validity of their own

[5] M. H. Seashore *et al.*, The effects of denial of early mother-infant interaction on maternal self-confidence, *J. Pers. Soc. Psychol.*, 26:369–78, 1973.

[6] Marshall H. Klaus *et al.*, Maternal attachment: Importance of the first post-partum days, *N. Engl. J. Med.*, 268:460–63, (Mar. 2) 1972.

ideas as well as to obtain suggestions from the nurse.

5. Allow both parents to give as much care to their infant as they wish. Teach skills they are unfamiliar with and provide opportunity for them to practice in a supportive environment. Be sincere in praising them for their progress. The nurse should keep in mind that there is no one best way to do most things. The way the mother does it is likely to be just as good as the standard hospital practice. Incidentally, mothers often need to be reminded of this regarding fathers. Many women discourage men from caring for infants because they "don't do it the way I do."
6. Be accepting of parents' emotions, the negative ones as well as the positive ones. The freedom to let off steam, cry, and feel discouraged without fear of condemnation is important for mental health.

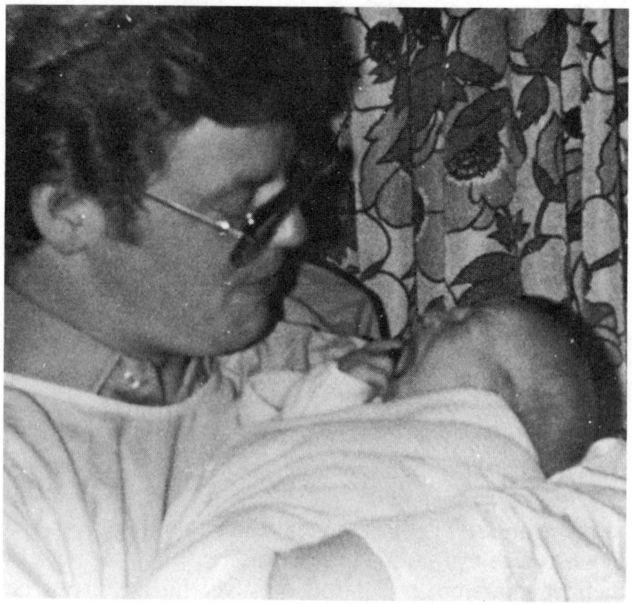

Figure 24–3. Father with his newly born son.

THE FATHER

Many times the father is the most forgotten member of the childbearing family. Unlike the mother and infant, he does not have pressing physical needs that necessitate contact with the traditional system of delivering obstetric care. He is stereotyped as a chain-smoking floor pacer who is quite out of place in a woman's world of birth and infants. Paying the bills has been seen as his chief contribution to the family. More recently he has been given the task of supporting the mother. Fathers are permitted in delivery rooms if the mother is awake and he is prepared to support her; they are encouraged to attend antepartum classes to help the mother. Little attention has been paid to meeting his own needs which arise from the role change to fatherhood.

Interest in the role of the father in the family and in relation to his children has flourished in the past decade, yet much remains to be learned.

Like a woman, a man's adaptation to parenthood depends in large measure on his experiences in his family as he was growing up and on the cultural expectations or norms for fathers in his society. In the United States at this time the trend appears to be toward an increasing involvement of fathers in pregnancy and in infant care. As more mothers enter the labor force, many fathers are assuming a greater share in the day-to-day responsibilities of childrearing. Nevertheless, the nurse should keep in mind that families vary widely in the ways they divide up the tasks of daily living. Assessment of the family interaction is important in determining how each member of the couple is adapting. If the man believes infants are women's work and the mother agrees, all is likely to go well. If the father wants to take a more active role in infant care but the mother is reluctant to give up any of her time with the infant, conflict may occur. Nursing care should be directed at providing the opportunity for both parents to begin parenting with the experts available as consultants. Often communication and role negotiation by the couple can be facilitated by discussing infant care with the nurse. When serious conflicts arise or the nurse feels unable to help, appropriate referrals should be made.

Many men feel isolated from their wives and infants for the first several months post partum. One father described himself as "the fifth wheel in the group." The mother spends much of her time with the infant, and, particularly if she is breast-feeding, has a relationship with the infant that may seem to exclude the father. She may be temporarily less interested in issues and activities outside the family and thus be a less interesting conversationalist. Sexual relationships may suffer due to tender episiotomy, fatigue, and night feedings. Mothers should be helped to understand the man's need for her love and support and for some time alone with her without any children.

SIBLINGS

Any right-minded preschooler would have to agree with the cartoon concept that a baby isn't nearly so much fun as a puppy. Baby brothers, or even baby sisters, can't do any good tricks. All they do is eat, sleep, cry, and mess their pants. When it comes to playing, they are a total loss. On top of that, they take up enormous amounts of mommy's time that she could otherwise spend much more profitably reading stories or playing ball. On the other hand, few children can resist a baby clinging to their finger. They don't know about grasp reflexes. To

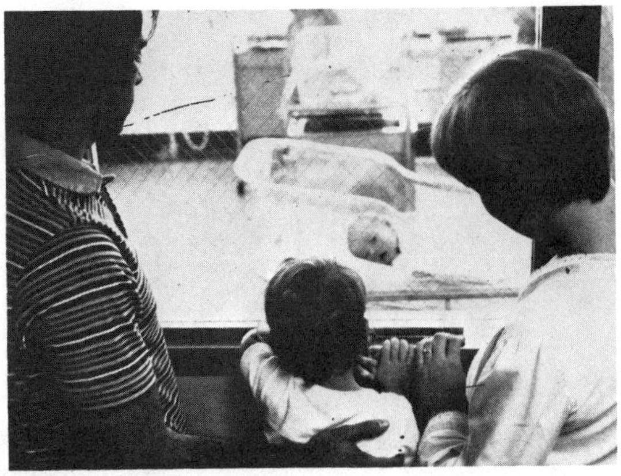

Figure 24-4. Parents helping their two-year-old get acquainted with his new sister.

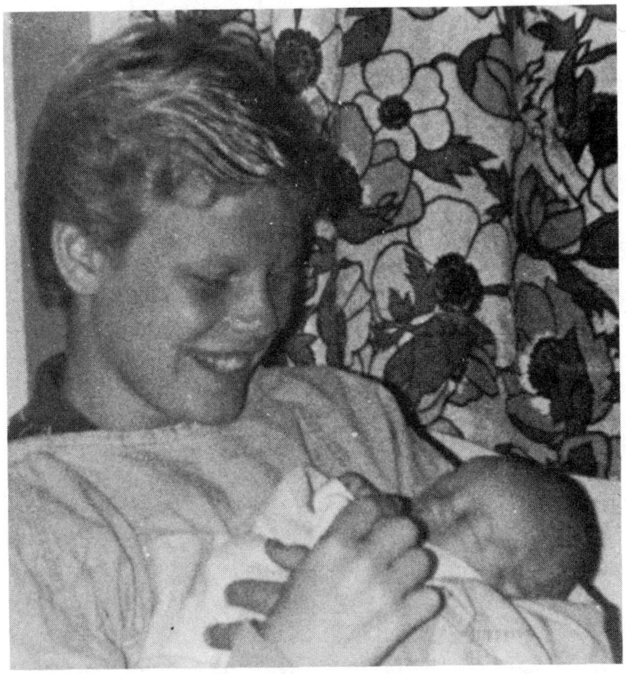

Figure 24-5. This young man looks pleased with his status as a new big brother.

them the baby is saying "I like you," because the baby wants to hold hands. And holding a baby and putting a cheek next to his soft, fuzzy hair is even better than hugging a teddy bear.

Even very young children can be helped to wash their hands and play some "games" with their babies which capitalize on the newborn's reflexes. For example, rubbing the baby's cheek will cause the baby to turn to look at you (rooting reflex); putting the back of your hand over the baby's mouth will result in sucking (sucking reflex); and shaking a baby rattle on one side will cause the baby to turn toward the sound. Of course, gentleness must always be emphasized.

Children, like their parents, need time to get acquainted with and become attached to the new member of the family. During pregnancy they should share the anticipation and preparation. By helping to put the baby clothes in the drawer and growing accustomed to the empty waiting crib, they begin to feel a pleasant expectation. Doll play and talking about what it will be like to have a baby in the house are ways of rehearsing behavior before the actual event happens. After the baby arrives, children enjoy touching, watching, and helping care for him. They also like to look at their own baby pictures to see if there is a resemblance to the new baby and to hear about what they were like when they were babies. Even very young children can be helped to observe the way the baby changes as he grows from day to day. They will soon come to applaud the new accomplishments of their baby in the same way their own accomplishments are applauded by others.

The resentment children feel toward new infants is created by their perceived loss of their valued position in the family. They are outraged at their mother for abandoning them to go to the hospital. When the family is reunited, some children exhibit their anger and frustration by having temper tantrums, regressing in toilet habits, refusing to follow bedtime routines, or any one of a number of disruptive behaviors. It is not uncommon for young children to ignore their mothers upon reunion, refusing to kiss her hello or even sit on her lap, retreating instead to Grandma or the babysitter. For a mother who has spent several days in the hospital very lonesome for her two-year-old, this can be a painful experience.

Helping parents understand normal child behavior and plan ahead for coping with it can do a great deal to minimize the stress for the whole family. It is important for parents to demonstrate to a child that he/she is still as loved as always and is still very special to them. It is usually necessary, especially with preschool-age children, to plan particular times to do things just with them.

Parents often need help dealing with problem behaviors during this time. Understanding the reason why a child is having tantrums or refusing to go to bed does not make it any easier to live with those behaviors. Neither does it mean parents should indulge the child. They must continue patiently to guide and teach him just as before the infant came. Just as a child must learn that he is no less loved and important because of the infant, he must also learn to share with his brother or sister. While love may be infinite and indivisible, parents' time and energy are not, toys are not, bedrooms are not. Learning to share is a hard but necessary part of growing up.

All children, regardless of age, experience some jealousy or sibling rivalry when a new infant joins the family. This is part of the role realignment that occurs throughout the family system in order to accommodate a new member. Changes are most marked, however, in a firstborn when a second child is born and in the "old baby" of the family when a third or subsequent infant is born.

PREPARATION FOR DISCHARGE FROM THE HOSPITAL

Planning for going home with the infant is begun well before delivery with the acquisition of a crib and preparation of the room. Nursing care during the antepartum period includes helping parents anticipate their needs for the time immediately after birth. Nevertheless, once the infant is born, it is necessary to review these plans and make necessary modifications. The nurse who is responsible for postpartum care should help the parents:

1. Evaluate their need for household help and determine how best to meet this need
2. Learn necessary infant care skills
3. Arrange for continued health supervision for both mother and infant
4. Anticipate some of the changes that will occur in their lives during the first three months at home
5. Learn about resources available to new parents in their community

Household Help

The need for household help during the first week or two after delivery is largely a matter of personal preference. A mother who has been ill, had a cesarean section, or is being discharged within a few hours of delivery may have less energy. Many families have a tradition of grandmothers coming to stay and help after an infant is born. Some couples prefer to have this time alone with their infant. It is becoming more acceptable for a father to get leave from his job or take vacation time when his new infant comes home.

If someone will be coming to help, the mother should give some thought to the division of labor. Generally it is best for the mother to care for her infant while the helper takes care of meals, laundry, and cleaning.

When the parents plan to manage without help, it is wise for them to decide what satisfactorily can be left undone and/or what shortcuts can be used. For example, they may consider diaper service or disposable diapers for a while to reduce the laundry and make use of convenience foods for some of their meals.

Teaching Infant Care Skills

The more infant care that the parents can perform in the hospital with the nurse available as a consultant, the more they have an opportunity to learn about their infant. In addition to learning how to hold, bathe, and dress their infant, procedures that seem complicated and sometimes cause anxiety, there is much more for parents to learn about the infant's care which is equally, or more, valuable. For example, they must learn to determine the meaning of the infant's cry, signs of hunger and satiety, methods of feeding and bubbling, number and type of stools considered normal; normalcy of regurgitation, sneezing, and hiccuping; methods of turning and positioning; and the value of cuddling and rocking the infant.

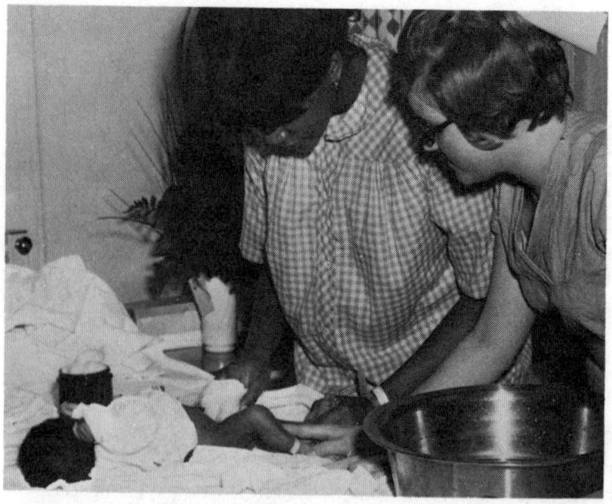

Figure 24–6. Mothers need an opportunity to practice infant care skills with the nurse available as a consultant.

Parents need help in learning to care for their infant from a nurse who can put them at ease and give them a feeling of self-assurance. It takes time for an inexperienced parent to develop skills. Encouragement that they are doing well and that they can meet their infant's needs will help them to feel at ease and gain confidence in their ability. To gain skill and confidence the parents need help with the infant's physical care and opportunities to make their own decisions regarding his needs. When they have been helped to find their own answers to questions and have been reassured that their judgment is good, they will be able to meet problems at home more easily.

Parent teaching may be both incidental and planned. Incidental teaching consists of explaining something "on the spot" in response to a specific question or situation. Planned teaching may be more formal. It is scheduled discussion of a particular topic, which may include a demonstration of a skill or a film. Teaching may be done on a one-to-one basis or with a group of parents. Individual teaching has the advantage of addressing the parent's particular needs and concerns in a manner tailored to their level of learning. It may encourage them to raise issues or ask questions that they would hesitate to do in a group. Group teaching is more economical and has the advantage of using the experiences of many people. Parents may learn as much from each other as from the nurse. In addition, they realize that they have fears and questions not unlike those of others.

Readiness to Learn

Regardless of whether teaching is incidental or planned, individual or in a group, the nurse must make an assessment of the parents' readiness to learn. Unless the information has significance for them, they will be unlikely to hear and remember what is being taught. It is often necessary to meet other needs of the parents before they will have the energy to attend to teaching about infant care. When a mother is physically uncomfortable or the couple has urgent concerns about financial affairs, they are likely to be distracted from instruction. Similarly, discussing the infant's bath while the mother is acutely anxious about getting her infant to suck well at breast will not be beneficial.

Level of Learning

The instruction itself should be adjusted to the individual ability of the learner. Care must be taken to use vocabulary that is understandable to the client and to proceed at a pace that allows for thorough comprehension. Repetition may be necessary from time to time. The method of instruction also should be considered. While some parents will learn readily from reading printed directions, others will need a verbal explanation, and still others will need to be shown how. Different topics may require different methods of instruction even for the same parents.

Evaluation

The nurse should be continually evaluating the amount of learning that is taking place. Asking the parents to repeat information back to the nurse is one way of ascertaining their understanding. Providing opportunities for return demonstrations of such manual skills as bathing or diapering is also a valuable means of evaluation.

Although it is by no means exhaustive, the following list contains many of the items of infant care commonly taught to parents.

1. *Feeding*. Holding the bottle so that air does not get into the nipple. Cleaning bottles and making formula. Positioning the infant for breast-feeding. Care of sore nipples. How to break the infant's suction on the breast. How to tell if the infant is getting enough to eat (Chapter 28).
2. *Bubbling or burping*. How often and in what position?
3. *Diapers*. Always keep safety pins closed and out of the infant's reach. Disposable diapers are more expensive but more convenient, especially for trips to grandma's house or pediatric office visits.
4. *Diaper rash*. Frequent change of diapers helps. Bottom should be washed off at each diaper change to remove irritants. Petroleum jelly (VASELINE) or vegetable shortening will protect the skin from moisture of urine. Fair-skinned infants may develop a rash from time to time even with the most conscientious care. Exposing the bottom to air is helpful as are several commercial oint-

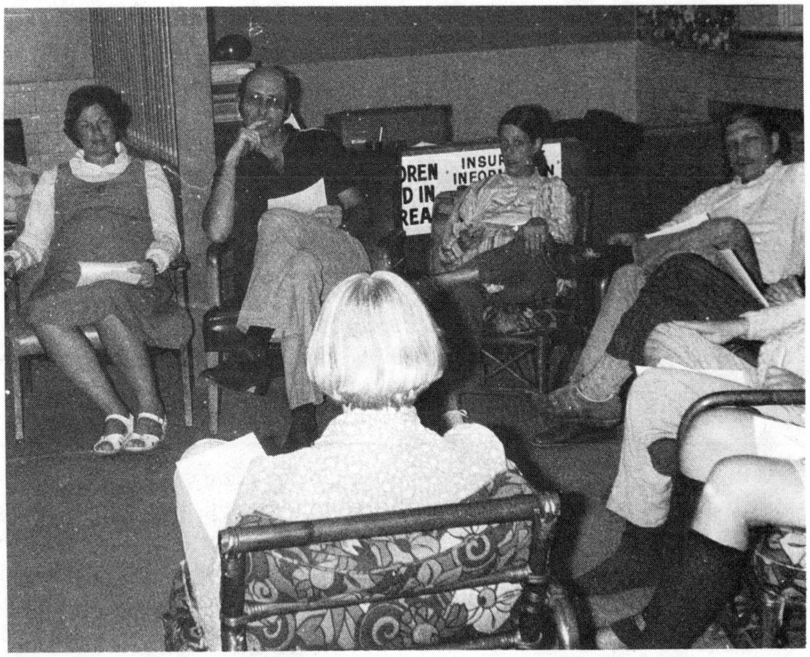

Figure 24-7. Photograph of parents' discussion group.

ments. Changing laundry soaps also may help sometimes.

5. *Bathing.* Although the bath demonstration is an honored ritual on many postpartum units, mothers usually will not have difficulty bathing their infants if they are taught how to hold them securely and are given an opportunity to practice with supervision. They should practice with equipment similar to that available in their homes, namely, a bar of soap, washcloth, towel, and basin or sink. The plastic bath basins many hospitals use for adult patients make fine infant bathtubs for the first month or two. The kitchen sink is often the ideal place to bathe an infant, since it is at a height that doesn't require bending and usually has a cabinet top next to it to lay the infant on to dry and dress. Until infants can sit alone, it is usually easier to wash them off as they lay on a towel and then lower them into the water for rinsing and playing. A bath need not be given daily but should be an enjoyable time for both parents and infant.
6. *Lotions and powders.* Not essential but enjoyable. Lotions should be mild and nonirritating. Rubbing them in over the infant's body provides pleasurable tactile stimulation. When using powder, care should be taken not to shake it freely over the infant so that the dust is not inhaled. It is best to shake some into the parent's hand and then smooth it onto the infant's skin, taking care to avoid accumulation in folds of skin where it will become moist, cake, and produce irritation. Powder is especially refreshing in warm weather. Cornstarch is an inexpensive alternative to powder.
7. *Umbilical cord.* Falls off in a week to ten days. Alcohol applied at the base of the cord will promote its drying. After the cord drops off, the mother may note a few drops of blood on the infant's clothes or bed covers for a day or so. The healing navel can be cleansed with alcohol. A protuberant navel may be indicative of an umbilical hernia. This benign condition will correct itself as the infant grows and the abdominal muscles strengthen.
8. *Pacifiers.* Very useful in meeting the nonnutritive sucking needs of many infants. Usually can be discontinued about four to six months of age as the infant gains more interests and has less need for sucking.
9. *Sleeping.* Infants usually sleep through the night by the time they are two or three months old. Parents can help minimize their own loss of sleep by teaching their infant that eating during the night is different from daytime eating. During the night the infant should be allowed to wake up completely before beginning to nurse. He should be fed with a minimum of talking and handling and put immediately back to bed. Most infants quickly will learn to go right back to sleep, particularly if the day feeding is accompanied by cuddling, talking, and playing, and time is spent awake when not eating.
10. *Crying.* This can be the most frustrating characteristic of infants, creating in parents feelings of helplessness and even panic. It is important to talk with parents in the hospital or even antepartally about how they think they will handle crying. They need to know that some infants cry more than others just because that is part of their individuality. If all the usual attempts to quiet the infant have failed (feeding, changing, rocking, talking to, and so on), letting the infant cry just for exercise may be necessary. Even a short period of crying can seem interminable to parents. Often it is useful to time the crying with the determination to permit it to continue ten minutes before trying additional measures. Most often the crying will cease before this time is up.
11. *Illness.* Because infants cannot complain of being ill in words, parents are concerned that they will not be able to tell when their infant is sick and should be seen by a physician. Several characteristics of infants make them susceptible to illness. These include (a) loose cardiac sphincter of the stomach, (b) short, straight eustachian tube which favors ear infections, (c) large proportion of body weight is fluid, which means they will dehydrate quickly, (d) tendency toward higher fevers than adults, (e) more likely to have febrile seizures, and (f) weight loss or slowed gain common with illnesses. The most common illnesses are acute infections. The most common symptoms are changes in behavior such as irritability or listlessness, loss of appetite, "cold" symptoms, and fever. Parents should know how to take their infant's temperature, what kinds of symptomatic home therapy can be undertaken (such as vaporizers), and should be encouraged to call the nurse or physician if they have any doubts about their infant's health.
12. *Taking the infant outside.* It is desirable to take an infant outside from time to time to permit some exposure to fresh air and sunshine as well as to give parents an opportunity to go out. Care should be taken that the infant is suitably dressed for the weather. In general he will be comfortable if dressed comparably to the parents. In warm weather protection against sunburn should be assured.

When traveling in a car the infant should be secured in a car seat which is fastened in place by the seat belts. The safest child restraint devices are those that have been crash tested. Most new models on the market since July 1, 1975, have been crash tested. However, some parents who may receive hand-me-downs or purchase items at garage sales should be cautious. Safety information is available in *Consumer Reports* at the public library as well as from the National Safety Council and some state health agencies.

THE FIRST THREE MONTHS AT HOME

It is impossible to predict how life will change for a given family as they mature as parents of a growing infant. Many families have similar experiences, however, and talking about these with new parents often helps them plan ways to help themselves.

Most mothers find the first months with a new infant to be very emotional ones. Mood swings are not unusual. The responsibilities of caring for a new infant occasionally seem overwhelming. Even if it is not her first infant, she may become frantic that she can't meet everyone's needs. Mothers should be warned that there will be times when they yearn to be childless again and hate the infant for robbing them of their freedom. Unless a woman realizes the normality of this feeling, she may be frightened and will certainly feel guilty and charge herself with being a bad mother. The relationship between the parents also can be strained during this time, particularly if their relationship was not a strong one to begin with.

To help parents begin problem-solving so that this time becomes a happy period for maturation as parents and as individuals, the nurse may discuss some of the following problems with them.

Organization of Time

The infant will take up quite a bit of time. In addition to the direct care of feeding, bathing, and so on, there will be more laundry and other tasks. At least for the first month the mother will require extra rest because of easy fatigability. Her husband and other children also will make demands on her time. If her mental health is to be maintained, she will need some time to herself to read a book or sew, work with her plants, or get out of the house for socialization.

Meeting all these needs will require some reordering of priorities. Some tasks will have to be left undone or done less frequently in order to make time for those things judged most important. A reliable babysitter can be an important asset. Some families can afford help to do housework or may have a willing friend or relative. Fathers often are willing to perform household chores in order to have some time for individual attention from their wives.

Sexuality

This is a frequent area of conflict between couples. Sexual gratification is often postponed during the last weeks of pregnancy. Now when the man desires intercourse, the woman may be tired and her perineum may be tender from the episiotomy and/or hemorrhoids. Intercourse also may be painful because of lack of estrogen-induced vaginal lubrication, especially if she is breast-feeding.

Women may be confused and embarrassed to find themselves sexually aroused by breast-feeding. At the same time sexual stimulation will result in milk leaking from the breast.

If the couple can talk to each other about their feelings and frustrations, they usually can solve their problems satisfactorily. Gentleness, time, and some water-soluble lubricant will resolve the perineal discomfort. Mutual love and a sense of humor will help much of the rest.

Couples should be aware that conception can occur even while the woman is lactating. If they wish to avoid another pregnancy at this time some form of contraception should be used.

Enjoying the Infant

In their zeal to prepare parents realistically for the frustrations of parenthood, professionals often forget to emphasize how enjoyable infants can be. They feel good when you hold them, they are cute to look at, and they grow in marvelous, fascinating ways. They are very tolerant of inexperienced parents, since they have never had parents before just as their parents have never had an infant before. Nurses should strive to increase the new parents' self-confidence to the point where they can relax and have fun with their infant.

Community Resources

Parents should be made aware of the community resources available to them. A directory listing the agencies, any eligibility requirements, and the services they offer would be a valuable service the hospital could provide postpartum patients.

In addition to professional health and counseling agencies, many communities have organized lay groups. Groups of parents with similar interests meet together to help each other. Examples of such groups include the LaLeche League for breast-feeding mothers, and groups for women who have had (or are going to have) cesarean sections, parents of twins, postpartum couples, parents of toddlers, and so on. These mutual support groups are also valuable for parents whose infant is in an intensive care nursery or who has an anomaly. Some groups, like those for parents of children with PKU or spina bifida, are organized on the national level and offer a variety of services to families.

PARENTS IN CRISIS

When Something Is "Wrong" with the Infant

Whenever any infant is born, the parents must resolve the loss of their fantasied, ideal child and form an attachment to the real child. The greater the discrepancy between the reality and the fantasy, the more difficult this task becomes. Anticipatory teaching during pregnancy can do much to help parents appreciate the appearance and behaviors of newborns, so their expectations are reasonably close to the reality of their own infant. In most cases, when a healthy infant is born, disappointments over sex and general appearance are overcome readily. However, when the infant is premature, sick, has an anomaly, or dies, the family suffers severe grief and is in a state of crisis for a period of time.

Different theorists have described various stages that individual families go through in response to a crisis. Initially there is a period of disorganization during which the usual patterns of behavior are inadequate. There are shock and disbelief that such a thing could have happened. Feelings of guilt, anger, and intense sorrow are common. During this time, a number of physical symptoms occur. There is a constricted, heavy feeling in the throat and chest; sighing and yawning are frequent due to a shortness of breath. There are feelings of exhaustion, emptiness, and unreality. Crying is frequent.

The second stage is one of relative equilibrium. This is a time of information-seeking and resource utilization. Anxiety is somewhat lessened and some problem-solving can begin with help. A stage of mobilization or action follows in which the individual or family works out new behavior patterns to resolve the crisis. Finally, there is reorganization. Ideally there will have been growth as a result of mastering the crisis so that the individual or family will emerge stronger and more mature. The stages of the crisis do not follow each other in a discrete sequence. There is considerable overlapping and often a person will move back and forth through several stages during a single day. Thus, information-seeking may be accompanied by anger and sorrow and then a period of disbelief or denial may follow.

The progress of families through crises may be modified by whether the event was expected or unexpected. Anticipated crises can be prepared for in advance and the impact often can be softened. Events that originate in or are caused by factors external to the family are generally less stressful, presumably because the burden of guilt is lessened. Intact families, characterized by common goals, mutual love and respect, and flexibility of roles, have more resources available to deal with stress and crisis. Similarly, families with strong kinship ties to an extended family generally fare better than isolated nuclear families. In addition, the way the family perceives the situation will influence its response and the ease with which it will be able to accept and cope with the crisis event. Finally, timely intervention by caring professionals can do much to facilitate the development of new coping strategies and the satisfactory resolution of the crisis situation.

The care of parents during a crisis with their newborn is very similar regardless of the nature of the newborn's problems. However, in order to highlight some of the differences, care is discussed separately for premature and/or sick infants, infants with anomalies, and infants who die. For a more complete discussion of this important topic the reader is referred to the books *Parent-Infant Bonding* by Marshall Klaus and John Kennell and to *Nursing Care for Parents at Risk* by Ramona Mercer.

Premature or Sick Infants

The birth of a premature infant always can be anticipated, at least for the duration of the mother's labor. In many cases, neonatal illness also can be predicted, as in the case of an Rh-sensitized fetus, an infant of a diabetic mother, or a fetus with intrauterine growth retardation or an abnormal fetal heart rate pattern. Thus, parents' concern for their infant precedes birth. Fearing the infant will die, parents may attempt to shield themselves from the pain of loss by remaining aloof from the infant. Anticipatory grief is common and may inhibit attachment to the infant even after the parents realize that their infant is going to get well.

Not only do parents themselves sometimes remain psychologically distant from their newborn, but the medical care system frequently imposes a physical separation of parents and newborn. As specialized, highly skilled, technical care is organized into regional centers, it becomes increasingly likely that the newborn will be given optimal care in a center some distance from the parents' home. To the extent that the birth of such infants can be predicted, their mothers should go to the center for delivery. This at least prevents complete separation of the mother and infant for the first several days of life. It is inevitable, however, that parents will have less contact with their premature or sick infant than they would have were the infant full term and healthy. Thus, it is a major responsibility of professionals who work in intensive care nurseries to help parents form realistic expectations of their infant's prognosis and to foster the early development of parent-infant attachment.

Both parents should see their infant as soon as possible even if only for a few seconds. If the mother is awake during delivery and the father is present, then they will, of course, see the infant at birth. Should the mother be anesthetized, the father may see the infant before she recovers from the anesthesia. Even a brief glimpse of the infant helps them to grasp the reality of the situation and often dispels fantasies about the infant's appearance that may be much more frightening than the actual situation. For example, one mother was surprised to see that her 32-week daughter was a complete, if miniature, baby. She had believed that, since she was premature, she was "unfinished" and would be missing some parts of her body.

If it becomes necessary to transfer the infant to a different hospital for care, it is preferable to transfer the mother as well, unless she is nearly ready for discharge. If she is not to be transferred, it is essential that she see and touch her infant before he leaves. The transport team from the intensive care nursery should take a few minutes to give her and the father some information about the nursery. This should be followed up with telephone communication on a regular basis until the mother is able to come to the nursery. The father frequently will accompany the infant to the new hospital.

From the very beginning parents should be encouraged to visit, touch, and care for their infant as much as they are able. Before they go into an intensive care nursery for the first time it is usually wise for the nurse or physician to explain a little of what they will see. The technical apparatus can be overwhelming even if their own infant is not gravely ill. It is usual for parents to be hesitant to touch a very small or sick infant, particularly if he is in an ISOLETTE and/or attached to various tubes and machines. Several visits may be required before some parents begin to touch their infant. It is important that this behavior be accepted without pushing the parents. (See Fig. 24-8.)

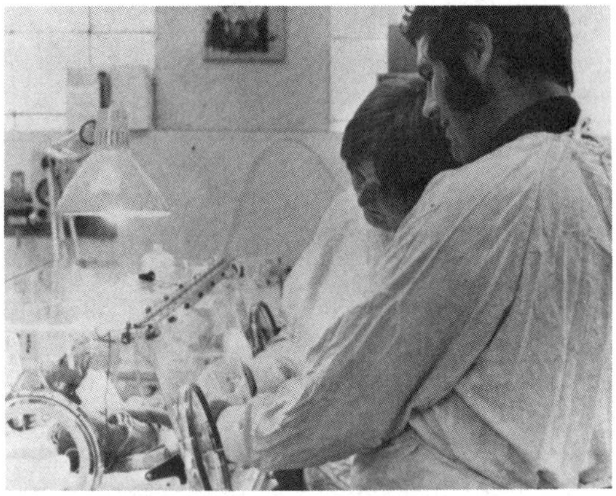

Figure 24-8. These parents are continuing the process of getting to know their premature son by touching him and participating in his tube feedings and other care. They quickly feel he belongs to them and not to the nursery. [Copyright October, 1975, The American Journal of Nursing Company. Reproduced from Mecca S. Cranley, When a high risk infant is born. *Amer. J. Nurs.*, 75 (10): 1696-1699, Oct. 1975.]

Discussions with the parents about the infant's prognosis always should be optimistic without giving false hope. They should be helped to realize that, although the infant requires special care for a time, this will not always be the case. As soon as he is well or as soon as he is older he can be treated like any healthy child. Of major help to parents is the identification of one nurse and one physician with whom they can relate during the entire hospitalization. This facilitates the development of a trusting relationship and permits consistency and continuity of care.

When a prolonged hospitalization is required, parents are not always able to visit daily. They may live some distance from the hospital, have other children, and so on. Daily telephone communication should be maintained, however. Not only medical progress but also individual behavior and growth and development should be described to the parents. The nurse should remember that in addition to the stress of a sick infant, the parents are coping with all of the other processes of the puerperium, plus family separation, financial stress, and perhaps many other factors. Attention should be paid to their rest and nutrition as well as to their feelings. They should be encouraged to talk and help each other, and appropriate social service referrals should be made whenever indicated.

Prior to discharge, plans should be made for the parents to spend an extended period of time with the infant, becoming familiar with him. Some hospitals have facilities for parents to live in for as long as necessary to become comfortable with their infant while consultants are readily available. Referral to community agencies is important to provide some assistance during the first several months at home.

Infants with Anomalies

It is paradoxical that, although virtually every pregnant woman worries that something will be wrong with her infant, when an anomaly does occur a common response is "I didn't think it could ever happen to me." The realization that their child is not perfect produces sorrow in all parents. The intensity of their response tends to be influenced by several factors in addition to their own personalities and backgrounds. Among these factors are:

1. Whether or not the defect is apparent from looking at the child (e.g., a cleft lip versus an internal, "invisible" anomaly)
2. The extent to which the defect can be corrected, if it can be corrected at all
3. Whether or not there is neurologic involvement; that is, to what extent will the child's growth and development and intelligence be impaired
4. Life expectancy of the child

In general, malformations that require long-term adaptations, especially if they include lifelong dependency on the parents, are the most difficult to accept. Defects of the head and face tend to produce stronger reactions than those of other parts of the body.

Early parent-infant contact is important when an infant is born with an anomaly just as it always is with a normal infant. Several studies have shown that parents report feeling better once they have seen their infant. They almost invariably say that the infant looks better than they had imagined. Once the parents feel they are ready to see their infant and then do so, a turning point seems to be reached in their crisis. The longer the contact is delayed, the greater the risk for maladaptive parenting. A case report will illustrate some of the tragedies that can occur.

> Mrs. R.'s second daughter was born early in the morning in a small community hospital with a severe bilateral cleft lip and palate. Although it was a normal vaginal delivery, she had general anesthesia. When she awoke and asked about her baby, the nurses evaded her questions. She was heavily sedated. Her husband was not permitted to visit, and she believed her baby to be dead. In the evening her physician told her of the cleft lip but encouraged her not to see the baby until after surgery. Although she asked to see the baby several times, she was not permitted to do so. The baby was concealed behind a screen in the small nursery. One nurse told Mrs. R., "You don't want to see her. She's such an ugly little thing it would only make you cry." Interestingly, the father was permitted to see the baby. Perhaps he was considered "stronger" and better able to "take it."
>
> On the second postpartum day the infant was transferred to a university medical center about six hours drive from the parents' home. On the day of her first lip surgery, ten days later, Mrs. R. first visited her. She was directed to a pediatric ward containing eight infants in identical cribs. She later described her feelings as she entered the ward: "I stopped in the door and just looked around. I suddenly realized that my very own baby was in that room and I couldn't even recognize her because I had no idea what she looked like. I wondered if I could ever be a mother to her."
>
> That child at ten years old is a very pretty little girl due to an unusually fine plastic repair. She is very bright and has no speech difficulties. Her mother refers to her as a tomboy who is "daddy's girl." In sharp contrast to her two sisters, she has always been encouraged to enter into her father's interests and activities. While her sisters take ballet lessons, she plays on the softball team. Although by no means an abused or disadvantaged child, she is obviously regarded as "different" by her mother.

Although the goal of crisis intervention is to help families achieve resolution, for some congenital malformations there only can be partial resolution because the parents are continually reminded of their misfortune by the presence of the child in the home. As the child grows, they are constantly faced with new challenges resulting from the malformation. The care of the newborn may be relatively easy compared to the needs of the growing child for mobility, education, social contacts, sexuality, and so on. These parents have been described by Olshansky as having "chronic sorrow."[7]

Parents Whose Infants Die

The death of a newborn introduces severe conflict. Birth is supposed to be an optimistic, joyful occasion, but now loss and sorrow have occurred. Nurses and physicians who choose perinatal practice are often unaccustomed to dealing with death and feel uncomfortable and inadequate to help. There is a temptation to gloss over the parents' grief with such statements as "It was probably for the best" or "You are lucky to have two healthy children at home." Mothers often are transferred from the maternity unit so other infants won't remind them of their loss and so they won't remind the staff.

These and other efforts to "protect" the parents from the impact of their loss are not beneficial, since they discourage the healthy expression of grief. Rather, parents should be helped to face the reality of the infant's death and to support each other in mourning. They need to cry, to express their anger and frustrations, and to talk about the infant and what has happened. Grieving for a dead infant is no different than grieving for the loss of any other loved person.

Parents should be offered an opportunity to see their infant after death, especially if the baby was stillborn or died before the parents could see him. Although this is a painful experience, it promotes healthy resolution of loss by making the death real. Religious and cultural traditions also play an important role in comforting the grieving parents.

Often the death of an infant is the couple's first close experience with death. Even if a parent or other close relative has died, this is very likely to be the first time they have had to make decisions about funerals, burial versus hospital disposal, autopsies, and so on. Therefore, in addition to psychologic support and comforting, they need some very practical information about their options, expenses involved, local laws that pertain, and so on.

Follow-up care of parents whose infant has died is important. Several weeks after the death parents may have many questions that did not occur to them during the disorganized time surrounding the death. This is often an appropriate time to review autopsy findings and to anticipate the need for any genetic counseling. It also permits an evaluation of the parents' progression through the grieving process. Other visits may be scheduled depending on the parents' needs. They should be aware that it is not uncommon for the grieving process to last for six to nine months or even a year. They

[7] S. Olshansky, Chronic sorrow: A response to having a mentally defective child, *Soc. Casework,* 43:190–93, 1962.

should be encouraged to ask for help whenever they feel the need. Professionals giving primary health care should be aware of the death and incorporate into the client's care plan a means of facilitating grief work.

SUMMARY

The puerperium is defined medically as the six weeks immediately following delivery. Psychosocially it extends through the first three to four months after birth.

Dramatic physiologic changes occur in the woman's body. The nurse must be able to assess the progress of these changes and evaluate their normality.

Equally dramatic psychosocial changes occur in the woman and in her family. The nurse must be aware of the usual pattern of these changes in order to foster parent-infant attachment, role adaptation, and family integration.

Parents require special nursing care when their infants are not full term and healthy if they are to master this crisis successfully and develop as competent parents.

REFERENCES AND SUGGESTED READINGS

Dean, Patricia G.; Morgan, Patricia; and Towle, Jeannine M., Making baby's acquaintance: A unique attachment strategy, *MCN,* 7(1):37-41, 1982.

Gromada, Karen, Maternal-infant attachment: The first step toward individualizing twins, *Matern. Child Nurs. J.,* 6(2): 129-34, 1981.

Hawkins-Walsh, Elizabeth, Diminishing anxiety in parents of sick newborns, *MCN,* 5(1):30-34, 1980.

Klaus, Marshall, and Kennell, John, *Parent-Infant Attachment,* 2nd ed., C. V. Mosby, St. Louis, 1982.

Lockhart, Beth, Childrearing patterns of young mothers: Expectations, knowledge and practices, *MCN,* 7(2):119-24, 1982.

Mercer, Ramona, *Nursing Care for Parents at Risk,* C. B. Slack, Thorofare, N.J., 1970.

——, The nurse and the maternal tasks of early post-partum, *MCN,* 6(5):341-45, 1981.

Mercer, R. T., A theoretical framework for studying factors that impact on the maternal role. *Nursing Research,* 30(2):73-77, 1982.

Newton, L. D., Helping parents cope with infant crying. *JOGN Nurs.,* 12(3):199-203, 1983.

Schroeder, Barbara D., Attachment and parenting despite lengthy intensive care, *MCN,* 5(1):37-41, 1980.

Ventura, J. N., Parent coping behaviors, parent functioning and infant temperament characteristics, *Nursing Research,* 31(5):269-273, 1982.

Wooten, Bonnie, Death of an infant, *MCN,* 6(4):257-60, 1981.

gressed until the mother became chronically ill and progressively weaker and frequently developed abscesses, which sometimes had to be incised and drained. Healing was often slow and painful, and destruction of breast tissue sometimes extensive. With present-day treatment the mother almost always recovers quickly.

Nursing Management

Preventive

Breast infections largely can be prevented by care of the breasts and nipples during the puerperium. The nurse may help to prevent this complication by cleanliness and gentleness in breast care, prevention of fissured nipples, treatment of fissures if they do occur, proper care of engorged breasts, and prompt reporting to the physician if any signs of infection develop.

Curative

Treatment generally consists of breast support, application of ice bags while the breast is indurated and painful, and administration of penicillin, or a combination of antibiotics. If treatment is instituted early, the infection usually subsides in a day or two. With the use of antibiotics the inflammation almost always resolves without abscess formation.

Controversy exists about whether or not to discontinue breast-feeding when mastitis occurs. Some authorities believe that it should be stopped immediately and the breasts allowed to "dry up." The rationale for this approach is that the less stimulation there is to the breasts, the more quickly the infection will disappear, and that the mastitis may recur later if nursing is continued. Others prefer to continue lactation to avoid the distention of the breasts that occurs when emptying of the breasts is stopped suddenly. In addition, if lactation is allowed to continue, the infant has the benefit of continued breast-feeding. Important factors in making this choice are the mother's wishes as well as her own general health and that of her infant. When lactation is to be continued, the nursing is temporarily stopped and the breast is emptied manually or by a pump. The milk is discarded during the time the mother has a fever. Breast-feeding usually can be resumed in one to three days.

CYSTITIS AND PYELITIS

The slight lesions which generally are present in the bladder mucosa following delivery favor development of cystitis, especially when catheterization is necessary or when residual urine, which becomes infected easily, is present. There are always stretching and trauma of the base of the bladder during labor and delivery. This causes mucosal edema and hyperemia. There is also a temporary loss of bladder tone, owing to pressure and minor injury, that makes the mother less sensitive to bladder fullness and gives her an increased bladder capacity. This may result in overdistention of the bladder, in complete inability to void, or in residual urine, thus predisposing to cystitis. The urethra is also subject to trauma during delivery with the result that voiding may be difficult or impossible. Primiparas and women who have had operative deliveries usually have more difficulty in emptying their bladder than women who previously have borne children or whose labor has terminated spontaneously.

As a preventive measure against cystitis it is important to observe the mother closely for evidence of a full bladder or residual urine. The distended bladder sometimes may be palpated above the symphysis pubis, or the uterine fundus may be felt laterally, having been pushed aside by the full bladder. Some mothers complain of discomfort and constant desire to void, some void small amounts frequently, and others have neither discomfort nor desire to void. With residual urine the mother frequently voids in small amounts, and, in a number of cases, the residual urine may be of sufficient quantity to make the bladder easily palpable. Since the bladder is less sensitive after delivery than under normal conditions, the mother may retain an undue amount of urine without discomfort.

Catheterization is deferred until the mother has been given opportunity to void spontaneously. If it does become necessary to catheterize, the procedure must be done very carefully since the chances of introducing bacteria from the vulva are great. When a mother is unable to void, some physicians recommend that an indwelling catheter be left in the bladder to avoid catheterization every few hours. Others believe that the indwelling catheter is as irritating as frequent catheterization and that the mother will regain tone more quickly if the bladder is allowed to fill. When an indwelling catheter is used, the nurse must use all possible precautions against organisms ascending up the inside of the catheter or alongside it.

Cystitis, then, is caused by bladder trauma, stagnant residual urine, and bacteria that have gained entrance to the bladder. Symptoms usually begin several days post partum. These patients often have suprapubic or perineal discomfort, frequent and painful urination, or a feeling of not having emptied the bladder completely. The temperature may rise to 37.8° C (100° F) or even to 38.3° C (101° F). Microscopic examination of a catheterized specimen will show pus cells, bacteria, and often red blood cells.

Treatment consists of making certain that the bladder is emptied completely, forcing fluids, and administering drugs to cure the bacteriuria. A culture of the urine is taken to determine the causative organism, and an anti-

Table 25-3. Summary of Postpartum Complications, Preventive and Curative Nursing Management

Complication	*Preventive Care*	*Curative Care*
Hemorrhage		
Uterine atony	Identification of women at increased risk Prevent anemia with diet and supplemental iron Avoid prolonged labor Supportive care to facilitate relaxation Appropriate timing of analgesia/anesthesia Use of oxytocin augmentation Minimize anesthesia time Monitor consistency of uterus q 15 min during immediate postpartum hour Teach woman to palpate her uterus for firmness Monitor vital signs and amount of lochia	Type and cross-match blood for women at high risk Massage uterus to stimulate contractions Administer oxytocic drugs IM or IV IV fluids and blood as dictated by degree of blood loss Treat for shock as appropriate Prophylactic antibiotics Good nutrition with iron supplementation as needed
Lacerations	Minimize use of forceps Careful inspection of reproductive tract immediately after delivery Repair of lacerations Monitor vital signs and amount of lochia	Locate and repair lacerations Provide volume replacement as needed (blood and other fluids) Prophylactic antibiotics Good nutrition with iron as needed
Retained placenta	Do not "force" expulsion of placenta, but promptly deliver separated placenta Inspect placenta carefully for intactness Monitor vital signs and amount of lochia	Manual examination of uterine cavity Oxytocic drugs to contract uterus and expel fragments Provide volume replacement as needed Prophylactic antibiotics Good nutrition with iron as needed
Puerperal infection	Strict aseptic technique Treat antepartal infections Correct antepartal anemia Prevent undue fatigue during labor with fluid and calories as needed Prevent hemorrhage	Isolation from other maternity patients Good nutrition: high protein, high caloric, high vitamin Increase fluids to 3000–4000 ml/24 hr Monitor temperature and other vital signs q 4 hr or more frequently Provide environment for rest and sleep Appropriate analgesia Oxytocic drugs Fowler's position to enhance draining of lochia Antibiotics
Venous thrombosis	Identify women at increased risk Prevention or early treatment of predisposing factors (see text) Encourage early ambulation and/or in-bed exercise Provide support stockings	Bed rest Monitor vital signs Hot, moist packs to affected leg Elevate foot of bed Support stockings Keep bed covers off foot and leg for comfort Administer anti-inflammatory drugs and analgesics Anticoagulant therapy Monitor clotting time If breast-feeding and receiving COUMADIN derivatives, vitamin K to infant
Mastitis	Instruct women in cleansing of breast and nipples during pregnancy and puerperium Inspect breasts and instruct women in inspection of breasts for lumps and "hot spots" Prevent nipple fissures or treat at once with ointment Good supportive bra Empty breasts at each feeding	Support breast with bra or binder Apply ice to breasts Discard milk from infected breast *while temperature is elevated* Antibiotics Monitor vital signs Give analgesia as needed Encourage rest and good nutrition
Urinary tract infections	Antepartal screening for asymptomatic bacteriuria Teach women good personal hygiene Promote frequent urination during labor Observe postpartally for overdistention of bladder Use measures to encourage voiding such as getting up to go to the toilet, running water, applying pressure over symphysis, and so on *If* catherization is required, strict asepsis	Monitor temperature and other vital signs q 4 hr or more often Force fluids Ensure complete emptying of bladder with each voiding Record intake and output Urine culture Antibacterial drugs

bacterial drug specific for the organism is administered for a few days with excellent results.

Postpartum pyelitis may recur after a previous infection or first appear post partum. The onset of symptoms is usually about the third day post partum, but may occur as late as the twenty-first day. The most frequent complaints are pain in the flank, frequency of urination, dysuria, chills, and fever. Microscopic examination of the urine shows pus cells and bacteria, most commonly the colon bacilli. The symptoms are similar to those occurring in antepartum pyelitis but less severe.

Treatment consists of increased fluid intake, bland diet, rest in bed, and administration of an antibacterial drug. Cultures of the urine are taken every four to eight weeks posttherapy to determine that it has become free of bacteria.

A summary of the preventive and curative treatments for the most common postpartum complications is contained in Table 25–3.

SUBINVOLUTION

When the uterus does not return to its usual size and consistency as rapidly as is normal, the condition is termed subinvolution. The uterus is larger and softer than it should be for the particular postpartum period, and the lochia is more profuse and brighter red in color. This condition may be due to retention of placental fragments or a part of the fetal membranes, or it may be caused by an endometritis. Treatment consists of administration of ergonovine and antibiotics or curettage as dictated by the patient's status.

MENTAL DISTURBANCES

Psychotic complications of pregnancy and the puerperium are relatively uncommon. They most frequently occur in women who have a history of previous psychiatric episodes. It is believed that pregnancy is merely the nonspecific precipitating crisis that triggers their illness.

Neurosis, on the other hand, is a relatively frequent accompaniment to the postpartum period. Some studies have indicated that as many as 25 percent of women experience "nervous symptoms" during the postpartum year. Undoubtedly many of these symptoms are regarded merely as idiosyncratic behavior by the woman and her family and do not appreciably disrupt their living patterns.

Perhaps as many as 4 or 5 percent of women experience a reaction strong enough to require psychiatric intervention. Depression is the most common manifestation of these neuroses, although it may take the form of anxiety states, phobias, obsessions, hypochondriasis, or other symptoms.

It is speculated that neurosis develops either as a reaction to the immediate circumstances of the new infant and family responsibilities, or that childbirth has brought to the surface deep-seated conflicts regarding the woman's own femininity and general self-concept. Symptoms rarely occur before one or two weeks post partum when the mother is home and the full weight of her new responsibilities has been felt. Women who are single and/or separated from their families are affected more frequently, suggesting the enormous importance of supportive significant others.

In situations where there is a solid family structure to initiate the woman into motherhood and give support to her and the new father as well as older siblings, this transition is likely to be easier. Such structures exist in diminishing numbers, however. For most women, the practice of limiting postpartum follow-up to a pelvic examination at six weeks after delivery is a disservice. In that period of time maladaptive behaviors can be well established.

Nurses who work with childbearing women should be alert for signs that the pregnancy or the infant is not being accepted. In addition, efforts should be made to assess the available support systems for each woman and to help her identify persons or agencies to whom she can turn for help. Facilitating good mental health is as important as preventing physical complications of pregnancy and the puerperium.

REFERENCES AND SUGGESTED READINGS

Eschenbach, D. A., and Wager, G. P., Puerperal infections, *Clin. Obstet. Gynecol.,* 23(4):1003–1037, 1980.

Herbert, W. N., Complications of the immediate puerperium, *Clin. Obstet. Gynecol.,* 25(1):219–232, 1982.

Lee, S. P. Postpartum emotional disorders, *Am. Fam. Physician,* 26(2):197–201, 1982.

Mercer, R. T., When the mother experiences a threat to her health. In Mercer, R. T., *Nursing care for parents at risk, C. B. Slack,* Thorofare, N. J., 1977, pp. 77–99.

Pritchard, J. A., and MacDonald, P. C., *Williams Obstetrics.* 16th ed. Appleton-Century-Crofts, N.Y., 1980.

Tentoni, S. C., and High, K. A., Culturally induced postpartum depression, *JOGN Nurs.,* 9(4):246–249, 1980.

PART FIVE

The Newborn

CHAPTER

26

Characteristics of the Normal Newborn

THE NURSE CARING for newborns needs an understanding of the infant's development at birth, the many adaptive changes that he must of necessity make to adjust to extrauterine life, and his needs during the adjustment period. The characteristics and physiology of newborns, mature and immature, and those born with deviations from normal intrauterine growth will be described in the following chapters. Insofar as feasible, the nurse's functions in the care of these infants will be described, but the nurse must determine the details of nursing care for the individual newborn through an evaluation of his specific needs.

BIOLOGIC ADJUSTMENTS IN THE NEONATAL PERIOD

The first four-week period after birth usually is designated as the *neonatal,* or newborn, period, although its chief characteristics pertain to the first two weeks of postnatal life. During this period the infant makes the physiologic adjustments necessary for the change from intrauterine to extrauterine life. The most drastic changes occur at the moment of birth, and many other important ones take place during the first day or two of life. Then adjustments continue at a somewhat slower rate, mostly during the first two weeks, but some are not complete for a month or more. The greatest mortality rate of any period in infancy and childhood occurs during the neonatal period. The incidence of morbidity is also high, especially during the first few days. In recognition of the unique dangers inherent in the first four weeks of life, students of obstetrics and pediatrics, of growth and development, and of biostatistics give them separate and important consideration.

At the time of birth an infant makes the most abrupt and complete changes in the environment and physiologic functions that he will make in his entire life. In a favorable intrauterine environment the fetus is supplied with the necessities for his development and survival. The fetus is kept at an optimal and even temperature and is protected from exertion and injury. At birth the fetus suddenly emerges from a very protective environment into one that is vastly different. The newborn must begin life immediately as an independent being who needs first and foremost to establish pulmonary ventilation and marked circulatory changes.

Many adaptive changes are necessary to extrauterine life, but those of the respiratory and circulatory systems are of first importance and must be rapid and radical.

Changes in function of all other body systems then can be established more slowly.

The hazards that the newborn may be presented with at birth and during the adjustment to extrauterine life must be anticipated and minimized if optimum possibilities are to be realized. Care must be directed toward providing the newborn with conditions that are most favorable to normal function, with minimal stress.

THE RESPIRATORY SYSTEM

The respiratory system must function immediately after birth if life is to be maintained. Loss of the placenta, through which gas exchange has taken place until birth, necessitates immediate and radical changes to permit the lungs to take over this function. Pulmonary ventilation must begin immediately after birth, and a marked increase in pulmonary circulation also must take place quickly.

Adequate maturation of the lungs is essential to extrauterine life. Of all the body organs, the stage of maturation of the lungs at birth is most crucial, since viability is not possible until the lungs are structurally developed to a degree of maturity sufficient to permit maintenance of good lung expansion and adequate exchange of gases. Development of the lungs rarely reaches an adequacy that will permit sufficient function to sustain life before the fetus is at least 26 weeks gestational age.

Structural Development of the Lungs

Structurally the lungs are in a continuous stage of development during fetal life and into childhood. Bronchi and canals first appear, and thereafter the potential air spaces develop. These air spaces, which eventually become alveoli, begin as small buds off the bronchi, grow in size, and later begin indentations and a thinning of their walls. During this progressive development of air spaces, the vascular portion of the lungs also develops more completely, with an ever-increasing number of capillaries extending toward and coming into close contact with the air spaces.

Beginning with the twenty-fourth week of fetal life, the air spaces of the lungs, the terminal air sacs, appear as saccules. As the saccules continue to develop, their membranes become thinner, and blood vessels grow closer to the membranes. By the twenty-sixth week of fetal life the thinness of the saccular membranes and the nearness of the blood vessels may be sufficient to maintain life if the fetus is born at this time. Until then the lung capillaries and the saccular membrane are not developed for sufficient exchange of gas. Up to the thirtieth week the fetal lung remains structurally immature, and there is little or no reserve for maintenance of extrauterine life if any condition develops that reduces optimum function. Beginning with the thirtieth week the reserve is better and the infant is able to increase ventilation to some extent should it become necessary.

Between the thirtieth and thirty-sixth weeks of fetal life, the saccules of the lung become increasingly indented, changing in structure from saccules to alveoli. The enlarging surface area of the air spaces, resulting from indentation, and the increase in number of blood vessels close to the alveoli give the lung more reserve and increases an infant's ability to maintain extrauterine life.

After the thirty-sixth week of fetal life, the air spaces of the lungs are true alveoli, and the lungs of an infant born at this time are structurally ready to function as well as those of a full-term infant. Lung development continues after birth, with alveoli increasing in number up to the age of eight years. Only one eighth to one sixth of the adult number of alveoli are present at birth, but the capacity for pulmonary gas exchange is very adequate in relation to body weight.

Lung Fluid

The fetal lung produces a considerable amount of fluid during the latter half of intrauterine development. This secretion is produced continuously and fills the fetal lung with fluid, partially expanding the air spaces. In addition, some of the fluid drains out of the lung into the amniotic fluid and some is swallowed. From 80 to 110 ml of fluid are present in the respiratory passages of a normal-term fetus at birth. This must be removed to provide for adequate movement of air in and out of the lungs. Some of the lung fluid, approximately one third, is squeezed out of the lungs during normal birth as the infant's chest is compressed in the passage through the birth canal. When the chest walls return to their normal position with release from the birth canal, their recoil draws air into the lungs to replace the fluid that was squeezed out. The remainder of the fluid is drawn back into the lungs with the first breath and is then absorbed into the bloodstream through the pulmonary capillaries and the pulmonary lymphatics. It is not known how quickly the fluid in the alveoli is absorbed, but under normal circumstances it is probably rapid. In a full-term, healthy infant the lungs may be cleared by the time the infant has taken a few breaths, or at least within the first hour after birth.

Infants who are immature and those who have had a complicated antenatal or delivery course may have a delay in clearing of their lung fluid. An immature infant does not have the lymphatics developed as well as a full-term infant and thus may have a decreased rate of fluid absorption from the lungs. Sometimes the birth process does not compress the chest walls and very little or no fluid is pushed out of the lungs. This is likely in delivery of a very small fetus through the birth canal and in birth by cesarean section. If the infant is asphyxiated at birth, having poor lung expansion, the pulmonary vascular resistance may be high, resulting in a decreased volume of blood flowing through the lungs and a delay in removal of fluid.

Pulmonary Surfactant

A surface-active material, called pulmonary surfactant, normally lines the alveoli of the lungs. Surfactant has the properties of changing surface tension as the surface area changes and of achieving a very low surface tension when the surface area becomes small. Surface tension between any two moist surfaces is normally strong and would be high between the moist alveolar surfaces without the presence of this surface tension–reducing material. For effective respiratory function in the newborn, it is thus essential not only that the potential air spaces of the lungs are developed to the stage at which inflation is possible, but also that the surface-active alveolar lining has been produced.

Surfactant is a substance produced by the alveolar lining cells of adults and infants and is secreted out onto the surface of the alveoli, forming a lining film. It is a complex of proteins and lipids, a lipoprotein, of which lecithin, a very important natural emulsifying agent, is a significant surface-active component. The time of appearance of surfactant in the fetal lung is somewhat uncertain, but it is probably present to some degree beginning at about the twenty-third week of development and perhaps sooner. Thereafter it is produced in increasing quantity and is usually present in sufficient amount for adequate lung function by the thirtieth week and in some infants enough may be present earlier. Around 35 weeks there is a surge in production of the major surfactant, lecithin, and an increase in its activity and stability.

See pages 247–48 for discussion of lecithin/sphingomyelin (L/S) ratio, where production of surfactant in the fetal lungs and measurement of its presence are described. Surfactant production sometimes can be stimulated and thus lung maturation accelerated by administration of corticosteroids to the mother if there is reason for concern of an early birth.

Pulmonary surfactant, owing to its property of reducing the cohesive force between the moist surfaces of the alveoli, is necessary to maintenance of good lung expansion. An absence or a deficiency in this surface-active film causes the surface tension at the air-fluid interface in the alveoli to be high and to become even higher as they retract during expiration. The result of this increasing surface tension is considerable retraction of the alveoli with each expiration. Such retraction greatly reduces the residual air that ordinarily is retained in the lungs at the end of expiration, and the lungs collapse more than they normally should with each expiration. This then requires greater than normal effort with the next inspiration in order to again fill the lungs, and each breath may require as much effort as the first breath of life.

Pulmonary surfactant not only has the property of achieving a low surface tension as the alveolar surfaces come closer together during expiration, but also of creating a constantly changing surface tension in each alveolus as its area changes. This has the effect of equalizing the pressure in alveoli of various sizes and preventing flow of air from one alveolus into another. It thereby prevents collapse of some alveoli and overdistention of others (Fig. 26–1).

Without surfactant and under the usual forces of surface tension, the collapsing force of the air and fluid interface in small alveoli is greater than in large ones. The collapsing force in the curved moist alveoli is determined by their size. Without surfactant this collapsing pressure increases as the radius of the curved surface decreases. A small alveolus with half the radius of a large one will have twice as much collapsing pressure in it as the large

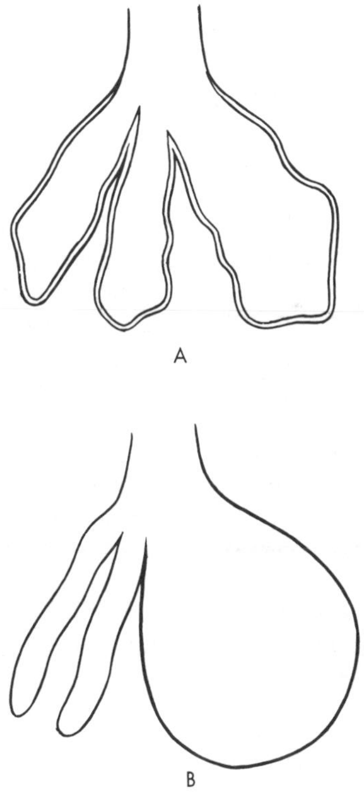

Figure 26–1. *A.* An alveolar lining film of a surface-active material, called pulmonary surfactant, is present. This keeps the surface tension in different-sized alveoli equal and prevents passage of air from a small alveolus to a larger interconnected alveolus. *B.* Without surfactant, the smaller alveoli, with the largest collapsing pressure, have emptied into the larger alveolus, which had a lower collapsing pressure, causing it to become over-distended. The result is atelectasis due to collapsed alveoli and interconnected overdistended ones.

one. When two or more alveoli are interconnected, the smaller alveolus with the largest collapsing pressure is likely to empty into the larger alveolus, which has a lower collapsing pressure. The small alveolus will then collapse and the large alveolus will become distended (Fig. 26–1). With inhalations the large alveoli may receive some of the air that might have entered the small alveoli if they were not collapsed. The result of this process is areas of atelectasis caused by collapsed alveoli and other areas of distended alveoli.

Surfactant has the property of bringing about a rapid variation in surface tension as the surface area changes. Specifically, it produces a decreasing surface tension as an area becomes smaller and an increasing surface tension as an area becomes larger. With a pulmonary surfactant film, as the surface area of an alveolus becomes smaller during expiration and the surfactant is compressed, it becomes more active and reduces the surface tension in the alveolus to a very low level. Then as the area of the alveolus becomes larger with expansion on inspiration and the surfactant is stretched, the surface tension in the alveolus becomes higher. Such increased surface tension tends to limit the extent to which alveoli become inflated, enhances their recoil, and prevents their overdistention. Owing to these changes in surface tension, brought about by pulmonary surfactant, the small alveoli, in which the film has produced a very low surface tension, will not deflate into the larger ones, where the surface-active film has caused the surface tension to be higher, and the alveoli will not completely collapse as they become very small on expiration.

In summary, pulmonary surfactant acts to stabilize respirations and to prevent atelectasis. This lining, which has the property of achieving a very low surface tension when compressed, prevents complete collapse of the alveoli with each expiration. Some residual air is then retained in the lungs at the end of expiration and they do not need to be reopened with each new breath. The property of surfactant to change surface tension as the area changes, creating very low surface tension in small alveoli and higher surface tension in larger alveoli, keeps the pressure in alveoli of different sizes equal. This averts passage of air from small to large alveoli and thereby prevents collapse of some alveoli and overdistention of others.

Fetal Breathing Movements

Fetal breathing movements *in utero* have been reported from time to time over the past 90 years, but most often they were disregarded or explained on the basis of some unusual stimulus. In the past it was felt that respiratory-like movements did not appear to be present to prepare the respiratory system for function after birth. However, there is now reason to know that the respiratory system does have practice before it must suddenly begin to function with considerable competence.

With the use of ultrasound equipment, fetal breathing movements can be observed. These movements have been detected as early as 11 weeks' gestation, but until the twentieth week they are very irregular; thereafter, the movements appear with more consistency.

The early movements are weak, episodic, and irregular and vary in depth and in rate from 30 to 90 times per minute. By 34 weeks' gestation the pattern of intrauterine respiratory movements has become regular, slower, more even, and the rate varies from 40 to 60 times per minute. Movement involves both the diaphragm and the intercostal muscles. Occasionally fetal respiratory movements are seen through the mother's abdominal wall.

Hypoglycemia and mild hypoxia will diminish or abolish fetal respiratory movements. Hypercapnia increases the movements. Gasping may occur in the fetus, especially during severe hypoxia and acidosis, and may cause the fetus, or the infant at the time of birth, to aspirate amniotic fluid.

Detection of normal intrauterine respiratory movements can be used as a valuable aid in determining the well-being of the fetus. Being unable to detect normal respiratory movements is not of equal value in diagnosis of fetal distress.

Respirations

Onset of breathing at birth is a continuation of previous breathing movements, with the addition of movement of air in and out of the lungs and exchange of gases in the lungs.

The exact mechanism by which onset of respiration is initiated is not certain. Sensory stimuli and chemical changes appear to exert an influence. It appears that the asphyxia normally present to varying degrees in all infants at birth is very important in initiation of the first breath in infants free of organic or physiologic dysfunction. Chemical changes in the blood—a lowered oxygen level, an increase in the carbon dioxide level, and a lowered pH—resulting from a brief period of asphyxia during delivery stimulate the respiratory center. However, if breathing is delayed for some reason, the asphyxia increases and may then depress instead of stimulate the respiratory center and resuscitation may be necessary. Also, the physical stimulation of the birth process and sudden change in the infant's environment (cold, touch, noise, pain, lights) may offer a stimulus to take the first breath. Boddy and Dawes say that if it is accepted that fetal breathing movements are normally present, an important question now is why breathing becomes continuous postnatally instead of remaining episodic as before birth.[1]

[1] K. Boddy and G. S. Dawes, Fetal breathing, *Br. Med. Bull,* 31:3–7, (Jan.) 1975.

A normal healthy infant, who is not depressed by medications administered to the mother or by the process of delivery, will have respiration established within one minute after birth, often taking the first breath within a few seconds after birth. A lusty cry usually accompanies establishment of respiration. The infant's first breath may require forceful contraction of the inspiratory muscles, mainly of the diaphragm, to overcome the fluid in the airways and the surface tension in the alveoli. Aeration of the lungs is rapid, however, occurring largely with the first breath, and continuing respiratory effort is normally not great.

The infant who begins to breathe normally immediately after birth will quickly overcome the effects of the transient asphyxia that normally develops during the birth process. With good oxygenation and excretion of carbon dioxide through the lungs, the oxygen tension rapidly rises to normal, the carbon dioxide tension quickly decreases, and the acid-base balance returns to relatively normal limits in the first hours of life. A delay in return to normal values is likely if the infant is asphyxiated at birth or becomes chilled after birth.

Respirations in the newborn should be quiet, accompanied by neither dyspnea nor cyanosis. The color of the infant's body is somewhat cyanotic at birth, but normally it becomes pink within a few minutes and remains so. Cyanosis of the hands and feet, and circumoral cyanosis, may persist for an hour or two, but thereafter these parts of the body also should be pink. Sluggish peripheral circulation or low body temperature may account for these areas of cyanosis.

The average respiratory rate is approximately 40 per minute. Breathing of the normal infant is regular in rhythm and without chest retraction, although the newborn on occasion normally may have short periods of irregularity in rhythm, momentary periods of apnea, and slight signs of chest retraction. Periodic breathing is common in prematures. A rate increase to over 60 or a decrease below 30 per minute may be serious, especially in the presence of other difficulty. Rate and rhythm of respirations normally are altered easily by stimuli and may vary with activity. Normal variations in respiratory function in the early hours of life are described on pages 547 and 548.

Respiratory movements of the newborn are carried out by the diaphragm and the abdominal muscles. There is very little thoracic movement. Pressure against the diaphragm from abdominal organs, especially if the infant has been placed in a position with the head and shoulders lower than the rest of the body, may limit excursion and cause the respirations to be shallow and rapid. If such positioning is used for drainage of mucus, careful observation is necessary to note if it interferes with the infant's respiratory movements and then to find the position of easiest respirations.

A newborn may have mucus in the nose, mouth, and oropharynx and may spit up or vomit stomach contents during the early hours of postnatal life. This mucus or fluid may cause episodes of gagging and occasionally choking, and the infant may need assistance to clear the respiratory tract.

Mucus is cleared from the infant's upper respiratory tract by suction. A soft bulb syringe removes mucus from the mouth effectively. When the mucus is far back, suction on a catheter may be indicated, since the catheter can be placed farther back in the throat than the bulb syringe. Deep suction, however, should be avoided, especially in the first five minutes of life because of vagal stimulation possibly causing cardiac arrhythmia. The mouth always must be cleared first, as stimulation of the nares may cause a reflex gasp and aspiration of oropharyngeal contents.

The Nose

The newborn's nose is small, shallow, and narrow; the openings into the nasal cavity are small. A delicate nasal mucous membrane causes the infant to sneeze vigorously and frequently, which helps to clear the tiny passages. Clear nasal passages are very important to the newborn because he normally breathes through the nose. Breathing through the mouth is very difficult for an infant, and nasal obstruction will cause considerable distress.

THE CIRCULATORY SYSTEM

At birth, when the placental circulation ceases and the infant's oxygen and carbon dioxide exchange must take place through the lungs, the pattern of circulation must change from a fetal to an adult type. Shifts in the circulatory system include a manyfold increase in pulmonary circulation, cessation of blood flow through the umbilical vessels and the placenta, and closure of the ductus arteriosus, the foramen ovale, and the ductus venosus. With cessation of the placental circulation, about 100 cm (40 in.) of low-resistance vascular channels are removed. Elimination of this low-resistance circuit causes a marked rise in the systemic vascular resistance. This rise takes place at the same time that the pulmonary vascular resistance is dropping. This results in orientation of pressure and pathways of circulation to the adult type. A review of fetal circulation, described on pages 107–109, may be helpful before study of changes in circulation at birth.

Changes in the circulatory system occur abruptly at birth, but all are not immediately complete. There is a short period of time, up to a day or two after birth, during which a small amount of blood may continue to flow through the ductus arteriosus and the foramen ovale, or, if these vessels have closed, they can reopen during this period, reversing some of the changes previously made. Since the circulation during this time of conversion from a fetal to an adult circulation has characteristics that are peculiar to it alone, being neither a fetal nor an adult pattern, it may be called a period of *transitional circulation*. The transition to an adult pattern of circulation in the normal-term infant is usually complete in a few days, when functional closure of the fetal structures becomes quite effective. Anatomic occlusion of fetal vessels is not complete for weeks or months, but functional closure is adequate to produce the necessary changes.

Changes in Pulmonary Blood Flow and Closure of the Ductus Arteriosus

It will be recalled that in fetal circulation a vessel termed the ductus arteriosus connects the pulmonary artery to the aorta (Fig. 6–11, page 109). Before birth, only about 10 percent of the blood that flows into the pulmonary artery passes through the lungs; the remainder bypasses the lungs by flowing into the ductus arteriosus and then directly into the aorta. Immediately after birth, when gas exchange must take place through the lungs, a great increase in pulmonary blood flow becomes essential. A marked alteration in circulation is brought about quickly *through changes in the lungs themselves,* in which resistance to blood flow is markedly lowered when the blood vessels dilate with aeration, and *through constriction of the ductus ateriosus.* With these changes all of the blood pumped into the pulmonary artery very soon will be conveyed to the lungs for exchange of gases instead of being shunted in considerable amount through the ductus arteriosus.

The ductus arteriosus constricts within a few minutes after birth, but functional closure is not immediately complete and a very small amount of blood may normally flow through this vessel for a few hours or a few days. This shunting of blood may follow the fetal pattern (from pulmonary artery to aorta) or it may take place in the opposite direction. Since the vessel is patent, blood flow from the aorta to the pulmonary artery (the reverse of fetal circulation) is temporarily possible. This takes place while the resistances of the pulmonary and systemic circulations are in transition. Shunting thus may take place in either direction, or at times it may be in both directions. With good ventilation, normal blood oxygen tension, and normal pH, the ductus arteriosus continues to constrict and shunting soon ceases.

Normal progression of the circulatory changes following birth may be slowed or interrupted by asphyxia and by alterations in normal acid-base balance. The ductus arteriosus responds to hypoxia and a reduced blood oxygen tension with a delay in closure, or a reopening of the vessel if it has already constricted. The pulmonary blood vessels are sensitive to changes in alveolar or arterial oxygen and carbon dioxide tension and to acidosis, but in contrast to the ductus arteriosus they are likely to constrict with a lowered blood Po_2 and pH. Constriction of the vessels reduces the pulmonary blood flow and the possibility of good gas exchange. A return to some of the features of a fetal type of circulation—increased pulmonary vascular resistance, decreased blood flow through the lungs, and consequently considerable shunting of blood from the pulmonary artery through the ductus arteriosus—may reach a dangerous degree and make oxygenation difficult. The respiratory and circulatory systems are associated so intimately in function that a deficiency in the function of one readily interferes with good function of the other.

Closure of the Foramen Ovale

The foramen ovale, the direct opening between the right and left atria of the heart, closes quickly after birth, but, similar to the ductus arteriosus, some shunting of blood may occur for the first few hours or few days. Closure of the foramen ovale is largely caused by pressure changes in the atria. Pressure in the left atrium is raised when the marked increase in pulmonary blood flow after birth brings about a large increase in venous return to the left atrium, and a rise in systemic resistance is brought about by cessation of placental circulation.

Pressure in the right atrium is lowered after birth. Aeration of the lungs decreases the pulmonary resistance and thus the pressure in the right atrium, and removal of the placental circulation decreases the amount of blood flowing through the inferior vena cava to the right atrium. With these changes in atrial pressures, the pressure in the left atrium is greater than that in the right and the valve over the foramen ovale closes. Blood that formerly passed from the right to the left atrium, through the foramen ovale (Fig. 6–11, page 109), now moves into the right ventricle, and from there to the lungs to be aerated.

If at any time during the transitional period of circulatory adjustment the right atrial pressure is raised or the left atrial pressure falls, there may be some reopening of the foramen ovale and a shunting of blood from right to left atrium. A small shunt may persist for a few hours or a day after birth without significant consequences. Greater shunting reduces effective cardiac function and oxygenation of blood. Asphyxia may cause a serious right-to-left shunt which may appear together with a shunt through the ductus arteriosus.

The Placenta, Umbilical Cord Vessels, and Ductus Venosus

Circulation through the placenta usually is interrupted by clamping the umbilical cord, but even without clamping this circulation would soon stop. The umbilical vessels constrict very soon after birth and the cord ceases to pulsate in five to ten minutes. The ductus venosus, the connecting vessel between the umbilical vein and the inferior vena cava, is sealed off after birth by the closing of a sphincter at the umbilical end. Although these vessels are constricted soon after birth, the umbilical vessels and ductus venosus are sufficiently patent for the first four to five days to permit insertion of a small polyethylene tube when this may become necessary for treatments such as infusion of fluids, frequent sampling of blood gases, and exchange blood transfusion. Final anatomic closure of these vessels occurs some days or weeks after birth.

The blood flow between the placenta and the infant reaches an equilibrium when a few minutes elapse between birth and the clamping of the umbilical cord or, if clamping is delayed, until pulsation of the cord has ceased. If the cord is clamped before the equilibrium, the blood volume of the infant will be increased or decreased depending upon the amount of blood that is in the infant and in the placenta at the moment of clamping. The infant's blood volume is increased by 30 to 50 ml, and the number of red blood cells are increased if the infant is held lower than the placenta before the cord is clamped. At present it is not certain if there is any value to the infant in an increased amount of blood, or if he may be at a disadvantage with an additional amount. Owing to the low-resistance placental reservoir, absorption of lung water by the pulmonary veins is enhanced if cord clamping can be delayed until the infant has taken the first breath.

Peripheral Circulation

The peripheral circulation of the newborn is somewhat sluggish. The hands and feet therefore may be somewhat cyanotic for an hour or two after birth. Peripheral circulation is often not sufficient to keep the infant's hands and feet as warm as the rest of the body, and circulatory instability may cause the skin to have a mottled appearance when exposed to air.

Heart

An infant's heart is relatively large at birth, is higher in the chest, and is in a more horizontal position than it is later in life. Its rate of growth slows after birth.

Transitory heart murmurs, which disappear in a few days and usually do not have pathologic significance, are heard in some newborn infants. Some of these murmurs are evidence of delayed closure of the fetal openings which ceased functioning at birth, the murmur being caused by leakage of blood through channels that have not yet been completely obliterated. Conversely, significant murmurs may not be present immediately after birth.

Variability in pulse rate is characteristic of the newborn. The pulse rate is affected by stimuli and is therefore under less environmental influence when counted during sleep. It is usually rapid, with an average of 120 to 140 beats per minute. It may increase to 180 beats per minute with crying or other activity and may drop to between 80 and 90 during sleep. Irregularity of rhythm of the pulse may follow the same pattern as that of the respiratory system—when the respirations are slow, the pulse may be slow, and when the respirations become rapid, the pulse also may become rapid. However, a persistent rate above 160 or below 110 may be indicative of problems.

Blood Pressure

Until recent development of an ultrasonic technique, blood pressure in the newborn was measured by an auscultation, palpation, or color change (flush) method. These methods are somewhat difficult to use in the newborn and are not precise. The conventional auscultation method is unreliable because the arteries of small infants seldom produce audible Korotkoff sounds, and the palpation and flush methods are only estimates of when the arterial walls open. The newer ultrasound (Doppler) method detects systole and diastole accurately, is more reliable, and is as simple to use as the conventional method with the stethoscope. It can detect very weak impulses and pick up sounds where the sphygmomanometer is unable to detect any blood flow. One other method of obtaining blood pressure measurements is by direct recording through an arterial catheter; this may be used in conditions in which an infant's illness requires an arterial catheter to be in place for checking of blood gases or for therapy. Good correlation has been shown between pressures obtained by the Doppler method and by intraarterial catheter.

With the Doppler ultrasonic-sphygmomanometer method the sphygmomanometer cuff is wrapped snugly around the limb and held in place by a strip of adhesive tape. The transducer, a substitute for the stethoscope, is placed under the cuff and applied to the skin directly over the brachial or popliteal artery where the Doppler signal is heard most clearly in the headphones. This sensor emits ultrasonic pulses when the arterial wall opens or closes under the inflated cuff. It yields Doppler shift signals that are converted to sound. With the cuff and transducer in position, the cuff is inflated to 20 to 30 mm Hg above the expected systolic pressure and then slowly deflated. The systolic pressure is heard when the cuff is sufficiently deflated to permit motion of the arterial wall. Between the systolic and diastolic pressures two signals, produced by the pulsating artery, are heard per cardiac cycle. At the diastolic pressure these signals merge and are heard as a change from a loud, sharp sound to a softer, muffled sound. Recognition of the sound changes at the diastolic pressure may be difficult. Frequently only the systolic pressure is read and recorded on neonates.

If the Doppler method of measuring blood pressure is not available, the color change (flush) method may be used. With the flush method the cuff is wrapped around an extremity either just above the wrist or just above the ankle, the extremity below the cuff is squeezed to blanch the distal area, the manometer is pumped to 120 to 140 mm Hg, and the manometer gauge is then allowed to fall 5 mm Hg/second, allowing perfusion of the extremity to take place. The pressure reading is noted at the time the extremity flushes, and the reading is recorded as the approximate mean diastolic-systolic pressure. If the reading is above 60 mm Hg or below 30, the procedure is repeated on a different extremity to rule out error or confirm finding.

For measurement of blood pressure the infant should be quiet, since activity will raise the blood pressure, and the cuff must be of proper size, covering about two thirds of the upper arm, or two thirds of the thigh if the latter is used as the site of measurement, and the bladder of the cuff should encircle the arm or leg completely. The pressure should be obtained at about heart level.

An infant's normal blood pressure varies somewhat with size and age. For example, the infant weighing under 2000 gm (4 lb, 7 oz) normally has a somewhat lower blood pressure than the over 3000-gm (6 lb, 10 oz) infant. An infant 10 days old normally has a higher blood pressure than he had at birth. Also the blood pressure is somewhat higher in the popliteal artery than in the brachial artery.

One of the general guidelines for recognizing hypotension is as follows:

- Full-term infants with systolic blood pressure less than 55
- Large preterm infants with systolic blood pressure less than 50
- Infants with systolic blood pressure less than 40[2]

A relatively recent study by investigators from the Cardiovascular Research Institute at the University of California at San Francisco resulted in some new standards for the first 12 hours of life. These values are as follows:

1. The lower limits of systolic blood pressure for an infant with a birthweight of 750 grams = 34 mm Hg.
2. The lower limit of systolic blood pressure for an infant with a birthweight of 1500 gm = 40 mm Hg.
3. The lower limits of systolic blood pressure for an infant with a birthweight of 3000 gm = 51 mm Hg.[3]

These values are somewhat lower than previously published, but the authors feel that they are more directly and accurately obtained figures. It should be pointed out that the blood pressure values are only for the first 12 hours of life.

BODY TEMPERATURE AND HEAT PRODUCTION

The growing fetus produces heat that must be dissipated. Under normal conditions the temperature of the fetus is approximately 0.5° C (0.9° F) above that of the mother, and the fetus gives up heat to the mother to maintain a steady body temperature. Most of this heat exchange takes place between fetal and maternal blood via the placenta. Some heat also may be conducted to the amniotic fluid and to surrounding maternal tissues. Although an infant's body temperature at birth is 0.5° C higher than the mother's, under the usual environmental conditions in the delivery room his body temperature may fall quickly after birth unless special precautions are taken to protect against heat loss. These precautions include providing the infant with a thermal environment that prevents heat loss from the body, conserving physical energy expenditures needed to maintain warmth, and avoiding the serious effects of the increase in metabolism that becomes necessary when the body must produce a large amount of heat. The premature or small infant is in greater danger of the potential consequences of cooling than is the full-term, normal-size infant.

Loss of Body Heat

The newborn infant loses body heat by evaporation, conduction, convection, and radiation. *Evaporation* can account for a large heat loss immediately after birth, when the infant's entire body is wet with amniotic fluid. Evaporation of this moisture removes heat from the body and rapidly lowers the temperature. In addition to evaporation, the infant may lose body heat to the cool environment of the delivery room by convection, conduction, and radiation, as described below (Fig. 26-2).

Unless the infant is adequately protected, the body temperature may fall to 94° F (34.4° C) or even as low as 92° F (33.3° C) as the amniotic fluid evaporates and heat is lost to the cool room. The skin temperature falls more rapidly than the deep body temperature (core temperature, ascertained by taking a rectal temperature), and may drop to 93° F (33.9° C) or 92° F (33.3° C) in 15 minutes. As heat from the inner body is conducted to the outside, the core temperature also falls but at a somewhat slower rate than the skin temperature. Immediately after birth, the skin temperature can fall as much as 0.5° F (0.3° C) per minute, especially in the

[2] Nancy Haddock, Blood pressure monitoring in neonates, *MCN*, 5:131–35, (Mar./Apr.) 1980.

[3] Hans T. Uersmold *et al.*, Aortic blood pressure during the first 12 hours of life in infants with birth weight 610 to 4220 grams. *Pediatrics*, 67:607, (May) 1981.

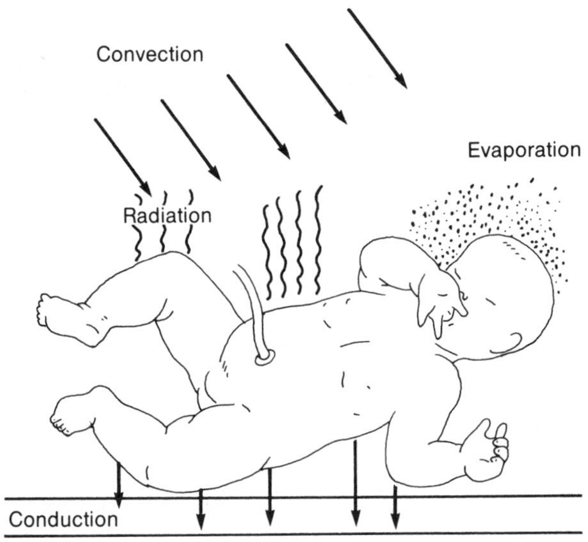

Figure 26–2. Four ways in which the newborn can lose body heat. Convection—movement of body heat to flow of cool air. Evaporation—heat loss as water vaporizes from skin and from lungs. Conduction—direct transfer of heat to surface on which the infant is lying. Radiation—heat loss from infant's body to cooler, more distant objects in room.

premature, and the body temperature as much as 0.3° F (0.1° C) per minute. The calculated heat loss with such a temperature drop is approximately 100 calories per pound per minute. Considering that an ounce of milk provides 20 calories, a loss of each 100 calories is equivalent to the calories that would be provided by 5 oz of milk.

The fall in body temperature at birth indicates that the infant's heat production is not sufficient to make up for heat loss in the immediate period after birth. The infant's heat production will quickly increase upon exposure to cold, but it may take many hours before the body temperature returns to normal unless the infant's heat loss is halted and he is placed in a heat-retaining environment.

Heat loss by ways other than evaporation must be considered both in the immediate period in the delivery room and also at a later time in the nursery. Since heat is transferred from one object to another, flowing from a warm body to a cooler one, the infant may lose heat by *convection* to the cool air in the delivery room and by *conduction* to the cool sheet or blanket on which the infant may be placed for clamping of the umbilical cord, stimulation of breathing, and sometimes identification and eye care. This heat loss is also significant if the infant is placed into blankets or an incubator that has not previously been warmed. When clothing and blankets are cool, heat will flow from the infant's body to the cool sheets or clothing, warming them.

As soon as the infant is dressed and placed into a warm nursery or into an incubator that is warm, heat loss by convection and conduction may become negligible. Clothing and covers help to insulate the infant and warm dry surfaces will not conduct heat away from the body.

Loss of body heat by *radiation* may account for a considerable amount of an infant's total heat loss. While loss of heat by convection is to the surrounding air and loss by conduction is through transfer of heat directly to the material touching the infant, radiation loss is to solid objects at a greater distance. Radiant heat given off by the infant's warm body travels through the air to the cooler objects in the room, where it is absorbed (Fig. 26–2). Radiant heat loss may continue during the days following birth, especially from an unclothed infant in an incubator. An incubator alone does not necessarily provide a constant thermal environment.

An infant's body temperature will vary in an incubator which is maintained at a constant temperature as conditions outside the incubator change, or if the temperature does not change, the infant is changing his metabolism for production of heat. When a window or an outside wall of a nursery becomes cooled at night, the infant's temperature will either drop or heat production must be greatly accelerated to maintain a normal temperature. The infant radiates heat from the body, through the air in the incubator, to the walls of the incubator, which are profoundly affected by the temperature of the windows or walls of the nursery. A warm incubator will provide comfort to the infant, but it does not protect him against variations in the environment outside the incubator.

An infant's temperature may rise to above normal when a source of heat in close proximity to the incubator, such as a radiator or sunshine through a window, warms the environment considerably. It may be necessary to move the incubator from such a source of radiant heat or to lower the incubator temperature to prevent overheating the infant.

Production of Body Heat

The newborn is capable of increasing heat production a considerable amount when he is cool and is thereby able to compensate for some or all of the heat loss from the body. An infant is able to generate heat (1) by shivering, (2) by metabolism of brown fat, and (3) by increasing the general metabolism. An infant with hypoxia or increased P_{CO_2} or under the influence of drugs will encounter difficulty in regenerating body heat (Table 26–1).

An immediate way of generating heat is by *shivering,* and a newborn quickly can begin to increase heat production in this way. He shivers when he is cold. An infant's shivering may not be as apparent as shivering is in an adult, but increased muscular activity, restlessness, crying, and at times intermittent shivering may be noticeable. A large infant is better able to produce heat

Table 26-1. Processes of Heat Control in the Newborn*

Mechanisms of Heat Loss	*Prevention of Heat Loss*
Evaporation—of moisture on body	Quickly dry off amniotic fluid
Convection—to surrounding air	Protect against cool drafts
Conduction—by direct transfer to cool material	Use warmed blankets to cover Place on warmed surface for care
Radiation—through the air to cooler objects in the room An incubator permits radiation of body heat to the environment outside the incubator	Insulate with warm clothes and blankets and/or Provide radiant heat and/or Depend on maternal body heat
Mechanisms of Heat Production	***Effects of Cooling and Increased Heat Production***
Increase in muscular activity and shivering	Increase in oxygen consumption Increase in glucose consumption Possible metabolic acidosis due to lactic acid from anaerobic metabolism
Increase in metabolic rate	Increased oxygen and glucose consumption and possible metabolic acidosis—as above General metabolic rate remains elevated for 7 to 10 days, even after warming
Metabolism of brown fat	Release of fatty acids which contribute to metabolic acidosis Possible inhibition of surfactant production because of a reduction in amount of glucose and available oxygen, and presence of acidosis
Mechanisms of Heat Conservation	***Protection of the Small Baby Handicapped in Heat Conservation***
Subcutaneous fat	Poorly developed in premature and SGA infants The infants need extra protection against heat loss
Flexed position to decrease surface	Premature infants have less tone than full-term and may not be able to assume a flexed position The relatively large surface of an infant's head and damp hair may require extra protection to reduce heat loss
Peripheral vasoconstriction	Present in prematures as well as full-term

*Mechanisms of heat loss, heat production, and heat conservation; the effects of these processes on the newborn; and actions that the nurse can take to reduce the serious consequences of chilling. Premature, small-for-gestational age, and sick infants are likely to be seriously handicapped by the effects of chilling because of low glycogen reserves, low reserves for increasing ventilation, and possibly preexisting acidosis. These infants have special needs for protection against heat loss.

by shivering than a small one, since a larger amount of muscle is available for this increased activity.

Metabolism of brown fat is an important source of heat production in the newborn. Brown fat is a unique kind of adipose tissue, which functions to produce heat under the stress of cooling. Each cell of brown fat has many small droplets of fat, in contrast to the single, much larger fat vacuole in cells of normal white adipose tissue. Brown fat has a rich nerve and blood supply. Its fat is metabolized quite easily and when it is used to produce heat, the cells may become partially or completely depleted of fat.

The newborn has a significant accumulation of brown fat. It is found in the interscapular region, in the posterior triangle of the neck, and in the axillae. When the infant is cooled, his autonomic nervous system stimulates the brown fat deposits to metabolize this fat, which produces heat. An infant who has a good accumulation of brown fat under cold stress will have a warmer skin temperature between the shoulders and over the nape of the neck than he does over other parts of the body. The warmer areas are where the skin lies over a layer of brown fat. This increased skin temperature reflects the heat being produced in the brown fat. The rich blood supply of brown adipose tissue helps to distribute the heat that is generated by metabolism of brown fat to other parts of the body.

The newborn responds to cooling with an *increase in metabolic rate*. The infant's thyroid gland is stimulated to hyperactivity when he is exposed to cold and his general metabolism increases considerably. There will be a delay of a few hours, and perhaps 12 to 24 hours, before the metabolic rate rises significantly, but thereafter, it will respond to cooling or warming of the body. Although an infant's general metabolism will decrease as he is warmed, the impact of the increase in metabolic rate that took place as a result of cooling at birth will continue for a week or more. The metabolism of an infant who was cooled at birth is higher than that of one who did not lose much body heat, and it remains elevated throughout the first week to 10 days of life.

Effects of Chilling on a Newborn

As infants who are cooled increase their metabolism, they must increase their oxygen consumption and their use of glucose and brown fat. These infants have a tendency to develop a metabolic acidosis and are in danger of being unable to produce pulmonary surfactant adequately.

As the infant *increases heat production, oxygen consumption rises sharply.* In a thermal environment in which the infant does not lose body heat and thus does not need to increase metabolism for heat production, oxygen consumption for the basic body needs is from 4 to 6 cc of oxygen per kilogram per minute. This is at a body temperature of 97.5 to 99° F (36.4 to 37.2° C). With a relatively small reduction in skin temperature, the infant begins to increase oxygen consumption, and as the infant cools to a considerable degree, oxygen need increases accordingly. When the skin temperature drops to between 94 to 95° F (34.4 and 35° C), the basal oxygen need is twice as high. This means a doubling of oxygen need with a drop of body temperature of 3° F (1.7° C). At a body temperature of 92° F (33.3° C) the infant needs three times as much oxygen to meet his basic needs (to remain alive) as he needs at a normal body temperature. Such a great increase in oxygen need may mean that supplemental oxygen may be necessary to maintain body temperature, or if the infant cannot breathe well, he may not be able to obtain enough oxygen to sustain life (Table 26–2).

Need for calories is high when heat production is high. As the infant is increasing his oxygen consumption, he is equally increasing his use of glucose. This means that when an infant's oxygen consumption is doubled or tripled, the utilization of glucose is likewise doubled or tripled. Although the normal full-term infant may have a reasonably large amount of glucose available (stored as glycogen), the small infant has only a small amount accessible in the body for increased metabolism.

With increased metabolism during cold stress, an infant can quickly exhaust the glycogen store of the body and become hypoglycemic. A small infant may use all of the glycogen in 4 to 6 hours, and the blood sugar will fall to a very low level. Under such conditions the infant may sustain brain damage, since brain cells are in need of glucose as well as oxygen for adequate development and function.

An infant who is cooled and in need of increasing the metabolism is likely to develop a metabolic acidosis quickly. This is particularly true if metabolic needs are higher than the amount of oxygen available to carry metabolism to completion. When more oxygen is required than can be supplied to the body, products of incomplete metabolism will accumulate.

Cooling quickly stimulates shivering and brown fat metabolism. Glucose is the source of energy for the shivering, and sometimes the glucose metabolism cannot be carried to completion owing to an inadequate supply of oxygen. This incomplete (anaerobic) metabolism leads to an accumulation of lactic acid. When brown fat is metabolized, fatty acids are released into the blood. The combined effect of fatty acids from the fat metabolism and lactic acid from the incomplete glucose metabolism is a lowering of blood pH, resulting in acidosis. The pH may drop even as low as 7.0 in the presence of considerable cooling and respiratory distress. A severe acidosis may interfere with essential body functions to a degree that is incompatible with life.

An infant *who is cool may not be able to produce surfactant well.* Pulmonary surfactant must be replaced continually. Its activity lasts only about 12 hours without replacement and, if production is halted, an infant can lose the surfactant present at birth within 12 hours or even in a shorter time. As a result of the loss the infant can progress to severe respiratory distress. The infant needs glucose and good oxygenation and a good circulation to produce surfactant well. Cooling may greatly reduce the amount of glucose and available oxygen, produce acidosis, and result in a decrease in circulation through the lungs. All these factors, especially when combined, inhibit production of surfactant (Table 26–2). A small infant is in greater danger of losing the ability to produce surfactant than a large one, since the small infant is handicapped by a low reserve of glycogen and a low reserve for increasing his ventilation.

A small infant or one who has respiratory distress is at a considerable disadvantage when the body is cooled. An infant who does not have good lung function or who has required resuscitation may not be able to meet the body's doubled or trebled oxygen need for the increased metabolism necessary for heat production. This infant already may have an acidosis from the respiratory difficulty and he is likely to have a superimposed cause for becoming more acidotic.

Table 26–2. Dangerous Effects of Chilling in the Newborn Period

1. Sharp rise in oxygen consumption; meeting the need for oxygen may even become unattainable
2. Sharp increase in utilization of glucose; glycogen stores may be quickly depleted. Hypoglycemia develops
3. Metabolic acidosis develops; quickly may become severe
4. Production of surfactant inhibited; respiratory distress may develop or progress

CLASSIFICATION ACCORDING TO GESTATIONAL AGE

As will be recalled from Chapter 5, "*Development of the Embryo and Fetus,*" a fetus develops physical characteristics, functional ability, and neuromuscular signs along predictable lines. A fetus' gestational age therefore could be judged from the signs of development he or she presented at birth, or if the gestational age were accurately known, the stage of development could be predicted.

Since some infants are born before full-term gestation and some others remain *in utero* for two to three weeks after full-term gestation, it is important to include gestational age assessment in a discussion on characteristics of the newborn.

An accurate assessment of gestational age is of great importance to the immediate clinical care of the newborn, since the problems, the needs, and the clinical course are very different for each group of infants—the preterm, the term, and the postterm infant.

In order to anticipate problems, gestational age may need to be speculated before birth by the use of a number of different criteria. Often estimation of the expected date of full-term gestation can be made fairly accurately by calculating from the day of onset of the mother's last menstrual period. The accuracy of this date is enhanced when it compares favorably with a clinical estimation of the duration of pregnancy from such signs as expected progression of the height of the uterine fundus at various stages of pregnancy and the time when the fetal heart is heard for the first time (see Chapter 9). Sometimes fetal maturity studies, carried out prenatally by examination of the amniotic fluid (pages 246–48) and by fetal biparietal diameter measurements (pages 250–52), are used to estimate gestational age, but these tests are better for assessment of maturity and size than of gestation. However, they do give supportive data.

After birth, the infant is examined for characteristics that can be used for a fairly accurate assessment of gestational age. Such an assessment can be detailed, or it can consist of looking at only a few characteristics.

It is obviously not as accurate to assess gestational age from observation of a few developmental characteristics as it is to use a larger number of parameters and a scoring system, and yet a quick appraisal of certain well-defined characteristics has clinical value. It is very useful to determine from a quick appraisal almost immediately after birth if the infant belongs to a term or preterm category of age. To make such a brief, sketchy evaluation of the infant, a few physical characteristics that easily can be assessed by quick observation are used. This usually means looking at sole creases, breast growth, ear cartilage development, and progress in development of the external genitalia. These characteristics and their stage of development at several gestational ages are shown in Figure 27–2, page 540.

These few clinical criteria, combined with information obtained prenatally, usually will suffice to place the infant tentatively into an appropriate gestational age category for beginning care. A more detailed examination later should be used to confirm or revise the original calculation of gestational age.

A detailed examination for assessment of gestational age is carried out by evaluation of a number of parameters. Such assessment is possible because certain physical characteristics of an infant and neurologic signs change predictably with increasing fetal age.

Since the mid-1960s a number of methods for assessing a newborn's age have been proposed. Some of these evaluations are based on external physical characteristics of the infant, some are based on neurologic examination, some use both external characteristics and neurologic criteria. A scoring system, developed by Dubowitz, Dubowitz, and Goldberg[4] in 1970, is often used for age assessment. The Dubowitz assessment score, which can be learned easily by the nursing staff, may be used at any time after birth. It is not influenced by the sleep-awake cycle of the infant. Since the Dubowitz system is rather detailed, some persons have selected a smaller number of criteria that are easier to determine and yet give an estimation that is accurate for clinical purposes.[5] The Ballard system is one such evaluation procedure and is described in Chapter 27.

The above detailed gestational age examination, called the Ballard system, is illustrated in Figure 27–3*A*, B, C. This system uses six neuromuscular maturity criteria that are mainly dependent on development of posture and muscle tone. Also used are six physical maturity criteria based largely on development of skin, breasts, ears, and genitalia. All these criteria are assessed and given a score for the stage of their development. The total score, obtained on all 12 criteria, is compared to a score chart that has been worked out to give an accurate assessment of gestational age in weeks.

The Ballard scoring system has been described as a rapid, simplified, clinical test of maturation, based on both physical and neurologic maturation. It is suggested that it is performed most reliably between 30 and 42 hours, giving the infant time to stabilize and adjust after the stress of birth.

With careful assessment and scoring, it should be possible to assess an infant's gestational age quite accurately, with no more than one to two weeks' error. It is then also possible to categorize him according to maturity status as follows:

[4] Lily M. S. Dubowitz, Victor Dubowitz, and Cissie Goldberg, Clinical assessment of gestational age in the newborn infant, *J. Pediatr.*, 77:1–10, 1970.

[5] J. L. Ballard, K. Kazmaier, and M. Driver, A simplified assessment of gestational age, *Pediatr. Res.*, 11:374, 1977.

Born at less than 26 weeks' gestation—immature infant

Born between 26 and 37 completed weeks of gestation—preterm or premature infant

Born between 38 and 42 weeks of gestation—term or mature infant

Born after 42 completed weeks of gestation—postterm infant

It should be noted that the division between preterm and term classification of infants has been variously given as 37 weeks' gestation and 38 weeks' gestation on the charts that are used. The World Health Organization definition of prematurity in 1961 stated that an infant born prior to 36 completed weeks of gestation was a premature. This put the division of preterm and term at 37 weeks' gestation. The American Academy of Pediatrics, Committee on Fetus and Newborn, in 1967, recommended the use of the words *preterm, term,* and *postterm* to indicate length of gestation, wishing to use terms referring to time alone rather than to imply evidence of maturity in classification. When the Colorado classification of newborn infants was devised, the words *preterm, term,* and *postterm* were used, and the division between preterm and term was placed at 38 weeks. (This is seen in Figure 26–3.) This classification differed from that of the World Health Organization for prematurity but was acceptable to the American Academy of Pediatrics, Committee on Fetus and Newborn.[6]

Several reasons were given for placing the division between preterm and term at 38 weeks. The distribution of births by gestational age is such that the peak birth rate is at 40 weeks' gestation, with 80 percent of births occurring between 38 and 42 weeks. Also there is evidence that seems to indicate that infants between 37 and 38 weeks are not as mature as term infants.[7] It is not now known if a different classification by gestational age may be necessary for other racial groups, but the present division seems satisfactory for now.

Intrauterine Growth in Weight and Length

For a number of years birthweight was used as a measure of a newborn's gestational age. Infants weighing 2500 gm (5 lb, 8 oz) or less were considered premature and those above a weight of 2500 gm as term infants. An infant with a period of gestation of less than 37 weeks also was classified premature, but the weight classification took priority for statistical purposes and for planning of public health programs. It then became increasingly evident that birthweight was not valuable for identifying gestational age. About one third of infants weighing under 2500 gm at birth are term infants, who for some reason have not grown according to a normal rate. Also, some infants who weigh over 2500 gm are prematures as far as aspects of development other than weight are concerned. From this it became apparent that birthweight alone cannot be used as a measure of maturity. The birthweight must be correlated with gestational age to be valuable in estimating the meaning of the weight and how it may relate to the infant's condition.

In 1961 the Expert Committee on Maternal and Child Health of the World Health Organization, in recognition of the fact that a large number of infants fell within the definition of prematurity who were apparently not premature, recommended that the concept of "prematurity" in the previous definition should give way to the term "low-birth-weight." This meant that the term *low birthweight* was to be given to all infants, regardless of gestational age, who weighed 2500 gm or less. It also meant that the term "premature" was reserved for infants born at less than 37 weeks' gestation (less than 36 completed weeks).

As the concept that an infant might be small because of intrauterine growth retardation was being accepted through studies by Gruenwald[8] and the necessity of relating birthweight to gestational age was becoming apparent, the Colorado intrauterine growth charts were being developed.[9, 10] These charts were used as a means of determining the appropriateness of an infant's weight in relation to gestational age.

Using an accurate measurement of birth weight and an accurate assessment of an infant's gestational age, the two values are placed on the chart shown in Figure 26–3 at the point where this infant's weight and weeks of gestation intersect. The weight chart of Figure 26–4 may be used instead of Figure 26–3, but it requires more interpretation by the user.

From the chart in Figure 26–3 the newborn can be categorized according to where the point of intersection of this infant's weight and weeks of gestation is found. The infant is thus categorized as appropriate (in weight) for gestational age (AGA), small for gestational age (SGA), or large for gestational age (LGA). At the same time the infant is identified as preterm, term, or postterm.

For further evaluation of a newborn's size in relation to gestational age, the length and head circumference also are measured and compared to percentiles of

[6] Lula O. Lubchenco, The high risk infant. *Major Probl. Clin. Pediatr.*, 14:2–3, 1976.

[7] *Ibid.*, pp. 2–4.

[8] Peter Gruenwald, Chronic fetal distress and placental insufficiency, *Biol. Neonat.*, 5:215–65, 1963.

[9] Lula O. Lubchenco, Charlotte Hansman, and Edith Boyd, Intrauterine growth in length and head circumference as estimated from live births at gestational ages from 26 to 42 weeks, *Pediatrics*, 37:402–408, (Mar.) 1966.

[10] Frederick C. Battaglia and Lula O. Lubchenco, A practical classification of newborn infants by weight and gestational age, *J. Pediatr.*, 71:159–63, (Aug.) 1967.

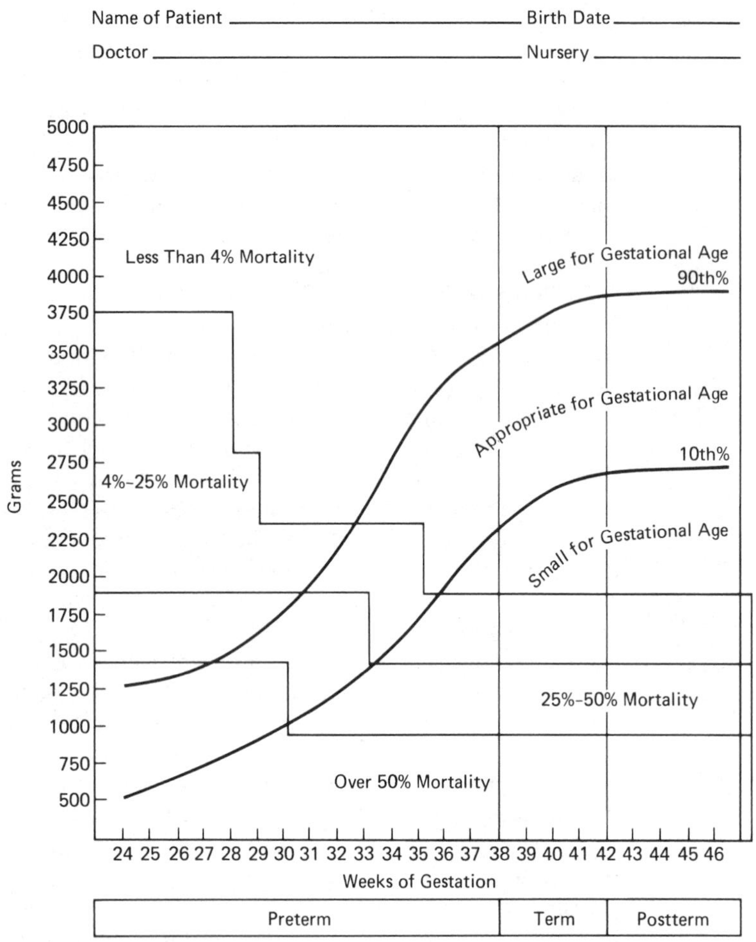

Figure 26–3. Each newborn can be classified by birth weight and gestational age with the use of this chart. It is easy to recognize the baby as large, appropriate, or small for his gestational age and provide him with the appropriate care immediately after birth. This illustration may be used as a wall chart in the nursery to provide for quick recognition of the "at-risk" baby. Neonatal mortality risk is also shown. (Reproduced from Frederick C. Battaglia, and Lula O. Lubchenco, A practical classification of newborn infants by weight and gestational age. *J. Pediatr.* 71:159–63, 1967, p. 161.)

measurements for infants of similar gestational age. Thus, a newborn's weight, length, and head circumference may be plotted on the intrauterine growth chart shown in Figure 26–4. From this chart the infant's relative weight, length, and head circumference may be observed. It is possible, using these data, to determine if all the measurements are appropriate for gestational age, if only growth in weight is affected, if both weight and length are small, or if all three measurements are small. In general, mild growth retardation affects only weight and somewhat more severe retardation affects both weight and length. Head size appears to be the last affected and when it is also small, retardation is severe, unless the infant is genetically of small size.

Use of a weight-length ratio helps to further identify the infant who is proportionately of good size or who may have considerable discrepancy between weight and length. The relationship of body weight to body length has been used primarily to detect infants with intrauterine growth retardation, but it also may be used to detect infants who are high risk because they are too heavy for their length.

The weight-length ratio helps to define the greater retardation in weight than in length and will show the severity of the malnourishment of the body tissues. It will also show whether a large infant with a weight above the ninetieth percentile has an excessive weight for size or if the infant's weight is reasonable in relation to the length. Infants who fall below the third percentile for dates are considered malnourished, and those who are above the ninety-seventh percentile for dates are overweight.

The weight-length ratio is especially useful when infants are near to or outside extremes of growth on any of the measurements on the intrauterine growth chart, and also when there is a discrepancy between percentile positions of weight, length, and head circumference. The ratio has the advantage of not being influenced by sex or by race.

Additional Comments on Weight and Length

The mean, or average, birthweight of full-term Caucasian babies is 3400 gm (7 lb, 8 oz). There are, however, wide variations in birthweights even of normal full-term infants. Approximately one half of all full-term infants weigh between 2950 gm (6 lb, 8 oz) and 3515 gm (7 lb, 12 oz). A full-term infant weighing 2500 gm (5 lb, 8 oz) or

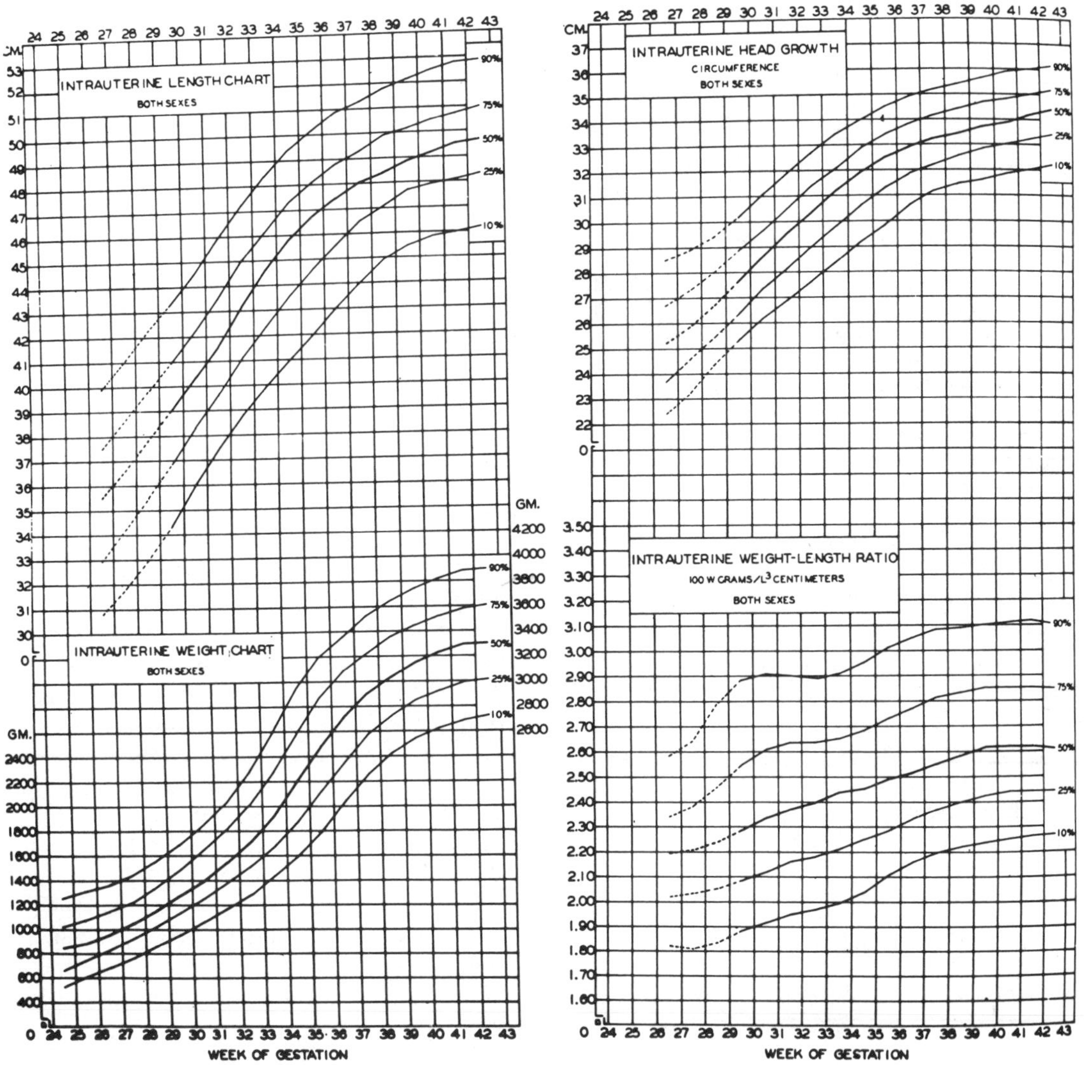

Figure 26–4. Percentiles of intrauterine growth in weight, length, head circumference, and weight-length ratio. This form is usually included as a part of the hospital record of each newborn. [Reproduced with permission from Lula O. Lubchenco, Charlotte Hansman, and Edith Boyd, Intrauterine growth in length and head circumference as estimated from live births at gestational ages from 26 to 42 weeks. *Pediatrics* 37:403–408 (Mar.) 1966, p. 404. Copyright American Academy of Pediatrics, 1966.]

less at birth is considered a low-birthweight infant. A weight of 4080 gm (9 lb) or over at full-term gestation is considered excessive in size. Excessive size may cause dystocia, increasing risk of injury to mother and fetus during delivery. Both low-birthweight infants and those of excessive size are considered high risk and require special observation and care in the nursery.

After 38 weeks' gestation male infants are larger than female infants, weighing an average of 200 gm (7 oz) more. The difference, although significant, is not differentiated on the intrauterine growth chart illustrated in Figure 26–4. The normal full-term weights of babies of non-Caucasian races (Negro, Oriental, Indian) are usually somewhat smaller than those quoted above.

An unexplained maternal factor regulates the genetic growth potential of a fetus. Given a normal healthy mother and fetus, the size of the infant will be within approximately a 20 percentile range of the mother's own birthweight. Barring disease processes that are likely to alter fetal growth, all infants born to a mother will be close to the percentile of her own birthweight, if the gestational age and the birthweight of each individual are considered in establishing the comparison. (See Fig. 26–4 for charting of birthweight against gestational age.) The hereditary influence of the father on size has an effect on the growth period after birth.

Physiologic Weight Loss

All infants lose weight during the first few days of life. The weight loss ranges between 5 and 10 percent of the birthweight. This decrease in body weight is caused by a

and fourteenth days, varying degrees of jaundice of the skin may be present.

Petechiae, accompanied by bluish discoloration of the skin, may be seen on the face for a day or two after delivery as a result of pressure during birth. Edema and extravasation of blood into the tissues of the buttocks and genitalia are seen frequently following a breech delivery because of pressure changes in the area lying over the cervical opening, as well as bruising of the tissues as the breech is pushed through the birth canal (Fig. 26-10).

Vernix caseosa, a greasy, white, cheeselike material, consisting of an accumulation of secretion from the sebaceous glands and including epithelial cells and lanugo hair, covers the skin at birth. This material may be present as a very thin covering or as a thick layer; it is especially heavy in folds and creases of the skin and between the labia. The vernix caseosa absorbs, rubs off on the clothing, or dries and falls off within the first day, except that present in the creases.

Lanugo hair, the downy covering that develops on the fetus during the fourth month and begins to disappear after the eighth lunar month of intrauterine life, may still be present on certain parts of the body, especially over the shoulders, back, earlobes, or forehead (Fig. 26-11). Most of the lanugo is lost during the first week of the neonatal period. The covering of the head varies from almost complete baldness to a growth of thick, dark hair extending over the temples; this hair later may be lost and replaced by a new growth. Eyebrows and eyelashes are present, but may be thin and very light in appearance.

An ample distribution of subcutaneous fat gives the full-term baby's skin a soft, elastic texture. The epidermis comes off in flakes during the first week or two of life, and peeling of the skin may be quite generalized. During this time the skin may be very dry, and fissures at the wrists and ankles are not uncommon (Fig. 26-12). Occasionally desquamation of the hands and feet is seen at birth.

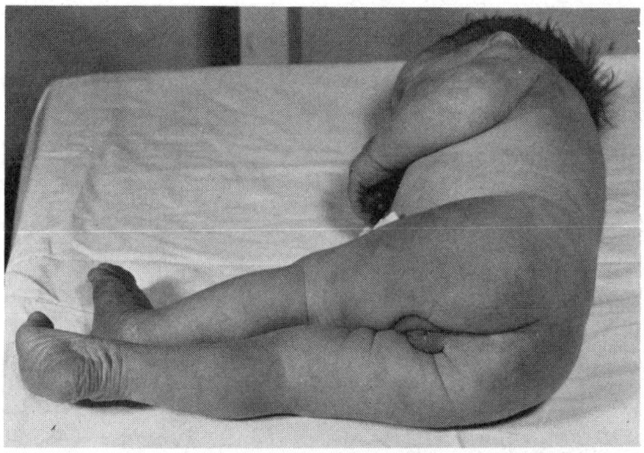

Figure 26-10. Infant delivered by breech extraction—age 18 hours. The legs continue to assume the intrauterine position by remaining in extension, with the toes pointing toward the shoulders. There are edema and extravasation of blood into the tissues of the buttocks and genitalia. This is the result of pressure changes in the area which presented at the cervical opening during labor and bruising of the tissues as the breech was pushed through the birth canal.

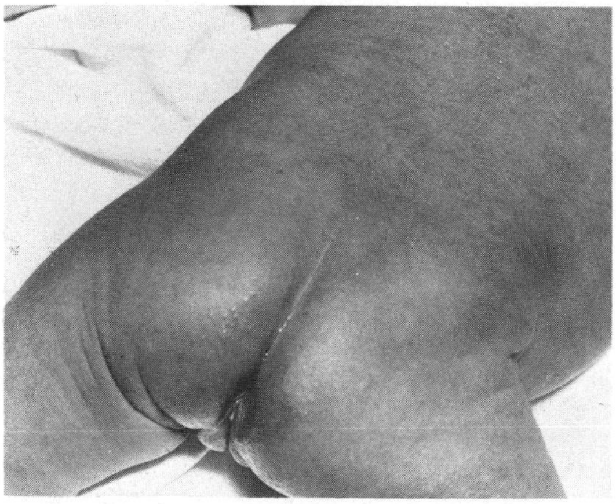

Figure 26-11. An infant's back covered with lanugo hair.

Milia, pinpoint-size white spots beneath the epidermis, may be seen over the nose and chin during the first one to two weeks. These spots are concretions of sebaceous material that has been retained in the ducts of the sebaceous glands.

The newborn infant's skin is very sensitive. Some infants have benign, self-limited eruptions, called *erythema toxicum* (erythema neonatorum). These eruptions appear as splotchy erythematous blotches, or as firm white papules or hivelike areas on an erythematous base (Fig. 26-13). On some infants they appear and disappear at intervals during the first few days of life, often following slight irritation from clothing or bathing or after a period of crying. Etiology of these eruptions is unknown. There are no apparent related systemic symptoms and treatment is not necessary.

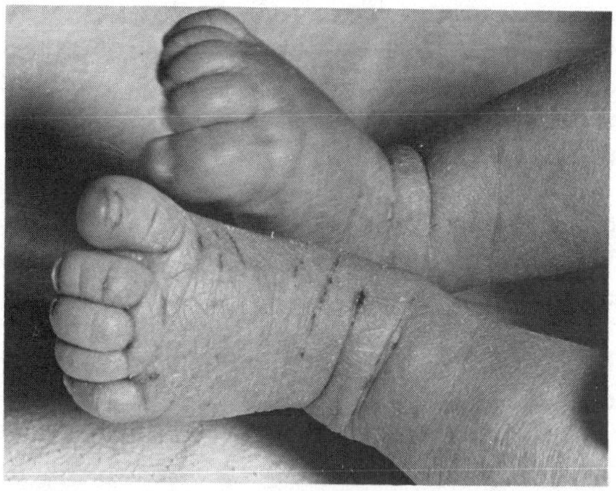

Figure 26-12. Dryness and cracking of the skin, which are often temporarily present in the newborn—this infant is 4 days old.

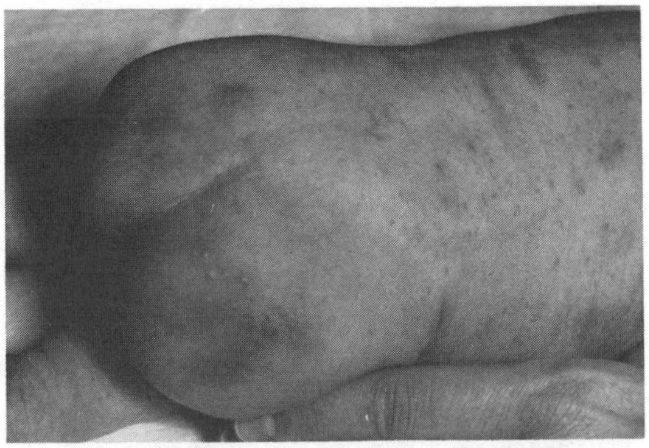

Figure 26–13. Erythema toxicum (erythema neonatorum) on the back of a newborn. Some infants develop these benign eruptions which appear as erythematous blotches or as firm pale-yellow or white papules on an erythematous base. They are likely to appear at intervals after slight irritation from clothing or bathing or after a period of crying.

The skin of the newborn is very thin and even minor irritations easily produce rashes and breaks in the skin. *Denuded areas* are seen following even minor, but frequent, irritation of one specific site. The active infant may rub some part of the body, mainly nose, knees, or toes, against the crib covers during crying and break the skin enough to cause active bleeding. The skin of the buttocks likewise is irritated easily, and if the infant has frequent stools, the buttocks may become quite raw and sore.

Flat *hemangiomatous areas,* light red in appearance, may be present on the upper eyelids, between the eyebrows, on the upper lip, or at the nape of the neck; these eventually fade and disappear between one and two years of age. *Papillomas* of the skin may be present; they are seen most frequently near or in front of an ear. Infants of black or Oriental parents and of parents from Mediterranean countries may have bluish pigmented areas, known as *mongolian spots,* on the back or the buttocks. Infants of dark-skinned races also may have areas of dark pigmentation in certain localized areas, especially over the genitalia and at the base of the nails.

Sweat glands are present over all of the skin, but infants usually do not sweat during the first one to two days of life. Sweating begins on the face at about the third day of life in full-term infants and later over other parts of the body. Sweating will vary markedly with ambient and body temperature, with activity, and with fever. *Sebaceous glands* are active up to and immediately after birth. Shortly thereafter, when maternal androgens are no longer present, they become quiescent and remain so until puberty.

Insensible water loss through the skin can be great in the newborn because the thin skin and relatively large body surface in relation to body mass permit a large loss. Fluid loss through the skin may be very significant in preterm infants and in infants under radiant warmers (page 614).

The infant's fingernails are well developed and may extend well beyond the tips of the fingers. The toenails are also well formed, but may appear embedded at the distal end.

UMBILICAL CORD

The umbilical cord begins to discolor and shrink soon after birth; within a few days the stump has shriveled and turned black, and a red line of demarcation has begun to appear at the juncture of the umbilical cord with the skin of the abdomen. This skin may extend just to the base of the cord, or it may extend up onto the cord a short distance. By the sixth to tenth day the cord has atrophied to a dry black string; it then sloughs off and leaves a small granulating area, which heals entirely in another week (Fig. 26–14). The amount of granulation tissue is determined by the amount of Wharton's jelly that was present in the umbilical cord. Occasionally there is a delay in separation of the cord into the third week of life, but this is not significant if the cord appears dry and healthy.

The blood vessels at the base of the umbilical cord are sealed off by the formation of thrombi, but final obliteration does not occur until toward the end of the neonatal period when the thrombi organize and the vessels become fibrous cords. Until this anatomic closure has occurred, the blood vessels are portals of entry to pathogenic organisms.

An umbilical hernia may develop, but strapping of the area is not recommended. A strap or abdominal band offers no benefits and may cause skin irritation or infection. The hernia usually disappears during the infant's first year.

HORMONE REACTIONS

Breast hypertrophy, uterine bleeding, and vulvar or prostatic hypertrophy may occur in newborn infants. These changes are produced by maternal or placental hormones that have been transmitted through the placenta and are present temporarily.

A number of those changes probably result from a dominant influence of maternal steroids, particularly estrogens, which are at a high level in the mother's blood just before labor. These easily cross the placenta. After birth the tissues of the newborn that were stimulated by the steroids soon regress to their normal state of development, and some of the changes that occur are caused by the sudden withdrawal of maternal hormones.

The moist, congested, external female genitalia,

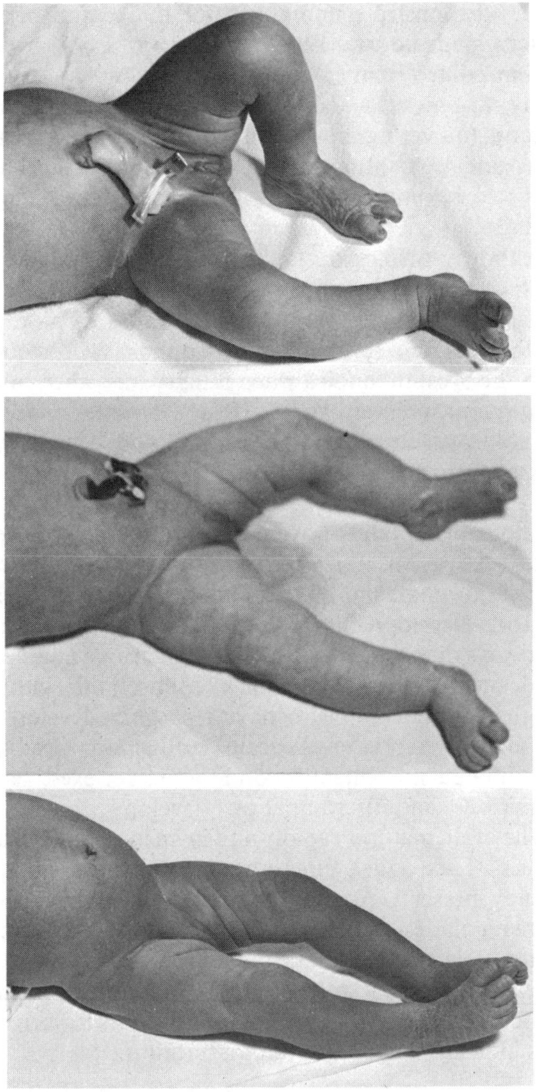

Figure 26–14. Mummification and separation of the umbilical cord. *Top:* Appearance of the umbilical cord six hours after birth. *Center:* Appearance of the umbilical cord four days after birth. *Bottom:* Appearance of the umbilicus one day after separation of the umbilical cord.

hymenal tags of tissue, and vaginal discharge, first watery and later a thick, white mucoid material, are a result of endocrine substances that affect the genital organs. The maternal hormones present in the fetus and their subsequent withdrawal and exhaustion following birth are considered responsible for the hypertrophied vaginal epithelium, resembling the adult type, which is present at birth, and for the desquamation and mucosal changes with regression to an infantile type of tissue, which takes place in two to three days. Within a week or two after birth, congestion of the genitalia has disappeared, and vaginal discharge decreases.

Bleeding from the vagina, which occurs in some in-

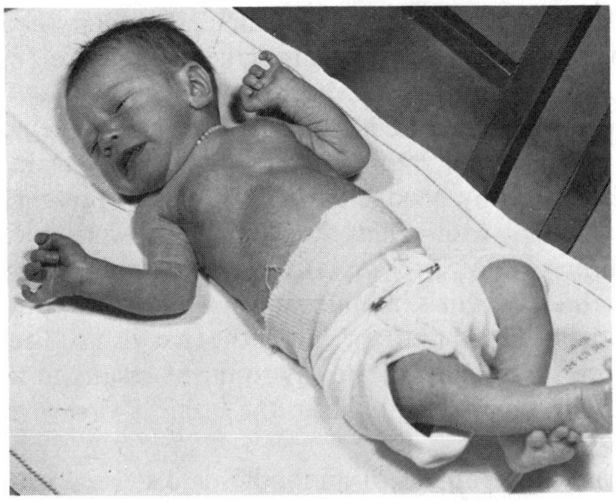

Figure 26–15. Breast engorgement in the newborn infant. Engorgement may occur in an infant of either sex during the first week of life.

fants during the first neonatal week, is also caused by a temporary imbalance in the endocrine system, which produces hyperemia of the pelvic organs and subsequent bleeding. This pseudomenstruation is considered physiologic, occurring because of the activity of the maternal hormones transmitted to the fetus *in utero* and subsequently withdrawn at birth.

Another manifestation of reactions produced by maternal hormones is breast enlargement, with swelling and tenseness; this may occur in infants of either sex during the first week of life (Fig. 26–15). A milky fluid, called witch's milk, may be secreted from the engorged breasts. Engorgement and secretion are much more pronounced in some infants than in others. They also disappear in approximately one month.

IMMUNITY

Antibodies to diphtheria and tetanus and antiviral immune bodies against measles, smallpox, mumps, poliomyelitis, and probably some other infectious diseases pass from the mother to the infant through the placenta, provided the mother herself has an immunity to the disease. There is very little or no inherited immunity to whooping cough or herpesvirus. This relative, not absolute, inherited passive immunity lasts for varying periods of time; for some infections the period of resistance may be very short, while for others it may be active for several months. The average half-life for the passively transferred IgG immunoglobulins is between 20 and 30 days. Their concentration in serum drops quite rapidly thereafter and reaches a low level between two and four months of age. This period is referred to as physiologic hypogammaglobulinemia. There is no immunity to many of the organisms to which the neonate is most apt to be exposed; for example, the staphylococcus and cold and flu viruses. This makes good asepsis essential in the care of all newborns.

In addition to providing protection for the newborn, the passively acquired IgG antibodies may interfere with active antibody production while they are present. Immunization with killed vaccines, however, such as diphtheria and pertussis, is usually begun at two to three months. Live virus immunization, with the exception of polio, is delayed until the end of the first year of life. Exposure to antigens in the environment results in an increase in gamma globulin in the infant's first years of life.

Placental transfer of antibodies is discussed on page 105, and deficiency of antibodies in the newborn is described on page 687.

THE NERVOUS SYSTEM

The brain of the newborn is in a period of rapid growth at the time of birth. The nerve cells, called neurons, are formed primarily between 10 and 18 weeks' gestation. The adult number of neurons is established quite early in the baby's development. After this period of neuronal development, a period of rapid brain growth begins. The brain growth spurt appears to start at about mid-pregnancy and continues well into the second postnatal year. Further gradual growth of the brain continues until its maturity is reached.

In the weeks and months immediately following birth the brain grows rapidly, and a number of functionally important processes take place. Glial cells, which form a protective and supportive framework for the nerves throughout the brain and spinal cord; dendrites, the short, thick protoplasmic projections of the nerve cell body that receive impulses; and synapses, junctions where two neurons come into functional contact, multiply and grow. Myelination progresses.

John Dobbing states:

> The demonstration that the human brain growth spurt is much more postnatal than was formerly thought creates a new opportunity to ensure one important positive . . . , by actively promoting good bodily growth at the time when this most important organ is passing through its own vulnerable period of growth.[12]

The newborn's motor coordination is quite sophisticated. Some of the behaviors are necessary for survival, and some have no apparent immediate usefulness. Many actions show good motor control; others demonstrate immaturity of the central nervous system and poor cerebral influence. Poor nervous system control makes the infant "jumpy"; he startles easily, at times the chin quivers, and frequently he has tremors (quivering movements) of short duration of the arms and legs. Much of the infant's motor behavior seems to be under control of the spinal cord and the medulla.

Although the nervous system is relatively immature at birth, cortical activity appears to have more influence on behavior than has been suspected in the past. The newborn is able to turn toward sounds, follow objects with the eyes, take food when hungry, cry when hungry or in pain, maintain good postural muscle tone, show spontaneous alertness and activity, and become quiet when comforted.

Certain behavior patterns, including those that regulate intrauterine movements, are present before the fetus is born, but it is after birth that behavior becomes more coordinated and comes under the higher levels of control. Development takes place rapidly. Soon certain pathways that control the activity of various muscles are used, nerve fibers make new connections with one another, more complex behavior patterns develop, and the higher cerebral levels begin to function. Gradually, coordinated movements, conditioned reflexes, habits, inhibitions, and discriminations develop.

The brain matures rapidly and in an integrated orderly process. Each added function is incorporated with those already present. As development proceeds, more and more regulation of behavior is taken over by the cerebral cortex. Generalized mass movements are replaced by specific individual responses. Rapid development of consciousness, arousal, and responsiveness to surroundings indicates ongoing brain maturation.

Reflexes

The baby is born with certain reflexes that are significant to note as evidences of normal development. Their presence or absence and the time at which they appear or disappear are indicative of progress. The manner in which they are used gives evidence of the functioning of the nervous system. For example, a weak or absent reflex may indicate the presence of a lesion in the central nervous system. Certain reflexes, which are evidences of immaturity, are normal only in the newborn infant. With normal development of the nervous system, they disappear in the first few months of extrauterine life.

An infant's reflex response may depend upon his behavioral state. While one response may be diminished when tested during light sleep, another may be checked during this state or deep sleep. Sucking may change a response. Some reflexes are present in all states. Some should not be tested when the infant is sleepy; an alert period may be the most desirable time to check reflexes.

[12] John Dobbing, The later development of the brain and its vulnerability, in *Scientific Foundations of Paediatrics,* edited by John A. Davis and John Dobbing. Heinemann Medical Books, London, 1974, p. 576.

Moro Reflex

The Moro reflex is a vestibular reflex that demonstrates an awareness of equilibrium in the newborn infant. It requires certain nerve tracts which are present and can be elicited at birth, unless there has been damage to either the central nervous system or the peripheral nerves.

The Moro reflex is tested when the infant is lying quietly. It is elicited more easily when the baby is undressed. A sudden stimulus, such as jarring of the table on which the infant lies, sudden jerking of the blanket, or a sudden change in position elicits the response. The infant stiffens the body, draws up the legs, and throws the arms up and out and then brings them forward as in an embrace position (Fig. 26–16). It may be noted that the infant also semiflexes the thumb and index finger of each hand, forming the shape of a C and extends the remaining fingers. The infant often begins to cry at the end of the embrace gesture. Movement of the arms is the most prominent feature of this reflex. Their movements should be symmetric. When one arm does not come forward, the possibility of an injury to the arm, the clavicle, or a nerve must be considered.

If the Moro reflex is absent at birth but present on the following day, its previous absence may have been caused by edema of the brain; the reflex returns when the edema subsides. If this reflex is present at birth but absent soon thereafter, increasing edema of the brain or slow bleeding due to intracranial hemorrhage is considered as a possible cause of its disappearance. If brain injury has occurred during delivery, the reflex is absent at birth and for the next several days; it will return, however, in three or four days if the damage is not too severe.

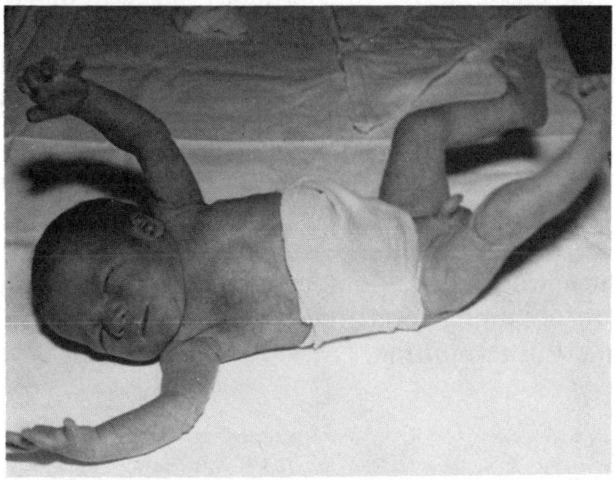

Figure 26–16. The Moro reflex. A sudden stimulus causes the infant to stiffen his body, draw up his legs, and throw his arms up and out. He will next bring his arms forward as in an embrace position and he may begin to cry. The response of the arms and legs is symmetric in the normal infant. The semiflexion of the thumb and index finger of each hand, forming the shape of a C, which normally occurs during the Moro reflex, can be seen on this infant's left hand. (Note the mottling of the skin, which is probably due to circulatory instability and exposure.)

The characteristics of the Moro reflex pattern depend upon gestational age. In the immature infant, below 30 weeks' gestation, the Moro reflex is not well developed and is barely apparent and easily exhaustible. The second phase of the reflex, the flexion component, becomes stronger as the infant matures; it is not fully developed until after 35 weeks' gestation. While checking the Moro reflex it is well to note separately the degree of abduction at shoulders and extension and flexion at elbows, and also the ease with which the reflex is elicited. The Moro reflex normally disappears two or three months after full term.

Tonic Neck Reflex (The Asymmetric Reflex)

The tonic neck reflex is a postural reflex in which the infant assumes a fencing position. When this reflex is present, it will be noted that, as the infant lies on the back and rotates the head to either side, the arm and leg on the side to which the head faces are partly or completely extended and the opposite arm and leg are flexed (Fig. 26–17). The tonic neck reflex develops in the fetus by 28 weeks, and it disappears in the newborn by the age of two or three months. The reflex is more marked and persists longer in spastic babies.

The Neck-Righting Response

If the head of a healthy full-term newborn is turned to one side, his trunk will follow. The receptors of the neck-righting reflex are located in the muscles and joints of the neck. It is present at birth and strongest at the age of three months. This reflex is the first of several that develop to help the infant to restore the normal position of the head in space and maintain the normal postural relationship of the head and trunk. Other righting reflexes will develop as the infant gets older to help to roll over, to get on his hands and knees, and to sit up.

Grasp Reflex

The grasp reflex is present in both the hands and the feet. The infant will grasp an object placed into his hands, hold on tightly for a short time, and then drop it (Fig. 26–18). The grasp of a full-term infant may be strong enough to support his weight and lift him to a standing position. Holding a finger firmly against the sole of the foot just below the toes will elicit a plantar grasp causing all of the toes to turn downward at the same time. Although grasping is a reflex at birth, it later becomes voluntary and purposeful. The reflex is strongest at full term, becomes much weaker by two

some instability of the various systems. This instability shows itself in many ways: tremors and quiverings, gagging, choking, poor sucking, regurgitation, irregular pulse, and hyperactivity during sleep, and even awakening every few minutes.

Within a few days to a week the effects of birth and sudden change of environment have been largely overcome. Molding of the head has receded; edema of the presenting part has disappeared; the face has become symmetric; temperature maintenance has improved; the respiratory, circulatory, and digestive systems are functioning better; and the posture is more relaxed. The normal newborn will have good color and good muscle tone, cry lustily, sleep approximately 20 hours a day, awaken only when hungry or uncomfortable, eat well, and gain weight steadily.

Newborns have been observed to be in different sleep and awake states which range from deep sleep to light sleep, to drowsy, to quiet awake, to active awake, to crying.

At about 28 weeks of gestation a fetus begins to show some degree of alertness that apparently is not present earlier. He can be aroused from sleep and will remain alert for a few minutes, and occasionally may show spontaneous alerting. By 32 weeks a newborn may alert spontaneously, the eyes may remain open for awhile, and roving eye movements appear. By 37 weeks alertness is increased and the newborn cries vigorously when awake. By full term the newborn has distinct sleep and awake periods and he responds well to stimuli.

When in a quiet awake (alert) state the normal newborn is likely to focus his eyes on faces and objects and to follow them even within a few hours after birth. He will respond to a variety of sounds and is likely to try to locate sounds.

Infants differ a great deal in how they respond to stimuli: how active they are, the amount they fuss and cry, how alert they are, and how easily they are quieted. Infants are capable of responding in an organized way in each state of sleep or awakeness and can control the kind of input they get from their environment. They can close out repeated, unwanted stimuli just as easily as they can respond to significant and interesting stimuli.

Most infants move easily from one state of consciousness to another. Some, however, do not move easily and smoothly between states and do not spend much time in some states. They sleep or they cry and spend little time in the drowsy or quiet awake states. Normal infants will differ considerably from one another in their behavior and therefore in the care that they need.

As the infant develops postnatally, he will reduce the total amount of time he sleeps, his sleep and wakefulness periods will lengthen, and he will shift from daytime to nighttime sleeping.

REFERENCES AND SUGGESTED READINGS

Avery, Gordon B. (ed.), *Neonatology,* 2nd ed., Lippincott, New York 1981.

Brazelton, T. Berry, *Neonatal Behavioral Assessment Scale, Clinics in Developmental Medicine,* No. 50, Spastics International Medical Publications, Heinemann Medical Books, London, and Lippincott, Philadelphia, 1973.

Desmond, Murdina M., *et al.* The clinical behavior of the newly born. I. The term baby, *J. Pediatr.,* 62:307–25, (Mar.) 1963.

Dubowitz, Lilly M.S.; Dubowitz, Victor; and Goldberg, Cissie, Clinical assessment of gestational age in the newborn infant, *J. Pediatr.,* 77:1–10, (July) 1970.

Gibes, Rita M., Clinical uses of the Brazelton neonatal behavioral assessment scale in nursing practice, *Pediatr. Nurs.* 7:23–26, (May/June) 1981.

Haddock, Nancy, Blood pressure monitoring in neonates, *MCN.,* 5:131–35, (Mar./Apr.) 1980.

Hughes, James G., *Synopsis of Pediatrics,* 5th ed. C. V. Mosby, St. Louis, 1980, Chap. 15.

Klaus, Marshall H., and Fanaroff, Avroy A., *Care of the High-Risk Neonate,* 2nd ed., W. B. Saunders, Philadelphia, 1979.

Korones, Sheldon B., *High-Risk Newborn Infants: The Basis for Intensive Nursing Care,* 3rd ed., C. V. Mosby, St. Louis, Mo., 1981.

Ludington-Hoe, Susan M., What can newborns really see? *Am. J. Nurs.,* 83:1286–89, (Sept.) 1983.

Mauer, Daphne, and Mauer, Charles E., Newborn babies see better than you think, *Psychol. Today,* 10:85–88, (Oct.) 1976.

Powell, Marcene, *Assessment and Management of Developmental Changes and Problems in Children,* 2nd ed., C. V. Mosby, St. Louis, Mo., 1981.

Prechtl, H. F. R., The behavioral states of the newborn infant. A review, *Brain Res.,* 76:185–212, 1974.

Rudolph, Abraham M., How the fetal circulation responds to stress, *Contemp. Ob./Gyn.,* 21:145–47, (June) 1983.

Scharping, Earlene M., Physiologic measurements of the neonate, *MCN.,* 8:70–73, (Jan./Feb.) 1983.

CHAPTER

27

Nursing Management of the Normal Newborn

NURSING MANAGEMENT OF the newborn begins with an appraisal immediately after birth of the infant's ability to make a satisfactory adjustment to extrauterine life. Repeated assessments are carried out in the following hours and days to determine the infant's gestational age, his stage of development, his ongoing adaptation to his environment, his general physical condition, and his behavioral abilities.

Assessment of the newborn's gestational age, physical condition and adaptation, and abilities is essential to providing the infant with appropriate care. The cumulative observations and assessment of the infant's first hours and days of life are used for planning care to meet the infant's needs and for assisting the parents in developing their approaches to his care.

Several tools have been developed as aids to a systematic assessment of the newborn for determining his stage of development and for assessing a number of different abilities. Included are the (1) Apgar score, (2) intrauterine growth charts, (3) scoring systems for clinical assessment of gestational age, (4) physical examination, and (5) Brazelton neonatal behavioral assessment scale. All these scales of development and observation will be needed to make a complete evaluation of a newborn's abilities and an appropriate plan of care.

CARE IN THE DELIVERY ROOM

Nursing care of the newborn begins with the infant's birth. In the period immediately after birth the infant must be assisted in establishing and maintaining respirations and must immediately be protected against heat loss and provided with warmth. Apgar scoring is done at 1 and 5 minutes; a quick appraisal is made of the infant's overall appearance and behavior, and the entire body is examined quickly for gross anomalies. After respirations have stabilized, the infant also may be examined for anomalies not grossly apparent. Suggestions for this examination as made by the American Academy of Pediatrics are described on page 540.

Appropriate identification of the infant and probably prophylactic treatment against gonorrheal ophthalmia also are included in the early care of the newborn. Depending on the mother's and infant's condition, the newborn is handed to the mother to look at and hold and examine as soon as possible. All the immediate care of the newborn given in the delivery room has been described on pages 410–24.

The Apgar Score

The Apgar score, described on page 412, is important as an initial screening tool and is used for assessment of the infant immediately after birth. It reflects the condition of the infant after the stress of labor and delivery, and it provides a quick assessment of those functions that must immediately begin adapting to extrauterine existence and are necessary to sustain life. From this score one can determine roughly the degree of alertness or depression of the infant after birth. In the Apgar assessment the immediate response of the cardiovascular and respiratory systems to extrauterine change is evaluated, and a perfunctory idea of the state of the lower centers of the nervous system can be obtained by observing the muscle tone and reflex irritability of the infant.

The Apgar score is important for early recognition of any problems. The 1-minute score is used to determine what kind of assistance, if any, an infant needs to adapt favorably to the new environment, and the 5-minute score gives an indication of the immediate capacity of the infant to respond to the stress of labor and delivery and the likelihood of problems in the early neonatal period. The Apgar score may be repeated in 5 and 10 minutes if indicated.

The Apgar score, done in the early minutes after delivery, is important as an initial assessment of the infant, but it has limited predictability of later abilities of the infant. Other assessment methods therefore also must be used for a complete evaluation of the infant. These will be described below.

Protecting the Infant Against Heat Loss

Delivery Room Care

Chilling of the infant after birth can be reduced considerably when immediate attention is given to minimizing his heat loss while in the delivery room. Proper care in the delivery room includes quickly drying the infant's body to reduce heat loss through evaporation of amniotic fluid, replacement of wet blankets with dry ones, and immediate care after birth in an incubator or under a radiant heater. This care is described on page 412.

When a newborn is moved from the delivery room to the nursery, he must be kept well covered with warm blankets. A full-term, healthy infant can be moved out of the delivery room with his mother and observed by both parents without undue cooling, if he is well covered. A corner of the blanket around the infant's head will reduce heat loss from the relatively large surface of his head and possibly from damp hair. When the mother holds her infant in skin-to-skin contact, her body is a source of considerable warmth, particularly when a blanket covers both mother and infant. When inspection of the newborn by his parents is done, careful attention must be given to ascertaining that the room is warm in order to prevent chilling while the infant is uncovered or that a radiant heat source is provided. A premature infant probably will need to be taken directly to the nursery. Transportation in a warmed incubator will protect him in transit.

Immediate Nursery Care

In the nursery the infant is placed in a warmed bassinet (or incubator) to provide warmth and help him to regain quickly a normal body temperature. Birthweight can be obtained by weighing the infant in a blanket and subtracting the weight of the blanket from the total weight. The infant's initial bath should be postponed until his respirations are stabilized and his body temperature has returned to around 36.7° C (98° F), which is likely to be three to four hours later. Physical examinations, laboratory procedures, x-rays, and other procedures that may be necessary in the first hours after birth and that require that the infant be exposed or undressed should be done under a heat lamp.

Incubator Care

A premature or low-birthweight infant, or a full-term infant who has been delivered with difficulty, is placed into an incubator in the nursery as quickly as possible after birth. The incubator is used for control of air temperature, humidity, and oxygen if necessary, and for close observation of the infant, since he does not need covers and clothing in an incubator (Fig. 27–1). When a premature birth is anticipated, the incubator should be warmed well in advance.

Maintenance of a constant air temperature in the incubator and in the nursery does not assure a constant thermal environment for the newborn. Other factors, such as the humidity of the air, the temperature of the walls and windows of the nursery, and the amount of covers over the infant, will influence his environmental conditions. Therefore, even an incubator temperature of 34 to 35° C (93 to 95° F) does not ensure that the infant will maintain a basal metabolic rate. An incubator helps to decrease heat loss from an infant, but it does not provide heat; the infant must produce his own body heat, unless he is provided with warmth from a source of radiant heat. See page 613 for additional ways in which to protect the preterm infant in an incubator against heat loss.

When one finds that an infant can maintain a constant normal body temperature in an incubator maintained at

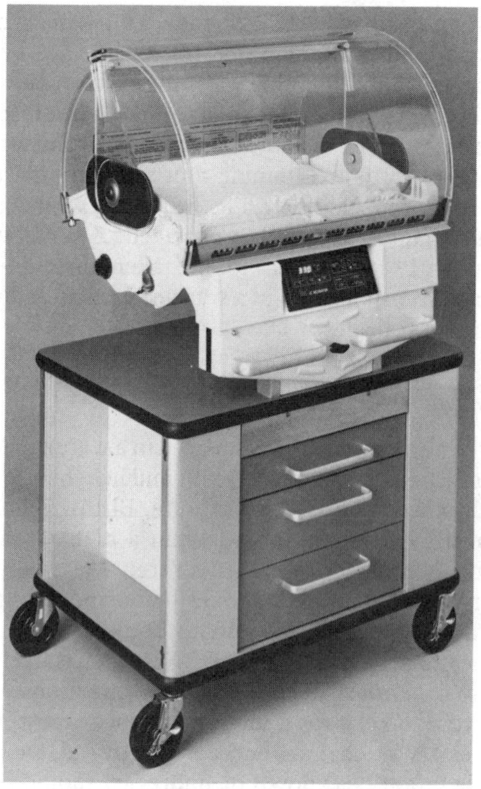

Figure 27-1. Ohio ® IC Incubator. Incubators are used for care of newborns who require more intensive care than the normal full-term infant. Environmental temperature and oxygen concentration can be regulated more easily in an incubator than in a bassinet, and the infant can be observed with ease. [Photograph courtesy of Ohio Medical Products (Division of Airco, Inc.), Madison, WI.]

a constant temperature, the assumption cannot be made that his thermal environment is satisfactory. The infant may be able to raise his metabolism sufficiently to produce adequate heat to maintain his body temperature even while he is radiating heat to his environment, but the cost to the infant of such heat production is likely to be great.

Radiant Heat

A source of radiant heat can be used to supply warmth to an infant. Placed above the bassinet or the roof of the incubator, the lamp will radiate heat to the infant. A radiant heater should be used when the newborn is first placed in the bassinet or incubator, and at any time that an infant cannot maintain a normal body temperature well, or when outside conditions indicate that the infant needs warmth. Such radiant heat helps to deliver warmth to the infant, reduces his metabolic rate, and serves to return his body temperature to normal more rapidly than with incubator or clothing protection alone.

The infant's metabolic rate increases or decreases rapidly with cooling or warming. Even while the infant's body temperature is still low, his metabolic rate and thus his oxygen need decrease when he is placed in a heat-gaining environment. A gradual rise in body temperature to normal will then take place without undue expenditure of energy.

When it becomes necessary to obtain blood samples and to begin intravenous fluids on the infant, he needs protection from covers, where possible, and heat from lamps. When treatments are necessary, it may be advisable to use an open-ended radiant warmer infant care table (page 613).

Need for radiant heat to the infant is lessened if the baby is clothed, if the incubator temperature is high, at 35° C (95° F) or above, and as he gets older.

Regulation of Incubator Temperature

An infant's surroundings should be such that he can maintain his body temperature between 36.4 and 36.7°C (97.5 and 98° F) axillary, or 36.7 and 37° C (98 and 98.6° F) rectally, without stress. The incubator should be placed against an inside wall of the nursery, since the temperature of that wall does not become as cool or fluctuate as much as an outer wall, and heat loss by radiation is likely less. Even with little exposure to cold surfaces outside the incubator, the temperature of the infant's incubator may need to be as high as 35.6 to 36.1° C (96 to 97°F) if his weight is under 1360 gm (3 lb) and 34.4 to 35.6°C (94 to 96° F) if he is somewhat larger. With clothes or blankets on the infant, or a heat lamp over the incubator, a somewhat lower incubator temperature soon may be satisfactory. Clothes, however, interfere with good visibility and are ordinarily not used while an infant in an incubator is in need of close observation. A transparent plastic shell heat shield will help to conserve heat (page 613).

A highly desirable method of regulating the warmth of an incubator is through maintenance of the infant's skin temperature at or near a normal body temperature. Many incubators are equipped with a skin thermistor probe, which may be taped to the exposed skin of either of the sides of the infant's abdomen. This probe monitors the skin temperature and, through a control mechanism, regulates the heater in the incubator to increase or reduce heat output in accordance with a predetermined setting for the desired skin temperature.

The temperature of the infant's skin appears to have considerable influence on his metabolic rate. Relatively small changes in skin temperature influence oxygen need. Oxygen consumption is relatively low when the abdominal skin temperature is maintained between 36.4 and 37.6° C (97.5 and 98° F). To maintain such a skin temperature, the control mechanism of the heater of the incubator, to which the skin thermistor is attached, may be set at 36.4° C (97.6° F). A small piece of gauze or cotton should be used to cover the skin probe to insulate it against air currents in the incubator and against direct radiant heat.

When a skin thermistor is not used, it is necessary to monitor the infant's body temperature frequently to determine his need for, and his response to, warmth. Every effort must be made to maintain a warm and stable environment through careful control of the incubator temperature and the surrounding area.

Under any circumstances, with or without control of the incubator temperature according to a desired skin temperature, it is important to monitor the infant's body temperature and his environment frequently and to be concerned that his surroundings are such that he does not lose body heat to the environment. When the infant does not need to expend extra energy to keep warm, his use of oxygen and calories for heat production can be kept at a minimum. The infant then will not develop the metabolic acidosis and the deficiency of surfactant production that can accompany increased metabolism and an inadequate supply of oxygen and glucose.

When an infant is placed into a heat-gaining environment, it is important to guard against too much warming as well as too little. A newborn does not tolerate overheating, since his metabolism then also rises. He is likely to become restless and begin to perspire when his body temperature rises to 37.5° C (99.5° F). Overheating is more likely to occur with a full-term infant who is placed in a heated bassinet for quick regain of normal body temperature, than with a premature in an incubator. A full-term infant, who is likely to be dressed or wrapped in blankets, may become too warm after an hour or two in a warmed bassinet. His body temperature must be monitored every 30 minutes so that the heat in his bassinet can be reduced when he is warm. After the body temperature of a full-term infant returns to normal, external heat ordinarily is not necessary.

NURSING CARE DURING THE TRANSITIONAL PERIOD

The greatest hazard in the postnatal period is during the first day of life. The nurse must watch the newborn very closely during this period in which he is making drastic adjustments to his environment. Since many neonatal problems begin in the first 6 to 8 hours after birth, the infant's care during this time should be given in a nursery area specially designated as recovery room or transitional care area. There the infant can be monitored closely during this transitional phase and for a longer period of time if necessary. In terms of time the transitional period is usually considered to be the first 6 to 8 hours after birth, but for some infants a longer time is necessary for their conditions to stabilize, with the transitional period extending to an upper limit of 24 hours.

Each infant, regardless of how normal his past history, must be observed closely. Every infant must be assumed to be at risk, at least from choking by mucus, and all must be closely observed. For some infants the risk of postnatal difficulty is particularly great. Conditions that may complicate the postnatal course include intrauterine fetal distress, apnea or hypoxia at birth, prolonged labor, difficult delivery, and complications of the mother during pregnancy, such as antepartum bleeding and diabetes. The nurse caring for newborns should be acquainted with the prenatal, labor, and delivery history of each infant for whose care she is responsible. Infants in whom difficulty is anticipated may be cared for in an incubator where they are more protected and also observed more easily than they are in a bassinet.

After it becomes apparent that the infant has made a good adjustment to extrauterine life, anywhere from 6 to 24 hours for the normal full-term infant, he can be cared for in his mother's room or in the central nursery.

Admission to the Nursery

Antenatal and Labor History

Immediately on admission of an infant to the nursery, the nurse will need to have some important information about the pregnancy and the labor and delivery. She will want to know the estimated gestational age according to the mother's history and other assessments that may have been made before delivery, any medical or obstetric complications, the mother's Rh factor and serology, when labor began, when the membrane ruptured, all medications given to the mother during labor (kind and amount), the fetal heart rate and pattern during labor, the Apgar score and any resuscitative efforts. Additional history can be obtained later.

Check on Physical Condition and Behavior

The infant's general overall appearance and behavior can be assessed during admission procedures. It is important to look at relative size of body, head, and extremities; to observe for the normally flexed posture, strong muscle tone, and symmetric, spontaneous movement of all extremities; to check for a normally pink-red color with perhaps cyanotic hands and feet, forceps marks or bruises, condition of the skin, edema, and a normally strong, vigorous, spontaneous cry.

An initial assessment of the infant's physical status, usually done by the nurse, is made immediately after birth, mainly through use of the Apgar score; auscultation of the chest and heart, and a quick appraisal of the appearance of the infant to rule out gross abnormalities and congenital anomalies. The American Academy of Pediatrics recommends that after the infant's condition has stabilized (usually in 5 to 10 minutes of age), he should be checked for several anomalies not grossly ap-

Table 27–1. Checklist for Abnormalities in Physical Development*†

1. The infant's breathing should be observed to see if he can breathe with his mouth closed. (Rule out choanal atresia.)
2. A soft tube should be passed through the mouth a sufficient distance to reach the stomach. (Rule out esophageal atresia.)
3. The gastric contents should be aspirated quantitatively. (More than 15 to 20 ml leads to suspicion of high intestinal obstruction.)
4. The patency of the anus should be checked by passing a soft catheter into the rectum if no meconium is seen.
5. The number of umbilical vessels should be counted. Three are normal.

*To be used very early in the postnatal period.
†American Academy of Pediatrics, *Standards and Recommendations for Hospital Care of Newborn Infants,* 5th ed. Evanston, Ill., 1971.

parent. The Academy suggests an early check for the five signs of anomalies listed in Table 27–1.

A few reflexes may be checked on admission. The Moro reflex and grasp reflex, valuable signs of normal behavior, should be elicited easily. The infant may demonstrate his sucking reflex by attempting to suck on his fist or on anything that comes near his mouth.

Other Items of Care on Admission

The infant's identification bracelets are checked to correlate the information on them with the chart records.

As was suggested on page 421, it is desirable to postpone prophylactic treatment of the eyes (which for many years was a traditional delivery room procedure) until admission of the infant to the nursery. If the treatment was not done in the delivery room, it should be carried out as a part of the admission regime. The method of prophylactic eye treatment is described on pages 420–21.

The umbilical cord stump and the surrounding skin are wiped with an antiseptic, usually with alcohol 60 percent, or with a bacteriostatic such as triple dye. The number of umbilical cord vessels can be checked at this time.

Blood on the infant's face and scalp may be washed off with a warm wet cloth or cotton balls. No further bathing is done until the infant has regained a stable normal body temperature or until after the second period of reactivity described below.

Vitamin K, usually ordered as a single dose of 1.0 mg, is given intramuscularly to prevent a transitory deficiency in blood coagulation.

Assessment of Gestational Age and Intrauterine Growth

Somewhere around the time the newborn is transferred from the delivery room to the nursery, his birthweight is obtained and recorded, his length usually is measured, and a gestational age assessment is made, at least from a brief set of criteria (Fig. 27–2). Later, and as indicated, a more detailed gestational age assessment, using the Ballard (Fig. 27–3*A, B, C, D, E*) or another system, can be done.

From the Ballard system of assessing age, 12 evaluation criteria are used. These are illustrated in Figure 27–3*A, B, C, D, E.* This system uses six neuromuscular

Gestational Age According to Clinical Criteria

Clinical Criteria		36 weeks and less	37 to 38 weeks	39 or more weeks
Sole creases		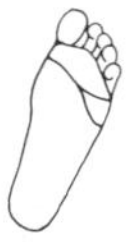 Anterior transverse crease only	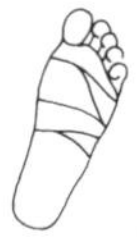 Occasional creases anterior two thirds	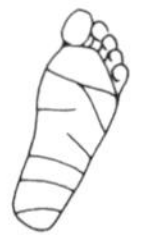 Sole covered with creases
Breast nodule diameter		2 mm	4 mm	7 mm or greater
Ear cartilage (pinna)		Little or no cartilage Ear returns slowly from folding	Some cartilage Ear springs back from folding	Stiffened with cartilage Firm erect ear
Scalp hair		Very fine Wooly or fuzzy	Very fine Wooly or fuzzy	Coarse, silky texture Each hair appears as a single strand
Genitalia	Male	Testes in canal, have not yet descended completely into scrotal sac Scrotum small with few rugae	Intermediate	Testes fully descended Scrotum full and pendulous with many rugae
	Female	Labia majora open	Labia majora open	Labia majora closed and cover labia minora and clitoris

Figure 18-4. Gestational age according to several well-defined characteristics and clinical criteria.

NEWBORN MATURITY RATING and CLASSIFICATION

ESTIMATION OF GESTATIONAL AGE BY MATURITY RATING

Side 1

Symbols: X - 1st Exam O - 2nd Exam

NEUROMUSCULAR MATURITY

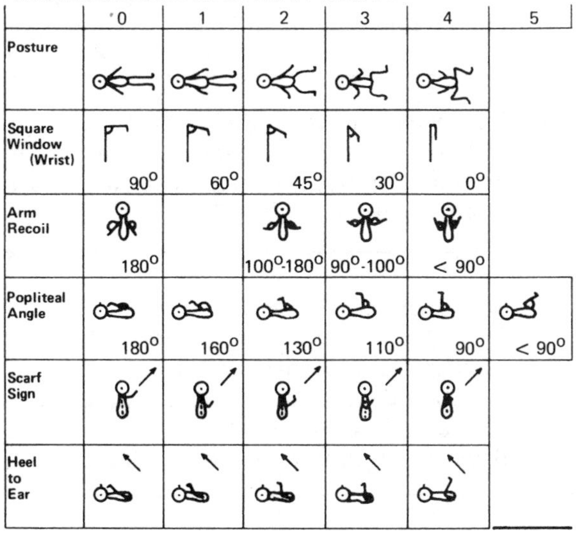

	0	1	2	3	4	5
Posture						
Square Window (Wrist)	90°	60°	45°	30°	0°	
Arm Recoil	180°		100°-180°	90°-100°	< 90°	
Popliteal Angle	180°	160°	130°	110°	90°	< 90°
Scarf Sign						
Heel to Ear						

PHYSICAL MATURITY

	0	1	2	3	4	5
SKIN	gelatinous red, trans-parent	smooth pink, visible veins	superficial peeling &/or rash, few veins	cracking pale area, rare veins	parchment, deep cracking, no vessels	leathery, cracked, wrinkled
LANUGO	none	abundant	thinning	bald areas	mostly bald	
PLANTAR CREASES	no crease	faint red marks	anterior transverse crease only	creases ant. 2/3	creases cover entire sole	
BREAST	barely percept.	flat areola, no bud	stippled areola, 1–2 mm bud	raised areola, 3–4 mm bud	full areola, 5–10 mm bud	
EAR	pinna flat, stays folded	sl. curved pinna, soft with slow recoil	well-curv. pinna, soft but ready recoil	formed & firm with instant recoil	thick cartilage, ear stiff	
GENITALS Male	scrotum empty, no rugae		testes descend-ing, few rugae	testes down, good rugae	testes pendulous, deep rugae	
GENITALS Female	prominent clitoris & labia minora		majora & minora equally prominent	majora large, minora small	clitoris & minora completely covered	

Scoring system: Ballard JL, *et al*: A Simplified Assessment of Gestational Age. Pediatr Res 11:374, 1977. Figures adapted from "Classification of the Low-Birth-Weight Infant" by AY Sweet in Care of the High-Risk Infant by MH Klaus and AA Fanaroff, WB Saunders Co, Philadelphia, 1977, p. 47.

Gestation by Dates ______________ wks

Birth Date __________ Hour __________ am pm

APGAR __________ 1 min __________ 5 min

MATURITY RATING

Score	Wks
5	26
10	28
15	30
20	32
25	34
30	36
35	38
40	40
45	42
50	44

SCORING SECTION

	1st Exam=X	2nd Exam=O
Estimating Gest Age by Maturity Rating	______ Weeks	______ Weeks
Time of Exam	Date ______ Hour ______ am pm	Date ______ Hour ______ am pm
Age at Exam	______ Hours	______ Hours
Signature of Examiner	______ M.D.	______ M.D.

A

Figure 27-3. *A, B, C, D, E.* Newborn Maturity Rating and Classification (Courtesy of Mead Johnson Nutritional Division).

ASSESSMENT OF NEUROMUSCULAR MATURITY

POSTURE With the infant supine and quiet, score as follows:	Arms and legs extended . . . . = 0 Slight or moderate flexion of hips and knees . . . . = 1 Moderate to strong flexion of hips and knees . . . . = 2 Legs flexed and abducted, arms slightly flexed . . . . = 3 Full flexion of arms and legs . . . . = 4
SQUARE WINDOW Flex the hand at the wrist. Exert pressure sufficient to get as much flexion as possible.	The angle between the hypothenar eminence and the anterior aspect of the forearm is measured and scored (see chart form). *Do not rotate the wrist.*
ARM RECOIL With the infant supine, fully flex the forearm for five seconds, then fully extend by pulling the hands and release.	Score arm reaction according to: Extended or random movements — 180° . . . = 0 Incomplete or partial flexion — 100-180° . . . . = 2 Increased flexion — 90-100° . . . . = 3 Brisk return to full flexion — $<$ 90° . . . . = 4
POPLITEAL ANGLE With the infant supine and the pelvis flat on the examining surface, the leg is flexed on the thigh and the thigh fully flexed with the use of one hand. With the other hand, the leg is then extended.	The angle attained is scored as indicated on the chart form.
SCARF SIGN With the infant supine, take the infant's hand and draw it across the neck and as far across the opposite shoulder as possible. Assistance to the elbow is permissible by lifting it across the body.	Score according to the location of the elbow: Elbow reaches the opposite anterior axillary line . . . . = 0 Elbow between opposite anterior axillary line and midline of thorax . . . . = 2 Elbow at midline of thorax . . . . = 3 Elbow does not reach midline of thorax . . . . = 4
HEEL TO EAR MANEUVER With the infant supine, hold the infant's foot with one hand and move it as near to the head as possible *without forcing it.* Keep the pelvis flat on the examining surface.	Score according to chart form.

B

odor. Greenish-yellow, curdy stools containing a small amount of mucus are normal in the young infant, and the stools may be loose during the first week or two of life if the infant is ingesting a large quantity of milk. Diarrhea must be considered if the stools are watery.

A minute amount of blood, which follows bowel irritation caused by ingested food or bacteria, may be present in the stools during the first few days and is not significant if the infant does not show any other signs of bleeding. Frank blood, either fresh or old, is abnormal and requires investigation. Blood may be found in the stools if the infant has nursed from a bleeding nipple.

The number of stools per day varies a great deal, tending to be more frequent in the breast-fed than in the formula-fed infant. There may be only one stool daily, but more frequently stools are passed from four to eight times a day in the early days of life. The infant possibly may have a small stool after each feeding. Later the stools become more infrequent. Constipation does not occur in the breast-fed infant and rarely with formula feedings. The mother is told of the number and kind of stools she may expect her infant to have and is advised to report watery stools to the physician.

Since urine is present in the bladder at birth, the infant frequently voids immediately after he is born, but emptying of the bladder may be delayed for 12 to 24 hours, and sometimes even longer. Many infants have voided within 8 hours, 50 percent have voided by 12 hours, and over 90 percent by 24 hours. There is need for concern if the infant has not voided by 48 hours.

The first urine voided, often shortly after birth, was formed *in utero* and is dilute. After the first voiding, which may be clear and pale, the urine appears cloudy and quite highly colored owing to more concentration and its rather high urate and mucus content. After fluid intake increases, the urine again becomes a pale-yellow color. It is practically odorless during infancy.

Uric acid excretion in the newborn is high; it may be deposited in crystal form in the kidneys and produce uric acid infarcts. As these uric acid crystals are passed in the urine, they may appear as red (brick-dust) spots on the infant's diaper and sometimes are confused with blood in the urine.

The number of voidings daily is recorded, and note is taken of amounts that appear either scanty or excessively large. Highly colored, concentrated urine, evidence of uric acid crystals, or observation of abnormal conditions such as blood is charted and reported to the physician. Efforts to increase fluid intake may be necessary when voiding is scanty and infrequent and when uric acid crystals are seen on the diaper.

Weight

The infant's weight usually is taken and recorded daily, ordinarily at bath time. In a warm nursery the average newborn may be weighed completely undressed without undue exposure, but small infants, under 2275 gm (5 lb), are protected against temperature changes by weighing them with their clothes on or wrapped in a blanket and the weight of the wrap deducted from the total weight.

While weighing the infant, adequate precautions must be taken to protect him from falling off the scales. An accident can be prevented by placing one end of the scales (the end toward which the infant's head will be placed) near but not against a wall and watching the infant carefully during the weighing instead of concentrating completely on balancing the scales.

The nurse compares the day's weight with the birthweight and with the weight of the previous day and reports to the physician any great weight loss during the first few days of life as well as a stationary weight or a very slow gain after the first week. The weight is recorded on the infant's hospital record each day and may be charted on a graph (Fig. 26–5, page 512).

The Physical Examination

A complete detailed physical examination may be done after the transition period either for the first time or as a repeat examination. The first physical examination should be done relatively early in the postnatal period, at least within the first 24 hours. Frequently such an examination is done by the physician. The nurse, however, is the only member of the health care team continuously with the infant and may be the only member available to appraise the infant in the first hours of life. Physical assessment skills have become increasingly important to the nurse, who is assuming increasing responsibility for evaluating the status of infants.

The nurse may do a physical assessment in order to plan appropriate care to assist the infant to make a good adjustment to extrauterine life, to determine any risk factors, and to notify the physician early of any abnormal findings in order to institute necessary medical management early. Nurse and physician physical assessment data may be much the same. As it is pooled and shared, optimum plans can be made for the infant for prevention of difficulty and protection against problems that could arise, for management of any problems present, for support of the infant's efforts in his adjustment, and for nurturance of his physical and emotional needs.

History

The obstetric history and the progress of the infant since birth are important sources of information before the actual physical examination is begun. The nurse will want to know the prepregnancy, pregnancy, and labor and delivery history, and about the adjustment the infant has made since birth.

Prepregnancy history should include maternal medical complications such as diabetes, hypertension, renal disease, thyroid disease, and how long the disease has existed and how it has been treated, including drugs. A history of any condition that is likely to alter the fetal environment is important. Pregnancy history also should include family history of congenital diseases and history of known drug abuse, child abuse, and psychiatric problems. If the mother has other children, information about the events of their birth and their present health is important. History of abortions or stillbirths also should be included.

Pregnancy history should include expected date of delivery; blood type and Rh factor; serology; history of any bleeding during pregnancy, of any blood pressure elevation; of any infection, and of all drugs or medications taken; weight before pregnancy and weight gain; amount of prenatal care; and data concerning fetal assessment, if such was done. It is also important to know if the pregnancy was planned.

Labor and delivery history should include length of gestation, kind and length of labor and type of delivery, all analgesic and anesthetic agents (how much and when), management of any maternal medical complications, time of rupture of membranes, meconium in amniotic fluid, fetal heart rate and pattern during labor, fetal pH if done, and any maternal fever or bleeding.

The infant's condition at birth, his Apgar score, any resuscitative efforts, gestational age and weight, and his extrauterine adjustment since birth must be included in the history.

Physical Examination

The physical examination must be done in a systematic, orderly manner to avoid overlooking some important observations. Modifications of approach may be necessary depending upon the "state" of the infant, but even modifications can be made in an orderly way. The value of the nurse's physical examination will depend upon her ability to differentiate between normal and abnormal findings and her knowledge of the range of normal for the newborn. A detailed record should be made of the findings of the physical examination in a way that will be useful to others.

The basic methods used in a physical examination of any individual are also used for the newborn. These include inspection, auscultation, palpation, and percussion. The methods should be used in that order, in the hope that the infant will not be disturbed and crying prior to auscultation. General inspection, observing the infant as a whole, and also local inspection, focusing on each anatomic region of the infant, will yield a great deal of information. Auscultation usually means listening with a stethoscope, but sounds such as noisy or grunting respirations and the quality of the infant's cry also may be included. Palpation, feeling by the sense of touch, can be used on every part of the body that is accessible to the examining fingers. Palpation is followed by percussion or tapping where appropriate.

The actual examination of the newborn is reviewed below, pointing out some of the observations that can be made and some of the common findings. No attempt has been made to cover all the possibilities of the examination and all the disorders that can be discovered. Experience gained by examination of many normal newborns will assist the nurse in identifying abnormalities when they arise.

GENERAL INSPECTION An overall inspection will show if the infant assumes the normally expected flexed posture, if he appears to have a normal, firm, strong muscle tone, and if he appears to have symmetric and easy movement of all of his extremities. He should not appear to be hypotonic or excessively jittery in response to stimuli. The infant's general size in relation to gestational age and the relative size of head, body, and extremities can be evaluated (Fig. 27-7A and B). General inspection should reveal any gross abnormalities. Characteristic facial features may lead to suspicion of Down's syndrome or other genetic disorders.

General inspection also includes looking at skin color for the normally pink or red color, with possibly bluish extremities, or for abnormalities such as ruddiness, pallor, cyanosis, or jaundice. Any abnormalities in respiration also may be observed. Effects of the birth process such as degree of molding of the head and ecchymosis may be observed. Facial expression may show an infant who is comfortable or one in distress. When the infant begins to cry, the quality and pitch of his cry may be evaluated.

HEART AND LUNGS Examination of the heart, lungs, and abdomen is done most easily while the infant is asleep or at least not crying. If the infant begins to cry, the examination may need to be postponed until he quiets.

Observation of the chest is made for the normal breathing pattern of diaphragmatic breathing with the abdomen rising and falling with inspiration and expiration, and for a normal respiratory rate of approximately 40 times per minute. Intercostal or xiphoid retractions, nasal flaring, expiratory grunt or sigh, and tachypnea are abnormal findings. It is also helpful to note if the chest appears high (hyperextended) or low (hypoextended) in the antero-posterior diameter. Auscultation is made for type of breath sounds, rales, rhonchi, and wheezes. The entire chest, both anterior and posterior, is examined. Sometimes auscultatory sounds are heard better if the infant is crying.

Localization and identification of chest sounds are very difficult in the newborn, and sometimes the sounds

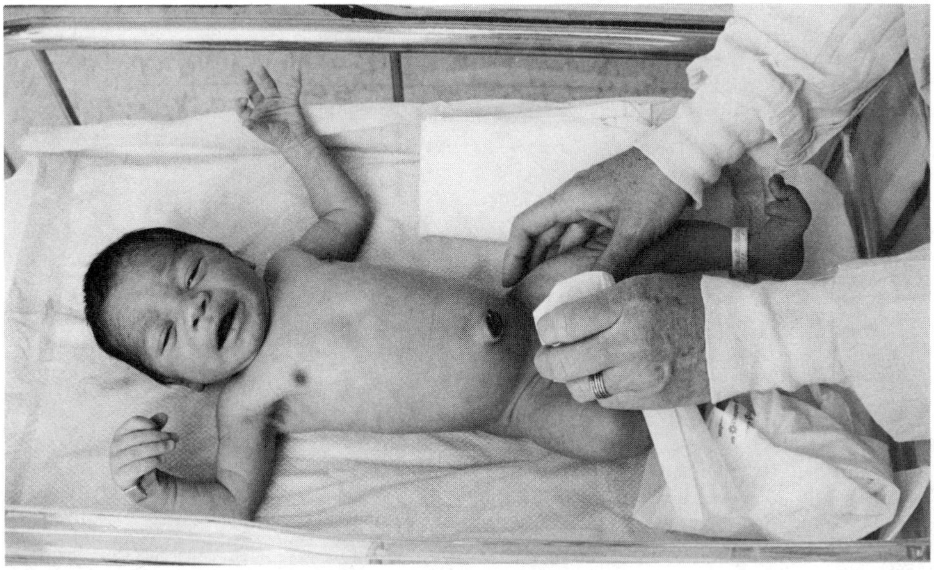

A

Figure 27–7. The nurse is performing a physical examination on this newborn. *A*. An overall inspection of this infant shows that he has firm, strong muscle tone. He responds with an active Moro reflex when he is touched. The relative size of his head, body, and extremities appear normal. His skin looks clear. The umbilical cord is drying. The genitalia will also be inspected.

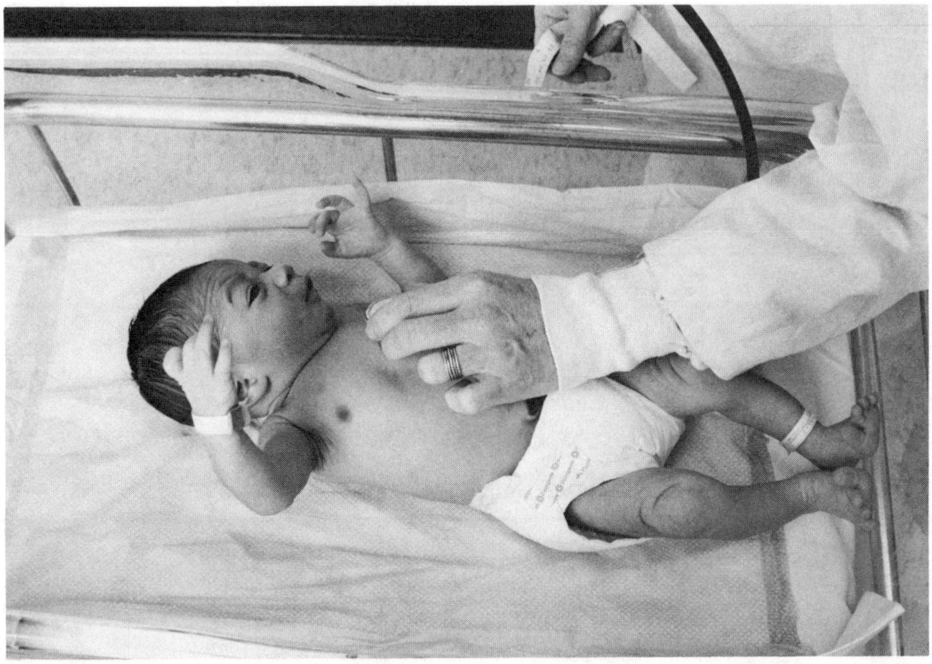

B

B. The infant's breasts are examined for size and development—one of the criteria for assessment of gestational age. The breasts are also examined for engorgement, an early hormonal reaction in some infants.

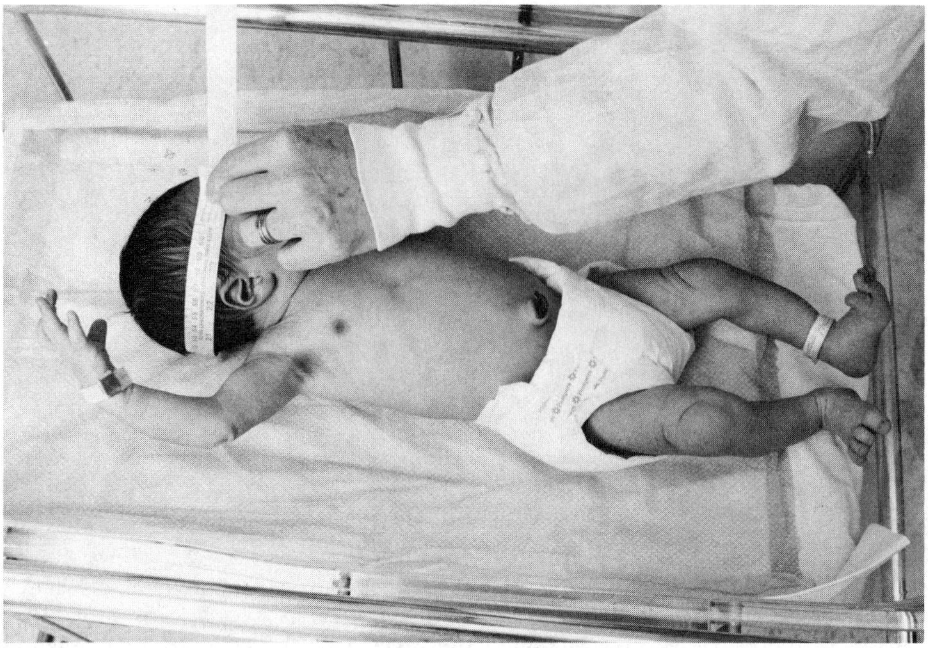

C

C. A measurement of the circumference of the head is made during a physical examination. This measurement is compared to normal measurements and also to measurement of the infant's chest.

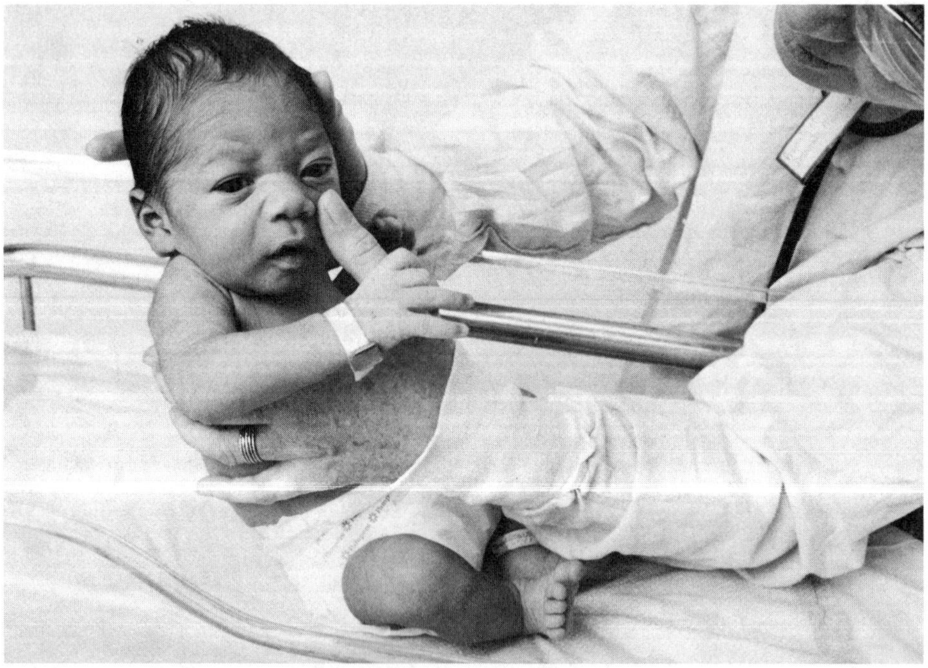

D

D. The infant's face is assessed for symmetry of features and the eyes, ears, nose, and mouth are inspected. Here the eyes are being examined for pupil reaction and for normal conjunctiva and cornea.

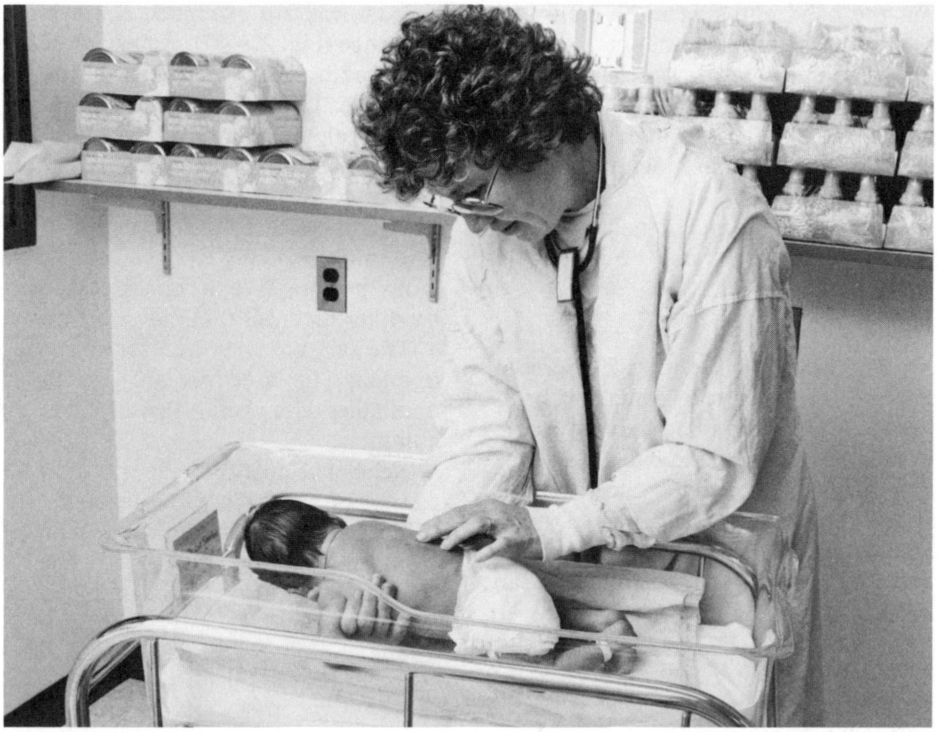

E

E. The infant's back is being inspected for skin color, turgor, elasticity, and any hemangiomatous areas, and it is palpated for normal spine development. [Courtesy of The Presbyterian Hospital in the City of New York. Photos by Elizabeth Marshall.]

are transmitted so well from an unaffected area of the lung to an affected one that the absence of sounds cannot be diagnosed. Auscultation of the newborn chest requires considerable experience.

The heart is examined for rate and rhythm of heartbeat, position of apical impulse, and intensity of heart sounds. Location of apical beat gives information about heart size and location. The apical impulse normally can be seen or palpated at the fifth intercostal space just left of the sternum. A shift in the mediastinum moves the apical impulse away from the affected side of the chest. Therefore a pneumothorax in the right chest moves the mediastinum to the left and the apical impulse farther to the left than normal. When the left chest is affected, the apical impulse is close to the midline of the chest or even to the right of midline.

By auscultation of the heart the first and second heart sounds can be heard clearly. They have been described as a rapid lubb-dubb or a toc-tic sound with the second sound being somewhat sharper and having a higher pitch than the first. Murmurs may be heard, but many are transient and disappear by the third day. Heart rate normally fluctuates from 100 to 180 beats per minute. Auscultation of the heart includes listening over the entire precordium, below the left axilla, and posteriorly below the scapula.

The femoral pulses are palpated by applying gentle pressure, perhaps using the middle finger, over the femoral canal. Decreased or absent femoral pulses indicate coarctation of the aorta. The brachial pulses also are palpated for equality with each other and with the femoral pulses.

ABDOMEN The abdomen is inspected for size and contour and for localized bulging. The abdomen is normally cylindrical in shape and there may be slight bulging between the recti muscles. The umbilical cord is inspected for normal drying or for redness and moistness, and it is examined for the presence of two arteries and one vein. Observation of only two vessels raises the suspicion of congenital anomalies elsewhere in the body.

Palpation of the abdomen for softness or tenseness and for masses should be done in a systematic manner, beginning in one of the quadrants and continuing to the others in a clockwise direction. Palpation may first be done lightly and then repeated with deeper pressure.

The edge of the liver of the newborn is normally palpated 1 to 2 cm below the right costal margin. The tip of the spleen sometimes can be felt in the normal newborn in the lateral portion of the left upper quadrant. Examination of the abdomen must include deep palpation for each kidney. With the infant in the supine position, a finger is placed at the posterior flank, the costovertebral angle, to provide upward pressure and the other hand presses down toward the finger at the posterior flank. The kidney can be felt as a small oval structure between the hand and finger. Normally the lower pole of each kidney is situated about 1 to 2 cm above the umbilicus. Kidneys below this level are enlarged. It is best to palpate the kidneys soon after birth, or at least before 4 to 6 hours have elapsed, since they can be felt much easier when the intestines have not yet filled with air.

If the infant has not passed meconium and if the anus has not been checked for patency, it may be done at this time.

HEAD AND NECK The head is inspected for degree of molding, for size, and for soft tissue edema and bruising. The circumference of the head is measured and compared to normal measurements of the chest. For measurement of the infant's head circumference, the tape should be placed over the most prominent part of the occiput and brought around to just above the eyebrows (Fig. 27-7C). Since head circumference is an important measurement of brain size and later measurements are good indicators of brain growth, the head circumference should be measured very carefully and accurately. To check on one's own measurements it is advisable to repeat the measurement a second and a third time.[4] Since measurement of the head may change as molding decreases, it is helpful to remeasure the head a few days later.

The anterior and posterior fontanels are palpated for size and depression or bulging, and then are measured, and the sutures between the cranial bones are palpated for amount of overlapping. For measurement of the anterior fontanel, the anteroposterior and transverse dimensions are measured with the fingers, and the size is recorded. The posterior fontanel also may be measured with a finger. In order to obtain an accurate measurement of the fontanels, the width of the examiner's fingers can be measured in centimeters.

Often the infant's chest is measured at the same time that the head is measured. For measurement of chest circumference, the measuring tape is placed at the lower end of the scapulas and brought around anteriorly directly over the nipple line. Three measurements are taken and the average is recorded.[5] Measurement of the abdominal circumference may also be taken at this time, placing the measuring tape around the infant's abdomen at the level of the umbilicus.

The infant's face is assessed for symmetry of the eyes, nose, and ears.

The eyes are checked for size, equality of pupils, reaction of pupils to light, the blink reflex to light, and edema and inflammation of the eyelids. The conjunctivas are checked for hemorrhage and inflammation and the corneas are examined for a bright and shiny appearance (Fig. 27-7D). A hazy, dull cornea is abnormal. The eyes are examined for the normal red reflex to check that there is no opacity between the lens and the retina and to rule out cataracts.

Examination of the eyes may be difficult in the newborn because the infant tends to keep his eyes closed. It usually is not helpful to attempt to hold the lids open. The infant is likely to open his eyes when he is rocked from the upright to the horizontal position a few times or by other methods that may alert him.

The ears are inspected for size, shape, position, and anomaly. Low-set ears are sometimes associated with anomalies elsewhere. Preauricular tags are relatively common.

Newborns must breathe through the nose, since they cannot ordinarily breathe through the mouth. Patency of the nares or unilateral choanal atresia can be checked by closing first one nostril and then the other, making sure the mouth is closed, and then observing respirations.

The mouth is checked especially for cleft palate. Visualization of the mouth is probably best when the infant is crying. Palpation with a finger also is done since a cleft of the hard palate with intact mucous membrane cannot be visualized. This is also an opportunity to evaluate the strength of the infant's suck.

The neck is inspected for webbing and palpated for presence of lymph nodes and masses.

The clavicles are palpated for crepitus, depressions, bony masses, or ridges to rule out fracture.

GENITALIA Examination of the male consists of looking for the position of the meatal opening and for any evidence of hypospadius and also inspecting the scrotum for size and symmetry, for hydrocele, and for undescended testicles. The testes should be palpated separately between the thumb and finger of one hand while the thumb and index finger of the other hand are placed together over the inguinal canal.

The female genitalia are examined for size of the labia majora and minora, for amount of protrusion of labia minora from majora, for clitoral size, and for fusion of the labia. Hymenal tags often are normally present, protruding from the vagina. A creamy, mucous vaginal discharge is normally present, and vaginal bleeding is seen occasionally.

SKIN The skin should be observed closely as each area of the body is examined. Color, consistency, turgor, elasticity, texture, hydration, and areas of desquamation are noted. The examiner is watchful for petechiae, areas of ecchymosis, hemangiomas, eruptions, hemorrhagic manifestations, inflammation, and nevi.

MUSCULOSKELETAL The spine is inspected and palpated for abnormal curvatures, for masses, tufts of hair over

[4] Marcene Erickson, *Assessment and Developmental Changes in Children,* C. V. Mosby, St. Louis, 1976, p. 25.

[5] *Ibid.,* p. 35.

the spine, spina bifida, and pilonidal sinus (Fig. 27-7E). The extremities are examined for gross deformities, for extra digits, for webbing, for clubfeet, and for range of motion.

The infant is examined for congenital dislocation of the hip by placing him supine, flexing the knees, and then abducting both of his hips and knees. Normally both knees can be brought down simultaneously to the examining table. A dislocated hip does not abduct well. Sometimes with dislocation a click can be heard and felt with this maneuver. Asymmetry of the buttock creases and unequal leg length when the infant lies on his abdomen also are present with dislocation.

NEUROLOGIC Some of the neurologic examination is accomplished throughout the physical examination as the infant is observed for respiratory movements, cardiac action, eye movements, posture and muscle tone, spontaneous activity, spontaneous alertness, the strength of the cry, and the response to stimuli. Fine, rapid tremors are normal, but large coarse tremors are suggestive of pathology.

A few of the infant's reflexes also may be checked to determine neurologic status. These usually include the Moro reflex, grasp, grasp and traction showing ability to bring the head up, standing and walking, and rooting and sucking.

More evidence concerning development of the central nervous system is obtained if a Brazelton neonatal behavior assessment is done.

Skin Care and Inspection

Care of the skin of the newborn during the hospital stay has changed from time to time. About 50 years ago the so-called "dry" technique of skin care began to replace the use of soap and water or oil baths, because there was evidence that the less handling the skin received, the less the irritation, and consequently the less the danger of infection. Thereafter, the hazard of staphylococcal infections among infants in newborn nurseries brought about another change. A bath with a liquid detergent containing 3 percent hexachlorophene often was used in an effort to reduce the rate of skin and nasal colonization by staphylococci and possibly reduce the incidence of skin infection.

Some years later a number of studies raised questions concerning the toxicity to the central nervous system of 3 percent hexachlorophene preparations when used daily for total body bathing of newborns. According to the *FDA Drug Bulletin,* December, 1971, the FDA and the Committee on Fetus and Newborn of the American Academy of Pediatrics have "jointly concluded that the use of hexachlorophene for total body bathing of infants in hospital nurseries or at home is not recommended." In its place the committee recommends the following procedures:

> At present we recommend dry skin care, washing with plain soap and water or tap water alone for skin care of the newborn infants. It should be emphasized that the most important factor in the transmission of infection from infant to infant is hand contact. This can be minimized by scrupulous hand washing before entering the nursery as well as just before and just after handling each infant. Either an iodophor preparation or 3% hexachlorophene emulsion is recommended.[6]

Following the above recommendations the question of a possible increase in staphylococcal infection was raised. Since then some hospitals have reported cases of staphylococcal infection, manifested mainly by a pustular dermatitis or impetigo. Where bacterial outbreaks have appeared, the FDA has permitted use of hexachlorophene temporarily for once-daily bathing of infants.

The "dry" technique is used between soap and water baths. It also may be used if a soap and water bath is postponed because of an infant's adverse condition or postponed until the infant has regained a normal temperature. Sometimes the "dry" technique is used throughout the infant's hospital stay. In this method of care, water or oil is not used on the infant's skin, with the exception of small areas that need special attention. As soon as possible after birth, blood on the infant's face and scalp is washed away with cotton balls or a soft washcloth dipped into warm water, and the infant is wrapped in a warm blanket. No attempt is made to wash or wipe off the vernix caseosa. To avoid undue chilling, the infant may be wrapped in the warm blanket before the blood is removed from the face and scalp.

The vernix acts as a vanishing cream and rubs into the skin or off onto the clothes within 12 to 24 hours. It remains for a longer time, however, in the creases and folds of skin where a heavy deposit may be found. Instead of being protected, these areas may become irritated if vernix is left indefinitely, therefore it should be removed in 24 to 48 hours.

The dry technique does not eliminate daily morning care. The only omission is use of soap and water or oil. Inspection of the condition of the skin and of the eyes, nose, mouth, ears, umbilicus, and genitalia must be done as thoroughly as any observation made during the more traditional bath. Special care must be taken to inspect the creases behind the ears, around the neck, in the axillae, and in the groin for skin irritation. The skin may become very dry and peel in large flakes after a few days, and dry cracks may appear around the wrists and ankles (Fig. 26-12). This drying is not significant except insofar as it causes the mother concern; the nurse explains that it is a temporary condition of the skin that does no harm and that after a few days the flakiness and cracks will

[6] U.S. Department of Health, Education, and Welfare, Public Health Service, Food and Drug Administration, *FDA Drug Bulletin,* Rockville, Md., December, 1971.

disappear. It is important for the nurse to note and report to the physician moist irritated areas, pustules, or water blisters which may be impetigo and therefore may need special attention.

The face is washed with clear, warm water and a soft washcloth, starting with the eyes and wiping from the inner canthus outward. The mouth area is washed clean of formula and mucus, and the outer ears and the creases behind the ears are washed and inspected for skin irritation. A cotton ball may be used to wash the face, but special care must be taken to moisten it completely to prevent cotton wisps from getting into the infant's eyes and nose, where they would produce irritation. For this reason, it is necessary to use a soft towel rather than a cotton ball for drying the face.

Care of the eyes, ears, and nose at bath time and of the umbilicus is described below.

After the face has been cleaned, the creases around the neck are wiped with warm water and they are inspected for irritation. The neck is difficult to clean because of several skinfolds, but these usually can be wiped fairly easily if the infant's head is hyperextended but supported in the back so that it does not fall back completely.

The vernix that collected in the axillae may be spread as cream to other parts of the body during the first day or two; after that the axillae are wiped with a wet cloth during daily morning care unless the skin in that area is dry.

The groin and buttocks are washed with warm water at bath time and each time the diaper is changed. Use of bland soap is often necessary to wash the buttocks and the crease between the buttocks to clean stool off completely. The external genitalia are cleaned as described below.

After a thorough inspection of the skin is completed, the infant is dressed in clean clothes, and he usually is ready for a feeding. Fingernails and toenails may need trimming if they extend beyond the ends of the fingers and toes.

SKIN IRRITATIONS Infants are very susceptible to skin irritation. They may develop a heat rash, especially in the neck region and in the groin, if they become too warm for even a short period of time. Occasionally pinpoint-or pinhead-size erythematous papules or vesicular lesions develop. Such irritations often are treated by washing the affected area and keeping it dry and by using less clothing. An infant may develop a chafing, called *intertrigo,* where two moist surfaces rub together, especially in the creases of the neck, in the axillae, and in the groin. These areas are also washed and kept as dry as possible, and cornstarch may be applied. Abrasions may occur on the heels, toes, or knees from kicking or rubbing against the sheets. Further irritation is prevented and healing takes place if the areas are bandaged. Although an infant's skin is very sensitive and frequently shows signs of minor insignificant irritations, the nurse must be alert for evidence of infection, which requires immediate treatment and precautions against spread to other infants.

Care of the Eyes, Nose, and Ears

In inspecting the eyes, edema of the lids and a purulent discharge from the eyes may be seen within a few hours after birth. This condition is a chemical conjunctivitis, which may be produced by the silver nitrate used in the eyes shortly after birth (Fig. 26–21). Small areas of subconjunctival hemorrhage, caused by changes in vascular tension during birth, may be present during the first week or two. They apparently do not leave defects.

An infant's eyes do not require daily care other than the removal of accumulated secretions in the corners of the eyes, using a soft washcloth and clean water. They should not be irrigated unless there is a conjunctival discharge. If it is necessary to irrigate the eyes, a physiologic salt solution may be used; the mother is given instructions in its preparation if its use at home becomes necessary or she may purchase it already prepared.

The newborn is an obligatory nose-breather and needs clear nasal passages, but his nose ordinarily does not need special attention because he sneezes vigorously and frequently to clear his own nasal passages. At birth and during the first hours of life when the infant may have mucus in the nose as well as the oropharynx, the nose is cleared with gentle suction on a catheter or a bulb syringe. If a small amount of mucus accumulates later and is well down in the nostrils, it may be possible to remove this with a twisted piece of cotton that has been moistened with water and the excess solution squeezed out. An applicator should not be used to clear the nose because of the danger of injury.

The ears are washed externally only. It is never advisable to introduce an applicator into the ear canals.

Care of the Umbilical Cord

Care of the umbilical cord immediately after birth has been described in Chapter 21. To avoid serious hemorrhage from the cord stump, it must be observed closely during the next 24 hours for evidence of bleeding; inspection may be necessary every one-half to one hour until it appears quite evident that bleeding will probably not occur. The danger of bleeding is greatest when the cord contains a large amount of Wharton's jelly, which shrinks and leaves a previously tight ligature or tight clamp loose. In some instances bleeding does not occur even when the ligature is loose because a blood clot has formed at the end of the cord stump. This clot may become loosened, however, with manipulation or movements of the infant, and bleeding may then occur. The quickest way to stop bleeding from the cord is to apply a sterile hemostatic forceps. This should be placed as far away from the abdominal wall as possible, allowing for adequate room to apply another ligature or clamp should the forceps in some way injure the cord itself and make hemostasis at this point impossible. After bleeding has been controlled with the hemostatic forceps, the nurse or doctor can apply another ligature or clamp, using aseptic technique.

In daily care of the umbilical area, it is important that asepsis be maintained until healing is complete. Until then, pyogenic bacteria can produce an infection that may even extend to the peritoneum, to the liver, or into the bloodstream. Careful hand washing before caring for the area is important. Moisture in the area should be kept at a minimum by avoiding putting the infant's diaper on so high that the cord is moist for long periods from a wet diaper. An umbilical cord dressing currently is not used.

Daily care of the umbilical cord often consists of wiping the stump and the area around the umbilicus with an antiseptic, sometimes several times a day. Alcohol, 60 percent, frequently is used. It also acts as a "drying" agent. Some physicians recommend painting the cord with a bacteriostatic such as triple dye or applying an antimicrobial agent such as bacitracin. After the cord drops off, further treatment may not be used or the granulating area may be cared for by wiping with an antiseptic until it is completely healed. This may take another few days. Until the area is healed, the infant's diaper should be applied low on the abdomen so that the umbilical cord remains dry.

As she cares for the cord, the nurse should note any signs of infection and report these to the physician immediately. There should be no odor or moistness of the cord while it is mummifying. If it is moist, which is indicative of a mild infection, or if there is a moist granulating area at the base of the cord with a slightly mucoid or purulent discharge, the physician orders a culture of the discharge to identify the organism and further treatment, sometimes application of an antibiotic ointment is ordered.

The mother should be instructed in the care of the umbilicus before the infant leaves the hospital. If the cord is still on, she is told that it soon will be found loose and that there probably will be a small amount of bloody discharge from the navel for a few days, but that the navel should appear more healed every day. She should be instructed concerning precautions to keep the area clean and advised not to give the infant a tub bath or to allow the navel to get wet until the scab has come off and the area is completely healed. It is advisable to give the mother an opportunity to care for the umbilicus before she leaves the hospital, especially if she has anxiety over care of the umbilical cord.

Care of the Genitalia

The external genitalia in the female are cleaned by gentle washing with soap and water; special care must be taken to separate the labia to remove secretion that may collect between the labia minora and majora. At birth there is a heavy layer of vernix caseosa between the labia, which may be washed away over a period of several days. It is impossible to remove all of this vernix at one time without vigorous effort; it is therefore better to remove a little each day by gently washing between the labia at bath time and whenever the buttocks are cleaned following a stool. This vernix, however, should be completely washed away by the time the infant is discharged from the hospital.

In the male the penis is cleaned of smegma over the exposed part of the glans. Ordinarily the foreskin cannot be retracted in the early days of life and it is pushed back only a very short distance. Until the physician has circumcised the infant or has retracted the foreskin for the first time, the nurse may retract it a short distance daily, only as far as this can be done easily, remove the smegma from the exposed part of the glans with water or oil, and then pull the skin back to its original position. Adherence of the skin to the glans usually will prevent the nurse from being able to retract the foreskin completely for the first time during the early days of life.

If the physician recommends early complete retraction, he may dilate the prepuce and draw it over the glans. After this first retraction the nurse may be instructed to continue the procedure daily and to use oil to clean the glans of smegma. After retraction the foreskin must be pulled back into its normal position, over the glans, within a few seconds, because its tightness will reduce circulation in the penis, cause edema, and soon make it impossible to draw it forward. A *paraphimosis* then would develop. Some physicians do not recommend complete retraction of the foreskin until the infant is several months old.

Circumcision

A circumcision, surgical removal of the foreskin of the penis, is frequently performed on the newborn. Circumcision is said to be done to make cleaning of the glans easier, to help prevent disturbances such as inflammation of the prepuce and the glans, and to lower the incidence of penile carcinoma and repeated infection. Others say that routine circumcision of newborns is not indicated and that the advantages claimed for circumcision are equally present in persons who practice good personal hygiene. A phimosis, a severe degree of narrowing of the foreskin, may necessitate circumcision.

The Committee on Fetus and Newborn of the American Academy of Pediatrics stated in 1971 that there are no valid medical indications for circumcision in the neonatal period. A later Committee undertook a review of the data to support arguments "pro" and "con" circumcision of the newborn, and found no basis for changing this statement.

Nevertheless, traditional, cultural, and religious factors play a part in the decision made by parents, pediatrician, obstetrician, or family practitioner on behalf of a son. It is the responsibility of the physician to provide parents with factual and informative medical options regarding circumcision. The final decision is theirs and should be based on true informed consent.[7]

Circumcision, when done, usually is performed before the infant is discharged from the hospital if his condition is good, which means that for the normal full-term infant, the operation is often done on the second or third day of life. This is at a time when physiologic hypoprothrombinemia ordinarily would be present, but it usually is not a problem because vitamin K_1 is often administered at birth to prevent a transitory deficiency in blood coagulation in the early days of life. A bleeding and coagulation time sometimes is indicated before the operation.

Sometimes a circumcision is performed immediately after birth, before the infant leaves the delivery room, if his condition is good. For most, this is inadvisable so early in life for at least two reasons. The infant is separated from his mother at a critical time of infant-maternal bonding, and the infant is subjected to loss of body heat to the cool environment of the delivery room unless special precautions are taken to provide warmth.

Jewish parents may wish to observe the religious rite of circumcision. Prayers are recited during the circumcision, and it may be performed by a rabbi who is called a *mohel.* Separate facilities are arranged for a ritual circumcision.

A circumcision usually is carried out on the obstetric unit. It is a sterile procedure; the physician uses sterile gloves, instruments, draping towels, and skin preparation solutions. The nurse restrains the infant for the operation on a U board, which holds the legs firmly separate, or she can restrain him very satisfactorily by grasping his legs and holding them firmly apart.

The infant should not be fed for an hour or more before operation because he may regurgitate his feeding during the operation. The procedure is frequently performed without anesthesia. (Anesthesia, if used, is administered locally.) Early operation is apparently not very painful, but the infant will cry, often because of the restraint as well as from discomfort of the operation. The nurse sometimes can comfort the infant during the procedure; a sterile nipple used as a pacifier may be quite effective.

[7] Committee on Fetus and Newborn, American Academy of Pediatrics, Report of the Ad Hoc Task Force on Circumcision, *Pediatrics,* 56:610–11, (Oct.) 1975.

The infant usually will stop crying as soon as he is removed from the restraints, but the nurse may continue comforting him by holding him for a short time. Perhaps the mother would provide the greatest source of comfort for the infant after his circumcision. There is no contraindication to feeding him after his circumcision if he appears hungry. The mother may appreciate the opportunity to give him his feeding, since she will have been anxious over her baby's operation.

After circumcision the nurse must watch the area for postoperative bleeding. If bleeding occurs, the nurse applies pressure to the operative site with sterile gauze and notifies the physician. The dressing on the operative area may be removed after the first voiding if it has been applied loosely; if it was applied firmly, it may remain in place for a day or two. The nurse should ascertain the physician's preference for aftercare. A sterile gauze to which sterile petroleum jelly has been applied may be placed over the penis each time the infant's diaper is changed. The mother may be instructed to continue this care at home until the operative area has healed sufficiently to prevent the diaper from adhering to it.

It may be necessary to retract regularly the foreskin that remains following a circumcision, after danger of bleeding is past, in order to prevent adhesions to the glans during the healing process. If adhesions do form, the physician will separate them later with a sterile probe or small forceps.

Care of the Buttocks

The groin and buttocks are washed with warm water each time the diaper is changed and sometimes bland soap is necessary. Some authorities recommend using petroleum jelly or an ointment for the diaper area, but others are opposed to such use during the hospital stay because they believe a moist skin is more susceptible to infection than one that is kept completely dry. When lubricants are used on the diaper area, they must be used from an individual container for each infant to avoid cross-contamination.

A change of the diaper before and after each feeding is sufficient for many infants, but some are uncomfortable from a wet diaper and wake up and cry between feeding times. Others may need more frequent changing because of an irritation of the skin in the diaper area.

Frequent diaper changes and careful cleaning of the buttocks of urine and stool are important in prevention of raw buttocks; such care is absolutely essential when there is evidence of skin irritation. If the buttocks become sore or the infant develops a diaper rash, an ointment such as petroleum jelly, zinc oxide, or one of several commercial preparations, such as vitamin A and D ointment or methylbenzethonium (DIAPARENE), may be applied; it helps keep the stool off the raw area and aids in the healing process.

Exposure of the buttocks for "air drying" is also advisable. Long periods of wet diapers and impervious materials such as plastic or rubber as diaper covers should be avoided. These permit bacteria to grow freely in the heat, moisture, and urine held next to the infant with no circulation of air. Exposure to air helps in healing; during exposure the infant's diaper is placed under him, but is not pinned on. The infant must be protected against chilling while exposed. Treatment may be alternated by exposing the buttocks to the air while the infant is asleep and applying an ointment when he is picked up to be fed.

Diapers need more attention than any other clothing because a *diaper rash* may develop from what is known as an ammoniacal diaper. A diaper rash consists of a diffuse redness of the buttocks and possibly also blisters and pustules and an irritation of the urethral orifice in the circumcised infant. Bacteria from stool decompose the urea in urine and liberate free ammonia; this causes the ammonia dermatitis. Some commercial antiseptic solutions used for diaper rinses have a marked bactericidal action and are useful in controlling the bacterial growth if directions are carefully followed, but boiling diapers is a safe and satisfactory means of killing the organisms. An ammonia dermatitis is usually not a problem in the hospital; in addition to adequate laundering, many hospitals autoclave all clothes used in the newborn nursery. Commercially laundered diapers are washed carefully to destroy bacteria and to ensure adequate rinsing to remove soap or detergent. Ordinary washing, however, does not destroy these bacteria, and the problem of ammonia dermatitis is most likely to appear when home-laundered diapers are used.

Everyone finds many uses for diapers; they often serve as sheets, or towels, or bibs. If diapers have not been boiled, it is unwise to use them for any area of the body other than the buttocks. Another safety reminder: it is never advisable to leave loose diapers or towels or plastic material at the head end of the infant's crib.

Feedings

Feeding of the infant, an important aspect of each day's care, will be described in the following chapter. Breast- and bottle-feeding and preparation of formula will be presented in detail.

Administration of Intramuscular Medication

Administration of intramuscular injections to newborns is described here because most infants receive vitamin K by that route and some infants need other medications by the intramuscular route.

Vitamin K, usually ordered as a single dose of 1.0 mg, is given intramuscularly, soon after birth, to prevent a transitory deficiency in blood coagulation.

The preferred intramuscular injection sites for infants are the muscles of the thigh. The gluteal region, a common site for intramuscular injections, is small and shallow in an infant; this relatively small area increases the possibility of injection in the vicinity of the sciatic nerve.

When the thigh is used for injection, one of two areas is satisfactory. The injection may be made into the large muscle at the upper third of the lateral aspect of the thigh or into the midportion of the anterior aspect of the thigh. For administration into the lateral area the infant is placed on his side, and his leg is held firmly while the injection is made. When the anterior aspect of the thigh is used, the infant is restrained during injection by placing him on his back, extending his leg, and making firm pressure on his knee. Use of the anterior injection site requires precaution against placing the needle toward the inner aspect of the thigh because of important nerves and blood vessels in that area.

Occasionally the infant's arm is used for injection, making the deltoid muscle the site of the injection. Care must be taken that the drug is injected into the muscle, and not into adjacent tissue. The deltoid muscle is used only when the thigh is not accessible or when the infant is receiving many repeated injections.

Prevention of Infection

Prevention of infection is an important part of planning for nursery care, and it is also the individual responsibility of everyone concerned with the care of the newborn. The first and foremost precaution is thorough hand washing whenever the infant is handled. An antiseptic detergent or a soap or detergent containing hexachlorophene is considered superior to other soap for nursery hand washing.

It is advisable for all persons who will care for newborns to carry out a 2- to 3-minute scrub with iodophor or hexachlorophene at the beginning of each shift. Thereafter the hands should be washed thoroughly with an antiseptic detergent and running water before and between handling infants, and before clean nursery equipment is handled. It is especially important that the hands are washed carefully before the infant is fed or the upper part of his body is handled after a diaper has been changed. Jewelry should not be worn by nursing staff. Adequate hand-washing facilities should be within easy reach of all bassinets.

Any time that any part of one's face or head (hair, eyes, ears, nose, mouth) is touched with one's hands, it is considered contaminated. The hands must be washed again before handling an infant. Persons caring for infants must develop a real awareness of this so that they do not unconsciously touch their face and hair.

To protect the infant from contact with uniforms, all persons wear a gown in the nursery. Nurses and auxiliary personnel wear a short-sleeved gown or scrub dress to permit washing to the elbows. The gown should be changed frequently enough to ensure cleanliness and at least once daily. Cover gowns may be left at each bassinet for staff use while handling an individual infant to prevent cross-contamination between infants. Routine wearing of masks in the nursery is not recommended. Masks become wet from the breath and, if occasionally worn, must be changed at least every one-half hour to be effective. Handling or adjusting of the mask means contamination of the hands and necessitates washing before anything else is handled. When masks are removed, they must immediately be discarded and not worn dangling around the neck.

During her stay in the hospital, the mother is taught the importance of washing her hands before handling her infant and after she has changed his diaper, by explanation of this precaution and reminders when necessary.

All personnel must be instructed not to enter the nursery when they develop any signs of an upper respiratory infection, diarrhea or other gastrointestinal upset, skin rashes, or any other infection. Hand washing, gowning, or masking precautions are not adequate in the presence of infection. It is essential that personnel remain away from the nursery until they have fully recovered from infectious disease. Similar signs of infection in the mother must be especially evaluated as to their seriousness.

All employees susceptible to rubella should be vaccinated. Vaccine should not be administered to pregnant women; conception should be avoided for three months after vaccination.[8]

As a safeguard against infection from outside sources the number of persons entering the nursery should be kept to a minimum, and people should be screened as to who may or may not enter.

The best possible physical facilities to make nursery care easy will help prevent spread of infection. Common bathing and dressing tables should not be used.

To prevent spread of infection from one infant to another, the nurse must observe all infants closely for evidence of infection. Any infant with a fever; frequent and loose stools; discharge from the umbilical area, the eyes, or the vagina; skin lesions; respiratory disease; or any other signs of infection should be isolated from the other infants by incubator or a separate room. The ISOLETTE incubator filters the air coming into it to protect the infant inside. It does not filter the air coming out to protect adjacent infants, but it does serve as protection of other infants by being a physical barrier that may remind caretakers of hand washing and infection dangers.

[8] American Academy of Pediatrics, and American College of Obstetricians and Gynecologists, *Guidelines for Perinatal Care,* American Academy of Pediatrics, Evanston, Il., and American College of Obstetricians and Gynecologists, Washington, D.C., 1983, p. 111.

When an infant becomes infected, parents should not be separated from the infant. They can be taught how to wash and gown when they visit.

Facilitating Parent-Infant Acquaintance

Facilitating maternal and paternal and infant bonding and assisting the parents in learning to know their infant and how to care for him are very important aspects of newborn care. This part of infant care is discussed in detail in Chapter 24. One way, that of making behavioral assessment of the infant and helping the parents to observe and interpret his behavior, is discussed below.

Clinical Use of Neonatal Behavioral Characteristics

Nurses should be aware of the observations that they can make using neonatal behavioral assessment tools or a modification thereof in the ordinary care of each newborn. It will help them assess the infant's responses to his care, assess their own reactions to his responses, anticipate and observe how the infant may or does affect his parents, and use this information to inform parents of their infant's behavior, help them to understand him, and plan for his individual care.

A behavioral assessment tool can be used very profitably with mothers or parents observing, or in discussion with parents, to demonstrate to them their infant's unique abilities. Nurses can, in addition, make a number of ongoing observations of the individual infant's sleep patterns, eating patterns, quieting and/or irritability characteristics, alerting behavior, and so on in their care of the infant while he is in the nursery and give this information to parents. Helping parents to understand and respond to their infant's individual temperament, characteristics, and needs is a very important contribution that can be made by professionals to the infant's future care and development.

Parents can be helped to learn about their infant's sleep and awake states, how quickly he changes states, how much he sleeps and alerts, why the alert state is the best time to feed him and play with him, when he needs to be picked up and consoled and when this may not be necessary.

Infants differ a great deal from one another in the length of their periods of sleep and wakefulness, in their eating cycle, in how rapidly and how smoothly they move from one state to another, how much they cry, how easily they are soothed. Some infants are neither readily awakened nor easily disturbed by noise or handling, while others are often wakeful and fussy and respond to minimal stimulation. A quiet infant may need periods of stimulation, and an excitable infant may need all sources of stimulation minimized and may need time for quieting. A fussy, crying infant will require a much different kind of care than one who is placid and easily soothed.

Cuddliness is a characteristic that most people like in an infant, and yet there are some infants that resist being held and cuddled. Parents with an infant that does not "settle in well" when held must be helped to understand that their infant's behavior is a part of his individual temperament, that he reacts in that way with other persons, and that his reaction is not a result of their care or a reaction to them personally. They need help to understand that such behavior happens to be the infant's preference.

By use of the behavioral assessment scale or some modification of it parents can learn that their infant is capable of alerting and turning toward their voice, of looking at them and fixating his eyes if they take care to get into his visual field, and of responding positively to gentle touch. The infant must be given time to respond. Parents can learn that the infant shows that he is attending to stimulation by such actions as quieting and settling down if he has been active, or by increasing his activity if he has been quiet, by visual fixation, by listening, by searching for the source of the stimulus. They can also learn how much their infant reacts to stimuli or closes it out.

Parents can learn about their infant's self-quieting efforts and that he should be given time to use them. They may learn that an infant is not necessarily hungry when he attempts to suck his fists.

Parents can learn of the various methods of soothing a crying infant, beginning with sight of face, voice, and touch, and moving to picking up and rocking as necessary. They can learn that picking up the infant and rocking him will not spoil him; he may need such help to quiet. Parents can be encouraged to search for a good method for their infant and what seems best for him. Parents' success in soothing their infant has a positive effect upon their feeling of competence. Table 27–2 lists a few of the behaviors that parents and nurses may wish to observe to help understand the individual infant's needs.

Table 27–2. Common Questions Concerning Newborn Behavior*

How clearly does the infant show he is asleep or drowsy or awake?
How does the infant act when he is hungry, or tired, or wet?
How does the infant act when he is satisfied?
How does the infant act when he is dressed and bathed?
When is the infant most likely to be fussy and crying?
How well does the infant quiet himself and in what ways?
How does the infant suck and feed? Does he spit up? Are there any special ways helpful in feeding him?
What are some of the reasons for the infant's crying? How can parents begin to interpret what he is trying to communicate by the cry?

*Questions parents and nurses may wish to consider in searching for an understanding of how to best meet an infant's needs.

It is apparent that there are many ways in which nurses, physicians, and parents can learn to understand an infant's individuality. An organized assessment form is a very useful way for the nurse to do a systematic observation of an infant's behavior. When the nurse has an understanding of the items usually assessed, she also will be alert to the behavior the infant demonstrates as she is giving daily care. All this information should be shared with parents to help them understand their infant's behavior and to interact with him in an effective way.

Table 27–3 summarizes the major goals of nursing management during the newborn infant's first few postnatal days and provides a number of suggestions for reaching these objectives.

BIRTH REGISTRATION

Registration of birth is of utmost importance to the infant. The law requires the physician, midwife, nurse, or other attendant at the birth to register, with the local registrar, the name of the child, the date of birth, the place of birth, names of the parents, and any other information that is requested. Proper blanks for registration of birth are obtained from the state department of health. All information must be accurately reported and legibly written. These records are permanently filed with the state bureau of vital statistics. A photographic copy of the birth certificate or some other form of notification of registration is sent to the parents.

A birth certificate is necessary for a number of reasons and must be retained throughout life. The following list of reasons is partial, but demonstrates the importance of this document: to prove place of birth; to prove parentage and legal dependency; to prove age for entrance to school, for right to vote, for right to marry, for social security; to prove right to inheritance of property; to obtain a passport; and for other legal purposes.

The parents should be told of their responsibility for receiving a photographic copy of the birth certificate, or a notice of registration, as absolute proof that their infant's birth has been registered.

DISCHARGE FROM THE HOSPITAL

Although the parents have had adequate instructions and some practice in the care of their infant during the hospital stay, it becomes necessary to adapt this learning to the care of the infant at home. Referral to a public health nursing agency, for one or more follow-up visits by a public health nurse, is valuable for parents who

Table 27–3. Summary of Nursing Care of the Newborn in the Early Days of Life

Goals	*Suggested Responsibilities*
Establish and maintain a patent airway and good oxygenation	Use postural drainage after birth Do Apgar score to check how infant has adjusted to birth Use oropharyngeal suction, oxygen, and stimulation if infant is sluggish. Resuscitative procedures if necessary Observe very closely for mucus and use oropharyngeal suction if indicated, especially during the period of transition Observe for apnea and cyanosis and be ready to stimulate and administer oxygen
Protect against heat loss from body	Dry off amniotic fluid immediately after birth Replace wet blankets with warm, dry ones Cover wet hair and head with a blanket Place infant under radiant heater, or in incubator, or in skin-to-skin contact with mother's body In nursery, place in heated bassinet until body temperature stabilizes at normal Do necessary procedures under a heat lamp or radiant heater. Postpone bath and any unnecessary procedure until body temperature is stable Avoid overheating of infant Monitor body temperature and temperature of incubator every 1/2 hour at first, then 1 hour, then 4 hours
Monitor vital signs	Respirations, heart rate, and blood pressure every 15 minutes for first hour, every 30 minutes for another hour, every 1 to 2 hours for next several hours or until stable Body temperature (axillary) every 30 minutes for 1 to 2 hours, and then every 2 to 4 hours until stable. Also record incubator temperature After transition period monitor vital signs once daily
Assess gestational age and intrauterine growth	Weigh and measure infant Do gestational age assessment from physical and neurologic signs Assess infant as to risk category and special needs
Assess physical condition and behavior	Brief physical examination in first hour Auscultate lungs and heart Check color, muscle tone, spontaneous vigorous cry, spontaneous symmetric movement, relative size of head, body, extremities Note color of skin—pink, cyanosis, pallor, jaundice Note bowel and bladder function Complete physical exam after infant stabilized
Protect against infection	Wash hands carefully before handling infant Avoid personnel with upper respiratory, skin, or gastrointestinal illness Protect infant's skin against intertrigo and diaper rash Prophylactic treatment of eyes soon after birth Keep umbilical area clean and dry—wipe with alcohol Be alert to early signs of infection in infant
Promote infant-parent attachment	Show infant to parents and allow them to hold him immediately after birth, if possible Permit parents to hold and examine infant during first hour or so after birth. Keep infant in warm room or provide a heat lamp Demonstrate to parents and discuss with them the infant's behavioral capabilities Provide for parents to learn to care for their infant
Provide adequate nutrition	Start feedings when infant shows signs of hunger Observe daily weight Feedings will be discussed in detail in next chapter

need or wish guidance at home. Such visits provide for assistance with problems that may arise at home and ensure continued nursing supervision for as long as necessary.

If the infant will not remain under the medical supervision of the physician who cared for him in the hospital following his discharge, continuing medical care is planned for by referral to the family physician or to a community agency maintaining a well-baby clinic. In some instances, where financial aid is needed, referral is also made to a family service agency.

REFERENCES AND SUGGESTED READINGS

American Academy of Pediatrics, and American College of Obstetricians and Gynecologists, *Guidelines for Perinatal Care,* American Academy of Pediatrics, Evanston, Il., and American College of Obstetricians and Gynecologists, Washington, D.C., 1983.

Auld, Peter A. M., Resuscitation of the newborn infant, *Am. J. Nurs.,* 74:68–70, (Jan.) 1974.

Avery, Gordon B. (ed.), *Neonatology,* 2nd ed., Lippincott, Philadelphia, 1981.

Ballard, J. L., *et al.,* A simplified assessment of gestational age, *Pediatr. Res.,* 11:374, 1977.

Boggs, Thomas R., Avoiding morbidity during the first 60 minutes of life, *Contemp. Ob/Gyn.,* 15:47–65, (May) 1980.

Brazelton, T. Berry, *Neonatal Behavior Assessment Scale, Clinics in Developmental Medicine,* No. 50, Spastics International Medical Publications, Heinemann Medical Books, London, and Lippincott, Philadelphia, 1973.

Buckner, Ellen B., Use of Brazelton neonatal behavioral assessment in planning care of parents and newborns, *JOGN Nurs.,* 12:26–30, (Jan./Feb.) 1983.

Clark, Ann L., Recognizing discord between mother and child and changing it to harmony, *MCN,* 1:100–106, (Mar./Apr.) 1976.

Clark, Ann L., and Affonso, Dyanne D., Infant behavior and maternal attachment: Two sides to the coin, *MCN,* 1:94–99, (Mar./Apr.) 1976.

Desmond, Murdina M., *et al.,* The clinical behavior of the newly born. I. The term baby, *J. Pediatr.,* 62:307–25, (Mar.) 1963.

Dubowitz, Lilly M. S.; Dubowitz, Victor; and Goldberg, Cissie, Clinical assessment of gestational age in the newborn infant, *J. Pediatr.,* 77:1–10, (July) 1970.

Grimes, David A., Routine circumcision reconsidered, *Am. J. Nurs.,* 80:108–109, (Jan.) 1980.

Haddock, Nancy, Blood pressure monitoring in neonates, *MCN,* 5:131–35, (Mar./Apr.) 1980.

Klaus, Marshall H., and Fanaroff, Avroy A., *Care of the High-Risk Neonate,* 2nd ed., Saunders, Philadelphia, 1979.

Klaus, Marshall H., and Kennell, John H., *Parent-Infant Bonding,* 2nd ed., C. V. Mosby, St. Louis, 1982, Chaps. 2 and 3.

Korones, Sheldon B., *High-Risk Newborn Infants: The Basis for Intensive Nursing Care,* 3rd ed., C. V. Mosby, St. Louis, 1981.

Lum, Sister Barbara; Batzel, Ruth Lortz; and Barnett, Elouise, Reappraising newborn eye care, *Am. J. Nurs.,* 80:1602–1603, (Sept.) 1980.

Ostwald, Peter F., and Peltzman, Philip, The cry of the human infant, *Sci. Am.,* 230:84–90, (Mar.) 1974.

Paukert, Sheryle, Maternal-infant attachment in a traditional hospital setting, *JOGN Nurs.,* 11:23–26, (Jan./Feb.) 1982.

Roberts, Joyce E., Suctioning the newborn, *Am. J. Nurs.,* 73:63–65, (Jan.) 1973.

Romanko, Monica V., and Brost, Bethea, Swaddling: An effective invention for pacifying infants, *Pediatr. Nurs.,* 8:259, (July/Aug.) 1982.

Stern, Leo, Clinical aspects of thermoregulation in the newborn, *Contemp. Ob/Gyn.,* 13:109–34, (March) 1979.

Sullivan, Rita; Foster, Jean; and Schreiner, Richard L., Determining a newborn's gestational age, *MCN,* 4:38–45, (Jan./Feb.) 1979.

Whaley, Lucille F., and Wong, Donna L., *Nursing Care of Infants and Children,* 2nd ed., C. V. Mosby, St. Louis, 1983.

Williams, Joann K., and Lancaster, Jean, Thermoregulation of the newborn, *MCN,* 1:355–60, (Nov./Dec.) 1976.

Zurawski, Glenn F., and Shnider, Sol M., How anesthetic drugs affect neonatal neurobehavior, *Contemp. Ob/Gyn.,* 17:179, (June) 1981.

CHAPTER

28

Infant Nutrition

THE NEWBORN INFANT may either be breast-fed or bottle-fed. Many factors enter into the decision of the method that will be used. Breast-feeding is the natural method of feeding the normal newborn and has certain advantages over artificial feeding, but if it is to be a satisfactory experience for both mother and infant, the mother must want to breast-feed her child. Assuming that the mother's and infant's conditions are satisfactory, breast-feeding usually will be successful if the mother has the desire to nurse her infant, and if she gets encouragement during the time the feeding is being established.

Breast-feeding is no longer necessary to maintain an infant's good health, or ensure his survival, as it was prior to development of satisfactory formula feedings, but it has important advantages. Breast milk is the natural and ideal food for the newborn infant. If the mother's diet is adequate, the infant receives from breast milk the nutrients necessary for growth during the early months of life, with the possible exception of sufficient vitamin D. Breast milk is readily digested and assimilated, and feeding difficulties are less frequent and usually less severe than with formula feedings.

Human breast milk has an optimum distribution of proteins, carbohydrates, and fats for infants. In addition, the protein, carbohydrate, and fat quality is especially suited to the infants' needs. Human milk also contains all the other nutrients the infant requires for growth and good nutrition. Supplementation of nutrients is not essential, at least for the first 4 to 6 months of age.

Human breast milk, particularly colostrum and early milk, contains a number of host-resistant factors, especially against upper respiratory and gastrointestinal infections. Breast milk contains secretory IgA and other immunoglobulins that provide protective antibodies for the gastrointestinal and respiratory tracts. It contains a growth factor of *Lactobacillus bifidus* that interferes with intestinal colonization of enteric pathogens, especially E. coli, and it inhibits staphylcocci with an antistaphylcoccal factor. Breast milk also contains lysozyme, lactoferrin, and many live leukocytes for phagocytosis.

Breast milk is clean, fresh, and readily available at the proper temperature. Breast-feeding eliminates the need for preparation of formula and warming of milk before the infant is fed. The milk flow from the breast is well regulated. The infant can suck at the breast until he is satisfied, and there is less tendency to attempt to control the food intake. Breast-feeding helps to meet the infant's and the mother's needs for close relationship if the mother wants to breast-feed her infant; if not, bottle-feedings may be more satisfactory for such close relationships.

FACTORS INFLUENCING METHOD OF FEEDING

Psychologic, sociologic, and physical factors enter into whether a mother breast-feeds her infant successfully or unsuccessfully or makes no attempt to breast-feed. Some mothers are very eager to breast-feed their infants; some nurse their infants, but feel that it makes little difference if they must change to bottle-feeding; some try to breast-feed even when they prefer to give bottle-feedings, and others are strongly opposed to breast-feeding. To some mothers this method of feeding seems repulsive or rather primitive, or they feel that it may be disfiguring or too tiring. Some mothers do not breast-feed because the custom in their community is to give bottle-feedings, especially since formula feedings have become safe and easy. Others believe that they may be criticized by relatives or friends who do not particularly approve of this method of feeding. In some cases the care of the infant by others will be easier if he is fed by bottle. Some women express the belief that their milk may not be good for the infant, or they think they will worry if they do not know exactly how much milk the infant is taking at each feeding.

The husband's interest and encouragement of a woman's desire to nurse her infant are very important to successful breast-feeding.

The attitude of the physician and nurse toward breast-feeding and the amount of assistance given to the mother in the early days while breast-feeding is being established often determine the mother's success in nursing. The mother may need a great deal of assistance at first, especially if she is insecure, or if her infant does not nurse well initially.

Breast-feeding is inadvisable or impossible in some instances because of the mother's or the infant's physical condition. Tuberculosis and certain acute infectious diseases, especially those to which an infant is particularly susceptible, such as certain viral or staphylococcal infections, are contraindications to breast-feeding. Other complications in the mother, such as heart disease, kidney disease, or syphilis, may be contraindications. In some cases of chronic disease and general debility, contraindication to breast-feeding is relative and depends on the mother's condition. If breast-feeding is started and the mother begins to show evidence of strain, it is discontinued. During acute illness of the mother, breast-feeding often must be discontinued temporarily.

Flat or inverted nipples may be impossible for the infant to grasp sufficiently to nurse. Fissured or cracked nipples may necessitate temporary discontinuance of nursing until the nipples heal. If mastitis develops, nursing is stopped temporarily or permanently discontinued.

The return of menstruation is not an indication for weaning, but the infant may have some colic, vomiting, or loose stools on the first day of the menstrual period. Pregnancy is an indication for weaning the infant because of the additional strain on the mother.

The infant's condition may be the factor determining the method of feeding. An immature infant or one with an abnormality, such as cleft lip or palate, may be unable to nurse. Sometimes, in these cases, the breasts are emptied by artificial means until the infant can nurse. The decision may depend on the mother's desire to continue lactation by artificial emptying of the breasts and also on the infant's disability and the period of time required for his recovery.

The prenatal period is the best time to discover the mother's attitude toward nursing her infant and to answer her questions concerning breast- and bottle-feeding. She will then have information for making decisions and plans.

A mother who is undecided about breast-feeding but who does not express adverse feelings often can be encouraged. Mothers often lack information, and they need the sanction of physicians and nurses. They may need help in deciding how to manage feedings when away from home for work or for social activities. Breast-feeding is not necessarily restricting, since a bottle-feeding can be given when the mother is away. The woman who is planning to return to work can be encouraged to breast-feed during the early weeks of the infant's life.

Any discussion with the mother concerning breast-feeding should encourage her to make her own decision. The advantages of breast-feeding should not be stressed to such a degree that the mother may develop a feeling of inadequacy or guilt if she decides not to breast-feed or if she cannot do so for a physical reason. If the idea of breast-feeding is repugnant to a woman, attempts to persuade her to breast-feed are unwise. Such efforts may lead to mental conflict and may inject or increase feelings of guilt.

An infant's nutritional needs can be met very satisfactorily with bottle-feedings and a good mother-child relationship can be established in many ways other than through breast-feeding.

NUTRITIONAL REQUIREMENTS

The goal of infant feeding should be a well-nourished infant, fed in a way that is satisfactory to the parents and the infant. To accomplish this, the infant may be either breast-fed or bottle-fed with a commercially prepared formula or an evaporated milk formula. The infant's diet should provide an adequate amount of water, calories, and essential nutrients for health and normal growth, and it should be easily digestible. Since the growth and nutritional status of the breast-fed infant is ordinarily excellent, the composition of breast milk is used as a standard for preparation of formulas for infants.

The *requirement* for a nutrient may be defined as the least amount of that nutrient that will promote an optimum state of health. The meaning of the terms "requirement" and "minimal requirement" is the same and the terms are sometimes used interchangeably. The *advisable intake* for a nutrient generally is set at values greater than the estimated requirement because of individual differences of infants and the various conditions that may influence the effect of the nutrient, such as genetic makeup of the infant, environment, activity, storage reserves, and influence of other nutrients.

The *recommended dietary allowances* (RDA), which are revised periodically by the Food and Nutrition Board, National Academy of Sciences, National Research Council differ further from the advisable intake. The RDA recommendations are at least equal to, and generally greater than, the advisable intake. The RDA recommendations are intended to serve as a general guide to provide an adequate nutritional intake for almost every healthy person.

Caloric Needs

Infants require a relatively large intake of food and fluids to cover basal metabolic needs and provide for growth. After an initial postnatal period of a few days, when a relatively small caloric intake appears to satisfy the infant, his caloric needs are high. By several days of age a baby needs 110 to 120 Calories (kilocalories) per kilogram of body weight per day (50 to 55 Calories per pound). Such caloric intake is necessary to provide energy for the infant's relatively high basal metabolic needs as compared with an adult, for his rapid growth and for his daily increasing activity during the neonatal period. An infant's increasing need for calories is shown by the daily increase in the amount of food that is necessary to satisfy him during his early days of life. Caloric needs vary greatly for different infant of the same age and size. The active infant, because of increased muscular activity, and the one who cries considerably use more energy than the quiet infant and thus require a higher caloric intake. Needs are based on weight gain, satiety, and general well-being. The very high caloric intake of the infant becomes more apparent when compared with an adult's caloric requirement of somewhere between 10 and 15 calories per pound of body weight.

There are so many variables involved in caloric needs of infants that it is difficult to state an ideal caloric intake for the newborn. The requirement of 120 kcal/kg/day is a rough rule of thumb of what is sufficient for growth for most infants. Optimal caloric intake should be supplied to the newborn to avoid any malnutrition. Too few calories cause tissue breakdown and divert all food substances into energy. On the other hand, overnutrition may contribute to adult obesity. It is difficult to define excessive intake, but it is well to be aware of the potential. Some infants will not gain weight on 120 kcal/kg/day and need to be fed a higher amount. Others, especially inactive infants, may gain satisfactorily on 90 kcal/kg/day. A weight gain of 15 to 30 gm (½ to 1 oz) per day is considered satisfactory and evidence of good growth.

The distribution of calories in the infant's food is important to well-being. That which seems appropriate for good nutrition for full-term infants and is recommended for full-size infants is as follows: 7 to 16 percent of calories to be derived from protein, 30 to 55 percent from fat, and the remainder from carbohydrate.[1] At least 1 percent of the calories should be supplied by the essential fatty acid, linoleic acid.

Human milk provides approximately 7 percent calories from protein; 55 percent from fat, and 38 percent from carbohydrate. Most commercially prepared formulas fed in the United States supply 9 to 15 percent of the calories from protein, 45 to 50 percent from fat, and the remainder from carbohydrate. An intake of protein of less than 6 percent of the caloric intake is likely to lead to protein deficiency. Extremely high fat content in the formula may lead to ketosis. Diets supplying less than 30 percent of the calories from fat or more than 65 percent of the calories from carbohydrate are believed possibly to be of low satiety, but little evidence for this is available.[2]

Fluid Needs

Fluid requirement per kilogram of body weight is greater in the infant than in the adult. The infant's increased muscular activity, caloric intake, and basal metabolism demand more water than he will need later in life. An adequate amount of fluid is thus essential to an infant's well-being. Infants have a relatively large percentage of body fluid, but their ability to withstand an inadequate fluid intake is not as efficient as that of an older child or an adult. In addition, infants need more water than older individuals for good excretion of solutes.

The normal newborn's need for fluid intake is between 150 and 200 ml per kilogram (2⅓ and 3 oz per pound) of body weight per 24 hours. Fluid intake also may be expressed in relation to caloric intake and would then be equivalent to 1.5 ml/kcal. That is the statement of the RDA recommendation. Need for fluid is very

[1] Samuel J. Foman, *Infant Nutrition,* 2nd ed. Saunders, Philadelphia, 1974, p. 473.

[2] *Ibid.*

great in hot weather and may increase to over 200 ml per kilogram of body weight (3 oz per pound) when the temperature is high.

The normal infant ordinarily will easily fulfill his own requirement by taking an adequate amount of breast milk or formula. Offers of water between certain feedings and later intake of orange juice add to the fluid intake of milk. Water must be given frequently if milk intake is inadequate because of poor appetite or poor sucking in the early days of life, if body fluids are lost due to heat, if the infant is under lights or a radiant heater, or if the newborn has a fever. It may be necessary to offer water between all feedings when need for fluid is great.

It is important to realize that between 70 and 90 ml of fluid per kilogram (1.2 and 1.5 oz per pound) of body weight is the minimal water requirement for a full-term normal newborn in a 24-hour period to protect him against dehydration. The much higher intake is advised to provide for a generous margin of safety.

When an infant gains poorly or gains excessively, the fluid and caloric intake should be calculated to determine the exact intake and to note how it compares with requirements.

Vitamins

When the mother is well nourished, the normal newborn can be expected to have adequate vitamin stores at birth. An infant's vitamin requirements are high, however, because of rapid growth, and vitamins are soon required to provide for good development of rapidly growing bones and tissues. Suggested daily allowances of some of the necessary vitamins are shown in Table 28-1. Recommended intakes of vitamins are estimates, which are generally higher than minimum requirements. In addition, intestinal absorption is not constant, and the vitamin content of natural food may vary considerably. The quantity of the various vitamins present in milk, both human and animal, will vary to some extent with maternal intake.

Vitamin A is present in large amount in human milk, cow's milk, and commercially prepared formulas. Many strained and chopped commercially prepared infant foods and many table foods fed to infants have a good supply of carotene. Vitamin A supplementation for infants therefore is not necessary under usual circumstances. Since vitamin A is stored in the liver, the average intake is more important than the daily intake.

The advisable intake of vitamin A has been tentatively set at 500 IU between birth and one year of age. This is twice the estimated requirement. The same intake is recommended for low-birthweight babies.

Since vitamin A has been used in excessive amounts and results in toxicity, a joint statement on the use and abuse of vitamin A was issued by the Committees on Drugs and on Nutrition of the American Academy of Pediatrics in 1971. These committees advise against the use of preparations providing more than 6000 IU/dose.[3]

Although it is unlikely that a normal infant in the United States who is receiving an adequate diet needs supplemental vitamin A, a deficiency of this vitamin is a common nutritional deficiency in most developing countries of the world. In countries where vitamin A deficiency is prevalent, animal fats are rarely eaten and the total dietary fat intake is so low that even if carotenes are present in the diet in moderate amounts, they are poorly absorbed.

[3] American Academy of Pediatrics, Committees on Drugs and on Nutrition, The use and abuse of vitamin A, *Pediatrics,* 48:655-56, (Oct.) 1971.

Table 28-1. Requirements, Advisable Intake, and RDA Recommendations for Selected Nutrients for Infant Diet

Daily Allowance—Birth to Six Months*

Nutrient	*Requirement (minimum)*	*Advisable*	*RDA Recommendation*
Water	70-90 ml per kg	150 ml per kg	1.5 ml per kcal
Calories	90-110 per kg	110-120 per kg	115 per kg
Protein	1.6 gm per 100 kcal	1.9 gm per 100 kcal	2.2 gm per kg
Vitamins			
A	250 IU	500 IU	1400 IU
D	100-200 IU	400 IU	400 IU
C	10 mg	20 mg	35 mg
Fluoride	—	0.25 mg	Fluoridation of water supply where indicated
Iron	6.7 mg	7 mg	10 mg

*Based on data obtained from Domenik Reina, Infant nutrition, *Clin. Perinatal.,* 2:373-39, (Sept.) 1975. RDA recommendations for all nutrients are listed in Food and Nutrition Board, National Academy of Sciences—National Research Council, *Recommended Daily Dietary Allowances,* revised, 1980.

Vitamin D is essential to the prevention of rickets. It is present in only small amounts in both breast milk and cow's milk, but cow's milk, evaporated milk, and commercially prepared formulas are well fortified with vitamin D. A daily intake of 400 IU of vitamin D is suggested as the advisable daily intake.

Use of a supplement is not advisable when dietary sources provide 400 IU daily, as may well be the case for the infant who is eating a large quantity of fortified formula or is taking a liter of fortified milk. In the United States most commercially prepared formulas, evaporated milk, and fresh whole milk are fortified with 400 IU of vitamin D per quart. Except for milk, few foods eaten by infants are fortified with vitamin D; therefore, if an infant's daily intake of vitamin D from milk or formula is below 400 IU, some supplementation to raise the infant's daily intake is advisable. However, excessive intakes (above 2000 IU per day) are dangerous and should be avoided.[4] A regular intake of vitamin D is important because it is poorly stored. Sunshine will fulfill some of the need for vitamin D, but ordinarily an infant under one year of age does not receive enough of the vitamin from this source.

Vitamin C is found in human milk in a quantity sufficient for the infant, provided the mother's diet is adequate, but cow's milk is low in this vitamin at all times, even when the milk is raw. Heat used to modify cow's milk for infant feeding destroys part of the vitamin C that is present, bringing the total amount even lower and making the addition of ascorbic acid important when bottle-feedings are given.

Commercially prepared formulas and fruit juices are fortified with vitamin C. The recommended dietary allowance of vitamin C is 35 mg daily. Two ounces of orange juice will provide the advisable daily intake of vitamin C for an infant; supplementation should be continued until the infant takes this amount of orange juice daily. There are no large body stores of vitamin C, and any excess is excreted in the urine.

Vitamin B complex is present in adequate amounts in human milk, cow's milk, and commercially prepared formulas. Deficiencies are rare in developed countries but may be severe in countries where rice gruel is substituted for milk a few weeks after birth. Toxicity is not a problem because the B-complex vitamins are only minimally stored in the body, and any excess is excreted in the urine.

Vitamin K intake is adequate after the first several days of life for the normal infant taking human milk, cow's milk, or commercially prepared formula. To avoid a vitamin K deficiency in the first few days of life, the newborn is given 0.5 or 1.0 mg of vitamin K_1 intramuscularly after birth (see page 517).

[4] Roslyn B. Alfin-Slater and Derrick B. Jelliffe, Nutritional requirements with special reference to infancy, *Pediatr. Clin. North Am., 24:6, (Feb.) 1977.*

Minerals

Most minerals are provided adequately by human milk, cow's milk, commercially prepared formulas, and other foods usually taken by infants. Iron and fluoride are exceptions. The need for iron and for fluoride and the fulfillment of these requirements are described on pages 600–601.

THE FIRST FEEDING

For the normal healthy infant who has good color, good muscle tone, and a lusty cry, evidence of hunger and desire to eat seem to be valid guides for offering the first feeding. Some infants seem to be ready to eat as soon as they are born, and some do not show hunger for several hours. It is desirable to feed each newborn according to his individual needs rather than according to an established routine. A scheduled time for a first feeding at a predetermined number of hours after birth requires some infants to wait long past their initial hunger, while others are offered a feeding when they are not ready to eat. (See also discussion on hypoglycemia on pages (671–74 in relation to first feedings.)

Many factors must be observed and considered in determining the time for offering the first feeding. The infant should be in good condition as determined by vital signs and general behavior. A newborn ordinarily shows signs of hunger by a search for food, sucking motions, and crying. When the mother plans to breast-feed, her condition should be assessed to ascertain if she is able and ready to nurse her infant. Type of delivery, analgesia during labor, and need for rest influence her readiness. The mother's desires and plans for feeding her infant are considered. Some mothers want to nurse their infants as soon as possible after birth, either in the delivery room or the recovery room. If mother and newborn are in good condition, this is a good time to begin breast-feeding. The infant is in his first period of reactivity, is alert and active, is likely to suck well at this time, and the feeding very likely will be successful. With an early feeding the infant will get early sucking experience, he will get some food from the colostrum that is present in the breast, the mother's breasts will be stimulated to begin producing milk, and the mother will have the satisfaction of a successful feeding.

If the infant is to be formula-fed, the first feeding may be postponed until the second period of reactivity, unless the infant is hungry or shows signs of hypoglycemia.

Often the first feeding, called a *test feeding* because it helps to assess the newborn's ability to swallow fluid, is

10 to 15 ml of sterile water followed by a 5 or 10 percent glucose solution. If the water feeding is regurgitated and aspirated, or if the infant cannot swallow because of an anomaly in the upper gastrointestinal tract, irritation of the respiratory tract may be less from water than from glucose or formula. Although water does not irritate the respiratory tract, there is always the possibility that aspiration of regurgitated fluids will include other gastric contents, including hydrochloric acid, which can cause severe irritation. After it has been ascertained that the infant can take fluid satisfactorily, breast- or formula-feedings are started.

The newborn may be satisfied with a very small amount of food at the first feeding. He often has a need to suck in addition to a need for food, and this desire to suck may be satisfied while he is taking his small feeding.

FREQUENCY OF FEEDING

Feeding schedules for infants, which often bring to mind schedules of every 3 or 4 hours are very unsatisfactory for normal newborns. These infants cannot easily fit into, or tolerate, a rigid schedule in either time of feeding or amount of food offered. Newborns are ready to eat and wish to be fed whenever they are hungry, which sometimes is every 2 hours or even sooner. At other times they may be entirely satisfied and not wish to eat until 5 or 6 hours have elapsed since the last feeding. Schedules require the infant who is alert and hungry before the scheduled feeding time to wait for his feeding and the one who is not hungry to be awakened and urged to take food.

Self-Demand Feedings

A self-regulating (self-demand) feeding schedule permits the infant to eat when he is awake and hungry and to take the amount of feeding that he wishes. This means that the interval between feedings may be from three to six hours and may even vary from every two to every eight hours. The individual newborn is likely to vary the schedule from day to day during the first week or two of life.

The normal newborn is a good judge of his need for food. Hunger wakes the infant and he begins to cry. If he is fed when he is hungry, eating is a pleasant experience. The infant also knows when he has had enough to eat. He will stop eating when he is satisfied and he should not be urged to take more food than he is eager to take. Prodded feedings are unpleasant, and it is not necessary for an infant to finish the last drop from a bottle. Pushing of breast feedings is a little less likely than bottle feedings because the actual amount of milk the infant has taken is not known.

With a rigid feeding schedule, an infant who is hungry early, but must wait until a certain approved time for feeding, may not eat well. The infant may have lost his feeling of hunger and he also may be exhausted from crying. When a sleeping infant is awakened to be fed, he may not eat well because he is not hungry enough to eat and he is not sufficiently awake. Sometimes the newborn does not wish to eat frequently, or in amounts that seem adequate, during the early days of life; the infant should not be prodded or patted too firmly in an effort to awaken him and to force him to eat more than he wishes. Even when he appears to be hungry, he may dawdle during the first few days; feedings should be offered with patience and calmness.

With breast-feeding it is especially important that the infant is ready to eat when he is put to the breast for nursing. When he does not have a desire to eat he is not likely to grasp the mother's nipple. The attempt at feeding is unpleasant for the infant, and, in addition, the mother may become concerned over the infant's lack of desire to eat and her ability to feed him.

Most normal newborns eat about six to eight times in a 24-hour period during the first week or two of life, with an occasional day or two of more frequent feedings. During the early days of life there may be considerable irregularity in an infant's need for food, both in the interval between feedings and in the amount of food taken. The infant may wish to have a feeding often on one day and less frequently on another, and sometimes he desires food at frequent intervals during a part of a day and at longer-spaced intervals during the rest of the day.

After three or four days of age many infants have several days on which they want to eat very frequently, sometimes as often as every two hours for at least several times in succession. This frequency will not continue, and the mother who is breast-feeding probably will be able to meet the needs by frequent nursing. The nurse, however, must observe the mother to ascertain that she is not becoming too tired and that her nipples do not become sore from frequent nursing. It may be possible to satisfy the infant occasionally with a pacifier, a drink of water, or other attention. Perhaps he does not really need food so often.

An infant establishes a fairly regular schedule after a week or two. As he gets a little older he usually takes from 3 to 4 oz of milk at each feeding and is satisfied for a three- to four-hour period.

BREAST-FEEDING

The various aspects of breast-feeding will be described below. In addition to a discussion of the factors important in breast milk secretion and the infant's sucking,

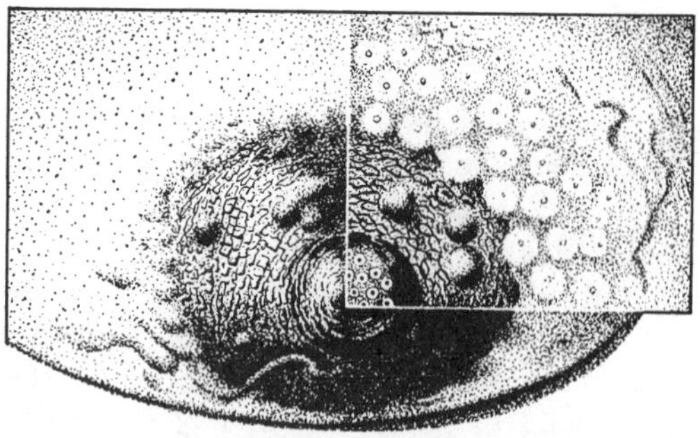

Figure 28–1. Front view of breast showing areola, tubercles of Montgomery, and orifices of milk ducts.

care of the breasts and nipples during lactation, and the nursing mother's health regime will be presented.

Anatomy and Physiology of Lactation

The secretory portion of each breast consists of 15 to 20 lobes of alveolar glandular tissue; each lobe has its own execretory duct opening into the nipple (Figs. 28–1 and 28–2). Each lobe is further subdivided into smaller lobes, or lobules, containing ducts opening into a larger duct. The lobules, in turn, are comprised of many acini or alveoli. These tiny sacs, or *alveoli,* lined with a single layer of cells which secrete milk, are the secretory portion of the breast. These secreting cells are surrounded by a capillary network.

Tiny ductules carry milk from the alveoli to the ducts of the lobules, which in turn open into the larger duct of the lobe; these lead to the nipple and open to its surface (Figs. 8–3, page 133 and 28–2). The walls of these ductules and ducts contain elastic and muscular tissue. Before it reaches the surface of the nipple, each large duct widens into a *lactiferous sinus,* a minute reservoir for milk (Figs. 8–3 and 28–2). These sinuses lie just behind and beneath the areolar part of the breast.

The clusters of alveoli or acini, uniting to form lobules with tiny ducts leading into the main duct of each lobule, closely resemble a bunch of grapes. The separate grapes correspond to the alveoli, their small stems to the tiny ducts that lead to a larger one, and the central stem of the grape cluster to the milk duct that opens through the nipple.

The size of the breasts largely depends on the amount of fatty tissue they contain and, therefore, is not indicative of ability to produce milk. Gross anatomy and development of the breasts have been described on pages 18 and 132.

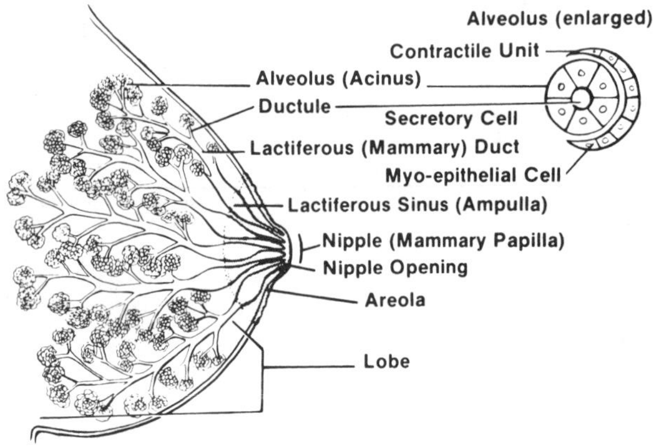

Figure 28–2. Schematic diagram of the breast. (Reproduced with permission from Jan Riordan, and Betty Ann Countryman, "The anatomy and psychophysiology of lactation." *JOGN Nurs.* 9:210–213, (July–Aug.) 1980.

Colostrum Secretion

There is little or no apparent change in the breasts during the first two or three days after the birth of an infant. In this early period, they secrete a small amount of thin, yellowish fluid called *colostrum.* Colostrum contains proteins, fat, sugar, salts, and water, but in different proportions than milk, having less fat and sugar than milk and a greater amount of protein and salts. Colostrum also contains large amounts of vitamins and antibodies. In addition, it contains cells with large masses of fat. These cells are called colostrum corpuscles and are secreting cells that have undergone fatty degeneration. The yellowish color is caused by a pigment.

The alveoli, ducts, and ampullae of the breasts are filled with colostrum at the time of delivery, and the alveolar cells continue to secrete colostrum at a slow rate. At the first few nursings the newborn receives the colostrum in the breasts in amounts varying from a few milliliters to ½ oz at each feeding.

Lactogenesis

The relatively small amount of colostrum in the breasts is replaced by milk on the second or third day after delivery. A major change in mammary gland function takes place during this time. The breasts begin to secrete a large volume of fluid, which gradually changes in composition from colostrum through a transitional fluid of early milk to mature milk by the end of about one week after delivery. This process, termed *lactogenesis,* is brought about by hormonal influences on the alveolar cells, biochemical changes in these cells, and circulatory changes in the breasts.

With delivery of the placenta and loss of its hormones, the hormonal milieu changes considerably. Estrogens and progesterone in the circulation fall to a low level. These hormones, especially the high level of progesterone, and lack of stimulation are believed to have inhibited milk secretion prior to delivery. As the level of placental hormones falls, secretion of a complex of lactogenic hormones from the anterior pituitary increases considerably. At the same time blood flow to the breasts increases, bringing more hormones and milk precursors to the alveolar cells. The lactogenic complex of hormones, which is made up of prolactin, somatotropin, ACTH, and probably TSH, causes cellular and biochemical mechanisms in the alveolar cells to secrete milk. ACTH and TSH act through the adrenal and the thyroid glands, respectively.

Lactogenesis is further promoted by the infant's sucking and by emptying of the breasts and relief of distention of the alveoli. As the alveoli are emptied, they can secrete more milk. Without emptying, true milk secretion will not develop. With regular emptying of the breasts, milk flows more freely and more abundantly with each nursing. The same complex of hormones that was necessary to start milk secretion is required for continuation of secretion.

The manner is which the breast milk comes in as well as the time of its appearance varies considerably in different women. Sometime between the second and fourth day after delivery, the breasts become heavy, full, and firm. Filling may be rapid, with a distinct change noticeable within a few hours, or it may be much more gradual.

Filling of the breasts often, but not necessarily, is accompanied by congestion or engorgement of the breasts. Engorgement lasts for a day or two and is likely to cause discomfort to varying degrees. Thereafter the congestion disappears, and although the milk supply steadily increases and the breasts are heavy with fullness from milk, they are not uncomfortable. Milk supply may increase rapidly during the first days following its initial secretion, or the increase may be very gradual. It even may be several weeks before the supply is adequate to fulfill the infant's needs completely.

Breast Engorgement

There is considerable variation in the degree of firmness of the breasts as well as in amount of discomfort the mother experiences at the time the milk comes in. Sometimes the breasts produce a large amount of milk without previous engorgement, but usually they become distended and tender to varying degrees and may become markedly uncomfortable. Sometimes the breasts become so full and tense that they are described as being "hard as boards." The distention may pull the skin so tight that it appears shiny. The skin also may be reddened and feel very warm in some areas, and distended veins may be visible. The mother may feel a throbbing in her breasts, with pain whenever they are touched or moved. If the tissues surrounding the nipples become taut, nursing becomes difficult because the infant cannot grasp the nipple and the areolar area adequately.

Engorgement disappears in 24 to 48 hours, and although the milk supply is increasing, the breasts become softer and more comfortable.

Engorgement of the breasts apparently is caused partly by an increased vascularity and partly by an increased accumulation of milk. There also may be secondary lymphatic and venous stasis if the milk cannot be removed. The amount of blood to the breasts increases quite suddenly sometime between the second and fourth postpartum days, and engorgement probably begins with a filling of the breasts with blood. As the breasts then fill with milk, the engorgement increases, especially if they cannot be emptied easily. It may be difficult to withdraw the milk because of occlusion of ducts by the congested tissues surrounding them and/or occlusion from blockage by earlier secretions which are viscous or have become thickened. Retention of milk in the alveoli causes them to become distended and to compress surrounding milk ducts. This compression interferes with the flow of milk. Secondary venous and lymphatic stasis may follow distention of the breasts with the milk that cannot be emptied.

Sometimes during this period of breast engorgement a hard, tender mass is felt in one or both axillae. This mass is glandular breast tissue which also becomes engorged and filled with milk. This congestion decreases in one or two days, and the lump gradually disappears as the milk in it dries up. An ice bag applied to the axilla helps relieve the discomfort.

Formerly it was believed that engorgement produced fever, but lactation is not an inflammatory process, and if there is fever at this time, some other cause (with rare exceptions) should be suspected.

While engorgement is present, measures are taken to keep the mother comfortable and also to empty her breasts to prevent a decrease in milk secretion. Discomfort is lessened or relieved by support of the heavy breasts, application of ice bags or warm water bottles or packs (whichever feels more comfortable to her), use of analgesic drugs as necessary for pain relief, and sometimes use of oxytocin. DARVON and aspirin or codeine and aspirin constitute the analgesics commonly used. Since the breasts do not remain uncomfortable for a long period, medication will only be needed for a very short time, and danger to the infant is minimal.

A breast support should be used as soon as the breasts become heavy. It should lift the breasts, suspending their weight from the shoulders, and should not put pressure on any area. Ordinarily the mother wears her brassiere for support, usually the nursing brassiere that she plans to wear throughout the period of lactation. A well-fitting brassiere is often very comfortable (Fig. 28–3).

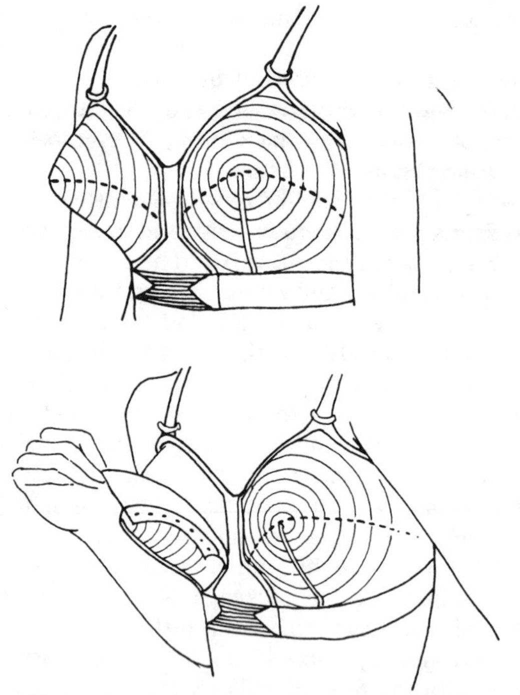

Figure 28–3. Nursing brassiere. Circular-stitched cups give extra support. Cup drops down for nursing.

Its front opening should be large enough to make it possible for the baby to grasp the mother's nipple without interference from the bra, or it should be possible to fold the cup of the bra down and out of the way without losing the support from the bra.

The pressure created by milk in the breasts can be relieved by emptying them, either by the infant's sucking if he can grasp the nipple or by a breast pump or manual expression if he cannot nurse well. A warm pack to the breasts, prior to attempts to empty them, may enhance the flow of milk and help bring relief of pressure from milk retention.

The mother needs reassurance that the discomfort of engorgement will subside in a day or two because she may think that the breasts will remain uncomfortable during the entire time that she nurses her infant and become discouraged with nursing. When the breasts become soft and comfortable, the mother then may think that her milk supply has decreased unless she is again assured that the breasts are normally comfortable even when they are functioning adequately.

Mechanisms in Lactation

For adequate lactation there must be both secretion of milk in the breasts and expulsion of milk from the breasts.

MILK SECRETION Secretion of milk begins two or three days after delivery and will continue for months if the breasts are frequently and sufficiently emptied. If little or no milk is withdrawn for a period of time, the milk that accumulates in the alveoli reaches a pressure level that inhibits secretion. If this back pressure in the alveoli is relieved inadequately over a period of several days, milk secretion decreases; if it is not relieved, milk secretion stops.

Frequent and complete emptying of the breasts stimulates production of milk, and the amount produced largely depends on the amount that is removed (Fig. 28–4).

Milk production often can be increased by nursing both breasts at each feeding time and by increasing the frequency of feedings, if they are not so frequent that the mother becomes tired. Milk production is slow in some

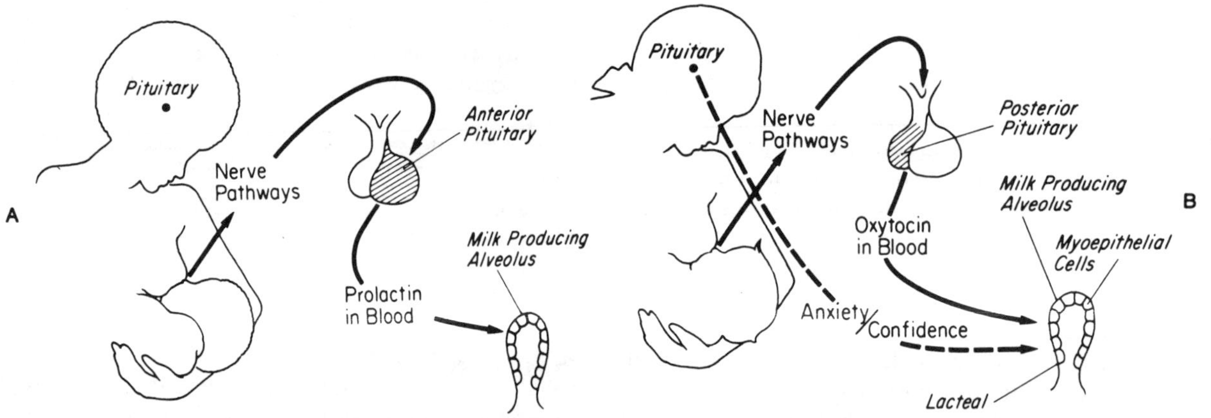

Figure 28–4. Key reflexes in lactation. A. Shows the prolactin reflex, a somatic response to sucking the breast, responsible for milk secretion (simplified). B. Represents the "let-down" or "milk-ejection" reflex, a psychosomatic reflex, impaired by anxiety and enhanced by confidence, responsible for moving milk from alveoli to terminal lacteals (simplified). Reproduced with permission from Derrick B. Jelliffe, and E. F. Patrice Jelliffe, "Breast is best: Modern meanings." *N. Engl. J. Med.* 297: 912–915, (Oct. 27) 1977.)

mothers, and persistence may be necessary to reach a level adequate to satisfy the infant's needs.

MILK EXPULSION The expulsion mechanism, also called the *let-down reflex,* must function adequately for proper emptying of the breast (Fig. 28–4). Initiation of the reflex by the infant's sucking on the mother's nipple, or by psychic factors, causes release of oxytocin from the posterior lobe of the pituitary gland. Sensory nerve endings in the breasts, mainly in the skin, are very sensitive to pressure, temperature, pain, and the infant's sucking. Afferent fibers from these nerves travel to and through the spinal cord and to the hypothalamus. Oxytocin is produced in response to impulses along the nerves and released into the circulation from the neurohypophysis (posterior lobe of the pituitary gland). Oxytocin then reaches the breast tissue through the circulation and causes the tissue surrounding the alveoli of the breasts to contract and propel the milk from the alveoli and the small ducts to the larger ducts opening through the nipple. From these large ducts the milk then can be removed by compression and suction. An active let-down reflex is important to maintenance of milk production. The milk expulsion reflex is easily conditioned and also easily inhibited in response to a number of other stimuli than sucking.

Some mothers experience a prickling or tingling sensation in the breasts before a feeding time. They report that they feel the milk coming in (not referring to the beginning of milk secretion) or that they feel the milk coming down. The mother may notice that milk begins to drip from her breasts at a time when she is anticipating giving a feeding or when she hears the infant cry. During a feeding time she may notice milk dripping from the breast opposite to the one from which the infant is sucking.

Worry, fatigue, pain, emotional conflicts, or other distractions interfere with the let-down reflex, and the infant gets less milk than he could if the reflex were functioning well. Nipple pain and painful uterine contractions sometimes make nursing difficult. To help prevent inhibition of the let-down reflex, the mother should be given adequate pain relief if she is uncomfortable, provided with a quiet and undisturbed atmosphere while nursing her infant, and given encouragement that the breast-feeding will be satisfactory. Inhibition of the let-down reflex over a period of time may result in breast-feeding failure (Fig. 28–5).

Fright, grief, anxiety, or any marked emotional disturbance may result in a decrease, perhaps only temporarily, in the quantity of milk that previously had been satisfactory.

Since emotions influence the secretion of milk in a number of ways, the first essential to successful breast-feeding appears to be a mother's real desire to nurse her infant. A desire to nurse, a state of good nutrition, adequate rest, and a relaxed attitude are important factors in establishing breast-feeding and in maintaining the secretion of an adequate supply. The psychic influence on the production of breast milk is so significant that emotional serenity and freedom from worry are especially important. A woman's lack of confidence in her ability to nurse, especially if quantity of milk is slow to increase, may have an adverse effect, and she needs frequent encouragement and reassurance that persistence will bring good results.

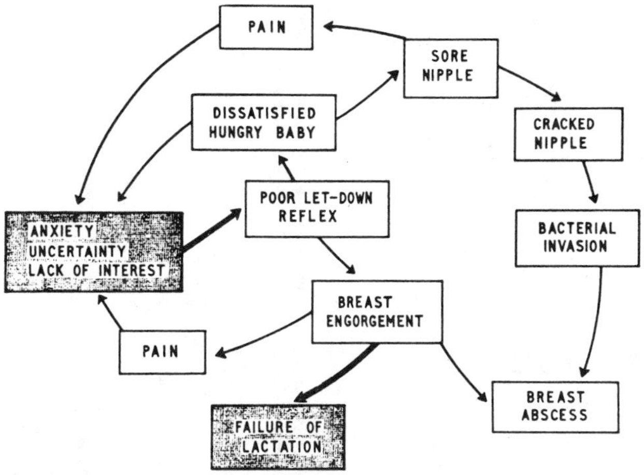

Figure 28–5. The "Anxiety-Nursing Failure Syndrome." (Reproduced with permission from Derrick B. Jelliffe, and E. F. Patrice Jelliffe, "Breast is best: Modern meanings." *N. Engl. J. Med.* 297:912–915, (Oct. 27) 1977.)

Oxytocin very occasionally is administered to a mother during early lactation to initiate milk flow and assist in the ejection of milk when the let-down reflex is inhibited, as in times of stress. Oxytocin may facilitate the flow of milk.

Oxytocin is available for administration as a spray into the nasal cavity, as well as in preparation for injection. It is absorbed readily into the blood from the nasal mucous membrane. It is provided in a plastic squeeze bottle and when used is sprayed into the nostril with a squeeze of the plastic container. A single spray, as a whiff, is made into one or both nostrils two or three minutes before the breast is nursed or pumped. The effectiveness of this treatment is not assured.

The Infant's Sucking

The infant obtains milk by taking the nipple well back in the mouth and closing the lips tightly around the breast tissue, compressing the lactiferous sinuses behind the areolar area to squeeze milk out (Fig. 28-6), and sucking the milk into his mouth and swallowing it.

For satisfactory nursing an infant must have the nipple well back in the mouth with the tongue pressing the nipple against the palate. When the nipple is far back in the infant's mouth, the gums press on the areolar area of

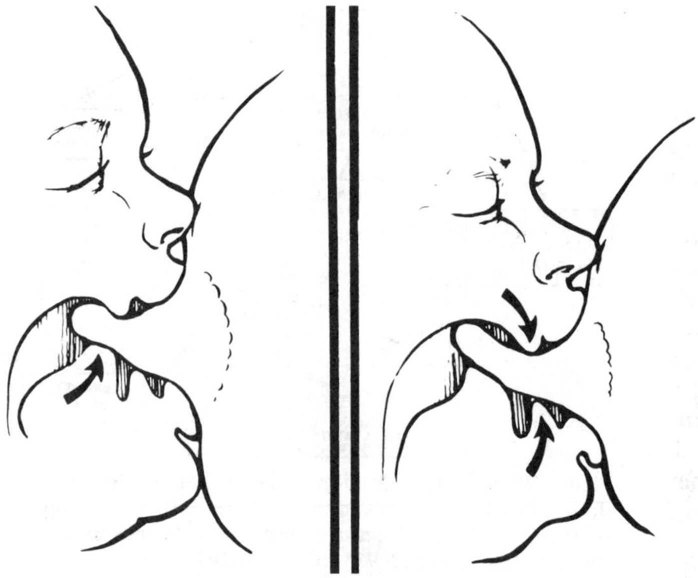

Figure 28–6. In breast-feeding, the tongue thrusts up and forward to grasp the nipple (left); the gums compress areola and the tongue moves backward creating negative pressure for suction (right). Lips are flattened against areola. Cheek muscles assist. (Reproduced with permission from Jan Riordan, and Betty Ann Countryman, "The anatomy and psychophysiology of lactation," *JOGN Nurs.* 9:210–213, (July-Aug.) 1980.)

the mother's breast and the lips can close tightly around the breast tissue to permit suction. Eminences across the inner part of the infant's lips are helpful in closing around the nipple. With his mouth firmly around the areolar area of the mother's breast, the infant empties the breast by compression and suction. As the infant nurses, his jaws move up and down and compress and empty the sinuses. Tongue action, which sucks the nipple back and presses it against the palate, and suction will complete removal of milk from the nipple. The milk is then swallowed. This action of compression, suction, and swallowing is continued rhythmically for a short period of time, followed by a few moments of rest, and then resumed. Periods of nursing interspersed with periods of rest are continued until satiety is reached.

An infant does not always take the mother's nipple properly, and although he goes through some of the movements used in nursing, he does not empty the breast satisfactorily. The infant may close his lips tightly around the nipple only and appear to suck vigorously. With this method very little milk is obtained, and the mother's nipple is apt to be injured by vigorous sucking. The infant also may attempt to suck with the tongue above the mother's nipple instead of underneath it; this too gives poor results.

If the infant has a good grasp on the nipple, he makes deep sucking movements with the muscles in his cheeks and frequent swallowing movements. When he does not have the nipple in his mouth properly, the jaws move up and down, but suction and swallowing movements are infrequent or absent.

When the infant nurses well, he usually sucks vigorously for a few minutes, stops a few moments to rest, and then sucks again. Some infants rest more frequently than others and some rest for several minutes at a time. The infant's nursing usually slows as his hunger decreases. He releases the nipple when his hunger and/or desire to suck is satisfied. Ordinarily the infant does not let go of the nipple during rest periods if he has a good grasp. If the infant releases the nipple frequently, he may not have it in the mouth properly, or he may need to do so to breathe. An infant normally breathes through the nose and can breathe easily during nursing if the nose is not obstructed. He will not have difficulty breathing when the nose is not tight against the breast tissue, provided it is not obstructed with secretions.

There are considerable individual differences in the ways in which infants nurse. These differences are described as follows by Dr. George R. Barnes, Jr., and coauthors:

1. "Barracudas": When put to the breast, these babies vigorously and promptly grasp the nipple and suck energetically for from 10 to 20 minutes. There is no dallying. Occasionally this type of baby puts too much vigor into his nursing and hurts the nipple. 2. Excited Ineffectiveness: These babies become so excited and active at the breast that they alternately grasp and lose the breast. They then start screaming. It is often necessary for the nurse or mother to pick up the baby and quiet him first, and then put him back to the breast. After a few days the mother and baby usually become adjusted. 3. Procrastinators: These babies often seem to put off until the fourth or fifth postpartum day what they could just as well have done from the start. They wait till the milk comes in. They show no particular interest or ability in sucking in the first few days. It is important not to prod or force these babies when they seem disinclined. They do well once they start. 4. Gourmets or Mouthers: These babies insist on mouthing the nipple, tasting a little milk and then smacking their lips, before starting to nurse. If the infant is hurried or prodded, he will become furious and start to scream. Otherwise, after a few minutes of mouthing he

settles down and nurses very well. 5. Resters: These babies prefer to nurse a few minutes and then rest a few minutes. If left alone, they often nurse well, although the entire procedure will take much longer. They cannot be hurried.

There are many babies who fall between these groups and others who fall into groups not described because they are less common. The above grouping serves merely to emphasize the fact that each baby nurses differently, and the course of the nursing will depend on the combination of the baby's nursing characteristics, the mother's personality, and the quality of help from the attending nurse. A calm mother with a "barracuda" will be quite a different matter from an anxious mother with an excited ineffective. It is accordingly advantageous to have the same nurse for both mother and baby; a nurse who knows both mother and baby can give more effective help.[5]

Assisting the Mother and Infant

The Early Feedings

If the pregnancy and the infant's birth have been relatively uncomplicated, the mother who plans to breast-feed should be allowed and encouraged to feed her infant as soon as possible after birth, often before she is moved from the delivery bed, and thereafter to do so whenever the infant seems hungry. Early and frequent breast-feeding is valuable for several reasons and is usually very satisfying to both mother and infant. The mother is eager and ready to see and handle and feed her baby at this time, and the infant is likely to suck well in this first period of reactivity. The infant's sucking reflex is very active and vigorous for the first 30 to 60 minutes after birth. When breast feeding is not started within an hour after birth, it is likely to be postponed to the second period of reactivity.

During the first few feedings the infant gets only a small amount of colostrum, but early breast-feeding, before the mature milk comes in, has several advantages. It appears to have a beneficial effect in early establishment of an adequate milk supply. It may lessen engorgement by keeping the milk ducts open through regular removal of colostrum and breast secretion, which minimizes distention of alveoli from an increased accumulation. If emptying of the breast is not begun before engorgement appears, emptying may be difficult.

Early breast-feeding accustoms both mother and infant to the nursing process. The mother learns how to handle her infant and to put him to the breast, and the infant learns how to take the mother's nipple. All newborns do not nurse well when first put to the breast; practice during the early days usually accustoms the infant to nurse well by the time the breasts secrete a larger amount of milk.

Attachment and bonding are thought to be enhanced by frequent and early contact of mother and infant while breast feeding at a time when both are in a sensitive period and very receptive to each other. Since newborns are in an alert state during the first hour or so after birth, breast-feeding at this time gives both mother and infant an opportunity for a very positive response to each other.

With early breast-feeding the infant has the advantage of receiving the immunological properties of colostrum early in his postnatal days. Another advantage of early feeding to the infant is stimulation of peristalsis of the gastrointestinal tract and early expulsion of meconium. This is important in facilitating excretion of bilirubin and reducing the development of jaundice. Bottle-fed infants are not as likely to be fed as early as breast-fed infants and possibly not as frequently.

Sucking on the nipples releases oxytocin, which promotes involution of the uterus, beneficial in the early days post partum. The mother is often aware of uterine contractions during nursing and sometimes becomes quite uncomfortable from them. Medication for pain relief may be necessary for comfort, both during and after the nursing period for the first day or two post partum. This discomfort sometimes makes the early nursing difficult and may inhibit let-down of breast secretion. These afterpains are most likely to appear in women who have had several children.

Starting the Infant to Nurse

Helping the mother breast-feed her infant is an important nursing skill. The nurse should be available to help the mother the first time she feeds her newborn and for as many times thereafter as is determined by the mother's and infant's need for assistance. Some mothers know how to make themselves and their infants comfortable during nursing, how to handle their infants with ease, and how to help them grasp the nipple. Others need help in all these methods. Many newborns grasp the mother's nipple easily and begin sucking immediately; others need assistance and urging.

In preparing to nurse her infant, the mother is advised to wash her hands and to assume a comfortable position. At first it may be easier for her to lie on her side with the head of the bed elevated slightly. Later she may wish to sit up, either in bed or in a chair. It is often easier for the nurse to assist a mother lying on her side than in an upright position. The mother is instructed to turn well over to her side so that the infant does not need to reach up to grasp the nipple. The mother may hold the infant in the curve of her arm, but care must be taken that he is not held in a cramped position. Sometimes the infant is more comfortable if he lies on the bed with the mother's arm securely around him.

After the infant has been handed to the mother, at-

[5] George R. Barnes, Jr., Anton N. Lethin, Jr., Edith B. Jackson, and Nilda Shea, Management of breast feeding, *JAMA,* 151:194, (Jan. 17) 1953.

milk in which the protein has been modified, being derived from less casein and more whey. This brings the protein content closer to that present in breast milk. Thus commercially prepared formulas are available with a whey content similar to that of breast milk and with a content similar to cow's milk.

Both human and cow's milk provides approximately 20 kcal/oz. This means that the infant who is eating well and having a satisfactory caloric intake will have an adequate fluid intake. However, with the higher protein content of cow's milk compared to human milk, the water reserve is larger in breast milk than in cow's milk. In prepared formulas the solute load is between that of breast milk and cow's milk but is usually brought closer toward that of breast milk. (See Table 28-2 for a comparison of human and cow's milk.)

The *protein content* of human milk is 1 to 1.5 gm percent, which provides approximately 8 percent of the calories. Cow's milk contains 3.3 gm percent protein and provides 16 percent of the calories in cow's milk. The higher protein content in cow's milk comes from its much higher casein content. Human milk has less casein but more whey protein.

The protein in commercially prepared formula may be "casein-based," providing 82 percent casein and 18 percent whey or "whey-based," providing 40 percent casein and 60 percent whey. The "whey-based" formulas are similar to human milk in relation to protein content, since human milk also provides 40 percent casein and 60 percent whey protein.

In addition to milk-based formulas, there are also formulas that have vegetable proteins as their major protein source, such as soy protein formulas. Soy-based formulas are used for infants who are sensitive or allergic to cow's milk protein, or who have difficulty digesting lactose, the sugar normally present in milk. Infants may need to drink soy-based formula for several months or they may be sensitive to cow's milk for only a period of days. An infant may be allergic to both milk formula and soy formula. For these infants a hypoallergenic formula is available. In such a formula not only the protein but also the fat and carbohydrate are modified.

Lactose is the sugar present in both human and cow's milk in a precentage of approximately 7 and 4.5, respectively. In commercially prepared, milk-based formulas carbohydrate in the form of lactose is added to bring the percentage of lactose to that found in human milk. Sometimes other sugars such as sucrose or glucose may be added.

The *fat content* of both human and cow's milk is

Table 28-2. Comparison of Human and Cow's Milk*

	Human Milk	*Cow's Milk*
Water and solid content	Same in both; 87 to 87.5 percent is water	
Calories	Same in both; 20 calories per ounce	
Protein	1 to 1.5 percent; 60 percent of this is lactalbumin, and 40 percent is casein	3.5 percent; 15 percent of this is lactalbumin, and 85 percent is casein
Carbohydrate (in form of lactose)	6.5 to 7.5 percent	4.5 to 5.0 percent
Fat(s)	Variable from time to time, but both have approximately 3.5 percent; differs qualitatively	
	Contains more olein, which is absorbed more readily	Contains more volatile fatty acids, which are irritating to the gastric mucosa
	Digestion of fat easy	Digestion of fat sometimes difficult
Minerals	0.15 to 0.25 percent	0.7 to 0.75 percent; contains more of all minerals with the exception of iron and copper
	Iron content is low in both milks, approximately: 1.5 mg/liter	0.5 mg/liter
Vitamins	Vary with maternal intake; vitamin content of cow's milk also may vary with cow's intake	
Vitamin A	Relatively large amount in both milks	
Vitamin B complex	Probably adequate in both milks	
Vitamin C	More is found in human milk	
Thiamine	Higher content in cow's milk	
Riboflavin	Higher content in cow's milk	
Vitamin D	Relatively small amount in both milks	
Vitamin E	Satisfactory level in breast milk	
Digestion	Cow's milk has a higher buffer content and therefore can absorb much more gastric acid than breast milk before it reaches the acidity necessary for digestion. The large amount of casein in cow's milk makes large, tough curds in the stomach as compared with the fine, easily broken-down curds of breast milk.	

*Since cow's milk is the most common substitute for human milk, a comparison of the constituents of each may be valuable in understanding why cow's milk is modified when used in infant formulas. The curd in cow's milk is altered and made smaller and less tough by boiling, pasteurization, homogenization, and by the heat necessary for making evaporated milk. These modification processes change the curd that is produced in the stomach either by altering the casein, or by homogenizing the fat, or by producing both changes, as in the evaporation process. Modification of cow's milk makes it more suitable for infant feeding.

variable, but generally averages 3.8 and 3.7, respectively. Fat provides about 50 percent of the calories in human milk and in formulas. The fat content of most formulas is similar. Fat in formula is provided primarily as vegetable and coconut fats. These fats are digested easily and well absorbed, and they contain acceptable amounts of linoleic acid, an essential fatty acid in the diet. Skim milk provides a high protein and carbohydrate intake, but has a very low content of essential fatty acids. Skim milk therefore should not be used as a formula for infant feeding.

Vitamins are added to commercially prepared formulas in an amount that will meet the requirements for the normal healthy baby who is eating well. Iron may be added to any one of the proprietary formulas; these formulas thus can be obtained with or without iron.

Feeding the Infant

As with breast-feeding, it is best to feed the bottle-fed infant when he is hungry, according to the infant's self-regulated schedule. The infant is prepared for his feeding by being made dry and comfortable and his bottle is prepared as necessary.

Moderately cold or room temperature formula usually is well tolerated by the infant. The temperature of the formula is relatively unimportant unless it is either too hot or too cold, but an infant's palate is very sensitive to temperature changes, and he usually likes the formula the same temperature each time. Commercially prepared, terminally sterilized formulas, which do not require refrigeration, allow for storage at room temperature. With use of such formula, warming is not necessary. When refrigerated formula is used, the bottle of formula usually is placed into a pan of warm water to remove the chill. A lavatory sink *should not be used* for warming formula since the bottle may become contaminated.

If the mother makes up one bottle of formula at a time (described later), she probably will not need to warm it. If a day's supply has been made, the bottle may be too cold as it comes from the refrigerator. It should not stand out for long, however, and is best warmed in a pan of water just prior to the feeding.

The infant is fed either by the mother or father or sometimes the nurse, being held throughout the entire feeding. The person offering the feeding should be pleasant and unhurried and sit in a comfortable chair.

The infant always should be held while he is being fed the bottle. "Propping" a bottle is dangerous because the infant may choke and aspirate milk. There is also the possibility that he may suck considerable air, which causes distention and discomfort, if he takes his feeding lying down. In addition, the infant gets more enjoyment from eating when he is held. The infant needs the closeness and security that accompany the feeding. The food, which quiets hunger pains, the feeling of being held, and a pleasant manner during feeding make his eating enjoyable. Although the infant's hunger will cease even when he receives the bottle lying down, he usually gets greater satisfaction if this feeding is received in a more comforting manner. Pleasure and satisfaction in eating may help to make adjustments to other situations easier.

The infant should be held in a semireclining position while eating so that the air he swallows is kept at the top of the stomach contents. To prevent swallowing of even more air than the infant ordinarily swallows while sucking, the bottle must be tilted enough to keep the nipple filled with milk at all times.

The infant may begin sucking as soon as the bottle is offered, or he may feel the nipple with his lips and take it and let go of it several times before he sucks well. Sometimes the infant raises the tongue when he takes the nipple. Although he may make sucking motions when his tongue is above the nipple, the sucking is ineffective, and the nipple must be gently manipulated or removed and replaced until it is above the tongue (Fig. 28–16).

The infant usually will suck well after he has a satisfactory start on his feeding, provided he is alert and hungry and the nipple holes are satisfactory. If the infant is obtaining formula, air bubbles can be seen going up into the bottle regularly. If air does not appear to enter the bottle, the nipple holes must be checked for clogging.

An infant usually takes the feeding in 15 to 20 minutes. Wide variations from this time may result from an unsatisfactory nipple. If the nipple holes are too small,

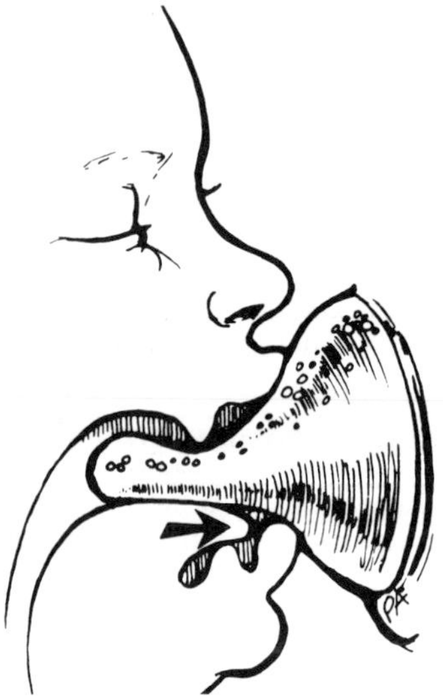

Figure 28–16. In bottlefeeding (above) the tongue is forward to control milk overflow from rubber nipple. Gums and lips cannot create compression. Air flows freely. Facial muscles are relaxed. (Reproduced with permission from Jan Riordan, and Betty Ann Countryman, "The Anatomy and Psychophysiology of Lactation." *JOGN Nurs.* 9:210–212, (July–Aug.) 1980.)

the infant may obtain very little milk even with vigorous sucking; the feeding may become too prolonged or the infant may become too tired to continue until he has obtained a satisfactory amount of formula. Some newborns cannot suck well on a new nipple, which is often stiff, and need a used nipple that has become softened or one that is made of soft rubber. If the nipple holes are too large, the infant may choke as the milk flows fast and may obtain the feeding so quickly that the desire to suck is not satisfied.

There are two kinds of openings for nipples; holes may be punctured in the end of the nipple, or a crucial incision (cross-cut) may be made at the end. Holes in the nipple should be large enough to permit milk to drop freely when the formula bottle is inverted, but not allow it to run in a stream. If the holes in a nipple are too small, they may be enlarged by slight burning of the rubber with the point of a fine needle heated to a red heat and quickly plunged through the end of the nipple. Several small holes are better than one large hole because there is less chance of complete plugging of the nipple.

The *cross-cut nipple* (crucial incision) has two 4-mm incisions, at right angles in the form of a cross, at the end of the nipple. Such an opening has a valvelike action, which opens as the infant sucks and closes as the pressure from the infant's mouth is released. The opening cannot be tested by inverting the formula bottle to observe the speed of the drops, but must rather be tested before the nipple is sterilized by milking the nipple on an inverted bottle of fluid.

Nipples used in a newborn nursery should not be touched after they have been sterilized. If a nipple becomes plugged while an infant is being fed or if the flow of milk is too rapid, a completely new unit—bottle of formula and nipple—should be used instead of a change of nipple. Additional bottles of formula should be available in the nursery to permit substitution of complete feeding units as frequently as necessary.

Raising an Air Bubble

When the infant's stomach is full, the sucking becomes slow and intermittent and the infant gradually falls asleep. The nipple may be taken away for a few minutes and then offered again to determine if he stopped sucking because of satisfaction or because of tiredness. Sometimes satiety seems to be reached when a large air bubble fills the stomach; the infant sucks with renewed interest after eructation of air.

Air is swallowed with milk during sucking; if the air is not eructed before the infant is placed in his bed, it will come up after he has been put down and bring milk along with it. Although the amount of milk thus vomited appears to be considerably larger than it actually is, owing to the air that comes up with the food, it may in some instances be necessary to feed the infant again.

To raise an air bubble from the infant's stomach (bubble the baby) he is held in an upright position, to allow the air to rise to the top of the stomach; his body is supported against the mother's or nurse's body or shoulder; and he is gently patted on the back. As the bubble comes up there is a definite belching noise. If the air has not come up after a two- to three-minute period, the infant can be held in a different position for five minutes and then held upright again; if a bubble is not raised during a second attempt, the infant may be put to bed, preferably on the right side or abdomen. It is then wise to attempt to raise an air bubble before the next feeding. An infant may not eructate air after each feeding, although the bottle-fed infant does so in most instances.

Bringing up the air bubble at the end of a feeding may be sufficient, especially with the breast-fed infant, but if an infant is known to swallow considerable air and ordinarily vomit before finishing a feeding, it may be necessary to stop once or twice during each feeding to attempt to raise the bubble.

Teaching the Mother

When an infant is bottle-fed, the mother ordinarily feeds him during the daytime hours so that she can become accustomed to his reactions and way of eating (Fig. 28–17). The night feedings usually are given in the nursery to allow the mother to obtain adequate rest. The mother needs assistance with the infant's feedings so that she can learn how to hold the infant, how to hold the bottle, to determine when the infant seems satisfied, and to gain experience with bubbling him.

The mother needs explanation that the amount of formula (or breast milk) that the infant wishes may increase each day for a week or more, but that he will not take exactly the same amount from the bottle at each feeding. When the infant ordinarily takes 4 oz at a time, he may stop after only 2 oz at some feedings; the bottle should not be jiggled to urge the infant to take more. It is also important for the mother to learn that caloric needs and gastric capacity vary greatly in infants of the same size and age and that her infant may not need the same amount that another infant of the same age will take. The question frequently asked, "How much should my baby be eating now?" gives the nurse an opportunity to explain the infant's ability to determine his needs.

Although the mother needs adequate instruction in how to raise the air bubble when she feeds her infant, she also needs reassurance that spitting-up of milk and some vomiting after a feeding are normal in the newborn and not always due to inadequate raising of the bubble. She may be told that vomiting decreases as the infant gets older and that it becomes significant only if it continues. Adequate bubbling, gentle handling after a feeding, and making certain that the infant's head is not lower than the rest of the body when he is put to bed all help to

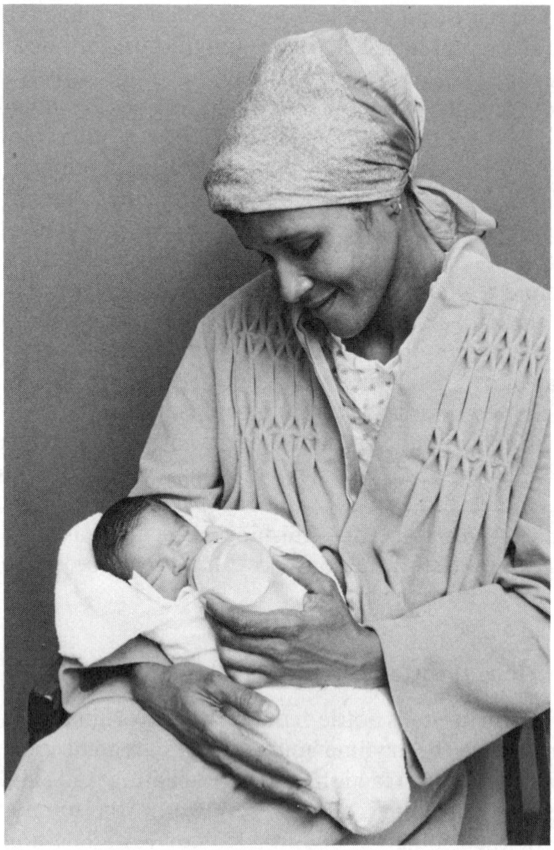

Figure 28–17. A mother giving her baby his bottle feeding. The bottle fed baby should be held for his feedings since it is the only safe way to feed him to prevent choking and aspiration of milk. The mother and the infant also need the closeness and cuddling that accompanies a feeding when the baby is being held. Mother and infant appear relaxed and happy. [Courtesy of The Presbyterian Hospital in the City of New York. Photo by Elizabeth Marshall.]

decrease regurgitation. Since the amount of food vomited is frequently less than it appears, the mother does not need to be concerned that the infant is not receiving an adequate amount of food unless he does not continue to gain weight. Persistent vomiting, of course, may have a serious underlying cause and also may result in a decrease in body fluids.

The mother needs reassurance that hiccuping is common after a feeding and is not significant. When the infant has hiccups, an attempt can be made once again to raise an air bubble, but further treatment is not necessary to try to stop hiccups; they soon will disappear.

Bottle-Feeding at Home

One of the many varieties of commercially prepared infant formulas or an evaporated milk formula prepared at home may be used for feeding the normal newborn who is to be bottle-fed. Fresh cow's milk, either whole or diluted or as reduced fat content milk, is not appropriate for newborn feeding.

Commercially prepared formula is available in powder form, in a liquid concentrate that requires dilution with water before it is fed to the infant, and in ready-to-feed mixture. The ready-to-feed formula may be purchased in 960-ml (32-fl oz) cans from which the formula is poured into feeding bottles, or it is available in 4-oz disposable bottles and nipples. The latter are expensive but convenient for certain purposes, as for use on a trip.

As to cost, ready-to-feed formula in the 960-ml cans is more expensive than the concentrated liquid which may be purchased in 385-ml (13-fl oz) cans. Ready-to-feed in small individual disposable nursing bottles is most expensive. Evaporated milk is the least expensive formula.

The formula used and the method of preparation may differ for the infant who is fed entirely by bottle from those recommended for preparation of an occasional bottle-feeding for the breast-fed infant. For the infant who is entirely on bottle-feedings, the formula is usually made by dilution of a commercially prepared concentrated formula or by mixing an evaporated milk formula as described below. For the infant who is breast-fed but needs an occasional bottle, a commercially prepared formula in powder form, which may be stored without refrigeration after opening, may be convenient. It is also possible that the parents will decide to purchase the ready-to-feed prepared formula in single bottle units for the occasional bottle-feeding.

Commercially Prepared Formulas

A large variety of prepared formulas are available for infant feeding in either liquid or powder form. Many of these preparations have a composition similar to that of breast milk; in some the composition is similar to that of breast milk with the exception of a higher percentage of protein; some have a relatively high-protein and low-fat content; and some have added iron. Vitamins have been added to prepared formulas, making it unnecessary to give the infant additional vitamins while he is eating commercially prepared formula.

Among commonly used commercially prepared cow's milk based formulas are ENFAMIL, SIMILAC, and SMA. Ready-to-feed formulas have been terminally sterilized in a closed system; refrigeration and subsequent warming are unnecessary. The ready-to-feed formulas may be prohibitive in cost for prolonged home use but often are desirable for an occasional bottle at any time that preparation of formula is difficult or impractical.

Formula Prepared at Home

Sometimes a formula which is completely home mixed is used for infant feeding instead of a commercially prepared formula. The home-mixed formula is prepared by combining three basic ingredients—evaporated milk, water, and sugar. The proportions of each ingredient are determined by the infant's caloric and fluid requirements. A formula prepared to approximately 20 calories per ounce usually fulfills the normal newborn's needs. Preparation of such a formula is described below.

MILK The kind of milk used in formula will depend on its safety and its digestibility by the infant. Unmodified milk should not be used because of its high bacterial count and because of the large, tough curd it produces.

The curd in cow's milk is altered and made smaller and less tough by boiling, pasteurization, homogenization, addition of acid or alkali, and by the heat necessary for making evaporated milk. These modification processes change the curd produced in the stomach either by altering the casein, or by homogenizing the fat, or by producing both of these changes, as in the evaporation process. Modification of cow's milk makes it more suitable for infant feeding.

Of the various modifications of cow's milk, evaporated milk is the kind recommended for bottle feeding during early infancy. It is readily available, is relatively inexpensive, may be stored without refrigeration in the unopened can, and is easy to use in infant formula. The process of evaporation of milk so alters the milk (alteration in casein and decrease in size of fat molecules) that the curd produced in the stomach from evaporated milk is small and soft. It is quite similar to that of breast milk.

Evaporated milk is decreased in volume to approximately one half of the original volume of whole milk; each fluid ounce of evaporated milk contains 44 calories. It is thus obvious that whole milk cannot be used as a substitute for evaporated milk, nor can evaporated milk be used in place of whole milk.

The amount of milk the infant needs varies from 1.5 to 2 oz of whole milk or ¾ to 1 oz of evaporated milk per pound of body weight in a 24-hour period, although this requirement may be less during the first two weeks of life. Protein requirements are fulfilled by ¾ oz of evaporated milk, but appetite may not be satisfied by this amount.

WATER The milk used in formula is diluted with water. Since most or all of a newborn infant's fluid intake is formula, the milk usually is diluted up to the amount that will fulfill the total fluid requirement for a 24-hour period.

SUGAR Sugar is often used in formula preparation. Sugar furnishes the calories that are needed because of the dilution of the milk. Many sugars are used satisfactorily. Lactose, which is the natural milk sugar, appears to have no advantage over other kinds and may even be less well tolerated. It may cause more flatulence because of its greater degree of fermentation. Cane sugar is obtained easily, is well tolerated by the normal infant, but is sweeter than other sugars. Combinations of maltose and dextrins are sometimes used; they digest and absorb more slowly than some of the other preparations and have a less sweet taste. Corn syrup has been used quite frequently. Many of the sugars contain 120 calories per ounce.

Honey should not be used as a source of sugar in formula. Honey may be contaminated with spores of the bacterium *Clostridium botulinum*.

One of several rules may be used to determine the quantity of sugar to add to a formula. One method is to add ½ oz sugar to the day's formula for the first two weeks of life, then 1 oz for four to six months, and then a gradual discontinuance until no sugar is added. Another rule that may be followed is to add slightly less than 1/10 oz of sugar per pound of the infant's body weight when an evaporated-milk formula is made. The amount of sugar added to a day's feeding should not exceed 1.5 oz.

To some extent the amount of sugar may be determined by the concentration of the formula, and also by the character of the infant's stools. In general, the more concentrated the formula, the less the amount of sugar the infant can tolerate. If the newborn develops loose stools, the amount of sugar in the formula may be reduced. Evaporated-milk formula is sometimes given without the addition of sugar, but the infant's caloric intake may not be adequate then.

In preparation of formulas it is important to know the variation in the number of tablespoons of sugar per ounce for the different kinds of sugars. If a tablespoon is used to measure the sugar for a formula, it is necessary to know the number of tablespoons per ounce of the particular kind of sugar that is used.[13]

Examples of Evaporated Milk Formulas

Using the above information for formula construction, a 24-hour supply of an evaporated-milk formula that may be considered adequate to meet the needs of a newborn weighing 3600 gm (8 lb) would be calculated as shown on page 596.

This formula may be divided into eight bottles, each containing 3 oz, or six bottles containing 4 oz, depending on the infant's preference for frequency and amount of feeding.

Since this formula furnishes 412 calories, an infant weighing 3600 gm (8 lb) receives 113 calories per kilo-

[13] Cane sugar—2 tbsp per ounce.
DEXTRI-MALTOSE—4 tbsp per ounce.
Dexin—6 tbsp per ounce.
Corn syrup—2 tbsp per ounce.

gram (51.5 calories per pound) in a 24-hour period if he takes all of the formula during that time. This formula also fulfills the infant's fluid needs.

The newborn will not take the total amount of this suggested formula in a 24-hour period during the first few days of life. He may not take more than 1 to 2 oz at each feeding during the early days. However, his need increases from day to day, sometimes slowly but sometimes rapidly, and he soon may want the full amount of formula. As the infant grows older, he will show dissatisfaction with the proportions of the original formula. Alterations in the formula are then made to satisfy hunger and to meet growth needs. A more concentrated formula usually is offered. As less water is added to formula, some of the infant's total fluid intake is furnished by orange juice and food high in water content and by drinking water between feedings.

Another recipe for evaporated milk formula, which may be used later, when the infant takes more food, is made as follows:

Evaporated milk	= 13 oz (one can)
Water	= 19 oz
Corn Syrup or Table sugar	= 2 tbsp

This formula is suitable in providing adequate caloric and nutrient intake for as long as the infant is fed formula. It does not need frequent changing in proportions, as was done in the past.

In using evaporated milk for formula it is important to use whole evaporated milk (not 2% or skim milk), and to check that it is vitamin A and D fortified. Condensed milk is not a substitute for evaporated milk, since it is made with sugar added to the milk.

For those mothers who wish to make only one bottle of evaporated milk formula at one time the recipe for an 8 oz bottle of formula is 3 oz of evaporated milk, 4 ½ oz of water, and 2 tsp of corn syrup. See "Single Bottle Method of Formula Preparation," p. 598.

Total fluid requirement (approximately 3 oz for each pound of body weight)	= 24 oz	
Total evaporated milk requirement (approximately 1 oz for each pound of body weight)	= 8 oz	
(8 oz of evaporated milk × 44 cal per oz)		= 352 cal
Amount of water to be added to the milk to make a total of 24 oz of formula	= 16 oz	
Sugar	= ½ oz	= 60 cal
Total	24 oz fluid	412 cal

Therefore, the formula prepared may read as follows:

Evaporated milk	= 8 oz
Water	= 16 oz
DEXTRI-MALTOSE	= 2 tbsp
or	
Corn syrup	= 1 tbsp

Note: Cane sugar is less likely to be prescribed than DEXTRI-MALTOSE or corn syrup because it so closely resembles salt in appearance that there is danger of mistakenly using salt instead of cane sugar in the formula. Such an error is likely to result in serious illness of the infant.

Cow's Milk Feeding

Whole cow's milk is not recommended for a feeding for an infant under 6 months of age. Pasteurized 2 percent milk, which in the past was used for the occasional bottle for the breast-fed infant, when a mother was not available to breast feed, is now considered inappropriate for feeding the infant. Milk that has not been heated to boiling produces a tough, cheesy curd that is hard to digest. This is in contrast to the soft, custard-like curd formed from formula or evaporated milk.

Undiluted cow's milk has a high solute load, derived from the protein and electrolyte content of the milk. Cow's milk contains approximately three times more protein, four times more calcium, six times more phosphorus, and three times more ash than human milk.

The Committee on Nutrition of the American Academy of Pediatrics states that more research is necessary before firm recommendations can be made concerning the age at which it is safe to introduce whole cow's milk in infants' diets, but that at present there is no convincing evidence that feeding whole cow's milk after 6 months is harmful if adequate supplementary feedings are given.

Until further studies are completed, the Committee makes the following recommendations for feeding infants 6 to 12 months old:

> Breast-feeding with appropriate supplementation is the preferred method of feeding infants 6 to 12 months old. . . .
>
> If breast-feeding has been completely discontinued and infants are consuming one third of their calories as supplemental foods consisting of a balanced mixture of cereal, vegetables, fruits, and other foods (thereby assuring adequate sources of both iron and vitamin C), whole cow's milk may be introduced. The amount fed should be limited to less than 1 L daily. Most infants who are not breast-fed should be consuming a significant portion of their calories from supplemental foods after they are 6 months old; those who are not should be given an iron-fortified formula.
>
> Reduced fat content milk is not recommended during infancy.[14]

Formula Preparation

Actual preparation of the formula may be by a terminal heat method, an aseptic method, or a clean method. Sometimes the method is determined by whether an entire day's supply is prepared at once or whether each bottle is prepared when needed (single bottle method).

Factors that are considered in advising the mother in a method are the kind of formula that will be used, the safety of the water, the availability of adequate refrigeration in the home, the mother's ability to utilize the method, and the number of bottles used each day. An occasional bottle may be prepared differently from those for total bottle feedings.

Regardless of method of preparation, care against contamination of the infant's food necessitates several general precautions. The person preparing the formula should always begin with careful handwashing with warm water and soap, and a clean towel should be used for drying the hands. The work counter and the sink must also be cleaned thoroughly with hot water and detergent and rinsed well with clean water.

All equipment used in preparation of the formula must be washed carefully in warm water and detergent and thoroughly rinsed—the bottles, nipples, measuring equipment, mixing bowls and spoons, can opener, and the tops of cans of formula or evaporated milk.

Adequate cleaning of bottles and nipples is very important to the safety of formula, especially that which is terminally heated. Cleaning is sometimes difficult because milk solids adhere to the inside of the bottle during heating of the formula. Bottles used daily without thorough cleaning will collect a milk film in which heat-resistant organisms, which can survive terminal heating, may build up and produce a contaminated formula. The bottle, nipple, and bottle cap should be rinsed under cold running water immediately after a feeding and then submerged in cold water to loosen milk solids and coagulated protein. After soaking, the bottles are washed in a warm detergent solution with a brush that reaches the bottom of the bottle so that all particles of formula that adhere to the glass are removed. A detergent is far superior to soap for cleaning formula bottles. Soap combines with milk casein to form a gummy substance that is difficult to remove from the surface of bottles, nipples, and utensils. The bottles are rinsed in hot running water until all detergent is removed, inspected in a good light to be certain that they are clean, and inverted to drain. Nipples and bottle caps should be cleaned in the same manner. A small brush may be used to reach the ball of the nipple or the nipple may be inverted for thorough cleaning. Water should be forced through the nipple holes.

Terminal Heat Method of Preparation

With the terminal heating method of formula preparation, the entire formula unit, consisting of a bottle filled with the milk mixture, nippled and capped, is exposed to a degree of heat that will destroy bacteria. The day's supply of formula is mixed in a clean container, the required amount for each feeding is poured into clean bottles, nipples and caps are loosely applied to the bottles, and the entire unit—bottles with formula, nipples, and caps—is placed into a large kettle with water 3 in. deep. The kettle is covered with a tight-fitting lid and the water is boiled for 25 minutes. Timing should not begin until the water is actually boiling. This means that the entire unit is heated at a temperature of 100°C (212°F) for 25 minutes with boiling water and steam in a water bath. This amount of heating kills pathogenic bacteria. It does not destroy spore formers, and nonpathogenic heat-resistant bacteria may survive. The bacterial count of the nonpathogenic bacteria is low enough to make the formula bacteriologically safe, but sterility cannot be assured in every bottle. Refrigeration of the formula is thus essential to keep the bacterial count low. The formula should be used within 48 hours.

At the end of 25 minutes of boiling the kettle is removed from the stove and allowed to stand covered—cooling—for about one hour. Thereafter the nipple caps are tightened and the bottles are placed in the refrigerator.

Terminal heating of a day's supply of formula is a very satisfactory method of preparation for either commercially prepared formula or evaporated milk formula. When using commercially prepared formula, either liquid or powder, the concentrated formula is diluted according to directions, poured into clean bottles, subjected to the heating process, and then refrigerated. The terminal heating method seems especially suitable for preparation of formula from evaporated milk, in which

[14] American Academy of Pediatrics, Committee on Nutrition, The use of whole cow's milk in infancy, *Pediatrics,* 72:253–255 (Aug.), 1983.

three ingredients are mixed. It may be easier to measure and mix milk, water, and sugar in the quantity necessary for a whole day's supply than in small amounts for a single bottle. An adequate number of bottles and adequate refrigeration and space for storage in the refrigerator are necessary to the method. Since the formula must be stored in the refrigerator, warming of each bottle before a feeding to remove the chill may be considered and adds an additional step in use of the method.

Aseptic Method of Preparation

In this method the bottles, nipples, caps, and all the measuring and mixing equipment used to make formula are sterilized before the formula is prepared. All of the equipment is placed into a large pan of water and boiled vigorously for 15 minutes. Since this makes a large load, the bottles, nipples, and nipple caps are usually boiled separately. Nipples are usually not boiled for more than 5 minutes, since they are likely to become very soft with longer sterilization. Tongs to be used as forceps for handling the equipment must also be boiled, being placed in a position that makes it possible for the mother to get at the handle easily without burning her hands and without contaminating the water.

For mixing the formula, the water to be used is boiled for 5 minutes and the can of formula concentrate or evaporated milk is washed before opening. Care is taken not to touch or contaminate any part of the bottles and nipples and measuring and mixing equipment that will come in contact with the formula. The bottles are filled with formula in the appropriate amount, nippled and capped, and refrigerated immediately. Any unused liquid formula or milk must also be covered, refrigerated, and used within 48 hours.

Clean Method of Preparation

When the infant gets older, and under desirable circumstances even in the newborn period, sterilization of bottles is not considered essential.

The mother is instructed to carefully wash, rinse, and drain the bottles. The day's supply of water is boiled and stored at room temperature. At feeding time an appropriate amount of boiled water and milk for a single feeding is poured into the clean bottle and fed immediately. When the water supply is safe, it is not essential to boil the water before it is added to the milk.

When evaporated milk or liquid formula concentrate is used, it is essential to refrigerate the remainder of the milk after the can has been opened. Powdered formula may be stored in the closed container in a dry place at room temperature.

Although the clean method of formula preparation does not require sterilization, it does require all of the precautions of careful hand washing, cleaning of work space and sink and equipment, and careful washing and rinsing of bottles and nipples as described previously.

A full day's supply of feeding bottles, filled and ready to use, can be prepared at one time by the clean method, instead of preparing each bottle as needed, but it seems best to use the single bottle method. Preparation of all of the bottles at one time requires immediate refrigeration of all the bottles and storage space in the refrigerator, and it means that some bottles are not used until 24 hours or more after preparation, giving bacteria a longer time to multiply.

Single Bottle Method of Formula Preparation

With the single bottle method only one bottle of formula is made at a time, being prepared just prior to the time it will be fed. Any one of the three methods described previously may be used for preparation of the single bottle. For the terminal heat method the nursing bottles are filled with an appropriate amount of water, nippled and capped, and terminally heated. A sufficient number of bottles of water for a day's supply are sterilized at one time and stored at room temperature until needed. At feeding time the appropriate amount of concentrated formula is added to one of the previously sterilized bottles of water. Instructions for preparation of a normal dilution formula, which provides 20 calories per ounce, are printed on the can of concentrated formula. The mother can determine from this the amount of water and the amount of concentrated formula, liquid or powder, that must be mixed for a normal concentration of formula.

For the aseptic method the bottles, nipples, and caps are sterilized by boiling. They are drained, allowed to dry, and stored until needed. A can of formula concentrate or evaporated milk is washed and opened. The appropriate amount of liquid is poured into the bottle, using the markings on the bottle for measurement. Assuming a safe water supply, an equal amount of fresh tap water is added for dilution. If indicated, the water must first be boiled. This formula should be fed within 30 minutes and discarded if it has not been used by 1 hour after preparation. The liquid formula concentrate or evaporated milk must be refrigerated immediately.

The single bottle preparation using the clean method has already been described.

In the single bottle method it is also important to prepare the bottle just prior to the time it will be fed. To prevent proliferation of bacteria, this is especially important when clean, instead of sterile, bottles are used.

Accuracy in mixing each bottle of formula is very important. This should be relatively easy when only two ingredients—concentrated formula and water—are used. It becomes somewhat more complex when the appropriate amount of evaporated milk, water, and sugar must be mixed. Evaporated milk formula can, however, be prepared in a single eight-ounce bottle by mixing evaporated milk, 3 oz; water, 4 ½ oz; and corn syrup or cane sugar, 2 tsp.[15]

A Few Precautions in Preparation and Use of Formula

1. When milk or commercially prepared liquid formula is used, it is essential to refrigerate the unused part of the milk after the can has been opened and to discard any unused amount within one day after the can is opened. Powdered formula may be stored in the closed container at room temperature in a dry place.
2. When an infant does not take all of the formula from the bottle, that which remains in the bottle always must be discarded after the feeding. It is unsafe to use the remaining formula for another feeding, even if the formula is refrigerated.
3. Nursing bottles and nipples should be rinsed immediately after use to prevent milk from drying on the surfaces. Terminally heated bottles also need to be soaked.
4. Formula should not be left standing at room temperature. When previously refrigerated it should be fed as soon as the chill is removed. Formula prepared in single bottles should be fed immediately after preparation.
5. Sometimes a mother who is breast-feeding has been told that she may use 2 percent milk for an occasional bottle-feeding interspersed with the breast-feeding. Some of these mothers stop breast-feeding soon after they are home, especially if they become discouraged because of poor lactation. They begin to feed the infant completely by bottle. In anticipation of such an event, these mothers should be told that 2 percent milk is not appropriate for a newborn and that they should contact their physician or nurse for formula instructions.
6. Overconcentrated formula imposes a high solute load on an infant which may lead to hyperosmolality and severe illness from dehydration and renal failure. Common offenders in this respect are improperly diluted powdered or evaporated milk. It is very important to make sure parents understand the instructions for formula preparation and also realize that an infant cannot tolerate milk that is more concentrated than the normal dilution.[16]

[15] Samuel J. Foman; Lloyd J. Filer, Jr.; Thomas A. Anderson; and Ekhard E. Ziegeler, Recommendations for feeding normal infants, *Pediatrics,* 63:52–59, (Jan.) 1979.

[16] Cyril A. L. Abrams *et al.,* Hazards of overconcentrated milk formula, *JAMA,* 232:1136-40, (June 16) 1975.

VITAMIN SUPPLEMENTS

Vitamin deficiency is rare in the United States where vitamin preparations usually are given to breast-fed infants and many of the newborns on bottle-feedings are given vitamin-fortified formula. In contrast, infants in developing countries may have severe vitamin lack. In these countries the fetuses may not receive adequate vitamins because of a maternal vitamin deficiency, breast-feeding may be discontinued early and other vitamin-poor foods are substituted, and vitamin supplementation may be lacking or inadequate.

Vitamins may be given in preparations that contain a single vitamin such as A or C or D, or they may be given in combination in a preparation that combines several vitamins.

A number of vitamin preparations containing vitamins A, C, and D, and also preparations that in addition include vitamin B complex, are available. If more than one vitamin is required, these multivitamin preparations usually are preferred as supplements, instead of separate administration of several vitamins. Concentrations in water-miscible vehicles are used to avoid danger of aspiration of oil.

Vitamin supplementation of an infant's milk feeding usually means the addition of vitamin D and sometimes vitamin C. Although human breast milk contains only a small amount of vitamin D, it appears that it is adequate for the normal infant fed by a well-nourished mother. *Vitamin D* is therefore not necessarily indicated, but may be recommended as a supplement of 400 IU daily if the mother's vitamin D intake has been questionable, if the infant gets very little exposure to sunlight (as may happen in winter when there are many short, cloudy days), and if the infant has a dark skin. Some authorities believe it is advisable to give all breast-fed infants a daily supplement of vitamin D, 400 IU, at least by 2 or 3 months of age.

Vitamin A was frequently used in the past as a supplement because it was often associated with vitamin D (as in cod liver oil). Vitamin A supplementation, however, does not seem indicated for the breast-fed infant.

An infant requires 35 mg of *vitamin C* per day. Vitamin C is probably not necessary for the breast-fed infant, however, since the mother will provide an adequate amount in her breast milk if her own intake is adequate. It is wise to inform the breast-feeding mother that it is important for her to drink 4 to 6 oz of orange juice per day. Infants fed a formula made from commercially prepared concentrate do not need vitamin C supplement. The formula provides approximately 35 mg of vitamin C per quart of formula.

Infants fed a home-prepared evaporated milk formula, require a supplement of vitamin C, 35 mg, or three oz of orange juice daily. Vitamin C is generally provided in a multivitamin combination along with vitamins A and D rather than as a single vitamin. The infant does not need additional vitamin D, since this is provided in the evaporated milk. He may even get an excessive amount of vitamin D if fed a multivitamin preparation and evaporated milk formula. It is therefore important to find a preparation only containing vitamin C or to feed the infant orange juice, 3 oz, daily. If the infant does not tolerate orange juice well, it is possible to use *infant-pack* apple juice, which is vitamin C fortified.

Commercially prepared formula concentrates have an appropriate amount of vitamin supplementation for infants. As long as infants are on such formula feedings they do not need additional vitamins. If and when infants are taken off formula and fed cow's milk after 6 months of age, the milk should be vitamin D fortified, and it is then also important to provide the infant with an adequate amount of food containing vitamin C.

FLUORIDE

Fluoride is a trace element deposited in the mineral of bones and teeth, increasing their hardness. It is considered important in the reduction of dental caries. Many communities have supplemented fluoride intake by adding it to drinking water. Other than fortified drinking water, infants receive very little fluoride from food or drink. Additional fluoride should not be given if the water supply contains an adequate amount because excess fluoride will cause mottling of the teeth. When drinking water is not fluoridated or when the infant is not taking drinking water because of complete breast-feeding, the physician may recommend administration of a fluoride beginning either shortly after birth or by 6 months of age. Use of fluoride for infants fed formula made from a commercial concentrate or from evaporated milk depends on the fluoride in the water that is used in mixing the formula. Ready-to-feed formulas, which a few parents may use for feeding their infant, are low in fluoride content. These require the same supplementation as for the breast-fed infant. The recommended dose of fluoride for the infant is 0.25 mg daily.

Desirable fluoride supplementation will depend on the fluoride content of the community water supply and upon the amount of that water consumed by the infant. No fluoride supplementation is recommended in communities in which the concentration of fluoride in drinking water is 0.3 ppm (parts per million) or more, if the infant is taking water daily.

Preparations of fluoride for infants generally contain 0.1 mg of fluoride per drop. This makes it convenient to adjust the dose as necessary. Parents must be cautioned about the importance of restricting dosage to the prescribed amount.

Combined fluoride-vitamin preparations are used widely and seem to be better accepted than fluoride preparation alone. The combined fluoride-vitamin supplement, however, makes it impossible to adjust the dose of fluoride without affecting the vitamin dose.

IRON

Iron is an essential nutrient for the body, being an important constituent of a number of enzymes as well as of hemoglobin. The means of providing infants with adequate iron intake is given serious consideration because iron deficiency has been found to be a common nutritional inadequacy of infants. The ordinary diet of an infant contributes a relatively small amount of iron requirement. Both human and cow's milk, which comprise a large portion of an infant's food intake, have a very small iron content. Other foods eaten in limited amounts during the first year ordinarily do not provide sufficient iron.

Over three fourths of the total iron content in the newborn's body at birth is present in the erythrocytes. There is only a small amount of iron stored in other tissues. The iron from the erythrocytes is retained in the body when the red blood cells break down, and it is reclaimed later for hemoglobin synthesis. The amount of iron available from this source will depend upon the initial hemoglobin mass. This amount may be inadequate to meet the infant's needs in later months if this initial hemoglobin level was somewhat low or if the infant was of low birthweight.

After birth the hemoglobin level falls steadily and the red blood cell count decreases. In the full-term infant recovery of erythrocyte and hemoglobin levels begins at about two months, when hematopoiesis resumes. In the premature infant, the physiologic anemia persists for a longer period of time. The premature has a smaller initial hemoglobin mass and this infant grows rapidly. The hemoglobin levels may remain depressed four months or longer. As hematopoiesis takes place, iron sources in the body are likely to be depleted, unless preventive measures have been taken. The infant's hemoglobin reading may fall to a level of anemia. Anemia, however, is only one manifestation of iron deficiency. By the time anemia appears, the deficiency also is affecting other tissues and organs.

Infants with low birthweight, full-term infants with a low initial hemoglobin level, and those infants who for some reason have sustained some blood loss are at risk of iron deficiency before one year. These infants may have special iron requirements during the first 18 months of life.

In the past it commonly had been thought that little or no iron was absorbed before three months of life. It is now known that iron will be efficiently absorbed when given to infants early in life and will be utilized in hemoglobin formation. Also, there appears to be no firm evidence that iron additives cause gastrointestinal disturbances in the infant, barring the rare exception. Therefore, the use of iron-fortified food (mainly milk and cereal) is considered advisable for prevention of iron deficiency in infants at risk.

The currently recommended intake of iron for normal full-term infants is at a dose of 1 mg/kg/day started no later than at four months of age. For premature infants and any others with special needs, the recommended intake is 2.0 mg/kg/day starting at two months or earlier. Formulas may provide anywhere from 0.1 mg to 1.5 mg/100 kcal. It is recommended that ordinary formulas should provide 0.15 mg/100 kcal and that iron-fortified formula should provide 1.0 mg/100 kcal. When the formula with the higher level of iron is prescribed for infants at risk of developing anemia, it should contain an ample amount of vitamin E and a moderate level of polyunsaturated fatty acids in order to reduce the possibility of vitamin E deficiency and hemolytic anemia.

Iron-fortified formula and/or iron-fortified baby cereal are readily available, convenient sources of iron and are preferable to the use of medicinal iron drops, unless there is a special reason to give the medicinal iron. Iron-fortified formula is generally prepared in such a way that when the infant takes an appropriate amount of formula for his size he will receive the appropriate amount of iron, the amount recommended for his size and maturity.

Iron-fortified infant cereal is prepared with electrolytic iron powder of small particle size, which is believed to be of high bioavailability. The iron-fortified cereal provides 7 mg of iron per 3 level tablespoons of dry cereal. This dry cereal diluted with milk or formula, makes a manageable serving and given daily provides the infant with an approximately correct amount of iron per day. According to Samuel J. Foman, M.D. and coauthors it is considered advisable to feed infants baby cereal daily from 5 to 6 months of age until 18 months of age. Iron-fortified cereals other than those specially prepared for infants should not be substituted for baby cereals for the first 18 months, since the iron used in the other cereals may not be of equal availability.[17]

Iron supplementation, generally recommended to begin at 4 months of age, can usually be safely delayed until 6 months of age in the breast-fed infant. Breast milk contains very little iron, but that which is present is absorbed better than the iron from other foods. Thus breast milk feedings help to delay depletion of the infant's iron stores. Adequate iron can probably be provided by 6 months of age by addition of cereal to the infant's diet.

[17] Samuel J. Foman, Lloyd J. Filer, Jr., Thomas A. Anderson, and Ekhard E. Ziegler, Recommendations for feeding normal infants, *Pediatrics,* 63:52–59, (Jan.) 1979.

Infants fed formula made from commercially prepared concentrate need iron supplementation after 4 months of age from either iron-fortified formula or iron-fortified cereal. Iron-fortified formula is sometimes used from the beginning for the bottle-fed infant. Once cereal feedings are adequate the infant does not also need iron-fortified formula.

For infants fed home-prepared evaporated milk formula, supplemental iron should be started at 4 months of age. Medicinal iron may need to be used until the infant takes an adequate amount of cereal.

Low-birthweight infants and those with an initial low iron level may require both iron-enriched formula and medicinal iron or iron-fortified vitamin preparations. Poisoning caused by accidental ingestion of medicinal iron is very serious and containers must be kept out or reach of other children.

INTRODUCTION OF SOLID FOODS

There has been a considerable amount of shifting back and forth over the years as to the appropriate time for adding food other than milk or formula to an infant's feeding. This additional food fed to infants is known as beikost. The time of adding "solid" food has varied anywhere from starting cereal around two weeks of age to feeding only milk for the first year of life.

Cereal is usually the first food added to an infant's diet. Many infants in the United States are fed beikost by at least two months of age. Early introduction of foods other than milk often seems to be the result of social pressure from friends or relatives who are feeding, or have fed, infant foods to their babies at an early age. The ready availability of commercially prepared baby food makes it easy to begin feeding "solid" foods early. Sometimes cereal is introduced very early in the belief that the infant will then sleep through the night. If the infant does sleep longer at night it may be due to his higher caloric intake. The question may then be asked: is it desirable for the infant to have such a long interval between feedings at an early age?

Current Recommendations

At the present time, recommendations by physicians and nutritionists for feeding infants, state that up to the age of 5 to 6 months breast feeding with a supplement of vitamin D, or commercially prepared formula provides the infant with a desirable total diet. After the age of 5 to 6 months "solid foods" are introduced according to the infant's developmental ability to take such food.

Samuel J. Foman, M.D. and coauthors have made the following recommendations:

> Breast-feeding with supplements of Vitamin D, iron, and fluoride provides a complete and highly desirable total diet for the infant until 5 or 6 months of age. . . .

Table 28–3. Overview of Developmental Patterns and Feeding Recommendations

	Birth	1 mo.	2 mo.	3 mo.	4 mo.	5 mo.	6 mo.	7 mo.	8 mo.	9 mo.	10 mo.	11 mo.	12 mo.	13 mo.	14 mo.	15 mo.	16 mo.
MOUTH PATTERN	Sucks only. Any "solids" will be sucked from the spoon and swallowed like liquids.			Beginning swallow pattern. Can transfer food from front of tongue to back.	Beginning of drooling.			Beginning chewing pattern; side-to-side motion of tongue and mashing food with jaws. Beginning tooth eruption.					Continuing maturation of biting, chewing, swallowing.				
HAND COORDINATION	Random motion of hands.				Hands beginning to go to mouth.		Palmar grasp. Urge to put anything in mouth continues and curiosity increases until about age three. Increases risk for poisoning throughout this time.	Pincer grasp beginning.	Demands spoon.		Can get spoon in mouth but generally turns it over. Usually finger feeds.		Beginning mastery of spoon—still spilling most times.			Spoon to mouth—with load intact!	
BODY CONTROL	Prone on back. Can raise head when on stomach. Rooting reflex.				Sits supported. Loses balance when reaches.		Sits unsupported. Can balance while manipulating with hands.	Begins to stand. Risk for falling from high chair is increased.		Continuing improvement in balance while sitting.							
DIGESTIVE PATTERN	Digestive enzymes present for milk. No drooling.							Gastric acid volume begins to increase.			Can handle balanced amounts of all reasonably soft, moderately-seasoned family food.						
NUTRITIONAL REQUIREMENTS	Relatively high nutrient requirement for rapid growth. Begin fluoride in some form: water or supplement.		Iron stores depleted in premature infants.			Iron stores begin to be depleted in term babies.		Begin learning to take food sources of vitamins A and C.		Gradually increasing proportion of adequate diet offered by foods other than milk feedng. Fruits and vegetables provide sources of vitamins A and C; meats etc. additional sources of protein, other nutrients; breads and cereal sources of B vitamins and iron.						All daily nutritional requirements provided by a mixed table food diet: 16–24 ounces milk 4 servings breads and cereals 4 servings fruits and vegetables Vitamin C source daily Vitamin A source three times weekly 2 servings meat, etc. to provide one ounce or equivalent.	
FEEDING GOALS	Milk feeding with proper supplementation. Fed from breast or bottle.	May introduce cup for breast-fed babies for relief feedings.	Iron supplementation for premies; iron drops or iron-fortified formula.			Begin iron-fortified cereal.	Introduce cup with mealtime.	Begin fruits and vegetables.	Begin table foods, including meats, etc., self-feeding with hands. Getting better at drinking from cup. Wants own spoon.		Begin self-feeding with cup. Allow weaning from bottle. Wean from breast if baby and parents are ready.		Beginning proficiency with spoon.			Primary source of nutrients and calories is table food and cup. Reasonably adept with spoon and cup. Can feed self with spoon, drink from cup. Weaned from bottle. Continuance of breast-feeding up to baby and parents.	

Each baby is an individual and will develop at his or her own rate. This chart gives the average age when behaviors might appear.
Source: Ellyn Satter, R.D., MSSW, Clinical Dietitian and Virginia Dykstal, R.N. certified pediatric nurse practitioner, "Feeding Your Infant and Toddler," Jackson Clinic, Madison, WI, Feb., 1983. Copyright 1983.

Table 28–4. Recommended Feeding Schedule During Infancy

*Basic Four Food Groups**	*Birth to 5 Months*	*4 to 7 Months*	*6 to 8 Months*	*7 to 10 Months*	*10 to 12 Months*
MILK FEEDING	Breastmilk with supplemental Vitamin D **OR** Commercial formula **OR** Evaporated milk formula with supplemental Vitamin C: 35 mg. Fluoridated (1 ppm) water should be used in making or reconstituting formula. For the breast-fed infant give .25 mg. fluoride per day.	Breastmilk with supplemental Vitamin D **OR** Commercial Formula **OR** Evaporated milk formula with supplemental Vitamin C. Continue Fluoride Source.	Breastmilk with supplemental Vitamin D **OR** Commercial Formula **OR** Evaporated milk formula with supplemental Vitamin C. Continue Fluoride Source.	Encourage Cup. May be using two kinds of milk. Recommended milks include: Breastmilk with supplemental Vitamin D. Commercial Formula. Evaporated milk diluted 1 to 1 with water. Whole pasteurized milk may be introduced toward age 10 months if the child is eating a variety of food from the four basic food groups and three meals a day.	Encourage cup. Use whole milk. Milk consumption may drop for a time until cup skills are better. Work toward 16–24 oz; too much can replace other nutritious food.
CEREAL AND BREAD (INFANT CEREAL)	**NONE**	Begin rice or barley iron-fortified baby cereal—powdered form—mixed with breast milk, formula, or diluted evaporated milk. You may offer cereal at anytime, but it should not reduce the milk intake as milk is still the most important food nutritionally at this stage. To get enough iron, eventual total should be ½ cup daily, after mixing. More is O.K.	Continue iron-fortified baby cereal. Depending on your baby's allergy risk, may begin wheat. Crackers, bread, pasta, "adult" breakfast cereals, rice are now acceptable and make good finger foods. Introduce new grains one at a time. These foods offer B vitamins, iron and energy and are an important part of the diet.	Continue iron-fortified cereal. Offer all breads, cereal, grain products from the family table. Allow self-feeding with hands. These often are preferred foods and eaten in relatively large quantities. This is OK as long as other foods are eaten in adequate amounts.	Continue iron fortified cereal until eighteen months. Should have total of 4 servings daily from the bread and cereal group. Use enriched or whole grain. Read the label. A serving is ¼ slice bread, 1–2 tablespoons cereal product such as rice and noodles. Many children eat more from this group. This is O.K.
FRUITS AND VEGETABLES (INCLUDING JUICE)	**NONE** Infant on evaporated milk formula may have 3 oz. orange juice as a Vitamin C source. However, some babies may be allergic to orange juice.	**NONE**	Begin introducing, one at a time, foods from this group as vitamin A and C sources. Fork mashed or milled table food is appropriate. Babies like fruit juice, but too much can replace other foods. Feed it from a cup to help you limit it to around 3 ounces. Use fresh, frozen, or infant pack fruits, juices and vegetables. Serve baby's unsugared and unsalted. One tablespoon is an adequate serving but more is O.K.	Finger foods from table. Make transition to pieces of cooked fruits and vegetables from the family table; still limit added sugar and salt. Allow self-feeding with hands. One tablespoon still adequate serving, more is O.K. Powdered and canned fruit drinks are not substitutes for fruit juices.	Table food diet to allow 4 servings per day, including juice. A serving at this age is 1–2 tablespoons, 3 oz. juice. Continue to limit juices. Include one vitamin C source daily. One good vitamin A source 3 times per week.
PROTEIN SOURCES (MEAT, FISH, POULTRY, LEGUMES, CHEESE, EGGS & PEANUT BUTTER)	**NONE**	**NONE** **Egg yolk is a poor source of iron: postpone until child may eat the whole egg.**	**NONE**	Begin gradually, as part of a mixed table food diet. Milled or finely cut meat. Casseroles, ground beef, eggs, fish, peanut butter, cooked dried beans, cheese, are all appropriate. Use cheese moderately as it offers similar nutrients to milk.	Two servings per day to provide a total of one ounce of meat or equivalent. Processed meats, (bacon, luncheon meats and hot dogs) are high in nitrate and salt. Limit to 2 to 3 times weekly.

*Times overlap as each infant progresses at his/her own rate. Generally it takes 4 to 6 weeks from beginning one food group to the next. Duration of breastfeeding varies greatly (depends on parents and baby). Serving sizes are minimums for nutritional adequacy. Many children eat more.
Source: Ellyn Satter, R.D., MSSW, Clinical Dietitian and Virginia Dykstal, R.N. certified nurse practitioner, "Feeding Your Infant and Toddler," Jackson Clinic, Madison, WI, Feb., 1983. Copyright 1983.

An iron-fortified commercially prepared formula is a complete food for infants and requires no supplements of vitamins or minerals. . . .

Evaporated milk formulas, used mainly because of economic considerations, represent an acceptable feeding for the infant less than 6 months of age. . . .

An infant fed an evaporated milk formula should receive supplements of vitamin C and iron. . . .

FEEDING AFTER AGE SIX MONTHS

Breast-feeding

It is reasonable to offer other foods beginning at 5 or 6 months of age. An iron-fortified cereal commercially prepared for infants should be introduced first. It is then no longer necessary to administer the iron supplement given previously. Vitamin D supplementation should be continued. Fluoride supplements should be provided in accordance with the fluoride content of the local water supply.

Bottle Feeding

As with the breast-fed infant, it is reasonable to introduce beikost to the bottle-fed infant at 5 to 6 months of age. By 7 months of age it seems reasonable to limit the quantity of milk or formula to approximately 900 ml (30 oz) daily.[18]

Tables prepared by Ellen Satter, clinical dietitian, and Virginia Dykstal, certified pediatric nurse practitioner, for the use of parents summarize how food appropriately offered can provide for both the nutritional and developmental needs of the infant.[19] Table 28-3 lists signals the infant will give when he is ready for advancing in eating style. Table 28-4 explains food selection in greater detail than in the first table. More detailed information is available in Ellyn Satter, *Child of Mine—Feeding with Love and Good Sense,* Palo Alto, CA, Bull Publishing, 1983.

REFERENCES AND SUGGESTED READINGS

American Academy of Pediatrics, Committee on Nutrition, Vitamin and mineral supplement needs in normal children in the United States, *Pediatrics,* 66:1015–20, (Dec.) 1980.

———Committee on Nutrition, Fluoride supplementation: Revised dosage schedule, *Pediatrics,* 63:150–52, (Jan.) 1979.

American Academy of Pediatrics, Committee on Nutrition, Nutritional needs of low-birth-weight infants, *Pediatrics,* 60:519–30, (Oct.) 1977.

———Commentary on breast feeding and infant formulas, including proposed standards for formulas, *Pediatrics,* 57:278–85, (Feb.) 1976.

———Committee on Nutrition, Iron supplementation for infants, *Pediatrics,* 58:765–68, (Nov.) 1976.

Avery, Gordon B. (ed.), *Neonatology,* 2nd ed., Lippincott, Philadelphia, 1981.

Beer, Alan E., and Billingham, Rupert E., Immunology and the breast, *Perinatology-Neonatology,* 5:13–18, (Jan./Feb.) 1981.

Foman, Samuel J., *et al.,* Recommendations for feeding normal infants. *Pediatrics,* 63:52–59, (Jan.) 1979.

Grams, Kathryn; Doucette, Joan Sheridan; Grassley, Jane; Davis, Kristine; Henderson, Kathryn J.; and Newton, Laura D., Special section on breast-feeding, *MCN,* 3:340–57, (Nov./Dec.) 1978.

Gulick, Elsie E., Informational correlates of successful breast feeding, *MCN,* 7:370–75, (Nov./Dec.) 1982.

Hambraeus, Leif, Proprietary milk versus human breast milk in infant feeding. *Pediatr. Clin. North Am.,* 24:17–36, (Feb.) 1977.

Harris, Stephanie G., and Highland, Joseph H., *Birthright Denied: The Risks and Benefits of Breast-Feeding,* Environmental Defense Fund, Washington, D.C., 1977.

Jelliffe, Derrick B., and Jelliffe, E. F. Patrice, "Breast is Best": Modern Meaning. *N. Engl. J. Med.,* 297:912–15, (Oct. 27) 1977.

Johnson, Nancy Winters, Breastfeeding at one hour of age, *MCN,* 1:12–16, (Jan./Feb.) 1976.

Kemberling, Sidney R., Supporting breast-feeding, *Pediatrics,* 63:60–63, (Jan.) 1979.

LaLeche League International, *The Womanly Art of Breast Feeding,* 3rd ed., LaLeche League International, Franklin Park, Ill., 1981.

Lawrence, Ruth A., *Breast Feeding: A Guide for the Medical Profession,* C. V. Mosby, St. Louis, 1980.

Milgrom, Henry; Sharp, Elizabeth S.; and Palmer, E. L., Colostrum and breast milk. Immune protection from Enteroviruses, *Perinatal Press,* 2:63–64, (May) 1978.

Pittard, William B., Breast milk immunology: A frontier in infant nutrition, *Am. J. Dis. Child.,* 133:83–87, (Jan.) 1979.

Riddick, Daniel H., All about the human breast, *Contemp. Ob/Gyn.,* 19:101–24, (Feb.) 1982.

Riordan, Jan, *A Practical Guide to Breast Feeding,* C. V. Mosby, St. Louis, 1983.

Riordan, Jan, and Countryman, Betty Ann, The anatomy and psychophysiology of lactation. Part II of a series on Basics of Breastfeeding, *JOGN Nurs.,* 9:210–13, (July/Aug.) 1980. Other articles in this series published in *JOGN Nurs.,* 9:273–83 and 9:357–66.

Satter, Ellyn, *Child of Mine. Feeding with Love and Good Sense,* Bull Publishing Co., Palo Alto, CA, 1983, Chapters 3, 5, 6 and 7.

Schlegel, Ann M. Observations on breast-feeding technique: Facts and fallacies, *MCN,* 8:204–208, (May/June) 1983.

Tibbetts, Edith, and Cadwell, Karin, Selecting the right breast pump, *MCN,* 5:262–64, (July/Aug.) 1980.

Vaughan, Victor C.; McKay, R. James; and Behrman, Richard E., *Nelson Textbook of Pediatrics,* 11th ed., W. B. Saunders, Philadelphia, 1979, pp. 190–207.

Wicklund, Sally, Special report. Drugs for two in lactation, *Am. J. Nurs.,* 82:1428–30, (Sept.) 1982.

Yu, V. Y. H., Effect of body position on gastric emptying in the neonate, *Arch. Dis. Child.,* 50:500–504, (July) 1975.

[18] Samuel J. Foman, Lloyd J. Filer, Jr., Thomas A. Anderson, and Ekhard E. Ziegler, Recommendations for feeding normal infants. *Pediatrics* 63:52–59 (Jan.) 1979.

[19] Ellyn Satter, R.D., MSSW, Clinical Dietitian and Virginia Dykstal, R.N., certified pediatric nurse practitioner, "Feeding Your Infant and Toddler," Jackson Clinic, Madison, WI, Feb. 1983. Copyright 1983.

CHAPTER

29

High-Risk Newborn Infants—Characteristics and Nursing Management

HIGH-RISK NEWBORNS are infants who need even more intense care in the first hours after birth than that described for the normal-term newborn and who most likely will need intense care for a much longer period of time. Predisposing factors that are likely to place the newborn into a high-risk category are conditions that exist within the infant at birth, such as immaturity and/or abnormal development or disease, and maternal and environmental conditions that have not permitted optimum fetal development or that make adjustment to extrauterine life difficult.

This chapter will deal with identification and care of infants who are born preterm (prematurely), infants of full-term gestation who are underweight, infants who are large for their gestational age, and infants who are born postterm. Certain illnesses and other abnormalities of newborns, which make them high risk, will be described in Chapter 30.

Accurate assessment of gestational age is necessary to distinguish true premature infants from full-term, low-birthweight infants, and to differentiate full-sized infants born prematurely from full-sized term babies. Methods of gestational age assessment have been described in Chapter 27, pages 540–46.

In order to plan appropriate care for a newborn, it is important to classify each infant by gestational age as being preterm, term, or postterm and also by weight as being appropriate-for-gestational age (AGA), small-for-gestational age (SGA), or large-for-gestational age (LGA). Looking at Figure 29-1, which has been adapted from Figure 26-3, page 510, it is apparent that an infant may be placed into one of nine groups of infants. He may be at term and appropriate for gestational age, or he may be at term and large-for-gestational age or small-for-gestational age. If the infant is preterm, he also will be classified as appropriate-for-, small-for-, or large-for-gestational age. The same three classifications for size also apply to the postterm infant.

A classification according to gestational age and birthweight, therefore, identifies infants at risk. The increased risk of morbidity and the type of morbidity are suggested by the group into which the infant falls. The neonatal mortality rate for these groups can be seen in Figure 26-3, page 510. It is apparent that an infant may

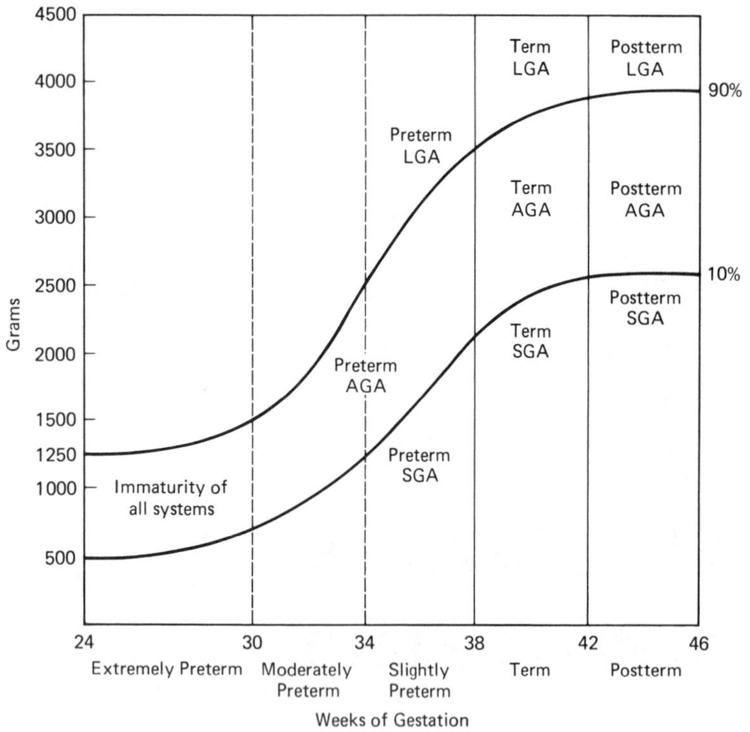

Figure 29–1. Classification of newborns by gestational age and by birth weight according to Figure 26–3, which was reproduced from Frederick C. Battaglia and Lulu O. Lubchenco, A practical classification of newborn infants by weight and gestational age *J. Pediatr.*, 71:159–63 (Aug.) 1967. This illustration identifies the nine groups of infants discussed in the text and also identifies degrees of prematurity of preterm infants. Problems common to the different groups of infants are listed in Table 29–1.

be small because he is preterm and, in addition to that, small-for-gestational age. Such a situation would put the infant at risk for both prematurity and poor intrauterine growth. Term and postterm infants may be identified in the same way. Birthweight and gestational age are the two parameters that can be used very effectively to identify the infant at risk. (See Fig. 29–1).

Term infants with a weight appropriate for gestational age are in the optimum range for both birthweight and gestational age. Given appropriate care, they should have the least number of problems, unless they have complications of such a nature as congenital anomalies or infection. The term infant, according to both the mother's dates and the clinical estimates, who has an appropriate intrauterine growth for gestational age, who is born to a mother without complications, and who does not have intrauterine anomaly or disease is considered a *low-risk infant.* Infants who fall into any of the other eight classifications require observation for problems specific to that category (Table 29–1).

Infants who are within the limits of appropriate weight but are close to the tenth percentile or the ninetieth percentile may have some of the problems of infants in the tenth or the ninetieth percentile groups. These infants are in the appropriate weight category, but they border on the risk category.

Infants who are appropriate for gestational age but are preterm or postterm will not have problems because of inappropriate weight, but they will have the special problems of immature infants and postterm infants.

Small-for-gestational-age infants are at special high risk. They may be preterm, term, or postterm. For some reasons, these infants have not developed appropriately *in utero* and they are growth-retarded. If the small-for-gestational-age infant is also preterm, the baby has the problems of both immaturity and inappropriate intrauterine growth.

When a small infant, under 2500 gm, is born, it is very important to identify the infant correctly, because the problems of the preterm infant are not the same as those of the infant who may be small because he is growth-retarded. For example, the preterm infant is susceptible to hyaline membrane disease because of immaturity of the lungs, whereas the SGA infant is likely to have mature lungs, especially if he is at term, but is susceptible to lung problems from birth asphyxia and aspiration pneumonia. The preterm infant may have nutritional problems because of immaturity of suck and swallow and of the gastrointestinal tract, while the SGA infant may be mature enough to take food and fluids well but have problems with hypoglycemia because of inadequate nutritional stores laid down *in utero.*

Large-for-gestational-age infants also may be term, preterm, or postterm. Frequently, the LGA infant has a diabetic mother. If the infant is preterm, he is predisposed to the problems of immaturity such as respiratory distress, jaundice, and bleeding, as well as the metabolic problems associated with the mother's diabetes. It is very important to the infant's care that he be recognized as a preterm infant so that his large size will not be

Table 29–1. Common Problems of Several Different Groups of Infants at Risk Because of Variations in Their Gestational Ages and Birthweights*

Preterm			*Term*	*Postterm*	*All Ages*
Extremely Preterm	*Moderately Preterm*	*Slightly Preterm*	*SGA*	*SGA, AGA, LGA*	*LGA*
Immaturity of all systems	Birth asphyxia Hyaline membrane disease Apneic spells Susceptible to retrolental fibroplasia Susceptible to body heat loss Feeding problems Jaundice Infection Necrotizing enterocolitis Patent ductus arteriosus	Temperature instability Slow to feed Slow to gain Prone to jaundice	Fetal distress Birth asphyxia and aspiration Meconium aspiration Hypoglycemia Cold stress Polycythemia	Postmaturity syndrome Fetal distress Birth asphyxia Meconium aspiration Hypoglycemia Cold stress Polycythemia Persistent fetal circulation	Hypoglycemia Polycythemia Trauma owing to mechanical problems at delivery RDS if preterm

* The importance of determining the proper classification of each infant at birth is apparent from the different problems that should be anticipated. It can be seen that even if a term, small-for-gestational-age infant and a preterm infant were of the same birthweight, they could have a list of very different management problems.

misleading and that he will receive care appropriate to the immaturity. This kind of infant often looks big enough to be treated as a term newborn unless he is identified as preterm through careful gestational age assessment.

Each category of infants has its own specific high-risk problems. Knowing how a newborn is classified helps caretakers to anticipate problems and prepare to treat them. (See Table 29–1). Good anticipatory care helps to reduce considerably the complications of the postnatal period and also the long-term complications.

The several different classifications of infants that have been described briefly above will now be discussed in greater detail.

THE PRETERM (PREMATURE) INFANT

The terms *preterm* and *premature* will be used interchangeably in this chapter. The term *low-birthweight* also is often used in speaking of a preterm infant, but since a low-birthweight classification includes both preterm and term babies under 2500 gm, it does not appear to identify the preterm infant specifically.

The preterm infant has a number of special problems because of the immaturity of his body systems, but the magnitude of these problems will depend to a considerable extent upon the degree of the infant's prematurity. Neonatal mortality rises progressively with increasing degree of immaturity.

In addition to identifying an infant as preterm, the degree of maturity also must be established. This can be done quite precisely by determining the infant's estimated weeks of gestation and using gestational age to identify the infant rather than the broad overall preterm categorization. For example, saying that "an infant is of 32 weeks' gestation" gives everyone involved in the infant's care an idea of his developmental stage and a basis for beginning to plan his care.

Degrees of Prematurity

Since different degrees of prematurity present different problems, preterm infants have been divided into three groups called extremely premature, moderately premature, and borderline premature.

Both Usher and Lubchenco consider infants born at less than 30 weeks' gestation as belonging in a group called *extremely premature* or *preterm*[1,2] These infants are at the borderline of viability and require sophisticated management to improve their chances of survival. Infants at these early gestational ages are likely to have a large number of complex interrelated problems. When at all possible, infants of less than 30 weeks' gestational age should be delivered in a hospital equipped to give intensive care from the moment of birth. These infants need

[1] Robert H. Usher, The special problems of the premature infant, in *Neonatology, 2nd* ed., edited by Gordon B. Avery, Lippincott, Philadelphia, 1981, pp. 230–61.

[2] Lula O. Lubchenco, The high risk infant, *Major Probl. Clin. Pediatr.*, 14:143, 1976.

optimum support to give them the best chance possible to survive with good physical and neurologic function and to prevent impairment of function through CNS damage. Within recent years the chances of survival for infants of 28 to 30 weeks' gestation have become reasonably good; for infants of 24 to 27 weeks, the outlook is improving but is still very poor.

The *moderately premature* infant is defined by Usher as one of 31 to 36 weeks' gestation.[3] Lubchenco defines the *moderately preterm infant* as one born between 30 to 34 weeks.[4] These infants have a number of physiologic handicaps and require the same care as the extremely premature infant, but their chances of survival are good. There is definitely an advantage for these infants to be born in a hospital that can provide intensive care from the beginning because optimum care must be intense and early.

The *borderline premature* is defined by Usher as an infant of 37 to 38 weeks' gestation.[5] Lubchenco defines the *slightly preterm infant* as one of gestational age from 34 to 38 weeks.[6]

The slightly preterm infant often looks like, and acts like, a full-term infant. These newborns have characteristics of both preterm and term infants. One half of these infants weigh over 2500 gm at birth. Although these infants progress reasonably well and neonatal mortality is low, it is important to recognize them as preterm and give them the care they need for their physiologic handicaps. Slightly preterm infants may need close attention to their environmental temperature, they may be slower to feed adequately at breast or bottle, they may be slower to gain weight, and they may be more prone to jaundice than full-term infants. Borderline prematures may not need the care of an intensive care nursery, but they need special observation and care if they are cared for in a low-risk nursery.

Causes and Prevention of Preterm Birth

Adequate antepartum care, started early and continued throughout pregnancy, is an important factor in prevention of preterm births. With good antepartum care, the mother is kept in the best possible health, and abnormal conditions are detected and treated as soon as they arise. This will help bring the mother and fetus to the end of pregnancy in the best possible condition.

Premature labor occurs without known cause in a fairly large number of cases. In others, such as multiple pregnancy, premature rupture of the membranes, placenta previa, and hydramnios, preventive measures against the cause are not known. Hospitalization of the mother, however, increases the infant's chance of survival, and with premature labor it may be possible to stop the labor long enough to give additional time for maturation of the infant's lungs. Delay of labor and enhancement of lung maturation are described on pages 247 and 272.

Conditions in which prevention of premature birth may be possible by early diagnosis and adequate treatment include the toxemias of pregnancy, syphilis, chronic diseases such as diabetes and cardiovascular-renal disease, incompetent cervical os, urinary tract infection, acute infectious diseases, and genital tract abnormalities. Syphilis is not the important cause of premature delivery that it was in the past because of earlier prenatal care and more effective treatment of the disease. Some premature births caused by genital tract abnormalities may be prevented by preconceptional examination and treatment. Certain fetal abnormalities, another factor in premature deliveries, may be prevented by advising the mother to avoid exposure to virus infections and drugs.

Premature induction of labor is sometimes necessary because of maternal complications, but it is performed as late as the mother's health and/or the fetal environment will permit in order to give the infant the longest possible intrauterine existence. In some of these cases pregnancy can be prolonged by hospitalization of the patient, which may improve the disease or slow its progress. However, recognition of the possibility of an adverse intrauterine environment for the fetus must be considered, and premature delivery may be in the best interests of the infant. Assessment of the fetal environment and fetal well-being is described on pages 245–56.

Incidence and Cause of Deaths

The incidence of premature births varies widely, ranging from 4 to 12 percent of the total births in different countries; in the United States the incidence is approximately 8 percent of all live births. Although the mortality rate of infants has decreased during the past 25 years, especially since the establishment of neonatal intensive care units, prematurity is still the leading cause of infant deaths. Most deaths of immature infants occur during the first month of life, with the first day being the most critical period. Approximately two thirds of all infant deaths in the first month of life are related to immaturity. Many deaths are caused by respiratory distress.

The mortality rate of premature infants is inversely proportional to gestational age and birthweight. Infants born prior to 28 weeks' gestation have a neonatal mortality rate that may be 50 percent or more. Thereafter the mortality rate decreases considerably as gestational age increases, especially if the infant has developed appropriately up to the time of birth. Postneonatal sequelae, especially of neurologic disorders, although still

[3] Usher, *op. cit.*

[4] Lubchenco, *op. cit.*, p. 145.

[5] Usher, *op. cit.*

[6] Lubchenco, *op. cit.*, p. 146.

showing a relatively high incidence, have diminished considerably since the advent of intensive care centers.

Effectiveness of premature care should be gauged by a reduction of sequelae in later life as well as by decreasing neonatal mortality rates. Reduction of sequelae is much more difficult to measure, but recent reports do indicate that about 90 percent of infants who were under 1500 gm (3 lb, 5 oz) at birth and survived are mentally and neurologically intact on follow-up examinations.[7]

Characteristics at Birth

Characteristics of the preterm infant will depend upon weeks of gestation at birth. They will range from a great deal of immaturity to characteristics similar in many respects to the full-term newborn. It can be anticipated when the infant is born preterm that he will have immaturity of all systems—pulmonary, cardiovascular, gastrointestinal, and renal—and that the infant will have problems with temperature control, with metabolic adjustments, and with jaundice. A number of the problems created by the infant's immaturity may be interrelated, and all require that the baby be given specialized care.

Development of the lungs and particularly of adequate production of surfactant is the major factor influencing a preterm infant's survival after birth. Without adequate and ongoing production of surfactant, the infant will develop respiratory distress syndrome, a common cause of severe illness and death of the preterm infant.

Since adequate respiratory function is absolutely essential to the infant's survival, the amount of surfactant produced by the fetal lung must be checked prior to a preterm delivery whenever time permits. This should make it possible either to provide intensive care to the mother to prolong her pregnancy and allow fetal lung maturation, or to facilitate lung maturation through administration of steroids to the mother. When time does not permit enhancement of further lung maturation, preparation must immediately be made for intensive care of the infant after birth.

Although lung maturation is vital to extrauterine survival, maturation of other systems is also of great importance. Unless the intrauterine environment is hostile, the longer the infant remains *in utero,* the greater his chances of survival. In some infants surfactant production in the lungs is adequate relatively early, at 35 weeks or less, but other systems may not mature at the same rapid rate. A mature L/S ratio does not mean a mature infant. If lung maturation is the only consideration prior to delivery, the infant may have a number of problems of other body systems because of their immaturity. It is important, therefore, to consider overall development of the infant whenever possible prior to a decision for a preterm delivery.

Externally the preterm infant appears thin and scrawny. The infant's weight is usually under 2500 gm (5 lb, 8 oz), the length is often under 47 cm (18½ in.), and the head circumference is frequently under 33 cm. Infants of 24 to 30 weeks' gestation usually weigh between 500 and 1500 gm (1 lb, 2 oz and 3 lb, 5 oz). Moderately preterm infants, of 31 to 36 weeks' gestational age, range in weight from 1500 gm for the smallest of these infants to over 2500 gm (5 lb, 8 oz), for the largest. Infants between 37 and 38 weeks' gestation weigh between 2500 and 3250 gm (5 lb, 8 oz and 7 lb, 3 oz). (See Figure 29-2*A*, *B*.)

The preterm head is usually round and it is relatively large. Growth of the head is rapid in fetal life compared with growth of the rest of the body, especially in the earlier months, and the head therefore is large in relation

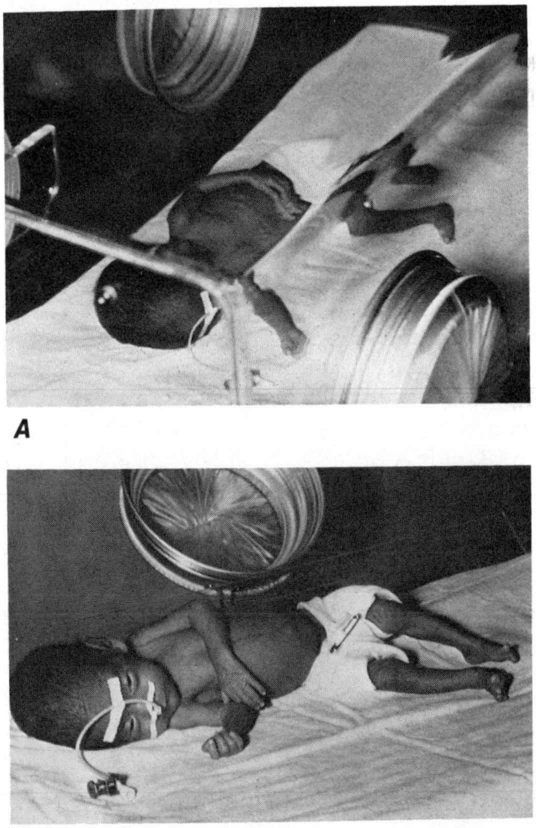

A

B

Figure 29-2. *A*. A premature infant, 23 days old, weighing 850 gm (1 lb 12 oz). Note the paucity of subcutaneous fat. (Distortions in the picture are a result of the curving glass of the incubator. It was considered unwise to open the incubator for the purpose of photography.) *B*. The same premature baby 3 weeks later. Note the large head as compared with the rest of the body. Blood vessels are visible through the thin skin of the abdomen. A polyethylene tube is in place for feedings.

[7] G. Rawlings, A. Stewart, E. Reynolds, *et al.*, Changing prognosis for infants of very low birth weight, *Lancet,* i:516, 1971.

to the body when the infant is born. There is a relatively large disproportion between the circumferences of the head and the thorax in the premature infant; that of the head usually being more than 3 cm greater than the chest circumference. The younger the infant, the greater the disproportion between head and chest size.

The preterm infant's neck and extremities are short, and his trunk is broad and long. The eyes are prominent, and the tongue is large. The ears are soft and flabby and hug the scalp. The thoracic cage is less rigid than that of the full-term infant; the abdomen is round and full, and hernias are common. The mammary glands are small, do not become engorged, and do not secrete milk. The genitalia are small.

The thin skin, through which the blood vessels can be seen readily is delicate, loose, and wrinkled, and has prominent lanugo hair. Increased jaundice is common; it appears earlier, is more severe, and lasts longer than in the full-term infant. Fingernails and toenails are soft but, contrary to popular belief, extend to the ends of the digits. Very little subcutaneous fat is present; this is true even when the infant is born close to the full gestation period, because fat is deposited rapidly in the last month of intrauterine life (Fig. 29-3). Body temperature is subnormal and may be markedly unstable.

There is a greater tendency toward respiratory distress in the preterm than in the full-term infant; this may be manifested by rapid respirations, dyspnea, attacks of cyanosis, and periods of apnea. There is a tendency to snuffles owing to mucus in the nose and large adenoids, which fill the nasopharynx.

The cardiovascular system may take hours or days to adjust to extrauterine life. The infant is susceptible to hypovolemia and hypotension. Perfusion of tissues and organs may be poor.

The infant may be inactive, and his cry is often feeble, whiny, and monotonous. Gagging, swallowing, and sucking reflexes are weak or absent. The infant has a lowered tolerance of the alimentary tract with a tendency to vomiting and diarrhea; abdominal distention is more common than in the full-term infant. The stools tend to be infrequent due to hypomotility of the intestinal tract; they are sometimes loose and frequent owing to lowered food tolerance, but may be so infrequent that they dry out and the infant becomes constipated. The preterm infant loses a larger amount of weight relatively than does the full-term infant, and he does not regain it as quickly as the normal infant.

Impairment of renal function and a poor water and acid-base metabolism may cause edema or dehydration, and acidosis. A heightened capillary fragility increases the tendency to hemorrhage, and defective hematopoiesis causes anemia.

Hepatic immaturity with bilirubinemia, hypoglycemia, coagulation defects, and hypoproteinemia is common in the early days of life. Interruption of pregnancy results in curtailment of placental transmission of minerals and vitamins and immune substances and thus may be the cause of rickets, anemia, and/or infection. Congenital malformations are believed to be more common in the premature infant.

When birth occurs before organs are well developed, it is not surprising that the mortality rate is high, and it is quite apparent that the premature infant requires expert medical and nursing care from the moment of birth.

Medical and Nursing Care

The delivery room and nursery should be ready at all times for emergency care for a newborn, with equipment for resuscitation and conservation of body heat, but when a woman is known to be in premature labor, it is possible to make additional plans and thereby avoid loss of time in instituting prompt treatment.

The pediatrician and the nursery staff should be notified of the impending birth so that they can begin

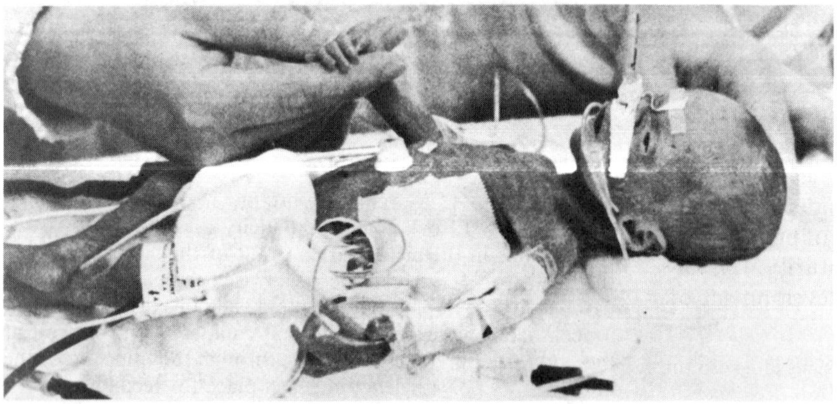

Figure 29-3. This infant was born at 24 weeks gestation, with a weight of 1 lb, 5 oz. (600 gm), and a length of 12 inches (30.5 cm). Her weight dropped down to 1 lb, 1 oz. (480 gm) before she started gaining. This life-size look at this infant, who is 18 days old on this picture, shows how tiny she really was. The mother's hands are in the picture and show how small the baby's head and hands are in comparison to the mother's hands. (Photograph courtesy of Carmen Hoxie and her parents and of Mr. L. Roger Turner, photographer, Wisconsin State Journal, Madison, Wisconsin.) See Figure 29-12 showing how the baby has grown and developed, making it possible for the parents to hold her.

preparations for the infant's care. Preparation should be made to reduce to a minimum the amount of time required to place the infant in an ideal environment. Plans can be made for extra personnel in the delivery room to give special attention to the newborn. This infant may need the undivided attention of a physician and a nurse in the delivery room and constant observation after he is moved to the nursery.

Care of the preterm infant will be described under broad headings covering common problems of the various systems, instead of as a progressive day-by-day observation and plan of care. Although the infant has several simultaneous immediate (and also more long-term) needs of the respiratory system, the cardiovascular system, and other systems, as well as thermal requirements, each system will be described in its immediate and also more long-term adjustments before another system is discussed.

Respiratory System

Asphyxia at Birth

Asphyxia at birth is commonly present in preterm infants. The more preterm the infant, the greater the chance of asphyxia. The immature respiratory center is the underlying cause of asphyxia, but causes of the premature delivery, such as antepartum bleeding, or complications of the delivery, such as breech presentation, also may contribute to difficulty in onset of breathing.

The principles of resuscitation, described on pages 410–19, apply to the preterm as well as the term infant. It is particularly important to anticipate impending asphyxia and to have personnel skilled in resuscitation present at a premature delivery. Trauma should be avoided by using the simplest measures first in resuscitation. Bag-and-mask resuscitation is often adequate to establish respirations, but endotracheal intubation may be necessary, especially with the extremely premature infant. Special care to provide adequate warmth during resuscitation is especially important for the preterm infant.

Periodic Breathing

Periodic breathing is a pattern of breathing in which there are periods of apnea of 5 to 10 seconds followed by periods of ventilation of 10 to 15 seconds at a rate of 50 to 60 per minute. The overall respiratory rate is 30 to 40 per minute. With such an irregular respiratory pattern, it is necessary to count the respirations for at least one full minute to obtain an overall rate and in some cases it is advisable to count for two minutes and divide by two. There is no change in heart rate or color during the period of apnea in periodic breathing, in contrast to the apneic episodes described below.

Periodic breathing occurs in up to 50 percent of preterm infants, depending upon the degree of immaturity. The more immature the infant, the more frequent the periodic breathing. After 36 weeks' gestation periodic breathing is much less frequent,[8] although it also may be present in full-term infants.

Apnea

Apnea usually is defined as a period of respiratory arrest of more than 20 seconds' duration and/or an arrest accompanied by bradycardia and cyanosis. Apneic spells should be distinguished from periodic breathing. Preterm infants are especially prone to apnea. With sustained monitoring, apneic spells can be detected in almost every newborn of less than 37 weeks' gestation, particularly those with birthweight of less than 1.25 kg.[9] With a conceptual age of more than 36 weeks, the frequency and severity of apneic spells decrease considerably.

Apneic spells do not occur during the first day after birth, but thereafter they are likely to increase during the first postnatal week. In very immature infants, the spells of apnea may occur for several weeks. Apneic spells may be accompanied by bradycardia and poor muscle tone, but not necessarily. Bradycardia and flaccidity are more likely when apnea is prolonged, but bradycardia also may occur from the beginning. Bradycardia also occurs without apnea.

Most apneic spells in preterm infants occur because of neuronal immaturity of the central respiratory control mechanisms. Apneic spells may present along with pressing or stretching such as occurs during or after feeding, particularly if the infant aspirated, during bowel movements, with lung disorders, and probably some other activities. Any adverse condition may interfere with the rhythmic breathing of the preterm infant, including hypoxia, hypoglycemia, hyperbilirubinemia, hypocalcemia, and others. Since adverse conditions can be heralded by apneic spells, they should be ruled out when apnea first appears.

The infant susceptible to apnea must be monitored for respiratory and/or heart rates with monitors that include an apnea alarm, so that apneic spells can be terminated. The time set for the alarm must be individualized for each infant according to how soon functional changes such as cyanosis and hypotonia are noted. This time will vary for different infants. Routine monitoring of all preterm infants under 34 weeks or below 2000 gm for 10 to 14 days, and until no apneic episodes have occurred for several days, is considered advisable.

The majority of apneic spells can be successfully terminated by gentle stimulation of the infant by touching,

[8] F. J. Schulte, Apnea, *Clin. Perinatal,* 4:65–76, (Mar.) 1977.

[9] *Ibid.*

rubbing the foot, gently stroking or patting the trunk, or just moving the infant slightly. To avoid opening the incubator frequently, the infant's mattress sometimes can be moved gently for stimulation from the outside. When resuscitative measures are necessary, use of a bag and mask with the same oxygen concentration the infant is receiving or with room air ordinarily is effective. A bag and mask should always be available in the incubator. For severe, prolonged, and repetitive apneic spells, artificial respiration may be considered.

Infants with apnea severe enough to treat are given theophylline. This drug is believed to abolish or reduce apnea by increasing alveolar ventilation through central stimulation.

Home monitoring of infants who have problems with prolonged infantile apnea has recently become available. Home monitoring is a very stressful undertaking for the parents and also very costly. Among the many issues that must be considered in relation to home monitoring is identification of infants who would benefit from such care.

Respiratory Distress Syndrome

Premature infants are especially susceptible to respiratory distress syndrome (hyaline membrane disease). This disease occurs in newborns who do not have an adequate amount of surface-active material for good postnatal pulmonary function. Surfactant may be deficient at birth because of extreme immaturity of the alveolar lining cells or because of diminished or impaired ongoing production.

Respiratory distress syndrome is most likely to develop in the extremely premature and moderately premature infants. Its incidence lessens with increasing maturity, but infants of borderline prematurity may develop the disease and should be observed carefully for signs of respiratory distress during the first 12 hours of life.

The signs and symptoms of hyaline membrane disease and its treatment are described along with other respiratory problems in Chapter 30.

Use of Oxygen

Administration of oxygen is often necessary to preterm infants because of their respiratory problems, but it requires precise control to avoid giving too much oxygen and to prevent the serious consequences of hyperoxia. Preterm infants, especially the more immature ones, are very susceptible to retinal arteriolar vasoconstriction and eye damage, resulting in partial or complete blindness (retrolental fibroplasia), if the Po_2 rises above 80 mm Hg. Use of oxygen and precautions in its administration are described on pages 649–54.

Thermal Regulation

Preterm infants are very susceptible to heat loss and to the effects of cooling. An infant has a large area from which to lose heat, since he has a large surface area in relation to body mass. This is even more pronounced in the preterm infant. Also, the thermal insulation of a newborn is low because of a relatively small amount of subcutaneous fat. A preterm infant has a very scant amount of subcutaneous fat and readily conducts heat from his warm inner body to his skin. The preterm infant, with rather poor muscle tone, is also apt to assume a more flaccid and stretched-out posture than a full-term newborn and thus expose much of his body surface to the environment. A preterm infant therefore becomes cooled even more quickly than a full-term infant of normal weight.

Heat production by shivering and muscular activity is difficult for the preterm infant because of his smaller muscles. These newborns also have only a very small supply of glycogen, since much of this is stored during the last six weeks of intrauterine life. They therefore may suffer from lack of sufficient available glucose when need for heat production is high. Also lung function is often poor, reducing available oxygen. With a small glycogen store and deficient oxygen supply, acidosis can develop early. The potential consequences of insufficient warmth are increased morbidity and mortality.

Ways of preventing heat loss immediately after birth have been described on page 412. The ways in which an infant loses body heat, the means by which he produces body heat, the effects of chilling, and the ways of preventing heat loss during daily care also have been described in detail on pages 504–507. The following discussion will highlight some of the important aspects of protection against heat loss in the preterm infant.

Since preterm and other low-birthweight infants must be protected against heat loss, they are cared for in an incubator until they have gained some weight and achieved stability. The incubator makes it possible to regulate the environmental temperature more easily and to take care of most of the infant's needs without removing him from that environment. It also makes it easier to maintain a desired oxygen concentration, and some automatically control circulation of air and regulate humidity as desired. The incubator can serve as an isolation unit. It filters the air coming into it, protecting the infant from the nursery environment and isolating him from others in the nursery. Several types of incubators are available, one of which is shown in Figure 29–4. (See also Figure 29–9 showing an infant being cared for in an incubator.)

It is important to note that an incubator alone does not protect the infant from radiant heat loss from his body. A warm incubator provides a warm air temperature, but does not protect against variations in the en-

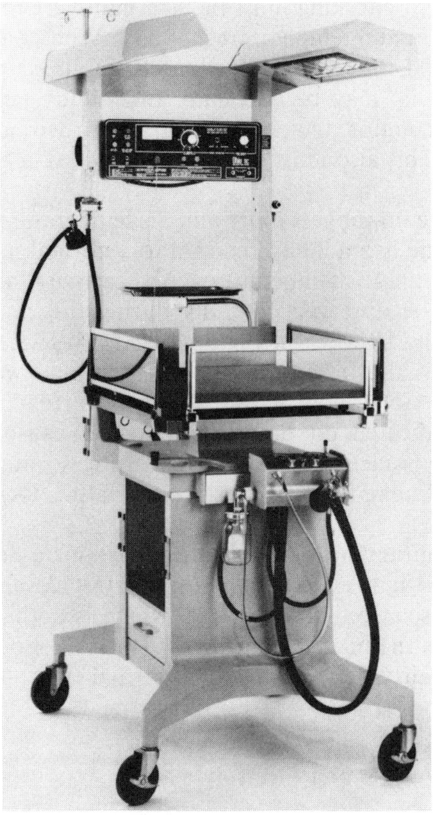

Figure 29-4. An incubator that is called a Neonatal Intensive Care Center. This "open incubator" provides an overhead radiant heater, of major importance in supplying warmth to the infant, and also provides ample space for personnel to work and care for the infant while he remains under the radiant heater. The incubator has equipment for aspiration of secretions and for administration of oxygen at either atmospheric or variable positive pressures. A normally breathing, as well as a distressed baby, will benefit from the protection that the heater of this incubator provides against loss of body heat to the cool environment. See also another kind of incubator in Figure 27-1, page 538. [Photograph courtesy of Ohio Medical Products (Division of Airco, Inc.), Madison, WI.]

vironment outside the incubator. The infant radiates heat from his body to the inside surface of the PLEXIGLAS cover in the incubator. The temperature of the PLEXIGLAS cover is affected not only by the incubator air temperature but also by the room temperature. Thus the temperature of the inside surface of the PLEXIGLAS may be very different from the temperature set on the incubator thermostat, and the radiant heat exchange between the infant and the PLEXIGLAS may be affected considerably by the room temperature. An infant can be protected from such radiant heat loss in several ways—by some control of the temperature outside the incubator, by a radiant heater over the roof of the incubator, by a heat shield, and by clothing.

Care can be taken that the temperature outside the incubator is not unduly cold. Incubators can be placed against inside rather than outside walls of the nursery and away from cold windows or air-conditioning vents. Likewise, it is important to watch that the incubator does not become overheated from sunlight through a window. Infants of full-term have a sweating response, but those below 36 weeks' gestation generally show a limited response, and below 30 weeks' gestation no sweating response. This means that overheating of the small preterm newborn is even more serious than it is in a full-term infant.

A radiant heater placed over the roof of the incubator will provide the infant with heat, keeping him from dissipating his own. A radiant heater is used when the infant is first placed in the incubator, at any time when outside conditions indicate that the infant needs warmth, and when it appears that the infant cannot easily maintain his own body temperature.

A heat shield, a transparent plastic shell, which is made of PLEXIGLAS, can be placed inside the incubator, over the infant, to conserve body heat. This second cover (the first cover is the incubator top or hood) is warmed by the incubator air, which is subject to the incubator's thermostat control, and is not influenced by the room temperature in the same way as the incubator hood or cover. The infant then radiates only to the warm inner plastic wall of the heat shield and not to the incubator walls.

Resistance to loss of body heat is considerably increased when the infant is cared for when clothed rather than naked. Infants often have been cared for in incubators without clothes on because it is easier to observe their color, breathing, and activities. It has been found, however, that the range within which an infant can be expected to maintain a normal body temperature without seriously increasing either heat production or evaporative water loss is very narrow for naked infants, and this range does not increase readily as the infant becomes older.[10] A clothed infant does not dissipate heat as easily as a nude one and thus has a wider range of a neutral thermal environment. This provides a larger latitude of safe environmental temperatures, and the consequences of any change in incubator temperature are not as great. When continuous observation of the infant is not required, it is advisable to put clothes on the infant or at least partially clothe him. Protection of the relatively large surface of an infant's head will reduce loss of body heat somewhat. Note the cap on the infant's head in Figure 29-11.

Often the small infant's incubator temperature is regulated by servo-controlled equipment, whereby the

[10] J. W. Scopes, Thermoregulation in the newborn, in *Neonatology, 2nd* ed., edited by Gordon B. Avery, Lippincott, Philadelphia, 1981, pp. 171-81.

heating device is regulated according to the infant's abdominal skin temperature (page 538). Use of the servo-control device may mask the onset of a febrile state and also the infant's inability to maintain his temperature. It is very important to compare the infant's temperature and the incubator temperature frequently when evaluating the infant.

An alternative to the convection type of incubator is the open-ended radiant warmer infant care table shown in Figure 29-4. These incubator warmers have been widely used for control of body temperature during resuscitation and other immediate care in the delivery room. Recently these radiant warmers more commonly are being used in the nursery for care of sick infants. The servo-controlled radiant warmer provides adequate thermal control, and it has the definite advantage of being open and providing easy accessibility to the infant. The unit is easy to maintain and easy to clean. Since the open warmer uses room air, it does not need a humidity reservoir, as an incubator sometimes does, which can become contaminated easily. There is some likelihood, however, of cross-contamination, and it is easier to forget hand washing while working with an infant on the radiant warmer table.

Studies have shown that there is an increase in insensible water loss in the infant being cared for on the radiant warmer.[11, 12] This could be a potential problem for a sick infant.

The American Academy of Pediatrics reports that radiant heaters in some cases have posed a problem of neonatal hyperthermia. The Academy states that serious overheating can result from mechanical failure of the controls, from dislodgement of the sensor probe attached to the infant's abdomen for monitoring skin temperature and regulation of the heater accordingly, or from manual operation without careful monitoring. Radiant heaters must be used with caution and the adequacy of safety mechanisms should be evaluated carefully.[13]

Radiant warmers have been used mostly for the care of very sick infants. When the infant is improving, he usually is moved to a convection-type incubator.

A preterm infant's temperature is checked on admission to the nursery and every 30 minutes until a proper balance between a normal body temperature and the warmth from the incubator has been established. Later the temperature is checked about every four hours. Frequency of checking must be determined by the infant's condition and temperature stability. When the infant is older and the temperature is well stabilized, a reading twice daily may be adequate. Both body temperature and incubator temperature are recorded after each check. This also must be done when the skin thermistor is used.

As the infant gets older and his temperature becomes stable, he is gradually changed to a normal nursery environment. His temperature, color, activity, and weight should be observed carefully during the change. The weight grid shown in Figure 29-5 may give some evidence of the infant's need for additional warmth. If he does not follow the steady upward trend in weight gain indicated on the weight grid, a cause must be sought. Sometimes the infant is using so much of his caloric intake for heat production that he does not gain weight.

The infant may need extra clothing or need to be wrapped in an extra blanket for additional warmth after he is discharged to his home, which is perhaps not as warm as the nursery, but by that time he should be adjusted fairly well to living in a normal environment.

Meeting Fluid and Electrolyte Needs

Fluid and electrolyte needs of any infant, especially when sick and unable to meet his own needs by ordinary oral intake, are an important aspect of clinical care of the newborn. The preterm newborn, who often is limited in the amount of fluid he can take orally, likely to have additional fluid losses, and often ill, is ordinarily in need of parenteral fluid therapy in the first days of life.

The total body water (TBW) ordinarily is divided into two major compartments: intracellular water (ICW) and extracellular water (ECW). Water constitutes a large portion of the body composition. With increasing gestational age the TBW gradually decreases from 94 percent at the third month of fetal life, to 80 percent at 32 weeks' gestation, to 78 percent at full-term gestation. At the same time a characteristic change takes place in the proportion of ECW and ICW. The ECW decreases from 60 percent of body weight at the fifth month of fetal life to about 45 percent at term. The ICW increases from 25 percent in the fifth month of fetal life to approximately 33 percent at full term. Then during the immediate postnatal period the ECW decreases rapidly from the 45 percent at birth to 39 percent at one week of age. This rapid change is the result of several physiologic changes, including an improvement in renal function.[14]

The electrolyte composition of the body fluid of an in-

[11] Kamio Yashiro, Forrest H. Adams, G. C. Emmanouildes, and M. E. Michey, Preliminary studies on the thermal environment of low-birth-weight infants, *J. Pediatr.*, 82:991–94, (June) 1973.

[12] Paul R. William and William Oh, Effects of radiant warmers on insensible water loss in newborn infants, *Am. J. Dis. Child.*, 128:511–14, (Oct.) 1974.

[13] American Academy of Pediatrics, Hyperthermia from malfunctioning radiant heaters, *Pediatrics*, 59, Part 2, *Neonatology Suppl.* 1041, (June) 1977.

[14] William Oh, Fluid and electrolyte management, in *Neonatology, 2nd* ed., edited by Gordon B. Avery. Lippincott, Philadelphia, 1981, pp. 643–60.

fant will depend upon gestational age. Per unit of body weight the preterm infant will have a larger extracellular ion content than the term infant simply because of more ECW. Conversely, the ICW electrolyte content of the preterm infant is lower because of the smaller ICW content. These facts must be kept in mind when electrolyte losses and replacement are considered in parenteral fluid therapy or in oral intake.

In determining fluid loss and replacement it is important to consider factors that affect fluid loss. A considerable amount of solute-free fluid is lost from the body through the skin and the lungs as insensible water loss (IWL). Many factors influence IWL in the infant. Immaturity is a large factor. Low-birthweight infants may have excess fluid losses because of increased water content in the skin, a thinner epidermis, and an increased skin permeability. The large bony surface ratio of the preterm infant in relation to body mass, the lesser amount of subcutaneous tissue, and the large exposed body surface because of the relaxed posture all increase IWL. Inefficient vasomotor control of peripheral vessels also may permit loss. Loss of body fluids will be greater in single-walled incubators than when a heat shield is used. Ambient temperature above the neutral thermal zone, radiant warmers, and bilirubin therapy lights increase water loss. Respiratory distress probably increases loss, but high ambient relative humidity will decrease loss. Activity of the infant, as, for example, with labored breathing, and expenditure of energy in other ways will increase fluid loss.

In calculating maintenance fluid for infants, the above-described insensible water loss must be taken into account. This is especially important when the infant's total fluid intake is by parenteral route instead of being somewhat influenced by the infant's desired intake. A prediction of the water required to replace IWL from the many factors involved cannot be precise, but a range in volume required has been established in some conditions.

Renal function in relation to fluid and electrolyte balance and endocrine control are both somewhat limited, especially when given a large challenge. An infant makes a slow diuretic response to a water load during the first three days of life. After about five days the infant can achieve maximum dilution, but the ability to excrete a water load is still slow. This is even more accentuated in the preterm infant. The urine of preterm infants does not reach the concentration of that of older children upon water deprivation. The low-birthweight infant has been shown to lose relatively large amounts of sodium. Renal water requirement cannot be estimated exactly, but it will depend upon the amount of solute excreted from the body. The amount of solute potentially to be excreted in the urine depends on the protein and electrolyte intake. Enough water to permit a urine flow of 50 to 100 ml per kilogram per day will not unduly stress renal concentration or dilution capacity, with a reasonable range of solute excretion.[15]

A newborn's hydration status may be estimated by several parameters. Body weight should be assessed at least daily, and if the infant is ill or requiring frequent changes in therapy, a record of weight may be necessary every 12 hours. Losses in excess of 10 percent of birthweight in the first three or four postnatal days are excessive.

In assessment of hydration status, tissue turgor also should be noted. This is only a rough estimate because of wide variations in the amount of subcutaneous fat in different infants, but a gross degree of dehydration would be detectable. With considerable dehydration the abdominal skin becomes very loose. Edema, as an early sign of overhydration, is detected easily from tissue turgor, at least in the low-birthweight infant. If dehydration becomes severe the infant may show a sunken fontanel, oliguria, and hypotension.

For fluid and electrolyte therapy it is necessary to estimate the amount of fluids and electrolytes lost and then to calculate fluid and electrolyte needs for daily physiologic maintenance, for replacement of past losses, and for replacement of any current abnormal losses if these are present. Careful monitoring must be done during fluid therapy and adjustments made on the results. A number of parameters requiring careful monitoring and suggested frequency of observations are listed in Table 29-2.

Calculation of fluid deficit for replacement is made on changes in body weight. The difference in weight is considered the fluid deficit. Other fluid loss will need to be estimated from clinical signs.

Estimates of electrolyte losses are made from measurement of serum electrolytes. Using serum sodium value as a criterion, dehydration can be classified as isotonic or isonatremic, when the serum sodium value is within the normal range of 136 to 143 mEq/liter, or it may be hypotonic or hyponatremic dehydration when the serum sodium value is below 130 mEq/liter, or it may be hypertonic or hypernatremic dehydration when the serum sodium value is above 150 mEq/liter. A careful clinical history of fever, diarrhea, vomiting, solute load of formula, and other ways in which fluids and electrolytes become unbalanced is also useful in estimating what kind of dehydration is present.

Calculation of Fluid and Electrolyte Needs[16, 17]

Calculation of fluids and electrolytes for maintenance is done on the basis of insensible water loss and urinary

[15] R. Neil Roy and John C. Sinclair, Hydration of the low-birth-weight baby, *Clin. Perinatol.*, 2:393–417, (Sept.) 1975.

[16] William Oh, Fluid and electrolyte therapy and parenteral nutrition in low birth weight infants, *Clin. Perinatol.*, 9:637–43, (Oct.) 1982.

[17] Harkavey, Kenneth L., Water and electrolyte requirements of the very low-birth-weight infant, *Perinatal Press*, 6:47–50, (Apr.) 1982.

Table 29-2. Information Useful for Preventing Fluid and Electrolyte Imbalance in the VLBW Infant*

Technique	*Frequency of Observation*	*Optimal Value*
Weight change	q 8–12 hr	− 1.5 to − 3.5%/d if < 72 hr old. 10–15% in the first week of life
Vascular volume		
Hematocrit	qd or PRN	Changes consistent with blood loss or gain
Blood pressure	q 1–2 hr	Gestational and postnatal age standards
Skin perfusion	q 1–2 hr	Capillary filling time 3 sec
Time to void	Continuously	95% within first 24 hr if no IV; 1–2 hr with IV
Serum		
Osmolarity	PRN	285–295 mOsm/kg H_2O
Electrolytes	q 8–12 hr	
Urine		
Specific gravity or osmolality	Each void	
Electrolytes	When serum electrolytes approach or exceed normal limits	
pH	Each void	

*Source: Kenneth L. Harkavey, Water end electrolyte requirements of the very low-birth-weight infant, *Perinatal Press,* 6:47–50, (Apr.) 1982.

loss. IWL and urinary loss depend upon energy expenditure, and theoretically fluid estimates for maintenance should be calculated on the basis of energy expended. In the newborn the relationships between energy expenditure and body weight are such that body weight can be used satisfactorily in calculations of fluid requirements. The IWL in the newborn has been established at an average of 30 to 35 ml per kilogram of body weight per 24 hours under normal, standard conditions. This fluid requirement definitely needs to be estimated upward when IWL is increased because of immaturity, high ambient temperature, radiant warmer, and other circumstances that cause excess loss of body fluids.

Water loss in the urine depends on the amount of solutes to be excreted by the kidneys. If 10 percent glucose is used for parenteral fluid and if maintenance electrolytes are added to the parenteral fluid, it is estimated that 45 ml of water per kilogram of body weight per 24 hours would provide for excretion of the solute load by the kidneys without posing a problem to the kidneys in regard to their concentrating ability.

The above calculations are the basis for the recommended amount of 75 to 80 ml of fluid per kilogram of body weight per 24 hours for *maintenance fluid* in the newborn during the first three days of life. The recommendation of 30 to 35 ml/kg/24 hours for IWL and 45 ml/kg/24 hours for urinary water loss adds up to 75 to 80 ml/kg/24 hours.

If the infant has an increased IWL because of one or several of the conditions mentioned above, fluid requirements are increased. Also when an infant is receiving oral formula feedings, the solute load to the kidneys is increased considerably, and the fluid requirement is likewise proportionately increased. This accounts for the higher fluid requirement for maintenance in infants as soon as these additional factors become operative. Fluid requirements are often up to 120 ml or even 150 ml per kilogram of body weight per 24 hours.

Electrolyte requirements for maintenance mainly involve the sodium (Na^+), potassium (K^+), and chloride (Cl^-) elements that are lost in the urine and the stool. Based on balance study data this amount is between 2 and 3 mEq per kilogram of body weight per 24 hours for each of the elements.

If there are concurrent fluid losses due to vomiting or diarrhea or other body fluids, the fluid is collected and measured, or estimated if necessary, and replaced in parenteral fluid. The solutes in the fluid that is lost also must be estimated and replaced.

Intravenous fluids are usually necessary in the first days of life of the preterm infant, especially in the very immature newborn or one who develops respiratory distress. The infant ordinarily is not able to take an adequate amount of fluid orally in the first days of life to meet his needs nor can he meet his caloric needs. Caloric needs exist immediately after birth and nutritional stores are deficient. Glycogen stores are very low in small infants and the need for glucose is urgent. Since fasting and thirsting have adverse effects quickly in a small infant, water and calories should be provided very early. Intravenous fluids are begun within a few hours after birth. Intravenous fluid therapy requires very close monitoring and frequent adjustments. Inappropriate management can easily lead to dehydration of the infant and inadequate caloric intake or it can lead to fluid overload, with a strong possibility that the infant may then develop a patent ductus arteriosus or/and necrotizing enterocolitis.

Fluid administration on the first day usually is given in an amount that will provide the maintenance requirements for IWL and renal loss—75 to 80 ml/kg/24 hours. If there is concern of overhydration, the amount of fluid used may be limited to 60 to 70 ml/kg/24 hours. The fluid administered in subsequent days usually is increased in amount. Fluid administration on subsequent days is guided by intake and output record, body weight, urine specific gravity, and serum electrolytes as described below. It does not appear that an attempt should be made to prevent entirely the normal physiologic weight loss of the first few days, but ignoring the loss could lead to dehydration.

Ten percent glucose usually is used for fluid administration at first. This will provide for some of the infant's glucose and caloric needs. Sodium chloride is added starting on the second day of age at a dose of 3 to 4 mEq/kg/24 hours. Potassium supplementation at 2 to 3 mEq/kg/24 hours is begun after 24 hours of age or after good urine output is established. If 10 percent glucose causes hyperglycemia, it will be necessary to give a lesser concentration. To achieve adequate caloric intake without fluid overload intravenous fat emulsions may be used to supplement the nutritional intake provided by the glucose. This provides additional calories without large amounts of fluid.

The volume of parenteral fluids to be given always should be calculated as to the amount needed by the infant in a 24-hour period. It should be administered at a constant rate over the period of 24 hours so as not to stress the infant with fluctuating amounts which may result in erratic blood glucose levels and dehydration. A constant infusion pump with a volumetric chamber is used in giving the fluids. Fluid needs are always reevaluated every 24 hours on the basis of previous monitoring results. If at some time loss of fluid occurs at an inconsistent rate, a reevaluation of need in 12 hours may be necessary.

The most common infusion site in infants is one of the superficial scalp veins. One of the peripheral veins of the dorsal aspect of either the hand or the foot or a vein in the antecubital fossa also may be used. It is difficult to immobilize the infusion needle in any site other than the scalp, and infiltration is more common. If the infant has an umbilical artery catheter in place for frequent monitoring of blood gases, the infusion may be given through the umbilical artery catheter, but usually only as long as another reason exists for use of an umbilical artery catheter.

Monitoring of the adequacy of parenteral fluid therapy must be done while parenteral fluids are being given. Monitoring includes a record of intake and output, body weight changes, urine specific gravity, serum electrolytes, blood urea nitrogen, and clinical assessment of hydration.

If the amount of fluid administered is inadequate, the urine volume will be reduced, the urinary specific gravity will be increased, and soon there will be a significant weight loss, and thereafter clinical signs of dehydration. If an excessive amount of fluid is being given, the urinary output will be large, and the specific gravity of the urine will be low. Soon fluid retention will lead to edema and weight gain. If overhydration is rapid, pulmonary edema and congestive heart failure can occur.

A good fluid balance is indicated by a stationary weight or an appropriate gain, a urinary specific gravity between 1.008 and 1.012, and no clinical evidence of edema. Weight is taken daily and sometimes twice daily. All urinary output is measured and recorded by weighing the diapers before and after they are applied. A normal range of volume of urine is between 35 and 40 ml/kg/24 hours in the first days and then increasing to between 50 and 100 ml. Urinary specific gravity is checked every 6 to 8 hours. Specific gravity of the urine is an accurate approximation of urinary solute excretion, except when there is significant glycosuria. Then a high specific gravity may reflect the presence of glucose rather than electrolytes. Daily serum electrolyte determinations will give evidence of electrolyte balance. A check of the urine for presence of glucose, and of the blood glucose by DEXTROSTIX, will provide evidence as to how well the infant is tolerating the amount of glucose in the infusion.

Parenteral fluids are continued in the small infant until the baby is able to ingest sufficient food and fluid to meet body needs for maintenance, for replacement of losses, and finally for growth.

Feeding the Preterm Infant

Feeding the preterm infant is made difficult by the lowered tolerance of the alimentary tract; weakness or absence of sucking and swallowing reflexes; relatively high caloric requirement, but a small stomach capacity; poor gag reflexes leading to aspiration; an incompetent esophageal cardiac sphincter; tendency to vomit and to develop abdominal distention; and decreased absorption of some of the essential nutrients. As with other aspects of care, the more immature the infant is, the more difficult the feeding problem.

Meeting the nutritional needs of the low-birthweight

baby very early is important for several reasons. Caloric needs exist immediately after birth. Water normally is lost to the environment by evaporation from the skin and the respiratory passages (IWL), and by excretion in the urine. IWL in the small infant may be very great. Fat and carbohydrate stores are deficient. Glycogen stores are very low in low-birthweight infants. Antenatal storage of substances such as minerals is low. The infant has a need to grow rapidly at this age, and malnutrition at this early neonatal period may inhibit normal central nervous system development.

Nutritional Requirements

The dietary needs of the preterm infant are those that will meet growth requirements for deposition of new tissue and maintenance requirements to replace the daily body losses. The adequacy of growth at present is judged according to increments in weight, length, and head circumference. What constitutes optimum nutrition is not clear, but in general an attempt is made to maintain growth within or above the percentiles at birth. It is expected that, with adequate growth, the infant will have an average weight gain of 30 gm each day after the first week or 10 days of life. A weight growth chart that has proven to be very satisfactory is shown in Figure 29-5. It is apparent from this figure that the extremely preterm infant may not begin weight gain as soon after birth as the larger preterm infant.

In planning feedings for the preterm newborn careful consideration must be given to gestational age as well as weight because the gastrointestinal capacity, metabolic rates, and fuel and water requirements will differ for different gestational ages. The caloric, water, electrolyte, mineral, and vitamin requirements of the preterm infant will depend on the rate of utilization and expenditure of substances, absorption of substances, excretion of substances, and body stores.

CALORIES Caloric requirements are usually met if the infant receives 120 kcal/kg (55kcal/lb) of body weight per day by the end of the first week of postnatal life. This recommended intake should be reached as soon as possible, but it usually takes a week to 10 days to achieve it. If the infant's metabolic rate is increased because of an environmental temperature outside the neutral thermal range, or increased muscular activity, or illness, the caloric requirements for growth increase. Caloric requirements for good growth must be found for the individual infant.

WATER The actual clinical requirements for water vary considerably, depending upon the condition of the infant. Fluid requirements and how such needs are met

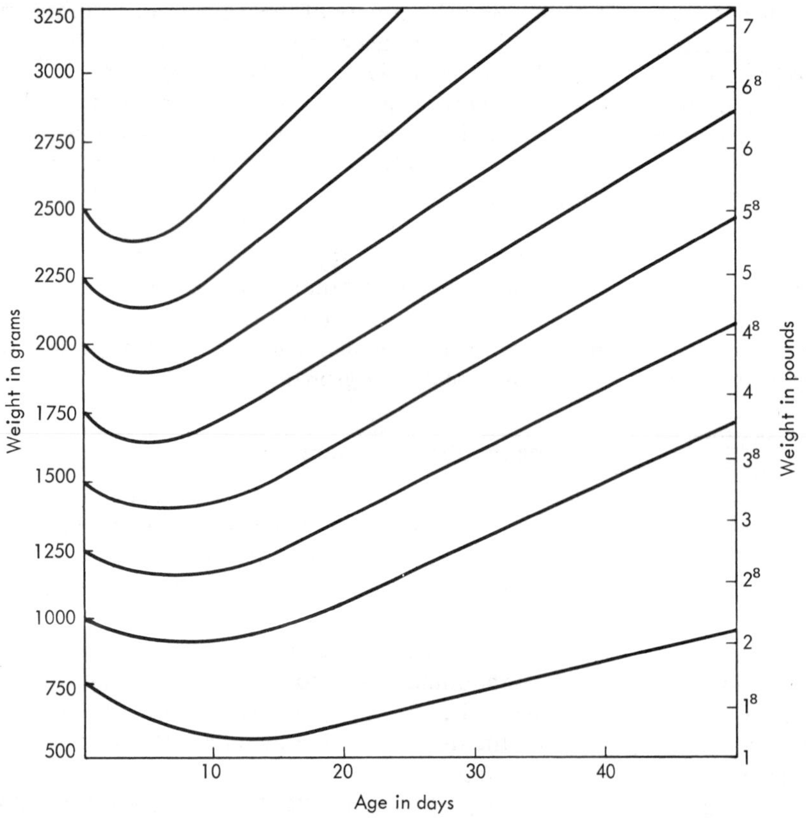

Figure 29-5. Premature weight chart. (Reproduced with permission from Joseph Dancis, John R. O'Connell, and L. Emmett Holt: A grid for recording the weight of premature infants. *J. Pediatr.*, 33:570-572 (Nov.) 1948, p. 571.)

prior to the time the infant is able to take sufficient oral fluids have been described above.

When the infant is able to fulfill his food requirements orally, he ordinarily obtains a sufficient amount of fluid in his formula.

Infants who receive between 120 and 180 ml of water per kilogram of body weight per day after several days, are usually in positive water balance. If the infant takes the necessary caloric intake of 120 kcal per kilogram per day, his fluid intake may be adequate. Some infants may be able to achieve this intake by three or four days after birth. Others, however, do not have the stomach capacity to take such a quantity of fluids orally at first and require intravenous fluids and calories for a number of days.

PROTEIN Protein requirements appear to be greater for preterm infants than the 2.2 gm/kg/day that is adequate for full-term infants. Currently 2.25 to 2.75 gm/kg/day of an appropriate protein is recommended for the preterm infant. Use of most any one of the commercial formulas, especially one prepared for preterm infants, or of human milk will meet this need if the infant can take the recommended amount of fluid and calories. See discussion on protein used in formulas and also on carbohydrate and fat on pages 590–92.

MINERALS In addition to daily requirements, the preterm newborn needs a diet high in calcium and phosphorus because the perinatal storage of many substances normally occurs during the last trimester of pregnancy. The infant born before full term has a low storage of calcium and phosphorus and a considerable need for these minerals because of rapid growth.

VITAMINS The premature infant's need for vitamins is high because of low antenatal storage and the demands made by rapid growth. Information concerning vitamin requirements of the premature is not complete, but prophylactic administration is considered important. The infant may not obtain enough vitamins in his milk, and then the daily requirement is given in the form of supplements.

Of particular importance are vitamins A, D, and C. The fat-soluble vitamins, A and D, may not be absorbed well from formula, especially when polyunsaturated vegetable fat has been used in preparation of the formula. Vitamin D is important for the absorption and use of calcium and phosphorus; it is thus very important early and in adequate amounts for preterm infants, who have a tendency to develop rickets.

Most commercially prepared formulas used for feeding preterm infants contain vitamin supplements, but the supplementation is adequate only when the infant takes about a liter of formula. Since this is quite obviously impossible for the small infant, vitamin supplementation is begun in 5 to 10 days.

Vitamins are given in a water-miscible preparation, which can be mixed with milk or water and given with the feedings. In the small, weak premature there is danger of aspiration if oil is used. TRI-VI-SOL or POLY-VI-SOL, 0.5 ml daily, is usually recommended in addition to the vitamins that the infant will receive from the commercial formula.

Vitamin K_1 is important in prothrombin formation and therefore in blood coagulation. It is administered at birth because the prothrombin value decreases in all infants during the first few days of life, thus increasing the blood clotting time. It is particularly valuable in prematures because of their tendency toward hemorrhage. Vitamin K_1 is administered prophylactically in a dose of 0.5 to 1.0 mg, by intramuscular injection, soon after the infant is born. One dose is usually adequate, except in special circumstances such as evidence of hemorrhage or suspicion of intracranial injury. Vitamin K_1 is administered with caution since excessive dosage may be harmful.

Vitamin E, a fat-soluble vitamin, among other properties, plays a role in hematopoiesis. An increase in the life span of red blood cells and in reticulocyte formation is correlated with the level of serum vitamin E. A deficiency in vitamin E increases red blood cell hemolysis, and a hemolytic anemia, characteristically seen in preterm infants at 6 to 10 weeks of age, has been associated with this deficiency. The infant especially needs supplementation of vitamin E when he is being given parenteral fat emulsion, and also when the infant has respiratory distress syndrome and is trying to overcome a surfactant deficiency.

Vitamin E absorption is poor in a preterm infant of less than 32 weeks' gestation, and its absorption has been shown to be decreased in prematures who also are receiving iron supplementation. The iron interferes with intestinal absorption of vitamin E.

Currently, the recommendation is to give vitamin E, 25 IU daily, and to delay giving supplemental iron until the third month in infants less than 36 weeks' gestation if that seems appropriate. Human milk is a better source of vitamin E than cow's milk.

IRON In anticipation of a late occurring iron-deficiency anemia, the preterm infant is given iron supplementation when the infant has attained vitamin E sufficiency, at about three months of age. Iron supplementation is given at 2 mg/kg/day beginning at two months or earlier during the first year either as medicinal iron in the form of FER-IN-SOL or through supplemented formulas and other iron-supplemented commercially prepared baby foods.

Feeding Schedule

Feedings in preterm infants, especially the very immature, used to be withheld for 48 hours or even much longer to give the infant an opportunity to come to tolerate feedings somewhat better. With this the threat of hypoglycemia was great, the infant was starved, and lost body fluids were not replaced. How early to begin feeding the newborn is no longer the serious decision it used to be because the infant now is given intravenous feedings until oral intake is adequate. Early oral feedings, however, will help the infant to begin to gain weight early.

Intravenous fluids usually are begun within the first hours after birth. Early intravenous fluids provide the infant with fluid and some calories and reduce the incidence of hypoglycemia, dehydration, and hyperbilirubinemia. An infusion of 10 percent glucose in water usually is used at first. If the infant will not be able to tolerate oral feedings early, other nutritional supplements will be added later.

The first oral feeding should be withheld until the infant has made a reasonable adaptation to extrauterine life. He should be breathing normally, have good color and muscle tone, and should be warm. The first feeding is usually a very small amount of sterile water—only 1 to 2 ml for the very small infant and possibly up to 4 to 5 ml for the infant weighing 2000 gm (4 lb, 7 oz). As in full-term infants, water is supposedly less injurious than glucose or milk if it is aspirated. Aspiration under any circumstances is serious, however, because of the lung irritation from the other gastric contents, including HCl. The first feeding may be given as early as three to six hours after birth, or it may be postponed for a day or even for several days. After the first water feeding, milk feedings are slowly begun.

The preterm infant's stomach capacity is very small at first. Overfeeding may lead to regurgitation or vomiting, abdominal distention, and respiratory embarrassment. Feedings therefore are given in small amounts and at frequent intervals.

For the very small infant, who ordinarily is not able to suck or take food orally, the early feedings are likely to be given by continuous drip. A nasogastric tube is put in place (see page 623) and attached to an infusion pump. Formula or breast milk, diluted with an equal amount of sterile water, is then given at 1 to 2 ml per hour with the pump. This amount of food is gradually increased as tolerated to full fluid needs and also gradually to full-strength formula or human milk. The increase in feeding may vary from every one to two days to every week or more, depending on the infant's tolerance.

When tolerated by the infant, a change is made from the continuous drip feeding to a small bolus of food every hour, to every two hours, to every three hours. Timing will depend upon the amount of food left in the stomach from the previous feeding, abdominal girth, and other signs of food tolerance. Rate of increase of quantity of food may vary from one milliliter every 3 to 4 hours to 1 ml every day, depending on infant's size and risks. Finally the infant is fed by nipple as tolerated and then begins a self-demand schedule.

Early feedings are always exploratory, and adjustments are made according to the infant's demonstration of ability to tolerate volume. Increases in volume of feeding will depend on the infant's ability to tolerate the amount offered. The nurse must observe the infant very closely during feedings for evidence of sufficiency. The small infant cannot indicate when he has had enough through refusal of food. Signs of distress such as difficulty in breathing, attacks of cyanosis, regurgitation or vomiting, and abdominal distention also must be observed closely and reported. "Spitting up" of feedings is unacceptable and may be harmful in a small infant in whom danger of aspiration is great. When this happens, the volume of formula must be reduced. The nurse must use her judgment in discontinuing a feeding before the entire amount is given or in omitting a feeding entirely if the infant has any signs of distress. Subsequent feedings are rescheduled after the physician has evaluated the infant's condition.

Kind of Food

Commercially prepared formulas generally are used to feed preterm infants beginning with a formula with a concentration of 20 kcal/30 ml (1 oz), probably diluting it at first with an equal amount of sterile water, making it one-half strength. Some of the formulas have a lactalbumin-to-casein ratio similar to that of breast milk (60:40) and, because of added demineralized whey, have a lower solute content. Calcium and phosphorus ratios are also closer to the 2:1 ratio present in breast milk.

When it is desirable to increase an infant's caloric intake without an increase in fluid volume, medium chain triglycerides (MCT) oil is given several times a day. Also, some special premature formulas contain medium chain triglycerides.

Although formulas that closely resemble breast milk are called humanized milk, they do not supply some of the factors found in breast milk that may be very important to the preterm infant. The immune globulins and the macrophages of colostrum and early breast milk either make or confer a certain amount of immunity to viral and bacterial infections. It may be that the protein quantity and quality, fat quantity and quality, immune substances, and low osmolality make human milk particularly suitable for the preterm infant.[18]

Although commercially prepared "humanized" for-

[18] Lewis A. Barness, Nutrition for the low birth weight infant, *Clin. Perinatol.*, 2:345–52, 1975.

mulas commonly are used to feed preterm infants, some physicians prefer to feed breast milk, at least to selected infants and for the early feedings, for the factors named above and for its easy digestibility and ready tolerance. If breast milk is available, it may be used for the early feedings.

To supply breast milk for early feedings, and for psychologic reasons if the mother wishes to nurse her infant, her lactation may be established and maintained by artificial emptying of the breasts until the infant is able to nurse at the breast.

Methods of Feeding

Preterm infants are fed by intermittent gavage feeding, indwelling nasogastric tube, indwelling nasojejunal tube, intravenous, or bottle, depending on their size and vitality, ability to suck, and tendency to respiratory distress. The safe way to feed a small premature is to start with an indwelling tube feeding or intermittent gavage, and when it is ascertained that the infant can suck well, make a change to bottle-feeding. A small infant may need tube feedings for a long period of time, this method being continued until he shows signs of sucking ability.

A fetus at the age of 24 weeks can swallow amniotic fluid quite well, and a preterm infant who has reached the age of 30 weeks can both suck and swallow. However, a preterm infant between 30 and 35 weeks frequently cannot fully integrate his swallowing mechanism with his sucking, and he may aspirate his feeding. (Actually such difficulty may arise with the full-term newborn.) Also, between 30 and 35 weeks' gestational age the infant has an increased tendency to vomit, and the mechanism for preventing gastric reflux remains immature. Anatomic capacity of the stomach is small, and emptying time of the stomach is slow.

Coordination between sucking and swallowing, and closing and opening of the epiglottis, develops at about 32 to 34 weeks' gestation. Prior to 32 weeks' gestation an infant should be fed by nasogastric or orogastric tube, at least in the beginning.

Between 32 and 36 weeks' gestational age, when offered a nipple, the infant may appear to suck well, but be unable to swallow well, or consistently, or in coordination with his respiration. The nurse must be watchful for such difficulty and proceed with feedings with caution.

The gag reflex of an infant is not complete prior to 32 weeks' gestation. Even if sucking is normal, the gag reflex still may be immature. This is another reason for tube feeding prior to 32 weeks.

Immature infants have an immature suck pattern for a period of time. After the first day or two of a transient immature suck pattern, mature infants have frequent prolonged periods of sucking bursts, with 10 to 20 sucks in each burst, and they often swallow during a sucking burst. The immature infant has instead short sucking bursts of 3 to 5 sucks and he swallows preceding or following the sucking bursts.[19] Development of sucking depends upon birthweight and degree of maturity, but an immature suck pattern may persist for some time. With such sucking the infant does not take large amounts of food in a short period of time. It is believed that this may be a developmental protective mechanism that prevents overloading of an esophagus not yet ready to transmit a large bolus. Suck and swallow improve with practice. Sucking is slowed by a stiff nipple, and sucking is not as effective with water or glucose as it is with milk.

In preparation for feeding and to avoid undue exposure, the infant at first is left in the incubator for feedings, but the upper part of his body is raised and supported in a semiupright position while he is fed. This position is maintained by elevating the head of the incubator mattress, if it is adjustable, to approximately a 30-degree angle or by support to the infant's head and shoulders with the nurse's hand. When the infant is able to maintain his temperature, he is wrapped in an extra blanket and held during his feedings.

INTERMITTENT GAVAGE FEEDING A gavage feeding is given through a catheter passed through the mouth, into the esophagus, to just above the cardiac end of the stomach. Formula is poured through a glass barrel of a syringe attached to the catheter.

The size of the catheter is somewhat determined by the size of the infant. For the very small infant a no. 5 French catheter is best, while for the infant weighing approximately 1500 gm (3⅓ lb) a no. 8 catheter is more satisfactory. The distance to which the catheter should be passed also is determined by the size of the infant; each infant, therefore, should have an individually measured catheter. The distance from the bridge of the infant's nose to the tip of the ensiform cartilage of the sternum is measured, and the catheter is marked at this point with a narrow strip of adhesive tape (Fig. 29-6). Two more marks may be made 2 and 4 cm above the first one for further guidance in passing the catheter, or catheters may be used that already have suitable marks on them for guides.

To prepare for the feeding, the catheter, previously measured, the sterile syringe, and warmed breast milk or formula are conveniently arranged. The infant is prepared for his feeding by changing his diaper so that he will be comfortable, and, to avoid handling after feeding, his temperature is taken if it is due to be checked. If the infant has gastric distention, he may be supported in a sitting position for a moment, and an attempt may be made to raise an air bubble. The infant

[19] Joyce Gryboski, Gastrointestinal problems in the infant, *Major Probl. Clin. Pediatr.*, 13:17–23, 1975.

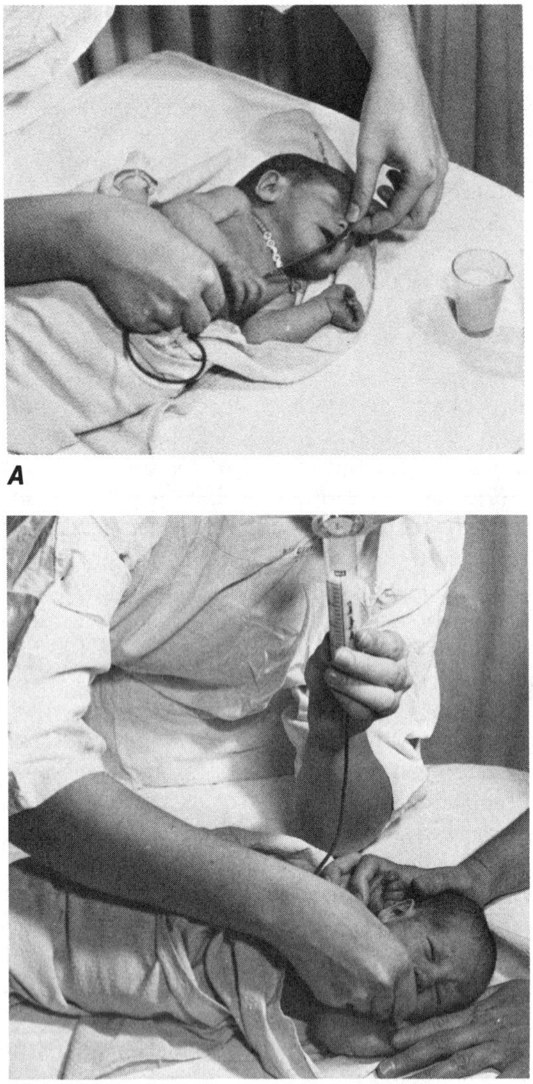

A

B

Figure 29–6. *A*. Measuring the distance from the bridge of the nose to the tip of the ensiform cartilage, to determine the exact length of gavage tube to be inserted. The tube is marked at this time. *B*. The tube, with the mark at the infant's lips, is held between the nurse's thumb and forefinger while her other fingers are in firm contact with the infant's chin. This assures the nurse that the tube will remain in the same position in the esophagus throughout the feeding. If the infant is active, it is advisible for a second person to hold his hands and head.

then is placed on his back on a flat surface with his head in a straight line and on a level with his body, and the catheter is passed through the mouth into the esophagus until the first mark is even with the infant's lips (Fig. 29–6). The catheter usually is passed without difficulty because it is almost impossible for it to enter the larynx, and there is little or no gagging or retching, owing to weakness or absence of reflexes. If the catheter does not enter the esophagus, it will turn on itself and come out of the mouth. A lubricant should not be used on the catheter because oil may drop into the pharynx.

Occasionally, bradycardia appears with passage of the feeding tube, often immediately on introduction of the tube, owing to a vagal response. If an infant shows a sensitivity to passage of a tube, an indwelling catheter may present fewer problems.

When the catheter is passed to the first mark, it is just above the cardiac opening of the stomach and is in the best position for the feeding. At this distance it does not stimulate the reflex at the cardiac opening and does not irritate the gastric mucosa. If gastric distention is present which could not be relieved by bubbling the infant before the catheter was passed, it becomes necessary to insert the catheter to the second or third mark so that it enters the stomach and allows the gas to escape. As soon as the stomach is entered, the gas can be heard coming through the tube. When indicated, the stomach contents may be aspirated at this time and then returned to the stomach. The catheter may be left in the stomach for the feeding or may be pulled out to the first mark on the tube so that its eye again rests in the esophagus (Fig. 29–7).

After the catheter has been inserted, the nurse waits a few moments to assure herself that it is not causing the infant distress. Then an accurately measured amount of the feeding is poured into the glass barrel of the syringe, which has been attached to the catheter, and the barrel is elevated to a level at which the formula will flow freely, but not rapidly. The time required for all of the feeding to be given is ordinarily the same as that required for a similar amount by bottle. The tube must be held in place throughout the feeding to ensure that it is not pulled out of its position in the esophagus, which would permit milk to spill into the mouth or pharynx (Fig. 29–6*B*).

Proper withdrawal of the catheter is important. The tube must be pinched firmly, or bent upon itself, preferably in two places, to prevent milk from dripping into the pharynx, and it is then withdrawn slowly and gently. The infant usually gasps as the tube is withdrawn, especially if it is done quickly, and he may aspirate food that is present in the pharynx.

The infant may be held in a sitting position or picked up immediately after the feeding and held up for a moment to raise air that may be present in the stomach, but the nurse must be careful not to flex his body in a manner that puts pressure on his stomach. It is not customary to bubble all premature infants after gavage, because they get very little air into the stomach with a tube feeding, and bubbling necessitates extra handling, but if the infant has been sucking on the tube or if he has a tendency to regurgitate, it may become necessary to pick the infant up. Elevating the head of the mattress for approximately 30 minutes following feeding allows for the escape of an air bubble. The infant is gently positioned after feedings, preferably on the right side or the abdomen, since the stomach empties more rapidly in the

Oral Catheter Insertion Procedure

1. Restrain infant in dorsal recumbent position with head hyperextended.

2. Select catheter of proper size (premature infants #8, term infants #8-10); check for patency, smoothness of tip.

3. Estimate distance from mouth to stomach by marking on catheter the distance from the bridge of the nose to the xiphoid process.

4. Moisten end of catheter in a medicine glass of sterile water.

5. Insert catheter. Open mouth with one hand and with the other hand gently push catheter over the tongue, down the esophagus and into the stomach.

6. If a whistling sound is heard, or if coughing, aphonia or cyanosis occurs during insertion, the tubing probably has entered the trachea and should be removed immediately and reinserted.

7. Check for correct placement of catheter.

- Invert free end of catheter into medicine glass of sterile water. If initial flow of air bubbles ceases, the catheter is in the stomach; if they are present with each respiration, the catheter is in the trachea. If no bubbles are observed, tubing may be plugged with mucus and should be removed and another catheter inserted.

- Aspirate for gastric contents using gentle suction to prevent trauma to the tissues.

- Place a stethoscope over the left upper quadrant of the abdomen. Quickly inject 1 to 2 cc of air into the catheter and listen for sound of air entering stomach.

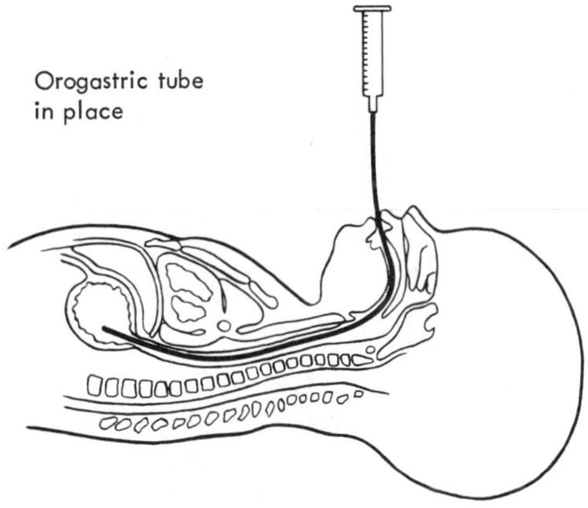

Figure 29-7. Intermittent infant gavage feeding; orogastric tube in place. (Reproduced with permission from Ross Inservice Aid No. 6, Ross Laboratories, Columbus, Ohio, 1963.)

prone or right lateral positions. For a change in position the infant may be placed on his left side midway between feedings.

INDWELLING NASOGASTRIC TUBE FEEDING An indwelling nasogastric tube feeding is a gavage feeding in which a tube is passed through the nostril into the stomach and left in place from one feeding to another (Fig. 29-8). This method is often preferable to introducing a tube into the esophagus for each feeding, since the very small infant can be fed frequently without the trauma and fatigue that may accompany frequent insertion of a gastric tube. With this method nurses are relieved of the responsibility of inserting a tube each time a feeding is done. Complications that may be encountered with an indwelling tube are a purulent rhinitis due to irritation from the tube and possibly some irritation of the esophagus or gastric mucosa.

A sterile polyvinyl tube, no. 5 French, 38 cm (15 in.) long, is used in most instances. The gastric end of the tube is closed and smooth, with openings along the side near its end; thus, the problem of irritation from the tip is not great. The proximal end of the tube attaches to a syringe; it also may be fitted with a stopper to use in closing the tube between feedings. Before the tube is inserted, it is measured and marked with a small piece of

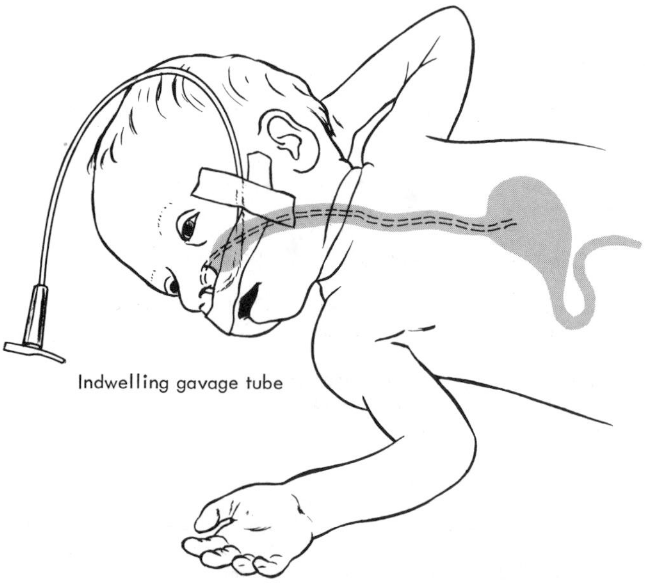

Figure 29–8. Indwelling gavage tube. (Reproduced with permission from Ross Clinical Aid No. 5, Ross Laboratories, Columbus, Ohio, 1960.)

adhesive tape at the approximate distance at which it will enter the stomach. Measurement for the adhesive marker is the distance from the xiphoid process to the tip of the ear lobe and from there to the nostril.

A knowledgeable nurse may insert the tube, passing it through the nostril as far as the marker. To make certain that the catheter has not entered the trachea, a stethoscope may be placed over the region of the stomach while a small amount of air is injected into the tube with a syringe, this air can be heard to bubble in the stomach. If the tube enters the trachea, the infant is apt to show signs of respiratory distress. The tube is secured to the infant's face with adhesive tape; it is necessary to secure it quite firmly since the infant may hook his fingers around the tube and pull it out. If the skin of the face shows signs of irritation from the adhesive tape, it may be protected with a prior application of tincture of benzoin.

The infant is positioned on his right side before each feeding is begun, and the head of the mattress, if it is adjustable, is elevated to approximately a 30-degree angle. The nurse then injects 1 cc of air into the tube and at the same time listens with a stethoscope for air entering the stomach, usually recognized by a growling sound. This gives assurance that the tube is still in the stomach. Next the air and any remaining food and fluids are aspirated to determine stomach emptying. This food and fluid are returned to the stomach and the amount deducted from the total feeding to be given to avoid overfeeding the infant. The feeding is then poured into a syringe barrel and allowed to flow into the stomach slowly by gravity, at about the rate the formula would be taken from a bottle. The infant must be watched carefully for signs of distress and the feeding discontinued if these become evident.

After the total prescribed or tolerated feeding has been introduced, 1 to 2 ml of sterile water are injected to clear the tube of milk. Then a stopper is placed into the end of the tube until the next feeding. The tube should be opened for a few minutes before each feeding is given to allow for escape of air that may be present in the stomach. This may be done by removing the stopper before preparation for the feeding is made.

The nasogastric tube is changed every three to five days, with the new tube being introduced into the opposite nostril. The infant may be given a rest without a tube for two to three hours if it is removed immediately after one feeding and reinserted just before the next.

Nasogastric feedings also may be given by a constant rather than an intermittent method through the use of a slow continuous gravity drip of the formula into the stomach or the use of an infusion pump. Residual gastric contents will need to be checked by aspiration, perhaps even every hour at first and then gradually lengthening the time interval to 2 to 3 hours and finally to 3 to 6 times daily. The formula supply and the syringe will need to be changed frequently, every 4 to 6 hours, so that it will not become contaminated with growing bacteria.

NASOJEJUNAL (TRANSPYLORIC) FEEDING With nasojejunal (NJ) feedings the infant is fed through a silicone or polyvinyl tube which has been passed through the nostril until its tip reaches the distal duodenum or the jejunum. The tube is passed through the infant's nostril into the stomach allowing for adequate length of tubing to pass through the pylorus into the duodenum. This may take a period of time. Placing the infant on the right side may facilitate passage of the tube. Fluid is aspirated through the tube and checked for pH frequently. When the pH of this fluid is found to be somewhere between 5 to 7, abdominal x-rays are taken to check on the position of the catheter tip. In most instances the tube will pass into the distal duodenum or the jejunum with time.

When the NJ tube is in the proper position, feedings are begun, usually with 5 percent glucose at first and then formula in gradually increasing amounts until the infant is receiving adequate daily fluid and caloric requirements in this manner. The feeding may be given in 10 to 15 ml amounts every two hours by slow drip, or a continuous infusion pump may be used. Care must be taken not to overload the jejunum with fluid at any one time. Initially the tube may be aspirated every hour to confirm placement and adequacy of gastrointestinal motility. A nasogastric tube may be placed to check on gastric residual and for regurgitation of food through the pylorus. The tubes are washed with 1 to 2 ml of water after a feeding is finished. As with continuous nasogastric feeding, when the continuous method of feeding is used, a fresh formula and fresh syringe must be used every four to six hours.

Nasojejunal feedings have their greatest advantage in

use for infants who have gastric limitations that do not permit an adequate quantity of feedings. They minimize the risk of regurgitation and aspiration because there is ordinarily no gastric pooling. NJ feedings have been used for very sick infants, infants on respirators, preterm infants with apnea requiring ventilation, and other small preterm infants. The NJ tube may be left in place for several weeks if necessary.

Reports about transpyloric feedings have been both favorable and cautionary. Weight gain of the infants fed by this method has been good. Complications have been encountered with use of NJ tubes. Duodenal perforation has been reported. It has been suggested that this is the result of the use of polyvinyl catheters, which harden after they have been in place for a short time. Silicone catheters, which remain soft, are thought to have a definite advantage.

Intravenous Supplementation of Oral Feedings

When an infant tolerates oral feedings but is not able to take a sufficient amount of nutrients in this manner, the feedings are likely to be supplemented with intravenous infusion. This involves giving an infusion of a supplementary nutrient mixture while at the same time feeding the infant by one of the gavage methods or by nipple.

Glucose, 10 percent, long has been used for supplementation of oral feedings and appears to be adequate when the infant will be able to take food relatively early. More recently glucose and amino acid mixtures or mixtures of glucose, amino acids, and lipid have been used when caloric intake via the gastrointestinal tract is unsatisfactory for a number of days.

One of the superficial scalp veins commonly is used for intravenous infusion in the newborn. A peripheral vein on the dorsal aspect of either the hand or the foot or an antecubital vein may be used.

Peripheral intravenous infusions require close observation for infiltration, which quickly will cause necrosis of tissue because of the hypertonicity of the solution used for intravenous feeding. Observation for thrombophlebitis and for infection is also important. Maintenance of the intravenous infusion over a period of time may become difficult.

Hyperglycemia may become a problem with intravenous glucose administration, especially in the very small infant who has a poor carbohydrate tolerance. Severe hyperglycemia could lead to cerebral dehydration and excess water loss because of osmotic diuresis. Glucose infusions for very small infants therefore are calculated in terms of milligram per kilogram per minute, or gram per kilogram per hour. Carbohydrate tolerance in these small infants appears to be no more than 6 gm/kg/day in the first day, rising to 10 to 12 gm/kg/day by the end of the first week. Blood and urine glucose determinations must be done two or three times daily until glucose tolerance limits are established. The glucose load will need to be determined accordingly.

Azotemia may develop if the intravenous solution provides excessive nitrogen intake. Careful check of each voiding for volume, specific gravity, glucose, and protein is valuable in monitoring the infant. A daily weight record is important.

An advantage of intravenous supplementation is that these infants can be fed small volumes orally until their stomachs can accept an adequate amount of food. The danger of aspiration thus is decreased. Weight gain of infants receiving a mixture of nutrients intravenously has been reported to be good.

BOTTLE-FEEDING A small, soft nipple is used for bottle-feedings. The nipple holes should be of such size that the milk drops slowly when the bottle is inverted, or a nipple with a crucial incision (cross-cut) may be used.

The infant should be held in the nurse's arm during feeding if he is permitted to be out of the incubator or supported in a semiupright position if he must be fed in the incubator. The bottle must never be propped. The infant usually will open his mouth when the nipple is touched to his lips. If his tongue is elevated against the roof of his mouth, the nipple may be pressed against his cheek and gently manipulated until he brings his tongue down so that the nipple can be placed above it. The infant may then "mouth" the nipple for awhile before he starts sucking. The nurse should stop the flow of milk frequently to coordinate with the infant's attempts to swallow. The infant should be allowed to rest at intervals during feeding, and sufficient time must be taken to bubble him both during and after the feeding. Elevation of the head of the mattress for approximately 30 minutes after feedings may prevent regurgitation of milk, and positioning on the right side is advisable.

During the first bottle feedings the infant may tire before the total feeding is taken. It is not wise to finish the feeding by gavage at this time because the infant may regurgitate as the tube is inserted. The feeding is halted when fatigue is observed, and the next feeding is given by gavage. The total duration of a bottle-feeding should not be more than 20 to 30 minutes. Substitution of a bottle for an occasional gavage feeding is resumed after several feedings because the infant's strength improves daily, and his ability to suck well will be strengthened by practice.

With all feedings the infant may need to be bubbled midway in the feeding and again at the end of the feeding. Bubbling may not be necessary when the very weak infant who does not suck is fed by tube, but should always be done at the end of a feeding as soon as the infant begins to suck on the tube, at which time he will swallow air. The infant who may not be removed from the incubator for feedings is bubbled by being held in a sitting position, supported with the nurse's hands.

To prevent regurgitation, and possibly aspiration, of milk following a feeding, the nurse must handle the infant very gently. It is advisable to place the infant on the right side or the abdomen after feedings, since the stomach empties more rapidly in the prone and right lateral positions than in the supine and left lateral positions.[20] This would be especially important for infants who have delayed gastric emptying time or who have difficulty in tolerating the volume of feeding that they require. A rolled towel tucked firmly behind the infant's back will provide support for the lateral position.

If the infant is placed on the right side after each feeding, he should be turned to the left side midway between feeding times to ensure adequate change of position. If the head end of the mattress has been raised, it is advisable to allow it to remain elevated at approximately a 30-degree angle for 30 minutes after feedings, as a further safeguard against regurgitation.

Further Suggestions

The infant must be watched carefully for regurgitation during the first one-half hour or so after each feeding, and the breathing pattern must be closely observed after feedings. Periodic breathing, or apnea, is likely to occur in small infants in about 15 minutes after feedings.

When formula is fed by continuous gravity drip or by infusion pump, great care must be taken to assure that fresh formula and a completely new unit are replaced frequently. As with milk, when formula becomes warm and exposed, it will quickly begin to grow bacteria, and it is likely to cause gastrointestinal problems.

A small infant who must be fed by tube should be offered a pacifier or a nipple to suck on as soon as he will and can make the effort. This may be offered during feedings and also between feedings. This will provide the infant with the pleasure and satisfaction of sucking, and it will strengthen his sucking ability. Nonnutritive sucking is also believed to favorably influence the premature infant's growth and development.[21]

Feeding should be an enjoyable experience. Even the tube-fed infant can be given some attention that may be satisfying during his feeding if he is talked to, patted, given an opportunity to suck, and rocked if that is permissible.

Parents should be given the opportunity to become involved in their infant's feedings as soon as the infant's condition permits and the parents feel able.

[20] Victor H. Yu, Effect of body position on gastric emptying in the neonate, *Arch. Dis. Child.*, 50:500–504, 1975.

[21] Judy C. Bernbaum *et al,* Nonnutritive sucking during gavage feedings enhances growth and maturation in premature infants, *Pediatrics,* 71:41–45, (Jan.) 1983.

Protection Against Exertion

The preterm infant needs rest and protection from exertion during the first hours after birth and probably longer if he is stressed by illness. Certain procedures must be done early, such as placing monitor leads and temperature probe and starting intravenous fluids, but if there is any care that can be postponed, rest will be very helpful to the infant. The infant needs much of his energy to adjust and adapt to his changed environment.

The infant's energy also can be conserved by helping him to maintain his respirations, body temperature, and fluid and electrolyte needs without stress. This care has been described, but as an example the reader is reminded of the great deal of energy an infant must use to maintain his body temperature if he becomes chilled.

In ongoing daily care the nurse should organize and plan the infant's care in a way that will reduce undue handling and stimulation and provide for periods of rest. The infant must be protected against becoming tired from too much activity at any one time. Careful observation of the infant's tolerance, and spacing of nursing care and procedures, can provide for appropriate periods of rest and activity. Care also must be taken that the infant is protected against unnecessary lights and noise and other stimulation that may waste energy.

The Infant's Parents

The preterm infant's parents will be gravely concerned over their small infant. If parents saw their infant briefly at birth, he most likely appeared very tiny and fragile. If, unfortunately, they did not see the infant before he was rushed to the nursery, it is hard to know how they imagine that he looks. When parents see the infant in the nursery, often at first from a distance, he is in an incubator, usually surrounded by physicians and nurses, and often by machines and equipment.

Parents need physician and nurse support to help them understand their infant's illness, all the mechanical equipment, and the care he is receiving, and they need a realistic explanation of his prognosis. Parents have a need to talk with their infant's caretakers frequently, and the caretakers should ask how they can help the parents. Parents should be invited and encouraged to go into the nursery to see their infant as soon as possible. They should be encouraged to see, touch, visit, and finally to care for their infant. They need a great deal of ongoing support, explanation of what is happening, and encouragement to have physical contact with their infant frequently. The parents need to be involved in the infant's care as soon as they feel able, and they should quickly be regarded as a part of the care team rather than visitors.

The first visit to a nursery intensive care unit can be

overwhelming and parents need preparation for it. Often their infant has at the least an intravenous infusion running, wires attached for monitoring, an oxygen hood or some other means for administration of oxygen, a radiant warmer or a heat shield, and possibly a feeding tube in place. Other machines and tubes may be attached to the infant. (See Fig. 29–9.) In addition to the previous preparation, the person caring for the infant can give parents further explanation at this time and answer their questions.

Parents should be encouraged to touch, talk to, and comfort their infant, but for some this may take a number of visits, especially if the infant is quite ill. Eventually they are encouraged to participate in much of their infant's care, including feeding, changing of diapers, and other care they feel able to carry out. In order to develop strong parent-child attachments the parents need the same opportunities for touch, eye-to-eye contact, and caretaking that are important with normal newborns. There may be some delay because of the infant's condition, but delay should be no longer than absolutely necessary. The nurse must help the parents to develop an acquaintance with their infant as early as possible.

The importance of early parent contact with their infant and the ways in which the nurse can promote parent-infant attachment is discussed in more detail for all newborns on pages 470–72.

If the mother had planned to nurse her infant, her breasts may be pumped to stimulate and maintain her milk supply so that she will be able to nurse her infant when he becomes strong enough. Ordinarily, arrangements can be made for the mother to pump her breasts at home, and plans may be made for her to bring the milk to the hospital for the infant's use. Later, of course, she can begin to nurse the infant. The mother who is supplying breast milk for her infant feels good about the valuable contribution she is making to her infant's care.

If at all possible, arrangement should be made for siblings to visit and see the infant through the nursery window to become acquainted, to ask questions, and to feel that they are getting to know the infant (Fig. 29–10). If family visiting is infrequent when an infant must remain in the hospital for a long time after the mother goes home, it is possible for the family to regroup (without the infant), and then it becomes difficult to find a place for the infant. When the mother is discharged from the hospital, frequent visiting, if distance permits, and telephone calls help to keep in close contact.

As time goes on parents need more and more direct contact with their infant if it is at all possible for them to spend such time at the hospital. They need to come to know their infant well, and the mother needs to develop confidence in her ability to care for her infant. As the infant improves, the mother should be able to give more and more of his care. Often arrangements can be made for her to spend a day, or several, at the hospital giving complete care to her infant before his discharge.

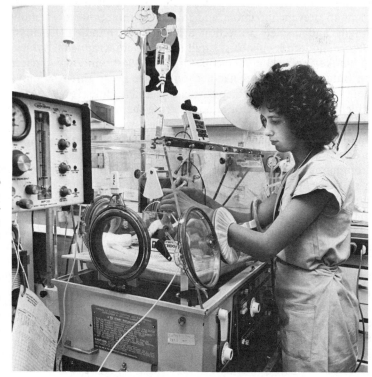

Figure 29–9. The infant in this incubator is receiving a number of treatments. A respirator can be seen to the left of the incubator. The infant is receiving an intravenous infusion and also feedings through an indwelling nasogastric feeding tube by a slow continuous method using an infusion pump. The formula is in the small flask hanging behind and above the respirator. The nurse is checking for gastric residual of formula. Oxygen is being given with an oxygen hood. An oxygen monitor is on the top of the incubator and the cardiac and respiratory monitor can be seen on the shelf against the wall. The lamp above the incubator can be used for radiant heat when necessary. It is apparent why parents may be overwhelmed by their baby's treatments and the technical apparatus, and why they need help in knowing how to visit and touch their baby.

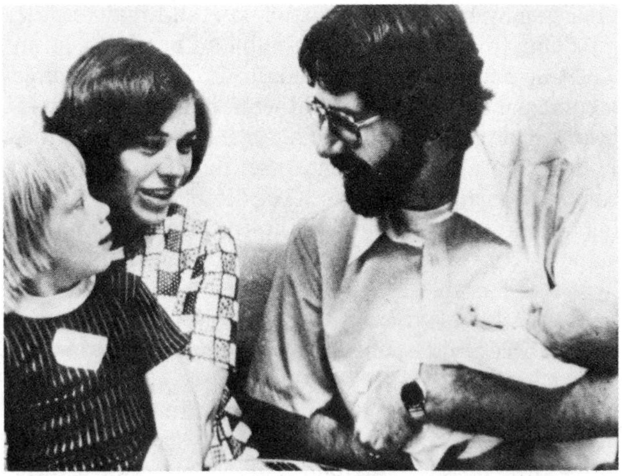

Figure 29–10. This infant has progressed very well and can now spend some time with her family. Mother and father and an older daughter are visiting and the parents are helping their older daughter to become acquainted with her sister. (Reprinted from the booklet *Special Care Nursery*, Madison General Hospital, Madison, WI, 1978. Photograph courtesy of Madison General Hospital and Ohio Medical Products, both of Madison, WI.)

Sensory Stimulation

Incubator care in the past has isolated the preterm infant from the frequent human contact and the tactile, visual, auditory, and kinesthetic stimulation that the full-term newborn ordinarily receives. It was previously felt that the small infant needed to be isolated from the environment to prevent infection, and that these infants were fragile and needed protection against being handled. Before modern incubators, small infants were wrapped in blankets, placed in an incubator with a glass window on only one side, and handled only once every three hours for diapering, temperature check, and feedings for which the infant was not removed from the incubator. With modern incubators the infant is less wrapped up, and is in an incubator that at least has PLEXIGLAS all around. This makes the infant somewhat less isolated from human stimulation, but an incubator environment is still very monotonous. The incubator separates the infant from much of the sensory stimulation that exists in the environment of the normal newborn, and if the infant is only diapered and fed as necessary, the amount of stimulation he receives will be very insufficient.

It is still true that the severely premature infant and the sick infant need to be protected against handling other than that which is absolutely necessary for essential care. All of the energy of these infants must be used for efforts at survival. However, when they show improvement and stability in their condition, they will profit from being given sensory stimulation.

Research within recent years has shown that newborns are much more capable of organized responses than previously had been assumed. It also has been observed that the preterm infant's ability to see, hear, smell, and respond to touch is quite good. Preterm newborns have been observed to gaze at the faces of the nurses who feed them, to respond to handling, and to quiet when someone talks to them.

Early stimulation of the preterm infant may come when parents visit if they are ready to touch, stroke, pat, and talk to the infant. Often parents will assume the *en face* position to look at the infant and thus visually stimulate him. A nursery mobile suspended from the roof of the infant's incubator at a focal plane about 8 to 9 in. from the infant's eyes will provide visual stimulation, and parents can be encouraged to bring other bright toys. (See Figure 29–11.)

Preterm infants can be removed from the incubator for feedings and extra stimulation as soon as they can maintain their body temperature while out of the incubator during a feeding. At feeding time they can be rocked, patted, talked to, and held in the position in which they can look at their caretaker's face. Holding the infant up for burping also gives him an opportunity to look around. Cuddling and burping can be a part of a gavage feeding as well as a breast- or bottle-feeding. This feeding and play are ideally done by the parents as frequently as they can be available, but are done by nurses when parents are not there. At times when parents are not available, nurses can offer sensory stimuli by talking to the infant, patting him, and managing to be in his visual field during care that involves diapering, temperature taking, feeding, and other care. Nurses should hold the infant for feedings as soon as that is permissible, and cuddle him and talk to him as they would during feeding of the normal newborns. Nurses and parents also may try to get the infant to follow their head movements with his eyes and to respond to their voices (Fig. 29–12).

Nurses are in a unique position to devise ways that will stimulate these small infants to respond. Nurses also have the information and the knowledge they need to decide when and how much stimulation should be given to each infant, making sure that there is a good balance between rest and activity.

When the preterm infant has matured enough to be moved to a regular bassinet, nurses need to continue to talk to, pick up, and play with these infants around feeding time. Parents should be urged to visit often. Early and frequent parent participation will strengthen the bond between parents and child.

Sensory stimulation should, of course, continue after the infant leaves the hospital. When parents have been involved in care that encourages sensory stimulation of their infant, they are likely to continue to do so at home, and the nurses can help them to understand the importance of this to their infant's continuing development.

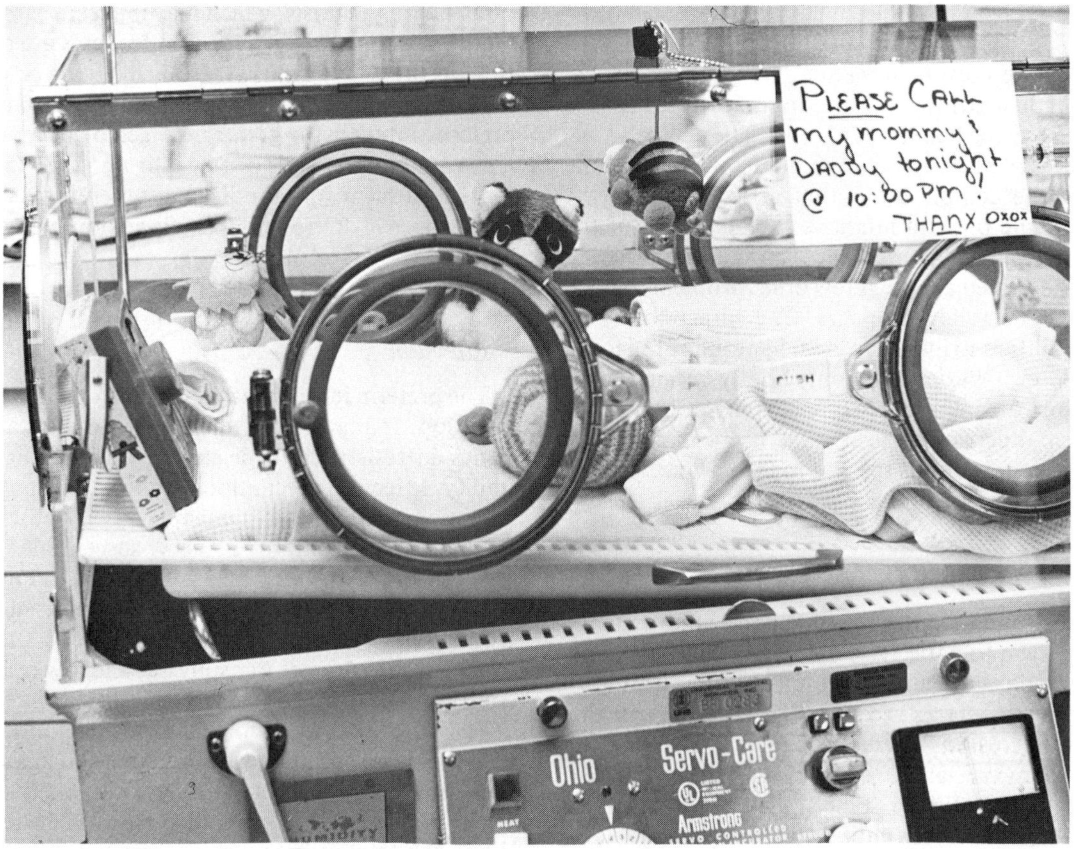

Figure 29–11. The infant in this incubator is progressing well. She no longer needs all of the special appartus for her care that is shown in Figure 29–9. She is in the incubator because she still needs protection against heat loss. Note that this baby is clothed and covered with a blanket and that she is wearing a stocking cap to reduce heat loss from the rather large surface of her head. This baby is being visited frequently by her parents, and they have brought several toys for her interest and stimulation.

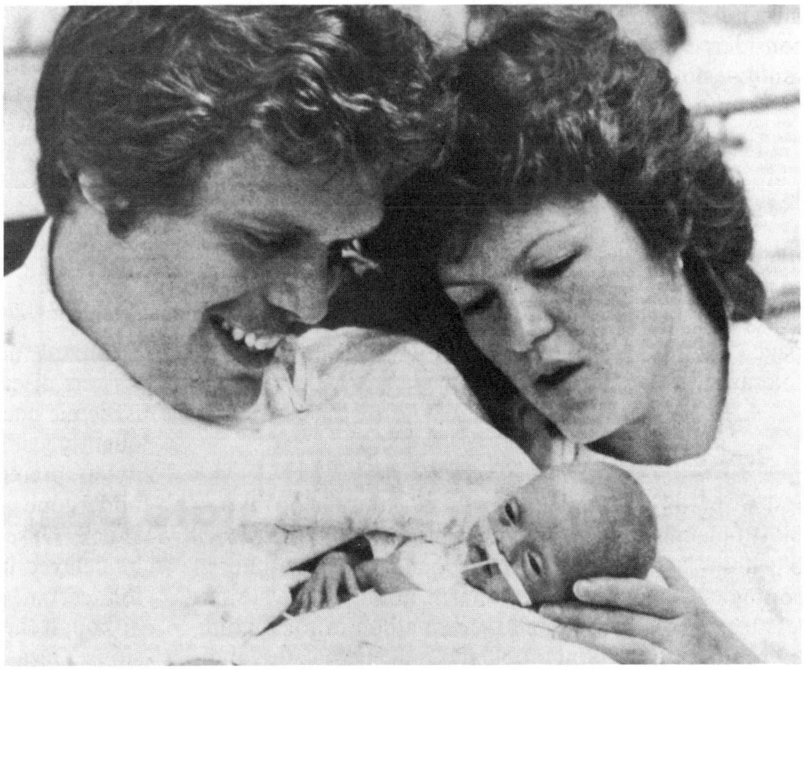

Figure 29–12. The infant, seen in Figure 29–3 has grown and developed at a rate that is normal for her gestational age. She is still very small, weighing only 3 lb, 2 oz (1400 gm). She is, however, progressing very well and may be out of the incubator while held by her parents. The parents, who have visited daily are delighted to be able to have closer contact with their daughter. (Photograph courtesy of Carmen Hoxie and her parents and of Mr. L. Roger Turner, photographer, Wisconsin State Journal, Madison, WI.)

Special Problems and Complications

Infants who are born preterm are likely to have special problems in their adjustment to extrauterine life because of their physiologic handicaps at birth. The degree of immaturity is very likely to determine the number and the severity of the complications that arise. Some of the problems of the preterm infant, especially those of the respiratory system, of thermal regulation, and of feeding have been described above. A few other problems will be discussed in the following pages. The susceptibility of the preterm infant to hypoglycemia, hyperbilirubinemia, and infection will be described only briefly because these complications are discussed in more detail in Chapter 30. Since patent ductus arteriosus and necrotizing enterocolitis are complications specific to the preterm infant, they will be described in this chapter.

Hypoglycemia

Preterm infants may become hypoglycemic, but not necessarily symptomatic. Hypoglycemia may occur in the hours or days after birth presumably as a result of low liver glycogen stores because of their early birth and because of increased metabolic demands after birth. Chilling, asphyxia, and respiratory distress will use glycogen stores quickly. Blood glucose should be checked every four hours until stable.

If intravenous glucose is started in the first hours in the preterm infant, as is recommended for fluid and caloric needs, the blood glucose level is likely to remain above a hypoglycemic level. In the preterm infant a blood sugar level below 30 mg/100 ml whole blood must be viewed with suspicion and a reading below 20 mg/100 ml whole blood (below 25 in plasma or serum) must be considered hypoglycemia and treated. If the preterm infant has not grown well *in utero,* being below the fiftieth percentile in weight, the likelihood of developing hypoglycemia may be greater.

Hyperglycemia

The extremely preterm infant may have a low carbohydrate tolerance and spill sugar into the urine when he receives above his tolerance in intravenous fluids. See page 625 for further discussion of carbohydrate tolerance.

Hyperbilirubinemia

The preterm infant is very likely to develop hyperbilirubinemia and is very vulnerable to the danger of free bilirubin. The preterm infant probably has less ability to conjugate bilirubin than the term infant does. He has less total serum protein and serum albumin for binding bilirubin than the term infant and is likely to have conditions such as acidosis, which may interfere with the binding of bilirubin. Also, since oral feedings are delayed or slow in preterm infants, there is likely to be a delay in evacuation of bilirubin-containing meconium. The preterm infant is in greater danger of developing kernicterus at lower levels of free bilirubin than the term infant. Treatment for jaundice must therefore begin early. See pages 677–82 for further discussion of hyperbilirubinemia.

Infection

The preterm infant must be carefully protected against infection. Immaturity of the infant's organs and a deficiency in resistance to disease give him a high susceptibility. Infection precautions, important in any nursery, discussed in Chapter 27, must be strictly observed.

The preterm infant is very susceptible to upper respiratory tract infections, septicemia, and meningitis. Every precaution should be taken to prevent infection from adults or through aspiration of food. Immaturity of the lungs, presence of asphyxia, and low resistance all contribute to the infant's susceptibility to infections.

The potential for an intrauterine infection, especially pneumonia, is greater in the preterm than in the term infant, because preterm births are more likely to be preceded by a prolonged period of ruptured membranes. When the fetal membranes rupture before labor in the term pregnancy, the mother either goes into labor quite promptly or labor is induced. With premature rupture of the membranes in a preterm pregnancy, the pregnancy is allowed to continue to permit further maturation of the fetus. With the membranes prematurely ruptured, there is danger of intrauterine infection and exposure of the fetus. See page 271 for management of rupture of membranes in a preterm pregnancy.

Clinical signs of infection are very difficult to evaluate in any newborn, and especially in the preterm infant. Any signs suggestive of infection will need to be investigated by laboratory means as described on page 687.

Necrotizing Enterocolitis

Neonatal necrotizing enterocolitis (NEC) is a very serious disease in the newborn that is characterized by ischemic necrosis of the gastrointestinal tract which frequently leads to perforation. The disease is seen primarily in preterm infants, especially in those who have undergone fetal distress and neonatal hypoxia and shock. Onset is usually in the first week of life but may be delayed into the second or third week. The right colon, cecum, and terminal ileum are most often involved, although the entire colon and small bowel may show lesions. Occasionally only small segments of the ileum are affected, but often large segments of bowel or even the entire bowel is involved.

With necrotizing entercolitis the involved area of the bowel is dilated and the serosal surface is hemorrhagic. Segments of intestine may become agglutinated. The mucosal surface has ulcerations and necrosis and is covered by a pseudomembranous formation of agglutinated inflammatory cells and necrotic epithelium. There is hemorrhage in the submucosa. An ileus develops with the disease. This leads to stasis of intestinal contents and proliferation of bacteria. Many times the bowel perforates; this may be in one place or in multiple places. Perforation of the thin, friable bowel is the most common and the most serious development. Peritonitis and generalized sepsis follow.

The cause of NEC is not certain, but two factors considered most strongly as an initial cause are ischemia of the intestines and the action of enteric bacteria. A period of fetal or neonatal hypoxia and/or systemic shock will bring about a reflexive response in which there is a redistribution of blood, which results in blood being shunted away from the peripheral, renal, and mesenteric vascular beds in order to supply and protect the brain and the heart from hypoxia. The resultant ischemia in the mesenteric vascular bed then may decrease the metabolism in the intestinal mucosa and damage intestinal cells to the point where they may decrease or stop their normal secretion of protective mucus. This exposes the intestinal mucosa to enzymatic autodigestion and allows bacterial invasion. Then, subsequent to the ischemia of the bowel brought about by the hypotension and hypoxia, there is bacterial invasion of the bowel.

When normal circulation is restored after an episode of ischemia, repair and regeneration of the bowel can take place. However, enteric bacteria and feedings may complicate the changes brought about by the ischemia of the bowel. Along with an adynamic ileus and stasis, there may be an overgrowth of bacteria. The gas-forming bacteria, which predominate, may invade the damaged areas of the bowel mucosa and produce gas blebs or small bubbly cysts in the bowel wall (pneumatosis). A third component—the availability of metabolic substrate (the feedings)—adds to the development and progress of the disease by providing good growth material for the bacteria.

The clinical picture of NEC includes the signs and symptoms that ordinarily could be expected to be associated with feeding and bowel problems. The infant may feed poorly and be lethargic. He is likely to have gastric retention because of prolonged gastric emptying. Abdominal distention, especially if associated with rigidity, should be of concern at once. Increase in abdominal distention can be observed by measurement of the abdomen every four to six hours. Ileus is likely to be present. Bowel sounds or their absence should be checked. A red or shiny abdominal skin may indicate peritonitis. Since the bowel is very friable, abdominal palpation should be done only with utmost care. If emesis occurs, it may be bile-stained. Stools become diarrheal and may be blood-streaked. A guaiac test should be done on the stools.

The infant with NEC may develop other signs of illness such as apneic episodes, thermal instability, jaundice, lethargy, and sometimes a shocklike condition.

X-ray of the abdomen of an infant with NEC shows intestinal distention with dilated loops of bowel and pneumatosis (air in the bowel wall). There also may be a pneumoperitoneum (free air in the peritoneum). Sometimes gas is seen in the portal vein, which is a very ominous sign.

From the above description it is apparent that NEC is a syndrome rather than a specific disease, being a constellation of clinical, radiologic, and pathologic signs.

The prognosis of necrotizing enterocolitis is very serious. When treatment is successful, it often depends on early recognition. Infants at risk require careful observation for signs that are ordinarily relatively nonspecific. As soon as any signs of NEC are detected, all enteric feedings are stopped and nasogastric suctioning is started. Intravenous fluid and electrolyte therapy is started, acid-base balance is carefully monitored and maintained, and the circulation is supported with blood and plasma as indicated. Antibiotics, parenterally and topically, are begun, wide spectrum at first, and possibly changed to others when results of blood, urine, and stool cultures are known. Abdominal x-rays are taken every four to six hours to watch for pneumoperitoneum, obstruction, or peritoneal fluid. A physical evaluation of the abdomen for evidence of perforation is done frequently.

When the infant's condition improves, feedings are begun cautiously after seven to 14 days of nasogastric suction and antibiotics. Feedings are not given earlier than one week and preferably much later. Until then parenteral fluids provide for nutrition. The stomach is kept empty with continuous suction. Antibiotics are given parenterally and locally through the stomach tube.

Surgery may become necessary. Indications for surgery include pneumoperitoneum, actual or impending perforation, peritonitis, and intestinal obstruction. All nonviable or acutely inflamed bowel is removed at surgery, and usually an ileostomy or a colostomy is done. Sometimes a large amount of bowel needs to be removed and malabsorption and short bowel syndrome become a problem. Long-term total intravenous alimentation is sometimes necessary for these infants.

Nursing observation of infants with NEC is very important both in recognizing early signs, which have been described above, and after a diagnosis is made in observing changes in the infant's condition. In addition the infant needs supportive care to decrease stress and to promote comfort.

The infant's abdominal area must be protected from trauma. The infant is best cared for without diapers, which put some pressure on the lower abdomen and also involve some pressure on the abdomen during diaper changes. Diapers may also obstruct good observation of the abdomen for any changes in condition. Since the infant is likely to have diarrhea, frequent cleaning of the buttocks and the adjacent area and ointment to the skin are important.

The abdominal area must also be protected from trauma by very careful handling of the infant, preferably not picking him up except when absolutely necessary. The infant needs comforting in other ways than by being held.

The abdomen must be watched carefully for signs of perforation of the bowel and for peritonitis, for reddening or shininess of the skin, and for increasing distention. Perforation of the bowel may be accompanied by signs of shock.

Vital signs must be observed closely. Blood pressure change may signal a problem. Apnea or other respiratory problems may suddenly appear. Since an infant on a respirator may not show these changes, he must be observed carefully for other signs. The body temperature may become unstable, and it may drop when shock develops. The temperature must be taken axillary, since taking rectal temperature is contraindicated. Other signs of shock such as change in pulse, change in color to pale or dusky, and limpness may appear.

As with any serious illness of an infant the parents will need support from the nurse. They need an explanation of the infant's condition, the reasons for treatment, and if surgery is done, an explanation of the anticipated postoperative course. They will need help with understanding how the ileostomy or colostomy functions, and assistance in learning to care for it unless an anastomosis is done before the infant goes home.

The role of breast milk in prevention of NEC has been, and is continuing to be, explored. Infants ordinarily do not develop this disease until they have been fed. There appears to be no clear evidence at this time, however, that breast milk may provide protection.

Since NEC is thought to be caused by an episode of compromised perfusion of the bowel and the result of many intestinal tract bacteria following ingestion of food, it appears that careful identification of infants at risk and caution in starting their feeding may be helpful in prevention or early diagnosis and treatment.

Patent Ductus Arteriosus

The ductus arteriosus, the large blood vessel that connects the pulmonary artery with the descending aorta during fetal life, ordinarily closes by constriction within hours in the normal infant. With the onset of respiration at birth the pulmonary vascular resistance is suddenly lowered and there is a large increase in pulmonary blood flow. Also, with clamping of the umbilical cord, and removal of the low-resistance placental circuit from the circulation, the systemic resistance increases. With the relative fall in the pulmonary vascular resistance and the rise in systemic vascular resistance, each of these resistances becomes nearly equal very soon after birth, with the pulmonary possibly being a little lower. This permits a small amount of blood flow from the systemic to the pulmonary circulatory system—a transitory left-to-right shunt. Normally this shunt is not large and with good oxygenation the ductus arteriosus soon constricts well. The ductus, however, does have the capacity to reopen during the first postnatal days if the Pao_2 drops below normal for any reason.

In preterm infants, and especially in those with respiratory distress syndrome, delayed closure or persistence of the ductus arteriosus is common. Persistence of a patent ductus arteriosus may occur in 40 to 50 percent of infants with a birth weight under 1500 gm (3 lb, 5 oz). Delay in closure probably is mainly due to (1) immaturity, there being insufficient development of the musculature, and (2) the hypoxemia associated with respiratory distress, which causes the ductus arteriosus to remain patent or to reopen in the early days after birth. Multiple other factors may have some influence.

When the ductus arteriosus is patent, shunting of blood can be from right to left, or from left to right, or bidirectional, depending upon whether the resistance is least in the pulmonary or in the systemic circulation. Persistent patency may lead to severe cardiorespiratory distress.

The more preterm an infant is, the less muscular are the pulmonary arterioles. This means that there is a greater difference between systemic and pulmonary resistance in the preterm than in the full-term infant and shunting from systemic to pulmonary circulation is likely to take place. Also, the hypoxia, common in preterm infants, is likely to delay closure of the ductus arteriosus. With these conditions a left-to-right shunt develops. (A small right-to-left or bidirectional shunt may occur in the first hour after birth.) When spontaneous closure of the ductus does not soon occur, but the shunting remains small, it may not cause any serious circulatory problems. If the shunting becomes significantly large, the left ventricle will become overloaded and congestive heart failure may develop.

Pulmonary vascular resistance continues a normal maturational decrease in the next several days and weeks after birth. As the pulmonary resistance decreases, there is an increase in blood flow into the pulmonary circulation if the ductus arteriosus is patent. This increase in blood flow through the lungs results in increased pulmonary venous return to the left side of the heart. As the volume of blood returning from the lungs increases, distention of the left ventricle increases and its stroke volume increases. If this process continues, the load on the left ventricle becomes increasingly greater. The ventricle may be able to maintain the increased stroke volume; if so, there will be no symptoms. If the heart becomes overextended, signs of cardiac failure appear.

When a patent ductus arteriosus is associated with respiratory distress, the infant may have respiratory problems because of the increased pulmonary blood flow in addition to those already present because of the status of the lung.

Diagnosis of a patent ductus arteriosus should be made prior to frank evidence of congestive failure. This permits early treatment. With left-to-right shunting through the ductus, an audible murmur develops, the basal heart rate gradually increases, the pulses become bounding so that the dorsalis pedis and palmar pulses may become perceptible, there is a wide pulse pressure, the apical cardiac impulse becomes hyperactive, pulmonary congestion develops, and peripheral edema becomes evident. Congestive pulmonary stress becomes manifest by tachypnea and chest retraction. Apneic spells may develop and increase in severity. Mild cyanosis may develop; it ordinarily is relieved easily by a small increase in ambient oxygen concentration, since the shunt is left to right and not right to left. Echocardiography helps to diagnose the extent of the shunting.

Treatment is likely to consist of administration of diuretics for removal of excess fluid, fluid intake restriction, oxygen as needed, maintenance of a normal blood pH, maintenance of adequate hemoglobin to ensure adequate oxygenation, and pharmacologic closure of the ductus by administration of indomethacin to inhibit prostaglandin synthesis. Prostaglandin has a relaxing effect on the ductus. With a prostaglandin inhibitor it is hoped that the ductus will close spontaneously with medical treatment. Sometimes surgical closure becomes necessary to prevent heart failure.

Complications of indomethacin therapy include transient renal dysfunction, hyponatremia, decrease in platelet aggregation, gastrointestinal and intracranial bleeding, and displacement of bilirubin from binding sites. According to Susan D. Foster care of the infant receiving indomethacin therapy should include the following:

> NURSING CONSIDERATIONS. During indomethacin administration—urine output and the infant's weight should be accurately recorded. Serum and urine electrolytes and BUN must be closely monitored. Because the PDA may not respond to indomethacin, or may reappear after initial closure, the nurse should continue to observe for the signs and symptoms of PDA and its complications.[22]

[22] Susan D. Foster, MCN Pharmacopoeia: Indomethacin: Pharmacologic closure of the ductus arteriosus, *MCN,* 7:171, (May/June) 1982.

Observation for bleeding tendency also becomes important.

Discharge from the Hospital

The preterm infant is usually ready for discharge from the hospital when he is able to maintain his temperature in an average environment, when he is able to eat well from a bottle or the breast and is gaining weight well, and when the mother demonstrates ability and confidence in providing care. Often this time coincides with the time the infant reaches a body weight of about 2250 gm (roughly 5 lb) and a gestational age of 36 to 37 weeks.

Conditions in the home may influence the time of discharge. The public health nurse is important in the transition from home to hospital. Arrangements are often made with a public health nursing agency to visit the home prior to the infant's discharge to help the parents prepare for the infant, and also for visits after he is home to give them further assistance with his care.

A social worker should be a member of the health care team that provides the infant's care. The social worker assists the family with adjustments that must be made in the hospital and in the home, and also with financial arrangements to cover the very high hospital and medical bills.

Physical and mental development of the preterm infant in general should be expected to coincide with that of a full-term infant only when the infant reaches the date when he would have been full-term. Since development is not likely to progress faster extrauterine than intrauterine, future evaluation of progress should be made from the expected full-term date rather than the date of the infant's birth.

THE SMALL-FOR-GESTATIONAL-AGE INFANT

The small-for-gestational-age (SGA) infant usually is defined as one whose birthweight is below the tenth percentile for a given gestational age. SGA also has been defined as a birthweight of more than two standard deviations below the mean for any given week of gestation. This corresponds to approximately the third percentile on the intrauterine growth curves. Defining small-for-gestational age in terms of low birthweight means that gestational age must be relatively closely assessed and that both birthweight and gestational age must be plotted on an intrauterine growth chart. With this definition a SGA infant may be preterm, term, or postterm. The unifying characteristic is a disproportionately small birthweight for gestational age.

Many small-for-gestational-age infants are full-term newborns whose birthweight falls below the tenth percentile on the intrauterine growth chart shown in Figure 29-1. This usually means that the term infant who is SGA weighs 2500 gm or less at birth. When weight was being used as a definition of prematurity, the SGA term infant was identified as a premature. Now that gestational age assessment is being used to identify the preterm infant, the full-term newborn of low birthweight is separated from the preterm and placed into a separate classification designated as term SGA. The full-term SGA infant can be thought of as a newborn who is mature but undergrown.

Many descriptive words or phrases have been used for infants who are growth-retarded—small-for-gestational age, small-for-dates, intrauterine growth retardation (IUGR), dysmature, chronic fetal distress, fetal malnutrition syndrome, pseudopremature. All these terms make some reference to factors of the fetal environment that do not permit the fetus to reach his growth potential as soon as should be expected. Of all the terms that have been used, SGA and IUGR will be used in the rest of this chapter.

The SGA infant may be small in weight only, or small in weight and length, or he may be below the tenth percentile in weight, length, and head circumference. The clinical picture of the infant is related to the duration, the intensity, and the time of onset of the growth-retarding influence. With undernutrition, weight is affected first, then there is a decrease in growth, indicated by a shortness in body length, and finally, if growth retardation is severe, the head circumference is affected. Sometimes, however, an infant is hereditarily of small size in all measurements.

When weight alone is diminished and length and head circumference are normal, it is felt that the factor that caused the fetus the distress that reduced its weight occurred only a few days or weeks prior to birth. When distress is of a longer standing, chronic nature, growth in body weight has been curtailed for weeks or months before birth, growth in length also has been retarded, and in extreme cases growth in head circumference was slowed.

Causes of Fetal Growth Retardation

Normal intrauterine growth for body weight, for length, and for growth of other organs is linear between 28 and 37 to 38 weeks of gestation. From 37 to 38 weeks growth of the fetus and placenta begins to fall off somewhat and no longer follows the straight line upward. When for some reason the fetus cannot follow this normal pattern, then growth falls off at some earlier time.

Fetal growth may be retarded either because the fetus is unable to grow normally in the presence of an adequate nutritional "supply line," or because a normal fetus does not receive adequate nutrition from the supply line.

Retardation of growth because of factors inherent in the fetus are caused by such problems as chromosomal aberrations (Down's and other trisomy syndromes), congenital anomalies, infections (rubella, toxoplasmosis, and so on), and perhaps other factors that cause subnormal development. A developmental abnormality in the fetus is likely to prevent normal growth of tissues and organs.

The supply line can be thought of as having a maternal and a placental component. Placental causes may be of a pathologic nature such as infarcts, or premature placental separation, or possibly some physiologic limitations, as, for example, being unable to supply adequately all fetuses of a multiple pregnancy. By and large, however, fetal and placental causes account for only a small proportion of fetal growth retardation. Maternal causes are therefore primarily the reason for fetal deprivation. In some cases the mechanism of fetal deprivation may not be known, and in other instances a primary abnormality of maternal circulation may be complicated by secondary pathologic changes in the placenta, but in general the search for cause of fetal deprivation should be made among maternal factors.[23]

Maternal undernutrition and diminished uterine blood flow are two maternal factors commonly considered. Studies done on animals have shown that dietary restrictions in mothers caused reduction in birthweight of offspring. Whether or not maternal malnutrition in human pregnancy has an appreciable effect is not clear. The role of chronic malnutrition, prior to conception, in causing IUGR is not well understood either. It is generally believed that the fetus will receive adequate nutrients from the mother if the mother has the necessary reserves. If continuing deprivation of some nutrient depletes maternal reserves, the fetus will be unable to get that nutrient. The effect on the fetus will depend upon how essential the particular deficient nutrient is to fetal growth.

Reduction of uteroplacental blood flow is thought to be a cause of IUGR, because maternal diseases that may cause a reduced placental blood flow are associated with IUGR. These include preeclampsia, chronic hypertensive vascular disease, and advanced diabetes. These conditions can result in significant lowering of fetal weight, and also in fetal mortality and neonatal morbidity. Among other maternal causes of IUGR are smoking, small stature, low maternal age, grand multiparity, inadequate prenatal care, and low socioeconomic class. In many instances the cause of small-for-gestational age cannot be identified.

Incidence and Significance of IUGR

Studies in the United States and Great Britain show that about one third of the infants with birthweight of less

[23] Peter Gruenwald, Introduction—The supply line of the fetus; Definitions relating to fetal growth, in *The Placenta and Its Maternal Supply Line,* edited by P. Gruenwald, University Park Press, Baltimore, Md., 1975, pp. 1–17.

than 2500 gm are not preterm but rather term SGA infants. The incidence of SGA births varies from 1.5 to 2 percent of all births.[24]

SGA is second only to preterm as a cause of perinatal mortality. The overall neonatal mortality for IUGR infants is 3.2 percent. This is less than the mortality rate for appropriately grown preterm but more than for appropriately grown term babies. An additional problem with SGA infants is a considerable increase in intrauterine fetal death. Death from intrapartum asphyxia in SGA babies is 10 times higher than for appropriately grown infants. Fourteen percent of all stillbirths and 6 percent of all neonatal deaths occur in infants whose birthweight is less than the third percentile for gestational age.[25]

Clinical Characteristics

The general appearance of the SGA infant varies from normal, at least at first glance, to one of general emaciation, which is more uncommon. The length and the head, chest, and abdominal circumferences often are less affected by fetal deprivation than the weight. Measurements other than weight may be normal or somewhat lower than normal for an appropriate-size baby of similar gestational age. The skull sutures may be wide secondary to failure of bone growth. The weight/length ratio is lower than normal. The length is likely to be 50 percent or more greater than the weight in SGA infants, indicating some degree of growth in length in excess of growth in weight. The weight-length ratio is useful for giving some indication of the duration of the malnutrition. Subcutaneous fat deposits and muscle mass may be quite low for maturity. The skin may be thin, loose, and with folds, and may be peeling, dry, and cracked. The umbilical cord may be thin.

Parameters of maturity—sole creases, hair texture, and ear cartilage—are similar to those of normal infants of the same gestational age. Breast size may be normal, or it may be considerably smaller owing to diminished growth of tissue.

Neurologic maturity ordinarily is not affected, and the examination is usually appropriate for actual gestational age. SGA infants are more advanced in motor ability, reflexes, alertness, and ability to take food than preterm infants of similar weight.

Chronic oxygen deprivation *in utero* in IUGR is likely to result in a higher hemoglobin concentration, high hematocrit, and higher erythrocyte count in these infants than in their gestational peers.

The SGA newborn has poor glucose control and may have both hyperglycemia and hypoglycemia. Thermoregulation is more limited than in appropriately grown term infants, but better than in premature infants of the same weight.

When growth retardation is severe, the SGA infant may have the appearance of the postmature infant described on page 637. SGA and postmaturity syndrome may be just a continuation of the same problem.

Neonatal morbidity and mortality are increased in infants with IUGR. Morbidity is likely to result from perinatal asphyxia, hypoglycemia, hyperbilirubinemia, and polycythemia.

Obstetric Management

Obstetric management of the SGA fetus will depend on suspicion of fetal growth retardation. This may be based on findings that the fundal height is not growing according to what should be expected for the period of gestation, that the uterus remains small, and that the mother is not gaining weight appropriately. On such suspicion it is important to recheck the estimate of gestational age, based on menstrual history and laboratory tests.

Rate of growth of the fetal head may be determined by serial biparietal diameter measurements. When the biparetal diameter grows less than optimal, the birthweight is also often low.

When the mother is known to have conditions that are likely to cause a reduced uteroplacental blood flow, such as chronic hypertensive vascular disease or diabetes, evaluations of placental function and fetal well-being are made during pregnancy. These include serial biparietal diameter measurements, estriol determinations, and weekly or semiweekly non-stress tests or oxytocin challenge tests or fetal activity determinations. These evaluations are described in Chapter 13.

Having the evaluations of fetal well-being and fetal maturity the physicians must make the decision if it is safe for the pregnancy to continue or if early delivery is advisable. The risks of a hostile, intrauterine environment must be balanced against the problems of early delivery. To avoid the risk of a premature infant who also has IUGR, maturity of the fetus should be attained before delivery whenever possible.

Intrapartum care must be managed carefully whenever IUGR is suspected. Continuous monitoring of the fetus during labor is very important. A fetus with IUGR does not tolerate labor well because the uterine contractions restrict uteroplacental blood flow sufficiently to augment any fetal hypoxia which already may be present. Fetal distress may develop early as shown by late decelerations and loss of beat-to-beat variability. Cesarean section delivery may be indicated to avoid further stress of labor.

With the great risk of birth asphyxia and aspiration in the SGA baby, it is important that the pediatrician or someone equally capable is present at delivery to carry out resuscitation and to give all other care for the infant immediately after birth.

[24] George Cassady, The small-for-date baby, in *Neonatology, 2nd* ed., edited by Gordon B. Avery. Lippincott, Philadelphia, 1981, p. 263.
[25] *Ibid.*

cess carbon dioxide in the blood, at least not in the early stages of the disease. In pulmonary disease of the newborn hypoxia is much more common than hypercapnia.

In some cases of uneven ventilation-perfusion ratios blood flow is decreased or bypasses alveoli that are ventilated. This results in an increased retention of carbon dioxide and an increase in arterial Pco_2. An elevated arterial Pco_2 is called hypercapnia or hypercarbia.

Sometimes, in response to stimuli or in an attempt to correct for lack of oxygen, hyperventilation occurs. With hyperventilation carbon dioxide is blown off in excess and the arterial Pco_2 decreases. In this circumstance, oxygen tension level may be normal or continue abnormally low, and the Pco_2 will also be low. This situation is almost always iatrogenic with bag-and-mask ventilation or the use of a respirator.

Blood samples for measurements of both arterial Po_2 and Pco_2 are very important laboratory tests that are used to determine the status of respiratory distress and the necessary treatment.[3] The Po_2 measurement is necessary to determine the extent of hypoxia, which cannot be judged by the infant's color. The presence of cyanosis will indicate hypoxia but not the degree. Often the infant already has had some of the ill effects of hypoxia by the time cyanosis appears, or else the infant's color may not change much even when hypoxia is relatively severe. The Pco_2 measurement is used to determine how well ventilation is taking place and also to measure how much carbon dioxide is collecting in the blood.

Poor alveolar ventilation, with resultant hypoxia, leads to abnormal biochemical and physiologic changes in the body. Tissue hypoxia results in anaerobic metabolism, which leads to metabolic acidosis. When adequate oxygen is not available, glucose is incompletely metabolized to lactic acid instead of to carbon dioxide and water. The lactic acid accumulates in the body, lowers the pH, and brings about a metabolic acidosis. Anaerobic glycolysis also depletes glycogen stores quickly because more glycogen is required for glucose production when oxygen is not available. Anaerobic metabolism is not very efficient and uses up a great deal of glycogen to produce energy. The result of all this is often hypoglycemia, especially when stores are small.

Cardiopulmonary Consequences of Altered Blood Gases

Constriction of the pulmonary arterioles and a reopening of the ductus arteriosus are other serious consequences of hypoxia. This situation is greatly accentuated if acidosis is also present. When the pulmonary arterioles constrict and the ductus arteriosus opens, there is pulmonary hypoperfusion with impairment of circulation through the lungs and a reestablishment of shunting of blood through the ductus arteriosus and also the foramen ovale. These changes are similar to some aspects of the fetal circulatory pattern. Blood flowing through the lungs is not well oxygenated, and some of the blood may return to the systemic circulation unoxygenated. Hypoxia worsens and hepatic and renal function may be suppressed.

Correction of Blood Gases

Oxygen is administered for treatment of hypoxia, and ventilation of the lungs is necessary if the infant is not able to move air in and out of the lungs adequately. With reoxygenation of the tissues, complete glucose metabolism is restored. Production of lactic acid decreases and pH improves with a lessening of metabolic acidosis. The pulmonary arterioles respond with less constriction, and the ductus arteriosus may close again. Circulation through the lungs improves.

Acid-Base Balance

Carbonic acid is one of the products of normal tissue metabolism. It is categorized as a volatile acid because it is converted constantly to carbon dioxide in the blood and eliminated in its gaseous state through the lungs. The respiratory system thus directly controls blood levels of carbonic acid. The concentration of carbonic acid in the blood is determined by the amount of carbon dioxide present (by the Pco_2), and the amount of carbon dioxide in the blood is dependent on the ventilatory ability of the lungs.

Ordinarily the respiratory center of the medulla responds quickly to the need to eliminate carbon dioxide from the body or to conserve it and directs the respiratory rate and depth accordingly. With respiratory disease, however, the lungs may not be able to eliminate carbon dioxide adequately. This retention of Pco_2 and its carbonic acid counterpart then results in an acidosis. Measurement of Pco_2 is very important therefore in helping to determine how much the retention of carbon dioxide is contributing to an acidosis. Similarly, if hyperventilation is contributing to excessive loss of carbon dioxide, the Pco_2 level will show that.

An acid-base equilibrium is normally maintained in the body and is necessary to normal function. Normal metabolism produces acids which must be neutralized and excreted from the body. These acids are volatile (carbonic acid, described above) and nonvolatile (or fixed) acids, principally lactic, sulfuric, and phosphoric acids. The nonvolatile acids are buffered in the blood and excreted through the kidneys. A buffer is a substance that combines chemically with excess acid or

[3] Pao_2 and $Paco_2$ refer to partial pressure of oxygen and carbon dioxide in arterial blood. The subscript "a" usually will not be used in this chapter because the measurements of these gases customarily are taken from arterial blood and the symbols "Po_2" and "Pco_2" are understood to mean partial pressure of oxygen and of carbon dioxide in arterial blood.

base to modify changes in the body acid-base balance. Normally, when nonvolatile acids, such as lactic acid, are added to the blood, their effect is minimized through the buffering activity of the bicarbonate–carbonic acid system. In this reaction lactic acid is buffered by sodium bicarbonate and converted to sodium lactate and carbonic acid. The sodium lactate is excreted by the kidneys and the carbonic acid by the lungs, as described above. Thus the respiratory center regulates the concentration of volatile acid, and the kidneys control the blood content of nonvolatile acid. The kidneys respond more slowly than the lungs but tend to carry compensatory mechanisms closer to completion.

Any serious illness in a newborn is likely to lead to an acid-base imbalance. Disturbance in acid-base equilibrium is described by a measurement of the acidity of the blood, known as the pH. Abnormalities may result in a lowered pH (acidosis) or an increased pH (alkalosis). The normal pH ranges from 7.35 to 7.45. For normal metabolic processes to take place, the acid-base balance must be kept within these very narrow limits. A pH below 7.25 clinically represents considerable acidosis. Although the range between normal and abnormal values is small in numbers, there is a tremendous difference in the acidity of the fluid where there is a small change in the numerical value of the pH.

Acidosis and alkalosis may be of respiratory or metabolic cause or a combination of both. Respiratory acidosis occurs when ventilation is inadequate and pulmonary gas exchange is decreased. Carbon dioxide is then retained in the blood, which means an increased Pco_2. Respiratory alkalosis occurs with excessive elimination of carbon dioxide during hyperventilation. The Pco_2 is then low. In newborns the cause of respiratory alkalosis is most frequently mechanical ventilation that is given above physiologic needs.

Metabolic (nonrespiratory) acidosis occurs when there is an increase in nonvolatile acids in the body because of overproduction of acids, or impaired renal excretion of acids, or excessive loss of the base that serves to buffer the acids in the body. In newborns this condition is most likely to occur when hypoxia leads to anaerobic metabolism and an overproduction of lactic acid.

Metabolic (nonrespiratory) alkalosis means an increased concentration of base (bicarbonate). In the newborn this condition most frequently is caused by administration of an abnormally large dose of sodium bicarbonate, sometimes used to correct acidosis. On occasion, repeated vomiting is a cause.

Sometimes acid-base disturbances are present even when the pH is normal or nearly so. In such instances the body tries to compensate for the abnormality through adjustment in lung or renal function. A normal ratio between the acid and base is partially or fully restored. The pH then may be normal or nearly so, but the values for the acid and base are abnormally high or abnormally low. This is called a compensated acidosis or alkalosis. The original source of the acid-base disturbance may still exist in this condition, and the correction of the pH may only be temporary.

The presence of acidosis or alkalosis is determined from pH measurement of the blood. The pH measures the hydrogen ion concentration after any buffer activity has taken place. The pH by itself does not indicate whether an abnormality in the pH is of respiratory or of metabolic origin. To determine its source, it is also necessary to measure the Pco_2 and the plasma bicarbonate of the blood. The plasma bicarbonate measures the total bicarbonate concentration, of which the normal values are between 20 and 25 mEq/liter. An example of using Pco_2 and plasma bicarbonate values to determine the cause of acidosis is as follows: a high Pco_2 and normal plasma bicarbonate in the presence of a low pH would mean an uncompensated respiratory acidosis, whereas a normal Pco_2 and low plasma bicarbonate with a low pH would mean an uncompensated metabolic acidosis.

Base excess (BE) or deficit is a value that is also important in management of the infant with acid-base imbalance. The base excess is a value that is calculated rather than measured directly. It may be expressed as a positive or negative value, with the negative value also referred to as base deficit. The base excess indicates in mEq/liter the amount of blood buffer base that remains after hydrogen ion is buffered. Normal values of base excess in newborns ranges from $+4$ to -4 mEq/liter.

Base excess can be calculated from a nomogram when hemoglobin and two of the following parameters are known—the blood pH, CO_2, plasma bicarbonate, or total carbon dioxide content of plasma. In the infant the pH and Pco_2 measurements are usually the ones used to calculate base excess.

Differential Diagnosis of Respiratory Distress

Respiratory distress in the first days of life may be caused by many conditions. Among these are hyaline membrane disease, aspiration, pneumonia, asphyxia, central nervous system depression, metabolic disturbances, tracheoesophageal fistula, cardiac problems, and many others. It is important to differentiate between pulmonary, cardiac, CNS, and metabolic causes.

Differential diagnosis can be very difficult, but often a complete history of past events and close observation of signs in the infant will give clues to a likely cause. For example, respiratory distress in a premature infant suggests hyaline membrane disease; a postmature infant or one who is stained with meconium-stained amniotic fluid it suggests aspiration; a history of premature rupture of the membranes and/or prolonged labor may mean pneumonia; excessive maternal analgesia and/or anesthesia may mean central nervous system depression in the infant; choking after feedings and history of hydramnios require search for tracheoesophageal fistula; and an infant's inability to breathe with the mouth closed suggests choanal atresia.[4]

A most useful and absolutely essential diagnostic aid is a chest x-ray, which at least will show or rule out such serious problems as a pneumothorax and a diaphragmatic hernia. When diagnosis is difficult, a number of laboratory procedures, an electrocardiogram, a lumbar puncture to look for central nervous system problems, and perhaps other tests may be indicated.

Common causes of respiratory distress are asphyxia at birth, hyaline membrane disease, transient tachypnea, and meconium aspiration. These will be described below.

Observation, Intervention and Nursing Care

Treatment of respiratory distress consists of a number of supportive measures and protection of the infant against further stress. It includes adequate oxygenation, assisted ventilation when indicated, correction of acid-base imbalance, adequate caloric and fluid intake, protection against heat loss, and provision for rest.

For some causes of respiratory distress there will be specific therapy, as, for example, the administration of antibiotics when an infant has pneumonia and aspiration of air from the chest when a pneumothorax is present. In addition, however, a number of the supportive measures described below are important in the treatment of respiratory distress from any cause. Administration of oxygen and assistance in ventilation are of major importance in coping with all respiratory problems.

Use of Oxygen

The most important consideration in treatment of infants with respiratory distress is to improve their oxygenation. This is necessary for adequate tissue oxygenation and normal cardiac output and renal perfusion. Without good oxygenation the fetal circulatory pattern will persist, lactic acid will be produced with its resultant acidosis, poor renal function will develop, and shock is likely to develop.

Oxygen can be both very beneficial and very hazardous to newborns, especially prematures, and it must be administered with great care. The desirable amount of inspired oxygen is that which will provide adequate tissue oxygenation without undue risk of damage to certain tissues from an excessive amount.

The oxygen tension or partial pressure is measured in millimeters of mercury. The partial pressure can be thought of as a driving force that determines the degree to which oxygen will move from plasma to tissues.[5] In normal adults the arterial Po_2 (Pao_2) is in the 90 to 100 mm range. Current information indicates that an arterial oxygen tension between 50 and 80 mm Hg is satisfactory in the newborn.[6] It should not exceed 100 mm Hg in the infant.

With hypoxia anaerobic metabolism takes place, lactic acid is produced, and acidosis develops. The ductus arteriosus and the lung arterioles are sensitive to arterial Po_2 and to blood pH levels. With hypoxia and acidosis the ductus arteriosus opens, and the lung arterioles constrict, raising pulmonary vascular resistance and reducing pulmonary blood flow. This induces further hypoxemia by adversely affecting the ventilation and perfusion in the lung. This leads to a reduction in surfactant synthesis. A vicious cycle is set up of hypoxia which leads to further pulmonary insufficiency, which leads to more severe hypoxia.

Clinical cyanosis is not ordinarily as useful a guide for need for oxygen in the infant as it is in the adult. In the newborn the Po_2 will be below 50 mm Hg and perhaps even much lower when cyanosis appears. The arterial partial pressure of oxygen will give a much closer idea of the amount of oxygenation of tissues.

Oxygen administration is used clinically when hypoxemia exists in order to improve or maintain oxygenation until the condition causing the hypoxemia is remedied. It is used therefore in asphyxia and resuscitation, in cardiopulmonary disorders, and in conditions where cerebral tissues are affected by such conditions as meningitis or intracranial hemorrhage.

Increase in oxygen concentration of inspired air (FIo_2) is used in respiratory distress syndrome where shunting in both ventilation and perfusion takes place and in pneumonia, where oxygen cannot diffuse well. The dose of oxygen is expressed as its fraction of inspired air (FIo_2).

Oxygen will act as a vasodilator when hypoxia has caused vasoconstriction. This generally happens at high concentrations of ambient oxygen resulting in a sudden jump in arterial Po_2. If oxygen then again is lowered rapidly and in large decrements, there may be a disproportionate fall in arterial Po_2 and vasoconstriction may follow. A gradual reduction in inspired oxygen concentration will minimize or avoid this flip-flop effect.

A patent ductus arteriosus, relatively common in prematures and also in respiratory distress syndrome, is more likely to close with high-oxygen breathing. Closure

[4] Mary Ellen Avery and Barry D. Fletcher, *The Lung and Its Disorders in the Newborn Infant,* 3rd ed., W. B. Saunders, Philadelphia, 1974, pp. 309–11.

[5] Leo Stern, The use and misuse of oxygen in the newborn infant, *Pediatr. Clin. North Am.,* 20:447, (May) 1973.

[6] W. Alan Hodson and William E. Truog, Special techniques in managing respiratory problems, in *Neonatology,* 2nd ed., edited by Gordon B. Avery, Lippincott, Philadelphia, 1981, p. 417.

is not likely to be permanent from this effect, however. It is important to add that, although hypoxemia should be corrected to enhance closure of the ductus, oxygen is not given to attempt closure in the absence of hypoxemia.

Since tissue hypoxia results in anaerobic metabolism and metabolic acidosis, the administration of oxygen will improve metabolism and help correct such acidosis.

Correction of acidosis will decrease pulmonary vascular resistance and promote closure of the ductus arteriosus. This diminishes right-to-left shunts and is followed by improved oxygen uptake. As a result, the blood Po_2 level is likely to rise far above normal during oxygen therapy as soon as the blood pH is corrected, unless the inspired oxygen concentration is decreased to levels appropriate to the infant's changing needs. Thus, frequent monitoring of inspired oxygen need must accompany correction of an acid pH.

Method of Administration

Oxygen is administered in concentrations between 21 and 100 percent, depending on the amount needed to keep the baby's Po_2 normal. (Room air contains 20.9 percent oxygen.) Very high inspired oxygen concentration may be necessary in some conditions to maintain adequate arterial oxygenation. Arbitrary limits such as 40 percent (formerly considered safe) cannot be set. Oxygen must be ordered and administered in percentage (concentration) rather than by liters per minute. Flow rates (liters per minute) to oxygen gauges give an indication of how much oxygen flow is required for various environmental oxygen concentrations, but they are not acceptable for guides to oxygen administration.

Several types of oxygen analyzers are available to monitor the percentage of oxygen. One kind requires manual sampling of the ambient oxygen concentration, which must be done at least every two hours. Another kind monitors the inspired oxygen continuously. High and low limits may be preset with an alarm system. Some equipment and respirators may have devices for regulating oxygen concentration, but they should not be relied upon totally.

Continuous transcutaneous measurements of arterial Po_2 and/or frequent measurements of arterial blood samples are necessary to determine the appropriate amount of inspired oxygen to be administered and to be able to decrease its concentration as soon as possible. Blood samples may be taken every 4, 8, or 12 hours depending on the severity of the infant's illness, the concentration of the inspired oxygen, and the ease or difficulty of obtaining blood.

Mixtures of oxygen and air may be administered by several methods including incubator, oxygen hood, face mask, and nasal prongs or endotracheal tube when the infant is given ventilatory assistance. When the ambient concentration does not need to be high it may be allowed to flow into the infant's *incubator*. The incubator, however, is ineffective for high concentration because the portholes need to be opened frequently for infant care. Concentration of oxygen greater than 30 percent cannot be maintained in incubators and flow is likely to be unsteady with opening of the portholes. If the lid of the incubator must be opened the oxygen will be dissipated very quickly. An *oxygen hood* around the infant's head permits better control of the oxygen concentration and allows a considerable amount of the care of the infant without disturbing the hood (Fig. 31–1A). A removable lid on the hood allows positioning and suctioning of the infant without loss of inspired oxygen concentration. Oxygen is heavier than air and is not lost easily. When an oxygen hood is used, gas flow through the hood should be at least 2 liters/min to prevent accumulation of carbon dioxide.[7]

Oxygen also may be given by *mask* (Fig. 31–1B), and when mechanical assistance to ventilation is necessary, it may be given by mask, by *nasal prongs,* or sometimes by *endotracheal tube*.

By whatever method oxygen is given, it must be humidified and warmed. The gas mixture is bubbled through water which may be warmed by a heating coil. Prolonged use of oxygen by mask is contraindicated. It is very likely to chill the infant even if the oxygen is warmed because the flow of oxygen from the mask over the infant's face results in considerable heat loss by convection. The oxygen hood has somewhat the same effect. A cap on the infant's head helps to protect it. Warming the oxygen is very important. Humidity and warmth also are extremely important with nasal prongs or endotracheal tube administration because the oxygen is then introduced directly over mucosal tissue. Dry air would increase evaporative fluid loss from the mucosa and augment evaporative heat loss. The mucosa also dries easily with dry air and secretions become thick and tenacious.

In relation to the exquisite thermal sensitivity of nerve ending in the skin of the face and the forehead Dr. Sheldon B. Korones warns:

"A constant blast of cold gas to the infant's face produces the responses to cold stress, even though the remainder of the body is in a thermoneutral environment, since thermal sensors of the face are more responsive than the skin sensors in any other part of the body."[8]

Blood Gas Monitoring

When oxygen is administered, frequent measurements of Po_2 are necessary to regulate the concentration of inspired oxygen. It must be administered in an amount that will return the Po_2 to normal but not raise it above

[7] *Ibid.*, p. 272.

[8] Sheldon B. Korones, *op. cit.* p. 224

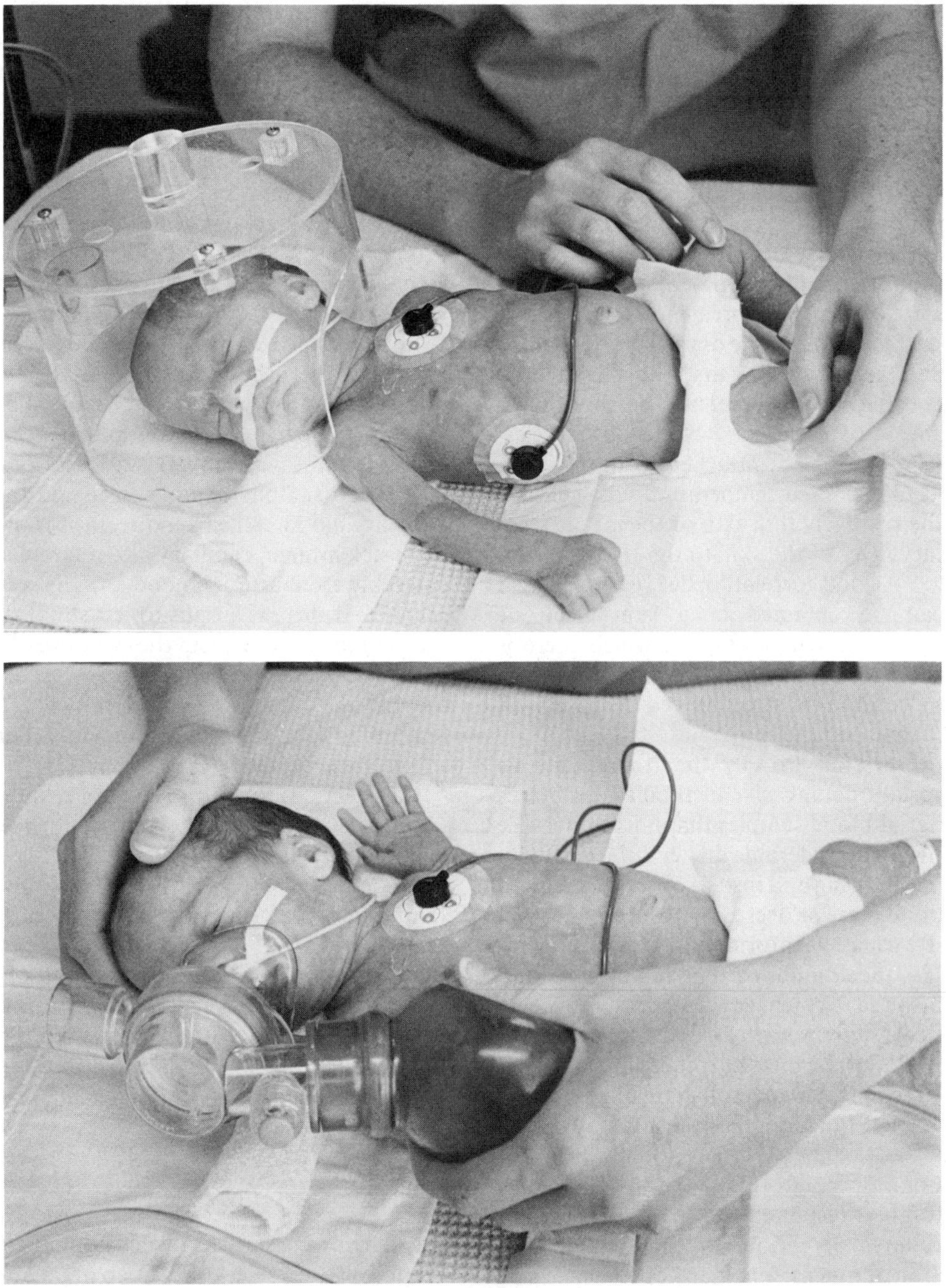

A

B

Figure 30–1. *A.* This infant is receiving oxygen by a clear plastic hood over his head. This makes it possible to have good control over his ambient oxygen concentration and permits giving much of the infant's care without disturbing the hood. Note that the baby's heart and respiratory functions are being monitored. *B.* This infant is receiving oxygen by face mask. The bag and mask may be used for assisted ventilation of the lungs if indicated. (Reprinted from the booklet *Special Care Nursery,* Madison General Hospital, Madison, WI, 1978. Photograph courtesy of Madison General Hospital and Ohio Medical Products, both of Madison, WI.)

normal. Requirements for oxygen may change very rapidly as ventilation and circulation through the lungs change. Every effort is made to maintain the Po_2 between 50 and 80 mm Hg.

The Pco_2 measurements are used to determine the amount of ventilation that is taking place. Since Pco_2 rises with hypoventilation and decreases with hyperventilation, it is the carbon dioxide tension of the blood, not the partial pressure of oxygen, that gives the correct indication of hypo- or hyperventilation. Carbon dioxide tension is an important measure in determining when ventilation needs assistance. Also when assisted ventilation is being used, the proper level of alveolar ventilation (as determined by the pressure, volume, and rate settings) is regulated on the basis of arterial Pco_2 measurements.

Blood gas monitoring can be done by transcutaneous Po_2 measurements, by indwelling arterial catheter, by intermittent puncture of accessible arteries, and by capillary sampling of blood. More than one method is likely to be used during the course of an infant's illness.

Noninvasive continuous monitoring of arterial Po_2 by transcutaneous Po_2 (tc Po_2) measurements is an excellent indirect method of monitoring the oxygen tension of the blood of an infant receiving oxygen. With this method blood Po_2 is measured transcutaneously on skin that is arterialized by means of a heated Po_2 electrode. The electrode for $tcPo_2$ monitoring is attached to the infant's skin and heated to a desired temperature. Oxygen diffuses through the relatively thin skin of the infant from the outer capillary layer of the skin to the electrode and measures the Po_2. A good correlation between $tcPo_2$ and arterial Po_2 can be obtained at a skin electrode temperature of 44°C, a temperature at which there is adequate vasodilation of the capillary bed under the electrode. The electrode must be moved every 2 to 4 hours to avoid damage to the skin.

Monitoring of arterial Po_2 by the transcutaneous route is an important noninvasive method that replaces the frequent arterial blood samples that must otherwise be drawn, often with considerable difficulty. It provides for continuous monitoring and instant observation of an infant's need for increase or decrease in ambient oxygen concentration. By using the information to optimum advantage it reduces the amount of time required to find the optimum inspired oxygen concentration, the best level of ventilatory support, the desired respirator setting, and the infant's response to procedures. It also helps to quickly recognize changes that are likely to take place if equipment malfunctions or if the infant develops complications.

Transcutaneous Po_2 monitoring makes it possible to know how the infant is responding to the effect of treatments, to procedures of various kinds, to positional changes, to suction of mucus, and many other aspects of care. Transcutaneous continuous monitoring makes it possible to know how the infant is responding at the instant the value is read. Handling of the infant and crying often cause hypoxemia. This can be seen in the $tcPo_2$ reading and the infant care can be modified, temporarily interrupted, or postponed until the $tcPo_2$ returns to normal. Blood sampling provides accurate information at the time the sample was taken, but it does not provide information about the intervals between samples.

Although continuous transcutaneous Po_2 monitoring is very valuable, it must be considered an adjunct rather than a substitute for intermittent blood sampling in a sick infant. It is still necessary to measure Pco_2 and pH from blood samples in sick infants and probably also arterial Po_2. Severe hypotension and perhaps other conditions may interfere with the accuracy of transcutaneous measurement.

Arterial blood samples are usually taken for Pao_2, $Paco_2$, and pH. The blood may be obtained from one of several sites. In very sick infants, who need frequent checks, a catheter may be inserted into the umbilical artery and left in place. Otherwise, blood samples may be collected from puncture of the temporal, brachial, or radial arteries. With good circulation, blood samples from a warmed heel or finger are acceptable for Pco_2 and pH. The heel or finger should be warmed with a warm, moist pack before the needle stick for obtaining the blood is made. The warmth dilates the capillaries and arterioles so that blood flows freely during collection. The blood sample then is considered to be arterialized capillary blood. When venous stasis is present, as it may be in sick infants, capillary blood samples may vary considerably from arterial blood and the results may be less reliable. If there is a right-to-left shunt through the ductus, a blood sample from the right radial artery, which is preductal and independent of the degree of shunt through the ductus, reflects more closely the oxygen content going to the brain and the eyes than a sample obtained from an umbilical artery.

Capillary blood samples are not reliable for Po_2 determinations. They do not correlate with arterial Po_2 levels. When a premature infant is receiving oxygen, which must be monitored carefully to avoid hyperoxia, blood samples for Po_2 certainly must be obtained from an artery.

Blood samples for blood gases and pH may be taken every 4 hours or somewhat more or less frequently, depending upon the stability of the infant's condition. They are also taken within 15 to 30 minutes after changes in ambient oxygen and after setting changes when assisted ventilation is used.

Hyperoxia

Oxygen has a toxic effect when administered in excess. It is known to adversely affect two organs, and it may have a detrimental effect on other tissues. The retina of the eye may be damaged when the arterial Po_2 rises too high, and the lungs are injured when the concentration of inspired oxygen is high and the period of administration is long.

Bronchopulmonary Dysplasia

The effect of oxygen on the lung appears to be a direct effect of irritation of the lung tissue by the oxygen. A condition called bronchopulmonary dysplasia develops. Changes in lung tissue result in collapse of alveoli, atelectasis, and thickening of alveolar and lung vascular structures. These toxic changes make the lungs less permeable to oxygen and further increase its need. These lung changes clearly show the need for careful assessment of an appropriate, not excessive, amount of oxygen administration to newborns through careful monitoring of arterial oxygen tension. It is important to note, however, that in spite of continuing risk of prolonged oxygen administration, its use may be essential to sustain the infant until he can survive without it.

The danger of high ambient oxygen, especially above 60 percent, is increased when used with endotracheal tube and mechanical ventilation. The exact relationship of these three factors in causation of this progressive chronic lung disease is not known.

In most instances bronchopulmonary dysplasia has been preceded by hyaline membrane disease. Once changes in the lung tissue develop and diffusion of oxygen from the alveoli to the capillaries is impaired, the problem in the lung may not resolve for months. With the passing weeks and months the inspired oxygen concentration and the ventilation pressure may need to be increased to maintain normal arterial blood gas levels. In advanced cases the lungs develop air cysts. Emphysema progresses and the lungs become greatly hyperinflated. Right ventricular problems are likely to develop.

Infants with BPD often require many months of hospitalization and some will die of respiratory or cardiac failure. In those infants who recover reduction in inspired oxygen concentration must be done very slowly until they can finally survive in room air. Recently a few oxygen-dependent infants have been cared for by their parents at home while they are recovering and being weaned from their increased oxygen need.[9]

Retrolental Fibroplasia

Retrolental fibroplasia, a retinopathy of prematurity, was discovered in 1942 as an acquired disease of premature infants. The disease is not present at birth; it results from too great exposure to oxygen. A high arterial concentration of oxygen (Po_2) causes changes in the immature retina of the premature and in the vitreous, and retinal detachment may follow. A retrolental (behind the lens) membrane forms as scar tissue develops (fibroplasia). The opaque tissue or grayish membrane behind the lens results in partial or complete blindness. Before prevention of this disease was known, it was a common cause of blindness in children.

By 1955 the cause of retrolental fibroplasia had been determined, and it is now a less common condition. Its frequency has been reduced by careful use of oxygen for hypoxia only, for the shortest time possible, and at the lowest concentration possible.

In rare cases retrolental fibroplasia occurs when oxygen has not been used or has been used only very briefly.

There appears to be considerable variability in arterial Po_2 at which the earliest phase of vasoconstriction of the retinal vessels occurs. Vascular spasm appears at less than 100 mm Hg in some infants. Degree of immaturity and perhaps other factors may contribute to this. The very early phase of vascoconstriction appears to be reversible. Watching for this early period by ophthalmoscopic examination may afford a means of early assessment of potentially toxic reactions in the retina to oxygen, and also another means of monitoring and controlling oxygen levels during the need for its administration.[10]

While prematures who are receiving continuous oxygen and are being monitored carefully appear to be quite safe against the effects of too much oxygen, small prematures who are resuscitated frequently from apneic episodes with a bag and mask connected to a direct oxygen line may be in danger of receiving too much oxygen. Some of these infants have a fairly normal cardiopulmonary function, do not have large right-to-left shunts of blood, and ordinarily are receiving little or no oxygen, but they have episodes of apnea. During resuscitation with bag and mask and oxygen they are exposed to very high oxygen concentrations which produce high levels of arterial Po_2. It therefore is highly recommended that a self-inflatable bag and mask be kept in the incubator and used with the incubator air for relief of apneic episodes in these infants so that the inspired oxygen concentration is not changed during the resuscitation procedure.[11]

Other Organs

There is increasing concern that vasospasm similar to that of the retinal vessels may occur during hyperoxia in other blood vessels of cerebral origin and thereby reduce the blood flow to other areas of the central nervous system. Certain adverse effects of excessive oxygen have been shown experimentally and suspected clinically, among which are changes in the renal tubules and an increased rate of destruction of red blood cells.

Oxygen Administration Summary

The desirable amount of inspired oxygen is that which maintains the infant's blood oxygen tension within safe effective limits. If an infant is breathing well and is of good color, he does not need oxygen therapy, regardless of how small he is. If the infant has respiratory distress, oxygen must be given in sufficient amount to maintain a normal arterial oxygen tension (50 to 80 mm Hg). The Po_2 should not exceed 100 mm Hg. Attempting to main-

[9] Marrianne Ruskay Glassanos, Infants who are oxygen dependent—sending them home, *MCN* 5:42–45, (Jan./Feb.) 1980.

[10] Leo Stern, *op. cit.*, p. 457.

[11] Leo Stern, *op. cit.*, p. 458.

tain the inspired oxygen concentration at 40 percent or less to avoid damage is not appropriate; 40 percent may be too much for some infants and too little for others. It is sometimes necessary to raise the inspired oxygen concentration to 60 or 80 percent and even higher to maintain an adequate arterial oxygen tension.

Optimum and reasonably safe use of oxygen requires accurate and careful monitoring of both the amount of oxygen in the blood and the concentration of oxygen in the inspired air. The concentration of inspired oxygen must be measured with an oxygen analyzer at least every one to two hours. The performance of the oxygen analyzer must be checked daily by calibration with room air and 100 percent oxygen. When possible, constant oxygen analyzers should be used.

A frequent adjustment in the concentration of inspired oxygen is made according to the infant's condition as determined by the arterial oxygen tension. The condition of infants requiring oxygen may improve rapidly. Under these circumstances, the inspired oxygen concentration should be lowered promptly, at least by 10 percent decrements at frequent intervals guided by blood gas measurements.

It is essential to chart both the inspired oxygen concentration, as measured by an oxygen analyzer, and the infant's color every time an adjustment in inspired oxygen concentration is made. The infant's muscle tone, which is a good indicator of blood pH, also should be noted. When changes are not frequent, charting is important at least every two hours.

Emergency Administration of Oxygen

The nurse should assume responsibility for rapidly increasing the inspired oxygen concentration if an infant's condition warrants it. This may happen if the infant has aspirated or becomes cyanotic for some other reason.

When the infant is a dusky color, his blood oxygen concentration is too low. His arterial Po_2 is below 50 mm Hg and perhaps even much lower. Since the ductus arteriosus and the lung arterioles are sensitive to blood Po_2 and pH levels, the ductus arteriosus may open and the lung arterioles may constrict if the Po_2 is less than 40 mm Hg. Shunting of blood then will follow. Therefore, when an infant is dusky, oxygen administration probably is best approached from the top. The oxygen flow should be turned high enough to rapidly flood the incubator, quickly achieving a high environmental concentration of oxygen for the infant, or oxygen may be given by bag and mask or from an oxygen tube held to the infant's face. A high inspired oxygen concentration is important at the beginning to raise the arterial Po_2 to a level where the pulmonary resistance will decrease and the ductus arteriosus will close. Small gradual increases of oxygen may not increase the blood Po_2 level enough to stop shunting of blood and an irreversible cycle of hypoxemia and shunting may result.

When facilities for blood gas determinations are available, these must be done promptly to determine the appropriate inspired oxygen percentage for continuing administration. In a clinical setting without facilities for measuring blood gas quickly, monitoring of oxygen need will have to be done by color, at least temporarily. As soon as the infant's color is pink, the concentration of inspired oxygen should be lowered in decrements of 10 percent every 30 minutes until the infant's color shows signs of becoming dusky. At this point the concentration of inspired oxygen is increased by 5 to 10 percent, which usually is a very rough approximation of the appropriate amount to maintain good oxygenation and still not cause hyperoxia.

If the infant becomes dusky after the concentration of inspired oxygen is decreased, raising the concentration slightly may result in return of a pink color. If color does not improve, it is necessary to increase the amount of inspired oxygen to a high level once again and then resume the gradual decrease as before. When it appears that the infant's color will remain good (one to two hours), the concentration of inspired oxygen is decreased further and then discontinued.

When supplemental oxygen is necessary for an immature infant, he should be cared for in a hospital in which inspired oxygen concentration can be regulated on the basis of blood gas measurements. Arrangements should be made for transfer of the infant to an intensive care facility as soon as possible.

Ventilatory Support

An infant may need assistance with ventilation in order to move adequately air in and out of the lungs, and/or to keep the alveoli from completely collapsing at the end of expiration.

The infant must move enough air in and out of the lungs to provide adequate oxygen to the tissues and to blow off enough carbon dioxide to avoid a buildup of this gas in the body. Assistance with moving air in and out of the lungs may be necessary (1) if breathing is not adequate in depth or frequency because of respiratory center depression, which may happen when maternal drugs cross the placenta; (2) if the baby becomes tired with breathing, as may happen with the increased work of breathing with hyaline membrane disease; and (3) if partial airway obstruction presents a problem, as may happen with aspiration of meconium. In any of these circumstances the infant is given ventilatory assistance until he has recovered from the underlying problem.

An infant sometimes needs assistance with breathing when the alveoli tend to collapse at the end of each breath owing to an insufficient amount of surfactant. In this circumstance the infant may have the ability to move air in and out of the lungs normally, but each breath is a great effort. In normal breathing some air is retained in the alveoli at the end of expiration, and the next breath can be taken with ease. With a deficiency in amount of surfactant the alveoli collapse at the end of expiration, and each breath requires as much, or almost as much, effort as the first breath. This is the situation in hyaline membrane disease. In this kind of respiratory difficulty areas of atelectasis develop, and there is also little reserve air left in the lungs between breaths. Also blood that flows through the atelectatic areas of the lungs does not become adequately oxygenated, and it returns to the left side of the heart with an inadequate supply of oxygen. This is termed right-to-left shunting of blood through the lungs. Assistance with the kind of breathing difficulty that permits collapse of alveoli involves some method that will help the infant to keep the alveoli open at the end of expiration.

If, along with respiratory difficulty because of collapsed alveoli, the infant also has trouble moving air in and out of the lungs because he is tired or has depressed respiration, he will need assistance with both problems at the same time. For assistance with ventilation an infant therefore may need a respirator that will provide (1) intermittent positive pressure ventilation (IPPV) to assist the infant to move air in and out of the lungs, or (2) a system that provides continuous distending airway pressure or continuous positive airway pressure (CPAP), which will counteract the tendency of the alveoli to collapse, or (3) a respirator that provides for the IPPV and also has a mechanism that will provide background CPAP or positive end expiratory pressure (PEEP) to help keep the alveoli open at end expiration. Several methods of ventilation are described below.

Bag and Mask

A bag and mask, with which air can be forced into the lungs when the bag is squeezed, is the simplest method of ventilation. The bag is attached to a face mask held firmly over the infant's face. The bag may be self-inflatable or flow-inflated. The self-inflatable bag returns to its original position after it is squeezed. It fills with the surrounding air, which means that it can be used anywhere. The flow-inflated bag is filled by being connected to a source of compressed air or oxygen.

The self-inflating bag has the advantage of not requiring a source of compressed air or oxygen, but it has several disadvantages. It is not possible to regulate accurately the oxygen concentration with this bag; most self-inflating bags do not deliver oxygen above 40 to 50 percent without an adaptor and may not deliver any air flow without being compressed; and they cannot be used to apply continuous positive airway pressure. The flow-inflated bag and mask setup should be capable of delivering any concentration of oxygen desired and can be used for continuous positive airway pressure and for intermittent positive pressure if desired and at various pressures and rates of ventilation as seems necessary. It should also permit heating and humidification of the gas, and have an escape valve for carbon dioxide. The bag should have a preset blow-off valve or a pressure gauge attached in order to enable the person using it to determine the amount of pressure delivered. The operator, however, must rely on clinical assessment rather than a blow-off valve for safety.

Bag and mask ventilation is a short term means of assisting ventilation. Bag breathing may be used for a number of reasons. It can be used for resuscitation in the delivery room for inflation of the lungs and delivery of oxygen to the baby (Fig. 21-11, p. 415), and it can be used at the bedside for infants who have spells of apnea. For infants in danger of respiratory difficulty a bag must always be available at the bedside in case of emergency. A bag and mask may be used in the nursery to support ventilation and to provide oxygen for the infant who is having some difficulty maintaining ongoing ventilation. In this respect it is used before need for mechanical ventilation is established.

When intermittent positive pressure ventilation (IPPV) is used, the mask is held firmly against the infant's face and the bag is squeezed in time with the infant's inspirations. When continuous positive airway pressure (CPAP) is used (with the flow-inflated bag), more gas is permitted to flow into the bag than is permitted to escape; pressure builds up in the system and is transmitted to the infant's airway and alveoli as the mask is held firmly against the infant's face. As the infant breathes spontaneously against this continuous positive pressure, the pressure helps to keep the alveoli from complete collapse at the end of each expiration. Continuous positive airway pressure and intermittent positive pressure ventilation can be used at the same time for the infant who needs that much ventilatory support. Since Po_2 rises significantly with ventilation, it is frequently necessary to ventilate with less oxygen concentration than has been used when the infant has been breathing spontaneously. Blood gas measurements are very important and must be done as quickly as possible.

When a bag and mask is used to help an infant move air in and out of his lungs, certain checks must be made for proper use of the bag. To avoid inadequate ventilation, the infant should be observed closely (1) for chest movement, especially of the apices, with each inspiration, (2) for improving pink color of the lips, and (3) for breath sounds with each inspiration. The ventilatory rate should be 40 to 60 times per minute, and the depth of ventilation should not be above that normally expected of the newborn. Any long-term ventilation requires frequent checking of blood gases and nasogastric tube for decompression of the stomach.

The bag and mask is most useful for short-term use and during transfer of an infant to an intensive care unit. Guidelines for bag and mask ventilation for short term use, as presented by Jerry Novak Mason, are shown in Table 30-1. For prolonged assisted ventilation, a more permanent arrangement is necessary. Machines or

Table 30-1. Suggested Methods of Emergency Hand Ventilation*

Condition	*Rate in Breaths per Minute (BPM)*	*Concentration of Inspired Oxygen (F_{IO_2})*	*Peak Pressure (cm H_2O pressure)*	*Positive End Expiratory Pressure—PEEP (cm H_2O pressure)*
Depressed neonate in delivery room (state of lungs unknown)	40–60	100%	Very first breath: 40–60 Other breaths: 16–25	0
Neonate with normal lungs (acute distress)	40–60	If witnessed deterioration, may try less than 100% If unwitnessed, 100%	16–20	0
Neonate with known diseased lungs (as initial stabilization before transport)	40–60	100%	16–25	Up to +5

*If efforts do not result in improvement of neonate's condition, other appropriate measures to be taken include (1) reassessment of airway (that is, need for suctioning and intubation); (2) emergency medicines including correction of hypovolemia; and (3) use of other bagging techniques such as increasing the F_{IO_2}, increasing the rate, using a PEEP or increasing the PEEP, and carefully increasing peak pressure (these techniques create increased risk of complications).

Source: Reprinted with permission from Terry Novak Mason, "A hand ventilation technic for neonates." *MCN* 7:366–69, (Nov./Dec.) 1982.

equipment that provide continuous distending airway pressure or intermittent positive pressure ventilation or both then are used.

Continuous Distending Airway Pressure

Continuous distending airway pressure, also called continuous transpulmonary pressure, is used quite extensively for treatment of respiratory distress syndrome, a common neonatal respiratory problem, which is described below. Continous distending airway pressure counteracts the tendency in this complication of the alveoli to collapse with each expiration and thus is helpful in improving oxygenation. The effects of continuous distending airway pressure are accomplished by continuous positive airway pressure (CPAP), or continuous negative pressure (CNP), or positive end expiratory pressure (PEEP).

With CPAP, a gas pressure greater than atmosphere is applied to the airway continuously during spontaneous breathing. With the CNP a pressure less than atmospheric is applied around the thorax during spontaneous breathing. With PEEP positive airway pressure is applied during the expiratory phase of breathing that is assisted mechanically. CPAP was introduced in 1971 to augment treatment of RDS.[12] Prior to that time artificial airway pressure had been used, but there were many difficulties in adapting it to small infants, and it was used only late in the disease.

Continous distending airway pressure achieves for the infant some of the beneficial effects that the infant achieves for himself when he grunts with expiration. With a grunt the end expiration is prolonged. This maintains the lung at a slightly larger volume for a longer period of time so that gas exchange can take place. This, plus rapid breathing, may prevent complete collapse of alveoli before the infant can take his next breath. The functional residual capacity of the lung thus remains more normal.

When constant distending pressure or end expiratory pressure is applied to the airway during respiration, the alveoli are kept from collapsing completely at end expiration. This improves gas exchange. As the terminal bronchioles and alveoli are kept open, functional residual capacity, that amount of air still remaining in the lungs at the end of the breath, is increased. This allows for continued diffusion of oxygen between breaths. Right-to-left shunting of blood past atelectatic areas also decreases. Blood pumped through the lungs reaches more aerated areas and can pick up oxygen much better. Arterial Po_2 increases significantly with continuous distending airway pressure. The exact mechanism by which the arterial Po_2 increases is not completely clear, since there is a significant increase in oxygenation even without a very significant change in total ventilation.

Continuous distending airway pressure is also likely to reduce the infant's work of breathing. When the alveoli do not collapse completely at the end expiration, they will reopen more easily with the next inspiration. The large amount of effort and energy the infant has been using to take each breath can be reduced. Signs of respiratory distress (retraction) improve.

With CPAP, an infant who is breathing spontaneously is attached to a system that applies a constant distending pressure to the airway. The pressure may be applied to the upper airway by means of a head hood, a face mask, or nasal prongs, or if it becomes necessary to

[12] G. A. Gregory *et al.*, Treatment of the idiopathic respiratory distress syndrome with continuous positive airway pressure, *N. Engl. J. Med.*, 284:1333–40, (June 17) 1971.

apply pressure to the lower airway, it is done by endotracheal tube. With CPAP, gas is brought into and held in a relatively closed system in a larger amount than is permitted to escape. The gas source should be able to supply any selected mixture of air and oxygen with warmth and humidification. Exhaust tubing and a means of regulating the amount of gas escaping help to regulate the amount of pressure in the system. A pressure relief valve, a pop-off, inserted into the system, is used to prevent extremely high pressures from accidentally occurring.

Continuous distending pressure is used most effectively in treatment of respiratory distress syndrome (hyaline membrane disease). Indications for its use vary somewhat, but there is fairly general agreement that a Po_2 below 50 mm Hg is unsatisfactory. CPAP may be instituted when it has become necessary to raise the concentration of oxygen the infant is breathing to 60 percent to try to maintain the Po_2 at 50 mm Hg. Sixty percent oxygen is an arbitrary choice, since it is not known what percentage of oxygen is toxic to the infant, and because of right-to-left shunting, higher concentrations of oxygen may not change Po_2 very much. High and prolonged concentration, however, is thought to be more toxic to the lung than the lower percentages.

The amount of carbon dioxide retention is also a factor in determining when ventilatory assistance should be given. A Pco_2 of greater than 70 mm Hg warrants ventilatory support in the form of intermittent positive pressure ventilation. When the Pco_2 is elevated but less than 70 mm Hg, other factors such as severity of distress, rate of rise of Pco_2, oxygen requirements, and presence of apneic spells are taken into consideration in a decision to provide assisted ventilation.[13]

Episodes of prolonged apnea that are accompanied by severe bradycardia or that do not respond to tactile stimulation require support of ventilation regardless of the blood gas values.[14]

All methods of continuous distending pressure have advantages and disadvantages; a number of these have been enumerated by Affonso and Harris.[15] It appears, however, that CPAP with nasal prongs is a widely used system.

CPAP must be regulated carefully for appropriate humidity and temperature and pressure of the gas. The air-oxygen mixture is passed through a humidifier and must be carefully observed for appropriate moisture. If the mixture is too dry, the infant's mucous membranes may become dry and thick; tenacious mucus may develop and block the airways. Suctioning of the airways may be necessary every two hours. Excessive humidification causes large droplets of fluid to form in the circuit, and these may get into the airway and cause distress.

The air-oxygen mixture is warmed so that it will not cause the infant to become chilled. Overheating, however, would cause hyperthermia.

The amount of CPAP pressure applied is critical and must be observed carefully. The goal is to apply just enough pressure to help open alveoli and keep them open, but not to overdistend any alveoli that already are considerably distended. Improvement in the infant's color and blood oxygen tension can be expected when the pressure level is appropriate. There should be little rise in arterial Pco_2. Blood gases must be monitored frequently, and the CPAP pressure must be checked periodically.

In thinking of levels of pressure in relation to ventilation, the following information may be a guide:

©3 cm H_2O = approximately the same pressure as is normally applied by the glottis.
6–8 cm H_2O = may prevent further atelectasis.
6–10 cm H_2O = general therapeutic range for keeping the alveoli from collapsing completely and preventing atelectasis.
□12–14 cm H_2O = not safe. Probably cannot be achieved with nasal prongs or with face mask.

The infant on CPAP must be observed constantly, since a change in condition may occur quickly. Observation includes looking for cyanosis or ruddiness, checking the heart rate, especially for bradycardia, observing the respiratory rate and pattern, and the infant's tone and activity.

The oxygen concentration in the air-oxygen mixture and the CPAP pressure are adjusted according to blood gas results. They are lowered as soon as the infant begins to improve, so that the infant will not be exposed to oxygen or to extra pressure over any unnecessary period of time.

CPAP sometimes leads to complications of pulmonary air leak or rupture of an alveolus, and reduction in venous return to the heart when airway pressure is too great. Alveoli may become overdistended, decreasing compliance, and eventually the high inspiratory pressure may cause an air leak into interstitial spaces. Air may reach the mediastinal area and cause a pneumomediastinum, or it may break through the pleura and result in a pneumothorax, with collapse of a portion of a lung. Difficulty with air leaks and its consequences may be suspected when the infant's condition suddenly worsens. He quickly develops tachypnea, cyanosis, decreased chest movement on one side, poor air or no air exchange on one side of the chest, displacement of heart sounds, and a general overall appearance of distress. Equipment must be available to remove air from the chest and establish chest drainage.

Some of the CPAP pressure is transmitted through the

[13] W. A. Hodson and W. E. Truog, *op. cit.*, p. 424.

[14] W. A. Hodson and W. E. Truog, *op. cit.*, p. 424.

[15] Dyanne Affonso and Thomas Harris, CPAP: Continuous positive airway pressure, *Am. J. Nurs.*, 76:570–73, (Apr.) 1976.

lungs to the mediastinum. As the lung compliance improves, more of the airway pressure reaches the mediastinum, where it may put pressure on the large vessels returning blood to the heart. This may obstruct venous blood return to the heart and lead to a decrease in cardiac output. The CPAP pressure should be reduced as soon as pressure on large vessels appears to be present.

Mechanical Ventilation

It sometimes happens that CPAP alone is not sufficient respiratory support, and the infant needs additional mechanical ventilation. Certain guidelines according to Jan Nugent are as follows: "Mechanical ventilation should be considered when apnea is protracted, when constant positive airway pressure has failed (Pao_2 is less than 50 mm Hg in 100% oxygen at distending pressures of 10 to 12 cm H_2O), or when blood gases reveal respiratory failure. Generally, a pH of less than 7.25, a Pao_2 of less than 50 mm Hg, and a $Paco_2$ of greater than 60 mm Hg in 60% oxygen indicate a need for some form of respiratory assistance."[16]

A respirator provides intermittent positive pressure ventilation (IPPV) to assist the infant to move air in and out of the lungs and also may have a built-in mechanism to provide the infant with positive end expiratory pressure (PEEP) or background CPAP. Such an arrangement makes it possible to assist the infant with adequately moving air in and out of the lungs and also with preventing complete collapse of the alveoli at the end of each expiration.

Respirators are now fairly versatile. This makes it possible to use a machine for IPPV alone or with PEEP or to use CPAP alone or with intermittent ventilation.

Intermittent mandatory ventilation (IMV) is another variation of a ventilator. This ventilator can be set for predetermined mandatory frequency of ventilation for the infant. The machine does not cycle in response to the infant's expiratory effort, but it does have a continuous flow of fresh gas through the circuit at the desired Fio_2. It is therefore possible for the infant to take extra breaths of fresh gas independent of the predetermined rate if he desires. The infant is thus able to superimpose his own breathing pattern over that provided by the ventilator.

Assisted ventilation with the machines described above is a specialized procedure that requires expertise in care and management of the infant and laboratory and x-ray facilities available at all hours. This type of care is given in neonatal care centers. A referral system should be available so that infants who develop respiratory distress can be transferred safely from community hospitals to specialized facilities. When respiratory distress can be anticipated, transfer of mother and infant to an intensive care center can sometimes be arranged prior to the infant's birth.

[16] Jan Nugent, Acute respiratory care of the newborn, *JOGN Nurs.* (Supplement): 31s–44s, (May/June) 1983.

Correction of Acid-Base Imbalance

Any serious illness in a newborn is likely to lead to an acid-base imbalance. An infant with respiratory distress is in danger of developing hypoxia, hypercapnia, and acidosis. Oxygen is used to correct hypoxia, and assisted ventilation may be necessary to correct hypercapnia. Acidosis, also needs correction as soon as possible. Respiratory acidosis is corrected by ventilation to reduce blood carbon dioxide levels. Metabolic acidosis is treated by improving oxygenation, by ascertaining that there is adequate perfusion of tissues, and in certain severe cases, with alkali therapy. Alkali treatment is only indicated when there is no response to ventilation and when other signs of distress, such as bradycardia, do not improve.

Since blood pH alone does not indicate whether an acidosis is of respiratory or metabolic origin, it is important to obtain a Pco_2 before therapy is started. Accumulation of carbon dioxide in the blood raises the Pco_2 and results in a rapid fall in blood pH, leading to a respiratory acidosis. If the acidosis is almost entirely of respiratory origin, as determined by an elevated Pco_2, therapy with sodium bicarbonate will not correct the acidosis and is then inappropriate treatment. In fact, administration of sodium bicarbonate is contraindicated with severe respiratory acidosis. Sodium bicarbonate gives off carbon dioxide, which these infants cannot blow off with their respirations, and their respiratory acidosis worsens. Mechanical ventilation is the only effective treatment for high Pco_2. Such ventilation is usually given when the Pco_2 is 60 mm Hg or over.

If the blood pH is low and Pco_2 is normal or nearly so, the acidosis is of metabolic origin. A combination of respiratory and metabolic acidosis is a common situation.

When acidosis is of metabolic origin and does not improve with oxygenation and adequate perfusion, intravenous administration of sodium bicarbonate may be used. The milliequivalent dose and the volume and route of administration of this base are determined on the basis of the degree of metabolic acidosis and the urgency for correcting the acidosis. Usually the base deficit is determined, and the dosage of sodium bicarbonate is calculated accordingly.

The base deficit can be calculated from a nomogram when the hemoglobin concentration, the blood pH, and the Pco_2 are known. With an acidosis this value will be a negative base excess or base deficit. The dosage of sodium bicarbonate to be given then is computed from a formula which states: mEq of sodium bicarbonate to be given = base deficit (mmEq/liter) × 0.3 × body weight in kilograms. The factor of 0.3 in this formula represents the approximate portion of the body weight that is made up of extracellular fluid.[17] It should be noted that there is some disagreement on the true bicarbonate space, the values ranging from 0.3 to 0.6 of body weight. Usually the 0.3 figure is used for calculation.

Sodium bicarbonate in the above concentration is available in ampuls of a 7.5 percent solution containing 0.88 mEq/ml. For ease of calculation for clinical use, the concentration of sodium bicarbonate in this solution may be considered to be 1.0 mEq/ml.[18] Sodium bicarbonate in the above concentration is hypertonic and may damage blood vessels if used undiluted and also will draw fluid into the vascular system. It therefore must be mixed with at least two times, and preferably five times its volume with water for injection. Some of the dosage may be injected over a period of several minutes and the remainder added to intravenous fluids, or all may be added to an intravenous fluid drip.

Dosage and timing of administration of sodium bicarbonate are done with great caution. Sodium bicarbonate can be the cause of very serious problems. Since carbon dioxide will be released from the sodium bicarbonate that is administered, and this also has to be eliminated through the lungs, ventilation must be good when sodium bicarbonate is given. If ventilation is poor, the carbon dioxide tension of the blood may rise, and respiratory acidosis will develop. This will produce a further reduction in the blood pH value.

Rapid administration of sodium bicarbonate may also present a problem by raising the serum osmolality to the high level that is associated with intraventricular hemorrhage. Hyperosmolar blood causes a shift of fluid from the extravascular space into the blood vessels. The blood vessels then become distended and the capillaries may rupture.

Treatment of Hypovolemia

Infants with respiratory distress, especially hyaline membrane disease, often have a low systemic blood pressure. Systemic hypotension will increase the right-to-left shunting of blood through the ductus arteriosus, especially when the pulmonary artery pressure is high. Infants with hypotension cannot be oxygenated properly and may develop shock.

When hypotension is present, it is dealt with by administration of albumin or plasma or small transfusions. Plasma and/or blood usually is given in any amount that equals 10 to 20 ml/kg of body weight. If hypotension was caused by blood loss, the infant may need up to 20 ml/kg for volume replacement.

Blood sampling for laboratory data, especially when done frequently, slowly reduces blood plasma and cell volume. A careful record must be kept of the amount of blood removed. Usually a small blood transfusion is given periodically to replace the blood that was removed for sampling.

Protection Against Heat Loss

An ambient temperature that is high enough to maintain the infant's body temperature at approximately 98° F (36.7° C) axillary or 98.6° F (37° C) rectal is crucial to the welfare of an infant with respiratory distress. If the infant must attempt to maintain a normal body temperature in an environment in which he loses body heat, the amount of oxygen needed to meet his increased metabolism for heat production is greatly increased. An infant with respiratory difficulties may not be able to meet the body's basal oxygen needs under such conditions. Even when the infant does increase his metabolic rate considerably, he may not be able to maintain his body temperature at a normal level while he is in a heat-losing environment. When oxygen needs cannot be met, the infant may need to change to anaerobic metabolism, which then may result in a buildup of lactic acid and metabolic acidosis.

To control the temperature environment, the infant may be placed in an incubator or on a neonatal intensive care unit (Fig. 29–4, page 613). On the open bed of the neonatal intensive care unit the infant is kept warm by a radiant heater. To maintain the body temperature between 98 and 98.6° F (36.7 and 37° C) (when the infant is in an incubator), the temperature in the incubator may need to be raised to 95° F (35° C) or above. It may be advisable to use a heat lamp over the roof of the incubator for radiant heat to the infant and, when possible, to use a skin thermistor for regulation of incubator temperature. A radiant heat lamp also is used to reduce heat loss during any procedure that increases exposure. When the infant is on an intensive care table, the skin thermistor is set to keep the skin temperature at 97.6° F (36.4° C), and care is taken to avoid drafts.

Nutrition

Adequate nutrition and good basic hydration are important for support in any disease. Intravenous fluids therefore are started very early in the disease to meet the infant's fluid requirements, to provide some caloric intake, and to ensure an adequate blood sugar level, which is often low in infants with respiratory distress.

Good basic hydration will vary, but in general, 140 to 160 ml per kilogram per 24 hours will maintain good water balance. For the first few days of fluid administration the average total fluid requirement is somewhat less (page 617). Excess water loss through the skin, especially when the infant is being cared for on an open bed heated by radiant lamps or through the kidneys because of di-

[17] Sheldon B. Korones, *op. cit.*, p. 176.

[18] Sheldon B. Korones, *op. cit.*, pp. 176.

uresis, may require a much higher fluid intake. A small infant with a large body surface and a small amount of subcutaneous tissue is in danger of evaporative water loss just as much as he is in danger of heat loss.

To recognize water loss the infant's skin turgor should be noted, the urinary output is measured by weighing the diapers or pads, and bodyweight is checked every 8 to 12 hours. Laboratory studies of urine specific gravity and serum electrolytes also aid in determining fluid need.

Ten percent glucose will prevent hypoglycemia and provide some calories, although not a sufficient amount to meet basal body needs. If the infant has a substantial amount of respiratory distress, and especially if he is a premature, his nutritional needs in the early days of life are often met by intravenous alimentation. Finally, when recovery is proceeding well, formula feedings by tube are begun with caution.

Glucose is offered as the first oral feeding and then a gradual change is made to milk feedings. Intravenous glucose is continued until the infant is able to take enough milk orally to meet his fluid and nutritional needs.

Parenteral Nutrition

Total parenteral nutrition is possible for infants who will be unable to take food over a prolonged period of time. This method of feeding infants has been proven useful for infants with gastrointestinal anomalies that require extensive surgery and for infants with chronic diarrhea and malabsorption syndromes and for those with necrotizing enterocolitis. It has increased survival of such critically ill infants significantly. Total parenteral alimentation has also been used to provide nutrition occasionally for infants with chronic respiratory failure.

With total intravenous alimentation the infant is given a constant infusion of a chemically complex mixture that meets the protein, caloric, water, electroyte, and vitamin needs for weight gain and positive nitrogen balance. The mixture is made up specifically for the individual infant each day and consists of protein hydrolysate or a mixture of pure crystalline amino acids to provide for amino acid needs, glucose to provide for calories, and minerals, vitamins, and appropriate electrolytes. Complete intravenous nutrition should include fat, a normal part of any diet, in order to avoid essential fatty acid deficiencies. INTRALIPID will provide calories without appreciably adding to the overall osmolality. Intravenous lipid cannot be mixed with glucose and amino acids, since the fat emulsion will break down. It is therefore given by "piggy-back" through a Y-connector so that it joins the glucose and amino acid mixture at the entry into the vein. When initiating use of fat emulsion it must be given slowly to observe for adverse reactions. INTRALIPID makes it possible to meet caloric needs with hyperalimentation of lower concentrations of glucose and protein, supplemented with INTRALIPID. This means that total alimentation by peripheral vein is possible.

The infusate is administered through an indwelling silastic catheter inserted into the superior vena cava via either the external or internal jugular vein or it is given through a peripheral vein. A constant infusion pump is used to maintain a constant rate of infusion. In general, the method of administering nutrition by catheter into the superior vena cava is used when it is anticipated that parenteral nutrition will be required for at least three weeks.

Peripheral infusion is made into one of the peripheral veins on the dorsal aspect of either the hand or the foot, or into one of the superficial veins of the scalp. Placing the needle and maintaining it in place often present a problem.

Initially the infusion fluid is started with low concentrations of glucose and protein. It is gradually increased to full caloric maintenance, which may not be attained before 7 to 10 days in low-birthweight babies.

Very careful monitoring of the infant is necessary during intravenous alimentation. All intake and output is recorded. The urine is examined for volume, specific gravity, protein, and glucose at each voiding. DEXTROSTIX for blood glucose is done at least every four hours. Blood glucose, electrolytes, BUN, serum proteins, hematocrit, and a number of other blood studies are done once, twice, or three times weekly. The infant's growth rate must be monitored carefully.

Complications of parenteral alimentation generally include sepsis, catheter-related problems, and metabolic problems. The infusion mixture promotes growth of certain organisms and fungi and must be mixed under strictly aseptic conditions. An indwelling catheter is placed in the operating room and is aseptically dressed and cared for thereafter. Strict adherence to placement and maintenance of the catheter reduces complications of malposition, dislodgement, and thrombosis.

Metabolic complications relate to the content of the parenteral solution. Hyperglycemia may occur owing to glucose intolerance. Acidosis may develop. Electrolyte imbalance may occur if the required amounts are misjudged, especially when infants have concomitant abnormal fluid losses. The blood urea nitrogen may become seriously elevated from excessive protein content, which must then be lowered.

Septic and metabolic complications appear to be less with use of a peripheral vein than with a central vein. Phlebitis and local complications from fluid extravasations and tissue sloughs may be a problem, and maintenance of influsion sites for an extended period of time becomes difficult. Infiltration of fluid will result in severe tissue slough if not discovered early.

Refeeding of the infant is begun with great caution and proceeds slowly with small amounts of food. Parenteral alimentation is discontinued very gradually, decreasing both the concentration and the amount of fluids as the infant increases his oral intake.

Stimulation of Sucking During Parenteral Alimentation

The infant who is on prolonged parenteral alimentation does not have the normal experiences of suck and swallow, hunger and relief of hunger by food, nor the taste and touch of food in his mouth. He will not receive the normal suck stimulation important to normal development unless a special effort is made to simulate feedings. The infant needs to be offered a pacifier and talked to, rocked, cuddled, and played with as he would be at a normal feeding time, or if he cannot be removed from the incubator, he can be given as much of this care as possible while in the incubator. Scheduled times at three- or four-hour intervals for feeding simulation will assure an appropriate amount of stimulation.

When the infant who has been on prolonged parenteral alimentation is permitted to begin feedings, he may take one or two more weeks to learn to develop a good suck-swallow pattern and to accept food and fluids from a nipple. If he resists taking fluids from a nipple, he is given feedings by dropper in very small amounts while he has a pacifier in his mouth. When he has learned to swallow fluid in this way, he can be offered a nipple. With the nurse's assistance and patience and effort the infant learns to take a small amount of food orally. Slowly the quantity can be increased. For an excellent discussion on nurses' techniques with feeding infants who have been on parenteral alimentation, as well as other aspects of care, the reader is referred to "Parenteral Alimentation," by Alice Conway and Tamara Williams.[19]

Position Changes

The infant with respiratory difficulty must have his position changed frequently to prevent pooling of secretions and thus hypostatic pneumonia, to maintain good ventilation, and to promote drainage of lung segments. The infant's position should be changed at least every hour, alternating between sides, prone, and supine positions.

The infant's own breathing ability may be improved when he is placed on his back with the bed elevated at the head at about a 30-degree angle. Since the cartilage in an infant's trachea is soft, and a head-forward position may compress the trachea, the infant's head should be slightly extended with a small towel under his neck and shoulders. Frequent checks are necessary to ensure that the small roll under the infant's shoulders does not slip under his head, causing it to flex. In this back position the diaphragmatic excursion may be better, the angle of the upper airway is reduced, and the upper air lobes may drain spontaneously.[20] This position, however, must not be used for more than one hour at a time.

Suction of Mucus

Removal of mucus and secretions from the respiratory tract is necessary for good ventilation. Suction with a catheter or a bulb syringe may be oropharyngeal, or through the nose, or through an endotracheal tube if one is in place. Keeping the infant's head straight or tipped back slightly during suctioning aids in getting suction to the respiratory tract.

In suctioning, the mouth always must be aspirated first. Putting a catheter in the nose is likely to stimulate the infant to inspire, and any secretions that are accumulated in the mouth and throat are likely to be aspirated. If a catheter is used for suction of the nostrils, it must be passed without force, using gentle rotation of the catheter between the thumb and forefinger to advance it. The catheter must be placed quickly without suction and then immediately withdrawn as intermittent suction is applied. Continuous suction is harmful to nasal and oral mucosa and may contribute to collapse of alveoli and developing atelectasis.

A newborn coughs infrequently, but secretions or stimulation with a suction catheter may stimulate a cough. Since the infant is likely to be unable to handle the mucus produced by the cough, the pharyngeal area should be suctioned immediately after a cough to avoid aspiration of the mucus back into the lungs.

Suctioning of an endotracheal tube should be intermittent and brief—5 to 10 seconds. Obstruction of an airway for a longer period of time is likely to produce bronchial spasm and hypoxia, vagal stimulation, and bradycardia and arrhythmia.

Bagging with slightly higher inspired oxygen percentage (5 to 10 percent higher than that being administered) before, during, and after suctioning may be indicated. Bagging with increased oxygen concentration helps to prevent a sudden dangerous drop in arterial oxygen tension during suctioning, and it decreases the likelihood of an adverse cardiac response. It is very advantageous to have $tcPo_2$ monitoring since the infant's reaction and arterial oxygen tension can be closely observed during suction. This will help determine the necessary oxygen administration.

Postural Drainage

For an infant with respiratory difficulty, postural drainage, positioning that uses gravity to drain bronchi,

[19] Alice Conway and Tamara Williams, Parenteral alimentation, *Am. J. Nurs.*, 76:574–77, (Apr.) 1976.

[20] Deon Dunn and Amber T. Lewis, Some important aspects of neonatal nursing related to pulmonary disease and family involvement, *Pediatr. Clin. North Am.*, 20:487, 1973.

may be implemented if symptoms indicate. It is especially useful in cases of prolonged endotracheal intubation and respirator care.

Gravity and pressure are the two main ways in which drainage of bronchial secretions can be facilitated so that gas exchange may be improved. For postural drainage the infant is placed into several different positions, at different times, so that gravity can move secretions from small bronchi to larger bronchi and to the trachea. Knowledge of the anatomy of the bronchi is essential to appropriate positioning.

Percussion with small plastic cups, followed by vibration, is a form of pressure that may be used to facilitate outward movement of bronchial secretions. These are special procedures in the newborn who presents special problems because of his very small tracheobronchial tree and his rapid respirations, especially when sick.

Persons caring for these infants must understand the principles of pulmonary therapy and must be able to carry it out quickly and efficiently to avoid undue fatigue in the infant. Bronchial drainage is fatiguing and stressful. Careful timing of the therapy and close monitoring of vital signs for the effects of treatment are essential. The nurse caring for the infant on an ongoing basis is likely to be the best person to do pulmonary therapy, knowing when the infant can tolerate treatment, how much, and how he responds to stress.[21]

Rest

Whereas the development of the normal infant is enhanced by stimulation, the sick newborn will not benefit and may well deteriorate from any stimulation in addition to the stress that already accompanies all the procedures that are necessary in his treatment. The sick infant usually is exposed to a number of intrusive procedures and a great deal of noise from the mechanical equipment. This causes excessive stimulation and loss of rest and sleep.

In an article written for the Neonatology Supplement of *Pediatrics* J. F. Lucey states:

> Picture yourself. . . . You're startled and frightened by loud, strange noises (beepers, voices, roaring respirators, telephones, radios, incubator noise). . . .
>
> You are sleep deprived. Everytime you doze off, somebody gets worried about you. They think you're in a coma. You have to be very careful to breathe *very* regularly. You're not allowed the multiple long pauses (15 seconds or more) of a sleeping, dreaming adult. If you do pause, a bell goes off, waking you up, and somebody slaps your feet or pulls your hair to see if you will or can cry. If you're exhausted or unresponsive, you're in trouble. If you have any jerky movements, you're suspected of having a convulsion.
>
> Every few hours somebody cuts your foot or sticks a needle into your scalp or one of your arteries. Your arms and legs are taped down to boards. Electrodes are attached to your chest. You're immobilized. . . .
>
> We all care "intensely" but in our zeal to care we may have become too enthusiastic and lost sight of the possible therapeutic value of rest, sleep, and quiet. . . .
>
> What should be done? Isn't all this "intensive care" very necessary? I believe it is, but I think we can minimize the stresses it places on babies by some simple changes in the techniques we use.
>
> Since the introduction of continuous transcutaneous oxygen tension monitoring, it has become apparent that the stress caused by such simple procedures as feeding, crying, suctioning, blood sampling, noise, physical examinations, lumbar punctures, and chest physiotherapy may cause repeated episodes of hypoxemia and hypertension. . . . We then find ourselves caught in a vicious circle as these iatrogenic episodes of hypoxemia result in more apnea, requiring more stressful handling and diagnostic studies.
>
> We have much to learn from studies utilizing the new techniques for continuous monitoring of heart rate, blood pressure, and arterial oxygen tension. One of the simplest and most effective things these studies may accomplish may be to remind us of the values of gentle handling and rest, which seem to have been forgotten.[22]

Intensive care surely will require that a number and a variety of procedures will need to be carried out and done so frequently, but these must be balanced insofar as possible with the infant's need for rest. The nurse plays an important role in planning care that provides for quiet periods which permit the infant the sleep that is also necessary for recovery.

As soon as the infant has recovered from his illness reasonably well and is ready and can tolerate stimulation he should be held, talked to, and played with, perhaps especially along with feedings. The parents can play an important role in holding the infant, feeding and playing with him at this time.

Disorders of Respiration

A number of causes of respiratory distress have been enumerated on page 643. A few of these conditions will be described in further detail. Since respiratory distress from any cause has many similar signs and symptoms and also requires similar care and intervention, that which already has been discussed will in general be applicable to the conditions described below.

ASPHYXIA AT BIRTH

A normal infant establishes respirations within one minute after birth, often taking his first breath within seconds after delivery. The chemical changes resulting

[21] *Ibid.*, p. 493.

[22] J. F. Lucey, Commentary. Is intensive care becoming too intensive, *Pediatrics,* 59, Part 2, Neonatology Suppl.: 1064–65, (June) 1977.

from the brief period of asphyxia during delivery stimulate the respiratory center, but if respirations do not begin almost immediately, the asphyxia increases, and it may then depress the respiratory center rather than stimulate it. If the condition is not quickly reversed, serious damage to tissues or death of the infant may occur.

Failure to breathe at birth, or failure to establish adequate respirations, is usually caused by three principal factors: intrauterine hypoxia, drugs, or central nervous system trauma. Infection of the fetus also may be a cause of distress. Many of the conditions enumerated under causes of respiratory distress on page 643, and also less common complications, lead to apnea or hypoxia through depression of the respiratory center. Sometimes the cause of distress originates in the respiratory tract as obstruction of the air passages. More than one condition that will cause apnea or hypoxia may exist at a time, but intrauterine asphyxia is a common cause.

The clinical condition of all newborns should be evaluated immediately after birth in order to institute resuscitative measures quickly if indicated.

The time of onset of sustained respirations with resuscitative measures depends on the duration and severity of previous asphyxia, the amount of depression from drugs administered to the mother, or the amount of trauma. An Apgar score below 4 indicates danger to the infant, and the longer the score remains low, the greater the danger. After resuscitation, scoring is repeated during the next 5 to 10 minutes for subsequent evaluation of the newborn. The infant also is examined for appraisal of his general condition.

Exposure of the infant should be reduced to a minimum during resuscitative procedures and the hours following. The infant should be kept as warm as possible while procedures are being carried out, and he should be placed in a heated incubator or bassinet as quickly as possible. The infant must be warmed to a skin temperature of 98° F as quickly as possible to reduce his metabolism and oxygen needs to their lowest level.

Subsequent care in the nursery depends on how rapidly and how well the infant establishes good pulmonary function, the cause of the respiratory difficulty, and the findings of the infant's general examination. The infant should be under intensive observation for further signs of respiratory distress, and for the effects of perinatal hypoxia and/or ischemia on other organs.

Numerous organ systems may be affected by an episode of intrauterine asphyxia, and this makes management of these infants potentially very complex. It is very important to evaluate the effects of asphyxia on the brain, since the brain is one of the vital organs that may be adversely affected by hypoxia and ischemia. The hypoxia occurs in association with the birth asphyxia. The ischemia, the diminished perfusion of the brain, usually is associated with the systemic hypotension that occurs with bradycardia, either prior to or after birth.

Some of the observations and care of infants following birth asphyxia are as follows:

1. *Respiratory:* The newborn with apnea at birth may have normal vital signs, remain alert, and cry spontaneously at intervals as soon as respirations are established, or he may continue for some time to show evidence of severe respiratory distress. Distress is characterized by rapid and labored respirations with chest retractions and cyanosis.

   When the infant has been narcotized as a result of deep maternal analgesia and anesthesia, he not only may have had difficulty in initiating breathing, but may continue to respond sluggishly even after crying. Skin stimulation and change of position at frequent intervals are necessary until the effects of the drug have worn off.

   Oxygen administration is continued if the infant continues with respiratory distress after respirations have been established.

   Even when the infant does not require further therapy for respiratory distress, he needs warmth and protection from exposure. Unessential care, such as a bath, can be postponed for many hours. The infant usually is kept in an incubator until his own body temperature can be maintained without stress.
2. *Vital signs* must be checked at least every hour. A check of heart and respiratory rate may be indicated every half hour.

   Blood pressure check and maintenance at normal are important aspects of care. The blood pressure should be taken at birth and every hour for the next 12 hours. The blood pressure should be maintained at normal range with use of fresh frozen plasma or plasma expander such as albumin given at 10 ml/kg.[23]
3. The *hematocrit* should be obtained soon after birth and repeated in 12 or 24 hours if indicated. If the mother had antepartum bleeding, the infant may have a low hematocrit. A hematocrit of 10 to 12 or lower requires administration of blood. Anemia may not be apparent, however, until after the first day. A hematocrit of 65 or greater is considered polycythemia and usually means that treatment by partial exchange transfusion is indicated.
4. The *blood sugar* should be checked as soon as possible after resuscitation and as frequently as indicated to assure that it remains within a normal range. The blood sugar value should be kept at 45 mg/100 ml or above. An asphyxiated infant, especially if small, if likely to become hypoglycemic very early. The infant quickly uses glycogen, and stores may be meager.

[23] A. W. Brann, Jr. and Francine D. Dykes, The effects of intrauterine asphyxia on the full-term neonate, *Clin. Perinatol.*, 4:149–61, (Mar.) 1977.

The brain must have glucose for its energy. A finding from animal data suggests that, even when the systemic blood sugar is normal or above normal in the asphyxiated patient, brain sugar may be less than normal. For this reason, blood sugar should be maintained above 45 mg/100 ml. Intravenous glucose solution is started early.[24]

5. *Fluids and acid-base balance:* Intravenous fluids of glucose may be given, at least during the first few hours after birth, and especially if the asphyxia has been severe. The infant who has been asphyxiated is not able to restore a normal acid-base balance as quickly as the infant who has breathed normally since birth, and he also quickly depletes his glycogen reserve. Glucose will promote recovery from the biochemical disturbances by helping to restore a normal acid-base balance and by replacing necessary glucose. Very occasionally sodium bicarbonate may be added to the intravenous glucose. The water will help to maintain a normal fluid balance.
6. *Renal function* should be assessed by careful measurement of urinary output, because a decrease in renal blood flow sometimes occurs during intrauterine asphyxia. Need for administration of fluids and electrolytes also may be determined by this assessment of renal function.
7. Observations for *cerebral effects* of asphyxia should include quality and variation in muscle tone, type of cry, presence and quality of sucking reflex, and clinical evidence of seizure activity. Any evidence of seizure activity must be evaluated promptly and treated (see page 702).

A great deal of consideration is now being given to determining if, and how much, brain swelling, along with resultant altered blood flow, occurs in the full-term asphyxiated infant, and how such swelling can be delineated and effectively reduced.

Prognosis

Prognosis following birth asphyxia depends on the degree of asphyxia and the length of time it existed. Delayed respirations may cause permanent damage to brain tissue. Postnatal complications in infants who had asphyxia at birth are greater than in those who had no respiratory difficulty.

The newborn infant at birth possibly may be able to tolerate anoxia and ischemia to a greater degree than an older individual, but this is not certain. The longer the period of insult, the greater the chances of damage to the central nervous system. Some infants apparently tolerate safely several minutes of apnea, while others have irreparable damage in a very short time. The length of time that anoxia and/or ischemia can be tolerated after birth is likely to be influenced by the amount of insult the infant suffered *in utero*.

Although the possibility of injury to brain cells during asphyxia is present, all asphyxiated infants do not later have manifestations of damage. If injury occurs, it may vary from a very mild degree that is quite inconspicuous to a severe defect in either motor control or intellectual ability, and may manifest itself in a variety of ways such as convulsions, mental deficiency, behavior problems, and cerebral palsy.

IDIOPATHIC RESPIRATORY DISTRESS SYNDROME OR HYALINE MEMBRANE DISEASE

Idiopathic respiratory distress syndrome (IRDS or RDS) and hyaline membrane disease (HMD) are terms often used synonymously. This is the most important cause of newborn respiratory distress, occurring mainly in prematures. It is a worldwide disease and an important cause of death in newborn infants. The disease develops in about one sixth of all premature infants, but the more immature the infant, the greater the incidence and the severity of the disease. It has carried about a 25 percent mortality rate, but survival is improving with modern treatment.

Respiratory distress syndrome appears in newborn infants who have a deficiency of the normal surfactant lining of the alveoli. The result of this deficiency is poor stability of aeration (see pages 499–500). The alveoli tend to collapse at the end of each expiration, retaining little or no residual air, and the infant has a generalized atelectasis. Atelectasis is the main pathologic alteration of this disease. The collapse of many of the alveoli reduces the amount of lung tissue capable of expansion and leads to marked respiratory distress. The infant needs to apply a large amount of pressure with each breath to try to open collapsed alveoli, and when they cannot be opened, the infant ventilates only a small portion of the lungs.

A material called a hyaline membrane, from which this disease derives its name, often forms in the alveoli and the bronchioles after the disease is in progress. The membrane does not appear until after several hours of breathing and is a consequence, rather than a cause, of the disease. The cause of the formation of the hyaline membrane, which is composed of protein high in fibrin and of cellular debris, is not known.

Immature infants and those who have suffered hypoxia before birth are highly susceptible to the neonatal respiratory distress syndrome. The disease appears in infants who have not reached an age where production of pulmonary surfactant is sufficient for adequate lung function and in those in whom production of surface-active lecithin is not sufficiently rapid to maintain

[24] *Ibid.*

alveolar stability. When conditions are unfavorable, either before or after birth, for ongoing rapid synthesis of surface-active lecithin, postnatal demands cannot be met. Surfactant can be depleted quickly, and, unless it is replaced continually, soon there will be a deficiency. The problem in respiratory distress syndrome is a very early birth when not enough stable lecithin has been produced or when there is an inability to meet the demands of postnatal respiratory adjustment by sufficiently rapid synthesis of surface-active pulmonary lecithin.

The inability to produce surfactant rapidly enough may be a result of pulmonary immaturity or factors that inhibit production. Production of surfactant is inhibited by any condition that interferes with good circulation through the lungs, reduces the amount of oxygen and glucose available to the lungs, and produces a low pH of the blood.

Asphyxia at any time, either before or after birth, interferes with good pulmonary circulation and adequate oxygenation and results in a lowering of the blood pH. Asphyxia owing to poor oxygenation *in utero* or difficulty in breathing after birth, quickly can inhibit production of surfactant. Chilling of the infant after birth may result in a reduction in the amount of available oxygen and glucose and in acidosis, thus also in the infant's ability to produce surfactant.

Maternal diabetes, maternal bleeding caused by placental separation, or any condition that causes intrauterine hypoxia carries an increased risk of respiratory distress in the infant. Such conditions, especially when coupled with prematurity, are likely to result in impairment of pulmonary surfactant production. Cesarean section seems to predispose to hyaline membrane disease, especially when it is done for fetal distress or maternal hemorrhage. In some families a familial factor appears to predispose to hyaline membrane disease, with a tendency for more than one infant in the same family to develop the respiratory distress syndrome. Boys are affected with hyaline membrane disease more than girls.

A deficiency in meeting the demands for production of surface-active lecithin seems to be self-limiting, and it disappears if supportive measures such as oxygen and correction of acid-base imbalance are provided and if the infant survives the first two or three days of the disease. Beginning about the third day of life, the capacity to form an alveolar surface film appears better, for reasons at present not clear. A spontaneous reversal to a normal condition of the lungs then occurs, and recovery from the instability of aeration takes place.

Progression of the Disease

Early Clinical Signs

Since loss of potential stability of aeration because of deficient pulmonary surfactant usually is present before birth, signs of difficulty will appear at birth or very soon thereafter. The infant may show definite signs of distress as soon as respirations are established, or his respirations and color may appear normal at first and his condition appear to be satisfactory. An asymptomatic period between birth and appearance of signs of distress, however, is apparently very short or nonexistent when the infant is carefully observed and evaluated. Very soon after birth, often within 5, 10, or 15 minutes, a moan or a grunt with respirations may be noticeable, and slight chest retraction is visible. As the condition progresses, signs of distress increase.

Respiratory distress is mild in some infants. In these infants signs of respiratory insufficiency gradually decrease after 12 to 24 hours, and recovery is rapid.

Later Clinical and Pathologic Signs

In many infants with hyaline membrane disease respiratory distress becomes progressively more serious. Chest retraction becomes severe owing to the large amount of effort that is necessary to inflate the lungs with each breath. The hard pull of the respiratory muscles on the soft thoracic cage causes marked indrawing of the intercostal spaces and of the sternum, and breathing may become seesaw. Grunting with expiration increases, and in severely affected infants expiration may be accompanied by a whimper or a cry. The respiratory rate rises to over 60 per minute within the first hours of life and may soon rise to 80 per minute or above. The work of the respiratory muscles is great, and they may not be able to function continuously as the disease progresses. Apneic periods and a decreasing respiratory rate may appear and are poor prognostic signs.

Since atelectasis is likely to increase during the disease, the infant's marked respiratory effort does not increase the adequacy of lung function. Cyanosis usually becomes apparent fairly early in the disease and is always present in severely affected infants.

The poor alveolor ventilation with hyaline membrane disease leads to abnormal biochemical and physiologic changes. The infant with respiratory distress is not able to correct the derangement in blood gases and the acidosis present at birth in the same manner in which the infant who breathes normally does. Poor lung function results in a decrease in arterial oxygen tension (Po_2), an increase in arterial carbon dioxide tension (Pco_2), and a lowering of the blood pH. A metabolic acidosis develops with the poor alveolar ventilation, may be superimposed on a respiratory acidosis, and causes the pH to fall considerably. As respiratory insufficiency continues or worsens, acidosis, both respiratory and metabolic, increases.

Pulmonary vascular resistance increases with abnormal blood gases and with acidosis. Shunting of blood through the ductus arteriosus and foramen ovale takes place. A persistent patent ductus arteriosus is fairly common. Considerable shunting of blood will contribute to a reduction in the arterial oxygen tension to a dangerously low level, making the infant's chance of survival poor. In addition to some of the blood bypassing the lungs by way of shunts through fetal blood vessels, all of the blood which does flow through the lungs may not be oxygenated. Some blood may be shunted through the atelectatic areas of the lungs and return to the systemic circulation unoxygenated. The progressive hypoxia in hyaline membrane disease may be caused by both poor ventilation of the lungs and this right-to-left shunting of blood through nonventilated areas of the lungs and through fetal vessels.

Increasing hypoxia and acidosis also lead to peripheral vasoconstriction. With poor peripheral circulation and possibly systemic hypotension the infant has a pale or an ashen-gray color.

Heat production in infants with hyaline membrane disease is low, and hypothermia, which is common in prematures, may be pronounced even in a relatively warm environment.

White, frothy mucus may be present in the respiratory tract.

Edema may develop with hyaline membrane disease, and there may be pitting in the extremities. Its cause is not known.

The infant with respiratory distress syndrome has poor muscle tone and is limp and unresponsive. Jittery movements owing to cerebral irritation sometimes appear. The infant typically assumes a position in which his thighs are widely abducted in a frog-leg position, his arms are flexed at the elbows, and his hands lie along each side of his head. This position may be related to the infant's immaturity as well as or instead of the respiratory distress.

It is apparent from the preceding description of hyaline membrane disease that it produces pulmonary, circulatory, and metabolic disturbances. A vicious cycle of events is likely with this disease. A deficiency in pulmonary surface-active lecithin leads to atelectasis and poor lung ventilation. This disturbance results in a lowered arterial oxygen tension, elevated carbon dioxide tension, and lowered pH and acidosis. The abnormal concentration of blood gases and the acidosis lead to pulmonary hypoperfusion, which in turn interferes with production of surface-lecithin (Fig. 30–2).

Babies who progress beyond the mild stage of the disease, in which recovery begins to be evident within 24 hours, will become progressively worse during the first 48 to 72 hours of life. Labored respiration becomes marked and the respiratory rate may continue to rise. If the respiratory and circulatory systems cannot meet the infant's needs, a severe anoxemia, a rising blood carbon dioxide tension, and a falling pH level may continue in

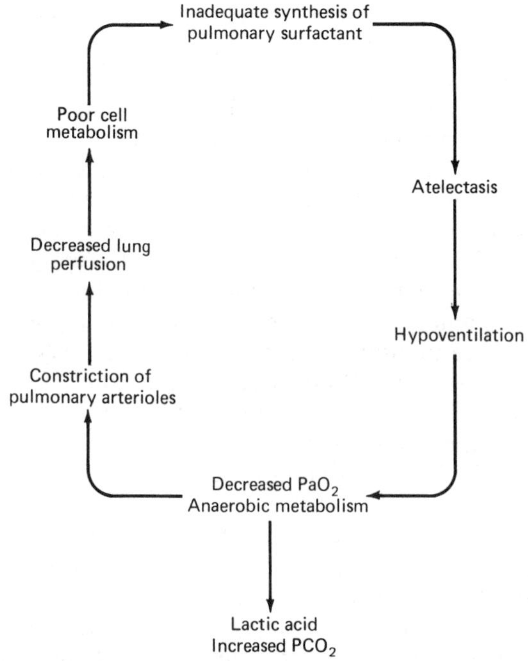

Figure 30–2. A vicious cycle of physiological disturbances in neonatal respiratory distress syndrome. Inadequate synthesis of pulmonary surfactant leads to atelectasis, a decrease in lung compliance, increased work in breathing, and decreased ventilation. Inadequate ventilation leads to hypoxia, hypercapnia, anaerobic metabolism, and acidosis. As a result of hypoxia and acidosis, the pulmonary arterioles constrict and the ductus arteriosus opens and pulmonary blood flow is decreased. Diminished pulmonary blood flow causes pulmonary ischemia and affects metabolism of the lung. This in turn decreases synthesis and secretion of pulmonary surfactant. The above sequence of events can start at any place in the cycle. For example, antepartum bleeding could lead to hypotension and reduced lung perfusion, asphyxia at birth could lead to hypoxia, hypercapnia, and acidosis, and hypoglycemia in the newborn could lead to poor alveolar cell metabolism. Each of these conditions and also others could start the cycle.

spite of therapy. The infant's color becomes an ashen cyanosis, and the respiratory rate may drop to 20 to 30 times per minute with long periods of apnea. If the infant succumbs, death usually occurs within 72 hours, mainly caused by respiratory failure.

Some infants survive even when they have had severe distress. When improvement takes place, it may be rapid and dramatic. Within 48 to 72 hours the infant is usually able to produce an adequate amount of pulmonary surfactant. With this, the alveoli become well aerated and the atelectasis disappears. The infant breathes easier by the third or fourth day of life and recovery proceeds rapidly. Long-term effects are not known. Survival is improving, and more information will become available.

Diagnosis

Hyaline membrane disease cannot be identified clearly by a clinical or laboratory finding, but diagnosis is inferred from clinical signs and symptoms, physical examination, and chest x-ray. A grunt with expiration very soon after birth, often within 15 minutes, chest retraction within the first hour of life, and a respiratory rate of over 60 per minute within a few hours suggest that great effort is necessary to ventilate the lungs. On chest x-ray the lungs show a fine mottling or granular appearance early in the disease and increased opacity later; the x-ray also shows air clearly present in the bronchi and shows hypoexpansion, which suggests atelectasis. A chest x-ray does not give conclusive evidence of the disease, but it aids in diagnosis and is important in ruling out other causes of respiratory distress.

Prevention

Preventive measures against hyaline membrane disease are those that help the infant to be born in optimum condition and assist him to make the transition to extrauterine life with minimum stress. These include prevention of premature birth, and optimum treatment of complications of pregnancy to protect the infant from intrauterine distress, if possible; protection against causes of asphyxia at birth, and protection against chilling at birth.

Prenatal identification of infants at risk of developing HMD through L/S studies is very important because delivery sometimes can be postponed until the lung matures, or if early delivery is likely or is indicated, glucocorticoids often can be given to accelerate lung maturation. The important finding that accurately predicts increasing fetal lung maturity is an increase in the concentration of lecithin in the amniotic fluid. Amniocentesis and measurement of the ratio of lecithin to sphingomyelin have been described on pages 246–48. When the concentration of lecithin is at least two times greater than the sphingomyelin, the probability of the infant developing HMD is very small.

Careful evaluation of the lung maturity of a fetus by L/S ratio is a necessary preventive measure prior to elective induction of labor or elective cesarean section. The L/S ratio is usually mature by 36 weeks' gestation, but it may be delayed until after 37 weeks. Lung maturation can be determined only by L/S ratio, and with such evaluation inadvertent delivery of an infant with immature lungs can be avoided. A "lung profile," a more detailed examination of the components of surfactant, may add to the information obtained about lung maturity prior to birth (see page 247).

Observation and Treatment

With careful observation of all infants immediately after birth, signs of respiratory difficulty can be detected very early. When the nurse recognizes early signs of respiratory distress and reports these to the physician immediately, the supportive care that the infant needs can be started before respiratory distress reaches a stage of serious physiologic disturbances. As the disease progresses, the nurse's continuous care of the infant often helps to avert serious difficulty if a sudden change in condition takes place, and her ongoing observations and reports to the physician provide an overall picture of the infant's progress and need for medical management.

Nursing care and observations of the infant with hyaline membrane disease can be inferred from the preceding description of the characteristics of the disease and its treatment. A brief comment on a number of these aspects of care follows.

Observation of vital signs and signs of respiratory distress must be made and recorded at hourly intervals at least. The infant's body temperature reading must be observed and the incubator temperature adjusted as necessary to raise the body temperature as quickly as possible to approximately 98° F (36.7° C) axillary or 98.6° F (37° C) rectally. Skin temperature, if possible, incubator temperature, and body temperature should be recorded.

The heart rate and respiratory rate must be observed closely. Monitoring machines may be used to monitor heart function and respirations, but these functions also must be closely observed visually and with the stethoscope. The blood pressure must be monitored carefully for variations from normal. A small newborn of 1000 to 2000 gm (2 lb, 4 oz to 4 lb, 7 oz) normally will have a blood pressure of approximately 50/30; one that weighs over 3000 gm (6 lb, 10 oz) will have a pressure of around 64/42.

Mucus must be suctioned from the respiratory tract as it appears, and the infant's position must be changed frequently to prevent hypostatic pneumonia.

Apneic spells must be observed, and if breathing does not resume readily, the nurse must stimulate and, if necessary, resuscitate the infant while the physician is called.

Treatment of infants with hyaline membrane disease is supportive. It is directed toward elimination or improvement of each abnormality in the cycle of events described above and includes careful regulation of the thermal environment, oxygen therapy, intravenous fluids to correct acidosis and provide for nutrition, continuous positive airway pressure or assisted mechanical ventilation, and protection from unnecessary exertion. Treatment must be started early in an attempt to avert major pathologic changes or to reverse changes before they become severe.

Treatment for HMD includes all of the therapies described for respiratory distress on pages 649–62. The most important consideration in treatment of infants with hyaline membrane disease is to improve oxygenation. This is essential for normal tissue oxygenation and for normal cardiac output and renal perfusion. Without good oxygenation anaerobic metabolism takes place and metabolic acidosis develops. Also, there will be pulmonary vasoconstriction and right-to-left shunting of blood. With hypoxia and acidosis, pulmonary hypoperfusion and fetal circulatory patterns will shunt considerable blood, which then does not become oxygenated.

The goal of oxygen administration is to maintain the Po_2 between 50 and 80 mm Hg. The infant is given enough oxygen to try to correct hypoxia, but great care must be taken to avoid hyperoxia and damage to the eyes and/or the lungs.

Continuous positive airway pressure (CPAP) is a very useful treatment for HMD. Current data suggest that the lung is unable to synthesize surface-active pulmonary surfactant in sufficient quantity when the alveoli collapse with each expiration and need to be reinflated with each inspiration. When such a condition exists, early use of CPAP is believed to conserve surfactant, or at least make its production possible by improving oxygenation. Continuous positive airway pressure has reduced effectively the severity of hyaline membrane disease and has reduced markedly the mortality rate.

Continuous positive airway pressure is usually instituted when it has become necessary to raise the concentration of inspired oxygen up to 60 percent or sometimes more in order to keep the Po_2 at 50 mm Hg.

The infant with hyaline membrane disease may become very tired from the constant effort to take each breath and then may need IPPV as well as CPAP. The amount of carbon dioxide retained, as measured by Pco_2, also determines use of ventilatory assistance. A Pco_2 of 60 mm Hg usually indicates need for assisted ventilation. Frequent and prolonged spells of apnea also indicate a need for ventilation.

Nutritional support is important for a sick infant for recovery as well as for growth. Intravenous fluids of glucose will be started early for fluid requirements, and if the infant is unable to take oral food for a number of days, nutrients of protein and fat are given intravenously. Careful regulation of intravenous fluids is required, and a careful record of intake and output is kept.

The infant with respiratory distress needs protection from all unnecessary handling and exertion. With the infant in an incubator many of the necessary observations can be made without undue handling. Baths should be limited to only those that are absolutely essential, and any unnecessary care should be omitted. The infant needs as much rest as possible.

Use of assisted ventilation and oxygen requires very special care and close observation of blood gases. Special care nurseries have the staff and the facilities to carry out the very sophisticated treatment that is now possible for these sick infants. Such treatment should be provided since it has effectively reduced the mortality of hyaline membrane disease in premature infants.

Since the infant with hyaline membrane disease is usually preterm, the care described for preterm infants on pages 610–29 is continued as the infant recovers from respiratory distress. A long period of hospitalization may yet be ahead for the immature infant after recovery from the respiratory problem.

TYPE II RESPIRATORY DISTRESS SYNDROME

Type II respiratory distress syndrome (RDS) bears resemblance to hyaline membrane disease, but has a different history, is more benign in its course, and has a good prognosis. This syndrome also has been called transient tachypnea of the newborn, transient respiratory distress of the newborn, aspiration syndrome, wet-lung disease, and perhaps other names.

Infants with type II RDS initially may have respiratory symptoms similar to those with hyaline membrane disease, although usually less severe. In the first hours after birth they develop tachypnea, retractions, grunting, and cyanosis. Respiratory rate may be normal or even depressed at first because many of these infants present a picture of oversedation at birth. They may be alert and appear to be in good condition at the moment of birth and have a good Apgar score because of the stimulation of birth and the environment. Then when stimulation decreases, the infant becomes sleepy and may hypoventilate, and have depression of cough, gag, and swallowing reflexes. Aspiration is a possibility. After a few hours, tachypnea appears, and respiratory rate may be as high as 100 per minute or even more.

Grunting respirations begin early. The amount of chest retraction will depend upon the extent of illness and the maturity of the infant, since the chest cage has more stability in the older infant than in the very immature. Flaring of the nostrils is often seen. Cyanosis is usually visible in room air.

A predisposition to this syndrome occurs in infants who are slightly preterm, showing some evidence of immaturity, and with a history of heavy maternal sedation. Sometimes there has been an episode of intrauterine asphyxia, as with maternal bleeding, and sometimes with cesarean section. The history is in contrast to that of HMD, which occurs in more immature infants who frequently have had a period of perinatal distress.

Whereas infants with HMD have a surfactant deficiency and widespread atelectasis, those with type II RDS are likely to have some problem with aspiration and a delayed absorption of lung fluid. (See page 498 for discussion on lung fluid.) Heavy sedation may result in the infant's failure to clear the airway well of mucus. Even when initial suctioning of the airways has been good, depressed gag, swallow, and cough reflexes may permit pooling of secretions in the tracheobronchial tree, especially if the infant is not observed carefully until he becomes reactive. If there has been some birth asphyxia, there also may be a delay in the normal changes in the circulatory pattern and a delay in the removal of lung fluid by the lymphatics. The chest x-ray shows hyperaeration and overexpansion of the lungs.

Respiratory distress with type II RDS usually lasts from 24 to 96 hours. Grunting and retraction last 24 to 48 hours, and tachypnea lasts somewhat longer. These infants need oxygen during their period of respiratory distress, perhaps even as high as 70 percent for a while, but oxygen need is not as progressive as with HMD. These infants can be hyperoxygenated easily, and they must be watched very carefully to avoid giving too much. Ventilatory assistance is rarely needed. Hypovolemia is rarely a problem. Intravenous glucose is given for calories and fluids.

Infants who have been sedated require careful observation of their respiratory function, resuscitation as necessary, and continuing observation in the nursery for accumulation of mucus and for ventilatory efforts, at least through their second period of reactivity. (See pages 547–52 for discussion of periods of reactivity and for observations and care during the transitional period.)

TRANSIENT TACHYPNEA OF THE NEWBORN

With transient tachypnea of the newborn (TTNB), the infant, either full term or preterm, has an unexplained, persistently high respiratory rate, up to 100 or more per minute. Cyanosis is not common, although the infant may need a small increase in percentage of inspired oxygen. Air exchange seems to be good, expiratory grunt generally is not heard, and intercostal retraction is usually minimal. An x-ray usually can be used to distinguish this condition from HMD and type II RDS. It has been suggested that this transient tachypnea is the result of slow absorption of lung fluid. The lung compliance would be decreased because of the additional fluid, and the rapid respirations would then minimize respiratory work. Aspiration of amniotic fluid or mucus also has been considered a cause.

The TTNB syndrome appears to be self-limiting. It resolves in several days. Careful monitoring of respiration and heart rate is necessary, at least at first, to distinguish this syndrome from more serious respiratory distress. Oral feedings may need to be withheld until tachypnea subsides in order to avoid aspiration.

DISTRESS FROM ASPIRATION OF MECONIUM

Aspiration of amniotic fluid containing meconium is apt to be followed by respiratory distress. Meconium may plug small air passages and is irritating to lung tissues. Following aspiration the lungs may have areas of atelectasis owing to obstruction and areas of consolidation, and the infant is susceptible to secondary infection of the lungs.

Aspiration of meconium may occur in any condition in which hypoxia causes the fetus to pass some meconium *in utero*. An infant with hypoxia is in danger of aspiration *in utero* or at birth. It therefore may follow any complication of pregnancy or labor that interferes with adequate fetal oxygenation. It may be associated with fetal growth retardation (SGA baby) and with postmaturity—conditions in which intrauterine hypoxia and passage of meconium may occur because of insufficient placental function. An infant with meconium-stained amniotic fluid and meconium-stained skin must be observed closely for signs of distress. The lungs may clear within 24 to 48 hours after aspiration of meconium, but distress may be severe enough to cause a serious illness that requires long-term respiratory assistance, and often it causes death.

The morbidity and mortality from meconium aspiration can be greatly reduced by carrying out tracheal suction before the meconium is pulled into the small air passages. The mechanism of meconium aspiration and prevention of airway obstruction by meconium has been described on page 638 in relation to the postmaturity syndrome.

If an infant does aspirate meconium, he is likely to have tachypnea and labored respirations, which may be gasping. Chest retraction is common. Significant hyperinflation of the chest is usually seen. The chest is enlarged, especially in the anteroposterior diameter, and there may be a prominent anterior sternal bulge. A chest x-ray shows areas of increased density and areas of overexpansion distributed throughout the lung. The infant may have considerable mucus, which may be meconium-stained. Pneumothorax is a complication of respiratory distress from meconium aspiration. A pneumothorax must be considered whenever there is an abrupt worsening in the infant's condition.

Management of respiratory distress from meconium aspiration will depend upon the clinical course. It will include oxygen, humidification, parenteral fluids, correction of acid-base imbalance, postural drainage and percussion, and perhaps other interventions. Antibiotics may be used if lung infection is suspected.

NEONATAL HEART DISEASE

Many and complex anatomic anomalies involving the heart and/or the great vessels may develop in the fetus. The heart goes through a very complicated developmental process, and a disturbance at any one of the series of changes may result in a congenital malformation.

Some cardiac problems in the newborn are critically

serious, complicated cardiac malformations, but others are caused by relatively less serious left-to-right shunts. Among important left-to-right shunt lesions are isolated ventricular septal defect, which is believed to account for between 30 and 40 percent of all congenital heart disease, atrial septal defect, and patent ductus arteriosus. Serious and sometimes fatal lesions include hypoplastic left ventricle syndrome, coarctation of the aorta, transposition of the great arteries, hypoplastic right ventricle syndrome, and tetralogy of Fallot. Lesions may involve persistent communication between pulmonary and systemic circulation, underdeveloped ventricles or pulmonary artery, stenosis of valves, constriction of vessels such as the aorta, and transposition of vessels. Various combinations of defects may exist.

Some defects are functional and disappear within a few months. Some remain but do not require treatment and do not produce a handicap. Some require surgery to support life, and some are so marked that they are incompatible with life. Congenital heart lesions may be accompanied by anomalies in other parts of the body.

Remarkable advances have been made in recent years in management of infants with heart disease. Diagnostic methods and corrective operative procedures for infants have become much more sophisticated and now are used in the neonatal period. Formerly early treatment was not the case. Centralization of services is necessary for the complex treatment that is now possible for infants with heart disease.

Congenital cardiac anomalies may present no problem until the circulatory adjustments after birth have taken place. Cardiac lesions are not detrimental to the fetus because they do not interfere with the fetal circulatory pattern. With birth and the radical change in the pattern of circulation, a defect in the development of the heart and/or the great vessels is likely to compromise the normal flow pattern and cause cardiac disease. Cardiac problems in the newborn frequently do not appear immediately after birth for several reasons. All the changes in circulation are not completed immediately after birth, and difficulty may not appear until these changes are more complete. Also, compensatory mechanisms may be established and function reasonably well for awhile, until their load becomes too great. The kind of malfunction and its extent will determine how and when signs and symptoms appear.

At birth, when the placental circulation is eliminated and its large low-resistance circuit is removed, the infant's total systemic vascular resistance increases. At the same time expansion of the lungs with air results in a considerable decrease in pulmonary vascular resistance. The result of the increase in systemic vascular resistance and the decrease in pulmonary vascular resistance is a nearly equal resistance in each system very soon after birth. A small amount of blood may flow from one circulation to another for a short time, but normally, with good oxygenation, the ductus arteriosus closes functionally within 10 to 15 hours. Also pressure changes in the atria close the foramen ovale after birth. Pressure in the left atrium is raised with the marked increase in pulmonary blood flow, and pressure in the right atrium is lowered as aeration of the lungs decreases the pulmonary vascular resistance and as removal of the placental circulation decreases the amount of blood flowing through the inferior vena cava to the right atrium.

The pulmonary circulation is not completely changed immediately after birth, but rather continues to undergo changes during the first six to eight weeks postnatally. In the first several days the pulmonary vascular resistance continues to decrease as the result of further expansion of alveoli. Then, in a normal maturational development, the pulmonary arterioles lose some smooth muscle and dilate still more, bringing about a further decrease in pulmonary arteriole pressure.

With the changes in circulatory resistances that take place at birth and thereafter, problems will arise if there is communication between the systemic and pulmonary circulations, as there is with a ventricular septal defect and a persistent patent ductus arteriosus. At first, when the pulmonary vascular resistance is still relatively high, flow across communication channels may not be great. As pulmonary resistance decreases, however, there is an increase of blood flow into the pulmonary circulation. As a result of such increase there is an increase in the pulmonary venous return to the left atrium and the left ventricle.

The action of the left ventricle will be related to the volume of blood that expands it. As the volume of blood returning from the lungs to the left ventricle increases, the ventricle increases its stroke volume. As pulmonary resistance increasingly falls during the first weeks of life, a greater and greater load is placed on the left ventricle as it works against the rising blood volume and as it tries to meet the systemic circulatory needs. As long as the ventricle can maintain its increased stroke volume or has time to develop hypertrophy, symptoms do not appear, but finally the ventricle becomes overworked and cardiac failure becomes apparent.[25] Any congenital heart lesion in which there is communication between the ventricles or great vessels is likely to show left ventricular failure in time, along with the decrease in pulmonary vascular resistance that occurs with normal maturation during the weeks after birth.

When congenital heart defects are the result of a narrowed opening that causes obstruction to blood flow, heart failure may develop because of the increased systolic pressure that is necessary to effect blood flow across the obstruction. If there is no time for a compen-

[25] Abraham M. Rudolph, Cardiac failure in children: A hemodynamic overview, *Hosp. Pract.*, 5:44–55, (July) 1970, p. 45.

satory hypertrophy to develop, the increased end-systolic volume will dilate the ventricle. As increase in end-diastolic pressure and volume then will occur, and the same problem of overextension and cardiac failure occurs that was described above for shunt lesions. It is because of this that infants with coarctation of the aorta or aortic stenosis develop heart failure almost immediately after birth. A large overload of pressure is applied to the left ventricle before it has had time to develop a compensating hypertrophy. When a lesion is small enough to allow time for adaptive growth, heart failure does not occur until late childhood or adult life.[26]

An elevated left ventricular pressure from either left-sided obstructive lesions or large left-to-right shunts causes an increase in left atrial and pulmonary venous pressure. The pressure may become high enough to cause more exudation of fluid through the pulmonary capillaries than can be removed by lymphatic drainage. Pulmonary edema then develops. Clinical evidence of pulmonary edema appears at lower pressures in infants than in adults.

Pulmonary edema is associated with increased rate and depth of respirations. Increased respiratory effort is the most common sign of heart failure in infants, since most cardiac defects that produce heart failure in infancy are associated with left-sided failure. Commonly, there are increased respiratory effort, mild cyanosis, decreased P_{O_2}, and slightly increased P_{CO_2}. When a heart murmur is not detected, it is difficult to differentiate the problem from respiratory disease, at least initially.

The majority of heart defects that produce heart failure in infants are associated with left-sided failure. When left-sided failure persists for some time, right-sided failure usually develops. Right-sided failure, however, may be primary, as with severe pulmonary stenosis or preductal coarctation of the aorta with patent ductus arteriosus. Right-sided failure does not commonly present with gross edema as in the adult. An early sign is enlargement of the liver. Another early sign of heart failure is increased perspiration, especially around the face and head, particularly noticeable during feedings.

Early recognition of heart disease is important to permit time for transfer of the infant to a specially equipped and staffed cardiac center, and time for cardiac evaluation for diagnosis, and then surgery as indicated. An infant with heart disease in the early days of life may deteriorate rapidly.

For reasons described above, signs and symptoms of heart disease may be absent in the infant, may occur occasionally, or may be constant in a mild or severe form. Signs and symptoms may occur because of a communication between the systemic and pulmonary circulation, or because of an increased load placed on the heart when it is necessary to force blood through narrow passages or stenotic valves.

Cyanosis is a common manifestation of congenital heart disease, but it may be absent or may not appear until later in life. Blueness of the infant's hands and feet is normal for a few hours after birth, but all other parts of his body should be pink. A persistence of cyanosis of the hands and feet after several hours, when oxygenation and circulation should be improved, is considered abnormal. It is suggestive of heart disease, pulmonary pathology, or occasionally birth injury. Cyanosis without pulmonary disease is usually caused by serious cardiac abnormality. Especially in the first week of life, cyanosis may be the only evidence of a cardiac lesion. Cyanosis, which is much more threatening than a murmur, is likely the result of impaired oxygenation because of edema fluid in the alveoli.

A persistent heart murmur is a common sign of a heart abnormality. A precordial murmur in the early neonatal period may be caused by delayed closure of one of the fetal openings. Therefore, it may not be significant unless is persists.

Respiratory symptoms commonly precede first detection of a murmur. Rapid, labored respirations, often 60 breaths per minute or more, may precede deterioration to dyspnea and congestive heart failure. Tachypnea requires investigation for respiratory or cardiac cause. When the infant with cardiac disease has predominantly respiratory symptoms, he may have congestive heart failure.

Edema may appear early or late.

An infant with cardiac disease may not take his feedings well.

Palpation of the femoral and brachial arteries for pulsation and comparison with each other may help to detect coarctation of the aorta before other signs develop. Pulsations in the femoral arteries are decreased or absent or significantly delayed in coarctation of the aorta because the circulation of the lower part of the body must, to a large extent, be carried on by a collateral circulation. Left brachial pulses may be decreased if the left subclavian arises at or below the coarctation.

While preparing for diagnosis by means of noninvasive diagnostic tools and further treatment, the infant with respiratory problems and edema is treated with administration of oxygen, diuretics, and digitalis.

HYPOGLYCEMIA

The importance of hypoglycemia in the newborn with its serious threat to the infant's welfare has come to be well recognized in recent years and has been found to be more common than previously thought. Hypoglycemia can be the cause of certain early postnatal problems such as a contributing cause of respiratory distress. Much more

[26] *Ibid.*, p. 47.

important, it may result in irreparable brain damage. Hypoglycemia is a serious threat to brain cells since the brain can use *only glucose* (not other sugars) for its energy and requires a constant supply. The amount of glucose available to the brain is directly related to the blood glucose concentration. When the blood glucose value is low, there is a real possibility of deprivation of glucose to cerebral tissues, possible permanent impairment of the cells, and residual neurologic defects. The effect upon the brain cells is likely to correlate with the duration of the hypoglycemia.

Since brain damage from hypoglycemia is preventable, the importance of early recognition of a low blood sugar in the newborn and prompt intervention to replace a blood glucose deficiency cannot be overemphasized. Dangerously long periods of hypoglycemia in any infant are unnecessary with current easy diagnostic procedures and knowledge of treatment.

Hypoglycemia may be defined as a significantly low level of *glucose* (*true sugar*) in whole blood on two reliable repeated examinations that measure the level of *true* blood sugar. Normal blood sugar values in newborns range from 45 to 100 mg/100 ml of blood. A value of 45 mg is considered slightly low and one that reaches a level of 100 mg slightly high. An average between these two values, such as 70 to 80 mg, comes near to an ideal level during the first several days of life. Less than 30 mg of glucose/100 ml of blood is regarded as hypoglycemia. This is considered to be harmful to the infant and may cause symptoms, described below, and will cause chemical brain damage if allowed to persist.

Stated in somewhat more detail, a common definition of neonatal hypoglycemia is as follows: a whole blood sugar level of less than 30 mg/100 ml (less than 35 mg in serum or plasma) in the first 72 hours of life, or of less than 40 mg (less than 45 mg in serum or plasma) after the third day, in full-term, full-size infants. In infants of low birthweight the lower figure of normal is 20 mg/100 ml in whole blood or 25 mg in plasma or serum. One low reading is adequate for initiating therapy, but two successive low readings should be used to establish a diagnosis if the infant is asymptomatic.[27]

Dr. Leo Stern states that the levels of blood sugar given above for a definition of hypoglycemia may be dangerously low for some infants. He states that blood glucose levels below 40 mg/100 ml in any infant should be corrected.[28]

During intrauterine life glucose is continuously transferred across the placenta from the maternal to the fetal circulation, supplying a major source of energy to the fetus. At birth, when the infant's energy demands increase, his glucose supply is suddenly cut off. The infant's immediate response to this change is rapid glycogenolysis, using the liver glycogen supply. In addition, fat deposits are mobilized for energy.

At birth the blood glucose level in the newborn is proportional to that of the mother; venous blood sugar values in the newborn are 70 to 80 percent of those of the mother's venous blood sugar level. Variations in values will depend upon maternal expenditures of energy during labor and administration of glucose to the mother during labor. The newborn's blood glucose level at birth will depend upon the mother's actual blood glucose level. After birth the newborn's blood glucose level falls with a rate varying with the baby's condition and expenditure of energy. In the normal newborn, the blood glucose reaches its lowest level sometime between 1½ and 3 hours of age and then averages around 45 to 50 mg/100 ml of blood. In the normal newborn, without undue postnatal stress, there is a gradual return to higher levels of blood glucose and a stability of values by 4 to 6 hours of age. A rise to 60 mg or more/100 ml of blood will occur if the infant has been kept warm; with cooling this value may only average 45 mg. In general, during the first 6 to 12 hours of life, normal infants who have not been fed will have blood sugar levels between 30 and 125 mg/100 ml of blood with average values of 60 mg/100 ml. After 72 hours most normal infants maintain a blood glucose level of 70 to 75 mg/100 ml of blood. At this age values below 40 mg/100 ml are considered hypoglycemic; values over 125 mg are also abnormal.

Return to normal blood glucose values in a few hours in the *normal* newborn occurs because the infant can make energy and glucose for himself in several ways. He can mobilize glycogen stored in the liver and convert it to glucose and mobilize fatty acids from fat stores and convert them into energy. Stress of low blood sugar increases release of epinephrine from the adrenal gland. The epinephrine mobilizes liver glycogen and inhibits pancreatic release of insulin. With less insulin the blood glucose level tends to remain up.

The level of blood glucose in a fasting newborn is the balance between the amount of liver glycogen that is mobilized and converted to glucose and the amount that is used for energy, vital body functions, and adjustments to extrauterine life. Respiratory distress at birth and chilling quickly use up a supply of glucose. Food and intravenous fluids can augment the body supply of glucose, but unless both glycogen stores and exogenous supply are adequate, the blood glucose level drops to below normal.

When feeding an infant is started, his blood sugar tends to rise, although fluctuations may remain wide. Early feedings thus would seem to be advantageous to most normal newborn infants.

[27] Marvin Cornblath, Disorders of carbohydrate metabolism, in *Diseases of the Newborn,* 4th ed., edited by Alexander J. Schaffer and Mary Ellen Avery, W. B. Saunders, Philadelphia, 1977, p. 519.

[28] Leo Stern, Comment on hypoglycemia, in *Care of the High-Risk Neonate,* edited by Marshall H. Klaus and Avroy A. Fanaroff, W. B. Saunders, Philadelphia, 1973, p. 170.

Hypoglycemia may occur in many conditions. In some infants hypoglycemia is considered idiopathic and may appear in apparently normal healthy newborns. In others, there are predisposing factors, mainly placental dysfunction and neonatal illness.

Hypoglycemia often has its onset with undernourishment *in utero.* Infants of low birthweight, either premature or full-term gestation, are very susceptible to hypoglycemia. Most of the liver glycogen reserve and the fat stores are built up late in pregnancy and normally increase with gestational age. An infant born prematurely does not yet have an adequate glycogen supply or fat store. Placental insufficiency, resulting in intrauterine growth retardation, often means failure of adequate liver glycogen storage and fat deposits, even when the pregnancy continues to full term, or the store once laid down may be depleted before birth. These infants usually are undernourished, and many are under the tenth percentile of birthweight for gestational age. An infant born to a mother with complications such as preeclampsia, renal disease, cardiac disease, or chronic infection must be considered susceptible to hypoglycemia. The postterm infant is likely to develop low blood glucose levels. Placental function is apt to decrease after full-term gestation, and the infant who remains *in utero* for 42 to 43 weeks or even longer begins to exhaust his stores to satisfy his nutritional needs before he is born. If any of the low-birthweight infants becomes cooled or has respiratory distress he rapidly uses up his meager stores. A small infant under optimal conditions is low on glucose reserves in 18 to 24 hours. If he became cooled he may be lacking reserves in six to eight hours, and if he also was asphyxiated, his reserve is likely to be very low in four hours.

A large infant, over the ninetieth percentile of birthweight for gestational age and the infant born of a diabetic mother are very susceptible to hypoglycemia. The problems of the infant of a diabetic mother are discussed separately below.

Among other conditions that lead to susceptibility to hypoglycemia are a hematocrit of over 65 percent, hypothermia, asphyxia, hypoxia, respiratory distress syndrome, infection, erythroblastosis, and any other condition that results in illness. Any stress condition that increases the metabolic rate requires additional glucose and is likely to deplete an infant's glycogen stores.

Symptoms

Symptoms of hypoglycemia are vague, subtle, and nonspecific to the disorder. It is especially important to be aware of the fact that hypoglycemia in the newborn may be asymptomatic and that diagnosis is made only by blood sugar determination. This makes it important to be alert to an infant's susceptibility and to screen any infant in question.

Among symptoms that may appear in an infant with hypoglycemia are increased respiration; apneic spells; cyanosis; tremors, twitching, and jitteriness, or apathy, limpness, listlessness, poor muscle tone and weak reflexes; unstable temperature regulation; eye rolling; high-pitched cry; and difficulty in feeding. Convulsive seizure may appear late. It is apparent that any of these symptoms may be caused by a number of other conditions.

Diagnosis

Diagnosis of hypoglycemia is made by blood glucose determinations. Since asymptomatic hypoglycemia may be significant, or symptoms may be vague, routine measurement of blood glucose on all low-birthweight infants, all other high-risk infants, and any apparently normal suspect infants is important. Duplicate screening is important for diagnosis and repeated monitoring must be done until it is certain that the infant's blood sugar level is remaining normal. The nurse has an important responsibility to recognize suspicious symptoms of hypoglycemia and to identify infants with increased risk in order that she may alert all individuals concerned with the infant's care. Such observation and reporting should ensure that rapid assessment and treatment, if indicated, will be fulfilled.

Infants in any risk category require routine screening at least at 1½, 3, and 6 hours after birth. In some nurseries all newborn infants in the nursery are screened between two and four hours of age.

In addition to a laboratory micromethod of testing blood sugar, a reagent test strip (Ames Company, DEXTROSTIX) may be used as a screening test. The DEXTROSTIX has an enzyme on the active end of the test strip that changes color when exposed to glucose. A drop of blood from a finger or heel puncture is put on the active end of the strip, washed off in exactly 60 seconds, and read immediately by comparison to a color chart. The color change of the test strip is proportional to the amount of glucose in the blood. The scale of color ranges from pale gray at 20 to 30 mg/100 ml blood through deepening shades of blue-gray when the amount of sugar in the blood is higher. The color distinguishes between glucose values of 20, 30, 45, 60, and 90 and higher mg/100 ml of blood. The color scheme is accurate, reliable, and dependable, at least at the lower levels of the scale. Laboratory studies may be necessary as follow-up when color changes are doubtful or when confirmation of results is desirable. (See Fig. 30–3).

The DEXTROSTIX enzyme test strip is very useful for occasional or frequent checks since it is readily available and easy to use. It may be used for frequent checks of infants "at-risk," or with suggestive symptoms, or for results of treatment, or for routine screening. Nurses can easily learn to use the DEXTROSTIX. Since timing is of

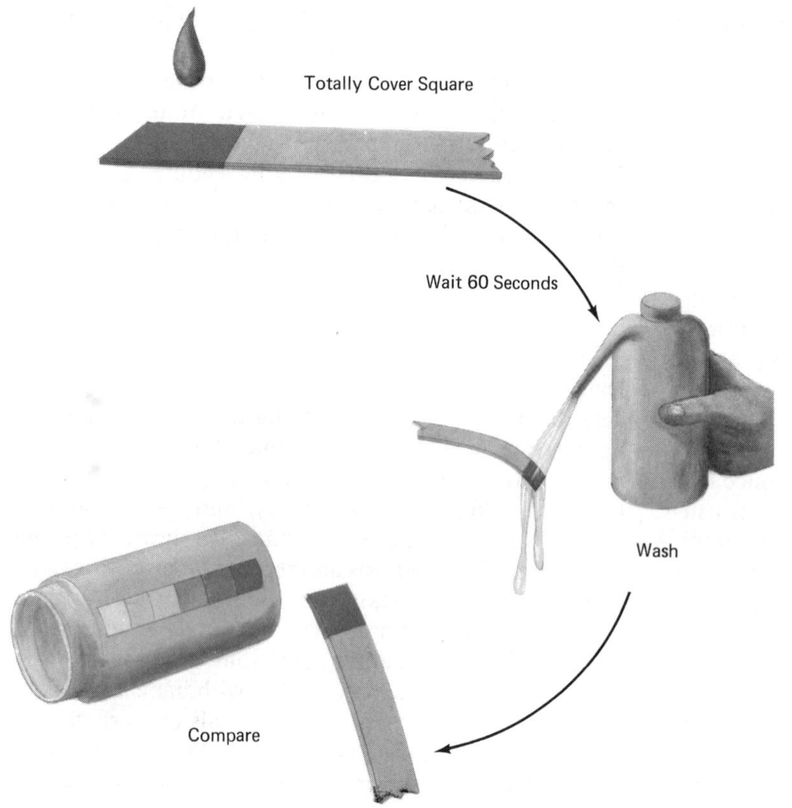

Figure 30–3. Method of testing blood sugar with a reagent test strip—the DEXTROSTIX. A large drop of blood is put on the reagent end of the test strip, covering it completely. After exactly 60 seconds the blood is washed off with water from a wash bottle and the color of the reagent end of the test strip is compared with a color chart. All directions must be carefully observed. Accurate timing is crucial to the accuracy of the results.

crucial important in the accuracy of the test, this precaution and all other directions must be observed carefully when the test is done. Some nurses feel more comfortable in using a short, small-gauge hypodermic needle instead of a lancet for the heel stick. The method of heel stick seems immaterial if a large drop of blood, sufficient to cover the entire reagent area, is obtained easily.

Treatment

Prompt administration of glucose usually will establish normal blood glucose levels. The method of administration will depend upon the infant's ability to suck and swallow. The amount and strength of the glucose solution to be given will be gauged by the blood sugar readings.

A large infant may be fed a 5 or 10 percent glucose solution orally as soon as his blood glucose value is found to be lower than 45 mg/100 ml of blood. He usually is given the amount of glucose he will take, which may vary from 10 to 30 ml of fluid. His blood sugar level may be monitored one-half hour after completion of his feeding to determine if sufficient amount of glucose was taken to raise his blood sugar level to normal. Since a hypoglycemic infant may lose his swallowing reflex, the nurse who feeds the infant must proceed with caution. The infant may not be able to take an oral feeding. A gavage feeding may be indicated.

For a small infant the glucose solution may be administered intravenously, usually by peripheral vein. A constant infusion pump will ensure a steady flow of solution as determined to meet the infant's requirement to maintain a good blood sugar level. A hypertonic glucose solution may be used at first. Blood glucose levels are monitored every one to two hours to determine his needs to maintain a normal level.

After an infant's blood glucose level has been raised, subsequent frequent assessments are important until it is determined that the level will remain normal. The cause of the hypoglycemia and presence or absence of complications will determine if normoglycemia will be established quickly or if observation and treatment over a period of several days are necessary. When tolerated, early oral or intravenous glucose feedings are soon followed by full formula feedings with glucose supplementation, if necessary.

In view of the frequency of hypoglycemia in newborns, delayed feedings, a common practice in the past, must be questioned seriously. It would appear that early bottle- or breast-feedings, if the infant can suck and swallow, or tube feedings or intravenous administration of glucose is important to all infants.

THE INFANT OF THE DIABETIC MOTHER

The infant born of a diabetic mother is susceptible to certain complications that require intensive care. The infant is usually large for gestational age, having received a great deal of glucose because of maternal hyperglycemia. However, some infants born of mothers with diabetes are small for gestational age because of insufficient placental perfusion. The fetus of a mother with diabetes is very vulnerable to maternal ketoacidosis. Congenital anomalies are more common than in the general population of newborns (see page 305). The possibility of intrauterine death during the last weeks of pregnancy raises concern, and preterm delivery is sometimes necessary. For delivery, labor is often induced and may be rather long, and the incidence of cesarean section delivery is increased.

In the past, these infants often were delivered prematurely, a few weeks before term, because of concern over intrauterine death. Currently it is possible to monitor closely placental function and fetal response to the intrauterine environment. This makes it possible to permit pregnancy to continue closer to term in a number of patients. Monitoring during labor also may show that a cesarean section is not necessary as frequently as it was done in the past.

An attempt is made to keep maternal blood glucose levels under 100 mg/100 ml of blood during labor or prior to cesarean section. This gives the fetus an opportunity to adjust to a lower glucose load with a decrease in insulin production and a decrease in hypoglycemia response after birth. It is advisable for the reader to review diabetes mellitus (its effects on mother and fetus and its management) on pages 301–309.

Unusual environmental conditions *in utero,* which lead to the need for marked postnatal adjustment, plus perhaps prematurity and sometimes long labor or cesarean section, result in two major serious difficulties in the newborn—hypoglycemia and respiratory distress. In addition, hypocalcemia and hyperbilirubinemia may present problems in these infants.

The fetus of a diabetic mother often grows to excessive size in weight and length. His size is inconsistent with his gestational age. A premature infant may be as large as, or larger than, a full term. Typically the infant is in the upper percentile on an intrauterine growth chart, unless the mother had some other condition that caused intrauterine growth retardation. The infant's abnormal weight is caused by an excess of fat and glycogen in his body tissues. Insulin does not transfer across the placental barrier freely, but glucose does. Since glucose passes from the mother's blood to the fetal circulation with ease, the hyperglycemia that is common in the mother keeps the blood glucose in the fetus at an abnormally high level much of the time. This elevated blood sugar level in the fetus exaggerates certain metabolic functions, particularly storage of glycogen and fat and increased insulin production. The excess glucose in converted into glycogen, which is stored in the liver and heart, and into fats, which are stored in fat depots. These large stores result in enlargement of the liver and heart, and in abundant subcutaneous fat. Increased blood sugar from the mother stimulates increased fetal insulin production, which does not cross the placenta to the mother, leaving the fetus with hyperinsulinemia.

In addition to excessive size, the infant of a diabetic mother may have a puffy, cushingoid appearance with round cheeks and short neck; enlarged heart, liver, and spleen; rapid irregular respirations; lethargy at times but an increased Moro reflex and irritability with slight stimulation; and at first a red, tense skin, which later shows jaundice.

James W. Farquhar has described the intrauterine environment and its effects, and the appearance of infants born of diabetic mothers, as follows:

> The infants are remarkable not only because, like fetal versions of Shadrach, Meshach and Abednego, they emerge at least alive from within the fiery metabolic furnace of diabetes mellitus, but because they resemble one another so closely that they might well be related. They are plump, sleek, liberally coated with vernix caseosa, full-faced and plethoric. The umbilical cord and the placenta share in the gigantism. During their first 24 or more extrauterine hours they lie on their backs, bloated and flushed, their legs flexed and abducted, their lightly closed hands on each side of the head, the abdomen prominent and their respiration sighing. They convey a distinct impression of having had such a surfeit of both food and fluid pressed upon them by an insistent hostess that they desire only peace so that they may recover from their excesses. And on the second day their resentment of the slightest noise improves the analogy, while their trembling anxiety seems to speak of intrauterine indiscretions of which we know nothing.[29]

If the mother's diabetes can be controlled carefully throughout pregnancy, the infant may not grow to be excessively large for his gestational age, but oftentimes management is very difficult even with excellent medical care and efforts on the part of the mother. Perhaps with the increasingly good control of maternal blood sugar that is now possible the fetuses of diabetic women will develop and attain a more normal intrauterine growth.

Regardless of size or gestational age the infant is treated as a premature or high-risk newborn and cared for in an intensive care unit. He usually is cared for in an incubator for good visibility of his condition and close control of his environment. Observation and treatment for respiratory distress and hypoglycemia are of major immediate concern.

Hypoglycemia

With birth the infant of the diabetic mother suffers from the sudden cut-off of the high glucose supplyfrom his mother and the stimulus that the pancreas received *in utero* to secrete a large amount of insulin. All newborns

[29] James W. Farquhar, The child of the diabetic woman, *Arch. Dis. Child.,* 34:76–77, 1959.

have a lowering of blood glucose. The infant of a diabetic, in addition, has a large amount of circulating insulin which will lower his blood glucose level more than normal. As liver glycogen is broken down to elevate the infant's blood glucose level, that elevation of blood glucose in turn causes a further large secretion of insulin, resulting in a still greater hypoglycemia. In many infants the glucose level quickly falls below 30 mg/100 ml of blood, and often goes below 20 mg or even lower during the first few hours, and often even within the first hour. The necessity for immediate blood sugar check after birth and continuing frequent checks is obvious.

In addition to abnormal hypoglycemia the infant of a diabetic mother may be unable to mobilize excess fat stores. Thus, with hypoglycemia and low serum levels of free fatty acids, the infant has a very small source of energy for certain tissue functions, especially for the glucose-dependent brain and for the heart, which utilizes free fatty acids.

Monitoring and treatment of the infant of a diabetic mother may be somewhat as follows. The blood sugar of the umbilical cord blood may be checked for a baseline. A DEXTROSTIX is done immediately on admission to the nursery and every one-half hour thereafter for three hours. Monitoring following this period may be determined by the infant's response and stability of blood sugar. Laboratory evaluation of blood sugar also may be done once or twice during the first three or four hours and oftener if indicated.

The infant must be given glucose, orally or intravenously, to keep his blood glucose level higher than 40 mg/100 ml of blood, even though elevation of blood glucose may stimulate further insulin production. For the infant who is able to suck and swallow well, oral feedings may be started. The infant usually can be fed at one hour of age offering formula of 20 kcal per 30 ml (1 oz) in an amount of 7 ml/kg by gavage or nipple, or the infant may be breast-fed. Possible loss of swallow reflex requires careful evaluation whenever oral feedings are offered. Intravenous administration of 10 percent glucose is started if the infant is unable to take oral feedings, if the DEXTROSTIX falls to 20 mg/100 ml or lower, if the DEXTROSTIX remains below 30 mg on two successive checks, or if the infant becomes symptomatic.

The infant of a diabetic mother is very susceptible to respiratory distress syndrome, regardless of whether he is premature or full term. The full-term infant's respiratory difficulty is often of metabolic origin. Hyperbilirubinemia is fairly common. Both of these complications are discussed elsewhere in this chapter. Hypocalcemia is a significant complication in infants of diabetic mothers. Many of the signs and symptoms of a low calcium level are nonspecific and similar to those of hypoglycemia. Diagnoses must be made by serum calcium determination. Treatment is administration of calcium gluconate.

NEONATAL HYPOCALCEMIA

Neonatal hypocalcemia may occur early, within the first two days after birth, or "late" when the infant is a week old. A serum calcium level below 7 mg/100 ml blood usually is considered a hypocalcemia.

The "early" hypocalcemia is thought to be caused by perinatal factors and is most likely to occur in preterm infants, infants who have had birth asphyxia, and infants of diabetic mothers. Late hypocalcemia occurs from dietary imbalance of calcium and phosphate.

The cause of hypocalcemia is not completely clear. Several factors are thought to exert an influence. There may be hypofunction of the parathyroid gland, especially in the preterm infant or in perinatal asphyxia or stress. This may lead to a decreased ability to excrete phosphate in the urine. During perinatal asphyxia tissue breakdown adds an additional phosphate load to the circulation. There also may be a maturational delay in responsiveness of the renal tubule to parathormone. This results in hyperphosphatemia with a secondary decrease in serum calcium level. Exchange transfusion with citrated blood temporarily binds ionized calcium, and rapid correction of acidosis with an alkali decreases the concentration of ionized calcium. It is the ionized calcium that is necessary for use by the cells.

The "late" hypocalcemia, sometimes called "seventh-day hypocalcemia," is usually secondary to a high phosphorus load in cow's milk formula. The immature neonatal parathyroid gland is not ready to handle the load. This condition does not occur with breast milk, which contain relatively less calcium and much less phosphate. Presently modified cow's milk formulas have significantly less phosphorus than is present in unmodified cow's milk. Commercially prepared formulas are likely to contain a calcium-phosphorus ratio very similar to that of breast milk, but an infant who is fed diluted evaporated milk or cow's milk may receive an imbalance of these minerals.

Clinically, the infant with hypocalcemia may show tremulousness, apneic spells, cyanosis, vomiting, and abdominal distention. Carpopedal spasm and convulsions may occur. Symptoms may be confused with those of hypoglycemia, respiratory problems, central nervous system problems, and narcotic withdrawal.

For diagnosis a measurement of serum calcium is made. A value below 7.0 mg/100 ml is considered hypocalcemia. Total calcium levels may drop to 3.0 mg or even lower in severe cases. Roughly about 50 percent of the total calcium is ionized and is available to the cells. The amount of ionized calcium will depend to some extent on the serum protein concentration and on pH.

Hypocalcemia is treated by intravenous administration of calcium gluconate at about 100 mg/kg/day. When symptoms are not dramatic and the infant can take medication orally, treatment may be by oral calcium preparation given in divided doses over 24-hour periods.

HYPERBILIRUBINEMIA

Hyperbilirubinemia in the newborn is an abnormal elevation in serum bilirubin level. It may be caused by an excessive breakdown of red blood cells resulting in accumulation of an unusual amount of indirect bilirubin, or by failure of metabolism of bilirubin to an excretable variety, or a combination of both causes.

Bilirubin is produced when red blood cells break down. Each gram of hemoglobin that is released with red blood cell breakdown gives rise to about 35 mg of bilirubin, which must be conjugated by the liver to be excreted. During fetal life bilirubin is removed from the fetal circulation by the placenta and detoxified and excreted by the mother. After birth the free bilirubin, termed indirect, unconjugated bilirubin, is transported to the infant's liver by serum albumin and there detoxified. Until it is converted, it is insoluble and cannot be excreted. In the liver the indirect bilirubin must be converted by the enzyme glucuronyl transferase to direct bilirubin (bilirubin glucuronide). Direct, conjugated bilirubin is nontoxic, water soluble, and easily excreted into the gastrointestinal tract and the urine. A number of conditions, discussed below, may interfere with adequate excretion of bilirubin. The reader may wish to review a discussion of bilirubin metabolism on pages 516–17.

The concern over hyperbilirubinemia in the newborn is that bilirubin is a toxic substance. Any bilirubin not bound to serum albumin is free to deposit in body tissues—skin, cardiac muscle, kidney, brain. Jaundice of the skin becomes apparent. However, jaundice of the nuclear masses of the brain, termed *kernicterus* (*bilirubin encephalopathy*), is the major concern, since it will leave residual brain damage. Clinical signs of kernicterus are shrill cry, poor sucking, increased lethargy, and later rigidity, spasms, and an opisthotonic position. The amount of unconjugated bilirubin deposited in the brain tissue determines the extent of the neurologic problems.

A nurse's astute observations are important in early discovery and treatment of hyperbilirubinemia. The nurse must observe each infant closely for any evidence of jaundice and report it to the physician promptly. Some infants are known to be at risk of accumulating excessive bilirubin, but any infant may retain an abnormal amount for any one of a number of reasons. For the infant's color to be judged well, he should be examined in sunlight or white fluorescent light. Yellow-white artificial lights and yellow walls or ceilings give a misleading color. The infant's skin should be blanched by firm pressure with the nurse's thumb or finger over a firm surface such as the forehead or sternum. The color of the underlying skin is observed as soon as the pressure is removed.

Jaundice begins at the face and advances downward on the body, proceeding from face to trunk to extremities and finally to the palms and soles. It is thus advisable to examine the infant undressed. The degree of jaundice and the extent of advancement then must be recorded and reported. Even infants with deeply pigmented skin can be inspected for jaundice of the nonpigmented palms and soles.

Hyperbilirubinemia of physiologic or pathologic jaundice is somewhat difficult to differentiate. In general, however, jaundice is considered abnormal if it appears in the first 24 hours of life, and if the serum bilirubin level rises above 12 mg/100 ml of blood in the full-term infant and 10 mg/100 ml of blood in the premature. A reading up to 12 mg/100 ml of blood often has been considered physiologic but may be pathologic at this level.

A committee on phototherapy in the newborn infant, established by the National Research Council, made the following statements in regard to risks of hyperbilirubinemia and tolerable limits of serum bilirubin levels. Their preliminary report was published in the *Journal of Pediatrics* in January, 1974.

> The risks of damage to the central nervous system related to hyperbilirubinemia are increased if jaundice is associated with a history of perinatal asphyxia, respiratory distress, hemolytic disease, acidosis, hypothermia, low serum albumin concentration, hypoglycemia, or a birth weight of less than 2000 gm. The relation of the serum concentration of bilirubin to that of albumin, for example, the relative saturation of the serum albumin with bilirubin, is probably more important than serum bilirubin concentration alone in determining the ultimate neurologic outcome.
>
> Serum bilirubin concentrations of 20 mg/100 ml or greater are associated with an increased incidence of kernicterus, particularly in infants with erythroblastosis. However, indirect-reacting bilirubin concentrations less than 20 mg/100 ml may also lead to death, neurologic abnormality, and retarded mental and motor development. In low-birth-weight infants, there is an increased risk of impaired neuromuscular development at bilirubin concentrations of 15 mg/100 ml or greater. About 17 percent of premature white infants and 8 percent of premature black infants can be expected to develop bilirubin concentrations greater than 15 mg/100 ml and thus to be at risk. The infants at greatest risk are those weighing less than 1500 gm as well as those with acidosis, hypoxia, hypoglycemia, starvation, hypoalbuminemia, cold stress, sepsis, or hemolysis and those taking drugs that compete with bilirubin for albumin-binding sites. In general, it is accepted practice to try to keep bilirubin concentrations below 15 mg/100 ml in the latter group and

below 20 mg/100 ml in all infants, whether full-term or not, even in the absence of the other complicating factors.[30]

In a study on advancement of dermal icterus[31] it was found that generally dermal icterus (1) was not discernible at serum bilirubin levels of less than 4 mg/100 ml, (2) was confined to the face and neck at serum bilirubin between 4 and 8 mg/100 ml, (3) progressed as far as the umbilicus at levels between 5 and 12 mg/100 ml, (4) reached the groin and upper thighs at serum bilirubin levels between 8 and 16 mg/100 ml, and (6) showed on the feet, hands, palms, and soles at serum bilirubin levels of 15 mg/100 ml or higher. Icterus of the hands and feet was present in all infants studied whose serum bilirubin level was greater than 18 mg/100 ml of blood.

Low-birthweight infants tended to become icteric to their palms and soles at lower levels than full-term infants; however, if the hands and feet were not involved, the serum bilirubin level did not exceed 18 mg/100 ml of blood. Some infants of low birthweight showed a more rapid progression of skin icterus than full-term infants. Variations in patterns of icterus in some low-birthweight infants make estimation of bilirubin level by inspection less useful, but progression of jaundice does indicate a rise and a leveling off of serum bilirubin level. Fading of jaundice took place gradually in all skin areas rather than in a progressive pattern.

The author of this report states that estimation of serum bilirubin by advancement of jaundice is not meant to replace laboratory determination of serum bilirubin. It does enable an astute observer to determine the extent of dermal icterus at a given time.

Cause, Course, and Evaluation

There are many causes of hyperbilirubinemia, some somewhat self-limiting and relatively easily treated, others of a serious nature. The accelerated breakdown of red blood cells in the newborn period makes hyperbilirubinemia a common problem. This breakdown results in an accumulation of indirect bilirubin. The enzymes in the liver, which detoxify bilirubin and make it excretable, may be deficient during the first few days of life. When hemolysis is excessive and bilirubin is not excreted, it accumulates in the blood and that which is not bound to albumin enters the tissues.

With either abnormal bilirubin production or inadequate liver function, the pigment accumulates. Most or all serum bilirubin is bound to albumin. The bound pigment cannot enter the brain, but the unbound can do damage. Anything that increases the amount of unbound bilirubin can increase its toxicity. In evaluation of the amount of serum bilirubin it is the bound amount that can be measured. It is not yet possible to measure the unbound bilirubin, which would be most useful. Also, the risk of kernicterus with a specific level of serum bilirubin is not known since many factors beside level determine when it enters the brain cells.

A large group of infants with jaundice of moderate degree have an idiopathic hyperbilirubinemia. The cause and mechanism of this are obscure. The chief problem may be a functional immaturity of the liver. This variety appears after the first 24 hours of life, usually on the second or third day. It should disappear in 7 to 10 days.

Enclosed bleeding, such as a cephalhematoma, considerable bruising from delivery, or central nervous system bleeding may produce significant amounts of bilirubin as this blood breaks down. Hemolytic disease due to Rh and ABO incompatibilities may be a serious cause of jaundice. These problems will be discussed later.

Bacterial infections lead to an increase in destruction of red blood cells. There is an increased incidence of hyperbilirubinemia in prematures and in infants of diabetic mothers. A metabolic disorder that produces hyperbilirubinemia is breast milk jaundice.

When jaundice is apparent, bilirubin and hemoglobin determinations are done promptly. These values are useful as baselines for further evaluation. The mother's and infant's blood types are obtained, a direct Coomb's test is done, and the mother is checked for antibodies. A physical examination of the infant is done. The mother and infant are checked for infection. Breast-feeding or late start of any feedings may be considered a cause.

Interferences with Bilirubin Metabolism

Most of the bilirubin is transported to the liver bound to albumin. However, the binding to albumin is decreased by acidosis, leaving more bilirubin free to deposit in tissues. Acidosis, and also hypoxia, hypoglycemia, infection, and prematurity are all factors that decrease the resistance of the brain cells to deposition of bilirubin. Thus acidosis not only leaves bilirubin free but also increases the danger of kernicterus.

A low serum albumin level, less than 3 gm/100 ml, is inadequate for ample binding sites, and again considerable free bilirubin is available to enter tissues. Bilirubin binding to albumin also may be affected by competition for binding sites by certain chemicals, such as some antibacterial drugs and vitamin K analogues. Also, free fatty acids compete with bilirubin for a binding site on albumin. It becomes apparent that when a considerable amount of bilirubin is unbound, kernicterus could occur with low levels of serum bilirubin,

[30] Committee on Phototherapy in the Newborn Infant, National Research Council, National Academy of Sciences, Preliminary report of the committee on phototherapy in the newborn infant, *J. Pediatr.*, 84:140–41, (Jan.) 1974.

[31] Lloyd I. Kramer, Advancement of dermal icterus in the jaundiced newborn, *Am. J. Dis. Child.*, 118:454–58, (Sept.) 1969.

even with levels normally considered within physiologic limits.

Certain factors may interfere with detoxification of bilirubin when it does reach the liver. Immaturity of the infant may decrease the amount of bilirubin converted. The enzyme glucuronyl transferase may be inhibited by other factors, two of which are novobiocin and a lipase or an inhibitor substance usually present in breast milk, but in a few women it is present in such large concentration that it inhibits the enzyme from conjugating bilirubin. The inhibition may be of short duration or severe and prolonged. With maturity of the conjugation mechanism the bilirubin level, which has been kept elevated by an inhibitor, falls in several days to two weeks. When an inhibitor is believed to be the problem, the infant usually is fed formula until the jaundice clears, and the mother is advised to empty her breasts artificially until she can resume nursing.

Treatment

From the foregoing discussion it is apparent that acidosis, hypoxia, and hypoglycemia must be corrected. Good hydration and early feedings are important. The infant must be examined carefully for infection and treated if indicated. Competitive drugs must be avoided. Serum albumin levels should be checked and albumin administered if it is low and if the serum bilirubin is high.

Early feedings facilitate bilirubin excretion by preventing reabsorption of some of the bilirubin that is present in the gastrointestinal tract at birth. Conjugated bilirubin, which has been excreted into the bowel, cannot be reabsorbed, but it can be converted back to unconjugated bilirubin by the activity of a deconjugating enzyme, β-glucuronidase, present in high concentration in the intestines of the newborn in the early days of life. The unconjugated bilirubin is then reabsorbed by the intestinal mucosa by way of an enterohepatic circulation and is thus recycled through the liver. Since feedings should stimulate gastrointestinal activity and hasten expulsion of meconium, early feedings are considered important in facilitating bilirubin excretion. It is thought that early feedings also may introduce bacteria into the intestines that will reduce bilirubin to urobilinogen.

Phototherapy

Phototherapy commonly is used for treatment of rising bilirubin levels. The infant is placed under a daylight fluorescent light, unclothed to ensure exposure of as much of his body as possible. The light may be placed over an incubator or a crib, depending on the infant's needs from the environment. This supplemental light lowers levels of serum bilirubin by (1) photooxidation of bilirubin in the tissues, and (2) increased excretion of unconjugated and conjugated bilirubin by the liver.

Dr. Jerold F. Lucey states that the current hypothesis is that the light from the phototherapy penetrates the skin and increases peripheral blood flow. This brings more bilirubin to the surface for photodestruction. The breakdown products are excreted rapidly by the liver and kidneys. Also, however, "the major effect of light is to increase, to a significant degree, excretion of *unconjugated bilirubin* by the liver." Since bilirubin ordinarily cannot be excreted by the liver without being conjugated, the light produces some change that cannot be adequately explained that allows the substance to be excreted directly.[32]

Phototherapy has a number of other effects, including vasodilation of the skin, increased insensible water loss, decreased gastrointestinal transit time, and sometimes skin rashes and bronzing of the skin.

Phototherapy increases considerably insensible water loss. This is believed to be due to increased peripheral blood flow, increased skin temperature, and increased evaporative heat loss. Infants on phototherapy frequently pass loose, green stools. The green color is caused by excretion of photodegradation products. The looseness is caused by increased water content associated with the decreased transit time. Stool water loss is increased. Diarrhea could be masked by this stool pattern.

An infant under phototherapy may develop a fine skin rash, described as a flea-bite dermatosis. Occasionally, phototherapy causes a transient bronze discoloration of the skin, serum, and urine. The pigment producing the bronze color has not been identified but is not believed to be harmful. A tanning effect (hyperpigmentation) has been noticed in black babies receiving phototherapy.

Phototherapy is a medical treatment that is useful in decreasing serum bilirubin levels, but has some probable hazard in its use. It therefore is carefully considered for use when the bilirubin is rising and other appropriate therapy is not available. The infant is checked prior to therapy for probable etiology of the hyperbilirubinemia, and certain guidelines for treatment are followed. A complete history and physical examination are done, looking for probable cause of increased bilirubin. Laboratory tests include at least total and direct bilirubin levels, hemoglobin or hematocrit, Rh factor and Coombs' test, smear for red blood cell morphology, reticulocyte count, serum albumin level, maternal and infant blood types, and antibody screen.

The level of indirect bilirubin is used as a guide for phototherapy. In general it is started when a full-term infant has an indirect bilirubin level above 15 mg/100 ml of blood. For the preterm baby phototherapy is used at lower values—at above 12 mg for the moderate preterm and above 8 mg for the very small preterm. These values may need to be adjusted downward when conditions ex-

[32] Jerold F. Lucey, Phototherapy: What it has to offer, *Contemp. Ob/Gyn.*, 6:51–52, (Nov.) 1975.

ist that interfere with bilirubin binding or that decrease the resistance of brain cells to deposition of bilirubin. This includes conditions such as acidosis, hypoxia, hypoglycemia, hypoalbuminemia, and use of other drugs. Phototherapy is not used as a prophylactic treatment and therefore is not started earlier than the values stated, except when the other conditions enumerated are present. Phototherapy may be used as an adjunct to exchange transfusion. More and more information is being gathered on phototherapy, and guidelines may change with a clearer understanding of its effects.

Nursing Observations and Care

The infant receiving phototherapy is completely undressed during treatment to expose as much of the body surface as possible. The infant may be restless at times without clothes on. The nurse may find that one position is more comforting than another and also may find other ways to quiet the infant. Some position changes, of course, must be considered.

A mask is used to cover the infant's eyes when under the light. Commercial masks of adequate thickness or of black felt ovals are available to fit the infant. It is important to be sure that the infant's eyes are closed before the mask is applied. The mask may need to be replaced frequently if the infant is restless. If a bandage is used instead of a mask for shielding the eyes, care must be taken that it is not too tight. Excessive pressure from the bandage may injure the eyes and excoriate the cornea if the infant can open his eyes under the bandage. Mothers often need reassurance that the infant's eyes have been closed under the mask for bandage. The eyes must be examined for discharge and for injury at frequent intervals. (See Fig. 30–4).

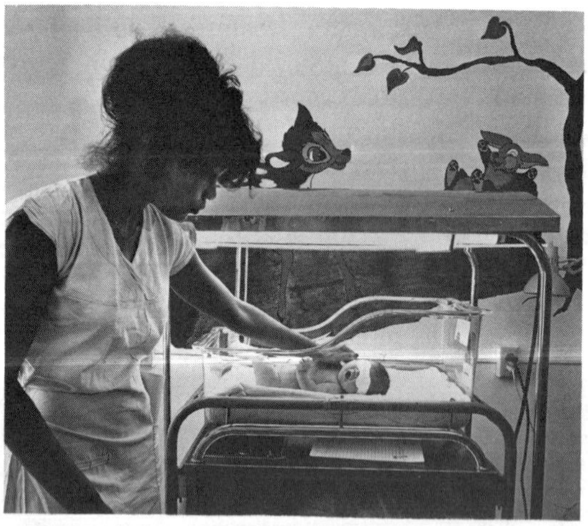

Figure 30–4. A three-day-old infant receiving photo-therapy for non-hemolytic hyperbilirubinemia. Note that the entire body is exposed, but that the eyes are protected by a mask.

For male infants the testes should be shielded from the bilirubin light. This can be done with a diaper.

The infant's vital signs should be observed and recorded every four hours. The temperature especially must be observed closely to be sure it is not elevated.

The infant must be observed carefully for chilling from drafts from air conditioning if he is in an open crib. An incubator must be observed carefully so that the temperature will not become too warm from the light above it. If an incubator with a servo-control is being used, care must be taken that the thermistor is not exposed to direct radiation.

Sensory stimulation is important to the infant. He is taken outside of the light and held for feedings, and his mask is taken off at that time to give him visual stimulation, skin care under the mask area, and inspection of his eyes. Mother-infant contact should be encouraged at feeding time and at other times if they wish. Parents must be kept informed of the infant's progress (Fig. 30–5). Treatment must never be started without first discussing this with the parents.

A careful record of intake and output must be kept. If the infant eats poorly or loses considerable fluid, glucose water is offered between regular formula- or breast-feedings to compensate for increased insensible water loss.

The bilirubin light must be kept in good condition. The lamps must be shielded adequately, and the bulbs need to be changed after a specified number of hours of use.

Follow-up Care

Direct and indirect-reacting serum bilirubin levels are monitored every 8 to 12 hours during treatment. It is important to know how fast the bilirubin is rising if such is the case and also to know when the trend is downward, since discontinuation of therapy will be determined by results. Since photodecomposition of the bilirubin will occur under lights, the lights must be turned off when the blood is drawn for evaluation. The serum bilirubin is also monitored 12 or 24 hours after therapy is discontinued to observe for possible rebound. The hematocrit should be monitored to detect anemia.

Exchange Transfusion

An exchange transfusion must be considered when the serum bilirubin level rises dangerously. It is difficult to determine the critical level of bilirubin for an individual infant since other relevant factors in the infant's condition are influential in bilirubin entry into the central nervous system. In general, however, an exchange transfusion is considered when the bilirubin level reaches 20 mg/100 ml of blood in the full-term, 16 mg/100 ml in the premature, or rises in excess of 0.5 mg/100 ml of blood

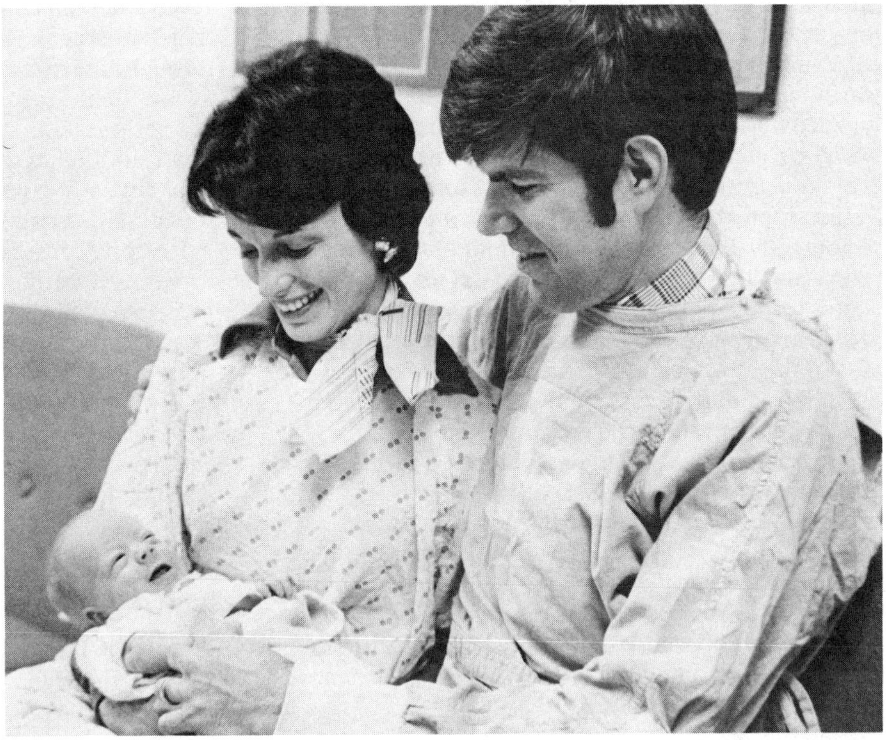

Figure 30–5. It is very important that the parents of a sick infant are given the opportunity to become acquainted with him. Physical contact is very important to both infant and parents. Parents are encouraged to visit and touch their baby frequently. As soon as the infant can be removed from his protective environment in the incubator for even short periods of time his parents can be encouraged to hold him. These parents and the baby appear to be delighted to have this time together. (Reprinted from the booklet *Special Care Nursery*, Madison General Hospital, Madison, WI, 1978. Photograph courtesy of Madison General Hosiptal and Ohio Medical Products, both of Madison, WI.)

per hour. Exchange transfusion is not without risk and is considered only when other treatments have not lowered the serum bilirubin.

Procedure

Fresh blood (*less than five days old*) is obtained. Older blood is undesirable since red cell breakdown releases potassium into the serum, which may cause an electrolyte imbalance, and old blood becomes acidotic. Heparinized blood is preferable because it eliminates the metabolic hazards of the acid-citrate-dextrose anticoagulant. Heparinized blood is especially important in very small infants and in those who are acidotic.

Aseptic technique is absolutely necessary. A disposable exchange transfusion set is required. The procedure is carried out on an open-ended radiant warmer infant care table. The infant needs careful regulation of warmth and may need oxygen.

To prepare the infant, his stomach is aspirated to prevent vomiting and aspiration, baseline vital signs are obtained, arrangements are made for continuous heart monitoring during the exchange, and restraint is made. Oxygen and suction equipment should be readily available.

The umbilical vein is the preferred route for an exchange transfusion and usually can be used for the first seven days. Thereafter the extent of thrombosis makes it unavailable, and it is usually necessary to use the femoral vein. A polyethylene or polyvinyl catheter is introduced into the umbilical vein for a distance of 6 to 8 cm until the catheter tip lies in the inferior vena cava. This catheter is attached to a stopcock, and blood is then withdrawn from the vein and injected into the vein with syringes.

The infant may have an increase in venous pressure and blood volume at birth, and an additional increase in blood volume with transfusion may be dangerous. The venous pressure therefore is checked at the beginning of the transfusion and periodically during the procedure. If the venous pressure exceeds 8 to 10 cm, the amount of blood injected may be slightly less than that removed for the first few times or until the venous pressure is normal. Entrance of air into the catheter while checking venous pressure must be guarded against.

The exchange of blood is made by alternately withdrawing and discarding from 10 to 20 ml of the infant's blood and replacing it with an equal amount of donor blood. As a syringeful of donor blood is injected, it mixes in the infant's circulation and some of the mixture then is removed with the next withdrawal of blood. A gradual replacement of the infant's blood thus is made. The exchange is proportional to the amount of blood added and removed. The infant's blood with its high bilirubin level is replaced gradually by donor blood. When an exchange is made with a volume of donor blood that is equal to twice the estimated blood volume of the infant (approximately 85 ml/kg body weight), most of the circulating blood at the end of the procedure is donor blood. The maximum volume exchanged is 500 ml of blood. This usually should take about 60 minutes; longer if the infant is very sick.

A small amount of calcium, 5 to 10 ml of a 10 percent calcium gluconate solution, may be administered in divided doses of 0.5 to 1 ml after each 100 ml of blood when citrated blood is used for exchange transfusion. This is given to overcome danger of tetany, which may result from depletion of serum calcium by the large amount of sodium citrate in the donor blood. When heparinized blood is used, it will affect the coagulation status of the infant for several hours. After use of heparinized blood, protamine sulfate may be given at the end of the transfusion, especially in sick infants in whom metabolism of heparin may be impaired.

Albumin sometimes is given intravenously prior to the transfusion, or it is added to the transfusion blood. The albumin is used to attract bilirubin, actually facilitating its movement from the tissues, and thus increasing its removal from the body with the transfusion.

Blood is collected at the beginning and end of the procedure for bilirubin and hemoglobin determination. A blood culture specimen also is collected at the end of the procedure. The umbilical vein catheter then is removed, and the umbilical cord is ligated.

Embolism with air or clots, electrolyte imbalance, and infection are known hazards of exchange transfusion but usually can be avoided with care. Cardiac arrest has occurred on occasion, but with careful monitoring and adequate resuscitation this can be avoided.

Careful observation by the nurse of the infant's vital signs and general behavior is essential both before and after transfusion. Incubator care of the infant is desirable to ensure a stable environment, proper concentration of oxygen if required, and easy observation. Vital signs must be monitored frequently, the umbilicus should be checked for bleeding, and the infant's activity and alertness observed. Any change in behavior suggestive of hypoglycemia, kernicterus, sepsis, and cardiac difficulty must be reported promptly. The infant usually is not fed orally for several hours. Blood sugar levels should be monitored closely in the first few hours after an exchange to check for rebound hypoglycemia. (The donor blood may have had a high glucose content that may have stimulated insulin production in the infant.) Further frequent serum bilirubin checks are required. A repeat exchange transfusion may become necessary.

HEMOLYTIC DISEASE OF THE NEWBORN (ERYTHROBLASTOSIS FETALIS)

Hemolytic disease of the newborn is a blood disturbance of late fetal or early neonatal life that may occur when there is a blood-group incompatibility between mother and infant. Incompatibility exists when the fetus possesses a red blood cell antigen, inherited from the father, that is absent in the mother. Fetal blood cells can pass through the placenta into the maternal circulation. When these blood cells are incompatible with the mother's blood, she may produce antibodies to them. These antibodies then pass through the placenta into the fetal circulation and there destroy fetal red blood cells, sometimes to a severe degree.

Hemolytic disease usually is caused by incompatibility between an Rh-positive fetus and an Rh-negative mother or between a blood group A or B fetus and its mother. Occasionally hemolytic disease is the result of blood antigens less common than the D antigen of the Rh factor or the A and B antigens of the major blood groups.

Development of maternal sensitization to fetal red cell antigens and transfer of the antibodies to the fetus, resulting in erythroblastosis has been described on pages 275–78.

Signs and Symptoms

The classic signs of hemolytic disease are anemia, jaundice, and edema. In the individual infant any one of these signs may predominate. The disease may be present in a mild or severe form or in any degree between these two extremes.

Clinical manifestations of hemolytic disease and laboratory findings are largely due to hemolysis of red blood cells caused by the antibody-antigen reaction, the resultant end products of hemolysis, and the great increase that takes place in blood production and extramedullary erythropoiesis because of the hemolysis.

Anemia may be present at birth or may develop anytime during the newborn period. Severe anemia at birth may cause congestive heart failure. In mild untreated cases anemia may become pronounced in a week or two and the infant's color become quite pale. However, erythrocytes may be destroyed so rapidly that even where there is only a slight suggestion of anemia at birth, it may become quite evident within 12 hours and profound within a day or two. The erythrocytes may decrease as rapidly as a million cells per microliter per day.

Immature red blood cells, appearing as nucleated cells, are found in the infant's blood in large number. This increased number of nucleated erythrocytes led to the term erythroblastosis fetalis for this disease. Since the presence of many nucleated erythrocytes is only one of several manifestations of this disturbance, the term "hemolytic disease," which better depicts the changes that occur, is considered preferable.

The normal infant has from 200 to 2000 nucleated red blood cells per microliter of blood, whereas the infant with hemolytic disease has from 10,000 to 100,000 and even 500,000 nucleated erythrocytes per microliter of blood during the first 48 hours of life. This means more than 10 and usually from 25 to 200 nucleated red blood cells per 100 white blood cells. Normally the number of nucleated erythrocytes should not exceed 10 per 100 white blood cells at any time during the newborn period. Nucleated red blood cells in the infant with hemolytic disease diminish and disappear within a few days after birth, but this finding does not mean an improvement in condition.

The *reticulocyte count,* which is normally not above 3 percent in the newborn, may be increased, sometimes to a high level. This count is often used as a criterion of severity of illness.

Jaundice rarely is seen at birth, but develops rapidly. It may appear within a few hours, or even within one hour, or sometime during the first day. Jaundice becomes increasingly deep and frequently masks the pallor of the anemia.

Serum bilirubin may be elevated above 3 mg/100 ml of blood at birth and accumulates rapidly thereafter. Levels of 30 to 40 mg/100 ml of blood, or even higher readings, may be reached in a few days if early treatment is not instituted.

The *liver* and *spleen* become *enlarged* owing to increased hematopoietic activity. They may be enlarged enough to be palpable at birth or may become palpable during the first week. Cardiac enlargement and murmurs may be present.

The *placenta* may be normal size, or it may be enlarged considerably, very edematous, and pale in color. The *vernix caseosa* may be normal, or it may have a golden-yellow color, and the amniotic fluid may be greenish-yellow.

Universal edema (hydrops fetalis) may develop. It usually is seen only in stillborn infants or in those who die within a few hours after birth. Fetal cardiac failure due to severe anemia may be a major cause of universal edema. The infant with hydrops fetalis is very waxy in appearance, has a large amount of fluid in all tissues, and has a very low hemoglobin level and red blood cell count.

Course

Hemolytic disease may be so mild that there are no clinical signs of illness, or it may result in such profound changes that death occurs *in utero*. Between these two extremes there are all degrees of illness. Many liveborn infants appear to be in good condition at birth, but rapidly show signs of illness. This course always must be anticipated.

Prognosis

In general, the chances of recovery for liveborn infants are good when treatment is adequate. After the first week prognosis is favorable, and there are no residual symptoms unless kernicterus developed, which may leave the infant with cerebral damage.

The first infant born after maternal sensitization has a fairly good prognosis. When a sensitized mother has once had a child with hemolytic disease, subsequent Rh-positive infants are in danger of developing severe symptoms, and the chances of a stillbirth are greatly increased.

Since fetal death may occur in the last weeks of pregnancy, delivery prior to term, but usually not before the thirty-sixth week, may be considered desirable if amniotic fluid analyses for the amount of bilirubin it contains indicate that the fetus is likely to be in jeopardy and if L/S studies show fetal lung maturity.

Diagnosis

Diagnosis of Rh incompatibility begins in the prenatal period. It is made tentatively before the infant is born with discovery of anti-Rh antibodies in the mother's blood and is confirmed after birth by determining that the infant is Rh positive. See page 278 for antepartum diagnosis and management.

When hemolytic disease is anticipated, the infant is checked carefully at birth for all signs of illness. Umbilical cord blood, from the placental end of the cord, is collected for determination of Rh type, blood group, Coombs' test, hemoglobin level, erythrocyte count, nucleated red blood cell count, reticulocyte count, and serum bilirubin. The infant is examined for skin color and general appearance, for color of the vernix caseosa, and for size of liver and spleen. The size and appearance of the placenta are noted.

The umbilical cord blood is immediately tested for Rh type and direct antiglobulin (Coombs') test. The direct Coombs' test is very important in diagnosis since it is positive when there are anti-Rh antibodies in the infant's blood, even in the absence of clinical evidence of disease. The test for Rh type is not always reliable since false-negative results may be obtained when anti-Rh antibodies attached to the infant's red blood cells interfere with Rh typing.

The direct Coombs' test reveals the presence of maternal antibodies attached to the red blood cells of an Rh-positive infant (Fig. 14–7, p. 277). Red cells of an infant with hemolytic disease may be coated with anti-Rh antibodies. These antibodies will cause hemolysis of the infant's cells, but also may interfere with the normal agglutinating activity of the typing serum. The infant's cells thus are not agglutinated with an anti-Rh serum under ordinary methods of testing and thus appear to be Rh negative. When the infant types Rh negative, it is necessary to exclude the possibility of a false Rh-negative reaction. This false reaction occurs when the maternal antibodies that have been absorbed on the sur-

ally can be made by passing a catheter into the esophagus. The catheter meets an obstruction and cannot be passed into the stomach. Some physicians pass a catheter into the stomach of each infant they examine shortly after birth and aspirate his stomach contents. In such instances the diagnosis is made shortly after birth. Hydramnios during pregnancy raises suspicion of a digestive tract obstruction and often leads to early investigation of patency of the esophagus. Radiology may be used to confirm diagnosis.

Respiratory distress followed by pneumonia usually develops early. The infant may aspirate the saliva that fills the upper pouch of the esophagus or aspirate a feeding if it is offered. Digestive secretions from the stomach may pass upward and enter the lungs through the fistulous tract. Although the tendency is to place an infant with excess secretions in a head-down position, any infant with a confirmed or suspected tracheoesophageal fistula should have the head elevated to at least a 30-degree angle to minimize upward passage of gastric secretions. Since the infant cannot be fed orally and early develops respiratory distress, surgery is done as early as possible.

The most common abnormality of the stomach is *hypertrophic pyloric stenosis,* resulting from hypertrophy of the musculature of the pylorus—chiefly of the circular muscles. This hypertrophy constricts the lumen of the pyloric opening and thus mechanically interferes with emptying of the stomach. This condition is much more common in male than in female infants.

Pyloric stenosis is not apparent in the immediate newborn period. Vomiting usually begins in the second or third week of life, occasionally in the first week. It becomes more frequent and increasingly projectile. The infant vomits during or shortly after a feeding. As a result of vomiting the infant does not obtain an adequate amount of food and fluid. He becomes dehydrated, loses weight, and becomes constipated.

Surgery almost always is necessary to correct pyloric stenosis. The hypertrophied muscles of the pylorus are split, without incision of the mucosa underneath.

Early signs of pyloric stenosis are similar to a *pylorospasm* not associated with hypertrophy of the muscles. Infants with pylorospasm are hyperactive, easily disturbed, and excited. They sleep little, awaken easily, and seem very tense. They vomit frequently during the first few weeks of life. Vomiting occurs suddenly and with considerable force. Slow, careful feeding and bubbling before, during, and after feedings may reduce vomiting.

Intestinal obstruction in a newborn may be complete or partial. It may be located at any level of the small or large intestine. It may be caused by stenosis, or atresia, or absence of a portion of the intestine. Evidence appears early, in the first day or two of life. Signs are vomiting, abdominal distention, abnormal meconium, which may be drier or lighter than normal, or absence of stools. Vomiting begins early and becomes more frequent and more severe. The character of the vomitus depends on the level of the obstruction. It may consist of milk and thin fluid only. If the obstruction is below the ampulla of Vater, it contains bile. When the obstruction is as far down as the lower ileum or the colon, fecal material is vomited.

Roentgenograms, even without contrast media, are valuable in diagnosis. There is marked distention of the bowel above the obstruction. Barium usually not is given because of danger of clogging the intestines.

Treatment of intestinal obstruction caused by congenital malformations is surgery. Its success will depend on the extent of the anomaly.

Imperforate anus may be caused by a persistent membrane over the anal opening with a normal anus just above the membrane, or there may be complete absence of the anus with the rectal pouch ending some distance above. Direct inspection may reveal the defect. The nurse may discover it when she attempts to take the infant's temperature. A slight depression may be seen where the anal opening should be located. Meconium will not be passed, and the infant may strain, cry, and appear restless. An x-ray will help to determine how much of the rectum or anus is absent.

Surgical correction is necessary. Perineal surgery may establish an opening, but sometimes a colostomy must be done first, followed later by correction of the rectal defect.

Atresia or stenosis of the anus or rectum may be complicated by a fistulous connection with the genitourinary tract.

A *diaphragmatic hernia,* which is a protrusion of the abdominal viscera, to varying degrees, into the thoracic cavity, may be congenital, caused by either an absence or a weakness of the diaphragmatic tissue. Symptoms, which include respiratory distress, vomiting, and other evidences of intestinal obstruction, may be present at birth or appear later. Treatment is surgery. It is performed early, before the intestines become distended.

Biliary tract developmental abnormalities, which obstruct the flow of bile into the intestinal tract, cause clay-colored or white stool, bile-stained urine, and early jaundice. The anomaly may or may not be amenable to surgery.

Genitourinary System

Malformations of the genitourinary tract are common, especially in male infants. The development of the genitourinary system is a very complicated process, and any interruption may result in a large variety of abnormalities. Many of these anomalies do not produce symptoms or disturb function. Some cause difficulty sometime later in life—perhaps at a time of stress on the system. Among the anomalies may be absence, aplasia, or duplication of the kidneys, ureters, or bladder; obstruction of ureters or urethra; and fistulas from the bladder and urethra to the rectum or vagina.

Bilateral renal agenesis, an absence of the kidneys and ureters, causes death within a few hours after birth. It is accompanied by characteristic facial features.

Congenital cystic, or polycystic, kidneys are the most common of kidney malformations. Many cysts, large or small, exist in one or both kidneys. They may not cause symptoms for several years and sometimes not until adult life. This condition will eventually impair kidney function, but it may not be recognized during the neonatal period unless the kidneys are greatly enlarged or irregular.

Exstrophy of the bladder is a partial or complete exposure of the bladder mucosa through an opening in the abdomen. When complete, this defect is caused by a failure of union of the abdominal wall, and anterior bladder wall, the symphysis pubis, and the urethra. The opening in the lower abdominal and anterior bladder wall exposes the posterior bladder wall and the ureters on the abdomen.

Ureteral transplants to the bowel and operative removal of the bladder may be necessary; plastic closure may be possible when the exstrophy is not complete. Other anomalies of the genitourinary tract and of the pelvic organs also may be present.

Phimosis is a narrowing of the preputial opening to a degree that makes it impossible to retract the foreskin. Ordinarily it does not interfere with urination, but the opening may be so small that straining is necessary during voiding. The stream of urine is small.

Hypospadias is an anomaly in which the urethra does not extend the entire length of the penis, but rather opens on its lower surface somewhere behind the glans. In severe cases it opens in the perineum. The tip of the penis is bent down. Treatment may not be necessary if the condition is not severe. In other cases a plastic operation may be performed. The urinary flow of these infants should be observed to make certain that the urethral opening is sufficiently large.

A *hydrocele,* an accumulation of fluid in the scrotum, making it a tense, fluctuating, translucent sac, may be congenital. Fluid may be present at birth or may accumulate later. Absorption of the fluid is usually spontaneous. A hydrocele may be accompanied by a hernia.

Undescended testicles make the scrotum appear small. If only one testis is undescended, a difference in size in the two sides of the scrotum is visible. The testes develop in the abdomen and normally descend into the scrotum during the last two months of fetal life. They may, however, remain in the inguinal canal, or even the abdominal cavity, for a longer period of time. Descent is usually spontaneous during the first few weeks of life or at any time up to the age of puberty. An undescended testicle may be associated with hernia.

Musculoskeletal System

Abnormal conditions of the musculoskeletal system may be caused by developmental defects and anomalies of bones and muscles, or they may be the result of an unusual fetal position *in utero.* Developmental defects may result in the absence of individual muscles, absence of individual bones, supernumerary fingers or toes, union of fingers and toes owing to either actual fusion of the bones or webbing of the skin only, and various other deformities.

As the fetus grows, it becomes more and more confined in the uterine cavity. It does not move around as easily as it did earlier in its development, and it may finally maintain a certain posture, at least of some parts of the body. When a certain part is firmly pressed against another bony part, abnormalities, mild or severe, may develop. Unusual positions may result in severe molding of various areas of the body, in asymmetric development, or in a deformity.

Examples of molding caused by pressure are abnormal positions of the feet, grooving of the chest owing to pressure of the arms against it, and asymmetry of the face from pressure of the chin against the shoulder or the chest. Developmental anomalies or position may cause shortening of muscles and result in contractural defects such as congenital clubfoot or torticollis.

The marked relaxation that characterizes the newborn period diminishes after one week, this being true especially of those muscles and joints that were stretched and strained by fetal position. They become restricted in motion. An example is resistance encountered to leg abduction in the potentially dislocated hip because the muscles splint an unstable hip joint. The joints and muscles that were not strained *in utero* remain pliant for a longer period of time.

Clubfoot (talipes) is the result of an unequal pull of muscles, producing a deformity in which the foot is turned at an abnormal angle (Fig. 30-6*A*). Intrauterine position or muscular imbalance is considered a possible cause. The condition is usually bilateral. Diagnosis is sometimes difficult because the foot of the newborn is often normally held in a position similar to a clubfoot.

Since muscular pull may increase the deformity as the muscles mature, corrective measures that change the direction of muscle pull are started early. The method of correction depends on the severity of the condition. One form of treatment consists of passive overcorrection of the position of the foot at frequent intervals during the day. This manipulation may be started before the infant leaves the hospital and is continued at home. The nurses and the mother may be instructed to pull the foot as far

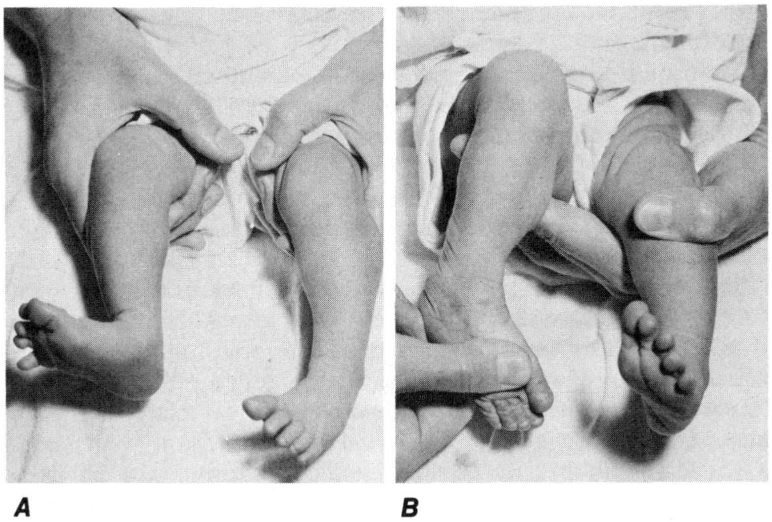

Figure 30–6. *A*. Talipes calcaneovalgus; right foot moderately resistant. *B*. Pulling the foot downward and inward to overcome the resistance. The nurses were instructed to manipulate the foot in this manner three or four times each time the baby was picked up to be care for, and the mother was instructed to continue this manipulation at home. If the resistance is not overcome by this treatment, casts will be applied.

as possible in the opposite direction and hold it in that position for a minute each time that the infant is handled (Fig. 30–6*B*). During manipulation the leg must be well supported under the calf and the knee must be flexed. This protects the lateral ligaments of the knee and the epiphysis of the tibia from strain. The entire foot must be supported to avoid merely bending it in the middle. Bending the foot alone does not correct the shortened heel cord and may result in a rocker foot deformity.

Plaster casts may be applied within a few days after birth. These are changed every one to three weeks to allow for growth of the foot and for further correction. Until the cast is thoroughly dry, care must be taken not to indent it with the fingers while handling the infant. It may be necessary to pick up the infant and hold him more than usual after application of the cast until he becomes used to it. After application of a cast, the upper leg and the toes must be watched for signs of circulatory impairment. The toes should be warm and a normal pink color—not pale, dark red, or blue. There should be no signs of swelling as indicated by pressure on the edges of the cast against the thigh or the toes. A waterproof material applied to the edge of the cast at the thigh will help to keep it clean of urine and stool.

Congenital dislocation of the hip is a displacement of the head of the femur from the acetabulum. It is much more common in the female than in the male infant and is more often unilateral than bilateral. Actual dislocation may be present at birth; however, it usually is not actually, but potentially, present. This means that there is in most instances an instability of the joint. This instability is present because the head of the femur is not well anchored into the acetabulum, which is shallow and cartilaginous instead of deep and ossified, and because the joint capsule has poor tone and is stretched. The surrounding muscles, by attempting to splint and protect this soft joint, are actually helping to produce the dislocation.

The femoral head, which is cartilaginous at birth but begins to have an ossification center at six weeks, remains cartilaginous much longer in these infants, unless treatment is begun early. As the muscles increase in strength and finally as the infant stands, the femoral head is pulled and displaced more and more, the head and the socket are malformed, and the head of the femur finally is completely dislocated.

Early recognition to permit early treatment is important in prevention of an actual dislocation. At the first examination of the infant, it may be difficult to recognize a potentially dislocated hip because of the great pliability of the joints of the newborn. By the age of one month and often earlier, muscular splinting is evident. The thighs resist abduction. When the normal infant is placed on his back with the knees flexed, his hips and knees can be abducted until they nearly reach the examining table. If a potential dislocation exists, abduction of the affected leg is possible only to one half of this distance. X-ray reveals a persistence of fetal cartilage.

The nurse caring for an infant with a potential dislocation may encounter some difficulty in moving one leg to the side when washing the groin or changing the diaper. Observation of inability to abduct the leg completely is reported to the physician. The infant also may be observed to move this leg less than the unaffected one. Other early signs of congenital dislocation of the hip, such as apparent shortening of the affected leg, a higher gluteal and inguinal fold, and an additional transverse crease in the thigh, may not be noticeable in the newborn period.

Early treatment of a potential dislocation of the hip is directed toward maintaining the affected leg in complete abduction. The muscle pull then directs the femoral head into the acetabulum, and the pressure thus created stimulates ossification.

A position of abduction may be achieved during the first two months by placing the infant in a prone position whenever he is put to bed and keeping his legs flexed and abducted while he is lying prone. The diaper can be pinned to the sheet to hold the legs in the desired position. Body weight helps to increase the degree of abduction. Another method of keeping the legs flexed and abducted is by the use of a Frejka splint. This consists of a square pillow placed against the infant's diaper and help snugly in place by suspenders or straps. The application of several diapers, in such a manner that there is a very heavy thickness in the center, is another method that may be used to keep the legs widely abducted. Extension of the leg should be avoided when handling the infant.

If treatment is not started early, it may need to be prolonged, and a body cast may be necessary. With early diagnosis and adequate treatment the infant may be able to walk at the average age.

The Skin

Nevi may be caused by a hyperplastic development of the blood and lymph vessels or of the epidermis and connective tissue. Nevi made up largely of blood vessels, known as *birthmarks,* are found on various parts of the body. While caring for the infant, the nurse should observe his skin closely for any unusual areas. Birthmarks may be flat or slightly raised. They may range in color from a light red to a darker red or to blue-black. They may or may not have a growth of hair. Birthmarks may be variously described. Some of the most common terms are port-wine mark, strawberry mark, and mole. Some lesions regress and disappear. Treatment varies considerably and may not be necessary at all.

The Eye

There are many congenital malformations of the eye. Among them are *congenital cataracts,* which may be caused by a rubella (German measles) infection in the mother in the first three months of pregnancy. This is an important time in the embryonic development of the eye, and the tissue may be particularly susceptible to the effects of the virus. If opacity of the lens is present at birth, it is usually noticeable early as the eyes are observed when the infant opens them in a fairly good light.

Syndromes Caused by Chromosomal Abnormalities

Since 1959, when it was discovered that Down's syndrome (mongolism) was caused by an extra chromosome in the body cells, certain other clinical conditions of previously unknown cause have been found to be associated with the presence of an abnormal number of chromosomes. These syndromes are linked with lack of or acquisition of an additional whole chromosome, or a portion of a chromosome, within the nucleus of a cell, which then continues to reproduce itself.

An irregular number of chromosomes is the result of one of several abnormalities that can occur during cell division, such as nondisjunction during maturation of the sex cells, translocation of a portion of a chromosome, or failure of a chromosome to divide during mitosis as the zygote or early embryo begins development. See pages 49–52 for a description of the mechanism by which alterations in chromosomal distribution may come about.

Some anomalies are linked with abnormalities in the number of sex chromosomes, others with autosomal abnormalities, or possibly a combination of both kinds (Figs. 4–9*B* and 4–11, pages 48 and 51). In some of the resulting syndromes the physical anomalies are multiple and severe and mental retardation is common. Among conditions caused by an abnormal number of sex chromosomes are rudimentary ovaries and failure to develop full female characteristics, termed Turner's syndrome, and incomplete development of male gonads and other male characteristics, known as Klinefelter's syndrome. Among anomalies linked with an autosome in triplicate are Down's syndrome, D_1 trisomy syndrome, and 18 trisomy syndrome, each resulting in a multiplicity of malformations. Lack of an autosome has not yet been found; this possibly may result in nonviability of the embryo.

Down's syndrome is the name recently suggested for the term *mongolism,* which has long been in use. In this condition mentality is severely retarded, and developmental defects of other tissues are common. Some of the physical characteristics of an individual with Down's syndrome are a small skull, eyes wide set with a lateral upward slope, protruding tongue, short nose with a flat bridge, mobile relaxed joints, poor muscle tone, and often cardiac malformations. Some of the characteristics are not distinct at birth, but become more obvious with age.

Down's syndrome is associated with an extra chromosome, trisomy for no. 21. The extra chromosome is apparently sometimes the result of nondisjunction and occasionally of translocation of no. 21 to another chromosome. There is also a type of Down's syndrome that results from a mosaic pattern, or mixed types, of body cells.

Phenylketonuria

Phenylketonuria (PKU) is a disease of a deficiency of the enzyme phenylalanine hydroxylase, which normally converts phenylalanine to tyrosine. Phenylalanine is an essential amino acid and is necessary for growth, but any excess that is ingested must be degraded, normally by conversion to tyrosine. An infant with phenylketonuria lacks this ability and any phenylalanine not incorporated into body tissues accumulates in the body and eventually spills into the urine.

With phenylketonuria there is progressive mental retardation unless the amount of phenylalanine presented to the tissues is limited to that which is essential. Dietary control must begin early to avoid brain damage. Diagnosis therefore must be made very early.

With PKU the serum phenylalanine level rises raidly after birth as the infant is fed milk. In most states blood is routinely collected on the day of the infant's discharge from the hospital for examination of an increased amount of phenylalanine. A few drops of heel-stick blood are placed on a filter paper for a Guthrie test. A diagnosis may be made with the test, or a suspicious rise in phenylalanine, which requires recheck, may be found.

An important precaution in the Guthrie test is to make certain that the infant has ingested a significant amount of protein for two or three days prior to the test. If the infant is discharged early, or if there has been feeding problems, or if the infant has vomited, the test may be falsely negative. In cases where feedings have not been sufficient before the infant goes home, the test should be done several days after the infant's discharge. The nurse is usually the person who knows best about the infant's food intake.

BIRTH INJURIES

Trauma during labor or delivery may involve any part of the newborn's body. Some injuries produce only a temporary change, while others cause permanent damage.

Soft-Tissue Injuries

Soft-tissue bruises usually occur in the presenting part of the fetus. Edema of tissues and discolored areas owing to an extravasation of blood into tissues may develop in part of the body that presents at the cervix and vaginal outlet at the time of delivery. This may be the scalp in vertex presentation (caput succedaneum and cephalhematoma), the face in face presentation, and the genitalia, buttocks, and feet in breech presentation (pages 512 and 521).

The face and scalp sometimes have reddened areas or abrasions owing to bruising from the obstetric forceps. Occasionally the face has petechial areas for a few days after birth. Subconjunctival hemorrhages may appear following spontaneous as well as instrumental deliveries. They are not considered serious and do not require treatment. Mothers frequently observe this reddened area in the white portion of the infant's eye and inquire about its significance.

Most soft-tissue injuries are not serious. The tissues return to normal in a few days, but should be protected from further trauma during recovery. Breakdown of blood in the tissues may produce hyperbilirubinemia if the bilirubin cannot be excreted rapidly.

Injury to Bones

Injury to bones occurs most frequently to the clavicle and the extremities, rarely to the skull, vertebrae, or ribs. The *clavicle* is the most common site of fractures. It is susceptible to injury when delivery of the shoulders is difficult, but may break during an apparently easy delivery. A fracture is suspected if there is limitation of movement of an arm, if the Moro reflex is unilateral, and if there is spasm of the sternocleidomastoid muscle. However, these signs are not always present. Crepitus may be felt on examination of the clavicle. A roentgenogram will confirm the diagnosis.

Treatment of a fractured clavicle usually consists of immobilization of the arm and shoulder on the affected side. The arm may be placed against the chest wall with the hand lying across the chest and held in place by wrapping a strip of stockinet material around the arm and chest. Complete immobilization is not always done. The infant should be handled carefully to prevent further trauma. When he is picked up, his shoulders should not be pressed toward the middle of the body. The arm on the affected side should not be put through a sleeve daily. When the arm is left out of the sleeve of the shirt or gown, clothing helps to partly immobilize it.

Healing of a clavicle fracture takes place without deformity. A large callus forms within a week and then gradually absorbs. When a fracture is not suspected, it may not be diagnosed until the callus is felt as a hard mass a week or more after birth.

A fracture of one of the extremities may occur if there is difficulty in delivery of an arm or a leg. Spontaneous movement of the involved extremity is limited, and the Moro reflex is not symmetric. These fractures heal rapidly. They heal without deformity when the extremity is immobilized in the corrected position.

Peripheral Nerve Injuries

Injury to peripheral nerves sometimes may occur during birth. The most common involves the *facial nerve*. Temporary paralysis of this nerve usually is caused by pressure on it during labor or pressure by a forceps blade during delivery. The affected side of the face is smooth, the eye may remain open, the corner of the mouth droops, and the forehead cannot be wrinkled. This condition is most obvious when the infant cries because the facial muscles on the affected side do not contract, and there is immobility of one side of the mouth. Only the unaffected side of the face moves, and the mouth is drawn to that side. The infant may have some difficulty in sucking during the first few days of life, but this is not always a problem.

Treatment of facial nerve injury is not necessary, but if the eye does not close, it must be protected from injury until it can close. If sucking is difficult for the first few days, it may be necessary to feed the infant with a medicine dropper or a small, soft nipple during this time. Prognosis is good. Improvement begins soon, and recovery is complete in a few weeks. Often this condition is quite transitory, and recovery is complete in a few days.

Brachial palsy is a partial or complete paralysis of certain muscles of the arm caused by trauma to nerve fibers of the brachial plexus. The brachial nerves may be injured by pressure, stretching, or actual severance. This injury may occur during delivery from a cephalic presentation when strong traction is exerted on the head during difficult delivery of the shoulders. It may follow breech delivery if traction is made on the brachial plexus as an arm is stripped over the head or if tension is placed on the brachial plexus in making traction.

The site of the injury determines which muscles are affected. The degree of paralysis, therefore, depends on the amount of nerve involvement. The upper arm, the lower arm, or the whole arm may be paralyzed. The Erb-Duchenne (upper arm) paralysis in which the upper part of the plexus (the fifth and sixth cervical nerves) is injured is the most common type. The arm lies limp at the side. It is in a position of extension and is rotated inward. The forearm is in such a position that the palm of the hand faces downward and may even face outward. The infant cannot elevate or abduct the arm. The wrist and hard are normal. The Moro reflex is absent on the affected side. Pain seems to be present at first. The lower arm type of paralysis, which is rare, occurs when the nerves of the lower part of the plexus are injured. The hand and wrist are then paralyzed. The whole arm may be involved, with symptoms of both upper and lower arm paralysis. The nurse caring for the newborn should observe any abnormal arm position or diminished arm movements.

Treatment is directed toward restoring function of the involved muscles and preventing contractures of the unaffected ones. Treatment is started as soon after birth as the condition is observed. At first the infant may be placed in a position that keeps his arm abducted and externally rotated and his elbow flexed. The arm is raised to shoulder height, and the elbow is flexed 90 degrees. This position may be maintained in one of several ways. A strip of muslin, tied to the head of the bassinet, may be brought down and tied around the wrist to hold the arm up. With another method the arm may be maintained in the desired position by placing it in a sling made of a folded towel pinned to the mattress. Sometimes the arm is held up by pinning the sleeve of the infant's gown or shirt to the mattress or the top of the crib after the arm has been positioned. Later a splint may be used to hold the arm in the desired position, and massage and exercise may be given. In dressing the infant, the arm should be supported at shoulder level. Clothing should be put on the affected arm first and taken off the affected arm last, and movement of the arm must be gentle.

Prognosis depends on the amount of trauma. If it is slight, caused by edema or hemorrhage around the nerve fibers, the condition soon improves. If the nerves are not lacerated, muscle power usually returns in a few months. Nerve laceration has a more serious prognosis.

Central Nervous System Injury

Injury to the central nervous system is the most serious form of birth injury. *Intracranial hemorrhage,* the most severe form of injury, may be caused by trauma or hypoxia during birth. The infant's head may be traumatized in a prolonged hard labor, in a difficult delivery, by mechanical injury with obstetric forceps, or in a precipitous labor and delivery.

The shape of the fetal head changes during labor to adapt to the maternal pelvis. Overlapping sutures and soft cranial bones make it possible for the head to accommodate to a pelvic canal of adequate size. Given time, the head usually can make extreme adjustments; when compressed in one direction, it will elongate in another. Excessive molding and overlapping of the cranial bones or sudden molding, however, may cause the meninges or sinuses to tear, resulting in bleeding to a small or large degree. The differences in pressure that cause a caput succedaneum to develop may at times affect the veins of the meninges and the brain in the same area. A short, apparently easy, labor and precipitous delivery are sometimes dangerous because blood vessels may break with sudden changes in pressure during the fetus's rapid passage through the birth canal.

Hypoxia and/or ischemia prenatally, during delivery, or following birth is a major cause of brain injury. Common causes of hypoxia prenatally are placenta previa, premature separation of the placenta, and complications of pregnancy. Among perinatal causes are hypotension, asphyxia during labor and delivery or at birth or in association with later respiratory distress. Hypoxia and hypercarbia produce vasodilation of the cerebral vessels and increased cerebral blood flow. Rapid infusion of fluids and use of hyperosmolar solutions may also present a problem.

Trauma to the brain varies in degree from mild to severe. It may be slight, with only edema and no bleeding. When there is bleeding, it may range from a minimal amount due to rupture of a few small vessels to a massive hemorrhage. Large hemorrhages are infrequent and usually fatal. Bleeding may occur from one or more of several sites. It may be subdural, subarachnoid, periventricular-intraventricular, over the cerebellar area, or into the brain substance itself.

Improved obstetric care has now greatly reduced traumatic births, especially those related to forcep deliveries and birth following an abnormal presentation. However, nontraumatic, spontaneous intracranial hemorrhages that occur particularly in preterm infants still remain a leading cause of neurologic morbidity.

The preterm infant is very susceptible to *periventricular-intraventricular* hemorrhage at birth because of the stage of development at that time. A highly vascularized structure, known as the subependymal germinal matrix, is present in the brain, most abundantly at the level of the foramen of Monro and the head of the caudate nucleus. This germinal matrix produces millions of neuronal and glial cells during the third to the sixth months of gestation that migrate to various parts of the cerebral hemispheres. The germinal matrix is most pronounced between 28 and 32 weeks' gestation and reaches a peak of vascularization at that time. After the peak period of vascularity involution begins and at term gestation few vessels remain.

The vessels in this subependymal germinal matrix are thin and fragile and poorly supported by connective tissue. A somewhat gelatinous material surrounds them. The origin of periventricular-intraventricular bleeding is believed to be from the vessels of the germinal matrix that become injured by hypoxic insults. The amount of hemorrhage may be very small and may remain in the germinal matrix, or it may extend into the ventricular system or it may extend into a cerebral hemisphere. The more preterm the infant the greater the chance of hemorrhage.

Signs of intracranial injury may be generalized and similar to those produced by several other conditions. Attacks of cyanosis, vomiting, listlessness, and poor sucking may be the only signs of cerebral irritation. These also may be due to other causes, such as respiratory distress and congenital heart disease. Included in signs of cerebral injury are irregular, difficult respirations; a pale, cold, clammy skin; cyanosis at intervals or continuously; an anxious expression, sometimes with the eyes open and staring; restlessness; failure to suck well; forceful vomiting; and a high-pitched cry. Localized muscular twitchings or generalized convulsions may occur several hours after birth. The infant is flaccid at first and in 12 to 14 hours becomes spastic. The fontanels may be tense; the pupils may be of unequal size; Foote's sign, an adderlike, rhythmic protrusion of the tongue, may be present; the neck and spine may become rigid; and the infant may assume an opisthotonic position.

Signs of intracranial injury may be present immediately after birth or may be delayed for several days. With massive hemorrhage there may be few signs, but death may occur soon after birth, or signs may be severe at or shortly after delivery. With slight hemorrhage, owing to rupture of small vessels, signs may develop gradually. Clinically the infant's condition may rapidly worsen or deterioration may be episodic with periods of apparent stability alternating with periods of worsening condition.

The difference in signs of cerebral irritation, cerebral edema, and intracranial hemorrhage is frequently only in degree of severity and length of time they are present. Slight trauma may give rise to mild signs. The infant may be sleepy and listless and suck poorly during the first few days of life. He usually recovers quickly and soon becomes alert, responds more readily, and begins to eat well. Cerebral edema is apt to give the same signs as mild hemorrhage, and it is frequently impossible to determine which is present. With edema the signs usually appear almost immediately after birth and last only three to four days. After this, improvement is rapid and recovery complete.

The Moro embrace reflex is checked on several succeeding days when intracranial injury is suspected. Absence of the reflex immediately after birth with a return in a few days is indicative of cerebral edema. It returns when the edema subsides. With hemorrhage the Moro reflex is often present for 24 to 48 hours after birth, then disappears and does not return until much later.

To test for increased pressure and for blood, a spinal puncture is done as an aid in diagnosis. It may relieve pressure. Interpretation of findings from a spinal puncture may be difficult. Absence of increased pressure does not exclude intracranial hemorrhage. Presence of blood does not confirm it, since the trauma of puncture may produce blood from injury of a vessel of the spinal canal. A subdural tap may be done. Spinal punctures may be repeated for serial removal of blood and spinal fluid as these are indicated.

Ultrasound is now a standard method of diagnosis; it is a method that can be used in the intensive care unit, that brings the equipment to the infant's bedside. Computerized transaxial tomography scanning (CAT scan) is also often used to pinpoint the site of hemorrhage and to determine its extent. It is also used to check for the presence or absence of posthemorrhagic hydrocephalus.

Treatment largely is directed toward keeping the infant quiet. Rest and a quiet environment may prevent stimulation of bleeding. The infant is handled as infrequently as possible and with utmost gentleness. Care that is not essential, such as bathing, is omitted.

The infant may need additional warmth. He sometimes needs oxygen. He usually is placed in an incubator for temperature control, administration of oxygen if necessary, and easy observation. Following difficult delivery, an infant, regardless of size, may be given premature care in an incubator until it is ascertained that his condition is good. Instead of lowering the head of the crib following birth, as is sometimes done for drainage

To this point, medicine has functioned as an intervention art rather than looking into how people develop. We must go back to the very beginning. Our concern must be multi-generational for the quality of life of the baby begins with the birth of the parents. Emphasizing prevention more than screening, the entire life span must be included. Medicine is but one aspect to be considered in health. The social, environmental and educational conditions must also become part of the evaluation.

Too many people are born without the opportunity to be born healthy. Not all of those people are in the traditional classifications of poor or poverty laden. Emotional considerations are vital.

Obstetricians and pediatricians have a crucial role in the determination of the productivity of the entire life span of an individual. In the early years—conception through 25 years—a lifetime must be planned. There is a great need for supportive services during this time. The middle years—25 to 65—involve growth and developmental tasks. The later years—65 and on—are the testing ground of perinatal endeavors. If a human being lives in this period without poverty of spirit, feeling important and loved until death, the perinatal work has been done well.

APPENDIX 2

The Pregnant Patient's Bill of Rights and Responsibilities

THE PREGNANT PATIENT'S BILL OF RIGHTS

American parents are becoming increasingly aware that well-intentioned health professionals do not always have scientific data to support common American obstetrical practices and that many of these practices are carried out primarily because they are part of medical and hospital tradition. In the last forty years many artificial practices have been introduced which have changed childbirth from a physiological event to a very complicated medical procedure in which all kinds of drugs are used and procedures carried out, sometimes unnecessarily, and many of them potentially damaging for the baby and even for the mother. A growing body of research makes it alarmingly clear that every aspect of traditional American hospital care during labor and delivery must now be questioned as to its possible effect on the future well-being of both the obstetric patient and her unborn child.

One in every 35 children born in the United States today will eventually be diagnosed as retarded; in 75% of these cases there is no familial or genetic predisposing factor. One in every 10 to 17 children has been found to have some form of brain dysfunction or learning disability requiring special treatment. Such statistics are not confined to the lower socioeconomic group but cut across all segments of American society.

New concerns are being raised by childbearing women because no one knows what degree of oxygen depletion, head compression, or traction by forceps the unborn or newborn infant can tolerate before that child sustains permanent brain damage or dysfunction. The recent findings regarding the cancer-related drug diethylstilbestrol have alerted the public to the fact that neither the approval of a drug by the U.S. Food and Drug Administration nor the fact that a drug is prescribed by a physician serves as a guarantee that a drug or medication is safe for the mother or her unborn child. In fact, the American Academy of Pediatrics' Committee on Drugs has recently stated that there is no drug, whether prescription or over-the-counter remedy, which has been proven safe for the unborn child.

The Pregnant Patient has the right to participate in decisions involving her well-being and that of her unborn child, unless there is a clearcut medical emergency that prevents her participation. In addition to the rights set forth in the American Hospital Association's "Patient's Bill of Rights," (which has also been adopted by the New York City Department of Health) the Pregnant Patient, because she represents TWO patients rather than one, should be recognized as having the additional rights listed below.

1. *The Pregnant Patient has the right,* prior to the administration of any drug or procedure, to be informed by the health professional caring for her of any potential direct or indirect effects, risks or hazards to herself or her unborn or newborn infant which may result from the use of a drug or procedure prescribed for or administered to her during pregnancy, labor, birth or lactation.
2. *The Pregnant Patient has the right,* prior to the proposed therapy, to be informed, not only of the benefits,

risks and hazards of the proposed therapy but also of known alternative therapy, such as available childbirth education classes which could help to prepare the Pregnant Patient physically and mentally to cope with the discomfort or stress of pregnancy and the experience of childbirth, thereby reducing or eliminating her need for drugs and obstetric intervention. She should be offered such information early in her pregnancy in order that she may make a reasoned decision.

3. *The Pregnant Patient has the right,* prior to the administration of any drug, to be informed by the health professional who is prescribing or administering the drug to her that any drug which she receives during pregnancy, labor and birth, no matter how or when the drug is taken or administered, may adversely affect her unborn baby, directly or indirectly, and that there is no drug or chemical which has been proven safe for the unborn child.
4. *The Pregnant Patient has the right* if Cesarean section is anticipated, to be informed prior to the administration of any drug, and preferably prior to her hospitalization, that minimizing her and, in turn, her baby's intake of nonessential pre-operative medicine will benefit her baby.
5. *The Pregnant Patient has the right,* prior to the administration of a drug or procedure, to be informed of the areas of uncertainty if there is NO properly controlled follow-up research which has established the safety of the drug or procedure with regard to its direct and/or indirect effects on the physiological, mental and neurological development of the child exposed, via the mother, to the drug or procedure during pregnancy, labor, birth or lactation—(this would apply to virtually all drugs and the vast majority of obstetric procedures).
6. *The Pregnant Patient has the right,* prior to the administration of any drug, to be informed of the brand name and generic name of the drug in order that she may advise the health professional of any past adverse reaction to the drug.
7. *The Pregnant Patient has the right* to determine for herself, without pressure from her attendant, whether she will accept the risks inherent in the proposed therapy or refuse a drug or procedure.
8. *The Pregnant Patient has the right* to know the name and qualifications of the individual administering a medication or procedure to her during labor or birth.
9. *The Pregnant Patient has the right* to be informed, prior to the administration of any procedure, whether that procedure is being administered to her for her or her baby's benefit (medically indicated) or as an elective procedure (for convenience, teaching purposes or research).
10. *The Pregnant Patient has the right* to be accompanied during the stress of labor and birth by someone she cares for, and to whom she looks for emotional comfort and encouragement.
11. *The Pregnant Patient has the right* after appropriate medical consultation to choose a position for labor and for birth which is least stressful to her baby and to herself.
12. *The Obstetric Patient has the right* to have her baby cared for at her bedside if her baby is normal, and to feed her baby according to her baby's needs rather than according to the hospital regimen.
13. *The Obstetric Patient has the right* to be informed in writing the name of the person who actually delivered her baby and the professional qualifications of that person. This information should also be on the birth certificate.
14. *The Obstetric Patient has the right* to be informed if there is any known or indicated aspect of her or her baby's care or condition which may cause her or her baby later difficulty or problems.
15. *The Obstetric Patient has the right* to have her and her baby's hospital medical records complete, accurate and legible and to have their records, including Nurses' Notes, retained by the hospital until the child reaches at least the age of majority, or, alternatively, to have the records offered to her before they are destroyed.
16. *The Obstetric Patient,* both during and after her hospital stay, has the right to have access to her complete hospital medical records, including Nurses' Notes, and to receive a copy upon payment of a reasonable fee and without incurring the expense of retaining an attorney.

It is the obstetric patient and her baby, not the health professional, who must sustain any trauma or injury resulting from the use of a drug or obstetric procedure. The observation of the rights listed above will not only permit the obstetric patient to participate in the decisions involving her and her baby's health care, but will help to protect the health professional and the hospital against litigation arising from resentment or misunderstanding on the part of the mother.

Endorsed by the International Childbirth Education Association

THE PREGNANT PATIENT'S RESPONSIBILITIES

In addition to understanding her rights the Pregnant Patient should also understand that she too has certain responsibilities. The Pregnant Patient's responsibilities include the following:

1. The Pregnant Patient is responsible for learning about the physical and psychological process of labor, birth and postpartum recovery. The better informed expectant parents are the better they will be able to participate in decisions concerning the planning of their care.
2. The Pregnant Patient is responsible for learning what comprises good prenatal and intranatal care and for making an effort to obtain the best care possible.
3. Expectant parents are responsible for knowing about those hospital policies and regulations which will affect their birth and postpartum experience.
4. The Pregnant Patient is responsible for arranging for a companion or support person (husbnd, mother, sister, friend, etc.) who will share in her plans for birth and who will accompany her during her labor and birth experience.
5. The Pregnant Patient is responsible for making her preferences known clearly to the health professionals involved in her case in a courteous and cooperative man-

ner and for making mutually agreed-upon arrangements regarding maternity care alternatives with her physician and hospital in advance of labor.

6. Expectant parents are responsible for listening to their chosen physician or midwife with an open mind, just as they expect him or her to listen openly to them.
7. Once they have agreed to a course of health care, expectant parents are responsible, to the best of their ability, for seeing that the program is carried out in consultation with others with whom they have made the agreement.
8. The Pregnant Patient is responsible for obtaining information in advance regarding the approximate cost of her obstetric and hospital care.
9. The Pregnant Patient who intends to change her physician or hospital is responsible for notifying all concerned, well in advance of the birth if possible, and for informing both of her reasons for changing.
10. In all their interactions with medical and nursing personnel, the expectant parents should behave towards those caring for them with the same respect and consideration they themselves would like.
11. During the mother's hospital stay the mother is responsible for learning about her and her baby's continuing care after discharge from the hospital.
12. After birth, the parents should put into writing constructive comments and feelings of satisfaction and/or dissatisfaction with the care (nursing, medical and personal) they received. Good service to families in the future will be facilitated by those parents who take the time and responsibility to write letters expressing their feelings about the maternity care they received.

All the previous statements assume a normal birth and postpartum experience. Expectant parents should realize that, if complications develop in their cases, there will be an increased need to trust the expertise of the physician and hospital staff they have chosen. However, if problems occur, the childbearing woman still retains her responsibility for making informed decisions about her care or treatment and that of her baby. If she is incapable of assuming that responsibility because of her physical condition, her previously authorized companion or support person should assume responsibility for making informed decisions on her behalf.

Prepared by Members of ICEA

APPENDIX 3

Clinical Laboratory Values in Pregnancy

Table 1. Hematologic Changes During Pregnancy

	Nonpregnant	*Pregnant*
Complete blood count		
Hemoglobin, gm/100 ml	12–16	10–14
Hematocrit, %	37–47	32–42
Red cell volume, ml	1600	1900
Plasma volume, ml	2400	3700
Red blood cell indexes	Normal	Normal
White blood cells, total, /mm^3	4500–10,000	5000–15,000
Polymorphonuclear cells, %	54–62	60–85
Lymphocytes, %	38–46	15–40
Erythrocyte sedimentation rate, mm/hr	<20	30–90
Coagulation system		
Bleeding time	Normal	Normal
Clotting time	Normal	Normal
Platelets, /mm^3	175,000–250,000	200,000–350,000
Prothrombin time	Control $\pm$ 3 sec	10% decrease
Fibrinogen, mg/100 ml	250	400
Factor VIII	Normal	3 $\times$ normal
Factors V, VII, IX, X	Normal	Moderate increase
Fibrinolytic activity	Normal	Moderate decrease
Erythropoietic system		
Serum iron, μg	75–150	65–120
Total iron-binding capacity, μg	250–450	300–500
Iron saturation, %	30–40	15–30
Vitamin B_{12}, folic acid, ascorbic acid	Normal	Moderate decrease

Table 2. Cardiovascular Changes During Pregnancy*

	Nonpregnant	*Pregnant*
Blood pressure, mm Hg	120/80	114/65
Peripheral resistance, dyne/sec-cm $^{-5}$	120	100
Venous pressure, cm H_2O		
Femoral	9	24
Antecubital	8	8
Pulse, rate/min	70	80
Stroke volume, ml	65	75
Cardiac output, liters/min	4.5	6
Circulation time (arm-tongue), sec	15–16	12–14
Blood volume, ml		
Whole blood	4000	5600
Plasma	2400	3700
Red blood cell	1600	1900
Plasma renin, units/liter	3–10	10–80
Chest x-ray		
Transverse diameter of heart	Normal	1–2 cm increase
Left border of heart	Normal	Straightened
Cardiac volume	Normal	70 ml increase
Electrocardiogram	Normal	15° left axis deviation
V_1 and V_2	Normal	Inverted T wave
V_4	Normal	Low T
III	Normal	Q + inverted T
aVr	Normal	Small Q

*32 to 36 weeks' duration.

Table 3. Changes in Renal Function During Pregnancy*

	Nonpregnant	*Pregnant*
Renal blood flow, ml/min	900	1200
Renal plasma flow (PAH†), ml/min	500	700
Glomerular filtration rate (creatinine clearance), ml/min	80–120	110–180
Blood urea nitrogen, mg/100 ml	10–18	4–12
Creatinine, mg/100 ml	0.6–1.2	0.4–0.9
Uric acid, mg/100 ml	2.0–6.4	2.0–5.5
Phenolsulfonphthalein excretion	Normal	Delayed
Fishberg concentration test	1.023	Often less
Urine glucose	Negative	Present in 20% of patients
Intravenous pyelogram	Normal	Slight to moderate hydroureter and hydronephrosis; R > L

*32 to 36 weeks' duration.
†PAH, para-aminohippuric acid.

Tables 1, 2, and 3 reproduced with permission from David W. Brewer, Jr. and Richard H. Aubry, The physiology of pregnancy, *Postgrad. Med.*, 52(6):110–14, (Dec.) 1972, and 53(1):221–26, (Jan.) 1973.

Table 4. Additional Laboratory Values

	Nonpregnant	*Pregnant*
Blood sugar		
Fasting, mg/100 ml	70–80	65
2-hour postprandial, mg/100 ml	60–110	Under 140 after a 100-gm carbohydrate meal is considered normal
Serum proteins		
Total, gm/100 ml	6.7–8.3	5.5–7.5
Albumin, gm/100 ml	3.5–5.5	3.0–5.0
Globulin, total, gm/100 ml	2.3–3.5	3.0–4.0
Thyroid		
Protein-bound iodine μg/100 ml	4.0–8.0	6.5–12.0
Thyroxine, μg/100 ml	3.4–6.4	5.5–10.0
Triiodothyronine, percent	25–38	12–25
Free thyroxine, μg/100 ml	1.2–1.6	0.9–1.4

APPENDIX 4

Clinical Laboratory Values in the Newborns

Constituent	*Normal Range*	*Comments*
pH	7.35–7.45 arterial, venous, or arterialized	Below 7.25 there is acidosis clinically
Pco_2, mm Hg	35–40 arterial, venous, or arterialized	45 is upper limit of normal
Po_2, mm Hg	50–80 arterial. capillary blood samples are not reliable	50 is lower limit of normal P_{O_2} should not exceed 100
Plasma bicarbonate, mEq/liter	20 to 25	
Base excess, mEq/liter	+4 to −4	
Hemoglobin, gm/100 ml	16–20 peripheral 14–17.0 venous	Less than 14.5 (capillary), Less than 13.0 (venous) = anemia 22.0 or more (venous) = polycythemia
Hematocrit, %	48–60	45 or less = anemia 65 or greater (venous) = polycythemia
Red blood cells, mm^3	4,000,000 to 6,000,000	
Reticulocytes, %	3–4 at birth 1–3 at 4 days 0–1 by 7 days	
WBC, mm^3	9,000 to 30,000 15,000 = mean	

Constituent	*Normal Range*	*Comments*
Differential	Preponderance of polymorphonuclear neutrophils until day 3–4; then lymphocytes predominate	After 72 hours a neutrophil count below 1,350 or over 8,800 should be regarded as sign of bacterial infection until proven otherwise†
Platelet count, mm^3	100,000–300,000	
Serum bilirubin		
Total, mg/100 ml	5–12 after 48 hours and for no longer than one week	Above 12 = pathologic Daily increment in excess of 5 mg/100 ml – 24 hr = pathologic
Direct, mg/100 ml	0.0–1.0	Exceeding 1.0–2.0 = pathologic
Blood chemistry		
Blood sugar, mg/100 ml	40–100 in whole blood 5 mg/100 ml must be added if values are done on serum rather than whole blood	Hypoglycemia In full term < 30 in first 72 hours < 40 after third day In low birthweight < 20
Serum calcium,		
mg/100 ml	8–10	Below 7 mg/100 ml or 3.5 mEq/liter = hypocalcemia
mEq/liter	4–5	
Serum magnesium,		
mg/100 ml	1.5–2.8	< 1.5 mg/100 ml = hypomagnesia
mEq/liter	1.5–2.5	
Serum sodium, mEq/liter	136–143	Below 130 = hyponatremia Above 150 = hypernatremia
Serum potassium, mEq/liter	3.8–6.5	Over 7.0 = hyperkalemia
Serum chloride, mEq/liter	95–105	
Total serum proteins, gm/100 ml	4.8–7.4 term 4.0–6.4 preterm	
Serum albumin, gm/100 ml	3.6–5.4 term 3.28–4.50 preterm	
Urine specific gravity	1.008–1.012	

*These values are an overall average normal. Laboratory values will vary with the gestational age, the postnatal age, and the birthweight of the infant. Laboratory data also may vary with individual laboratories.

†Frank A. Oski, Hematologic problems, in *Neonatology,* edited by Gordon B. Avery, Lippincott, Philadelphia, 1975, p. 415.

APPENDIX 5

Conversion Table for Newborn Weights

	OUNCES															
POUNDS	*0*	*1*	*2*	*3*	*4*	*5*	*6*	*7*	*8*	*9*	*10*	*11*	*12*	*13*	*14*	*15*
0	0	28	57	85	113	142	170	198	227	255	284	312	340	369	397	425
1	454	482	510	539	567	595	624	652	680	709	737	765	794	822	851	879
2	907	936	964	992	1021	1049	1077	1106	1134	1162	1191	1219	1247	1276	1304	1332
3	1361	1389	1418	1446	1474	1503	1531	1559	1588	1616	1644	1673	1701	1729	1758	1786
4	1814	1843	1871	1899	1928	1956	1985	2013	2041	2070	2098	2126	2155	2183	2211	2240
5	2268	2296	2325	2353	2381	2410	2438	2466	2495	2523	2552	2580	2608	2637	2665	2693
6	2722	2750	2778	2807	2835	2863	2892	2920	2948	2977	3005	3033	3062	3090	3119	3147
7	3175	3204	3232	3260	3289	3317	3345	3374	3402	3430	3459	3487	3515	3544	3572	3600
8	3629	3657	3686	3714	3742	3771	3799	3827	3856	3884	3912	3941	3969	3997	4026	4054
9	4082	4111	4139	4167	4196	4224	4253	4281	4309	4338	4366	4394	4423	4451	4479	4508
10	4536	4564	4593	4621	4649	4678	4706	4734	4763	4791	4820	4848	4876	4905	4933	4961
11	4990	5018	5046	5075	5103	5131	5160	5188	5216	5245	5273	5301	5330	5358	5387	5415
12	5443	5472	5500	5528	5557	5585	5613	5642	5670	5698	5727	5755	5783	5812	5840	5868
13	5897	5925	5954	5982	6010	6039	6067	6095	6124	6152	6180	6209	6237	6265	6294	6322
14	6350	6379	6407	6435	6464	6492	6521	6549	6577	6606	6634	6662	6691	6719	6747	6776
15	6804	6832	6861	6889	6917	6946	6974	7002	7031	7059	7088	7116	7144	7173	7201	7229

To convert pounds and ounces to grams, multiply the pounds by 453.6 and the ounces by 28.35 and add the two sums.
To convert grams into pounds and decimals of a pound, multiply the grams by 0.0022.
To convert grams into ounces, divide the grams by 28.35.

APPENDIX 6

Conversion Table for Newborn Lengths

Inches	*Centimeters*	*Inches*	*Centimeters*
10	25.4	17	43.2
10½	26.7	17½	44.5
11	27.9	18	45.7
11½	29.2	18½	47.0
12	30.5	19	48.3
12½	31.8	19½	49.5
13	33.0	20	50.8
13½	34.3	20½	52.1
14	35.6	21	53.3
14½	36.8	21½	54.6
15	38.1	22	55.9
15½	39.4	22½	57.2
16	40.6	23	58.4
16½	41.9	23½	59.7
		24	60.9

To convert inches to centimeters, multiply inches by 2.54 or divide inches by 0.394.

To convert centimeters to inches, multiply centimeters by 0.394 or divide centimeters by 2.54.

APPENDIX 7

Equivalent Temperature Readings of Celsius and Fahrenheit

°C	°F	°C	°F	°C	°F	°C	°F
0	32.0	35.8	96.4	37.4	99.3	39.0	102.2
		35.9	96.6	37.5	99.5	39.1	102.4
34.0	93.2	36.0	96.8	37.6	99.6	39.2	102.6
34.2	93.6	36.1	96.9	37.7	99.8	39.3	102.7
		36.2	97.2	37.8	100.0	39.4	102.9
34.4	93.9	36.3	97.3	37.9	100.2	39.5	103.1
34.6	94.3	36.4	97.5	38.0	100.4	39.6	103.3
		36.5	97.7	38.1	100.6	39.7	103.5
34.8	94.6	36.6	97.9	38.2	100.8	39.8	103.6
35.0	95.0	36.7	98.0	38.3	100.9	39.9	103.8
35.2	95.4	36.8	98.2	38.4	101.1	40.0	104.0
35.4	95.7	36.9	98.4	38.5	101.3		
		37.0	98.6	38.6	101.5	100	212
35.5	95.9	37.1	98.8	38.7	101.7		
35.6	96.1	37.2	99.0	38.8	101.8		
35.7	96.3	37.3	99.1	38.9	102.0		

1. To convert Celsius readings to Fahrenheit, multiply by 1.8 and add 32.
2. To convert Fahrenheit readings to Celsius, subtract 32 and divide by 1.8

OR

3. To convert Celsius readings to Fahrenheit, multiply by 9/5 and add 32.
4. To convert Fahrenheit readings to Celsius, subtract 32 and multiply by 5/9.

Index

A

B

C

D

E

I

M

O

P

Q

S

T

U

V

W

X

Y

Z